Greek Alphabet

A	α	Alpha	N	ν	Nu
B	β	Beta	Ξ	ξ	Xi
Γ	γ	Gamma	O	o	Omicron
Δ	δ	Delta	Π	π	Pi
E	ϵ	Epsilon	P	ρ	Rho
Z	ζ	Zeta	Σ	σ	Sigma
H	η	Eta	T	τ	Tau
Θ	θ	Theta	Υ	υ	Upsilon
I	ι	Iota	Φ	ϕ	Phi
K	κ	Kappa	X	χ	Chi
Λ	λ	Lambda	Ψ	ψ	Psi
M	μ	Mu	Ω	ω	Omega

PHYSICAL CONSTANTS

	cgs units	SI units
Acceleration of gravity, g	980.665 cm sec^{-2}	9.80665 m s^{-2}
Avogadro's number, N	6.0221×10^{23} mole^{-1}	6.0221×10^{23} mole^{-1}
Boltzmann constant, $k = R/N$	1.38066×10^{-16} erg deg^{-1} molecule^{-1}	1.38066×10^{-23} J K^{-1}
1 calorie (gram calorie)	4.1840×10^{7} erg	4.1840 J
Electronic charge, e (electron volt)	4.8030×10^{-10} esu 1.6022×10^{-20} emu 1.6022×10^{-19} coulombs (C)	1.6022×10^{-19} C
Faraday, F	96,485 coulomb Eq^{-1} 23,000 cal volt^{-1} Eq^{-1}	96,485 C mole^{-1}
Gas constant, R	8.3143×10^{7} erg deg^{-1} mole^{-1} 1.9872 cal deg^{-1} mole^{-1} 0.0821 liter atm deg^{-1} mole^{-1}	8.3143 J K^{-1} mole^{-1}
1 liter atmosphere	24.22 cal	
1 atmosphere	1.01325×10^{6} dyne cm^{-2} 760 mm Hg = 760 torr	101,325 Nm^{-2}
1 bar	0.987 atm = 10^{6} dyne cm^{-2}	100,000 Nm^{-2}
1 kilobar (kbar)	987 atm	10^{8} Nm^{-2}
Planck's constant, h	6.6262×10^{-27} erg sec	6.6262×10^{-34} J s
Velocity of light in a vacuum, c	2.99792×10^{10} cm sec^{-1}	2.99792×10^{8} m s^{-1}
Volume, ideal gas at STP	22.414 liter mole^{-1}	22.414×10^{-3} m^{3} mole^{-1}

$\ln (\log_e) = \log_{10} \times 2.303$
Ice point, 0° C = 273.15° K
Temperature conversion: (°F − 32)/180 = °C/100

Circle: circumference, $C = 2\pi r = \pi D$
area, $A = \pi r^2 = (\frac{1}{4})\pi D^2$
Sphere: area, $A = 4\pi r^2 = \pi D^2$
Volume, $V = (\frac{4}{3})\pi r^3 = (\frac{1}{6})\pi D^3$

Physical Pharmacy

Physical Pharmacy

PHYSICAL CHEMICAL PRINCIPLES IN THE PHARMACEUTICAL SCIENCES

Alfred Martin, Ph.D.
Emeritus Coulter R. Sublett Professor
Drug Dynamics Institute,
College of Pharmacy,
University of Texas

with the participation of
PILAR BUSTAMANTE, Ph.D.
Titular Professor
Department of Pharmacy
and Pharmaceutical Technology,
University Alcala de Henares,
Madrid, Spain

and with illustrations by
A. H. C. CHUN, Ph.D.
Associate Research Fellow
Pharmaceutical Products Division,
Abbott Laboratories

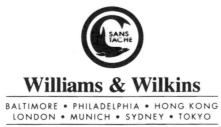

Williams & Wilkins

BALTIMORE • PHILADELPHIA • HONG KONG
LONDON • MUNICH • SYDNEY • TOKYO

A WAVERLY COMPANY

Williams & Wilkins
351 West Camden Street
Baltimore, Maryland 21201-2436 USA

Rose Tree Corporate Center
1400 North Providence Road
Building II, Suite 5025
Media, Pennsylvania 19063-2043 USA

Executive Editor: George H. Mundorff
Production Manager: Thomas J. Colaiezzi
Project Editor: Denise Wilson

Library of Congress Cataloging-in-Publication Data

Martin, Alfred N.
    Physical pharmacy : physical chemical principles
in the pharmaceutical sciences / Alfred Martin ; with
the participation of Pilar Bustamante and with
illustrations by A.H.C. Chun.—4th ed.
        p. cm.
    Includes index.
    ISBN 0-8121-1438-8
    1. Pharmaceutical chemistry. 2. Chemistry,
Physical and theoretical. I. Bustamante, Pilar.
II. Title.
    [DNLM: 1. Chemistry, Pharmaceutical. 2.
Chemistry, Physical.   QD 453.2 M379p]
    RS403.M34 1993
    541.3′024′615—dc20
    DNLM/DLC   92-49751
    for Library of Congress   CIP

PRINTED IN THE UNITED STATES OF AMERICA

Print No. 10 9 8 7 6

Dedicated to my parents
Rachel and Alfred Martin, Sr.,
my wife, Mary, and my sons,
Neil and Douglas.

Preface

The fourth edition of *Physical Pharmacy* is concerned, as were earlier editions, with the use of physical chemical principles as applied to the various branches of pharmacy. Its purpose is to help students, teachers, researchers, and manufacturing pharmacists use the elements of mathematics, chemistry, and physics in their work and study. The new edition has been updated and revised to reflect a decade of current advances, concepts, methods, instrumentation and new dosage forms and delivery systems.

Two chapters in the third edition—Introductory Calculus and Atomic and Molecular Structure—have been removed. The calculus chapter has been replaced by an appendix that provides necessary rules of differentiation and integration. The space made available by these deletions has allowed extensive revision in other chapters: Complexation and Protein Binding, Kinetics, Interfacial Phenomena, Colloids, Rheology, and Coarse Dispersions. The chapter on Drug Product Design has been rewritten and expanded to reflect the many advances in controlled drug delivery systems over the past two decades. The problems at the end of the chapters have been varied and considerably increased in number.* This new and revised edition will bring readers up-to-date with the last 10 years of progress in the physical and chemical foundations of the pharmaceutical sciences.

The author acknowledges the outstanding contributions of Professor Pilar Bustamante to the preparation of this fourth edition with regard to originating new problems and writing a major part of Chapter 19, Drug Product Design. The time and professional devotion she gave to the revision process, in a variety of ways, was exceptional. Dr. A. H. C. Chun prepared most of the

illustrations, as he has skillfully done for each of the editions. Dr. Stephen Baron, who checked the problems in the first edition, has again assisted in reviewing the problems and in reading galley proof for the fourth edition.

The author expresses his appreciation for additional contributions to this book by Dr. R. Bodmeier, University of Texas; Dr. Peter R. Byron, Virginia Commonwealth University; Dr. S. Cohen, Tel-Aviv University, Israel; Dr. T. D. J. D'Silva, Rhone-Poulenc; Dr. J. B. Dressman, University of Michigan; Dr. J. Keith Guillory, University of Iowa; Dr. V. D. Gupta, University of Houston; Dr. Bhupendra Hajratwala, Wayne State University; Dr. E. Hamlow, Bristol–Meyers Squibb; Dr. A. J. Hickey, University of Illinois at Chicago; S. Jarmell, Fisher Scientific; Dr. A. E. Klein, Oneida Research Services; Dr. A. P. Kurtz, Rhone-Poulenc; Dr. Z. Liron, Tel-Aviv University, Israel; Dr. T. Ludden, U.S. Federal Food and Drug Administration; Dr. James McGinity, University of Texas; B. Millan-Hernandez, Sterling International, Caracas, Venezuela; Dr. Paul J. Niebergall, Medical University of South Carolina; Dr. Robert Pearlman, University of Texas; Dr. R. J. Prankerd, University of Florida; H. L. Rao, Manipal, India; Dr. E. G. Rippie, University of Minnesota; T. Rossi, Fisher Scientific; Dr. Hans Schott, Temple University; Dr. V. J. Stella, University of Kansas; Dr. Felix Theeuwes, Alza Corporation; Dr. K. Tojo, Kyushu Institute of Technology, Japan; and Dr. J. Zheng, Shanghai Medical University.

Recognition is also given for the use of data and reference material found in the Merck Index, 11th Edition, Merck, 1989; the U.S. Pharmacopeia, XXII-NF XVII, U.S. Pharmacopeial Convention, 1990;

*The percent increase in figures, tables, and so on in the 4th edition of *Physical Pharmacy* as compared with those in the 3rd edition is as follows:

	Figures	Tables	References	Equations	Examples	Problems
% Increase	12	2	45	17	32	107

and the CRC Handbook of Chemistry and Physics, 63rd Edition, CRC Press, 1982. The author acknowledges with thanks the use of problems patterned after some of those in J. William Moncrief and William H. Jones, *Elements of Physical Chemistry*, Addison-Wesley, 1977; Raymond Chang, *Physical Chemistry with Applications to Biological Systems*, 2nd Edition, Macmillan, 1981; and David Eisenberg and Donald Crothers, *Physical Chemistry with Application to the Life Sciences*, Benjamin/Cummings, 1979.

The suggestions and assistance of Dean J. T. Doluisio and colleagues at the University of Texas are acknowledged with thanks. Much of the work by the author was made possible by the professorship provided by Coulter R. Sublett.

Dr. Pilar Bustamante is grateful to Dean Vicente Vilas, to Professor Eugenio Selles, and to her colleagues at the University Alcala de Henares, Madrid, Spain, for their support and encouragement during the many hours of revision work.

George H. Mundorff, Executive Editor; Thomas J. Colaiezzi, Production Manager; and Dorothy A. Di Rienzi, Project Editor of Lea & Febiger have been patient, sympathetic, and helpful during the revision for the fourth edition of *Physical Pharmacy*.

Austin, Texas   ALFRED MARTIN

Contents

1
Introduction

Dimensions and Units
Some Elements of Mathematics

Statistical Methods and the Analysis of Errors

The pharmacist today more than ever before is called upon to demonstrate a sound knowledge of pharmacology, organic chemistry, and biochemistry and an intelligent understanding of the physical and chemical properties of the new medicinal products that he or she prepares and dispenses.

Whether engaged in research, teaching, manufacturing, community pharmacy, or any of the allied branches of the profession, the pharmacist must recognize the need to borrow heavily from the basic sciences. This stems from the fact that pharmacy is an applied science, composed of principles and methods that have been culled from other disciplines. The pharmacist engaged in advanced studies must work at the boundary between the various sciences and must keep abreast of advances in the physical, chemical, and biologic fields to understand and contribute to the rapid developments in his own profession.

Pharmacy, like many other applied sciences, has passed through a descriptive and an empiric era and is now entering the quantitative and theoretic stage.

The scientific principles of pharmacy are not as complex as some would believe, and certainly they are not beyond the understanding of the well-educated pharmacist of today. In the following pages, the reader will be directed through fundamental theory and experimental findings to practical conclusions in a manner that should be followed easily by the average pharmacy student.

The name *physical pharmacy* has been associated with the area of pharmacy that deals with the quantitative and theoretic principles of science as they apply to the practice of pharmacy. Physical pharmacy attempts to integrate the factual knowledge of pharmacy through the development of broad principles of its own, and it aids the pharmacist, the pharmacologist, and the pharmaceutical chemist in their attempt to predict the solubility, stability, compatibility, and biologic action of drug products. As a result of this knowledge, the pharmaceutical scientist is in a better position to develop new drugs and dosage forms and to improve upon the various modes of administration.

This course should mark the turning point in the study pattern of the student, for in the latter part of the pharmacy curriculum, emphasis is placed upon the application of scientific principles to practical professional problems. Although facts must be the foundation upon which any body of knowledge is built, the rote memorization of disjointed "particles" of knowledge does not lead to logical and systematic thought. The student should strive in this course to integrate facts and ideas into a meaningful whole. In the pharmacist's career, he or she frequently will call upon these generalizations to solve practical pharmaceutical problems.

The comprehension of course material is primarily the responsibility of the student. The teacher can guide and direct, explain and clarify, but facility in solving problems in the classroom and the laboratory depends largely on the student's understanding of theory, recall of facts, ability to integrate knowledge, and willingness to devote sufficient time and effort to the task. Each assignment should be read and outlined, and assigned problems should be solved outside the classroom. The teacher's comments then will serve to clarify questionable points and aid the student to improve his or her judgment and reasoning abilities.

DIMENSIONS AND UNITS

The properties of matter are usually expressed by the use of three fundamental dimensions: length, mass, and time. Each of these properties is assigned a definite *unit* and a *reference standard*. In the metric system, the units are the centimeter (cm), the gram (g), and the second (sec); accordingly, it is often called the *cgs* system. A reference standard is a fundamental unit

TABLE 1–1. *Fundamental Dimensions and Units*

Dimension (Measurable Quantity)	Dimensional Symbol	CGS Unit	SI Unit	Reference Standard
Length (*l*)	L	Centimeter (cm)	Meter (m)	Meter
Mass (*m*)	M	Gram (g)	Kilogram (kg)	Kilogram
Time (*t*)	T	Second (sec)	Second (s)	Atomic frequency of Cesium 133

relating each measurable quantity to some natural or artificial constant in the universe.

Measurable quantities or dimensions such as area, density, pressure, and energy are compounded from the three fundamental dimensions just referred to. In carrying out the operation of measurement, we assign to each property a dimension that is expressed quantitatively in units. Thus the quantities of length, area, and volume are measured in the dimension of length (L), length squared (L^2), and length cubed (L^3), respectively corresponding to the unit of cm, cm^2, and cm^3 in the cgs system. The fundamental dimensions, units, and reference standards are given in Table 1–1.

The International Union of Pure and Applied Chemistry (IUPAC) has introduced a *Système International* or *SI units* in an attempt to establish an internationally uniform set of units. *Physical Pharmacy* generally uses the cgs or common system of units. However, since SI units appear with increasing frequency in research articles and are found in some textbooks, they are introduced to the student in this chapter. They are also used in Chapter 4 and to some extent elsewhere in the book. SI units are listed in Tables 1–1 and 1–2, and some appear inside the front cover of the book under *Physical Constants*.

Length and Area. The dimension of length serves as a measure of distance and has as its reference standard the *meter*. It is defined as follows:

$$1 \text{ meter} = 1.65076373 \times 10^6 \lambda_{\text{Kr-86}}$$

in which $\lambda_{\text{Kr-86}} = 6.0578021 \times 10^{-7}$ m is the wavelength in vacuo of the transition between two specific energy levels of the krypton-86 atom. Prior to this definition, the meter was arbitrarily defined as the distance between two lines on a platinum–iridium bar preserved at the International Bureau of Weights and Measures in Sèvres, France. The unit of length, the centimeter, is

one hundredth of a meter, the common dimensions and multiples of which are found in Table 1–2. In the microscopic range, lengths are expressed as micrometers (μm), nanometers (nm), and angstroms, A, sometimes written Å. Units are often multiplied by positive and negative powers of 10 to indicate their magnitude, the micrometer being 1×10^{-3} millimeters or 10^{-4} cm, the nanometer 0.001 μm, and the angstrom 0.1 nm or 10^{-8} cm. Although the micrometer (μm) is the preferred term for 0.001 mm in modern textbooks on colloid chemistry, the practice is sometimes to use the older and more familiar term, micron (μ). Similarly, the nanometer has replaced the millimicron (mμ). The student should be familiar with the prefixes (see Table 1–2) accompanying units such as mass, volume, and time. For example, a nanosecond, or ns, is 10^{-9} second; a megaton (Mton) is 10^6 tons. Area is the square of a length and has the unit of square centimeters (sq. cm or cm^2).

Volume. The measurable quantity, volume, is also derived from length. Its reference standard is the *cubic meter*; its cgs unit is one millionth of this value or 1 cubic centimeter (cc or cm^3). Volume was originally defined in terms of the *liter*, the volume of a kilogram of water at 1 atmosphere pressure and 4° C, and was meant to be equivalent to 1000 cm^3. Owing to the failure to correct for the dissolved air in the water, however, the two units do not compare exactly. It has since been established that 1 liter actually equals 1000.027 cm^3. Thus, there is a discrepancy between the milliliter (one thousandth of a liter) and the cubic centimeter, but it is so slight as to be disregarded in general chemical and pharmaceutical practice. Volumes are usually expressed in milliliters in this book, abbreviated ml or mL, in conformity with the U.S. Pharmacopeia and the National Formulary; however, cubic centimeters are used in the book where this notation seems more appropriate.

The pharmacist uses cylindric and conical graduates, droppers, pipettes, and burettes for the measurement of volume; graduates are used more frequently than the other measuring apparatus in the pharmacy laboratory. The flared conical graduate is less accurate than the cylindric type, and the use of the flared graduate should be discouraged except for some liquids that need not be measured accurately. The selection of the correct graduate for the volume of liquid to be measured has been determined by Goldstein et al.[1]

TABLE 1–2. *Fractions and Multiples of Units*

Multiple	Prefix	Symbol
10^{12}	tera	T
10^9	giga	G
10^6	mega	M
10^3	kilo	k
10^{-3}	milli	m
10^{-6}	micro	μ
10^{-9}	nano	n
10^{-12}	pico	p

Mass. The standard of mass is the kilogram. It is the mass of a platinum–iridium block preserved at the Bureau of Weights and Measures. The practical unit of mass in the cgs system is the gram (g), which is one thousandth of a kilogram. Mass is often expressed as the weight of a body. The balance is said to be used for "weighing," and the standard masses are known as "weights." The proper relationship between mass and weight will be considered under the topic of force.

To weigh drugs precisely and accurately, the pharmacist must understand the errors inherent in operating a balance. A Class A balance, used for the compounding of prescriptions, is serviceable only if kept in good working condition and checked periodically for equality of arm length, beam rider accuracy, and sensitivity. These tests are described in the booklet by Goldstein and Mattocks.[2] Furthermore, a good balance is of no use unless an accurate set of weights is available.

Density and Specific Gravity. The pharmacist frequently uses these measurable quantities when interconverting between mass and volume. Density is a derived quantity since it combines the units of mass and volume. It is defined as mass per unit volume at a fixed temperature and pressure and is expressed in the cgs system in grams per cubic centimeter (g/cm³). In SI units, density is expressed as kilograms per cubic meter.

Specific gravity, unlike density, is a pure number without dimension, however, it may be converted to density by the use of appropriate formulas.[3] Specific gravity is defined as the ratio of the density of a substance to the density of water, the values for both substances being determined at the same temperature unless otherwise specified. The term *specific gravity*, in light of its definition, is a poor one; it would be more appropriate to refer to it as *relative density*.

Specific gravity is defined more often for practical purposes as the ratio of the mass of a substance to the mass of an equal volume of water at 4° or at some other specified temperature. The following notations are frequently found to accompany specific gravity readings: 25°/25°, 25°/4°, and 4°/4°. The first figure refers to the temperature of the air in which the substance was weighed; the figure following the slash is the temperature of the water used. The official pharmaceutical compendia use a basis of 25°/25° to express specific gravity.

Specific gravity may be determined by the use of various types of pycnometers, the Mohr–Westphal balance, hydrometers, and other devices. The measurements and calculations are discussed in elementary chemistry, physics, and pharmacy books.

Other Dimensions and Units. The derived dimensions and their cgs and SI units are listed in Table 1–3. Although the units and relations are self-explanatory for most of the derived dimensions, force, pressure, and energy require some elaboration.

Force. One is familiar with force in everyday experience as a push or pull required to set a body in motion. The larger the mass of the body and the greater the required acceleration, the greater the force that one must exert. Hence, the force is directly proportional to the mass (when acceleration is constant) and to the acceleration (when the mass is constant). This may be represented by the relation

$$\text{Force} \propto \text{Mass} \times \text{Acceleration} \qquad (1\text{--}1)$$

This proportionality is converted to an equality, that is, to an equation or mathematical expression involving an equal sign, according to the laws of algebra, by the introduction of a constant. Accordingly, we write

$$f = k \times m \times a \qquad (1\text{--}2)$$

in which f is the force, k is the *proportionality constant*, m is the mass, and a is the acceleration. If the units are chosen so that the constant becomes unity (i.e., has the value of 1), the well-known force equation of physics is obtained:

$$f = m \times a \qquad (1\text{--}3)$$

The cgs unit of force is the *dyne*, defined as the force that imparts to a mass of 1 g an acceleration of 1 cm/sec².

The reader should recall from physics that weight is the force of gravitational attraction that the earth

TABLE 1–3. *Derived Dimensions and Units*

Derived Dimensions	Dimensional Symbol	CGS Unit	SI Unit	Relationship to Other Dimensions
Area (A)	L^2	cm²	m²	the square of a length
Volume (V)	L^3	cm³	m³*	the cube of a length
Density (ρ)	ML^{-3}	g/cm³	kg m⁻³	mass/unit volume
Velocity (v)	LT^{-1}	cm/sec	m s⁻¹	length/unit time
Acceleration (a)	LT^{-2}	cm/sec²	m s⁻²	length/(time)²
Force (f)	MLT^{-2}	g cm/sec² or dyne	kg m s⁻² = J m⁻¹ = N	mass × acceleration
Pressure (p)	$ML^{-1}T^{-2}$	dyne/cm²	N m⁻² = kg m⁻¹s⁻² = Pa	force/unit area
Energy (E)	ML^2T^{-2}	g cm²/sec² or erg	kg m² s⁻² = N m = J	force × length

Key: N = newton, or kilogram × meter × second⁻²; Pa = pascal, or newton × meter⁻²; J = joule; in this table, m = meter, not mass; L = length; T = time; M = mass.

*The cubic meter is a large volume, so that volume is often expressed in SI units as decimeter cubed (dm³) which is equal to 1000 cm³.

exerts on a body, and it should be expressed properly in force units (dynes) rather than mass units (grams). The relationship between weight and mass can be obtained from equation (1–3). Substituting weight w for force and g for acceleration, the equation becomes

$$w = m \times g \qquad (1-4)$$

Although the gravitational acceleration of a body varies from one part of the earth to another, it is approximately constant at 981 cm/sec^2. Substituting this value for g, the weight of a 1-g mass is calculated from equation (1–4) as follows:

$$w = 1 \text{ g} \times 981 \text{ cm/sec}^2$$

and

$$w = 981 \text{ g cm/sec}^2 \text{ or } 981 \text{ dynes}$$

Therefore, the weight of a body with a mass of 1 gram is actually 981 dynes. It is common practice to express weight in the mass unit, grams, since weight is directly proportional to mass; however, in problems involving these physical quantities, the distinction must be made.

The SI unit of force is the newton (N), which is equal to one kg m s^{-2}. It is defined as the force that imparts to a mass of 1 kg an acceleration of 1 m/sec^2 (see Table 1–3).

Pressure. *Pressure* may be defined as force per unit area; the unit commonly used in science is dyne/cm^2. Pressure is often given in atmospheres (atm) or in centimeters or millimeters of mercury. This latter unit is derived from a measurement of the height of a column of mercury in a barometer, which is used to measure the atmospheric pressure. The equation from elementary physics used to convert height in a column of mercury or another liquid into pressure units is

$$\text{pressure (dyne/cm}^2) = \rho \times g \times h \qquad (1-5)$$

where ρ is the density of the liquid in g/cm^3 at a particular temperature, g is the acceleration of gravity 980.665 cm/sec^2, and h is the height in cm of the column of liquid. At sea level, the mean pressure of the atmosphere supports a column of mercury 76 cm (760 mm) or 29.9 inches in height. The barometric pressure may be translated into the fundamental pressure unit, dyne/cm^2, by multiplying the height, $h = 76$ cm, times 1 cm^2 cross-sectional area by the density ρ of mercury, 13.595 g/cm^3, at 0° to give the mass and multiplying this by the acceleration of gravity, $g = 980.7$ cm/sec^2. The result divided by cm^2 is 1.0133×10^6 dyne/cm^2 and is equal to 1 atm. This series of multiplication and division is expressed simply by equation 5.

In the SI system, the unit of pressure (or stress) is the newton divided by the meter squared (Nm^{-2}) and is called the pascal (Pa), (see Table 1–3).

Example 1–1. Convert the pressure of a column of ethyl alcohol 76 cm Hg (760 mm Hg) high to a pressure at sea level and 0° C (standard pressure) expressed in *(a)* dyne/cm^2 and *(b)* pascals (Pa). The density (ρ) of ethanol at 0° C is 0.80625 g/cm^3.

(a) To obtain the standard pressure in dyne/cm^2, one uses equation (1–5) with the density $\rho = 0.80625$ g/cm^3, the acceleration of gravity g at sea level as 980.665 cm/sec^2, and the height h of the column of mercury as 76.000 cm Hg.

$$\text{Pressure} = 0.80625 \text{ g/cm}^3 \times 980.665 \text{ cm/sec}^2 \times 76.000 \text{ cm}$$
$$= 6.00902 \times 10^4 \text{ dyne/cm}^2$$

(b) To obtain the standard pressure in pascals (Pa), we use SI units in equation (1–5):

$$\text{Pressure} = \left(0.80625 \text{ g/cm}^3 \times \frac{\text{kg}}{10^3\text{g}} \times \frac{(10^2)^3\text{cm}^3}{1\text{m}^3}\right)^*$$
$$\times \left(980.665 \text{ cm/sec}^2 \times \frac{\text{m}}{100 \text{ cm}}\right) \times \left(76.000 \text{ cm} \times \frac{\text{m}}{100 \text{ cm}}\right)$$
$$= 6.00902 \times 10^3 \text{ kg m}^{-1} \cdot \text{s}^{-2} \text{ (or N} \cdot \text{m}^{-2}, \text{ or Pa)}$$

*1 meter = 10^2 cm; therefore, 1 m^3 = $(10^2)^3$cm^3 = 10^6cm^3.

Work and Energy. Energy is frequently defined as the condition of a body that gives it the capacity for doing work. The concept actually is so fundamental that no adequate definition can be given. Energy may be classified as kinetic energy or potential energy.

The idea of energy is best approached by way of the mechanical equivalent of energy known as *work* and the thermal equivalent of energy or *heat*. When a constant force is applied to a body in the direction of its movement, the work done on the body equals the force multiplied by the displacement, and the system undergoes an increase in energy. The product of force and distance has the same dimensions as energy, namely ML^2T^{-2}. Other products also having the dimensions of energy are pressure × volume, surface tension × area, mass × velocity^2, and electric potential difference × quantity of electricity.

The cgs unit of work, also the unit of kinetic and potential energy, is the erg. It is defined as the work done when a force of 1 dyne acts through a distance of 1 centimeter:

$$1 \text{ erg} = 1 \text{ dyne} \times 1 \text{ cm}$$

The erg is often too small for practical use and is replaced by the joule (J) (pronounced *jewel*), which is equal to 10^7 ergs:

$$1 \text{ joule} = 1 \times 10^7 \text{ erg}$$

In carrying out calculations in the cgs system involving work and pressure, work must be expressed in ergs and pressure in dynes/cm^2. When using the SI or any other system, consistent units must also be employed.

Heat and work are equivalent forms of energy and are interchangeable under certain circumstances. The thermal unit of energy in the cgs system is the gram calorie (small calorie). Formerly it was expressed as the amount of heat necessary to raise the temperature of 1 gram of water from 15° to 16° C. The small calorie is now defined as equal to 4.184 joules. The large or kilogram calorie (kcal) equals 1000 small calories. The SI unit for energy or work is the joule (J), which is seen in Table 1–3 to be equivalent to the newton × meter (N m).

Temperature. Temperature is assigned a unit known as the degree. On the centigrade and the Kelvin or absolute scales, the freezing and boiling points of pure water at 1 atm pressure are separated by 100 degrees. Zero degree on the centigrade scale equals 273.15° on the Kelvin scale.

SOME ELEMENTS OF MATHEMATICS

The student should become familiar with the fundamental concepts of mathematics that are frequently used in the physical sciences and upon which are based many of the equations and graphic representations encountered in this book.

Calculations Involving dimensions. Ratio and proportions are frequently used in the physical sciences for conversions from one system to another. The following calculation illustrates the use of proportions.

Example 1–2. How many gram calories are there in 3.00 joules? One should first recall a relationship or ratio that connects calories and joules. The relation 1 cal = 4.184 joules comes to mind. The question is then asked in the form of a proportion: If 1 calorie equals 4.184 joules, how many calories are there in 3.00 joules? The proportion is set down, being careful to express each quantity in its proper units. For the unknown quantity, an "X" is used.

$$\frac{1 \text{ cal}}{4.184 \text{ joules}} = \frac{X}{3.00 \text{ joules}}$$

$$X = \frac{3.00 \text{ joules} \times 1 \text{ cal}}{4.184 \text{ joules}}$$

$$X = 0.717 \text{ cal}$$

A second method, based on the requirement that the units as well as the dimensions be identical on both sides of the equal sign, is sometimes more convenient than the method of proportions.

Example 1–3. How many gallons are equivalent to 2.0 liters? It would be necessary to set up successive proportions to solve this problem. In the method involving identity of units on both sides of the equation, the quantity desired, X (gallons), is placed on the left and its equivalent, 2.0 liters, is set down on the right side of the equation. The right side must then be multiplied by known relations in ratio form, such as 1 pint per 473 ml, to give the units of gallons. Carrying out the indicated operations yields the result with its proper units.

$$X \text{ (in gallons)} = 2.0 \text{ liter} \times (1000 \text{ mL/liter})$$
$$\times (1 \text{ pt/473 mL}) \times (1 \text{ gal/8 pt})$$
$$X = 0.53 \text{ gal}$$

One may be concerned about the apparent disregard for the rules of significant figures (p. 11) in the equivalents such as 1 pint = 473 mL. The quantity of pints can be measured as accurately as that of milliliters, so that we assume 1.00 pint is meant here. The quantities 1 gallon and 1 liter are also exact by definition, and significant figures need not be considered in such cases.

Exponents. The various operations involving exponents, that is, the powers to which a number is raised, are best reviewed by studying the examples set out in Table 1–4.

TABLE 1–4. *The Rules of Exponents*

$a \times a \times a = a^3$	$a^2/a^4 = a^{2-4} = a^{-2} = \dfrac{1}{a^2}$
$a^2 \times a^3 = a^{2+3} = a^5$	$a^2/a^2 = a^{2-2} = a^0 = 1$
$(a^2)^3 = a^2 \times a^2 \times a^2 = a^6$	$a^{1/2} = \sqrt{a}$
$\left(\dfrac{a}{b}\right)^3 = a^3/b^3$	$a^{1/2} \times a^{1/2} = a^{1/2+1/2} = a^1 = a$
$a^5/a^2 = a^{5-2} = a^3$	$a^{2/3} = (a^2)^{1/3} = \sqrt[3]{a^2}$
$a^5/a^4 = a^{5-4} = a^1 = a$	

Logarithms. The equality

$$10^3 = 1000 \tag{1–6}$$

is expressed in logarithmic notation as:

$$\log_{10} 1000 = 3 \tag{1–7}$$

The exponent 3 to which the base 10 is raised to give 1000 in equation (1–6) is referred to as the logarithm of 1000. The number 1000 is known as the *antilogarithm* of the number 3. In general, if b, raised to the power x, gives the number a, then the logarithm to the base b of a is x:

$$b^x = a \tag{1–8}$$
$$\log_b a = x \tag{1–9}$$

When 10 is used as the base, the logarithm is known as the *common* or *Briggsian* logarithm, whereas the number 2.71828 . . . , designated as e, is used as the base for the *natural* or *Napierian* logarithms. The quantity e is important in the theoretic development of the physical and biochemical sciences and is discussed in some detail by Daniels.[4] It is the sum of the series 1 + 1 + 1/2! + 1/3! + 1/4! . . . in which ! denotes a factorial number that is defined as the product of the positive integers between 1 and the number. Thus, 2! = 1 × 2, 3! = 1 × 2 × 3 = 6, and 4! = 1 × 2 × 3 × 4 = 24. The common logarithms are designated by the symbol $\log_{10}$ or simply as log, while the natural logarithms are written as $\log_e$ or ln.

Although one usually has access to a hand calculator for obtaining the logarithms of numbers, it sometimes happens that one has only a table of common logarithms (see the back cover of this book). To convert from one system to another, particularly from the natural to the common logarithm, the following formula is used:

$$\ln a = 2.303 \log a^* \tag{1–10}$$

Equation (10) may be derived as follows. Let

$$\log a = x \tag{1–11}$$

so that

$$a = 10^x \tag{1–12}$$

*The conversion factor, 2.303, is more accurately expressed as 2.302585.

and taking the natural logarithm, equation (1–12) becomes

$$\ln a = \ln 10^x = x \ln 10 \qquad (1\text{–}13)$$

Now $\ln 10 = 2.303$, and equation (1–13) becomes

$$\ln a = 2.303\, x \qquad (1\text{–}14)$$

Substituting the identity $x = \log a$ from equation (1–11) into equation (1–14) gives the desired formula.

The application of logarithm is best demonstrated by considering several examples. In the expression,

$$\log 60.0 = 1.778$$

the digit 1 to the left of the decimal point in the logarithm is known as the *characteristic* and signifies that the number 60.0 belongs to that class of numbers with a magnitude of 10^1 and thus contains two figures to the left of the decimal point. The quantity 0.778 of the logarithm is known as the *mantissa* and is found in the table of common logarithms. It is often convenient to express the number 60.0 by writing it with one significant figure to the left of the decimal point, 6.00, multiplied by 10 raised to the first power, viz., 6.00×10^1. The exponent of 10 then gives the characteristic, and the value in the logarithm table gives the mantissa directly.

This method may be used to obtain the logarithm of 6000 from a table as follows. The number is first written as 6.000×10^3 if it is accurate to four significant figures. The characteristic is observed to be 3, and the mantissa is found in the table as 0.778. Hence,

$$\log 6000 = 3.778$$

For decimal fractions that frequently appear in problems involving molar concentration, the following method is used. Suppose one desires to know the logarithm of 0.0600. The number is first written as 6.00×10^{-2}. The characteristic of a number may be positive or negative; the mantissa is always positive. The characteristic in this case is -2 and the mantissa is 0.778. Hence,

$$\log 0.0600 = -2 + 0.778 = -1.222$$

Finding the number in a table when the logarithm is given, that is, obaining the *antilogarithm*, is shown by the following example. What is the value of a if $\log a = 1.7404$? The characteristic is 1 and the mantissa is 0.7404. From the table of logarithms, one finds that the number corresponding to a mantissa of 0.7404 is 5.50. The characteristic is 1, so the antilogarithm is 5.50×10^1 or 55.0.

Let us find the antilogarithm of a negative number, -2.699. Recalling that the mantissa must always be positive, we first separate the logarithm into a negative characteristic and positive mantissa:

$$-2.699 = -3.00 + 0.301$$

This transformation is easily seen in Figure 1–1, in

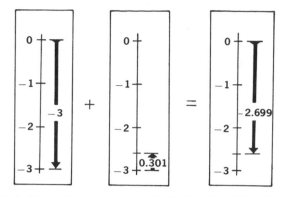

Fig. 1–1. Schematic representation for finding the antilogarithm of a negative number.

which -2.699 corresponds to going down the scale in a negative direction to -3 and coming back up the scale 0.301 units in the positive direction. Actually, by this process, we are subtracting 1 from the characteristic and adding 1 to the mantissa, or to the quantity

$$-2.699 = (-2) + (-0.699)$$

we subtract and add 1 to yield

$$(-2 - 1) + (-0.699 + 1) = -3 + 0.301$$

The result $(-3 + 0.301)$ is sometimes abbreviated to $(\bar{3}.301)$, in which the minus sign above the 3 applies only to the characteristic. $\bar{3}$ is commonly referred to as "bar three." It has been the practice in some fields, such as quantitative analysis, to use the form in which 10 is added and subtracted to give

$$\bar{3}.301 = 7.301 - 10$$

For physical chemical calculations and for plotting logarithms of numbers, it is more convenient to use the form -2.699 than one of the forms having a mixture of negative and positive parts. For use with logarithm tables, however, the mixed form is needed. Thus, in order to obtain the antilogarithm, we write the logarithm as $\bar{3}.301$. The number corresponding to the mantissa is found in the logarithm table to be 2.00. The characteristic is observed to be -3, and the final result is therefore 2.00×10^{-3}.

We have dealt with logarithms to the base 10 (common logarithms) and to the base $e = 2.71828\ldots$ (natural logarithms). Logarithms to any other positive number as the base, b, may also be obtained. The formula used for this purpose is

$$\log_b(a) = \log_e(a)/\log_e(b) \qquad (1\text{–}15)$$

To obtain the logarithm of the number $a = 100$ to the base $b = 37$, we substitute in equation (1–15):

$$\log_{37}(100) = \ln(100)/\ln(37) = 1.2753$$

One may also use common logs on the right side of the equation:

$$\log_{37}(100) = \log_{10}(100)/\log_{10}(37) = 1.2753$$

TABLE 1–5. *Rules of Logarithms*

$\log ab = \log a + \log b$	$\log \dfrac{1}{a} = \log 1 - \log a = -\log a$
$\log \dfrac{a}{b} = \log a - \log b$	$\log a^2 = \log a + \log a = 2 \log a$
$\log 1 = 0$ since $10^0 = 1$	$\log \sqrt{a} = \log a^{1/2} = \frac{1}{2} \log a$
	$\log a^{-2} = -2 \log a = 2 \log \dfrac{1}{a}$

These formulas allow one to obtain a logarithm to a base b for any whole or fractional positive number desired. *Problem 1–12* is an exercise involving the change from one logarithmic base to another.

As seen in the table of exponents (Table 1–4), numbers may be multiplied and divided by adding and subtracting exponents. Since logarithms are exponents, they follow the same rules. Some of the properties of logarithms are exemplified by the identities collected in Table 1–5.

Variation. The scientist is continually attempting to relate phenomena and establish generalizations with which to consolidate and interpret experimental data. The problem frequently resolves itself into a search for the relationship between two quantities that are changing at a certain rate or in a particular manner. The dependence of one property, the *dependent variable y*, on the change or alteration of another measurable quantity, the *independent variable x*, is expressed mathematically as

$$y \propto x \qquad (1-16)$$

which is read: "*y* varies directly as *x*," or "*y* is directly proportional to *x*." A proportionality is changed to an equation as follows. If *y* is proportional to *x* in general, then all pairs of specific values of *y* and *x*, say y_1 and x_1, y_2 and x_2, . . . , are proportional. Thus

$$\frac{y_1}{x_1} = \frac{y_2}{x_2} = \cdots \qquad (1-17)$$

Since the ratio of any *y* to its corresponding *x* is equal to any other ratio of *y* and *x*, the ratios are constant, or, in general

$$\frac{y}{x} = \text{constant} \qquad (1-18)$$

Hence, it is a simple matter to change a proportionality to an equality by introducing a *proportionality constant*, *k*. To summarize, if

$$y \propto x$$

then

$$y = kx \qquad (1-19)$$

It is frequently desirable to show the relationship between *x* and *y* by the use of the more general notation,

$$y = f(x) \qquad (1-20)$$

which is read: "*y* is some function of *x*." That is, *y* may be equal to $2x$, to $27x^2$, or to $0.0051 + \log(a/x)$. The functional notation, equation (1–20), merely signifies that *y* and *x* are related in some way without specifying the actual equation by which they are connected. Some well-known formulas illustrating the principle of variation are shown in Table 1–6.

Graphic Methods. Scientists are not usually so fortunate as to begin each problem with an equation at hand relating the variables under study. Instead, the investigator must collect raw data and put them in the form of a table or graph to better observe the relationships. Constructing a graph with the data plotted in a manner so as to form a smooth curve often permits the investigator to observe the relationship more clearly, and perhaps allows expression of the connection in the form of a mathematical equation. The procedure of obtaining an empiric equation from a plot of the data is known as *curve fitting* and is treated in books on statistics and graphic analysis.

The magnitude of the independent variable is customarily measured along the horizontal coordinate scale called the *x* axis. The dependent variable is measured along the vertical scale or the *y* axis. The data are plotted on the graph, and a smooth line is drawn through the points. The *x* value of each point is known as the *x* coordinate or the *abscissa*, the *y* value is known as the *y* coordinate or the *ordinate*. The intersection of the *x* axis and the *y* axis is referred to as the *origin*. The *x* and *y* values may be either negative or positive.

The simplest relationship between two variables, where the variables contain no exponents other than one (*first-degree equation*), yields a straight line when plotted on rectangular graph paper. The straight-line or linear relationship is expressed as

$$y = a + bx \qquad (1-21)$$

in which *y* is the dependent variable, *x* is the independent variable, and *a* and *b* are constants. The constant

TABLE 1–6. *Formulas Illustrating the Principle of Variation*

Measurement	Equation	Dependent Variation	Independent Variable	Proportionality Constant
Circumference of a circle	$C = \pi D$	Circumference, C	Diameter, D	$\pi = 3.14159 \ldots$
Density	$M = \rho V$	Mass, M	Volume, V	Density, ρ
Distance of falling body	$s = \frac{1}{2}gt^2$	Distance, s	Time, t^2	Gravity constant, $\frac{1}{2}g$
Freezing point depression	$\Delta T_f = K_f m$	Freezing point depression, ΔT_f	Molality, m	Cryoscopic constant, K_f

b is the *slope* of the line; the greater the value of b, the steeper the slope. It is expressed as the change in y with the change in x or $b = \dfrac{\Delta y}{\Delta x}$; b is also the tangent of the angle that the line makes with the x axis. The slope may be positive or negative depending on whether the line slants upward or downward to the right. When $b = 1$, the line makes an angle of 45° with the x axis (tan 45° = 1), and the equation of the line may then be written

$$y = a + x \qquad (1\text{-}22)$$

When $b = 0$, the line is horizontal (i.e., parallel to the x axis), and the equation reduces to

$$y = a \qquad (1\text{-}23)$$

The constant a is known as the *y intercept* and signifies the point at which the line crosses the y axis. If a is positive, the line crosses the y axis above the x axis; if negative, it intersects the y axis below the x axis. When a is zero, equation (1–21) may be written,

$$y = bx \qquad (1\text{-}24)$$

and the line passes through the origin.

The results of the determination of the refractive index of a benzene solution containing increasing concentrations of carbon tetrachloride are found in Table 1–7. The data are plotted in Figure 1–2 and are seen to produce a straight line with a negative slope. The equation of the line may be obtained by using the two-point form of the linear equation,

$$y - y_1 = \frac{y_2 - y_1}{x_2 - x_1}(x - x_1) \qquad (1\text{-}25)$$

The method involves selecting two widely separated points (x_1, y_1) and (x_2, y_2) on the line and substituting into the two-point equation.

Example 1–4. Referring to Figure 1–2, let 10.0% be x_1 and its corresponding y value 1.497 be y_1; let 60.0% be x_2 and 1.477 be y_2. The equation then becomes

$$y - 1.497 = \frac{1.477 - 1.497}{60.0 - 10.0}(x - 10.0)$$

$$y - 1.497 = -4.00 \times 10^{-4}(x - 10.0)$$

$$y = -4.00 \times 10^{-4}\,x + 1.501$$

The value -4.00×10^{-4} is the slope of the straight line and corresponds to b in equation (1–21). A negative

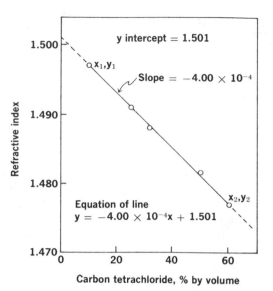

Fig. 1–2. Refractive index of the system benzene-carbon tetrachloride at 20° C.

value for b indicates that y decreases with increasing values of x as observed in Figure 1–2. The value 1.501 is the y intercept and corresponds to a in equation (1–21).* It may be obtained from the plot in Figure 1–2 by *extrapolating* (extending) the line upwards to the left until it intersects the y axis. It will also be observed that

$$\frac{y_2 - y_1}{x_2 - x_1} = \frac{\Delta y}{\Delta x} = b \qquad (1\text{-}26)$$

and this simple formula allows one to compute the slope of a straight line. The use of *statistics* to determine whether data fit the slope of such a line and its intercept on the y axis is illustrated later in this chapter.

Not all experimental data form straight lines when plotted on ordinary rectangular coordinate paper. Equations containing x^2 or y^2 are known as *second-degree* or *quadratic equations*, and graphs of these equations yield parabolas, hyperbolas, ellipses, and circles. The graphs and their corresponding equations may be found in standard textbooks on analytic geometry.

Logarithmic relationships occur frequently in scientific work. The data relating the amount of oil separating from an emulsion per month (dependent variable, y) as a function of the emulsifier concentration (independent variable, x) are collected in Table 1–8.

The data from this experiment may be plotted in several ways. In Figure 1–3, the oil separation y is plotted as ordinates against the emulsifier concentration x as abscissas on a rectangular coordinate grid. In

TABLE 1–7. *Refractive Indices of Mixtures of Benzene and Carbon Tetrachloride*

(x) Concentration of CCl$_4$ (volume %)	(y) Refractive Index
10.0	1.497
25.0	1.491
33.0	1.488
50.0	1.481
60.0	1.477

*The y-intercept, 1.501, is of course the refractive index of pure benzene at 20° C. For the purpose of this example we assume that we were not able to find this value in a table of refractive indices. In handbooks of chemistry and physics the value is actually found to be 1.5011 at 20° C.

TABLE 1–8. *Emulsion Stability as a Function of Emulsifier Concentration*

Emulsifier (% Concentration) (x)	Oil Separation (mL/month) (y)	Logarithm of Oil Separation (log y)
0.50	5.10	0.708
1.00	3.60	0.556
1.50	2.60	0.415
2.00	2.00	0.301
2.50	1.40	0.146
3.00	1.00	0.000

Figure 1–4, the logarithm of the oil separation is plotted against the concentration. In Figure 1–5, the data are plotted on semilogarithm paper, consisting of a logarithmic scale on the vertical axis and a linear scale on the horizontal axis.

Although Figure 1–3 provides a direct reading of oil separation, difficulties arise when one attempts to draw a smooth line through the points or to extrapolate the curve beyond the experimental data. Furthermore, the equation for the curve cannot be obtained readily from Figure 1–3. When the logarithm of oil separation is plotted as the ordinate, as in Figure 1–4, a straight line results, indicating that the phenomenon follows a logarithmic or exponential relationship. The slope and the y intercept are obtained from the graph, and the equation for the line is subsequently found by use of the two-point formula:

$$\log y = 0.85 - 0.28x$$

Figure 1–4 requires that we obtain the logarithms of the oil-separation data before the graph is constructed and, conversely, that we obtain the antilogarithm of the ordinates to read oil separation from the graph. These inconveniences of converting to logarithms and antilogarithms may be overcome by the use of semilogarithm paper. The x and y values of Table 1–8 are plotted directly on the graph to yield a straight line, as seen in

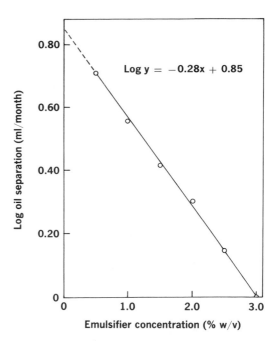

Fig. 1–4. A plot of the logarithm of oil separation of an emulsion vs. concentration on a rectangular grid.

Figure 1–5. Although such a plot ordinarily is not used to obtain the equation of the line, it is convenient for reading the oil separation directly from the graph. It is well to remember that the ln of a number is simply 2.303 log of the number. Therefore, logarithmic graph scales may be used for ln as well as for log plots.

Computers and Calculators. Computers are used widely in industry, government, business, education, and research and touch the lives of nearly everyone in one way or another. Computers may be divided into analog and digital machines. Digital computers deal

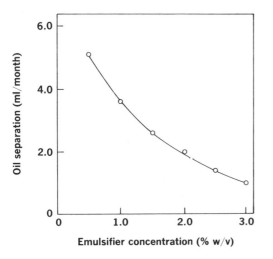

Fig. 1–3. Emulsion stability data plotted on a rectangular coordinate grid.

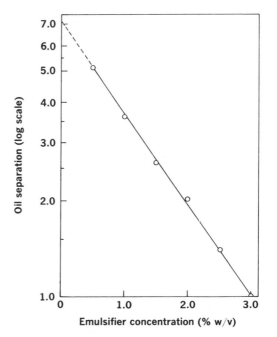

Fig. 1–5. Emulsion stability plotted on a semilogarithmic grid.

with numbers much like desk and hand-held calculators do. The modern calculator is provided with registers for the storage of data and a central core that can be programmed with mathematical instructions to carry out most mathematical functions. The programmable calculator, like the computer, also has a decision-making capacity through its ability to determine whether a number is larger than zero (positive), smaller than zero (negative), or equal to zero. The computer differs from the calculator in that it is faster, capable of greater storage, and more versatile.

The analog computer, unlike the digital computer, handles mathematical problems using voltages to represent variables such as concentration, pressure, time, and temperature. If the problem can be written as a differential equation (Examples A–9, A–12, p. 599), the solution is obtained by expressing the equation in voltages, capacitances, and resistances and then causing the voltage to vary with time as determined by the differential equation. The solution to the problem appears as a graphic plot on a recorder or is displayed as a tracing on an oscilloscope screen. The analog computer is composed of tens or hundreds of amplifiers that are used for the mathematical operations of addition, multiplication, and so on. The amplifiers are connected by the operator into a circuit that represents the differential equation at hand. Each amplifier corresponds to one step in the chemical, physical, or mechanical process under consideration. The analog computer is used in engineering to simulate the spring action on the axles of an automobile or the movement of a skyscraper in a high wind. It has been used to calculate the absorption, distribution, and elimination constants for a drug that is administered to a patient and to plot the curves for uptake and excretion. Today the digital computer can also calculate such values and prepare graphs with facility, and the popularity of the analog computer has diminished in pharmacy in recent years.

Currently, the microcomputer and the hand-held calculator are of great interest in small business and education and for personal use. The microcomputer, at a price within reach of the average individual, is more powerful today than the large institutional computers of the 1960s.

Programs may be written for large electronic computers and microcomputers in a number of languages, the most popular of which are FORTRAN, BASIC, PASCAL, C, and C++. Even some hand-held calculators can now be programmed in BASIC.

It will profit the student to become familiar with BASIC and/or FORTRAN and with the operation of an institutional or personal microcomputer. A hand-held calculator will be useful for working the problems at the ends of the chapters of this book. A programmable calculator is particularly convenient to obtain the slopes and intercepts of lines and for carrying out a repetitive sequence of mathematical operations. For example, in the chapter on solubility, if one desires to calculate the

minimum pH for complete solubility of a series of 10 acidic drugs of known pK_a values, it is simpler and faster to program the calculator than to carry out a number of repetitive steps for each of the 10 drugs.

Significant Figures. A significant figure is any digit used to represent a magnitude or quantity in the place in which it stands. The number zero is considered as a significant figure except when it is used merely to locate the decimal point. The two zeros immediately following the decimal point in the number 0.00750 merely locate the decimal point and are not significant. However, the zero following the 5 is significant since it is not needed to write the number; if it were not significant, it could be omitted. Thus, the value contains three significant figures. The question of significant figures in the number 7500 is ambiguous. One does not know whether any or all of the zeros are meant to be significant, or whether they are simply used to indicate the magnitude of the number. To express the significant figures of such a value in an unambiguous way, it is best to use exponential notation. Thus, the expression 7.5×10^3 signifies that the number contains two significant figures, and the zeros in 7500 are not to be taken as significant. In the value, 7.500×10^3, both zeros are significant, and the number contains a total of four significant figures. The significant figures of some values are shown in Table 1–9.

The significant figures of a number include all certain digits plus the first uncertain digit. For example, one may use a ruler, the smallest subdivisions of which are centimeters, to measure the length of a piece of glass tubing. If one finds that the tubing measures slightly greater than 27 cm in length, it is proper to estimate the doubtful fraction, say 0.4, and express the number as 27.4 cm. A replicate measurement may yield the value 27.6 or 27.2 cm so that the result is expressed as 27.4 ± 0.2 cm. When a value such as 27.4 cm is encountered in the literature without further qualification, the reader should assume that the final figure is correct to within about ±1 in the last decimal place, which is meant to signify the mean deviation of a single measurement. However, when a statement is given in the official compendia (U.S. Pharmacopeia and National Formulary) such as "not less than 99," it means 99.0 and not 98.9.

Significant figures are particularly useful for indicating the precision of a result. The precision is limited by

TABLE 1–9. *Significant Figures*

Number	Number of Significant Figures
53.	2
530.0	4
0.00053	2
5.0030	5
5.3×10^{-2}	2
5.30×10^{-4}	3
53000	indeterminate

the instrument used to make the measurement. A measuring rule marked off in centimeter divisions will not produce as great a precision as one marked off in 0.1 cm or mm. One may obtain a length of 27.4 ± 0.2 cm with the first ruler and a value of, say, 27.46 ± 0.02 cm with the second. The latter ruler, yielding a result with four significant figures, is obviously the more precise one. The number 27.46 implies a precision of about 2 parts in 3000, whereas 27.4 implies a precision of only 2 parts in 300.

The absolute magnitude of a value should not be confused with its precision. We consider the number 0.00053 mole/liter as a relatively small quantity because three zeros immediately follow the decimal point. But these zeros are not significant and tell us nothing about the precision of the measurement. When such a result is expressed as 5.3×10^{-4} mole/liter, or better as 5.3 (± 0.1) $\times 10^{-4}$ mole/liter, both its precision and its magnitude are readily apparent.

In dealing with experimental data, certain rules pertain to the figures that enter into the computations:

1. In rejecting superfluous figures, increase by 1 the last figure retained if the following figure rejected is 5 or greater. Do not alter the last figure if the rejected figure has a value of less than 5. Thus, if the value 13.2764 is to be rounded off to four significant figures, it is written as 13.28. The value 13.2744 is rounded off to 13.27.

2. In addition or subtraction, include only as many figures to the right of the decimal point as there are present in the number with the least such figures. Thus, in adding 442.78, 58.4, and 2.684, obtain the sum and then round off the result so that it contains only one figure following the decimal point:

$$442.78 + 58.4 + 2.684 = 503.684$$

This figure is rounded off to 503.9.

Rule 2 of course cannot apply to the weights and volumes of ingredients in the monograph of a pharmaceutical preparation. The minimum weight or volume of each ingredient in a pharmaceutical formula or a prescription should be large enough that the error introduced is no greater than, say, 5 in 100 (5%), using the weighing and measuring apparatus at hand. Accuracy and precision in prescription compounding is discussed in some detail by Brecht.[5]

3. In multiplication or division, the rule commonly used is to retain the same number of significant figures in the result as appear in the value with the least number of significant figures. In multiplying 2.67 and 3.2, the result is recorded as 8.5 rather than as 8.544. A better rule here is to retain in the result the number of figures that produces a percentage error no greater than that in the value with the largest percentage uncertainty.

4. In the use of logarithms for multiplication and division, retain the same number of significant figures in the mantissa as there are in the original numbers.

The characteristic signifies only the magnitude of the number and accordingly is not significant. Since calculations involved in theoretic pharmacy usually require no more than three significant figures, a four-place logarithm table yields sufficient precision for our work. Such a table is found on the inside back cover of this book. The hand calculator is more convenient, however, and tables of logarithms are used less frequently today. Logarithms to nine significant figures are obtained by the simple press of a button on the modern hand calculator.

5. If the result is to be used in further calculations, retain at least one digit more than suggested in the rules just given. The final result is then rounded off to the last significant figure.

STATISTICAL METHODS AND THE ANALYSIS OF ERRORS

If one is to maintain a high degree of exactitude in the compounding of prescriptions and the manufacture of products on a large scale, one must know how to locate and eliminate constant and accidental errors insofar as possible. Pharmacists must recognize, however, that just as they cannot hope to produce a perfect pharmaceutical product, neither can they make an absolute measurement. In addition to the inescapable imperfections in mechanical apparatus and the slight impurities that are always present in chemicals, perfect accuracy is impossible because of the inability of the operator to make a measurement or estimate a quantity to a degree finer than the smallest division of the instrument scale.

Error may be defined as a deviation from the absolute value or from the true average of a large number of results. Two types of errors are recognized: *determinate* (constant) and *indeterminate* (random or accidental).

Determinate Errors. Determinate or constant errors are those that, although sometimes unsuspected, may be avoided or determined and corrected once they are uncovered. They are usually present in each measurement and affect all observations of a series in the same way. Examples of determinate errors are those inherent in the particular method used, errors in the calibration and the operation of the measuring instruments, impurities in the reagents and drugs, biased personal errors that, for example, might recur consistently in the reading of a meniscus, in pouring and mixing, in weighing operations, in matching colors, and in making calculations. The change of volume of solutions with temperature, while not constant, is, however, a systematic error that also may be determined and accounted for once the coefficient of expansion is known.

Determinate errors may be combated in analytic work by the use of calibrated apparatus, by the use of blanks and controls, by using several different analytic procedures and apparatus, by eliminating impurities, and by carrying out the experiment under varying conditions. In pharmaceutical manufacturing, determinate errors may be eliminated by calibrating the weights and other apparatus and by checking calculations and results with other workers. Adequate corrections for determinate errors must be made before the estimation of indeterminate errors can have any significance.

Indeterminate Errors. Indeterminate errors occur by accident or chance, and they vary from one measurement to the next. When one fires a number of bullets at a target, some may hit the "bull's eye," while others will be scattered around this central point. The greater the skill of the marksman, the less scattered will be the pattern on the target. Likewise, in a chemical analysis, the results of a series of tests will yield a random pattern around an average or central value, known as the *mean.* Random errors will also occur in filling a number of capsules with a drug, and the finished products will show a definite variation in weight.

Indeterminate errors cannot be allowed for or corrected because of the natural fluctuations that occur in all measurements.

Those errors that arise from random fluctuations in temperature or other external factors and from the variations involved in reading instruments are not to be considered accidental or random. Instead, they belong to the class of determinate errors and are often called *pseudoaccidental* or *variable determinate* errors. These errors may be reduced by controlling conditions through the use of constant-temperature baths and ovens, the use of buffers, and the maintenance of constant humidity and pressure where indicated. Care in reading fractions of units on graduates, balances, and other apparatus can also reduce pseudoaccidental errors. Variable determinate errors, although seemingly indeterminate, can thus be determined and corrected by careful analysis and refinement of technique on the part of the worker. Only errors that result from pure random fluctuations in nature are considered truly indeterminate.

Precision and Accuracy. *Precision* is a measure of the agreement among the values in a group of data, while *accuracy* is the agreement between the data and the true value. Indeterminate or chance errors influence the precision of the results, and the measurement of the precision is accomplished best by statistical means. Determinate or constant errors affect the accuracy of data. The techniques used in analyzing the precision of results, which in turn supply a measure of the indeterminate errors, will be considered first, and the detection and elimination of determinate errors or inaccuracies will be discussed later.

Indeterminate or chance errors obey the laws of probability, both positive and negative errors being equally probable, and larger errors being less probable than smaller ones. If one plots a large number of results

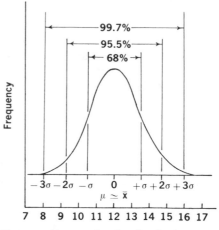

Fig. 1–6. The normal curve for the distribution of indeterminate errors.

having various errors along the vertical axis against the magnitude of the errors on the horizontal axis, a bell-shaped curve, known as a *normal frequency distribution curve,* is often obtained, as shown in Figure 1–6. If the distribution of results follows the normal probability law, the deviations will be represented exactly by the curve for an infinite number of observations, which constitute the *universe* or *population.* Whereas the population is the whole of the category under consideration, the *sample* is that portion of the population used in the analysis.

The Arithmetic Mean. When a normal distribution is obtained, it follows that the arithmetic mean is the best measure of the central value of a distribution; that is, the mean represents a point corresponding closest to the "bull's eye." The theoretic mean for a large number of measurements (the universe or population) is known as the *universe* or *population mean* and is given the symbol μ (mu).

The arithmetic mean $\overline{X}$ is obtained by adding together the results of the various measurements and dividing the total by the number N of the measurements. In mathematical notation, the arithmetic mean for a small group of values is expressed as

$$\overline{X} = \frac{\Sigma(X_i)}{N} \qquad (1\text{--}27)$$

in which Σ is the Greek capital letter sigma standing for "the sum of," X_i is the ith individual measurement of the group, and N is the number of values. $\overline{X}$ is an estimate of μ and approaches it as the number of measurements N is increased.

Measures of Dispersion. After having chosen the arithmetic mean as the central tendency of the data, it is necessary to express the dispersion or scatter about the central value in a quantitative fashion so as to establish an estimate of variation among the results. This variability is usually expressed as the *range,* the *mean deviation,* or the *standard deviation.*

The range is the difference between the largest and the smallest value in a group of data and gives a rough idea of the dispersion. It sometimes leads to ambiguous results, however, when the maximum and minimum values are not in line with the rest of the data. The range will not be considered further.

The average distance of all the hits from the "bull's eye" would serve as a convenient measure of the scatter on the target. The average spread about the arithmetic mean of a large series of weighings or analyses is the mean deviation δ of the population.* The sum of the positive and negative deviations about the mean equals zero; hence, the algebraic signs are disregarded in order to obtain a measure of the dispersion.

The *mean deviation d* for a sample, that is, the deviation of an individual observation from the arithmetic mean of the sample, is obtained by taking the difference between each individual value X_i and the arithmetic mean $\overline{X}$, adding the differences without regard to the algebraic signs, and dividing the sum by the number of values to obtain the average. The mean deviation of a sample is expressed as

$$d = \frac{\Sigma|X_i - \overline{X}|}{N} \qquad (1-28)$$

in which $\Sigma|X_i - \overline{X}|$ is the sum of the absolute deviations from the mean. The vertical lines on either side of the term in the numerator indicate that the algebraic sign of the deviation should be disregarded.

Youden[6] discourages the use of the mean deviation since it gives a biased estimate that suggests a greater precision than actually exists when a small number of values are used in the computation. Furthermore, the mean deviation of small subsets may be widely scattered around the average of the estimates, and accordingly, d is not particularly efficient as a measure of precision.

The standard deviation σ (the Greek lower case letter sigma) is the square root of the mean of the squares of the deviations. This parameter is used to measure the dispersion or variability of a large number of measurements; for example, the weights of the contents of several million capsules. This set of items or measurements approximates the *population* or the *universe*, and σ is therefore called the *standard deviation of the universe*.** Universe standard deviations are shown in Figure 1–6.

As previously noted, any finite group of experimental data may be considered as a subset or sample of the population; the statistic or characteristic of a sample from the universe used to express the variability of a subset and supply an estimate of the standard deviation of the population is known as the *sample standard deviation* and is designated by the small letter *s*. The formula is

$$s = \sqrt{\frac{\Sigma(X_i - \overline{X})^2}{N}} \qquad (1-29)$$

For a small sample the equation is written

$$s = \sqrt{\frac{\Sigma(X_i - \overline{X})^2}{N - 1}} \qquad (1-30)$$

The term $(N - 1)$ is known as the *number of degrees of freedom*. It replaces N to reduce the bias of the standard deviation s, which on the average is lower than the universe standard deviation.

The reason for introducing $(N - 1)$ is explained as follows. When a statistician selects a sample and makes a single measurement or observation, he or she obtains at least a rough estimate of the mean of the parent population. This single observation, however, can give no hint as to the degree of variability in the population. When a second measurement is taken, however, a first basis for estimating the population variability is obtained. The statistician states this fact by saying that two observations supply one *degree of freedom* for estimating variations in the universe. Three values provide two degrees of freedom, four values provide three degrees of freedom, and so on. Therefore, we do not have access to all N values of a sample for obtaining an estimate of the standard deviation of the population. Instead, we must use 1 less than N or $(N - 1)$, as shown in equation (1–30). When N is large, say $N > 100$, one may use N instead of $(N - 1)$ to estimate the population standard deviation, since the difference between the two is negligible.

Modern statistical methods handle the small sample quite well; however, the investigator should recognize that the estimate of the standard deviation becomes less reproducible and, on the average, becomes lower than the universe standard deviation as fewer samples are used to compute the estimate.

A sample calculation involving the arithmetic mean, the mean deviation, and the estimate of the standard deviation follows.

Example 1–5. A pharmacist received a prescription for a patient with rheumatoid arthritis calling for seven divided powders, the contents of which were each to weigh 1.00 gram. To check his skill in filling the powders, he removed the contents from each paper after filling the prescription by the block-and-divide method and then weighed the powders carefully. The results of the weighings are given in the first column of Table 1–10; the deviations of each value from the arithmetic mean, disregarding the sign, are given in column 2; and the squares of the deviations are shown in the last column. Based on the use of the mean deviation, the weight of the powders may be expressed as 0.98 ± 0.046 gram. The variability of a single

---

*The population mean deviation is written as

$$\delta = \frac{\Sigma|X_i - \mu|}{N}$$

where X_i is an individual measurement, μ is the population mean, and N is the number of measurements.

**The equation for the universe standard deviation is

$$\sigma = \sqrt{\frac{\Sigma(X_i - \mu)^2}{N}}$$

TABLE 1-10. *Statistical Analysis of Divided Powder Compounding Technique*

	Weight of Powder Contents (grams)	Deviation, (Sign Ignored) $|X_i - \overline{X}|$	Square of the Deviation $(X_i - \overline{X})^2$
	1.00	0.02	0.0004
	0.98	0.00	0.0000
	1.00	0.02	0.0004
	1.05	0.07	0.0049
	0.81	0.17	0.0289
	0.98	0.00	0.0000
	1.02	0.04	0.0016
Total	$\Sigma = 6.84$	$\Sigma = 0.32$	$\Sigma = 0.0362$
Average	0.98	0.046	

powder may also be expressed in terms of percent deviation by dividing the mean deviation by the arithmetic mean and multiplying by 100. The result is 0.98 ± 4.6%; of course, it includes errors due to removing the powders from the papers and weighing the powders in the analysis.

The standard deviation is used more frequently than the mean deviation in research work. For large sets of data, it is approximately 25% larger than the mean deviation, that is, $\sigma = 1.25 \delta$.

The statistician has estimated that owing to chance errors, about 68% of all results in a large set will fall within one standard deviation on either side of the arithmetic mean, 95.5% within ±2 standard deviations, and 99.7% within ±3 standard deviations, as seen in Figure 1-6.

Goldstein[7] selected 1.73 σ as an equitable tolerance standard for prescription products, whereas Saunders and Fleming[8] advocated the use of ±3 σ as approximate limits of error for a single result.

In pharmaceutical work, it should be considered permissible to accept ±2 s as a measure of the variability or "spread" of the data in small samples. Then, roughly 5 to 10% of the individual results will be expected to fall outside this range if only chance errors occur.

The estimate of the standard deviation in *Example 1-4* is calculated as follows:

$$s = \sqrt{\frac{0.0362}{(7 - 1)}} = 0.078 \text{ gram}$$

and ±2 s is equal to ±0.156 gram. That is to say, based upon the analysis of this experiment, the pharmacist should expect that roughly 90 to 95% of the sample values will fall within ±0.156 gram of the sample mean.

The smaller the standard deviation estimate (or the mean deviation) the more *precise* is the compounding operation. In the filling of capsules, precision is a measure of the ability of the pharmacist to put the same amount of drug in each capsule and to reproduce the result in subsequent operations. Statistical techniques for predicting the probability of occurrence of a specific deviation in future operations, although important in

pharmacy, require methods that are outside the scope of this book. The interested reader is referred to treatises on statistical analysis.

Whereas the average deviation and the standard deviation can be used as measures of the *precision* of a method, the difference between the arithmetic mean and the *true* or *absolute* value expresses the error that can often be used as a measure of the *accuracy* of the method.

The true or absolute value is ordinarily regarded as the universe mean μ—that is, the mean for an infinitely large set—since it is assumed that the true value is approached as the sample size becomes progressively larger. The universe mean does not, however, coincide with the true value of the quantity measured in those cases in which determinate errors are inherent in the measurements.

The difference between the sample arithmetic mean and the true value gives a measure of the accuracy of an operation; it is known as the *mean error*.

In *Example 1-5*, the true value is 1.00 gram, the amount requested by the physician. The apparent error involved in compounding this prescription is

$$E = 1.0 - 0.98 = +0.02 \text{ gram}$$

in which the positive sign signifies that the true value is greater than the mean value. An analysis of these results shows, however, that this difference is not statistically significant, but rather is most likely due to accidental errors.* Hence, the accuracy of the operation in *Example 1-5* is sufficiently great that no systemic error can be presumed. We may find on further analysis, however, that one or several results are questionable. This possibility is considered later. If the

---

*The deviation of the arithmetic mean from the true value or the mean of the parent population can be tested by use of the following expression:

$$t = \frac{\overline{X} - \mu}{s/\sqrt{N - 1}}$$

In this equation, t is a statistic known as Student's t value, after W. S. Gosset, who wrote under the pseudonym of "Student." The other terms in the equation have the meaning previously assigned to them.

Student's t Values for Six Degrees of Freedom

Probability of a plus or minus deviation greater than t

	0.8	0.6	0.4	0.2	0.02	0.001
t value	0.27	0.55	0.91	1.44	3.14	5.96

Substituting the results of the analysis of the divided powders into the equation just given, we have

$$t = \frac{\overline{X} - \mu}{s/\sqrt{N - 1}} = \frac{0.98 - 1.00}{0.08/\sqrt{6}} = \frac{-0.02}{0.033} = -0.61$$

Entering the table with a t value of 0.61, we see that the probability of finding a ± deviation greater than t is roughly equal to 0.6. This means that in the long run there are about 60 out of 100 chances of finding a t value greater than −0.61 by chance alone. This probability is sufficiently large to suggest that the difference between the mean and the true value may be taken as due to chance.

arithmetic mean in *Example 1-5* were 0.90 instead of 0.98, the difference could be stated with assurance to have statistical significance, since the probability that such a result could occur by chance alone would be small.* The mean error in this case is

$$1.00 - 0.90 = 0.10 \text{ gram}$$

The *relative error* is obtained by dividing the mean error by the true value. It may be expressed as a percentage by multiplying by 100, or in parts per thousand by multiplying by 1000. It is easier to compare several sets of results by using the relative error rather than the absolute mean error. The relative error in the case just cited is

$$\frac{0.10 \text{ gram}}{1.00 \text{ gram}} \times 100 = 10\%$$

The reader should recognize that it is possible for a result to be precise without being accurate, that is, a constant error is present. If the capsule contents in *Example 1-5* had yielded an average weight of 0.60 gram with a mean deviation of 0.5%, the results would have been accepted as precise. The degree of accuracy, however, would have been low since the average weight would have differed from the true value by 40%. Conversely, the fact that the result may be accurate does not necessarily mean that it is also precise. The situation can arise in which the mean value is close to the true value, but the scatter due to chance is large. Saunders and Fleming[8] observe that "it is better to be roughly accurate than precisely wrong."

A study of the individual values of a set often throws additional light on the exactitude of the compounding operations. Returning to the data of *Example 1-5*, we note one rather discordant value, namely, 0.81 gram. If the arithmetic mean is recalculated ignoring this measurement, one obtains a mean of 1.01 grams. The mean deviation without the doubtful result was 0.02 gram. It is now seen that the divergent result is 0.20 gram smaller than the new average or, in other words, its deviation is 10 times greater than the mean deviation. A deviation greater than four times the mean deviation will occur purely by chance only about once or twice in 1000 measurements; hence, the discrepancy in this case was probably caused by some definite error in technique. This rule is rightly questioned by statisticians, but it is a useful though not always reliable criterion for finding discrepant results.

---

*When the mean is 0.90 gram, the *t* value is

$$t = \frac{0.90 - 1.00}{0.08/\sqrt{6}} = \frac{-0.10}{0.033} \approx -3$$

and the probability of finding a *t* value greater than −3 as a result of chance alone is found in the *t* table to be about 0.02, or 2 chances in 100. This probability is sufficiently small to suggest that the difference between the mean and the true value is real, and the error may be computed accordingly.

TABLE 1-11. *Refractive Indices of Mixtures of Benzene and Carbon Tetrachloride*

(x) Concentration of CCl$_4$ (volume %)	(y) Refractive Index
10.0	1.497
26.0	1.493
33.0	1.485
50.0	1.478
61.0	1.477

Having uncovered the variable weight among the units, one can proceed to investigate the cause of the determinate error. The pharmacist may find that some of the powder was left on the sides of the mortar or on the weighing paper or possibly was lost during trituration. If several of the powder weights deviated widely from the mean, a serious deficiency in the compounder's technique would be suspected. Such appraisals as these in the college laboratory will aid the student in locating and correcting errors and will help the pharmacist to become a safe and proficient compounder before entering the practice of pharmacy. Bingenheimer[9] has described such a program for students in the dispensing laboratory.

Linear Regression Analysis. The data given in Table 1-7 and plotted in Figure 1-2 clearly indicate the existence of a linear relationship between the refractive index and volume percent of carbon tetrachloride in benzene. The straight line that joins virtually all the points can be drawn readily on the figure by sighting the points along the edge of a ruler and drawing a line that can be extrapolated to the *y* axis with confidence.

Let us suppose, however, that the person who prepared the solutions and carried out the refractive index measurements was not skilled and, as a result of poor technique, allowed indeterminate errors to appear. We might then be presented with the data given in Table 1-11. When this is plotted on graph paper, an appreciable scatter is observed (Fig. 1-7) and we are unable, with any degree of confidence, to draw the line that expresses the relation between refractive index and concentration. It is here that we must employ better means of analyzing the available data.

The first step is to determine whether or not the data in Table 1-11 should fit a straight line, and for this we calculate the *correlation coefficient*, *r*, using the following equation:

$$r = \frac{\Sigma(x - \overline{x})(y - \overline{y})}{\sqrt{\Sigma(x - \overline{x})^2 \, \Sigma(y - \overline{y})^2}} \qquad (1-31)$$

When there is perfect correlation between the two variables (i.e., a perfect linear relationship), $r = 1$. When the two variables are completely independent, $r = 0$. Depending on the degrees of freedom and the

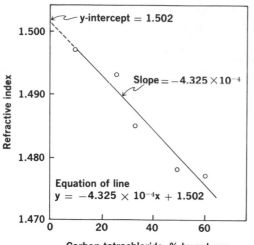

Fig. 1–7. Slope, intercept, and equation of line for data in Table 1–11 calculated by regression analysis.

y	$(y - \bar{y})$	$(y - \bar{y})^2$
1.497	+0.011	0.000121
1.493	+0.007	0.000049
1.485	−0.001	0.000001
1.478	−0.008	0.000064
1.477	−0.009	0.000081
$\Sigma = 7.430$	$\Sigma = 0$	$\Sigma = \overline{0.000316}$

$\bar{y} \div 1.486$

$(x - \bar{x})(y - \bar{y})$
−0.286
−0.070
+0.003
−0.112
−0.225
$\Sigma = \overline{-0.690}$

Substituting the relevant values into equation (1–31) gives

$$r = \frac{-0.690}{\sqrt{1606.0 \times 0.000316}} = -0.97*$$

From equation (1–32)

$$b = \frac{-0.690}{1606.0} = -4.296 \times 10^{-4}$$

and finally, from equation (1–33)

the intercept on the y axis = 1.486

$$-4.315 \times 10^{-4} (0 - 36)$$

$$= +1.502$$

Note that for the intercept, we place x equal to zero in equation (1–31). By inserting an actual value of x into equation (1–33), we obtain the value of y that should be found at that particular value of x. Thus, when $x = 10$,

$$y = 1.486 - 4.315 \times 10^{-4} (10 - 36)$$

$$= 1.486 - 4.315 \times 10^{-4} (-26)$$

$$= 1.497$$

The value agrees with the experimental value, and hence this point lies on the statistically calculated slope drawn in Figure 1–7.

Multiple Linear and Polynomial Regression. Regression for two, three, or more independent variables may be performed, using a linear equation:

$$y = a + bx_1 + cx_2 + dx_3 + \cdots \quad (1-34)$$

chosen probability level, it is possible to calculate values of r above which there is significant correlation and below which there is no significant correlation. Obviously, in the latter case, it is not profitable to proceed further with the analysis unless the data can be plotted in some other way that will yield a linear relation. An example of this is shown in Figure 1–4, in which a linear plot is obtained by plotting the *logarithm* of oil sepration from an emulsion against emulsifier concentration, as opposed to Figure 1–3, in which the raw data are plotted in the conventional manner.

Assuming that the calculated value of r shows a significant correlation between x and y, it is then necessary to calculate the slope and intercept of the line using the equation:

$$b = \frac{\Sigma(x - \bar{x})(y - \bar{y})}{\Sigma(x - \bar{x})^2} \quad (1-32)$$

in which b is the *regression coefficient*, or slope. By substituting the value for b in equation (1–33), we can then obtain the y intercept:

$$\bar{y} = y + b(x - \bar{x}) \quad (1-33)$$

The following series of calculations, based on the data in Table 1–11, will illustrate the use of these equations.

Example 1–6. Using the data in Table 1–11, calculate the correlation coefficient, the regression coefficient, and the intercept on the y axis.

Examination of equations (1–31), (1–32), and (1–33) shows the various values we must calculate, and these are set up as shown:

x	$(x - \bar{x})$	$(x - \bar{x})^2$
10.0	−26.0	676.0
26.0	−10.0	100.0
33.0	− 3.0	9.0
50.0	+14.0	196.0
61.0	+25.0	625.0
$\Sigma = 180.0$	$\Sigma = 0$	$\Sigma = 1606.0$

$\bar{x} = 36.0$

---

*The theoretic values of r when the probability level is set at 0.05 are:

Degrees of freedom ($N - 2$):

	2	3	5	10	20	50

Correlation coefficient, r:

	0.95	0.88	0.75	0.58	0.42	0.27

In *Example 1–6*, ($N - 2$) = 3 and hence the theoretic value of $r = 0.88$. The calculated value was found to be 0.97, and the correlation between x and y is therefore significant.

For a power series in x, a polynomial form is employed:

$$y = a + bx + cx^2 + dx^3 + \cdots \quad (1-35)$$

In equations (1–34) and (1–35), y is the dependent variable, and a, b, c, and d are regression coefficients obtained by solving the regression equation. Computers are used to handle these more complex equations, but some hand-held calculators, such as the Hewlett Packard HP41C, are programmed to solve multiple regression equations containing two or more independent variables. The r^2 used in multiple regression is called the square of the multiple correlation coefficient and is given the symbol R^2 in some texts to distinguish it from r^2, the square of the linear correlation coefficient. Multiple regression analysis is treated by Draper and Smith.[10]

References and Notes

1. S. W. Goldstein, A. M. Mattocks, and U. Beirmacher, J. Am. Pharm. Assoc., Pract. Ed. **12**, 421, 1951.
2. S. W. Goldstein and A. M. Mattocks, *Professional Equilibrium and Compounding Precision*, a bound booklet reprinted from the J. Am. Pharm. Assoc., Pract. Ed. April-August 1951.
3. *CRC Handbook of Chemistry and Physics*, 63rd Edition, CRC Press, Boca Raton, FL., 1982–83, p. D-227.
4. F. Daniels, *Mathematical Preparation for Physical Chemistry*, McGraw-Hill, New York, 1928.
5. E. A. Brecht, in *Sprowls' American Pharmacy*, L. W. Dittert, Ed., 7th Edition, Lippincott, Philadelphia, 1974, Chapter 2.
6. W. J. Youden, *Statistical Methods for Chemists*, R. Krieger, Huntington, N.Y., Reprint of original edition; 1977, p. 9.
7. S. W. Goldstein, J. Am. Pharm. Assoc., Sci. Ed. **38**, 18, 131, 1949; ibid., **39**, 505, 1950.
8. L. Saunders and R. Fleming, *Mathematics and Statistics*, Pharmaceutical Press, London, 1957.
9. L. E. Bingenheimer, Am. J. Pharm. Educ. **17**, 236, 1953.
10. N. Draper and H. Smith, *Applied Regression Analysis*, Wiley, New York, 1980.
11. N. C. Harris and E. M. Hemmerling, *Introductory Applied Physics*, McGraw-Hill, New York, 1972, p. 310.
12. M. J. Kamlet, R. M. Doherty, V. Fiserova-Bergerova, P. W. Carr, M. H. Abraham and R. W. Taft, J. Pharm. Sci. **76**, 14, 1987.
13. W. Lowenthal, *"Methodology and Calculations,"* in *Remington's Pharmaceutical Science*, A. R. Gennaro, Editor, Mack Publishing, Easton, PA., 1985, p. 82.

Problems

1–1. The density ρ of a plastic latex particle is 2.23 g cm^{-3}. Convert this value into SI units.

Answer: 2.23×10^3 kg m^{-3}. (See Table 1–3 and the physical constants on the inside front cover of the book for cgs and SI units.)

1–2. Convert 2.736 nm to cm.

Answer: 2.736×10^{-7} cm

1–3. Convert 1.99×10^4 Å^3 into (nanometers)^3.

Answer: 19.9 nm^3

1–4. The surface tension (γ) of a new synthetic oil has a value of 27.32 dyne cm^{-1}. Calculate the corresponding γ value in SI units.

Answer: 0.02732 N m^{-1} = 0.02732 J m^{-2}

1–5. The work done by the kidneys in transforming 0.1 mole of urea from the plasma to the urine is 259 cal. Convert this quantity into SI units.

Answer: 1084 J

1–6. The body excretes HCl into the stomach in the concentration of 0.14 M at 37° C. The work done in this process is 3.8×10^{11} erg. Convert this energy into the fundamental SI units of kg m^2 s^{-2}. M stands for molarity.

Answer: 3.8×10^4 kg m^2 s^{-2}

1–7. The gas constant R is given in SI units as 8.3143 J °K^{-1} mole^{-1}. Convert this value into calories.

Answer: 1.9872 cal °K^{-1} mole^{-1}

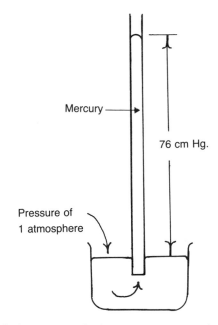

Fig. 1–8. Owing to atmospheric pressure, mercury rises to a height of 76 cm, as demonstrated here.

1–8. Convert 50,237 Pa to torrs or mm Hg, where 1 atm = 760 mm Hg = 760 torrs.

Answer: 376.8 torrs

1–9. Convert an energy of 4.379×10^6 erg into SI units.

Answer: 0.4379 J

1–10. A pressure of 1 atmosphere will support a column of mercury 760 mm high at 0° C (Fig. 1–8). To what height will a pressure of 1 atm support a column of mineral spirits at 25° C? The density of mineral spirits (mineral oil fraction) at 25° C is 0.860 g/cm^3. Express the results both in feet and in millimeters of mineral spirits. *Hint:* See *Example 1–1*.

Answer: 12010 mm of mineral spirits (or 39 ft)

1–11. How high can an ordinary hand-operated water pump (Fig. 1-9) lift a column of water at 25° C above its surface from a water well? How high could it lift a column of mercury at 25° C from a well filled with mercury? The density of mercury at 25° C is 13.5340 g cm^{-3}.

Answer: According to Harris and Hemmerling,[11] "since atmospheric pressure at the sea level is approximately 34 ft of water the most perfect pump of this type could not lift water more than 34 ft from the water level in the well." The same argument applies in the case of mercury.

1–12. Derive equation (1–15), shown on page 6 and used in this problem. Choose a base b for a logarithmic system. For the fun of it, you may pick a base $b = 5.9$ just because your height is 5.9 feet. Set up a log table with $b = 5.9$ for the numbers 1000, 100, 10, 0.1, and 0.001.

Answer: For the number 0.001 you would obtain $\log_{5.9}(0.001) = -3.8916$

1–13. According to Boyle's law of ideal gases, the pressure and volume of a definite mass of gas at a constant temperature are given by the equation $PV = k$ or $P = k(1/V)$, in which P is the pressure in atmospheres and V is the volume in liters. Plot the tabulated data so as to obtain a straight line and find the value of the constant k from the graph. Express the constant in ergs, joules, and calories.

Data for *Problem 1–13*

P (atm)	0.25	0.50	1.0	2.0	4.0
V (liters)	89.6	44.8	22.4	11.12	5.60

Answer: $k = 22.4$ liter atm, 2.27×10^{10} ergs, 2.27×10^3 joules, 5.43×10^2 cal

1–14. The distance traveled by a free-falling body released from rest is given by the equation $s = (1/2)gt^2$. Plot the accompanying data so as to obtain a straight line and determine the value of g, the

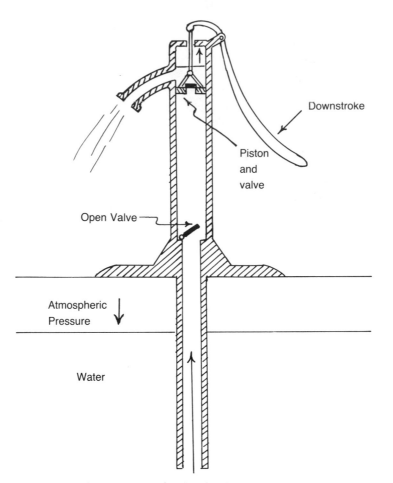

Fig. 1–9. An old-fashioned hand-operated water pump, showing the piston and valves required to lift the water from the well.

acceleration due to gravity. From the graph, obtain the time that has elapsed when the body has fallen 450 feet.

Data for *Problem 1–14*

s (ft)	0	16	64	144	256	400
t (sec)	0	1	2	3	4	5

Answer: $g = 32$ ft/sec; $t = 5.3$ sec

1–15. The amount of acetic acid adsorbed from solution by charcoal is expressed by the Freundlich equation, $x/m = kc^n$, in which x is the millimoles of acetic acid adsorbed by m grams of charcoal when the concentration of the acid in the solution at adsorption equilibrium is c mole/liter, and k and n are empirical constants. Convert the equation to the logarithmic form, plot $\log(x/m)$ vs. $\log c$, and obtain k and n from the graph.

Data for *Problem 1–15*

Millimoles of acetic acid per gram of charcoal (x/m)	Concentration of acetic acid (mole/liter) (c)
0.45	0.018
0.60	0.03
0.80	0.06
1.10	0.13
1.50	0.27
2.00	0.50
2.30	0.75
2.65	1.00

Answer: $k = 2.65$; $n = 0.42$

1–16. The equation describing the effect of temperature on the rate of a reaction is the Arrhenius equation,

$$k = Ae^{-\frac{E_a}{RT}} \tag{1–36}$$

in which k is the reaction rate constant at temperature T (in degrees absolute), A is a constant known as the Arrhenius factor, R is the gas constant (1.987 cal mole^{-1} deg^{-1}), and E_a is known as the energy of activation in cal mole^{-1}. Rearrange the equation so as to form an equation for a straight line (see equation (1–19)) and then calculate E_a and A from the following data:

Data for *Problem 1–16*

$t(°C)$	40	50	60
k	0.10	0.25	0.70

Hint: Take the natural logarithm of both sides of the Arrhenius equation.

Answer: $E_a = 20,152$ cal mole^{-1}; $A = 1.13 \times 10^{13}$ sec^{-1}

1–17. (a) Convert the equation, $F^N = \eta' G$ into logarithmic form, where F is the shear stress or force per unit area, G is rate of shear, and η' is a viscosity coefficient. N is an exponent that expresses the deviation of some solutions and pastes from the Newtonian viscosity equation (see Chapter 17, in particular pp. 454 and 456). Plot $\log G$ versus $\log F$ (common logarithms) from the table of experimental data given below, and solve for N, the slope of the line. On the same graph plot $\ln G$ vs. $\ln F$ (natural logarithms) and again obtain the slope, N. Does the value of N differ when obtained from these two lines?

(b) Directly plot the F and G values of the table on 1-cycle by 2-cycle log–log paper (i.e., graph paper with a logarithmic scale on both the horizontal and the vertical axes). Does the slope of this line yield the coefficient N obtained from the slope of the previous two plots? How can one obtain N using log–log paper?

(c) Regress $\ln G$ vs. $\ln F$ and $\log G$ vs. $\log F$ and obtain N from the slope of the two regression equations. Which method, (a), (b), or (c), provides more accurate results?

Data for *Problem 1–17*

G (sec^{-1})	22.70	45.40	68.0	106.0	140.0	181.0	272.0
F (dyne/cm^2)	1423	1804	2082	2498	2811	3088	3500

Hint: Convert G and F to ln and to log and enter these in a table of G and F values. Carry out the log and ln values to four decimal places.

Partial Answer: **(c)** $\log G = 2.69 \log F - 7.1018$; $r^2 = 0.9982$
$N = 2.69$, $\eta' = $ (antilog 7.1018) $= 1.26 \times 10^7$
$\ln G = 2.69 \ln F - 16.3556$; $r^2 = 0.9982$
$N = 2.69$; $\eta' = $ antiln(16.3556) $= 1.27 \times 10^7$

1–18. In the equation

$$-\frac{ds}{dt} = ks \qquad (1\text{-}37)$$

s is the distance a car travels in time t and k is a proportionality constant. In this problem the velocity ds/dt is proportional to the distance s to be covered at any moment. Thus the speed is not constant, but rather is decreasing as the car reaches its destination, probably because the traffic is becoming heavier as the car approaches the city. The equation may be integrated to solve for k, knowing the distance s at time t and the total distance, s_0. Separating the variables and integrating between the limits of $s = s_o$ at $t = 0$ and $s = s$ at $t = t$ yields

$$-\int_{s_o}^{s} \frac{ds}{s} = k \int_{0}^{t} dt \qquad (1\text{-}38)$$

$(-\ln s) - (-\ln s_o) = kt$ and $\ln s = \ln s_o - kt$, or in terms of common logs, $\log s = \log s_o - \dfrac{kt}{2.303}$. The quantity 2.303 must be used because $\ln s = 2.303 \log s$, as shown on p. 5.

Knowing the remaining distance, s, at several times, one obtains k from the slope, and the total distance s_0 from the intercept

Data for *Problem 1–18*

s (km)	259.3	192.0	142.3	105.4
t (hr)	1	2	3	4

Compute s_0 and k using ln and log values with the data given in the table above. Discuss the advantages and disadvantages in using natural logarithms (ln) and common logarithms (log) in a problem of this kind. Why would one change from ln to log when plotting data, as some workers do?

Answer: Using ln, $k = 0.300$ hr^{-1}; $\ln s_0 = 5.8579$; $s_0 = 350$ km. Using log, $k = 0.300$ hr^{-1}; $\log s_0 = 2.5441$; $s_0 = 350$ km.

1–19. After preparing a prescription calling for six capsules each containing three grains of aspirin, you remove the contents completely and weigh each. The weights are 2.85, 2.80, 3.02, 3.05, 2.95, and 3.15 grains. Compute the average weight of the contents of the capsules, the average deviation, and the standard deviation. One gram is equal to 15.432 grains (gr.)

Answer: Av. wt. = 2.97 grains; Av. dev. = 0.103 grain; stand. dev. = 0.13 grain.

1–20. (a) Using the data in Table 1–7 and the least-squares method, calculate the slope and the intercept for the linear relationship between refractive index and percent by volume of carbon tetrachloride. Calculate the correlation coefficient, r.

(b) Use the data in Table 1–8 and the least-squares method to obtain the equation of the line plotted in Figure 1–4. Calculate the correlation coefficient, r. Compare your results with the equation shown in Figure 1–4. Explain why your results using the statistical least-squares method might differ from the equation shown in Figure 1–4.

Answers: **(a)** Compare your least-square results with those found in Figure 1–2, which were obtained by use of equation (1–23). $r^2 = 0.9998$.

(b) $r^2 = 0.9986$; $\log y = 0.843 - 0.279 \, x$

1–21. According to a principle known as Trouton's rule the molar heat of vaporization, ΔH_V (cal/mole) of a liquid divided by its boiling point (T_b) on the Kelvin scale at atmospheric pressure should equal a constant, approximately 23. If this rule holds, a plot of ΔH_V of a number of liquids against their absolute boiling points, T_b, should fall on a straight line with a slope of 23 and an intercept of 0:

$$\Delta H_V = 0 + 23 T_b$$

(a) Plot ΔH_V versus T_b on rectangular coordinate paper using all the data points given in the table. With a least-squares linear regression program, obtain the slope and the intercept. Draw a line on the graph corresponding to the equation $\Delta H_v = 23 T_b$.

Data for *Problem 1–21*

Compound	T_b(°K)	ΔH_V (cal mole^{-1})	$\Delta H_V/T_b$ (cal °K^{-1} mole^{-1})
Propane	231	4,812	20.8
Ethyl ether	308	6,946	22.6
Carbon disulfide	320	6,787	21.2
Hexane	342	7,627	22.3
Carbon tetrachloride	350	8,272	23.6
Cyclohexane	354	7,831	22.1
Nitrobenzene	483	12,168	25.2

(b) Repeat the regression, removing nitrobenzene from the data.

(c) Repeat the analysis using the following combinations of data (nitrobenzene is not used in any of these):

(1) Propane
Carbon disulfide
Hexane
Cyclohexane

(2) Propane
Ethyl ether
Carbon disulfide
Hexane
Cyclohexane

(3) Propane
Carbon tetrachloride
Carbon disulfide
Hexane

(d) Compare the slopes you obtain in (a), (b), and (c1), (c2), and (c3). Which one compares best with the Trouton value of 23? Why did you get a slope in (a) quite different from the others?

(e) Does this approach we have used, employing the equation $\Delta H_v = 23 \, T_b$ and linear regression analysis, appear to be a convincing proof of the Trouton rule? Can you suggest another approach to test the validity of the Trouton principle in a more convincing way? (Hint: What result would you expect if you plotted $\Delta H_v/T_b$ on the vertical axis against T_b on the horizontal axis?) Regardless of the method used, the results would probably have been much improved if a large number of organic liquids had been chosen to test the Trouton principle, but in a student problem this approach is not practical.

Answers: (using a Casio hand calculator):
(a) $r^2 = 0.9843$; slope = 29.46; intercept = -2272
(b) $r^2 = 0.9599$; slope = 26.14; intercept = -1255
(c) (1) $r^2 = 0.9914$; slope = 24.65; intercept = -921.5
(2) $r^2 = 0.9810$; slope = 24.57; intercept = -839
(3) $r^2 = 0.9639$; slope = 27.0; intercept = -1517

1–22. A series of barbituric acids, disubstituted at the 5,5 (R_a, R_b) position, is tested for hypnotic action against rats. The relative activity required to produce hypnosis is measured for each derivative. It is presumed that this hypnotic activity, dependent variable y, may be linearly related to the logarithm of the *partition coefficient*, log K (see Chapter 10, p. 237 for a definition of K) as the independent variable x for each barbituric acid derivative. The observed activity

Data for *Problem 1-22*

| Derivative | | | | Relative Activity (RA) | | |
R_a	R_b	K	log K	Observed	Calculated	% Difference
Ethyl,	ethyl	4.47		2.79		
Ethyl,	phenyl	26.3		3.12		
Ethyl,	amyl	141.3		3.45		
Ethyl,	butyl	44.7		3.33		
Ethyl	isobutyl	28.2		3.28		
Allyl,	cyclopentyl	97.7		3.67		
Ethyl,	1-methyl-amyl	281.8		3.60		
Ethyl,	isoamyl	89.1		3.50		
Ethyl,	cyclopentyl	61.7		3.45		
Allyl,	1-methyl-butyl	143.3		3.83		

and partition coefficient for each disubstituted barbiturate derivative are as in table above. Calculate the log K values and enter them in the space under the log K heading. Plot the observed relative activities vs. log K values and obtain the slope of the line, using two widely spaced points. Determine the intercept. Then, using linear regression, determine the slope and the intercept by the least-squares method and calculate r, the correlation coefficient. Obtain the least-squares equation of the line and use it to obtain the calculated relative activity for each compound. Enter these calculated activities in the table and record the percent difference between observed and calculated relative activities for each compound.

Answer: $r = 0.9089$; $r^2 = 0.8262$; RA $= 2.472 + 0.5268 \log K$. For the (ethyl, ethyl) derivative, the calculated activity using the least-squares equation is 2.81, which is -0.7% different from the experimental value. Incidentally, the linear relationship found between activity and log K signifies that the more nonpolar the barbiturate derivative (as measured by the partition coefficient), the more active it is as a hypnotic agent in rats. The term r^2 has more significance than the correlation coefficient r; and r^2 of 0.8262 means that 82.62% of the barbiturate data are explained by the linear equation obtained in this problem.

(This problem came from C. Hansch, *Biological Correlations—The Hansch Approach*, American Chemical Society, 1972, pp. 30, 33. The data are from H. A. Shonle, A. K. Keltch and E. E. Swanson, J. Am. Chem. Soc. **52**, 2440, 1930. Calculated values are given by C. Hansch, A. R. Steward, S. M. Anderson and D. Bentley, J. Med. Chem. **11**, 1, 1968. The regression equation calculated here is slightly different from the result found in *Biological Correlations* because we have used only 10 of the 16 data points.)

1-23. The anesthetic activity of nine aliphatic ethers was plotted against the logarithm of the partition coefficient, log K. Log 1/C is used as a measure of anesthetic action, C being the molar concentration of each drug. A plot of the data was not linear but rather appeared to be quadratic, suggesting the need for a parabolic equation of the form

$$\log 1/C = a + b(\log K) + c(\log K)^2$$

The observed activity (log 1/C) and the log partition coefficient for each of the substituted aliphatic ethers are found in the table. Plot log 1/C on the vertical axis and log K on the horizontal axis of rectangular coordinate paper to observe the parabolic nature of the curve.

Using a polynomial regression program, available on a personal computer, fit the data points with a parabolic polynomial equation,

$$y = a + bx + cx^2$$

to obtain r^2, the y-intercept, and the regression coefficients b and c. Substitute the values of log K and $(\log K)^2$ in the parabolic equation

Data for *Problem 1-23:* Anesthetics in Mice*

Aliphatic Ether	Observed Activity $(\log 1/C)^\dagger$	Log Partition Coefficient $(\log K)$
Methyl cyclopropyl	2.85	0.75
Methyl isobutyl	3.00	1.00
Methyl butyl	3.15	1.27
Ethyl tert-butyl	3.25	1.50
Propyl isobutyl	3.33	1.75
Methyl amyl	3.40	2.03
Ethyl isoamyl	3.45	2.35
Di-sec-butyl	3.43	2.57
Diisobutyl	3.35	2.90

*These data are not real but rather were arbitrarily chosen to show an example of a quadratic (parabolic) relationship. See W. Glave and C. Hansch, J. Pharm. Sci. **61**, 589, 1972, Table I, for the actual data.
†The observed activity is recorded as the ED_{50} in mice.

to back-calculate the nine values of log 1/C. Compare these calculated values with the observed anesthetic activities found in the table for each substituted ether. If the value of r^2, called the multiple correlation coefficient when associated with multiple regression, is nearly 1.000 and the percent difference between observed and calculated log 1/C is small, you can assume that the polynomial equation you have chosen provides a satisfactory fit of the data.

Answer: $r^2 = 0.9964$

$$\log 1/C = 2.170 + 1.058(\log K) - 0.223(\log K)^2$$

1-24. Kamlet et al.[12] found that the logarithmic solubility (log S) of solutes in brain tissue was related to several physical properties according to the model

$$\log S = a + b(V/100) + c\pi + d\beta$$

where V is the intrinsic (van der Waals) molar volume, π is a parameter that measures solute polarity and polarizability, and β expresses the hydrogen bond acceptor basicity character of the solutes. The equation above is treated by multiple linear regression, where the dependent variable is log S and the three independent variables are V/100, π, and β.

(a) Using the data below and a computer program or a hand calculator (Hewlett-Packard 41V, for example) that provides the calculations for multiple linear regression of three independent variables, compute the square of the correlation coefficient, r^2, the y-intercept, a, and the regression coefficients b, c, and d.

Data for *Problem 1-24*

Solutes*	log S	V/100	π	β
Methanol	1.13	0.405	0.40	0.42
Ethanol	0.69	0.584	0.40	0.45
2-Propanol	0.33	0.765	0.40	0.51
1-Propanol	0.12	0.748	0.40	0.45
Isobutyl alcohol	−0.31	0.920	0.40	0.45
Acetone	0.36	0.734	0.71	0.48
2-Butanone	−0.06	0.895	0.67	0.48
$(C_2H_5)_2O$	−0.31	1.046	0.27	0.47
Benzene	−0.93	0.989	0.19	0.10
$CHCl_3$	−0.53	0.805	0.38	0.10

*Selected values from Table I of Kamlet et al.[12]

Data for *Problem 1-25*

t (°C)	Density (g/cm³)*
10	0.9997026
12	0.9995004
14	0.9992474
16	0.9989460
18	0.9985986
20	0.9982071

*The reader is referred to the latest handbooks for tables of values for the density of water. The values above were obtained from the *CRC Handbook of Chemistry and Physics*, 63rd Edition, pp. F5 and F6.

(b) Use the equation you obtained in part (a) to back-calculate the log S values for the 10 cases, and compare them with the experimentally determined log S values (those found in the table). Give the percent error

$$\frac{\log S_{(exper.)} - \log S_{(calc.)}}{\log S_{(exper.)}} \times 100$$

in the 10 calculated log S values. Do these percentage errors appear to be reasonable for a multiple linear regression? Discuss this point with the instructor and with your colleagues. (See Y. C. Martin, *Quantitative Drug Design*, Marcel Dekker, New York, 1978, pp. 194–198, to determine how well your multiple linear equation fits the data.)

Partial Answer: **(a)** Using a personal computer or a hand calculator capable of multiple linear-regression analysis, the square of the correlation coefficient is found to be $r^2 = 0.9811$ and the equation is

$$\log S = 1.3793 - 2.5201(V/100) - 0.1216\pi + 1.8148\beta$$

1-25. The specific gravity of alcohol is determined by measuring the mass (weight) of alcohol at 15.56° C and comparing it to the mass (weight) of an equal volume of water, taken as the standard at 15.56° C. The temperature 15.56° C is used because many years ago the United States government settled on a temperature of 60° F (15.56° C) for its testing of alcoholic products.[13]

To obtain the mass of an equal volume of water, one must know the density of water at the standard temperature, 15.56° C. The density of water at various temperatures, as found in handbooks of chemistry, is tabulated below.

Plot the data and obtain an equation that will reproduce the points on the curve most accurately. If the curve is not linear, it may require the use of a quadratic or a cubic equation to represent the data:

$$\text{Density} = a + bt + ct^2$$

or

$$\text{Density} = a + bt + ct^2 + dt^3$$

Some scientific calculators (such as HP41, TI56, and Casio) and personal computers are provided with multiple regression programs.

Using the equation that best fits the data, calculate the density of water at 15.56° C. Attempt to read the density at 15.56° C directly from the graph. Which method of obtaining the density of water appears to be more accurate, calculation or direct reading?

Using your equation and direct reading from the graph, obtain the density of water at 25° C and at 37° C. Compare your results with those from a chemistry handbook. Is it safe to extrapolate your results obtained from the range of 10° to 20° C to obtain values at 25° and 37° C?

Partial Answer: The cubic equation gives the density at 25° C = 0.9970524 g/cm³; the *CRC Handbook*, p. F5, gives the density at 25° C = 0.9970479 g/cm³.

1-26. Using the data in *Problem 1-15*, compute the correlation coefficient r and the regression coefficient b (n in *Problem 1-15*).

Answer: $r = 0.9995$; $b = 0.432$. The use of a programmed hand calculator or a personal computer will provide these results. The problem may also be done by hand, following the instructions on pages 11 through 16.

2
States of Matter

BINDING FORCES BETWEEN MOLECULES

In order for molecules to exist in aggregates in gases, liquids, and solids, *inter*molecular forces must exist. An understanding of intermolecular forces is important in the study of pharmaceutical systems and follows logically from a detailed discussion of *intra*molecular bonding energies. Cohesion, or the attraction of like molecules, and adhesion, or the attraction of unlike molecules, are manifestations of intermolecular forces. A knowledge of these forces is important for an understanding not only of the properties of gases, liquids, and solids, but also of interfacial phenomena, flocculation in suspensions, stabilization of emulsions, compaction of powders in capsules, and the compression of granules to form tablets.

Repulsive and Attractive Forces. When molecules interact, both repulsive and attractive forces operate. As two molecules are brought close together, the opposite charges in the two molecules are closer together than the like charges and cause the molecules to attract one another. When the molecules are brought so close that the outer charge clouds touch, the molecules repel each other like rigid elastic bodies.

Thus attractive forces are necessary in order that molecules cohere; repulsive forces are necessary in order that the molecules do not interpenetrate and annihilate one another. Moelwyn-Hughes[1] points to the analogy between human behavior and molecular phenomenon. Just as the actions of humans are often influenced by a conflict of loyalties, so molecular behavior is governed by attractive and repulsive forces.

Repulsion is due to the interpenetration of the electronic clouds of molecules and increases exponentially with a decrease in distance between the molecules. At a certain equilibrium distance, about 3 or 4 $\times$ 10^{-8} cm (3 or 4 angstroms), the repulsive and attractive

forces are equal. At this position, the potential energy of the two molecules is a minimum and the system is most stable (Fig. 2–1). This principle of minimum potential energy applies not only to molecules but to atoms and to large objects as well.

Under the following headings are discussed the various types of *attractive* intermolecular forces.

Van der Waals Forces. Dipolar molecules frequently tend to align themselves with their neighbors, so that the negative pole of one molecule points toward the positive pole of the next. Thus, large groups of molecules may be associated through weak attractions known as *dipole–dipole* or Keesom forces. Permanent dipoles are capable of inducing an electric dipole in nonpolar molecules (which are easily polarizable) in order to produce *dipole–induced dipole*, or Debye, interactions, and nonpolar molecules can induce polar-

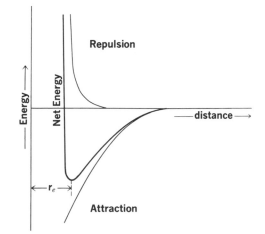

Fig. 2–1. Repulsive and attractive energies and net energy as a function of the distance between molecules. Note that a minimum occurs in the net energy because of the different character of the attraction and repulsion curves.

TABLE 2–1. *Intermolecular Forces and Valence Bonds*

Bond type	Bond Energy (approx.) (kcal//mole)
Van der Waals Forces and Other Intermolecular Attractions	
Dipole–dipole interaction, orientation effect, or Keesom force	
Dipole–induced dipole interaction, induction effect, or Debye force	1–10
Induced dipole–induced dipole interaction, dispersion effect, or London force	
Ion–dipole interaction	
Hydrogen bonds: O—H · · · O	6
C—H · · · O	2–3
O—H · · · N	4–7
N—H · · · O	2–3
F—H · · · F	7
Primary Valence Bond	
Electrovalent, ionic, heteropolar	100–200
Covalent, homopolar	50–150

ity in one another by *induced dipole–induced dipole*, or London, attractions. This latter force deserves additional comment here.

The weak electrostatic force by which nonpolar molecules such as hydrogen gas, carbon tetrachloride, and benzene attract one another was first recognized by London in 1930. The *dispersion* or London force is sufficient to bring about the condensation of nonpolar gas molecules so as to form liquids and solids when molecules are brought quite close to one another. In all three types of van der Waals forces, the potential energy of attraction varies inversely with the distance of separation, r, raised to the sixth power; that is, r^6. The potential energy of repulsion changes more rapidly with distance, as shown in Figure 2–1. This accounts for the potential energy minimum and the resultant equilibrium distance of separation, r_e.

These several classes of interaction, known as van der Waals forces* and listed in Table 2–1, are associated with the condensation of gases, the solubility of some drugs (Chapter 10), the formation of some metal complexes and molecular addition compounds (Chapter 11), and certain biologic processes and drug actions. The energies associated with primary valence bonds are included for comparison.

Ion–Dipole and Ion–Induced Dipole Forces. In addition to the dipolar interactions known as van der Waals forces, other attractions occur between polar or nonpolar molecules and ions. These types of interactions

account in part for the solubility of ionic crystalline substances in water, the cation for example attracting the relatively negative oxygen atom of water and the anion attracting the hydrogen atoms of the dipolar water molecules. Ion–induced dipole forces are presumably involved in the formation of the iodide complex,

$$I_2 + K^+I^- \rightarrow K^+I_3^- \qquad (2–1)$$

Reaction (2–1) accounts for the solubility of iodine in a solution of potassium iodide.

Hydrogen Bonds. The interaction between a molecule containing a hydrogen atom and a strongly electronegative atom such as fluorine, oxygen, or nitrogen is of particular interest. Because of the small size of a hydrogen atom and its large electrostatic field, it can move in close to the electronegative atom and form an electrostatic type of union known as a *hydrogen bond* or *hydrogen bridge*. Such a bond, discovered by Latimer and Rodebush[2] in 1920, exists in ice and in liquid water; it accounts for many of the unusual properties of water, including its high dielectric constant, abnormally low vapor pressure, and high boiling point. The structure of ice is a loose three-dimensional array of regular tetrahedra with oxygen in the center of each tetrahedron and hydrogen atoms at the four corners. The hydrogens are not exactly midway between the oxygens, as may be observed in Figure 2–2. Roughly one sixth of the hydrogen bonds of ice are broken when water passes into the liquid state, and essentially all the bridges are destroyed when it vaporizes. Hydrogen bonds also exist between some alcohol molecules, carboxylic acids, aldehydes, esters, and polypeptides.

The hydrogen bonds of formic acid and acetic acid are sufficiently strong to yield *dimers* (two molecules attached together), which can exist even in the vapor state. Hydrogen fluoride in the vapor state exists as a hydrogen bonded polymer $(F—H . . .)_n$, where n can have a value as large as 6. Several structures involving hydrogen bonds are shown in Figure 2–2. The dashed

---

*The term *van der Waals forces* is often used loosely. Sometimes all combinations of intermolecular forces among ions, permanent dipoles, and induced dipoles are referred to as van der Waals forces. On the other hand, the London force alone is frequently referred to as the van der Waals force since it accounts for the attraction between nonpolar gas molecules, as expressed by the a/V^2 term in the van der Waals gas equation. In this book, the three dipolar forces of Keesom, Debye, and London are called van der Waals forces. The other forces such as ion-dipole and the hydrogen bond (which have characteristics similar both to ionic and dipolar forces) are designated appropriately where necessary.

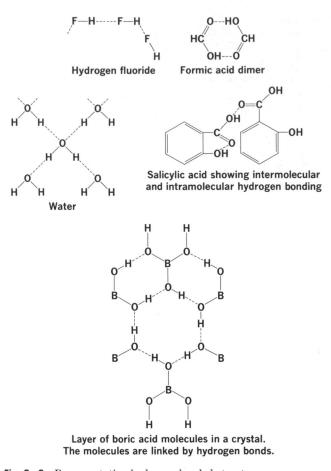

Layer of boric acid molecules in a crystal.
The molecules are linked by hydrogen bonds.

Fig. 2–2. Representative hydrogen-bonded structures.

lines represent the hydrogen bridges. It will be noticed that *intra-* as well as *inter*molecular hydrogen bonds may occur (cf. salicylic acid).

Bond energies serve as a measure of the strength of bonds. Hydrogen bonds are relatively weak, having a bond energy of about 2 to 8 kcal/mole as compared with a value of about 50 to 100 kcal for the covalent bond and well over 100 kcal for the ionic bond. The metallic bond, representing a third type of primary valence, will be mentioned in connection with crystalline solids.

The energies associated with intermolecular bond forces of several compounds are shown in Table 2–2. It will be observed that the total interaction energies between molecules are contributed by a combination of orientation, induction, and dispersion effects. The na-

ture of the molecules determines which of these factors is most influential in the attraction. In water, a highly polar substance, the orientation or dipole–dipole interaction predominates over the other two forces, and solubility of drugs in water is influenced mainly by the orientation energy or dipole interaction. In hydrogen chloride, a molecule with about 20% ionic character, the orientation effect is still significant, but the dispersion force contributes a large share to the total interaction energy between molecules. Hydrogen iodide is predominantly covalent, and its intermolecular attraction is supplied primarily by the London or dispersion force.

The ionic crystal sodium chloride is included in Table 2–2 for comparison to show that its stability, as reflected in its large total energy, is much greater than that of molecular aggregates, and yet the dispersion force exists in such ionic compounds even as it does in molecules.

STATES OF MATTER

Gases, liquids, and crystalline solids are the three states of matter. The molecules, atoms, and ions in the solid state are held in close proximity by intermolecular, interatomic, or ionic forces. The particles of the solid can oscillate only about fixed positions. As the temperature of a solid substance is raised, the particles acquire sufficient energy to disrupt the ordered arrangement of the lattice and pass into the liquid form. Finally, when sufficient energy is supplied, the molecules pass into the gaseous state. Solids with high vapor pressures, such as iodine and camphor, can pass directly from the solid to the gaseous state without melting. This process is known as *sublimation*, and the reverse process, that is, recondensation to the solid state, may be referred to as *deposition*.

Certain asymmetric molecules frequently exhibit a fourth phase, more properly termed a *mesophase* (Greek, *mesos*, middle), which lies between the liquid and crystalline states. This so-called *liquid crystalline* state is discussed later.

THE GASEOUS STATE

Owing to vigorous and rapid motion, gas molecules travel in random paths, frequently colliding with one another and with the walls of the container in which they are confined. Hence, they exert a *pressure*—a force per unit area—expressed in dynes per cm². Pressure is also recorded in atmospheres or in millimeters of mercury because of the use of the barometer in pressure measurement. Another important characteristic of a gas, its *volume*, is usually expressed in liters or cubic centimeters. The temperature involved in gas equations is given in absolute or Kelvin degrees

TABLE 2–2. *Energies Associated with Molecular and Ionic Interactions*

Compound	Interaction in kcal/mole			
	Orientation	Induction	Dispersion	Total Energy
H_2O	8.69	0.46	2.15	11.30
HCl	0.79	0.24	4.02	5.05
HI	0.006	0.027	6.18	6.21
NaCl	—	—	3.0	183

(°K). Zero degrees on the centigrade scale is equal to 273.15° K.

The Ideal Gas law. The student may recall from general chemistry that the gas laws were formulated by Boyle, Charles, and Gay-Lussac. Boyle's law relates the volume and pressure of a given mass of gas at constant temperature.

$$P \propto \frac{1}{V}$$

or

$$PV = k \qquad (2-2)$$

The law of Gay-Lussac and Charles states that the volume and absolute temperature of a given mass of gas at constant pressure are directly proportional.

$$V \propto T$$

or

$$V = kT \qquad (2-3)$$

These equations can be combined to obtain the relationship

$$\frac{P_1 V_1}{T_1} = \frac{P_2 V_2}{T_2} \qquad (2-4)$$

which should be familiar to the student. In equation (2–4), P_1, V_1, and T_1 are the values under one set of conditions and P_2, V_2, and T_2 the values under another set.

Example 2–1. In the assay of ethyl nitrite spirit, the nitric oxide gas that is liberated from a definite quantity of spirit and collected in a gas burette occupies a volume of 30.0 mL at a temperature of 20° C and a pressure of 740 mm of mercury. What is the volume at 0° C and 760 mm Hg? (We assume that the gas behaves ideally.)

$$\frac{740 \times 30.0}{(273 + 20)} = \frac{760 \times V_2}{273}$$

$$V_2 = 27.2 \text{ mL}$$

From equation (2–4) it is seen that PV/T under one set of conditions is equal to PV/T under another set, and so on. Thus, one reasons that although P, V, and T change, the ratio PV/T is constant and can be expressed mathematically as

$$\frac{PV}{T} = R$$

or

$$PV = RT \qquad (2-5)$$

in which R is the constant value for the PV/T ratio of an ideal gas. This equation is correct only for 1 mole (i.e., 1 gram molecular weight) of gas; for n moles it becomes

$$PV = nRT \qquad (2-6)$$

Equation (2–6) is known as the *general ideal gas law*, and since it relates the specific conditions or state, that is, the pressure, volume, and temperature of a given mass of gas, it is called the *equation of state* of an ideal gas. Real gases do not follow the laws of Boyle and of Gay-Lussac and Charles as ideal gases are assumed to do. This deviation will be considered in a later section.

The *molar gas constant R* is highly important in physical chemical science; it appears in a number of equations in electrochemistry, solution theory, colloid chemistry, and other fields, in addition to its appearance in the gas laws. To obtain a numeric value for R, let us proceed as follows. If 1 mole of an ideal gas is chosen, its volume under standard conditions of temperature and pressure (STP) (i.e., at 0° C and 760 mm Hg) has been found by experiment to be 22.414 liters. Substituting this value in equation (2–6), we obtain

1 atm × 22.414 liters = 1 mole × R × 273.16° K

$$R = 0.08205 \text{ liter atm/mole deg}$$

The molar gas constant may also be given in energy units by expressing the pressure in dyne/cm² (1 atm = 1.0133×10^6 dyne/cm² as calculated on p. 4 and the volume in the corresponding units of cm³ (22.414 liters = 22,414 cm³). Then

$$R = \frac{PV}{T} = \frac{(1.0133 \times 10^6) \times 22,414}{273.16°}$$

$$= 8.314 \times 10^7 \text{ erg/mole deg}$$

or, since 1 joule = 10^7 erg

$$R = 8.314 \text{ joules/mole deg}$$

The constant can also be expressed in cal/mole deg, employing the equivalent, 1 cal = 4.184 joules.

$$R = \frac{8.314 \text{ joules/(mole deg)}}{4.184 \text{ joules/cal}} = 1.987 \text{ cal/mole deg}$$

One must be particularly careful to use the value of R commensurate with the appropriate units under consideration in each problem. In gas law problems, R is usually expressed in liter atm/mole deg, whereas in thermodynamic calculations it usually appears in the units of cal/mole deg or joule/mole deg.

Example 2–2. What is the volume of 2 moles of an ideal gas at 25° C and 780 mm Hg?

(780 mm/760 mm atm⁻¹) × V =

2 moles × (0.08205 liter atm/mole deg) × 298° K

$$V = 47.65 \text{ liters}$$

Molecular Weight. The approximate molecular weight of a gas can be determined by use of the ideal gas law. The number of moles of gas n is replaced by its equivalent g/M, in which g is the grams of gas and M is the molecular weight:

$$PV = \frac{g}{M} RT \qquad (2-7)$$

or

$$M = \frac{gRT}{PV} \qquad (2-8)$$

Example 2–3. If 0.30 g of ethyl alcohol in the vapor state occupies 200 mL at a pressure of 1 atm and a temperature of 100° C, what is the molecular weight of ethyl alcohol? Assume that the vapor behaves as an ideal gas.

$$M = \frac{0.30 \times 0.082 \times 373}{1 \times 0.2}$$

$$M = 46.0 \text{ g/mole}$$

The two methods most commonly used to determine the molecular weight of easily vaporized liquids such as alcohol and chloroform are the *Regnault and Victor Meyer* methods. In the latter method, the liquid is weighed in a glass bulb; it is then vaporized and the volume is determined at a definite temperature and barometric pressure. The values are finally substituted in equation (2–8) to obtain the molecular weight.

Kinetic Molecular Theory. The equations just given have been formulated from experimental considerations. The theory that was developed to explain the behavior of gases and to lend additional support to the validity of the gas laws is called the *kinetic molecular theory*. Some of the more important statements of the theory are the following:

1. Gases are composed of particles called *molecules*, the total volume of which is so small as to be negligible in relation to the volume of the space in which the molecules are confined. This condition is approximated in actual gases only at low pressures and high temperatures, in which case the molecules of the gas are far apart.

2. The particles of the gas do not attract one another but rather move with complete independence; again, this statement applies only at low pressures.

3. The particles exhibit continuous random motion owing to their kinetic energy. The average kinetic energy E is directly proportional to the absolute temperature of the gas, or $E = \frac{3}{2}RT$.

4. The molecules exhibit perfect elasticity, that is, there is no net loss of speed after they collide with one another and with the walls of the confining vessel, which latter effect accounts for the gas pressure. Although the net velocity, and therefore the average kinetic energy, does not change on collision, the speed and energy of the individual molecules may differ widely at any instant.

From these and other postulates, the following *fundamental kinetic equation* is derived:

$$PV = \tfrac{1}{3}nm\overline{c^2} \qquad (2-9)$$

where P is the pressure and V the volume occupied by any number n of molecules of mass m having an average velocity $\bar{c}$.

Using this fundamental equation, the root mean square velocity $(\overline{c^2})^{1/2}$ (usually written μ) of the mole-

cules in an ideal gas can be obtained.* Solving for $\overline{c^2}$ in equation (2–9) and taking the square root of both sides of the equation leads to the formula

$$\mu = \sqrt{\frac{3PV}{nm}} \qquad (2-10)$$

Restricting this case to 1 mole of gas, PV becomes equal to RT from the equation of state (2–5), n becomes Avogadro's number N, and N multiplied by the mass of one molecule becomes the molecular weight M. The root mean square velocity is therefore given by

$$\mu = \sqrt{\frac{3RT}{M}} \qquad (2-11)$$

Example 2–4. What is the root mean square velocity of oxygen (molecular weight, 32.0) at 25° C (298° K)?

$$\mu = \sqrt{\frac{3 \times 8.314 \times 10^7 \times 298}{32}} = 4.82 \times 10^4 \text{ cm/sec}$$

Since the term nm/V is equal to density, we may write equation (2–10) as

$$\mu = \sqrt{\frac{3P}{d}} \qquad (2-12)$$

In other words, the rate of diffusion of a gas is inversely proportional to the square root of its density. Such a relation confirms the early findings of Graham, who showed that a light gas diffused more rapidly through a porous membrane than did a heavier one.

The van der Waals Equation for Real Gases. The fundamental kinetic equation (2–9) is found to compare with the ideal gas equation, since the kinetic theory is based on the assumptions of the ideal state. However, real gases are not composed of infinitely small and perfectly elastic nonattracting spheres. Instead, they are composed of molecules of a finite volume that tend to attract one another. These factors affect the volume and pressure terms in the ideal equation, so that certain refinements must be incorporated if equation (2–5) is to provide results that check with experiment. A number of such expressions have been suggested, the *van der Waals equation* being one of the best known of these. For 1 mole of gas, the van der Waals equation is written as

$$\left(P + \frac{a}{V^2}\right)(V - b) = RT \qquad (2-13)$$

For the more general case of n moles of gas in a container of volume V, equation (2–13) becomes

$$\left(P + \frac{an^2}{V^2}\right)(V - nb) = nRT \qquad (2-14)$$

---

*Note that the root mean square velocity $\sqrt{\overline{c^2}}$ is not the same as the average velocity, $\bar{c}$. This can be shown in a simple example where c has the three values 2, 3, and 4. $\bar{c} = (2 + 3 + 4)/3 = 3$, whereas $\mu = \sqrt{\overline{c^2}}$ is the square root of the mean of the sum of the squares or $\sqrt{(2^2 + 3^2 + 4^2)/3} = \sqrt{9.67}$ and $\mu = 3.11$.

TABLE 2–3. *The van der Waals Constants for Some Gases*

Gas	a liter^2 atm/mole^2	b liter/mole
H_2	0.244	0.0266
O_2	1.360	0.0318
CH_4	2.253	0.0428
H_2O	5.464	0.0305
Cl_2	6.493	0.0562
$CHCl_3$	15.17	0.1022

The term a/V^2 accounts for the *internal pressure* per mole resulting from the intermolecular forces of attraction between the molecules: b accounts for the incompressibility of the molecules, that is, the *excluded volume*, which is about four times the molecular volume. It will be seen in Chapter 10 that internal pressure is also used to describe the cohesive forces in liquids. Polar liquids have high internal pressures and serve as solvents only for substances of similar internal pressures. Nonpolar molecules have low internal pressures and are not able to overcome the powerful cohesive forces of the polar solvent molecules. Mineral oil is immiscible with water for this reason.

When the volume of a gas is large, a/V^2 and b become insignificant with respect to P and V, respectively. Under these conditions, the van der Waals equation for 1 mole of gas reduces to the ideal gas equation, $PV = RT$, and at low pressures, real gases behave in an ideal manner. The values of a and b have been determined for a number of gases. Some of these are listed in Table 2–3. The weak van der Waals forces of attraction, expressed by the constant a, are those referred to in Table 2–1.

Example 2–5. A 0.193-mole sample of ether was confined in a 7.35-liter vessel at 295° K. Calculate the pressure produced using *(a)* the ideal gas equation and *(b)* the van der Waals equation. The van der Waals a value for ether is 17.38 liter^2 atm mole^{-2}; the b value is 0.1344 liter mole^{-1}. To solve for pressure, the van der Waals equation may be rearranged as follows:

$$P = \frac{nRT}{V - nb} - \frac{an^2}{V^2}$$

(a)

$$P = \frac{0.193 \text{ mole} \times 0.0821 \text{ liter atm/deg mole} \times 295 \text{ deg}}{7.35 \text{ liter}}$$

$$= 0.636 \text{ atm}$$

(b)

$$P = \frac{0.193 \text{ mole} \times 0.0821 \text{ liter atm/deg mole} \times 295 \text{ deg}}{7.35 \text{ liter} - (0.193 \text{ mole}) \times (0.1344 \text{ liter/mole})}$$
$$- \frac{17.38 \text{ liter}^2 \text{ atm/mole}^2 \,(0.193 \text{ mole})^2}{(7.35 \text{ liter})^2}$$

$$= 0.626 \text{ atm}$$

Example 2–6. Calculate the pressure of 0.5 mole of CO_2 gas in a fire extinguisher of 1 liter capacity at 27° C using the ideal gas equation and the van der Waals equation. The van der Waals constants can be calculated from the critical temperature T_c and critical pressure P_c (see Liquefaction of Gases for definition):

$$a = \frac{27R^2T_c^2}{64\,P_c} \quad \text{and} \quad b = \frac{RT_c}{8P_c}$$

The critical temperature and critical pressure of CO_2 are 31.0° C and 72.9 atm, respectively.

Using the ideal gas equation,

$$P = \frac{nRT}{V} = \frac{0.5 \text{ mole} \times 0.0821 \text{ liter atm/deg mole} \times 300.15 \text{ deg}}{1 \text{ liter}}$$

$$= 12.32 \text{ atm}$$

Using the van der Waals equation,

$$a = \frac{27 \times (0.0821 \text{ liter atm/deg mole})^2 \times (304.15 \text{ deg})^2}{64 \times 72.9 \text{ atm}}$$

$$= 3.608 \text{ liter}^2 \text{ atm/mole}^2$$

$$b = \frac{(0.0821 \text{ liter atm/deg mole}) \times 304.15 \text{ deg}}{8 \times 72.9 \text{ atm}}$$

$$= 0.0428 \text{ liter/mole}$$

$$P = \frac{nRT}{V - nb} - \frac{an^2}{V^2}$$

$$= \frac{(0.5 \text{ mole} \times 0.0821 \text{ liter atm/deg mole}) \times 300.15 \text{ deg}}{1 \text{ liter} - (0.5 \text{ mole} \times 0.0428 \text{ liter/mole})}$$
$$- \frac{3.608 \text{ liter}^2 \text{ atm/mole}^2 \times (0.5 \text{ mole})^2}{(1 \text{ liter})^2}$$

$$= 11.69 \text{ atm}$$

THE LIQUID STATE

Liquefaction of Gases. When a gas is cooled, it loses some of its kinetic energy in the form of heat, and the velocity of the molecules decreases. If pressure is applied to the gas, the molecules are brought within the sphere of the van der Waals interaction forces and pass into the liquid state. Because of these forces, liquids are considerably denser than gases and occupy a definite volume. The transitions from a gas to a liquid and from a liquid to a solid depend not only on the temperature, but also on the pressure to which the substance is subjected.

If the temperature is elevated sufficiently, a value is reached above which it is impossible to liquefy a gas, irrespective of the pressure applied. This temperature, above which a liquid can no longer exist, is known as the *critical temperature*. The pressure required to liquefy a gas at its critical temperature is the *critical pressure*, which is also the highest vapor pressure that the liquid can have. The further a gas is cooled below its critical temperature, the less pressure is required to liquefy it. Based on this principle, all known gases have been liquefied.

The critical temperature of water is 374° C or 647° K, and its critical pressure is 218 atm, while the corresponding values for helium are 5.2° K and 2.26 atm. The critical temperature serves as a rough measure of the attractive forces between molecules, for at temperatures above the critical value, the molecules possess sufficient kinetic energy so that no amount of pressure can bring them within the range of attractive forces that cause the particles to "stick" together. The high critical values for water result because of the strong dipolar forces between the molecules and particularly the hydrogen bonding that exists. Conversely, helium molecules are attracted only by the weak London force, and, consequently, this element must be cooled to the extremely low temperature of 5.2° K before it can be liquefied. Above this critical temperature, helium remains a gas no matter what the pressure.

Methods of Achieving Liquefaction. One of the most obvious ways to liquefy a gas is to subject it to intense cold by the use of freezing mixtures. Other methods depend on the cooling effect produced in a gas as it expands. Thus, suppose we allow an ideal gas to expand so rapidly that no heat enters the system. Such an expansion, termed an *adiabatic* expansion, may be achieved by carrying out the process in a Dewar, or vacuum, flask, which effectively insulates the contents of the flask from the external environment. The work that has to be done to bring about expansion therefore must come from the gas itself at the expense of its own heat energy content. As a result, the temperature of the gas falls. If this procedure is repeated a sufficient number of times, the total drop in temperature may be sufficient to cause liquefaction of the gas.

A cooling effect is also observed when a highly compressed *nonideal* gas expands into a region of low pressure. In this case, the drop in temperature results from the energy expended in overcoming the cohesive forces of attraction between the molecules. This cooling effect is known as the *Joule–Thomson effect* and differs from the cooling produced in adiabatic expansion, in which the gas does external work. To bring about liquefaction by the Joule–Thomson effect, it may be necessary to precool the gas before allowing it to expand. Liquid oxygen and liquid air are obtained by methods based on this effect.

Aerosols. As mentioned earlier, gases can be liquefied by increasing pressure, provided we work below the critical temperature. When the pressure is reduced, the molecules expand and the liquid reverts to a gas. This reversible change of state is the basic principle involved in the preparation of pharmaceutical aerosols. In such products, a drug is dissolved or suspended in a *propellant*, a material that is liquid under the pressure conditions existing inside the container but that forms a gas under normal atmospheric conditions. The container is so designed that, by depressing a valve, some of the drug-propellant mixture is expelled owing to the excess pressure inside the container. If the drug is nonvolatile, it forms a fine spray as it leaves the valve orifice; at the same time, the liquid propellant vaporizes off. The propellant used in these products is frequently a mixture of fluorinated hydrocarbons, although other gases, such as nitrogen and carbon dioxide, are increasingly used. By varying the proportions of the various propellants, it is possible to produce pressures within the container ranging from 1 to 6 atm at room temperature. Alternate fluorocarbon propellants that do not deplete the ozone layer of the atmosphere are presently under investigation (Byron, Dalby et al.[3]).

The containers are filled either by cooling the propellant and drug to a low temperature within the container, which is then sealed with the valve, or by sealing the drug in the container at room temperature and then forcing the required amount of propellant into the container under pressure. In both cases, when the product is at room temperature, part of the propellant is in the gaseous state and exerts the pressure necessary to extrude the drug, while the remainder is in the liquid state and provides a solution or suspension vehicle for the drug.

The formulation of pharmaceuticals as aerosols is continually increasing, since the method frequently offers distinct advantages over some of the more conventional methods of formulation. Thus, antiseptic materials can be sprayed onto abraded skin with the minimum of discomfort to the patient. More significant is the increased efficiency often observed and the facility with which medication can be introduced into body cavities and passages. These and other aspects of aerosols have been considered by Pickthall et al.[4] and Sciarra.[5] Byron and Clark[6] have studied drug absorption from inhalation aerosols and provided a rather complete analysis of the problem. The USP XXII, 1990, includes a discussion of metered-dose inhalation products and provides standards and test procedures (see USP XXII, pp. 1556, 1689, and 1857, and a list of aerosol monographs on p. 2001).

One product, ethyl chloride, cools sufficiently on expansion so that, when sprayed on the skin, it freezes the tissue and produces a local anesthesia. This procedure is sometimes used in minor surgical operations.

Vapor Pressure of Liquids. Translational energy of motion (kinetic energy) is not distributed evenly among molecules; some of the molecules have more energy and hence higher velocities than others at any moment. When a liquid is placed in an evacuated container at a constant temperature, the molecules with the highest energies break away from the surface of the liquid and pass into the gaseous state, and some of the molecules subsequently return to the liquid state, or condense. When the rate of condensation equals the rate of vaporization at a definite temperature, the vapor becomes saturated and a dynamic equilibrium is established. The pressure of the saturated vapor* above the liquid is then known as the *equilibrium vapor pressure*. If a manometer is fitted to an evacuated vessel containing the liquid, it is possible to obtain a record of

---

*A gas is known as a *vapor* below its critical temperature. A less rigorous definition of a *vapor* is a substance that is a liquid or solid at room temperature and that passes into the gaseous state when heated to a sufficiently high temperature. A *gas* is a substance that exists in the gaseous state even at room temperature. Menthol and ethanol are vapors at sufficiently high temperatures; oxygen and carbon dioxide are gases.

the vapor pressure in millimeters of mercury. The presence of a gas, such as air, above the liquid would decrease the rate of evaporation, but it would not affect the equilibrium pressure of the vapor.

As the temperature of the liquid is elevated, more molecules approach the velocity necessary for escape and pass into the gaseous state. As a result, the vapor pressure increases with rising temperature, as shown in Figure 2–3. Any point on one of the curves represents a condition in which the liquid and the vapor exist together in equilibrium. As observed in the diagram, if the temperature of any of the liquids is increased while the pressure is held constant, or if the pressure is decreased while the temperature is held constant, all the liquid will pass into the vapor state.

Clausius–Clapeyron Equation: Heat of Vaporization. The relationship between the vapor pressure and the absolute temperature of a liquid is expressed by the Clausius–Clapeyron equation (the Clapeyron and the Clausius–Clapeyron equations are derived in Chapter 3):

$$\log \frac{p_2}{p_1} = \frac{\Delta H_v (T_2 - T_1)}{2.303 R T_1 T_2} \qquad (2-15)$$

in which p_1 and p_2 are the vapor pressures at absolute temperatures T_1 and T_2, and ΔH_v is the *molar heat of vaporization*, that is, the heat absorbed by 1 mole of liquid when it passes into the vapor state.

Heats of vaporization vary somewhat with temperature. For example, the heat of vaporization of water is 539 cal/g at 100° C; it is 478 cal/g at 180° C, and at the critical temperature, where no distinction can be made between liquid and gas, the heat of vaporization becomes zero. Hence, the ΔH_v of equation (2–15)

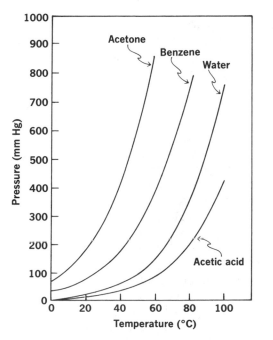

Fig. 2–3. The variation of vapor pressure of some liquids with temperature.

should be recognized as an average value, and the equation should be considered strictly valid only over a narrow temperature range. The equation contains additional approximations, for it assumes that the vapor behaves like an ideal gas and that the molar volume of the liquid is negligible with respect to that of the vapor.

Example 2–7. Compute the vapor pressure of water at 120° C. The vapor pressure p_1 of water at 100° C is 1 atm, and ΔH_v may be taken as 9720 cal/mole for this temperature range.

$$\log \frac{p_2}{1.0} = \frac{9720 \times (393 - 373)}{2.303 \times 1.987 \times 393 \times 373}$$

$$p_2 = 1.95 \text{ atm}$$

The Clausius–Clapeyron equation can be written in a more general form,

$$\log p = -\frac{\Delta H_v}{2.303 R} \frac{1}{T} + \text{constant} \qquad (2-16a)$$

or in natural logarithms,

$$\ln p = -\frac{\Delta H_v}{R} \frac{1}{T} + \text{constant} \qquad (2-16b)$$

from which it is observed that a plot of the logarithm of the vapor pressure against the reciprocal of the absolute temperature results in a straight line, enabling one to compute the heat of vaporization of the liquid from the slope of the line.

Boiling Point. If a liquid is placed in an open container and heated until the vapor pressure equals the atmospheric pressure, the vapor is seen to form bubbles that rise rapidly through the liquid and escape into the gaseous state. The temperature at which the vapor pressure of the liquid equals the external or atmospheric pressure is known as the *boiling point*. All the absorbed heat is used to change the liquid to vapor, and the temperature does not rise until the liquid is completely vaporized. The pressure at sea level is about 760 mm Hg; at higher elevations, the atmospheric pressure decreases and the boiling point is lowered. At a pressure of 700 mm Hg, water boils at 97.7° C; at 17.5 mm Hg, it boils at 20° C. The change in boiling point with pressure may be computed by using the Clausius–Clapeyron equation.

The heat that is absorbed when water vaporizes at the normal boiling point (i.e., the heat of vaporization at 100° C) is 539 cal/g or about 9720 cal/mole. For benzene, it is 91.4 cal/g at the normal boiling point of 80.2° C. These quantities of heat, known as *latent heats of vaporization*, are taken up when the liquids vaporize and are liberated when the vapors condense to liquids.

The boiling point may be considered as the temperature at which thermal agitation can overcome the attractive forces between the molecules of a liquid. Therefore, the boiling point of a compound, like the heat of vaporization and the vapor pressure at a definite temperature, provides a rough indication of the magnitude of the attractive forces.

The boiling points of normal hydrocarbons, simple alcohols, and carboxylic acids increase with molecular weight, since the attractive van der Waals forces become greater with increasing numbers of atoms. Branching of the chain produces a less compact molecule with reduced intermolecular attraction, and a decrease in the boiling point results. In general, however, the alcohols boil at a much higher temperature than saturated hydrocarbons of the same molecular weight because of association of the alcohol molecules through hydrogen bonding. The boiling points of carboxylic acids are still more abnormal because the acids form dimers through hydrogen bonding that can remain even in the vapor state. The boiling points of straight-chain primary alcohols and carboxylic acids increase about 18° C for each additional methylene group. The rough parallel between the intermolecular forces and the boiling points or latent heats of vaporization is brought out in Table 2–4. Nonpolar substances, the molecules of which are held together predominantly by the London force, have low boiling points and low heats of vaporization. Polar molecules, particularly those such as ethyl alcohol and water, which are attached through hydrogen bonds, exhibit high boiling points and high heats of vaporization.

Other properties of liquids, such as surface tension and viscosity, are discussed in Chapters 14 and 17, respectively.

SOLIDS AND THE CRYSTALLINE STATE

Crystalline Solids. The structural units of crystalline solids, such as ice, sodium chloride, and menthol, are arranged in fixed geometric patterns or lattices. Crystalline solids, unlike liquids and gases, have definite shapes and an orderly arrangement of units. Gases are easily compressed, whereas solids, like liquids, are practically incompressible. Crystalline solids show definite melting points, passing rather sharply from the solid to the liquid state. The various crystal forms are divided into six distinct crystal systems. They are, together with examples of each, cubic (sodium chloride), tetragonal (urea), hexagonal (iodoform), rhombic (iodine), monoclinic (sucrose), and triclinic (boric acid).

TABLE 2–4. *Normal Boiling Points and Heats of Vaporization*

Compound	Boiling Point (°C)	Latent Heat of Vaporization (cal/g)
Helium	−268.9	6
Nitrogen	−195.8	47.6
Propane	−42.2	102
Methyl chloride	−24.2	102
Isobutane	−10.2	88
Butane	−0.4	92
Ethyl ether	34.6	90
Carbon disulfide	46.3	85
Ethyl alcohol	78.3	204
Water	100.0	539

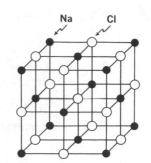

Fig. 2–4. The crystal lattice of sodium chloride.

The units that constitute the crystal structure can be atoms, molecules, or ions. The sodium chloride crystal, shown in Figure 2–4, consists of a cubic lattice of sodium ions interpenetrated by a lattice of chloride ions, the binding force of the crystal being the electrostatic attraction of the oppositely charged ions. In diamond and graphite, the lattice units consist of atoms held together by covalent bonds. Solid carbon dioxide, hydrogen chloride, and naphthalene form crystals composed of molecules as the building units. In organic compounds, the molecules are held together by van der Waals forces and hydrogen bonding, which account for the weak binding and for the low melting points of these crystals. Aliphatic hydrocarbons crystallize with their chains lying in a parallel arrangement, while fatty acids crystallize in layers of dimers with the chains lying parallel or tilted at an angle with respect to the base plane. Whereas ionic and atomic crystals in general are hard and brittle and have high melting points, molecular crystals are soft and have low melting points.

Metallic crystals are composed of positively charged ions in a field of freely moving electrons, sometimes called the *electron gas.* Metals are good conductors of electricity because of the free movement of the electrons in the lattice. Metals may be soft or hard and have low or high melting points. The hardness and strength of metals depend in part on the kind of imperfections, or *lattice defects*, in the crystals.

X-Ray Diffraction. X-rays are diffracted by crystals just as visible light is dispersed into a color spectrum by a ruled grating (i.e., a piece of glass with fine parallel lines of equal width drawn on it). This is due to the fact that x-rays have wavelengths of about the same magnitude as the distance between the atoms or molecules of crystals. The x-ray diffraction pattern is photographed on a sensitive plate arranged behind the crystal, and by such a method the structure of a crystal may be investigated. Employing a later modification of this principle, involving reflection of the x-ray beam from the atomic planes of the crystal, it has become possible to determine the distances of the various planes of the crystal lattice. The structure of various compounds can be determined in this way.

Where whole crystals are unavailable or unsuitable for analysis, a powder of the substance may be

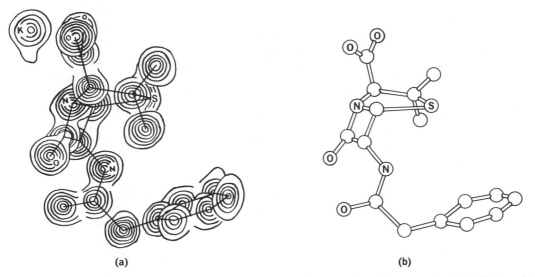

(a)   **(b)**

Fig. 2–5. *(a)* Electron density map of potassium benzylpenicillin. (Modified from G. L. Pitt, Acta Cryst. 5, 770, 1952.) *(b)* A model of the structure that can be built from analysis of the electron density projection.

investigated. Comparing the position and intensity of the lines on such a diagram with corresponding lines on the photograph of a known sample allows one to conduct a qualitative and a quantitative chemical analysis.

The electron density and, accordingly, the position of the atoms in complex structures such as penicillin may be determined from a mathematical study of the data obtained by x-ray diffraction. The electron density map of crystalline potassium benzylpenicillin is shown in Figure 2–5. The elucidation of this structure by x-ray crystallography paved the way for the later synthesis of penicillin by the organic chemist. Certain aspects of x-ray crystallography of pharmaceutical interest have been reviewed by Biles[7] and by Lien and Kennon.[8]

Melting Point and Heat of Fusion. The temperature at which a liquid passes into the solid state is known as the *freezing point*. It is also the *melting point* of a pure crystalline compound. The freezing point or melting point of a pure crystalline solid is strictly defined as the temperature at which the pure liquid and solid exist in equilibrium. In practice, it is taken as the temperature of the equilibrium mixture at an external pressure of 1

atm; this is sometimes known as the *normal freezing* or *melting point*.

The heat absorbed when a gram of a solid melts or the heat liberated when it freezes is known as the *latent heat of fusion*, and for water at 0° C it is about 80 cal/g (1436 cal/mole). The heat added during the melting process does not bring about a change in temperature until all of the solid has disappeared, since this heat is converted into the potential energy of the molecules that have escaped from the solid into the liquid state. The normal melting points of some compounds are collected in Table 2–5, together with the molar heats of fusion.

Changes of the freezing or melting point with pressure may be obtained by using one form of the Clapeyron equation. It is written

$$\frac{\Delta T}{\Delta P} = T\frac{V_l - V_s}{\Delta H_f} \qquad (2\text{–}17)$$

in which V_l and V_s are the molar volumes of the liquid and solid, respectively. Molar volume (volume in cm^3 per mole) is computed by dividing the gram molecular weight by the density of the compound. ΔH_f is the molar heat of fusion—that is, the amount of heat absorbed when 1 mole of the solid changes into 1 mole of liquid, and ΔT is the change of melting point brought about by a pressure change of ΔP.

Water is unusual in that it has a larger molar volume in the solid state than in the liquid state ($V_s > V_l$) at the melting point. Therefore, $\Delta T/\Delta P$ is negative, signifying that the melting point is lowered by an increase in pressure. This phenomenon can be rationalized in terms of *Le Chatelier's principle*, which states that a system at equilibrium readjusts so as to reduce the effect of an external stress. Accordingly, if a pressure is applied to ice at 0° C, it will be transformed into liquid water, that is, into the state of lower volume, and the freezing point will be lowered.

TABLE 2–5. *Normal Melting Points and Molar Heats of Fusion of Some Compounds*

Substance	Melting Point (°K)	Molar Heat of Fusion ΔH_f (cal/mole)
H_2O	273.15	1440
H_2S	187.61	568
NH_3	195.3	1424
PH_3	139.4	268
CH_4	90.5	226
C_2H_6	90	683
n - C_3H_8	85.5	842
C_6H_6	278.5	2348
$C_{10}H_8$	353.2	4550

Handwritten notes at top: $1 J = 10^7$ ergs $1 J = 1 Nm = 1 Pa$ $1 atm = 1.013 \times 10^5 Pa$ $1 L \cdot atm = 10^{-3} m^3 \times 101,325 \frac{Nm}{(Pa)}$

Example 2–8. What is the effect of an increase of pressure of 1 atm on the freezing point of water (melting point of ice)?

At 0° C, $T = 273.16°$ K, $\Delta H_f \cong 1440$ cal/mole, the molar volume of water is 18.018, and the molar volume of ice is 19.651, or $V_l - V_s = -1.633$ cm^3/mole. To obtain the result in deg/atm, using equation (2-17), we first convert ΔH_f in cal/mole into units of erg/mole by multiplying by the factor 4.184×10^7 erg/cal

1440 cal/mole $\times$ 4.184 $\times$ 10^7 erg/cal

$$= 6025 \times 10^7 \text{ erg/mole or } 6025$$

$$\times 10^7 \text{ dyne cm/mole}$$

Then multiplying the equation by the equivalent, 1.013×10^6 dyne/cm^2 per atmosphere (p. 4), gives the result in the desired units.

$$\frac{\Delta T}{\Delta P} = \frac{273.16 \text{ deg} \times (-1.633 \text{ cm}^3/\text{mole})}{6025 \times 10^7 \text{dyne cm/mole}}$$

$$\times 1.013 \times 10^6 \text{ dyne/cm}^2 \text{ atm}$$

$$\frac{\Delta T}{\Delta P} = -0.0075 \text{ deg/atm}$$

Hence, an increase of pressure of 1 atm lowers the freezing point of water by about 0.0075°, or an increase in pressure of about 133 atm would be required to lower the freezing point of water 1°. (When the ice-water equilibrium mixture is saturated with air under a total pressure of 1 atm, the temperature is lowered an additional 0.0023°.) Pressure has only a slight effect on the equilibrium temperature of *condensed systems* (i.e., of liquids and solids). The large molar volume or low density of ice (0.9168 g/cm^3 as compared with 0.9988 g/cm^3 for water at 0° C) accounts for the fact the ice floats on liquid water. The lowering of the melting point with increasing pressure is taken advantage of in ice skating. The pressure of the skate lowers the melting point and thus causes the ice to melt below the skate. This thin layer of liquid provides lubricating action and allows the skate to glide over the hard surface. Of course, the friction of the skate also contributes greatly to the melting and lubricating action.

Example 2–9.* According to *Example 2–8*, an increase of pressure of 1 atm reduces the freezing (melting) point of ice by 0.0075°. To what temperature is the melting point reduced when a 90-lb boy skates across the ice? The area of the skate blades in contact with the ice is 0.085 cm^2.

In addition to the atmospheric pressure, which may be disregarded, the pressure of the skates on the ice is the mass (90 lb = 40.8 kg) multiplied by the acceleration constant of gravity (981 cm/sec^2) and divided by the area of the skate blades (0.085 cm^2).

$$\text{Pressure} = \frac{40,800 \text{ g} \times (981 \text{ cm/sec}^2)}{0.085 \text{ cm}^2}$$

$$= 4.71 \times 10^8 \text{ dyne/cm}^2$$

Changing to atmospheres (1 atm = 1.01325×10^6 dyne/cm^2) yields a pressure of 464.7 atm. The change in volume ΔV from water to ice is 0.018 liter/mole − 0.01963 liter/mole, or −0.00163 liter/mole for the transition from ice to liquid water.

Use equation (2–17) in the form of a derivative:

$$\frac{dT}{dP} = T\frac{\Delta V}{\Delta H_f}$$

For a pressure change of 1 atm to 464.7 atm when the skates of the 90-lb boy touch the ice, the melting temperature will drop from 273.15° K (0° C) to T, the final melting temperature of the ice under the skate blades, which converts the ice to liquid water and facilitates the lubrication. For such a problem we must put the equation in the form of an integral; that is, integrating between 273.15° K and T caused by a pressure change under the skate blades from 1 atm to (464.7 + 1) atm:

$$\int_{273.15°K}^{T} \frac{1}{T} \, dT = \frac{\Delta V}{\Delta H_f} \int_{1 \text{ atm}}^{465.7 \text{ atm}} dP$$

$$\ln T - \ln(273.15) = \frac{-0.00163 \text{ liter mole}^{-1}}{1440 \text{ cal mole}^{-1}} \frac{24.2 \text{ cal}}{1 \text{ liter atm}} (P_2 - P_1)$$

In this integrated equation, 1440 cal/mole is the heat of fusion, ΔH_f of water in the region of 0° C, and 24.2 cal/liter atm is a conversion factor (see the front leaf of the book) to convert cal to liter atm. We now have

$$\ln T = (-2.74 \times 10^{-5}\text{atm}^{-1})(465.7 - 1 \text{ atm}) + \ln(273.15)$$

$$T = 269.69° \ K$$

The melting temperature has been reduced from 273.15° K to 269.69° K, or a reduction in melting point of 3.46° K by the pressure of the skates on the ice.

A simpler way to do the ice-skating problem is to realize that the small change in temperature, -3.46° K, occurs over a large pressure change of about 465 atm. Therefore, we need not integrate, but rather may obtain the temperature change ΔT per unit atmosphere change, ΔP, and multiply this value by the actual pressure, 464.7 atm. Of course, the heat of fusion of water, 1440 cal mole^{-1}, must be multiplied by the conversion factor, 1 liter atm/24.2 cal, to yield 59.504 liter atm.

$$\frac{\Delta T}{\Delta P} = \frac{T\Delta V}{\Delta H_f} = \frac{(273.15° \text{ K})(0.0180 - 0.0196) \text{ liter mole}^{-1}}{59.504 \text{ liter atm mole}^{-1}}$$

$$\frac{\Delta T}{\Delta P} = -0.00734° \text{ K/atm}$$

For a pressure change of 464.7 atm, the decrease in temperature is

$$\Delta T = -0.00734° \text{ K/atm} \times 464.7 \text{ atm}$$

$$= -3.41° \text{ K}$$

as compared with the more accurate value, −3.46° K.

Melting Point and Intermolecular Forces. The heat of fusion may be considered as the heat required to increase the interatomic or intermolecular distances in crystals, thus allowing melting to occur. A crystal that is bound together by weak forces generally has a low heat of fusion and a low melting point, whereas one bound together by strong forces has a high heat of fusion and a high melting point.

Paraffins crystallize as thin leaflets composed of zig-zag chains packed in a parallel arrangement. The melting points of normal saturated hydrocarbons increase with molecular weight, because the van der Waals forces between the molecules of the crystal become greater with an increasing number of carbon atoms. The melting points of the alkanes with an even number of carbon atoms are higher than those of the hydrocarbons with an odd number of carbon atoms, as observed in Figure 2–6. This phenomenon presumably is due to the fact that alkanes with an odd number of carbon atoms are packed in the crystal less efficiently.

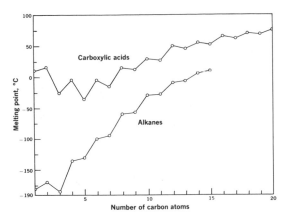

Fig. 2–6. The melting points of alkanes and carboxylic acids as a function of carbon chain length. (Modified from C. R. Noller, *Chemistry of Organic Compounds*, 2nd Ed., Saunders, Philadelphia, 1957, pp. 40, 149).

The melting points of normal carboxylic acids also show this alternation, as seen in Figure 2–6. This can be explained as follows. Fatty acids crystallize in molecular chains, one segment of which is shown in Figure 2–7. The even carbon acids are arranged in the crystal as seen in the more symmetric structure I, whereas the odd numbered acids are arranged according to structure II. The carboxyl groups are joined at two points in the even carbon compound; hence, the crystal lattice is more stable and the melting point is higher.

The melting points and solubilities of the xanthines of pharmaceutical interest, determined by Guttman and Higuchi,[9] further exemplify the relationship between melting point and molecular structure. Solubilities, like melting points, are strongly influenced by intermolecular forces, as will be discussed later in Chapter 10. It will be observed by reference to Table 2–6 that methylation of theophylline to form caffeine, and lengthening of the side chain from methyl (caffeine) to propyl in the 7 position results in a decrease of the melting points and an increase in solubilities. These effects presumably are due to a progressive weakening of intermolecular forces.

Polymorphism. Some elemental substances, such as carbon and sulfur, may exist in more than one crystal-

TABLE 2–6. *Melting Points and Solubilities of Some Xanthines**

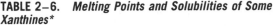

Basic structure

Compound	Melting Point (°C uncorrected)	Solubility in Water at 30° C (mole/liter $\times 10^2$)
Theophylline (R = H)	270–274	4.5
Caffeine (R = CH$_3$)	238	13.3
7-Ethyltheophylline (R = CH$_2$CH$_3$)	156–157	17.6
7-Propyltheophylline (R = CH$_2$CH$_2$CH$_3$)	99–100	104.0

From D. Guttman and T. Higuchi, J. Am. Pharm. Assoc., Sci. Ed. **46, 4, 1957.*

line form and are said to be *polymorphic*. Polymorphs generally have different melting points, x-ray diffraction patterns, and solubilities, even though they are chemically identical.

Nearly all long-chain organic compounds exhibit polymorphism. In fatty acids, this results from different types of attachment between the carboxyl groups of adjacent molecules, which in turn modify the angle of tilt of the chains in the crystal. The triglyceride, tristearin, proceeds from the low-melting metastable alpha (α) form through the beta prime (β′) form and finally to the stable beta (β) form, having a high melting point. The transition cannot occur in the opposite direction.

Theobroma oil or cacao butter is a polymorphous natural fat. Since it consists mainly of a single glyceride, it melts to a large degree over a narrow temperature range (34°–36° C). Theobroma oil is capable of existing in four polymorphic forms, the unstable gamma form melting at 18°, the alpha form melting at 22°, the beta prime form melting at 28°, and the stable beta form melting at 34.5° C. Riegelman[10] has pointed out the relationship between polymorphism and the preparation of cacao butter suppositories. If theobroma oil is heated to the point at which it is completely liquefied (about 35° C), the nuclei of the stable beta crystals are destroyed and the mass does not crystallize until it is supercooled to about 15° C. The crystals that form are the metastable gamma, alpha, and beta prime forms, and the suppositories melt at 23° to 24° C or at ordinary room temperature. The proper method of preparation involves melting cacao butter at the lowest possible temperature, about 33° C. The mass is sufficiently fluid to pour, yet the crystal nuclei of the stable beta form are not lost. When the mass is chilled in the mold, a

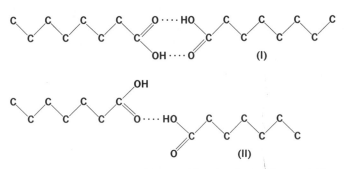

Fig. 2–7. Configuration of fatty acid molecules in the crystalline state. (Modified from A. E. Bailey, *Melting and Solidification of Fats*, Interscience Publishers, New York, 1950, p. 120.)

stable suppository, consisting of beta crystals and melting at 34.5° C, is produced.

Polymorphism has achieved significance in recent years owing to the fact that different polymorphs exhibit different solubilities. In the case of slightly soluble drugs, this may afffect the rate of dissolution. As a result, one polymorph may be more active therapeutically than another polymorph of the same drug. Aguiar et al.[11] have shown the polymorphic state of chloramphenicol palmitate to have a significant influence on the biologic availability of the drug. Khalil et al.[12] reported that form II of sulfameter, an antibacterial agent, was more active orally in humans than form III, although marketed pharmaceutical preparations were found to contain mainly form III.

Polymorphism can also be a factor in suspension technology. Cortisone acetate has been found to exist in at least five different forms, four of which were found to be unstable in the presence of water and which change to a stable form.[13] Since this transformation is usually accompanied by appreciable caking of the crystals, these should all be in the form of the stable polymorph before the suspension is prepared. Heating, grinding under water, and suspension in water are all factors that affect the interconversion of the different cortisone acetate forms.[14]

It is difficult to determine the crystal structure and molecular conformations of different polymorphs of a single drug, and the reports of such work are not common. Azibi et al.[15] studied two polymorphs of spiperone, a potent antipsychotic agent used mainly in the treatment of schizophrenia. The chemical structure of spiperone is shown in Figure 2–8a, and the molecular conformations* of the two polymorphs, I and II, are shown in Figure 2–8b. The difference between the two polymorphs is in the positioning of the atoms in the side chains, as seen in Figure 2–8b, together with the manner in which each molecule binds to neighboring spiperone molecules in the crystal. The results of the investigation showed that the crystal of polymorph II is made up of dimers (molecules in pairs), whereas polymorph crystal I is constructed of nondimerized molecules of spiperone. In a later study, Azibi et al.[16] examined the polymorphism of a number of drugs to ascertain what properties cause a compound to exist in more than one crystalline form. Differences in intermolecular van der Waals forces and hydrogen bonds were found to produce different crystal structures in antipsychotic compounds such as haloperidol (Fig. 2–9) and bromperidol. Variability in hydrogen bonding also contributes to polymorphism in the sulfonamides.[17]

Goldberg and Becker[18] studied the crystalline forms of tamoxifen citrate, an antiestrogenic and antineoplas-

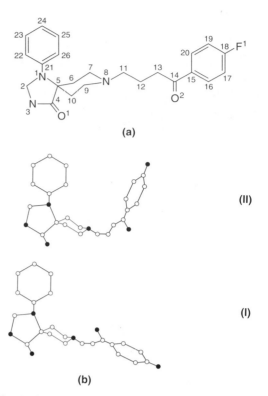

Fig. 2–8. *(a)* Structure and numbering of spiperone. *(b)* Molecular conformation of two polymorphs I and II of spiperone. (M. Azibi, et al., J. Pharm. Sci., **72**:232, 1983. Reproduced with permission.)

tic drug used in the treatment of breast cancer and postmenopausal symptoms. The structural formula of tamoxifen is shown in Figure 2–10. Of the two forms found, the stable polymorph, referred to as *form B*, is held in its molecular conformation in the solid state by hydrogen bonding. One carboxyl group of the citric acid moiety donates its proton to the nitrogen atom on an adjacent tamoxifen molecule to bring about the hydrogen bonding and to stabilize the molecular crystal of form B. The other polymorph, known as *form A*, is a metastable polymorph of tamoxifen citrate, its molecular structure being less organized than that of the stable B form. An ethanolic suspension of polymorph A spontaneously rearranges into polymorph B.

Lowes et al.[19] made physical, chemical, and x-ray studies of carbamazepine. Carbamazepine is used in the treatment of epilepsy and trigeminal neuralgia (severe pain in the face, lips, and tongue). The β polymorph of the drug can be crystallized from solvents of high dielectric constant, such as the aliphatic alcohols. The α polymorph is crystallized from solvents of low dielectric constant, such as carbon tetrachloride and cyclo-

---

*The arrangement of the atoms in a particular stereoisomer gives the *configuration* of a molecule. On the other hand, *conformation* refers to the different arrangements of atoms resulting from rotations about single bonds.

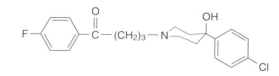

Fig. 2–9. Haloperidol.

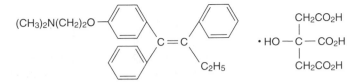

(CH₃)₂N(CH₂)₂O ... C=C ... C₂H₅ · HO—C—CO₂H

Fig. 2–10. Tamoxifen citrate.

hexane. A rather thorough study of the two polymorphic forms of carbamazepine was made using infrared spectroscopy (p. 89), thermogravimetric analysis (p. 49), hot-stage microscopy, dissolution rate (p. 330–332), and x-ray powder diffraction (p. 30). The hydrogen-bonded structure of the α polymorph of carbamazepine is shown in Figure 2–11a, together with its molecular formula (Fig. 2–11b).

Estrogens are essential hormones for the development of female sex characteristics. When the potent synthetic estrogen ethynylestradiol is crystallized from the solvents acetonitrile, methanol, and chloroform saturated with water, four different crystalline solvates are formed. Ethynylestradiol has been reported to exist in several polymorphic forms. However, Ishida et al.[20] have now shown from thermal analysis, infrared spectroscopy, and x-ray studies that these forms are crystals containing solvent molecules and thus should be classified as *solvates* rather than as polymorphs. Solvates are sometimes called *pseudopolymorphs*.[21]

Other related estradiol compounds may exist in true polymeric forms.

Behme et al.[22] reviewed the principles of polymorphism with emphasis on the changes that the polymorphic forms may undergo. When the change from one form to another is reversible, it is said to be *enantiotropic*. When the transition takes place in one direction only—for example, from a metastable to a stable form—the change is said to be *monotropic*. Enantiotropism and monotropism are important properties of polymorphs, as described by Behme et al.[22]

The transition temperature in polymorphism is important because it helps to characterize the system and determine the more stable form at low temperatures. At their transition temperatures, polymorphs have the same free energy, identical solubilities in a particular solvent, and identical vapor pressures. Accordingly, plots of logarithmic solubility of two polymorphic forms against $1/T$ provide the transition temperature at the intersection of the extrapolated curves. Often the plots are nonlinear and cannot be extrapolated with accuracy. For dilute solutions, in which Henry's law (p. 109) applies, the logarithm of the solubility ratios of two polymorphs can be plotted against $1/T$, and the intersection at a ratio equal to unity gives the transition temperature.[23] This temperature can also be obtained from the phase diagram of pressure versus temperature and by using differential scanning calorimetry.[24] An example of the solubility method is given as *Problem 2–20*.

Biles,[25] as well as Haleblian and McCrone,[26] have discussed in some detail the significance of polymorphism and solvation in pharmaceutical practice.

Amorphous Solids. Amorphous solids may be considered as supercooled liquids in which the molecules are arranged in a random manner somewhat as in the liquid state. Substances such as glass, pitch, and many synthetic plastics are amorphous solids. They differ from crystalline solids in that they tend to flow when subjected to sufficient pressure over a period of time, and they do not have definite melting points. In Chapter 17, it will be learned that the rheologist classifies as a solid any substance that must be subjected to a definite shearing force before it fractures or begins to flow. This force, below which the body shows elastic properties, is known as the *yield value*.

Amorphous substances, as well as cubic crystals, are usually *isotropic*, that is, they exhibit similar properties in all directions. Crystals other than cubic are *anisotropic*, showing different characteristics (electric conductance, refractive index, rate of solubility) in various directions along the crystal.

It is not always possible to determine by casual observation whether a substance is crystalline or amorphous. Beeswax and paraffin, although they appear to be amorphous, assume crystalline arrangements when heated and then allowed to cool slowly. Petrolatum, as already mentioned, contains both crys-

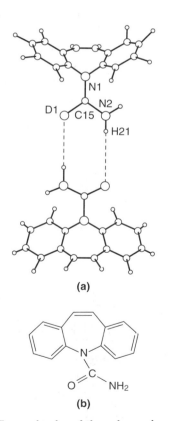

(a)

(b)

Fig. 2–11. *(a)* Two molecules of the polymorph, α-carbamazepine, joined together by hydrogen bonds. (M. M. J. Lowes, et al., J. Pharm. Sci., **76:**744, 1987. Reproduced with permission.) *(b)* Carbamazepine.

talline and amorphous constituents. Some amorphous materials, such as glass, may crystallize after long standing.

Whether or not a drug is amorphous or crystalline has been shown to affect its therapeutic activity. Thus, the crystalline form of the antibiotic novobiocin acid is poorly absorbed and has no activity, whereas the amorphous form is readily absorbed and therapeutically active.[27]

THE LIQUID CRYSTALLINE STATE

Three states of matter have been discussed thus far in this chapter: gas, liquid, and solid. A fourth state of matter is the *liquid crystalline* state or *mesophase*. The term *liquid crystal* is an apparent contradiction, but it is useful in a descriptive sense since materials in this state are in many ways intermediate between the liquid and solid states.

Structure of Liquid Crystals. As seen earlier, molecules in the liquid state are mobile in three directions and can also rotate about three axes perpendicular to one another. In the solid state, on the other hand, the molecules are immobile, and rotations are not possible.

It is not unreasonable to suppose, therefore, that intermediate states of mobility and rotation should exist, as in fact they do. It is these intermediate states that constitute the liquid crystalline phase, or mesophase, as the liquid crystalline phase is called.

The two main types of liquid crystals are termed *smectic* (soap- or grease-like) and *nematic* (thread-like). In the smectic state, molecules are mobile in two directions and can rotate about one axis (Fig. 2–12*a*). In the nematic state, the molecules again rotate only about one axis but are mobile in three dimensions (Fig.

2–12*b*). A third type (cholesteric crystals) exist but may be considered as a special case of the nematic type.

The smectic mesophase is probably of most pharmaceutical significance since it is this phase that usually forms in ternary (or more complex) mixtures containing a surfactant, water, and a weakly amphiphilic or nonpolar additive (see Chapter 18).

In general, molecules that form mesophases (1) are organic, (2) are elongated and rectilinear in shape, (3) are rigid, and (4) possess strong dipoles and easily polarizable groups. The liquid crystalline state may result either from the heating of solids (thermotropic liquid crystals) or from the action of certain solvents on solids (lyotropic liquid crystals). The first recorded observation of a thermotropic liquid crystal was made by Reinitzer in 1888 when he heated cholesteryl benzoate. At 145° C, the solid formed a turbid liquid (the thermotropic liquid crystal), which only became clear, to give the conventional liquid state, at 179° C.

Properties and Significance of Liquid Crystals. Because of their intermediate nature, liquid crystals have some of the properties of liquids and some of solids. For example, liquid crystals are mobile and thus can be considered to have the flow properties of liquids. At the same time they possess the property of being birefringent, a property associated with crystals. In birefringence, the light passing through a material is divided into two components with different velocities and hence different refractive indices.

Some liquid crystals show consistent color changes with temperature, and this characteristic has resulted in their being used to detect areas of elevated temperature under the skin that may be due to a disease process. Nematic liquid crystals are sensitive to electric fields, a property used to advantage in developing display systems. The smectic mesophase has applica-

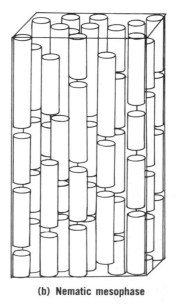

(a) Smectic mesophase

(b) Nematic mesophase

Fig. 2–12. Liquid crystalline state. *(a)* Smectic structure; *(b)* nematic structure.

tion in the solubilization of water-insoluble materials. It also appears that liquid crystalline phases of this type are frequently present in emulsions and may be responsible for enhanced physical stability owing to their highly viscous nature.

The liquid crystalline state is widespread in nature, with lipoidal forms found in nerves, brain tissue, and blood vessels. Atherosclerosis may be related to the laying down of lipid in the liquid crystalline state on the walls of blood vessels. The three components of bile (cholesterol, a bile acid salt, and water), in the correct proportions, can form a smectic mesophase, and this may be involved in the formation of gallstones. Bogardus[28] applied the principle of liquid crystal formation to the solubilization and dissolution of cholesterol, the major constituent of gallstones. Cholesterol is converted to a liquid crystalline phase in the presence of sodium oleate and water, and the cholesterol rapidly dissolves from the surface of the gallstones.

Nonaqueous liquid crystals may be formed from triethanolamine (TEA) and oleic acid with a series of polyethylene glycols or various organic acids such as isopropyl myristate, squalane, squalene, and naphthenic oil as the solvents to replace the water of aqueous mesomorphs. Triangular plots (pp. 43, 45, 46) were used by Friberg et al.[29] to show the regions of the liquid crystalline phase when either polar (polyethylene glycols) or nonpolar (squalene, etc.) compounds were present as the solvent.

Ibrahim[30] studied the release of salicylic acid as a model drug from lyotropic liquid crystalline systems across lipoidal barriers and into an aqueous buffered solution.

Finally, liquid crystals have structures that are believed to be similar to those in cell membranes. As such, liquid crystals may function as useful biophysical models for the structure and functionality of cell membranes.

Friberg has written a monograph on liquid crystals.[29] For a more detailed discussion of the liquid crystalline state, refer to the review by Brown,[31] which serves as a convenient entry into the literature.

PHASE EQUILIBRIA AND THE PHASE RULE

The Phase Rule. J. Willard Gibbs is credited with formulating the *Phase Rule*, a useful device for relating the effect of the least number of independent variables (e.g., temperature, pressure, and concentration) upon the various phases (solid, liquid, and gaseous) that can exist in an equilibrium system containing a given number of components. The phase rule is expressed as follows:

$$\mathbf{F} = C - P + 2 \qquad (2\text{--}18)$$

in which **F** is the number of degrees of freedom in the system, C the number of components, and P the number of phases present.

Looking at these terms in more detail, we may define a *phase* as a homogeneous, physically distinct portion of a system that is separated from other portions of the system by bounding surfaces. Thus, a system containing water and its vapor is a two-phase system. An equilibrium mixture of ice, liquid water, and water vapor is a three-phase system.

The *number of components* is the smallest number of constituents by which the composition of each phase in the system at equilibrium can be expressed in the form of a chemical formula or equation. The number of components in the equilibrium mixture of ice, liquid water, and water vapor is one, since the composition of all three phases is described by the chemical formula H_2O. In the three-phase system, $CaCO_3 = CaO + CO_2$, the composition of each phase can be expressed by a combination of any two of the chemical species present. For example, if we choose to use $CaCO_3$ and CO_2, we can write CaO as ($CaCO_3 - CO_2$). Accordingly, the number of components in this system is two.

The *number of degrees of freedom* is the *least* number of intensive variables (temperature, pressure, concentration, refractive index, density, viscosity, etc.) that must be fixed to describe the system completely. Herein lies the utility of the phase rule. Although a large number of intensive properties are associated with any system, it is not necessary to report all of these to define the system. For example, let us consider a given mass of a gas, say, water vapor, confined to a particular volume. Even though this volume is known, it would not be possible for one to duplicate this system exactly (except by pure chance) unless the temperature, pressure, or another variable is known that may be varied independently of the volume of the gas. Similarly, if the temperature of the gas is defined, it is necessary to know the volume, pressure, or some other variable to define the system completely. Since we need to know two of the variables to define the gaseous system completely, we say that the system has two degrees of freedom. This is confirmed by the phase rule since, in this instance, $\mathbf{F} = 1 - 1 + 2 = 2$.

Next consider a system comprising a liquid, say water, in equilibrium with its vapor. By stating the temperature, the system is completely defined because the pressure under which liquid and vapor can coexist is also defined. If we decide to work instead at a particular pressure, then the temperature of the system is automatically defined. Again, this agrees with the phase rule because equation (2–18) is now $\mathbf{F} = 1 - 2 + 2 = 1$.

As a third example, suppose we cool liquid water and its vapor until a third phase (ice) separates out. Under these conditions the state of the three-phase ice–water–vapor system is completely defined, and the rule is $\mathbf{F} = 1 - 3 + 2 = 0$; in other words, there are no degrees of freedom. If we attempt to vary the particu-

TABLE 2–7. *Application of the Phase Rule to Single-Component Systems*

System	Number of Phases	Degrees of Freedom	Comments
Gas, liquid, or solid	1	$F = C - P + 2$ $= 1 - 1 + 2 = 2$	System is *bivariant* ($F = 2$) and lies anywhere within the *area* marked vapor, liquid, or solid in Figure 2–13. We must fix two variables, e.g., p_2 and t_2, to define system *D*.
Gas–liquid, liquid–solid, or gas–solid	2	$F = C - P + 2$ $= 1 - 2 + 2 = 1$	System is *univariant* ($F = 1$) and lies anywhere along a *line* between two phase regions, i.e., *AO, BO,* or *CO* in Figure 2–13. We must fix one variable, e.g., either p_1 or t_2, to define system *E*.
Gas–liquid–solid	3	$F = C - P + 2$ $= 1 - 3 + 2 = 0$	System is *invariant* ($F = 0$) and can lie only at the *point* of intersection of the lines bounding the three phase regions, i.e., point *O* in Figure 2–13.

lar conditions of temperature or pressure necessary to maintain this system, we will lose a phase. Thus, if we wish to prepare the three-phase system of ice–water–vapor, we have no choice as to the temperature or pressure at which we will work; the combination is fixed and unique.

The relation between the number of phases and the degrees of freedom in one-component systems is summarized in Table 2–7. The student should confirm this data by reference to Figure 2–13, which shows the phase equilibria of water at moderate pressures.

The student should appreciate that as the number of components increases, so do the degrees of freedom. Consequently, as the system becomes more complex, it becomes necessary to fix more variables to define the system. The greater the number of phases in equilibrium, however, the fewer the degrees of freedom. Thus:

liquid water + vapor

$$F = C - P + 2$$
$$= 1 - 2 + 2$$
$$= 1$$

liquid ethyl alcohol + vapor

$$F = C - P + 2$$
$$= 1 - 2 + 2$$
$$= 1$$

liquid water + liquid ethyl alcohol + vapor mixture

$$F = C - P + 2$$
$$= 2 - 2 + 2$$
$$= 2$$

(*Note:* Ethyl alcohol and water are completely miscible both as vapors and liquids.)

liquid water + liquid benzyl alcohol + vapor mixture

$$F = C - P + 2$$
$$= 2 - 3 + 2$$
$$= 1$$

(*Note:* Benzyl alcohol and water form two separate liquid phases and one vapor phase. Gases are miscible in all proportions; water and benzyl alcohol are only partially miscible. It is therefore necessary to define the two variables in the completely miscible [one-phase] ethyl alcohol–water system, but only one variable in the partially miscible [two-phase] benzyl alcohol–water system.)

Systems Containing One Component. We have already considered a system containing one component, namely, that for water, which is illustrated in Figure 2–13 (not drawn to scale).

The curve *OA* in Figure 2–13 is known as the *vapor pressure curve*. Its upper limit is at the critical temperature, 374° C for water, and its lower end terminates at 0.0098° C, called the *triple point*. Along the vapor pressure curve, vapor and liquid coexist in equilibrium. This curve is identical with the curve for water seen in Figure 2–3. Curve *OC* is the sublimation curve, and here vapor and solid exist together in equilibrium. Curve *OB* is the melting point curve, at which liquid and solid are in equilibrium. The negative slope of *OB* shows that the freezing point of water decreases with increasing external pressure, as we have already found in *Example 2–8*.

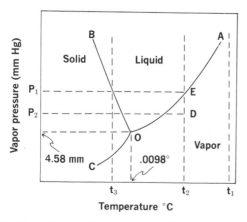

Fig. 2–13. Phase diagram for water at moderate pressures.

The result of changes in pressure (at fixed temperature) or changes in temperature (at fixed pressure) becomes evident by referring to the phase diagram. If the temperature is held constant at t_1, where water is in the gaseous state above the critical temperature, no matter how much the pressure is raised (vertically along the dotted line), the system remains as a gas. At a temperature t_2 below the critical temperature, water vapor is converted into liquid water by an increase of pressure, since the compression brings the molecules within the range of the attractive van der Waals forces. It is interesting to observe that at a temperature below the triple point, say t_3, an increase of pressure on water in the vapor state converts the vapor first to ice and then at higher pressure into liquid water. This sequence, vapor → ice → liquid, is due to the fact that ice occupies a larger volume than liquid water below the triple point. At the triple point, the three phases are in equilibrium, that is, they all have the same vapor pressure at this temperature of 0.0098° C.

As was seen in Table 2–7, in any one of the three regions in which pure solid, liquid, or vapor exists, and $P = 1$, the phase rule becomes

$$\mathbf{F} = 1 - 1 + 2 = 2$$

Therefore we must fix two conditions, namely temperature and pressure, to specify or describe the system completely. This statement means that if one were to record the results of a scientific experiment involving a given quantity of water, it would not be sufficient to state that the water was kept at, say, 76° C. The pressure would also have to be specified to define the system completely. If the system were open to the atmosphere, the atmospheric pressure obtained at the time of the experiment would be recorded. Conversely, it would not be sufficient to state that liquid water was present at a certain pressure without also stating the temperature. The phase rule tells us that the experimenter may alter two conditions without causing the appearance or disappearance of the liquid phase. Hence, we say that liquid water exhibits two degrees of freedom.

Along any three of the lines, where two phases exist in equilibrium, $\mathbf{F} = 1$ (see Table 2–7). Hence, only one condition need be given to define the system. If we state that the system contains both liquid water and water vapor in equilibrium at 100° C, we need not specify the pressure, for the vapor pressure can have no other value than 760 mm Hg at 100° C under these conditions. Similarly, only one variable is required to define the system along line OB or OC.

Finally, at the triple point where the three phases—ice, liquid water, and water vapor—are in equilibrium, we have seen that $\mathbf{F} = 0$.

As already noted, the triple point for air-free water is 0.0098° C; whereas the freezing point (i.e., the point at which liquid water saturated with air is in equilibrium with ice at a total pressure of 1 atm) is 0° C. In increasing the pressure from 4.58 mm to 1 atm, the freezing point is lowered by about 0.0075° (*Example 2–8*). The freezing point is then lowered an additional 0.0023° by the presence of dissolved air in water at 1 atm. Hence, the normal freezing point of water is 0.0075° + 0.0023° = 0.0098° below the triple point. In summary, the temperature at which a solid melts depends on the pressure. If the pressure is that of the liquid and solid in equilibrium with the vapor, the temperature is known as the triple point; whereas if the pressure is 1 atm, the temperature is the normal freezing point.

Condensed Systems. We have seen from the phase rule that in a single-component system, the maximum number of degrees of freedom is two. This situation arises when only one phase is present, that is, $\mathbf{F} = 1 - 1 + 2 = 2$. As will become apparent in the next section, a maximum of three degrees of freedom is possible in a two-component system, for example, temperature, pressure, and concentration. To represent the effect of all these variables upon the phase equilibria of such a system, it would be necessary to use a three-dimensional model rather than the planar figure used in the case of water. Since, in practice, we are only concerned with liquid and/or solid phases in the particular system under examination, we frequently choose to disregard the vapor phase and work under normal conditions of 1 atm pressure. In this manner, we reduce the number of degrees of freedom by one. In a two-component system, therefore, only two variables (temperature and concentration) remain, and we are able to portray the interaction of these variables by the use of planar figures on rectangular coordinate graph paper. Systems in which the vapor phase is ignored and only solid and/or liquid phases are considered are termed *condensed systems*. We shall see in the later discussion of three-component systems that it is again more convenient to work with condensed systems.

Two-Component Systems Containing Liquid Phases. We know from experience that ethyl alcohol and water are miscible in all proportions, whereas water and mercury are, for all practical purposes, completely immiscible regardless of the relative amounts of each present. Between these two extremes lies a whole range of systems that exhibit partial miscibility (or immiscibility). Such a system is phenol and water, and a portion of the condensed phase diagram is plotted in Figure 2–14. The curve *gbhci* shows the limits of temperature and concentration within which two liquid phases exist in equilibrium. The region outside this curve contains systems having but one liquid phase. Starting at the point *a*, equivalent to a system containing 100% water (i.e., pure water) at 50° C, the addition of known increments of phenol to a fixed weight of water, the whole being maintained at 50° C, will result in the formation of a single liquid phase until the point *b* is reached, at which a minute amount of a second phase appears. The concentration of phenol and water at

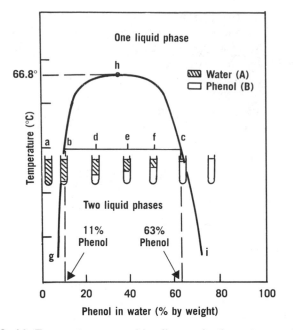

Fig. 2–14. Temperature-composition diagram for the system consisting of water and phenol. (From A. N. Campbell and A. J. R. Campbell, J. Am. Chem. Soc. 59, 2481, 1937).

which this occurs is 11% by weight of phenol in water. Analysis of the second phase, which separates out on the bottom, shows it to contain 63% by weight of phenol in water. This phenol-rich phase is denoted by the point c on the phase diagram. As we prepare mixtures containing increasing quantities of phenol, that is, as we proceed across the diagram from point b to point c, we form systems in which the amount of the phenol-rich phase (B) continually increases, as denoted by the test tubes drawn in Figure 2–14. At the same time, the amount of the water-rich phase (A) decreases. Once the total concentration of phenol exceeds 63%, at 50°, a single phenol-rich liquid phase is formed.

The maximum temperature at which the two-phase region exists is termed the *critical solution,* or *upper consolute, temperature.* In the case of the phenol–water system, this is 66.8° (point h in Fig. 2–14). All combinations of phenol and water above this temperature are completely miscible and yield one-phase liquid systems.

The line bc drawn across the region containing two phases is termed a *tie line;* it is always parallel to the base line in two-component systems. An important feature of phase diagrams is that all systems prepared on a tie line, at equilibrium, will separate into phases of constant composition. These phases are termed *conjugate phases.* For example, any system represented by a point on the line bc, at 50° C, separates to give a pair of conjugate phases whose composition is b and c. The *relative amounts* of the two layers or phases vary, however, as seen in Figure 2–14. Thus, if we prepare a system containing 24% by weight of phenol and 76% by weight of water (point d), at equilibrium we have two liquid phases present in the tube. The upper one, A, has

a composition of 11% phenol in water (point b on the diagram) while the lower layer, B, contains 63% phenol (point c on the diagram). Phase B will lie below phase A since it is rich in phenol and phenol has a higher density than water. In terms of the relative weights of the two phases, there will be more of the water-rich phase A then the phenol-rich phase B at point d. Thus:

$$\frac{\text{weight of phase } A}{\text{weight of phase } B} = \frac{\text{length } dc}{\text{length } bd}$$

The right-hand term might appear at first glance to be the reciprocal of the proportion one should write. The weight of phase A is greater than phase B, however, because point d is closer to point b than it is to point c. The lengths dc and bd can be measured with a ruler in centimeters or inches from the phase diagram, but it is frequently more convenient to use the units of percent weight of phenol as found on the abscissa of Figure 2–14. For example, since point $b = 11\%$, point $c = 63\%$, and point $d = 24\%$, the ratio $dc/bd = (63 - 24)/(24 - 11) = 39/13 = 3/1$. In other words, for every 10 g of a liquid system in equilibrium represented by point d, one finds 7.5 g of phase A and 2.5 g of phase B. If, on the other hand, we prepare a system containing 50% by weight of phenol (point f, Fig. 2–14), the ratio of phase A to phase $B = fc/bf = (63 - 50)/(50 - 11) = 13/39 = 1/3$. Accordingly, for every 10 g of system f prepared, we obtain an equilibrium mixture of 2.5 g of phase A and 7.5 g of phase B. It should be apparent that a system containing 37% by weight of phenol will, under equilibrium conditions at 50° C, give equal weights of phase A and phase B.

Working on a tie line in a phase diagram enables us to calculate the *composition* of each phase in addition to the weight of the phases. Thus, it becomes a simple matter to calculate the distribution of phenol (or water) throughout the system as a whole. As an example, let us suppose that we mixed 24 g of phenol with 76 g of water, warmed the mixture to 50°, and allowed it to reach equilibrium at this temperature. On separation of the two phases, we would find 75 g of phase A (containing 11% by weight of phenol) and 25 g of phase B (containing 63% by weight of phenol). Phase A therefore contains a total of $(11 \times 75)/100 = 8.25$ g of phenol, while phase B contains a total of $(63 \times 25)/100 = 15.75$ g of phenol. This gives a sum total of 24 g of phenol in the whole system. This equals the amount of phenol originally added and therefore confirms our assumptions and calculations. It is left to the reader to confirm that phase A contains 66.75 g of water and phase B 9.25 g of water. The phases are shown at b and c in Figure 2–14.

Applying the phase rule to Figure 2–14 shows that with a two-component condensed system having one liquid phase, $\mathbf{F} = 3$. Because the pressure is fixed, $\mathbf{F}$ reduces to 2, and it is necessary to fix both temperature and concentration to define the system. When two liquid phases are present, $\mathbf{F} = 2$; again, pressure is fixed. We need only define temperature to completely define the system, since **F** reduces to 1.* From Figure 2–14, it is seen that if the temperature is given, the compositions of the two phases are fixed by the points at the ends of the tie lines, for example, points *b* and *c* at 50° C. The compositions (relative amounts of phenol and water) of the two liquid layers are then calculated by the method already discussed.

The phase diagram is used in practice to formulate systems containing more than one component where it may be advantageous to achieve a single liquid phase product. For example, the handling of solid phenol, a necrotic agent, is facilitated in the pharmacy if a solution of phenol and water is used. A number of solutions, containing different concentrations of phenol, are official in several pharmacopeias. Unless the freezing point of the phenol–water mixture is sufficiently low, however, some solidification may occur at a low ambient temperature. This will lead to inaccuracies in dispensing as well as a loss of convenience. Mulley[32] determined the relevant portion of the phenol–water phase diagram and suggested that the most convenient formulation of a single liquid phase solution was 80% *w/v*, equivalent to about 76% *w/w*. This mixture has a freezing point of about 3.5° compared with Liquefied Phenol, USP, which contains approximately 90% *w/w* of phenol and freezes at about 17° C. It is not possible, therefore, to use the official preparation much below 20° C, or room temperature; the formulation proposed by Mulley from a consideration of the phenol–water phase diagram therefore is to be preferred. A number of other binary liquid systems of the same type as phenol and water have been studied, although few have practical application in pharmacy. Some of these are water–aniline, carbon disulfide–methyl alcohol, isopentane–phenol, methyl alcohol–cyclohexane, and isobutyl alcohol–water.

Figure 2–15 illustrates a liquid mixture that shows no upper consolute temperature but instead has a *lower* consolute temperature below which the components are miscible in all proportions. The example shown is the triethylamine–water system. Figure 2–16 shows the phase diagram for the nicotine-water system, which has both a lower and an upper consolute temperature. Lower consolute temperatures arise presumably because of that interaction between the components that brings about complete miscibility only at lower temperatures.

Two-Component Systems Containing Solid and Liquid Phases: Eutectic Mixtures: We shall restrict our discussion, in the main, to those solid–liquid mixtures in

which the two components are completely miscible in the liquid state and completely immiscible as solids, that is, the solid phases that form consist of pure components. Examples of such systems are salol–thymol and salol–camphor.

The phase diagram for the salol–thymol system is shown in Figure 2–17. Notice that there are four regions: (*i*) a single liquid phase; (*ii*) a region containing solid salol and a conjugate liquid phase; (*iii*) a region in which solid thymol is in equilibrium with a conjugate liquid phase; and (*iv*) a region in which both components are present as pure solid phases. Those regions containing two phases (*ii*, *iii*, and *iv*) are comparable to the two-phase region of the phenol–water system shown in Figure 2–14. Thus it is possible to calculate both the composition and relative amount of each phase from a knowledge of the tie lines and the phase boundaries.

Suppose we prepare a system containing 60% by weight of thymol in salol and raise the temperature of

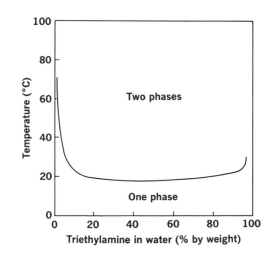

Fig. 2–15. Phase diagram for the system triethylamine–water showing lower consolute temperature.

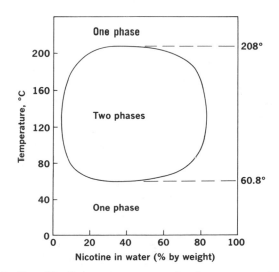

Fig. 2–16. Nicotine–water system showing upper and lower consolute temperatures.

---

*The number of degrees of freedom calculated from the phase rule if the system is not condensed is still the same. Thus, when one liquid phase and its vapor are present, **F** = 2 − 2 + 2 = 2; it is therefore necessary to define two conditions: temperature and concentration. When two liquids and the vapor phase exist, **F** = 2 − 3 + 2 = 1, and only temperature need be defined.

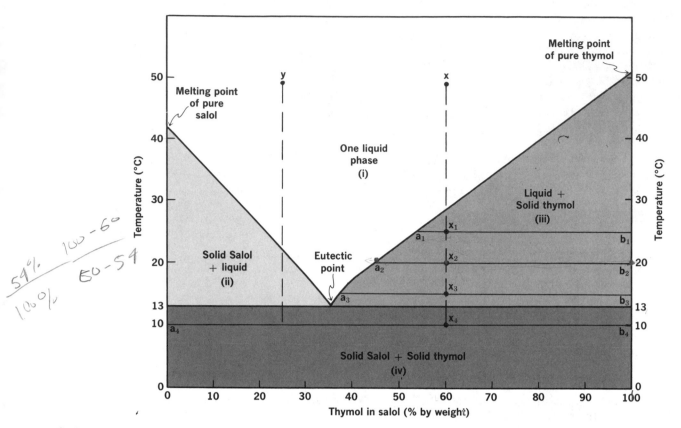

Fig. 2–17. Phase diagram for the thymol–salol system showing the eutectic point. (Data from A. Siedell, *Solubilities of Organic Compounds*, 3rd Ed., Vol. 2, Van Nostrand, New York, 1941, p. 723.)

the mixture to 50° C. Such a system is represented by point x in Figure 2–17. On cooling the system, the following sequence of phase changes is observed. The system remains as a single liquid until the temperature falls to 29° C, at which point a minute amount of solid thymol separates out to form a two-phase solid–liquid system. At 25° C, system x (denoted in Fig. 2–17 as x_1) is composed of a liquid phase, a_1 (composition 53% thymol in salol) and pure solid thymol, b_1. The weight ratio of a_1 to b_1 is $(100 - 60)/(60 - 53) = 40/7$, that is, $a_1:b_1 = 5.71:1$. When the temperature is reduced to 20° C (point x_2), the composition of the liquid phase is a_2 (45% by weight of thymol in salol), while the solid phase is still pure thymol, b_2. The phase ratio, $a_2:b_2 = (100 - 60)/(60 - 45) = 40/15 = 2.67:1$. At 15° C (point x_3), the composition of the liquid phase is now 37% thymol in salol (a_3) and the weight ratio of liquid phase to pure solid thymol ($a_3:b_3$) is $(100 - 60)/(60 - 37) - 40/23 = 1.74:1$. Below 13° C, the liquid phase disappears altogether and the system contains two solid phases of pure salol and pure thymol. Thus, at 10° C (point x_4), the system contains an equilibrium mixture of pure solid salol (a_4) and pure solid thymol (b_4) in a weight ratio of $(100 - 60)/(60 - 0) = 40/60 = 0.67:1$. As system x is progressively cooled, the results indicate that more and more of the thymol separates as solid.

A similar sequence of phase changes is observed if system y is cooled in a like manner. In this case,

however, the solid phase that separates at 22° C is pure salol.

The lowest temperature at which a liquid phase can exist in the salol–thymol system is 13° C, and this occurs in a mixture containing 34% thymol in salol. This point on the phase diagram is known as the *eutectic point*. At the eutectic point, three phases (liquid, solid salol, and solid thymol) coexist. The eutectic point therefore denotes an invariant system for, in a condensed system, $F = 2 - 3 + 1 = 0$.

Mixtures of salol and camphor show similar behavior. In this combination, the eutectic point occurs with a system containing 56% by weight of salol in camphor at a temperature of 6° C. Several other substances form eutectic mixtures (e.g., camphor, chloral hydrate, menthol, and betanaphthol).

Lidocaine and prilocaine, two local anesthetic agents, form a 1:1 mixture having a eutectic temperature of 18° C. The mixture is therefore liquid at room temperature and forms a mixed local anesthetic that may be used for topical application. Further work showed that the liquid eutectic can be emulsified in water, opening the possibility for topical bioabsorption of the two local anesthetics[33,34] (see Chapter 18, pp. 505–506).

Solid Dispersions. Eutectic systems are one example of solid dispersions. The solid phases constituting the eutectic each contain only one component and the system may be regarded as an intimate crystalline *mixture* of one component in the other. A second major group of solid dispersions is the *solid solution*, in which each solid phase contains both components, that is, a solid solute is *dissolved* in a solid solvent to give a mixed crystal.

There is widespread interest in solid dispersions since they offer a means of facilitating the dissolution, and frequently, therefore, the bioavailability, of poorly soluble drugs when combined with freely soluble "carriers" such as urea. This increase in dissolution rate is achieved by a combination of effects, the most significant of which is reduction of particle size to an extent that cannot be readily achieved by conventional comminution approaches. Other contributing factors include increased wettability of the material, reduced aggregation and agglomeration, and a likely increase in solubility of the drug owing to the presence of the water-soluble carrier. Consult reviews by Chiou and Riegelman[35] and Goldberg[36] for further details. Refer also to Chapter 19 for a discussion of newer solid dosage forms and devices.

Phase Equilibria in Three-Component Systems. In systems containing three components but only one phase, $F = 3 - 1 + 2 = 4$ for a noncondensed system. The four degrees of freedom are temperature, pressure, and the concentrations of two of the three components. Only two concentration terms are required because the sum of these subtracted from the total will give the concentration of the third component. If we regard the system as condensed and hold the temperature constant, then $F = 2$, and we can again use a planar diagram to illustrate the phase equilibria. Since we are dealing with a three-component system, it is more convenient

to use triangular coordinate graph paper, although it is possible to use rectangular coordinates.

The various phase equilibria that exist in three-component systems containing liquid and/or solid phases are frequently complex and beyond the scope of the present text. Certain typical three-component systems will be discussed here, however, because they are of pharmaceutical interest.

Rules Relating to Triangular Diagrams. Before discussing phase equilibria in ternary systems, it is essential that the reader become familiar with certain "rules" that relate to the use of triangular coordinates. It should have been apparent in discussing two-component systems that all concentrations were expressed on a weight-weight basis. This is because, while being an easy and direct method of preparing dispersions, such an approach also allows the concentration to be expressed as mole fraction or molality. The concentrations in ternary systems are accordingly expressed on a weight basis. The following statements should be studied in conjunction with Figure 2–18.

1. Each of the three corners or apexes of the triangle represent 100% by weight of one component (A, B, or C). As a result, that same apex will represent 0% of the other two components. For example, the top corner point in Figure 2–18 represents 100% of B.

2. The three lines joining the corner points represent two-component mixtures of the three possible combinations of A, B, and C. Thus the lines AB, BC, and CA are used for two-component mixtures of A and B, B and C, and C and A, respectively. By dividing each line into 100 equal units, the location of a point along the line can be directly related to the percent concentration of one

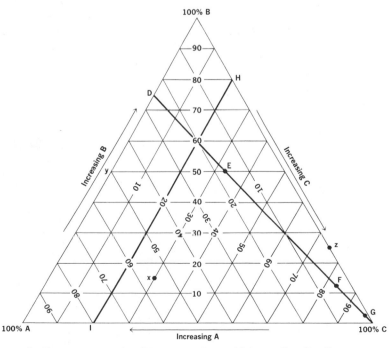

Fig. 2–18. The triangular diagram for three-component systems: preparing and interpreting the diagram.

component in a two-component system. For example, point *y*, midway between *A* and *B* on the line *AB*, represents a system containing 50% of *B* (and hence 50% of *A* also). Point *z*, three quarters of the way along *BC*, signifies a system containing 75% of *C* in *B*.

In going along a line bounding the triangle so as to represent the concentration in a two-component system, it does not matter whether we proceed in a clockwise or counterclockwise direction around the triangle, provided we are consistent. The more usual convention is clockwise and has been adopted here. Hence, as we move along *AB* in the direction of *B*, we are signifying systems of *A* and *B* containing increasing concentrations of *B*, and correspondingly smaller amounts of *A*. Moving along *BC* towards *C* will represent systems of *B* and *C* containing more and more of *C*; the closer we approach *A* on the line *CA*, the greater will be the concentration of *A* in systems of *A* and *C*.

3. The area within the triangle represents all the possible combinations of *A*, *B*, and *C* to give three-component systems. The location of a particular three-component system within the triangle, for example, point *x*, may be undertaken as follows.

The line *AC*; opposite apex *B*, represents systems containing *A* and *C*. *B* is absent, that is, *B* = 0. The horizontal lines running across the triangle parallel to *AC* denote increasing percentages of *B* from *B* = 0 (on line *AC*) to *B* = 100 (at point *B*). The line parallel to *AC* that cuts point *x* is equivalent to 15% *B*; consequently, the system contains 15% of *B* and 85% of *A* and *C* together. Applying similar arguments to the other two components in the system, we can say that along the line *AB*, *C* = 0. As we proceed from the line *AB* towards *C* across the diagram, the concentration of *C* increases until at the apex, *C* = 100%. The point *x* lies on the line parallel to *AB* that is equivalent to 30% of *C*. It follows, therefore, that the concentration of *A* is 100 − (*B* + *C*) = 100 − (15 + 30) = 55%. This is readily confirmed by proceeding across the diagram from the line *BC* toward apex *A*; point *x* lies on the line equivalent to 55% of *A*.

4. If a line is drawn through any apex to a point on the opposite side (e.g., line *DC* in Fig. 2–18), then all

systems represented by points on such a line have a constant ratio of two components, in this case *A* and *B*. Furthermore, the continual addition of *C* to a mixture of *A* and *B* will produce systems that lie progressively closer to apex *C* (100% of component *C*). This effect is illustrated in Table 2–8, in which increasing weights of *C* have been added to a constant-weight mixture of *A* and *B*. Note that in all three systems, the ratio of *A* to *B* is constant and identical to that existing in the original mixture.

5. Any line drawn parallel to one side of the triangle, for example, line *HI* in Figure 2–18, represents ternary systems in which the proportion (or percent by weight) of *one* component is constant. In this instance, all systems prepared along *HI* will contain 20% of *C* and varying concentrations of *A* and *B*.

Ternary Systems with One Pair of Partially Miscible Liquids. Water and benzene are miscible only to a slight extent, and so a mixture of the two usually produces a two-phase system. The heavier of the two phases consists of water saturated with benzene, while the lighter phase is benzene saturated with water. On the other hand, alcohol is completely miscible with both benzene and water. It is to be expected, therefore, that the addition of sufficient alcohol to a two-phase system of benzene and water would produce a single liquid phase in which all three components are miscible. This situation is illustrated in Figure 2–19, which depicts such a ternary system. It might be helpful for the student to consider the alcohol as acting in a manner comparable to that of temperature in the binary phenol–water system considered earlier. Raising the temperature of the phenol–water system led to complete miscibility of the two conjugate phases and the formation of one liquid phase. The addition of alcohol to the benzene–water system achieves the same end but by different means, namely, a solvent effect in place of a temperature effect. There is a strong similarity between the use of heat to break cohesive forces between molecules and the use of solvents to achieve the same result.

In Figure 2–19, let us suppose that *A*, *B*, and *C* represent water, alcohol, and benzene, respectively. The line *AC* therefore depicts binary mixtures of *A* and

TABLE 2–8. *Effect of Adding a Third Component (C) to a Binary System Containing A (5.0 g) and B (15.0 g)*

| Weight of Third Component C Added (g) | Final System | | | Ratio of A to B | Location of System in Figure 2–18 |
	Component	Weight (g)	Weight (%)		
10.0	A	5.0	16.67	3:1	point *E*
	B	15.0	50.00		
	C	10.0	33.33		
100.0	A	5.0	4.17	3:1	point *F*
	B	15.0	12.50		
	C	100.0	83.33		
1000.0	A	5.0	0.49	3:1	point *G*
	B	15.0	1.47		
	C	1000.0	98.04		

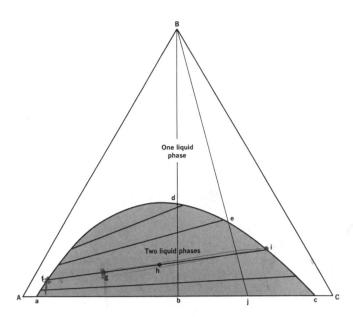

Fig. 2–19. A system of three liquids, one pair of which is partially miscible.

C, while the points *a* and *c* are the limits of solubility of *C* in *A* and *A* in *C*, respectively, at the particular temperature being used. The curve *afdeic*, frequently termed a *binodal curve* or *binodal*, marks the extent of the two-phase region. The remainder of the triangle contains one liquid phase. The tie lines within the binodal are not necessarily parallel to one another or to the base line, *AC*, as was the case in the two-phase region of binary systems. In fact, the directions of the tie lines are related to the shape of the binodal, which in turn depends on the relative solubility of the third component (in this case, alcohol) in the other two components. Only when the added component acts equally on the other two components to bring them into solution will the binodal be perfectly symmetric and the tie lines run parallel to the base line.

The properties of tie lines discussed earlier still apply, and systems *g* and *h* prepared along the tie line *fi* both give rise to two phases having the compositions denoted by the points *f* and *i*. The relative amounts, by weight, of the two conjugate phases will depend on the position of the original system along the tie line. For example, system *g*, after reaching equilibrium, will separate into two phases, *f* and *i*: the ratio of phase *f* to phase *i*, on a weight basis, is given by the ratio *gi:fg*. Mixture *h*, half way along the tie line, will contain equal weights of the two phases at equilibrium.

The phase equilibria depicted in Figure 2–19 shows that the addition of component *B* to a 50:50 mixture of components *A* and *C* will produce a phase change from a two-liquid system to a one-liquid system at point *d*. With a 25:75 mixture of *A* and *C*, shown as point *j*, the addition of *B* leads to a phase change at point *e*. Naturally, all mixtures lying along *dB* and *eB* will be one-phase systems.

As we saw earlier, $F = 2$ in a single-phase region, and so we must define two concentrations to fix the particular system. Within the binodal curve, *afdeic*, $F = 1$ and we need only know one concentration term, since this will allow the composition of one phase to be fixed on the binodal curve. From the tie line, we can then obtain the composition of the conjugate phase.

Effect of Temperature. Figure 2–19 shows the phase equilibria in a three-component system under isothermal conditions. Changes in temperature will cause the area of immiscibility, bounded by the binodal curve, to change. In general, the area of the binodal decreases as the temperature is raised and miscibility is promoted. Eventually, a point is reached at which complete miscibility is obtained and the binodal vanishes. To study the effect of temperature on the phase equilibria of three-component systems, a three-dimensional figure, the triangular prism, is frequently used (Fig. 2–20b). Alternatively, a family of curves representing

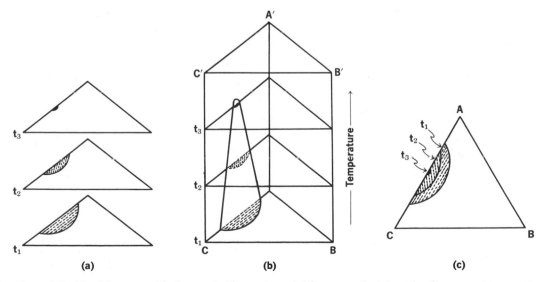

Fig. 2–20. Alterations of the binodal curves with changes in temperature. *(a)* Curves on the triangular diagrams at temperatures t_1, t_2, and t_3. In *(b)* is depicted the three-dimensional arrangement of the diagrams in the order of increasing temperature. The sketch in *(c)* represents the view one would obtain by looking down from the top of *(b)*.

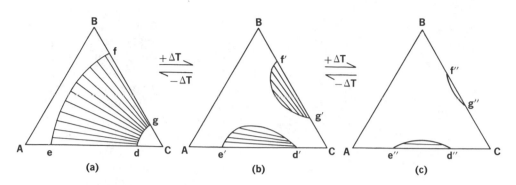

Fig. 2–21. Effect of temperature changes on the binodal curves representing a system of two pairs of partially miscible liquids.

the various temperatures may be used, as shown in Figure 2–20c. The three planar sides of the prism are simply three-phase diagrams of binary-component systems. Figure 2–20 illustrates the case of a ternary-component system containing one pair of partially immiscible liquids (A and C). As the temperature is raised, the region of immiscibility decreases. The volume outside the shaded region of the prism consists of a single, homogeneous, liquid phase.

Ternary Systems with Two or Three Pairs of Partially Miscible Liquids. All the previous considerations for ternary systems containing one pair of partially immiscible liquids still apply. With two pairs of partially miscible liquids, there are two binodal curves. The situation is shown in Figure 2–21b, in which A and C as well as B and C show partial miscibility; A and B are completely miscible at the temperature used. Increasing the temperature generally leads to a reduction in the areas of the two binodal curves and their eventual disappearance (Fig. 2–21c). Reduction of the temperature expands the binodal curves, and, at a sufficiently low temperature, they meet and fuse to form a single band of immiscibility as shown in Figure 2–21a. Tie lines stilll exist in this region, and the usual rules apply. Nor do the number of degrees of freedom change—when P = 1, **F** = 2; when P = 2, **F** = 1.

Systems containing three pairs of partially miscible liquids are of interest. Should the three binodal curves meet (Fig. 2–22a), a central region appears in which *three* conjugate liquid phases exist in equilibrium. In this region, D, which is triangular, **F** = 0 for a condensed system under isothermal conditions. As a

result, *all* systems lying within this region consist of three phases whose compositions are always given by the points x, y, and z. The only quantity that varies is the relative amounts of these three conjugate phases. Increasing the temperature alters the shapes and sizes of the regions, as seen in Fig. 2–22b and 2–22c.

We shall meet phase diagrams in later chapters (Chapters 10 and 15) in which their application in certain pharmaceutical systems will be discussed.

THERMAL ANALYSIS

As noted earlier in this chapter, a number of physical and chemical effects can be produced by temperature changes, and methods for characterizing these alterations upon heating or cooling a sample of the material are referred to as *thermal analysis*. The most common types of thermal analysis are differential scanning calorimetry (DSC), differential thermal analysis (DTA), thermogravimetric analysis (TGA), and thermomechanical analysis (TMA). These methods have proved valuable in pharmaceutical research and quality control for the characterization and identification of compounds, determination of purity, polymorphism[19,20] solvent and moisture content, stability, and compatibility with excipients.

In general, thermal methods involve heating a sample under controlled conditions and observing the physical and chemical changes that occur. These methods measure a number of different properties, such as melting point, heat capacity, heats of reaction, kinetics

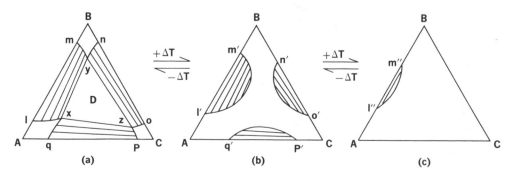

Fig. 2–22. Temperature effects on a system of three pairs of partially miscible liquids.

of decomposition, and changes in the flow (rheologic) properties of biochemical, pharmaceutical, and agricultural materials and food. The methods are briefly described, with examples of applications. Differential thermal analysis has been used more frequently in the past than DSC principally because the DTA instrument appeared earlier on the market and is less expensive. Differential scanning calorimetry is more useful in the research laboratory because its measurements can be related more directly to thermodynamic properties. It appears that any analysis which can be carried out with DTA can be done with DSC, the latter being the more versatile technique. `

Differential Scanning Calorimetry. In differential scanning calorimetry (DSC), a sample and reference material are placed in separate pans and the temperature of each pan is increased or decreased at a predetermined rate. When the sample (e.g., benzoic acid) reaches its melting point, 122.4° C, it remains at this temperature until all the material has passed into the liquid state, because of the endothermic process of melting. A

temperature difference therefore exists between benzoic acid and a reference, indium (mp = 156.6° C), as the temperature of the two materials is raised gradually through the range 122° to 123° C. A second temperature circuit is used in DSC to provide a heat input to overcome this temperature difference. In this way the temperature of the sample, benzoic acid, is maintained at the same value as the reference, indium. The difference is heat input to the sample, and the reference per unit time is fed to a recorder and plotted as dH/dt versus the average temperature to which the sample and reference are being raised. The differential heat input is recorded with a sensitivity of $\pm$ 0.1 millicalories per second, and the temperature range over which the instrument operates is $-175°$ to 725° C. The data collected in a DSC run for a compound such as benzoic acid are shown in the thermogram in Figure 2–23. The DSC-3 instrument is depicted schematically in Figure 2–24. The panel with its controls and temperature readout are shown, together with dials for preset temperature and rates of temperature change. The unit

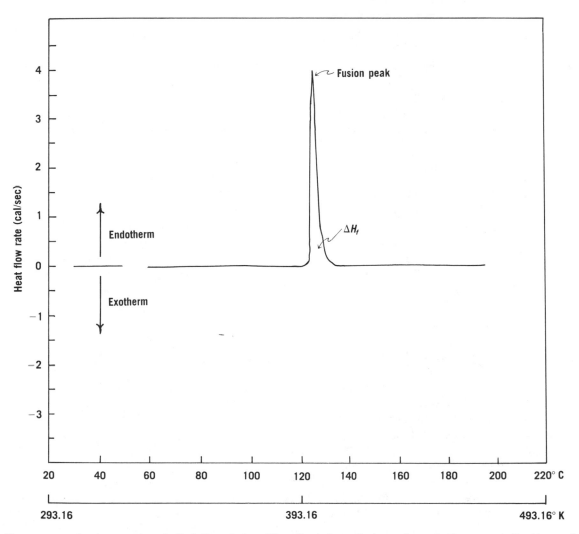

Fig. 2–23. Thermogram of a drug compound. Endothermic transitions (heat absorption) are shown in the upward direction, and exothermic transitions (heat loss) are plotted downward. Melting is an endothermic process, whereas crystallization or freezing is an exothermic process. The area of the melting peak is proportional to the heat of fusion, ΔH_f.

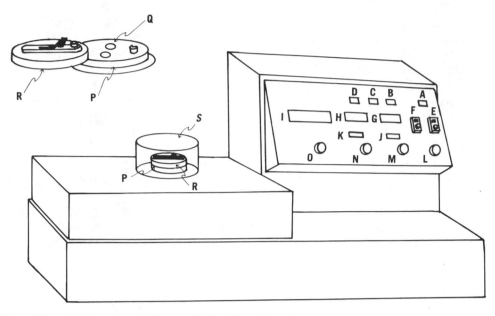

Fig. 2–24. Perkin Elmer differential scanning calorimeter, DSC-3. The dials and windows on the console at the right are used to program the increasing and decreasing temperature at definite rates and to set the baseline of the thermogram, which is plotted on an X–Y recorder. The left section of the instrument is the heating unit, with two sample holders, Q, in the heating block P. The sample cover R is closed and the heating unit is covered by a draft shield, S, during a run.

on the left provides uniform heating and cooling and contains the sample and reference in appropriate pans in the sample enclosure. A thermogravimetric analyzer (TGA) and a thermomechanical analyzer (TMA) may be added to the basic instrument. A data station may also be added to process the thermal data. The DSC-4 is slightly different in appearance from the DSC-3 shown in Figure 2–24.

Although DSC is used most widely in pharmacy to establish identity and purity, it may be used to obtain heat capacities and heats of fusion, referred to in Chapters 3 and 10. It is also useful for preparing phase diagrams to study the polymorphs discussed in this chapter, and for carrying out the kinetics of decomposition of solids (Chapter 12). Differential scanning calorimetry, as well as other thermal analytic methods, has a number of applications in biomedical research and food technology. Guillory and associates[37] have explored the applications of thermal analysis, DSC and DTA in particular, in conjunction with infrared spectroscopy and x-ray diffraction. Using these techniques, they have characterized various solid forms of drugs, such as sulfonamides, and have correlated a number of physical properties of crystalline materials with interactions between solids, dissolution rates, and stabilities in the crystalline and amorphous states.

Differential scanning calorimetry has found increasing use in standardization of the lyophilization process.[38] Crystal changes and eutectic formation in the frozen state can be detected by DSC (and by DTA) when the instruments are operated below room temperature.

For additional references to the use of DSC in research and technology, contact the manufacturers of differential thermal equipment for complete bibliographies.[39]

Differential Thermal Analysis. In differential thermal analysis (DTA), both sample and reference material are heated by a common heat source (Fig. 2–25) rather than the individual heaters used in DSC (Fig. 2–26). Thermocouples are placed in contact with the sample and reference in DTA to monitor the difference in temperature between the sample and reference as they are heated at a constant rate. The temperature difference between sample and reference is plotted against time, and the endotherm as melting occurs (or exotherm as obtained during some decomposition reactions) is represented by a peak in the thermogram.

Although DTA is a useful tool, a number of factors may affect the results. The temperature difference, ΔT, depends, among other factors, on the resistance to heat flow, R. R in turn depends on temperature, nature of the sample, and packing of the material in the pans. Therefore, it is not possible to directly calculate

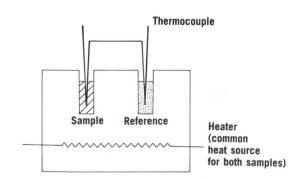

Fig. 2–25. Common heat source of DTA with thermocouples in contact with the sample and reference material.

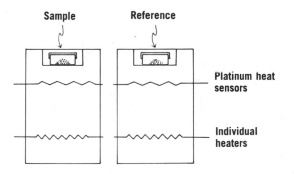

Sample **Reference**

Platinum heat sensors

Individual heaters

Fig. 2–26. Separate heat sources and platinum heat sensors used in DSC.

energies of melting, sublimation, and decomposition, and DTA is used as a qualitative or semiquantitative method for calorimetric measurements. The DSC, although more expensive, is needed for accurate and precise results.

Thermogravimetric and Thermomechanical Analyses.
Changes in weight with temperature (thermogravimetric analysis, TGA) and changes in mechanical properties with temperature (thermomechanical analysis, TMA) are used in pharmaceutical engineering research and in industrial quality control.

In TGA, a vacuum recording balance with a sensitivity of $0.1~\mu g$ is used to record the sample weight under pressures of 10^{-4} mm to 1 atmosphere. The changes in hydrated salts such as calcium oxalate, $CaC_2O_4 \cdot H_2O$, with temperature are evaluated using TGA, as discussed by Simons and Newkirk.[40]

The characterization by TGA of bone tissue associated with dental structures was reported by Civjan et al.[41] Thermogravimetric analysis also may be used to study drug stability and the kinetics of decomposition.

Thermomechanical analysis (TMA) measures the expansion and extension of materials or changes in viscoelastic properties, and heat distortions, such as shrinking, as a function of temperature. By use of a probe assembly in contact with the test material, any motion due to expansion, melting, or other physical change delivers an electric signal to a recorder. The furnace, in which are placed a sample and a probe, controls the temperature, which may be programmed over a range from $-150°$ to $700°$ C. The apparatus serves essentially as a penetrometer, dilatometer, or tensile tester over a wide range of programmed temperatures. Humphries et al.[42] have used TMA in studies on the mechanical and viscoelastic properties of hair and the stratum corneum of the skin.

References and Notes

1. E. A. Moelwyn-Hughes, *Physical Chemistry*, 2nd Ed., Pergamon, New York, 1961, p. 297.
2. W. M. Latimer and W. H. Rodebush, J. Am. Chem. Soc. **42**, 1419, 1920. According to Schuster et al., *Hydrogen Bond*, Vol. III, North Holland, New York, 1976, the concept of the hydrogen bond was first introduced by T. S. Moore and T. F. Winmill, J. Chem. Soc. **101**, 1635, 1912.
3. P. R. Byron, J. Pharm. Sci. **75**, 433, 1986; R. N. Dalby, P. R. Byron, H. R. Shepherd and E. Popadopoulous, Pharm. Technol. **14**, 26, 1990.
4. J. Pickthall, *The General Aspects of Aerosols, A Symposium*, Pharm. J. **193**, 391, 1964.
5. J. J. Sciarra, J. Pharm. Sci. **63**, 1815, 1974.
6. P. R. Byron and A. R. Clark, J. Pharm. Sci. **74**, 934, 939, 1985.
7. J. A. Biles, J. Pharm. Sci. **51**, 499, 1962.
8. E. J. Lien and L. Kennon, in *Remington's Pharmaceutical Sciences*, 17th Ed., Mack, Easton, Pa., 1975, pp. 176–178.
9. D. Guttman and T. Higuchi, J. Am. Pharm. Assoc., Sci. Ed. **46**, 4, 1957.
10. S. Riegelman, in R. A. Lyman and J. B. Sprowls (Eds.), *American Pharmacy*, 4th Ed., Lippincott, Philadelphia, 1955, Chapter 18.
11. A. J. Aguiar, J. Kro, A. W. Kinkle and J. Samyn, J. Pharm. Sci. **56**, 847, 1967.
12. S. A. Khalil, M. A. Moustafa, A. R. Ebian and M. M. Motawi, J. Pharm. Sci. **61**, 1615, 1972.
13. R. K. Callow and O. Kennard, J. Pharm. Pharmacol. **13**, 723, 1961.
14. J. E. Carless, M. A. Moustafa and H. D. C. Rapson, J. Pharm. Pharmacol. **18**, 1905, 1966.
15. M. Azibi, M. Draguet-Brughmans, R. Bouche, B. Tinant, G. Germain, J. P. Declercq and M. Van Meerssche, J. Pharm. Sci. **72**, 232, 1983.
16. M. Azibi, M. Draguet-Brughmans and R. Bouche, J. Pharm. Sci. **73**, 512, 1984.
17. S. S. Yank and J. K. Guillory, J. Pharm. Sci. **61**, 26, 1972.
18. I. Goldberg and Y. Becker, J. Pharm. Sci. **76**, 259, 1987.
19. M. M. J. Lowes, M. R. Caira, A. P. Lotter and J. G. Van Der Watt, J. Pharm. Sci. **76**, 744, 1987.
20. T. Ishida, M. Doi, M. Shimamoto, N. Minamino, K. Nonaka and M. Inque, J. Pharm. Sci. **78**, 274, 1989.
21. M. Stoltz, A. P. Lötter and J. G. Van Der Watt, J. Pharm. Sci. **77**, 1047, 1988.
22. R. J. Behme, D. Brooks, R. F. Farney and T. T. Kensler, J. Pharm. Sci. **74**, 1041, 1985.
23. W. I. Higuchi, P. K. Lau, T. Higuchi and J. W. Shell, J. Pharm. Sci. **52**, 150, 1963.
24. J. K. Guillory, J. Pharm. Sci. **56**, 72, 1967.
25. J. A. Biles, J. Pharm. Sci. **51**, 601, 1962.
26. J. Haleblian and W. McCrone, J. Pharm. Sci. **58**, 911, 1969; J. Haleblian, J. Pharm. Sci. **64**, 1269, 1975.
27. J. D. Mullins and T. J. Macek, J. Am. Pharm. Assoc., Sci. Ed. **49**, 245, 1960.
28. J. B. Bogardus, J. Pharm. Sci. **72**, 338, 1983.
29. S. E. Friberg, C. S. Wohn and F. E. Lockwood, J. Pharm. Sci. **74**, 771, 1985; S. E. Friberg, *Lyotropic Liquid Crystals*, American Chemical Society, Washington, D.C., 1976.
30. H. G. Ibrahim, J. Pharm. Sci. **78**, 683, 1989.
31. G. H. Brown, Am. Scientist **60**, 64, 1972.
32. B. A. Mulley, Drug Standards **27**, 108, 1959.
33. A. Brodin, A. Nyqvist-Mayer, T. Wadsten, B. Forslund and F. Broberg, J. Pharm. Sci. **73**, 481, 1984.
34. A. Nyqvist-Mayer, A. F. Brodin and S. G. Frank, J. Pharm. Sci. **74**, 1192, 1985.
35. W. L. Chiou and S. Riegelman, J. Pharm. Sci. **60**, 1281, 1971.
36. A. H. Goldberg, in L. J. Leeson and J. T. Carstensen (Eds.), *Dissolution Technology*, Academy of Pharmaceutical Science, Washington, D. C., 1974, Chapter 5.
37. J. K. Guillory, S. C. Hwang and J. L. Lach, J. Pharm. Sci. **58**, 301, 1969; H. H. Lin and J. K. Guillory, J. Pharm. Sci. **59**, 972, 1970; S. S. Yang and J. K. Guillory, J. Pharm. Sci. **61**, 26, 1972; W. C. Stagner and J. K. Guillory, J. Pharm. Sci. **68**, 1005, 1979.
38. J. B. Borgadus, J. Pharm. Sci. **71**, 105, 1982; L. Gatlin and P. P. DeLuca, J. Parent. Drug Assoc. **34**, 398, 1980.
39. E. I. Dupont, Instrument Division, Wilmington, Del. 19898; Fisher Scientific, Instrument Division, Pittsburgh, Pa. 15219; Mettler Instrument, Hightstown, N.J. 08520; Perkin Elmer, Norwalk, Conn. 06859.
40. E. L. Simons and A. E. Newkirk, Talanta, **11**, 549, 1964.
41. S. Civjan, W. J. Selting, L. B. De Simon, G. C. Battistone and M. F. Grower, J. Dent. Res. **51**, 539, 1972.
42. W. T. Humphries, D. L. Millier and R. H. Wildnauer, J. Soc. Cosmet. Chem. **23**, 359, 1972; W. T. Humphries and R. H. Wildnauer, J. Invest. Dermatol. **59**, 9, 1972.

43. R. C. Weast and M. J. Astle, Eds., *CRC Handbook of Chemistry and Physics*, 63rd Edition, CRC Press, Boca Raton, Fla., 1982–83, p. D-197.
44. J. K. Guillory, J. Pharm. Sci. **56**, 72, 1967.

Problems*

2–1. A weather balloon rises 2 miles into the upper atmosphere. Its volume at ground level is 2.50 liters at 1 atm pressure and 24° C. What is its final volume if the atmospheric pressure is 8.77×10^{-3} atm and the temperature is −44.7° C at the 2-mile position?

Answer: 219 liters

2–2. An air bubble is blown by a fish at the bottom of an aquarium tank and it rises to the surface. As in the case of the weather balloon, *Problem 2–1*, its volume increases as the pressure on the bubble decreases. The bubble has a radius of 0.1 cm at the bottom of the tank where the pressure is 1.3 atm and the temperature is 14° C. At the surface of the tank the pressure is 750 torrs and the temperature is 27° C. What is the radius of the bubble when it comes to the surface of the tank? For the equation for the volume of a sphere, see the inside front cover of the book.

Answer: The volume of the bubble at the bottom of the tank is 4.19×10^{-3} cm³. The radius of the bubble increases from 0.1 cm to 0.11 cm as the bubble rises to the surface.

2–3. Calculate the volume in liters of 1 mole of nitrogen gas at 400 atm and 0° C, using the ideal gas equation. Give the answer in mL of N_2.

Answer: 56 mL

2–4. If 0.50 g of a drug in the vapor state occupies 100 mL at 120° C and 1 atm pressure, what is its approximate molecular weight?

Answer: 161 g/mole

2–5. The Air Protection Laboratory in a large city isolated a new gaseous pollutant that was found to exert a pressure of 1.17 atm when 6.07 gram of the substance was confined in a 2.0-liter vessel at 28° C. **(a)** What is the molecular weight of the pollutant? **(b)** If the pollutant is known by chemical test to be a sulfur compound, what do you suppose the compound might be?

Answers: **(a)** 64.1 g/mole; **(b)** the molecular weight should provide a strong clue.

2–6. Nitrous oxide (N_2O), U.S.P., is used for the rapid induction of anesthesia (80% N_2O, 20% O_2) and at lower percentages for maintenance anesthesia. **(a)** Using the ideal gas equation, compute the molecular weight of this gas, given that 1 liter at 0° C and 760 mm Hg pressure weighs 1.97 g. Check your results using a table of atomic weights. **(b)** Compute the root mean square velocity, μ, of N_2O. **(c)** Use equation (2–12), p. 26, to compute the density ρ of N_2O at 1 atm and 0° C.

Answers: **(a)** 44.15 g/mole; **(b)** 3.9×10^4 cm/sec; **(c)** density $= 2 \times 10^{-3}$ g/cm³

2–7. An auto tire is inflated to 30 psi gauge pressure (1 atm = 14.7 pounds per square inch and the total air pressure is the tire gauge pressure plus 14.7 psi) on a day when the outside temperature is 10° C. After running on the highway for several hours the temperature of the air in the tire has risen to 26° C. **(a)** What is the pressure in the tire at this time, assuming that the volume of the tire does not change appreciably with temperature? **(b)** Refer to a table of conversion factors in a handbook of chemistry to assure yourself that 1 atm = 14.7 lb/in.² (actually 14.6959 lb/in.²). Express the value, 14.7 lb/in.², in the SI units of Pascals. **(c)** Would it be wise to release some air from the car tires after traveling for hours during August in the

Southwest? How high can the pressure in a tire become before it is in danger of blowing out?

Answers: **(a)** 47.23 psi; gauge pressure = 32.5 psig.; **(b)** 14.69594 lb (avoirdupois)/in.² $= 101,325$ kg m^{-1} s^{-2} $= 101,325$ N m^{-2} $= 101,325$ Pa; **(c)** check with your local service station attendant.

2–8. An experimenter wishes to determine the partial pressure of chloroform required to anesthetize a 28.0-gram mouse in a 2.37-liter container at 20° C. If 2.00 cm³ of $CHCl_3$ is introduced into the closed vessel through a valve, what is the partial pressure of the $CHCl_3$ in the container? Assume complete evaporation of the chloroform. Calculate the partial pressure using both **(a)** the ideal gas equation and **(b)** the van der Waals equation. Assuming the density of the mouse to be about 1 g/cm³, calculate its volume in liters and subtract this from the volume of the vessel to obtain the volume available to the chloroform vapor. The density of liquid chloroform at 20° C is 1.484 g/cm³, so 2.00 cm³ $\times$ 1.484 g/cm³ $=$ 2.968 g and since the molecular weight of chloroform is 119.4 g/mole, 2.096 g $\div$ 119.4 g/mole $=$ 0.0249 mol of chloroform in the vessel. The van der Waals a and b values for $CHCl_3$ are given in Table 2–3.

Answers: **(a)** 0.256 atm or 194.3 torr; **(b)** 0.254 atm or 193.3 torr

2–9. A 0.193-mole sample of ether was confined in a 7.35-liter vessel at 295.15° K. Calculate the pressure produced using **(a)** the ideal gas equation and **(b)** the van der Waals equation. The van der Waals a value for ether is 17.38 liter² atm mole^{-2}; the b value is 0.1344 liter mole^{-1}. To solve for pressure the van der Waals equation may be rearranged as follows:

$$P = \frac{nRT}{V - nb} - \frac{an^2}{V^2}$$

Answers: **(a)** 0.636 atm; **(b)** 0.626 atm

2–10. Equations for calculating the van der Waals constants a and b are the following:

$$a = \frac{27\,R^2\,T_c^2}{64\,P_c}; \quad b = \frac{R\,T_c}{8\,P_c}$$

where T_c is the *critical temperature* and P_c is the *critical pressure*. The critical temperature and critical pressure, respectively, for chloroform are $T_c = 263°$ C and $P_c = 54$ atm. R is expressed in units of liter atm °K^{-1} mole^{-1}. Calculate the a and b values for chloroform. Check your results against the values given in Table 2–3.

Answers: $a = 15.12$ liter² atm mole^{-2}; $b = 0.1019$ liter mole^{-1}

2–11. A small household fire extinguisher of 0.80-liter capacity contains CO_2 at a pressure of 12.3 atm and 25° C. **(a)** What is the weight of the CO_2 in kg in the extinguisher? **(b)** What is the volume of this mass of CO_2 at 25° C when the pressure is reduced to 1 atm? **(c)** Compare your result with that obtained from the density of gaseous CO_2 at 25° C (density = 0.001836 g/cm³). CO_2 is a gas, not a liquid, at atmospheric pressure. The molecular weight of CO_2 is 44.01 g/mole.

Answers: **(a)** 0.0177 kg; **(b)** 9.84 liter; **(c)** 9.64 liter

2–12. The vapor pressure of water at 25° C is 23.8 mm Hg. The average heat of vaporization between 25° and 40° C is about 10,400 cal/mole. Using the Clausius–Clapeyron equation, calculate the vapor pressure at 40° C. The experimentally determined value is 55.3 mm Hg.

Answer: 55.2 mm Hg

2–13. The vapor pressure of ethyl alcohol is 23.6 torr at 10° C, 78.8 torr (mm Hg) at 30° C, and 135 torr at 40° C. Using equation (2–16a) plot log P vs. $1/T$ (ln P of equation (2–16b) may be used instead of log P and the factor 2.303 will then not be needed), and obtain the vapor pressure of ethyl alcohol at 20° C. What is the heat of vaporization, ΔH_v, at this temperature?

Answer: From the graph, the vapor pressure P is 43.7 torr; $\Delta H_v = $ 10,282 cal/mole. Using linear regression, $\Delta H_v = 10,267$ cal/mole and $P = 43.9$ mm. The heat of vaporization ΔH_v of ethyl alcohol in the *CRC Handbook of Chemistry and Physics*, 67th Edition, is 9673.9 cal/mole.

---

*Problems 2–1 and 2–2 are modified from R. Chang, *Physical Chemistry with Applications to Biological Systems*, 2nd Edition, Macmillan, New York, 1977, p. 23. *Problems 2–8, 2–11, 2–15*, and *2–17* are modified from J. W. Moncrief and W. H. Jones, *Elements of Physical Chemistry*, Addison-Wesley, Reading, Mass., 1977, pp. 7, 9, and 97, respectively. *Problems 2–7 and 2–18* are modified from Chang, ibid, pp. 24 and 162, and from Moncrief and Jones, ibid, pp. 79 and 92, respectively.

2–14. (a) The vapor pressure of water at 100° C is 76 cm Hg and at 90° C it is 52.576 cm Hg.[43] Using the Clausius–Clapeyron equation, calculate the heat of vaporization ΔH_v of water in cal/mole within this temperature range.

(b) For 20° C and 30° C the vapor pressures of water are 17.535 mm Hg and 31.824 mm Hg, respectively. What is the heat of vaporization ΔH_v within this temperature range? Give the results in cal/mole.

(c) At 5° C and 10° C the vapor pressures of water are 6.543 mm Hg and 9.209 mm Hg, respectively. What is the heat of vaporization ΔH_v of water within this range of temperatures? Express the result in cal/mole.

(d) The results of (a), (b), and (c) may suggest that one obtains, and should use in further calculations, different ΔH_v values for water within these three temperature ranges. To test this suggestion, prepare a table of these six vapor pressures and their corresponding temperatures recorded in Kelvin degrees. Using equation (2–16), regress log P versus $1/T$ and obtain the overall ΔH_v for the temperature range of 5° to 100° C. (Be careful to use consistent units throughout the problem.) Finally, answer the question: Does ΔH_v have a single value over the temperature range from 5° to 100° C, or is it better represented by different values over the three temperature ranges considered in this problem?

Answers: (a) 9922 cal/mole; (b) 10,525 cal/mole; (c) 10,698 cal/mole; (d) ΔH_v (5° to 100° C) = 10,310 cal/mole; $r^2 = 0.9999$

2–15. A group of hikers decide to climb a mountain and heat cans of beans and some sausages when they reach the summit, using backpacker stoves. The mountain is 3500 meters high (11,500 ft), at which height the atmospheric pressure is 506 mm Hg. The temperature at this time of year is −15° C (5° F) at the mountain top.

The heat of vaporization of butane and propane, two volatile compounds used as fuel for backpacker stoves, are 5318 and 4812 cal/mole, respectively; and their normal boiling points (at sea level) are −0.50° C and −42.1° C.

It may be noted that flammable liquids such as butane and propane will not vaporize and ignite at temperatures below their boiling points and cannot serve as cooking stoves at lower temperatures. (a) Compute the boiling point of butane and propane at the top of the mountain. Changes in temperature with vapor pressure are dealt with using the Clausius–Clapeyron equation. (b) Could either the butane or propane stove be used at the top of this mountain? (c) Can water be "boiled" on the mountain top to prepare coffee for the hikers? The heat of vaporization of water is 9717 cal/mole and its boiling temperature is 100° C at 1 atm.

Partial Answer: (a) Butane, −11.30° C; propane, −50.73° C

2–16. Isoflurane and halothane are nonflammable volatile liquids used for general anesthesia. (a) What is the vapor pressure p' of isoflurane at room temperature, 25° C? The heat of vaporization $\Delta H_v'$ of isoflurane is 6782 cal/mole at its boiling point. The vapor pressure p' for isoflurane at its normal boiling point, 48.5° C, is 1 atm according to the definition of the normal boiling point. (b) What is the heat of vaporization $\Delta H_v''$ of halothane within the temperature range 20° C to its boiling point, 50.2° C? The vapor pressure p'' of halothane at 20° C is 243 mm Hg. These two general anesthetics are slightly greater in vapor pressure than ether (ether, $p = 217$ torr at 20° C). But of much greater importance, they are nonflammable whereas ether is highly flammable. (c) What other advantages does halothane have over ether as a general anesthetic? Consult a book on pharmacology.

Answers: (a) $p' = 329.3$ torr; (b) $\Delta H_v'' = 7112$ cal/mole

2–17. (a) What pressure is necessary to keep butane as a liquid in a container on a day when the storeroom temperature is 104° F. The heat of vaporization of butane is 5318 cal/mole, and the boiling point at 1 atm is −0.50° C.

(b) Repeat the problem using propane as the volatile liquid. The ΔH_v of propane is 4811.8 cal/mole and its boiling point at 1 atm (normal boiling point) is −42.1° C.

(c) From results in (a) and (b) conclude whether you can keep these gases as liquids at 104° F in plastic containers. The maximum safe pressure for plastic containers is 1.75 kg/cm². Can these volatile compounds be kept in aluminum containers that have a maximum safe pressure of 4.2 to 4.9 kg/cm²? (One atmosphere = 1.033 kg/cm².)

Answers: (a) 3.56 atm; (b) 15.60 atm; (c) to keep propane as a liquid at 104° F requires a pressure above 15.6 atm or 16.2 kg/cm². Neither plastic nor aluminum containers are satisfactory for propane.

2–18. If the skate blade of a 175-lb man on ice is 12 in. long and 1/64 in. thick and the heat of fusion of water (ice) is 6025 J/mole, what is the melting point change that produces liquid water under the skate allowing the liquid to lubricate the skate? The molar volume of liquid water (its molecular weight divided by its density) is 0.018 liter and the molar volume of ice is 0.01963 liter. (a) Carry out the calculations, using SI units and the integrated form of the Clausius–Clapeyron equation,

$$\int_{273.15°K}^{T} \frac{1}{T}\, dT = \frac{\Delta V}{\Delta H_f} \int_{P_1}^{P_2} dP$$

(b) Repeat, using the approximation

$$\frac{\Delta T}{\Delta P} = T\frac{\Delta V}{\Delta H_f}$$

Answers: (a) $\Delta T = -0.470°$ K; (b) $\Delta T = -0.468°$ K

2–19. When a solid that exists in more than one crystalline form is subjected to the relatively high pressure of a tablet machine it might favor transformation to a denser polymorphic form.

Sulfathiazole can be obtained in at least two polymorphic forms, I and II, I being the lower energy state at room temperature. The densities are 1.50 g/cm³ (form I) and 1.55 g/cm³ (form II). The transition temperature $I \rightarrow II$ is 161° C and the heat of transition ΔH_t is 1420 cal/mol.[44] (a) What is the effect of a normal pressure of 1 atm on the transition temperature of sulfathiazole from form I to form II? The molecular weight is 255.32 g/mole. Use equation (2–17), p. 31, substituting ΔH_f, V_l, and V_s with ΔH_t and the molar volumes of the two polymorphs.

(b) What is the transition temperature when form I is compressed in the tablet machine at 2812 kg/cm² (2757.6 bar)? Would form I be stable during the tableting process? (One bar = 14.5038 pounds/in.² and 1 kg/cm² = 14.223343 pounds/in.²)

Answer: (a) Using equation (2–17), $\frac{\Delta T}{\Delta P} = -0.041$ °K/atm; (b) 49.4°C. If the temperature during processing were greater than 50° C, form I might change to form II.

2–20. The temperature of transition T from one polymorphic form to another can be obtained from solubility data as explained on page 35. The solubilities m_1 and m_2 of sulfathiazole, forms I and II, at several temperatures are given in the table below. Plot the $\ln(m_2/m_1)$ on the vertical axis against $1/T$, (°K⁻¹), on the horizontal axis, and compute the transition temperature for the transformation, form I → form II.

Data for *Problem 2–20*

T (°C)	$1/T$ (°K⁻¹) × 10³	ln (m_2/m_1)
31.50	3.01	0.2562
19.80	3.11	0.3501
14.00	3.20	0.4243
9.93	3.30	0.5198
8.15	3.37	0.5552
7.10	3.41	0.6125

*From G. Milosovich, J. Pharm. Sci. **53**, 484, 1964.

Ln(m_2/m_1) is the natural logarithm of the ratios of the solubilities, m_2 and m_1, of the two polymorphic forms. Obtain the linear least-square fit of the line. Recognizing that ln(m_2/m_1) must be 0 when $(m_2/m_1) = 1$, read the value of $1/T$ (and hence T) from the graph when $\ln (m_2/m_1) = 0$. Or, better, from the least-squares equation, calculate the value of $1/T$, and therefore of T, when $\ln(m_2/m_1)$ is 0.

Answer: $0 = -2.34 + 864.5(1/T)$; $T = 369.4°$ K

2–21. A mixture containing 21% by weight of phenol in water (see Fig. 2–14) is prepared and allowed to come to equilibrium at 30° C. The two liquid phases that separate contain 7% and 70% of phenol, respectively. If the total weight of the original mixture was 135 g, calculate (a) the weight of each phase at equilibrium, and (b) the actual weight of water, in grams, in each phase.

Answers: (a) 30 g; 105 g; (b) 9.00 g; 97.65 g

2–22. A and B are two partially miscible liquids. The following mixtures (percent by weight) all formed two liquid phases below, and one liquid phase above, the temperature noted (in other words, these are temperatures at which two-phase systems became one-phase systems).

Data for *Problems 2–22* and *2–24*

A (% w/w)	B (% w/w)	Temperature (°C)
20	80	10
30	70	22
40	60	34
50	50	39
60	40	38
70	30	32
80	20	22
90	10	10

Plot these results on rectangular coordinate paper and describe accurately the phase changes observed as A is continually added to B at a temperature of (a) 25° C and (b) 45° C.

Answers: (a) There is a single liquid phase up to 31% w/w of A present, at which point two liquids are formed (compositions are 31% w/w A and 78% w/w A). As more A is added, the amount of the second phase B decreases while that of the first phase A increases. When the system exceeds 78% w/w A at 25° C the two phases disappear and the system again becomes one phase. (b) At 45° C, we are above the region of immiscibility, and hence a single phase exists for all combinations of A and B.

2–23. If a liquid mixture containing A (20 g) and B (30 g) is prepared and allowed to come to equilibrium at 22° C, (a) what are the compositions of the two phases present and (b) what is the weight of each phase? See *Problem 2–22.*

Answers: (a) 30% w/w A and 70% w/w B; 80% w/w A and 20% w/w B. These are conjugate phases; (b) 40 g of A and 10 of B g

2–24. Using the table of data in *Problem 2–22*, plot % A on the horizontal axis versus temperature (°C). Ten grams of a mixture containing equal weights of A and B at 50° C are cooled to 10° C. (a) At what temperature will a phase change be observed; (b) at 10° C, how much B must be added to produce a single phase; (c) at 10° C, how much A must be added to produce a single-phase system? See *Problem 2–22.*

Answers: (a) 39° C; (b) 15 g B (to produce a system containing 20% w/w A and 80% w/w B); (c) 40 g A (to produce a system containing 90% w/w A and 10% B)

2–25. Plot the following points on triangular coordinate paper for a mixture of three liquids. The area bounded by the binodal curve contains two liquid phases in equilibrium; the area outside the binodal curve contains one liquid phase.

Data for *Problems 2–25, 2–26,* and *2–27*

A (% w/w)	B (% w/w)	C (% w/w)
84	11	5
78	12	10
70	14	16
63	16	21
55	19	26
45	25	30
40	30	30
32	39	29
26	48	26
22	55	23
17	65	18
14	75	11
12	81	7
9	89	2

When a liquid system containing A (45 g), B (40 g), and C (15 g) was prepared and allowed to reach equilibrium, analysis of one phase gave the following data: A = 84% w/w; B = 11% w/w; C = 5% w/w. (a) From your knowledge of tie lines in binodal areas, what is the composition of the conjugate phase? (b) What is the weight of each of these two conjugate phases? The total weight of the components is 100 g.

Answers: (a) Approximately 21% w/w of A, 58% w/w of B, and 21% w/w of C. (b) 38 g; 62 g

2–26. Using the data given in *Problem 2–25*, you are required to formulate a 5-g single-phase solution containing 50% w/w B and 35% w/w C that is to be diluted to 100 g with A immediately prior to use. (a) What is the sequence of phase changes observed as A is progressively added? (b) What is the composition of the final system?

Answers: (a) A single liquid phase system contains approximately 30% w/w A, 41% w/w B, and 29% w/w C when a second liquid phase separates. When the composition of the system is 81% w/w A, 11% w/w B, and 8% w/w C, the system will revert to one liquid phase. (b) 95.75 g A, 2.5 g B, and 1.75 g C

2–27. Based on the data given in *Problem 2–25*, a system containing A (45 g), B (40 g), and C (15 g) was prepared and allowed to attain equilibrium. (a) How much of a mixture containing 30% w/w C and 45% w/w A would you need to add to produce a single-phase system from the two-phase system? (b) What would be the composition of this one-phase system? Suppose you now add increasing amounts of B to this phase, (c) how much B must you add before you produce a single-phase system again? (d) What is the composition of this phase? (e) Finally, you add A in increasing amounts; what amount of A must you add to produce a single-phase system? (f) What will be its composition? *Note:* When you add increasing amounts of a component, or a mixture of components, you prepare systems that lie on a straight line directed to the point that represents the mixture you are adding. Thus, if you continually add A to any mixture, you will eventually finish up at point A on the diagram.

Answers: (a) 60.0 g (27.0 g A and 33.0 g C); (b) 45% w/w A, 25% w/w B, and 30% w/w C; (c) 440 g B; (d) 12% w/w A, 80% w/w B, and 8% w/w C (approximately); (e) 4022 g A; (f) 89% w/w A, 10% w/w B, and 1% w/w C (approximate)

3
Thermodynamics*

The First Law of Thermodynamics
Thermochemistry
The Second Law of Thermodynamics

The Third Law of Thermodynamics
Free Energy Functions and Applications

Thermodynamics is concerned with the quantitative relationships between heat and other forms of energy, including mechanical, chemical, electric, and radiant energy. A body is said to possess *kinetic energy* because of its motion or the motion of its parts (i.e., its molecules, atoms, and electrons), and to possess *potential energy* by virtue of its position or the configuration of its parts. It is not possible to know the absolute value of the energy of a system; it is sufficient to record the changes in energy that occur when a system undergoes some transformation. Mechanical energy changes are expressed in ergs or joules and heat changes in calories. Count Rumford in 1798 and James Joule in 1849 showed the relationship between mechanical work and heat. Today the calorie, as defined by the United States National Bureau of Standards, is equal to 4.1840×10^7 ergs of 4.1840 joules, so that work and heat can be expressed in the same units.

Energy can be considered as the product of an *intensity factor* and a *capacity factor*. Stated more explicitly, the various types of energy may be represented as a product of an intensive property independent of the quantity of material, and the differential of an extensive property that is proportional to the mass of the system. For example, the mechanical work done by a gas on its surroundings is PdV, and the work performed by the molecules in the surface of a liquid against the surface tension is $\gamma \, dA$. Some of the forms of energy, together with these factors and their accompanying units, are given in Table 3–1.

Thermodynamics is based on three "laws" or facts of experience that have never been proved in a direct way. Various conclusions, usually expressed in the form of mathematical equations, however, may be deduced from these three principles, and the results consistently agree with observation. Consequently, the laws of thermodynamics, from which these equations are obtained, are accepted as valid for systems involving large numbers of molecules.

THE FIRST LAW OF THERMODYNAMICS

The first law is a statement of the conservation of energy. It states that, although energy can be transformed from one kind into another, it cannot be created or destroyed. Put another way, the total energy of a system and its immediate surroundings (which together are often referred to as an *isolated system*) remains constant during any operation. This statement follows from the fact that the various forms of energy are equivalent, and when one kind is formed, an equal amount of another kind must disappear. The present relativistic picture of the universe, expressed by Einstein's equation,

Energy = (mass change) × (velocity of light)^2

suggests that matter can be considered as another form of energy, 1 gram being equal to 9×10^{20} erg. These enormous quantities of energy, while involved in nuclear transformations, are not important in ordinary chemical reactions.

According to the first law,

$$\Delta E = Q - W \qquad (3-1)$$

---

*The student will find the subject of this chapter presented in a most readable form in the following books. G. Pimentel and R. Spratley, *Understanding Chemical Thermodynamics*, Holden-Day, San Francisco, 1969; B. H. Mahan, *Elementary Chemical Thermodynamics*, Benjamin/Cummings, Menlo Park, Calif., 1963; L. K. Nash, *Elements of Chemical Thermodynamics*, 2nd Edition, Addison-Wesley, Menlo Park, Calif., 1970; R. P. Bauman, *Introduction to Equilibrium Thermodynamics*, Prentice-Hall, Englewood Cliffs, N.J., 1966. Clear definitions of thermodynamic terms and discussions of concepts are found in A. M. James, *A Dictionary of Thermodynamics*, Wiley, New York, 1976.

53

TABLE 3–1. *Intensity and Capacity Factors of Energy*

Energy Form	Intensity or Potential Factor (Intensive Property)	Capacity or Quantity Factor (Extensive Property)	Energy Unit Commonly Used
Heat (thermal)	Temperature (deg)	Entropy change (cal/deg)	Calories
Expansion	Pressure (dyne/cm^2)	Volume change (cm^3)	Ergs
Surface	Surface tension (dyne/cm)	Area change (cm^2)	Ergs
Electric	Electromotive force or potential difference (volts)	Quantity of electricity (coulombs)	Joules
Chemical	Chemical potential (cal/mole)	Number of moles	Calories

in which ΔE is the increase in internal energy, Q the heat absorbed, and W the work done by the system. It should be noted that an input of heat is usually necessary before work can be done *by* a system. Conversely, work done *on* a system usually is accompanied by the evolution of heat. The convention followed in writing the first law is to give heat input as a positive quantity $+Q$ and work output as a negative quantity $-W$. The converse is to give heat output as a negative quantity $-Q$ and work input as a positive quantity $+W$. Internal energy results from the motions of the molecules, electrons, and nuclei in a system and depends on the *measurable properties:* pressure, volume, and temperature. Any two of these variables must be specified to define the internal energy. For an infinitesimal increase in the energy dE, equation (3–1) is written

$$dE = q - w \qquad (3-2)$$

in which q is the heat absorbed and w is the work done during the small change of the system. Capital letters, Q and W, are used for heat and work in equation (3–1) to signify finite changes in these quantities. Lower case q and w in equation (3–2) signify infinitesimal changes.

Changes of internal energy, rather than a knowledge of the absolute energy value (which, incidentally, cannot be determined), is the concern of thermodynamics. The finite change of internal energy is written

$$\Delta E = E_2 - E_1 \qquad (3-3)$$

in which E_2 is the energy of the system in its final state, say 1 g of water at 1 atm and 10° C, and E_1 is the energy of the system in its initial state, say 1 g of water at 5 atm and 150° C.

Exact and Inexact Differentials. dE is an exact differential and is written

$$dE = \left(\frac{\partial E}{\partial P}\right)_T dP + \left(\frac{\partial E}{\partial T}\right)_P dT \qquad (3-4)$$

The internal energy depends only on the initial and final conditions of, say, pressure and temperature and not on the manner in which these factors are varied. This fact is stated as follows: The increase in energy, $\Delta E = E_2 - E_1$, is independent of the "path" followed in going from state 1 to state 2.

We will come back to a consideration of the term *path* in a later paragraph, but first let us clarify the word

state. The term *thermodynamic state* means the condition in which the measurable properties have a definite value. The state of 1 g of water at E_1 may be specified by the conditions of, say, 1 atm pressure and 10° C and the state E_2 by the conditions of 5 atm and 150° C. Hence, the states of most interest to the chemist ordinarily are defined by specifying any two of the three variables, temperature, pressure, and volume; however, additional independent variables sometimes are needed to specify the state of the system. Any equation relating the necessary variables—for example, $V = f(T,P)$—is an *equation of state*. The ideal gas law and the van der Waals equation are equations of state. The variables of a thermodynamic state are known as *thermodynamic properties*. E, V, P, and T all belong to this class. In the study of interfacial phenomena, surface area also becomes one of the thermodynamic properties necessary to characterize the system completely. On the other hand, both the heat absorbed q and the work done w depend on the manner in which the change is conducted. Hence, q and w are not exact differentials, and heat and work are not, in these circumstances, thermodynamic properties.

To clarify the statement that the change in energy of a process does not depend on the path, whereas the heat absorbed and the work done vary with the means used to carry out the process, let us take the example of transporting a box of equipment from a camp in a valley to one at the top of the mountain. Here we are concerned with potential energy rather than internal energy of a system, but the principle is the same. We can haul the box to the top of the mountain by a block and tackle suspended from an overhanging cliff and produce little heat by this means. We can drag the box up a path, but more work is required and considerably more heat is produced owing to the frictional resistance. We can carry the box to the nearest airport, fly it over the spot, and drop it by parachute. It is readily seen that each of these methods involves a different amount of heat and work. The change in potential energy depends only on the difference in the height of the camp in the valley and the one at the top of the mountain, and it is independent of the path used to transport the box.

Although a number of variables, such as chemical composition, refractive index, and dielectric constant, can be specified, they are not all independent. In order to fix the internal energy, we need specify only two of the independent variables, pressure, volume, and temperature, in a closed system.

A *closed system* is one that may exchange heat and work but not *matter* with its surroundings. An *open system*, on the other hand, involves a transfer of matter in addition to the exchange of heat and work. If two immiscible solvents, for example, water and carbon tetrachloride, are confined in a closed container and iodine is distributed between the two phases, each phase is an open system, yet the total system made up of the two phases is closed, for it does not exchange matter with its surroundings. The discussion here is first restricted to reversible changes occurring in closed systems. Open systems are considered in a later section.

Isothermal and Adiabatic Processes. When the temperature is kept constant during a process, the reaction is said to be conducted *isothermally*. An isothermal reaction may be carried out by placing the system in a large constant-temperature bath so that heat is drawn from or returned to it without affecting the temperature significantly. When heat is neither lost nor gained during a process, the reaction is said to occur *adiabatically*. A reaction carried on inside a sealed Dewar flask or "vacuum bottle" is adiabatic since the system is thermally insulated from its surroundings. In thermodynamic terms, it can be said that an adiabatic process is one in which $q = 0$, and the first law under adiabatic conditions reduces to

$$w = -dE \qquad (3-5)$$

According to equation (3–5), when work is done by the system, the internal energy decreases, and since heat cannot be absorbed in an adiabatic process, the temperature must fall. Here, the work done becomes a thermodynamic property dependent only on the initial and final states of the system.

Reversible Processes. Imagine the hypothetic case of water at its boiling point contained in a cylinder fitted with a weightless and frictionless piston. The apparatus is immersed in a constant-temperature bath maintained at the same temperature as the water in the cylinder. By definition, the vapor pressure of water at its boiling point is equal to the atmospheric pressure, and if the pressure is 1 atm, the temperature is 100° C. The process is an isothermal one, that is, it is carried out at constant temperature. If the external pressure is decreased slightly, the volume of the system increases, and the vapor pressure falls. Water then evaporates to maintain the vapor pressure constant at its original value, and heat is extracted from the bath to keep the temperature constant and bring about the vaporization.

On the other hand, if the external pressure is increased slightly, the system is compressed and the vapor pressure rises. Some of the water condenses to reestablish the equilibrium vapor pressure, and the liberated heat is absorbed by the constant-temperature bath. If the process could be conducted infinitely slowly so that no work is expended in supplying kinetic energy to the piston, and if the piston is considered to be frictionless so that no work is done against the force of friction, all the work is used to expand or compress the vapor. Then, since this process is always in a state of virtual thermodynamic equilibrium, being reversed by an infinitesimal change of pressure, it is said to be *reversible*. If the pressure on the system is increased or decreased rapidly, or if the temperature of the bath cannot adjust instantaneously to the change in the system, the isolated system is not in the same thermodynamic state at each moment, and the process cannot be reversible.

Although no real system can be made strictly reversible, some are nearly so. One of the best examples of reversibility is that involved in the measurement of the potential of an electrochemical cell using the potentiometric method (p. 193).

Maximum Work. The work done by a system in an isothermal process is at a maximum when it is done reversibly. This statement can be shown to be true by the following argument. No work is accomplished if an ideal gas expands freely into a vacuum, where $P = 0$, since any work accomplished depends on the external pressure. As the external pressure becomes greater more work is done by the system, and it rises to a maximum when the external pressure is infinitesimally less than the pressure of the gas, that is, when the process is reversible. Of course, if the external pressure is continually increased, the gas is compressed rather than expanded and work is done *on* the system rather than *by* the system in an isothermal reversible process.

Work of Expansion Against a Constant Pressure. Let us first discuss the work term, considering only that work resulting from an expansion or compression of a gas against a *constant* opposing pressure, P.

Imagine a vapor confined in a hypothetic cylinder fitted with a weightless, frictionless piston of area A, as shown in Figure 3–1. If a constant external pressure P is exerted on the piston, the total force is $P \times A$, since $P =$ force/area. The vapor in the cylinder is now made

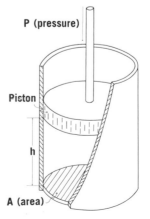

Fig. 3–1. Cylinder with weightless and frictionless piston.

to expand by increasing the temperature, and the piston moves a distance h. The work done against the opposing pressure is

$$W = \underset{\substack{\uparrow \\ \text{total} \\ \text{force}}}{P \times \overbrace{A \times h}^{\text{increase in volume}}} \qquad (3\text{--}6)$$

Now $A \times h$ is the increase in volume, $\Delta V = V_2 - V_1$, so that, at constant pressure,

$$W = P\,\Delta V \qquad (3\text{--}7)$$

$$W = P(V_2 - V_1) \qquad (3\text{--}8)$$

Example 3–1. A gas expands by 0.5 liter against a constant pressure of 0.5 atm at 25° C. What is the work in ergs and in joules done by the system?

$$W = P\,\Delta V$$
$$1 \text{ atm} = 1.013 \times 10^6 \text{ dyne/cm}^2$$
$$W = (0.507 \times 10^6 \text{ dyne/cm}^2) \times 500 \text{ cm}^3$$
$$= 2.53 \times 10^8 \text{ ergs} = 25.3 \text{ J}$$

The following example demonstrates the kind of problem that can be solved by an application of the first law of thermodynamics.

Example 3–2. One mole of water in equilibrium with its vapor is converted into steam at 100° C and 1 atm. The heat absorbed in the process (i.e., the heat of vaporization of water at 100° C) is about 9720 cal/mole. What are the values of the three first-law terms, Q, W, and ΔE?

The amount of heat absorbed is the heat of vaporization, given as 9720 cal/mole. Therefore,

$$Q = 9720 \text{ cal/mole}$$

The work W performed against the constant atmospheric pressure is obtained by using equation (3–8), $W = P(V_2 - V_1)$. Now V_1 is the volume of 1 mole of liquid water at 100° C, or about 0.018 liter. The volume V_2 of 1 mole of steam at 100° C and 1 atm is given by the gas law, assuming that the vapor behaves ideally:

$$V_2 = \frac{RT}{P} = \frac{0.082 \times 373}{1} = 30.6 \text{ liters}$$

It is now possible to obtain the work,

$$W = P(V_2 - V_1) = 1 \times (30.6 - 0.018) =$$
$$30.6 \text{ liters atm/mole} = 741 \text{ cal/mole}$$

The internal energy change ΔE is obtained from the first-law expression

$$\Delta E = Q - W = 9720 - 741 = 8979 \text{ cal/mole}$$

Therefore, of the 9720 cal of heat absorbed by 1 mole of water, 741 cal are employed in doing work of expansion or "$P\,\Delta V$ work" against an external pressure of 1 atm. The remaining 8979 cal increase the internal energy of the system. This quantity of heat supplies potential energy to the vapor molecules, that is, it represents the work done against the intermolecular forces of attraction. Internal energy includes not only potential energy due to intermolecular forces, but also rotational, vibrational, and translational kinetic energy of the atoms and the energy of the electrons that constitute the molecules.

Ideal Gases and the First Law. An ideal gas has no internal pressure, and hence no work need be done to separate the molecules against their cohesive forces when the gas expands. We therefore can write

$$\left(\frac{\partial E}{\partial V}\right)_T = 0 \qquad (3\text{--}9)$$

Equation (3–9) suggests that the internal energy of an ideal gas is a function of the temperature only, which is one of the conditions needed to define an ideal gas in thermodynamic terms.

It follows from this discussion that for an ideal gas involved in an isothermal process ($dT = 0$), dE is equal to zero, and the first law becomes

$$q = w \qquad (3\text{--}10)$$

Thus the work done in the isothermal expansion of an ideal gas is equal to the heat absorbed by the gas.

Isothermal Work of Expansion Against a Variable Pressure. Since the external pressure is only infinitesimally less than the pressure of an ideal gas in an isothermal expansion, the external pressure can be replaced by the pressure of the gas $P = nRT/V$ in the equation

$$\int dW_{\max} = nRT \int_{V_1}^{V_2} \frac{dV}{V}$$

$$W_{\max} = nRT \ln \frac{V_2}{V_1}$$

$$= 2.303 nRT \log \frac{V_2}{V_1} \qquad (3\text{--}11)$$

Equation (3–11) gives the heat absorbed as well as the maximum work done in the expansion, because $Q = \Delta E + W$, and ΔE is equal to zero for an ideal gas in an isothermal process. The maximum work in an isothermal reversible expansion may also be expressed in terms of pressure, since, from Boyle's law, $V_2/V_1 = P_1/P_2$ at constant temperature. Therefore, equation (3–11) can be written

$$W_{\max} = 2.303 nRT \log \frac{P_1}{P_2} \qquad (3\text{--}12)$$

Example 3–3. What is the maximum work done in the isothermal reversible expansion of 2 moles of an ideal gas from 1 to 5 liters at 25° C?

$$W_{\max} = 2.303 \times 2 \times 1.987 \times 298.2 \times \log 5 = 1908 \text{ cal}$$

Expressing R as 8.3143 J° K^{-1} mole^{-1} we obtain the answer in SI units:

$$W_{\max} = 2.303 \times 2 \times 8.3143 \times 298.2 \times \log 5 = 7982 \text{ J}$$

Heat Content (Enthalpy). When work of expansion is done at *constant pressure*, $W = P\,\Delta V = P(V_2 - V_1)$ by equation (3–7), and under these conditions, the first law may be written

$$\Delta E = Q_P - P(V_2 - V_1) \qquad (3\text{--}13)$$

in which Q_P is the heat absorbed at constant pressure. Rearranging,

$$Q_P = E_2 - E_1 + P(V_2 - V_1) \qquad (3\text{--}14)$$

$$= (E_2 + PV_2) - (E_1 + PV_1) \qquad (3\text{--}15)$$

The term $E + PV$ is called the *heat content* or *enthalpy* H. The increase in heat content ΔH is equal to the heat absorbed at constant pressure by the system. It is the heat required to increase the internal energy and to perform work of expansion as seen by substituting H in equation (3–15),

$$Q_P = H_2 - H_1 = \Delta H \qquad (3\text{--}16)$$

and writing equation (3–13) as

$$\Delta H = \Delta E + P\,\Delta V \qquad (3\text{--}17)$$

For an infinitesimal change, one can write

$$dQ_P = dH \qquad (3\text{--}18)$$

The heat absorbed in a reaction carried out at atmospheric pressure is independent of the number of steps and the mechanism of the reaction. It depends only on the initial and final conditions. We will take advantage of this fact in the section on thermochemistry.

It should also be stressed that $\Delta H = Q_P$ only when nonatmospheric work (i.e., work other than that against the atmosphere) is ruled out. When electric work, work against surfaces, or centrifugal forces are considered, we must write

$$\Delta H = Q_P - W_{\text{nonatm}}$$

Heat Capacity. The *molar heat capacity C* of a system is defined as the heat q required to raise the temperature of 1 mole of a substance by 1 degree. Since C varies with temperature, it is better to define it for an infinitely small change of temperature

$$C = \frac{q}{dT} \qquad (3\text{--}19)$$

A system at constant volume, for example, a gas confined in a calorimeter, does no PV work since $dV = 0$, and the first law becomes

$$dE = q_v \qquad (3\text{--}20)$$

Thus, the molar heat capacity C_v at constant volume can be defined as

$$C_v = \frac{q_v}{dT} = \left(\frac{\partial E}{\partial T}\right)_v \qquad (3\text{--}21)$$

which states that C_v is the ratio of the increase in energy content or the heat absorbed at constant volume to the increase of temperature. The partial notation is used because E is a function of volume as well as of temperature, and the volume is being held constant in this case.

When the pressure rather than the volume is held constant, as, for example, when a reaction proceeds in an open container in the laboratory at essentially constant atmospheric pressure, a heat capacity C_P at constant pressure is defined. Since $q = dH$ at constant

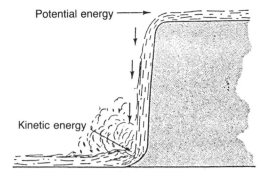

Fig. 3–2. Schematic of a waterfall showing its potential and kinetic energy. (Modified from H. E. White, *Modern College Physics*, 5th Ed., Van Nostrand, New York, 1966, p. 90, reproduced with permission of the copyright owner.)

pressure according to equation (3–18), the molar heat capacity C_P at constant pressure is written

$$C_P = \frac{q_P}{dT} = \left(\frac{\partial H}{\partial T}\right)_P \qquad (3\text{--}22a)$$

and for a change in heat content between product and reactant,

$$\Delta H = H_{\text{product}} - H_{\text{reactants}}$$

equation (3–22a) may be written

$$\left[\frac{\partial(\Delta H)}{\partial T}\right]_p = \Delta C_p \qquad (3\text{--}22b)$$

where $\Delta C_p = (C_p)_{\text{product}} - (C_p)_{\text{reactants}}$. Equation (3–22b) is known as the *Kirchhoff equation*.

Example 3–4.* A waterfall (Fig. 3–2) is often used in physics and thermodynamics as an example of a change from potential energy to kinetic energy or heat. At the top of a 200-ft (200 ft × 30.48 cm/ft = 6096 cm) waterfall, 1 g of water possesses the potential energy

$$E = mgh$$

or

$$1 \text{ g} \times (981 \text{ cm sec}^{-2} \times 6096 \text{ cm}) = 0.598 \times 10^7 \text{ g cm}^2 \text{ sec}^{-2}$$

$$0.598 \times 10^7 \text{ erg} = 0.598 \text{ joule} = 0.143 \text{ cal}$$

The potential energy, mgh, at the top of the falls is converted completely into heat (kinetic) energy, $Q = mc\Delta T$, at the bottom, where c is the specific heat of the water. Specific heat is the heat Q required to raise the temperature of 1 g of a substance by 1° C. Thus we have a relationship between the top and bottom of the falls:

$$mgh = mc\Delta T$$

in which the masses cancel, leaving

$$\Delta T = gh/c$$

$$= \frac{981 \text{ cm sec}^{-2} \times 6096 \text{ cm}}{1 \text{ cal g}^{-1} \text{ deg}^{-1}} = \frac{0.598 \times 10^7 \text{ g cm}^2 \text{ sec}^{-2} \text{ (erg)}}{\text{cal deg}^{-1}}$$

$$= \frac{0.598 \text{ joule}}{\text{cal deg}^{-1}} = \frac{0.143 \text{ cal}}{\text{cal deg}^{-1}}$$

$$\Delta T = 0.143° \text{ K} = 0.143° \text{ C}.$$

---

*After J. W. Moncrief and W. H. Jones, *Elements of Physical Chemistry*, Addison-Wesley, Reading, Mass., 1977, p. 18.

TABLE 3-2. *Modified First-Law Equations for Processes Occurring under Various Conditions*

Specified Condition		Process	Common Means for Establishing the Condition	Modification of the First Law, $dE = q - w$, Under the Stated Condition	
(a) Constant heat	$q = 0$	Adiabatic	Insulated vessel, such as a Dewar flask	$dE = -w$	(a)
(b) Reversible process at constant temperature	$dT = 0$	Isothermal	Constant-temperature bath	$w = w_{max}$	(b)
(c) Ideal gas at constant temperature	$(\partial E/\partial V)_T = 0$ $dT = 0$	Isothermal	Constant-temperature bath	$dE = 0$ $\therefore q = w$	(c)
(d) Constant volume	$dV = 0$	Isometric (isochoric)	Closed vessel of constant volume, such as a bomb calorimeter	$w = PdV = 0$ $\therefore dE = q_v$	(d)
(e) Constant pressure	$dP = 0$	Isobaric	Reaction occurring in an open container at constant (atmospheric) pressure	$dH = q_P$ $\therefore dE = dH - P\,dV$	(e)

Thus the potential energy of the water at the top of the waterfall has been converted completely into kinetic energy at the bottom, which is exhibited as an increase in temperature $\Delta T = 0.143°$ C. In *Modern College Physics*, Professor White states "All the available energy at the top of a waterfall is potential. At the bottom it is kinetic" (see Fig. 3–2).

In this process, no heat Q is exchanged with the surroundings and no work is done, so the net change in energy, by the first law, is zero:

$$\Delta E = Q - W = 0$$

William Thomson,* an important contributor to the development of thermodynamics (who later became Lord Kelvin) recalled how in the summer of 1847 he met Joule on a vacation in the Alps. James Joule, who had studied the relationship between work and heat and for whom the unit of energy was named, was on his honeymoon in the mountains. When Thomson met him, Joule had left his bride behind in the carriage and with a long and accurate thermometer in hand was attempting to measure the temperature at various heights of a waterfall. It is unlikely that Joule was successful in this crude attempt, particularly since we see in Example *3–4* that the temperature change is indeed small even for a very high waterfall. Joule would no doubt have done better to set aside his science experiments and pay more attention to his bride on their honeymoon in the beautiful Alps.

Summary. Some of the special restrictions that have been placed on the first law up to this point in the chapter, together with the resultant modifications of the law, are brought together in Table 3–2. A comparison of the entries in Table 3–2 with the material that has gone before will serve as a comprehensive review of the first law.

*D. Eisenberg and D. Crothers, *Physical Chemistry with Applications to the Life Sciences*, Benjamin/Cummings, Menlo Park, Calif., 1979, p. 93.

THERMOCHEMISTRY

Heat may be absorbed or evolved in physical and chemical processes, and the reactions are referred to as *endothermic* when heat is absorbed and *exothermic* when heat is evolved. Thermochemistry deals with the heat changes accompanying isothermal chemical reactions. These are usually carried out at atmospheric (essentially constant) pressure, and the heat absorbed is equal to the increase in heat content (i.e., $Q_P = \Delta H$). If the reaction is carried out at constant volume, then $Q_V = \Delta E$. In solution reactions, the $P\,\Delta V$ terms are not significant, so that $\Delta H \cong \Delta E$. This close approximation does not hold, however, for reactions involving gases.

In the reaction

$$C_{(s)} + O_{2(g)} = CO_{2(g)}; \qquad (3-23)$$

$$\Delta H°_{25°C} = -94{,}052 \text{ cal}$$

the subscripts represent the physical states, (s) standing for solid and (g) for gas. Additional symbols, (l) for liquid and (aq) for dilute aqueous solution, will be found in subsequent thermochemical equations. $\Delta H°_{25°C}$ is the *standard heat of reaction* for the process at 25° C. The negative sign accompanying the value for ΔH in equation (3–23) signifies that heat is evolved, that is, the reaction is exothermic. Equation (3–23) states that when 1 mole of solid carbon (graphite) reacts with 1 mole of gaseous oxygen to produce 1 mole of gaseous carbon dioxide at 25° C, 94,052 cal are liberated. This means that the reactants contain 94,052 cal in excess of the product, so that this quantity of heat is evolved during the reaction. If the reaction were reversed and CO_2 were converted to carbon and oxygen, the reaction would be endothermic. It would involve the absorption of 94,052 cal, and ΔH would have a positive value. When the pressure is not specifically stated, it is assumed, as it is in this case, that the reaction is carried out at 1 atm.

Heat of Formation. Equation (3–23) gives the *standard heat of formation* of carbon dioxide from its elements. The heat content of 1 mole of carbon dioxide is 94,052 cal less than the heat content of its elements in the *standard* or *reference state* of 25° C and 1 atm pressure. The state of matter or allotropic form of the elements also must be specified in defining the standard state. The heat contents of all elements in their standard states are arbitrarily assigned values of zero. Consequently, the heat involved in the formation of a compound from its elements is the *heat of formation* of the compound. The heat of formation of carbon dioxide is −94,052 cal. The heats of formation of a number of compounds have been determined, and some of these are found in Table 3−3.

Heat of Combustion. The heat involved in the complete oxidation of 1 mole of a compound at 1 atm pressure is known as the *heat of combustion*. The compound is burned in the presence of oxygen in a sealed calorimeter to convert it completely to carbon dioxide and water. The combustion of methane is written

$$CH_{4(g)} + 2O_{2(g)} = CO_{2(g)} + 2H_2O_{(l)};$$

$$\Delta H_{25° C} = -212.8 \text{ kcal} \quad (3-24)$$

This result can also be obtained from the heats of formation of reactants and products, since

$$\Delta H_{reaction} = \Sigma \, \Delta H_{products} - \Sigma \, \Delta H_{reactants} \quad (3-25)$$

in which the terms on the right are the heats of formation of the products and reactants. According to the National Bureau of Standards data (Table 3−3), the heat of formation of $CH_{4(g)}$ (methane$_{[g]}$) is −17.889; $CO_{2(g)}$, −94.052; and $H_2O_{(l)}$, −68.317 kcal/mole at 25° C. Since oxygen $O_{2(g)}$ is an element, it has a heat of formation of zero.

Employing equation (3−25),

$$\Delta H_{25° C} = [-94.052 + 2(-68.317)]$$

$$-(-17.889) = -212.797 \text{ kcal}$$

Note the 2 molecules of water, $2H_2O_l$, requiring that its standard heat of formation, −68.317, be multiplied by 2.

In the year 1840, Hess showed that since ΔH depends only on the initial and final states of a system, thermochemical equations for several steps in a reac-

tion can be added and subtracted to obtain the heat of the overall reaction. The principle is known as *Hess's law of constant heat summation* and is used to obtain the heats of reactions that are not easily measured directly. If one desires to obtain $\Delta H_{25° C}$ for a reaction that cannot be carried out in a calorimeter, he or she may proceed as illustrated in the following example.

$$C_{(s)} + O_{2(g)} = CO_{2(g)}; \; \Delta H_{25° C} = -94.052 \text{ kcal}$$

$$CO_{(g)} + \tfrac{1}{2}O_{2(g)} = CO_{2(g)}; \; \Delta H_{25° C} = -67.636 \text{ kcal}$$

Subtracting the second equation and its heat of combustion from the first yields the desired result:

$$C_{(s)} + \tfrac{1}{2}O_{2(g)} = CO_{(g)}; \; \Delta H_{25° C} = -26.416 \text{ kcal} \quad (3-26)$$

Differential and Integral Heats of Solution. When a mole of a solute is dissolved, the heat absorbed or liberated is not a constant quantity but varies with the concentration of the solution. Two kinds of heats of solution are recognized: differential or partial, and integral or total.

The *differential heat of solution* is the heat effect produced when 1 mole of a solute is dissolved in a large quantity of a solution of a definite concentration. No appreciable change in concentration results when the solute is added, and the heat change is thus obtained at the specified concentration. Differential heat of solution can be defined, in an equivalent way, as the heat change that occurs when an infinitely small amount of solute is dissolved in a definite quantity of solution. Since the amount of solute is infinitesimal, no change in concentration would result.

The *integral heat of solution* is the effect obtained when 1 mole of a solute is dissolved in a definite quantity of pure solvent, say 1000 g of water, to yield a solution.

Differential and integral heats of solution are not generally equal. In the case of differential heat, the process is conducted so that concentration does not change when the solute is added. The heat effects depends only on the conversion of the crystalline solute to the dissolved state, and the solvent is in essentially the same state before and after the dissolution of the solute. In integral heat, both the solute and the solvent are affected during the process.

Heats of hydration, mentioned on page 230, may be calculated from integral heats of solution. As seen in Figure 10−6, anhydrous sodium sulfate dissolves in water with the liberation of heat, because the heat of hydration is more than sufficient to disintegrate the crystal. The already hydrated $Na_2SO_4 \cdot 10 H_2O$, on the other hand, dissolves with the absorption of heat because no hydration energy is available to overcome the crystal energy. In the thermodynamic considerations of dissolution (solubility of a drug in a solvent, chapter 10) the heat term involved is a partial or differential heat of solution.

Heats of Reaction from Bond Energies. Heats of reaction may be estimated from covalent bond energies, found in

TABLE 3−3. *Standard Heats of Formation at 25° C**

Substance	$\Delta H°$ (kcal/mole)	Substance	$\Delta H°$ (kcal/mole)
$H_{2(g)}$	0		
$H_{(g)}$	52.09	Methane$_{(g)}$	−17.889
$O_{2(g)}$	0	Ethane$_{(g)}$	−20.236
$O_{(g)}$	59.16	Ethylene$_{(g)}$	12.496
$I_{2(g)}$	14.88	Benzene$_{(g)}$	19.820
$H_2O_{(g)}$	−57.798	Benzene$_{(l)}$	11.718
$H_2O_{(l)}$	−68.317	Acetaldehyde$_{(g)}$	−39.76
$HCl_{(g)}$	−22.063	Ethyl alcohol$_{(l)}$	−66.356
$HI_{(g)}$	6.20	Glycine$_{(g)}$	−126.33
$CO_{2(g)}$	−94.052	Acetic acid$_{(l)}$	−116.4

**From Rossini et al., *N.B.S. Circulars* No. C461 and 500.*

books on thermodynamics listed in the footnote on the first page of this chapter. In the reaction

$$H_2C{=}CH_2 + Cl{-}Cl \rightarrow Cl{-} \overset{\overset{\displaystyle H}{|}}{\underset{\underset{\displaystyle H}{|}}{C}} {-} \overset{\overset{\displaystyle H}{|}}{\underset{\underset{\displaystyle H}{|}}{C}} {-}Cl$$

a $C{=}C$ bond is broken (requiring 130 kcal), a $Cl{-}Cl$ bond is broken (requiring 57 kcal), a $C{-}C$ bond is formed (liberating 80 kcal), and two $C{-}Cl$ bonds are formed (liberating 2×78 or 156 kcal). Thus the energy ΔH of the reaction is

$$\Delta H \div 130 + 57 - 80 - 156 = -49 \text{ kcal}$$

Since 1 calorie = 4.184 joule, -49 kcal is expressed in SI units as -2.05×10^5 J.

Additional Applications of Thermochemistry. Thermochemical data are important in many chemical calculations. Heat of mixing data can be used to determine whether a reaction such as precipitation is occurring during the mixing of two salt solutions. If no reaction takes place when dilute solutions of the salts are mixed, the heat of reaction is zero.

The constancy of the heats of neutralization, obtained experimentally when dilute aqueous solutions of various strong acids and strong bases are mixed, has shown that the reaction involves only

$$H^+_{(aq)} + OH^-_{(aq)} = H_2O_{(l)};$$
$$\Delta H_{25° C} = - 13.6 \text{ kcal} \quad (3{-}27)$$

No combination occurs between any of the other species in a reaction such as

$$HCl_{(aq)} + NaOH_{(aq)} = H_2O_{(l)} + Na^+_{(aq)} + Cl^-_{(aq)}$$

since HCl, NaOH, and NaCl are completely ionized in water. In the neutralization of a weak electrolyte by a strong acid or base, however, the reaction involves ionization in addition to neutralization, and the heat of reaction is no longer constant at about -13.6 kcal/mole. Since some heat is absorbed in the ionization of the weak electrolyte, the heat evolved falls below the value for the neutralization of completely ionized species. Thus, a knowledge of ΔH of neutralization permits one to differentiate between strong and weak electrolytes.

Another important application of thermochemistry is the determination of the number of calories obtained from various foods. The subject is discussed in books on food and nutrition.

THE SECOND LAW OF THERMODYNAMICS

Heat flows spontaneously only from hotter to colder bodies, and a steam engine can do work only with a fall in temperature and a flow of heat to the lower temperature. No useful work can be obtained from heat at constant temperature. Gases expand naturally from higher to lower pressures, and solute molecules diffuse from a region of higher to lower concentration. These spontaneous processes will not proceed in reverse without the intervention of some external agency. Although spontaneous processes are not thermodynamically reversible, they can be carried out in a nearly reversible manner by an outside agency. Maximum work is obtained by conducting a spontaneous process reversibly; however, the frictional losses and the necessity of carrying out the process at an infinitely slow rate preclude the possibility of complete reversibility in real processes.

The first law of thermodynamics simply observes that energy must be conserved when it is converted from one form to another. It has nothing to say about the probability that a process will occur. The second law refers to the probability of the occurrence of a process based on the observed tendency of a system to approach a state of energy equilibrium. The energy that may be freed for useful work in a gas, liquid, or solid, or any reaction mixture, is known as the *free energy* of the system. The free energy decreases as a physical or chemical reaction proceeds. In general, *spontaneous processes at constant temperature and pressure are accompanied by a loss in free energy*, and this decrease signifies the natural tendency for the transformation to occur.

When a substance melts, it passes from a condition of low heat content and a highly ordered arrangement to a condition of higher heat content and more randomness. This change from orderliness to randomness is said by the physical chemist to represent an increase in the *entropy* of the system. The energy that is used to increase the randomness or, as Gibbs, one of the founders of thermodynamics, once referred to it, the "mixed-upness" of a system is obviously not available for other purposes, such as useful work. All forms of energy are made up of two terms: an *intensity factor* and a *capacity factor*, as shown in Table 3–1. Temperature is the intensity factor and entropy change is the capacity factor of heat energy.

The Efficiency of a Heat Engine. An important consideration is that of the possibility of converting heat into work. Not only is heat isothermally unavailable for work; *it can never be converted completely into work.*

The spontaneous character of natural processes and the limitations on the conversion of heat into work constitute the second law of thermodynamics.

Falling water can be made to do work, owing to the difference in the potential energy at the two levels, and electric work can be done because of the difference in electric potential (emf). A heat engine (such as a steam engine) likewise can do useful work by using two heat reservoirs, a "source" and a "sink," at two different temperatures. Only part of the heat at the source is converted into work, however, the remainder being returned to the sink (which, in practical operations, is often the surroundings) at the lower temperature. The fraction of the heat Q at the source converted into work W is known as the *efficiency* of the engine:

$$\text{efficiency} \equiv \frac{W}{Q} \qquad (3-28)$$

The efficiency of even a hypothetical heat engine operating without friction cannot be unity, for W is always less than Q in a continuous conversion of heat into work, according to the second law of thermodynamics.

Imagine a hypothetical steam engine operating reversibly between an upper temperature T_2 and a lower temperature T_1. It absorbs heat Q_2 from the hot boiler or source, and by means of the working substance, steam, it converts the quantity W into work, and returns heat Q_1 to the cold reservoir or sink. Carnot (1824) proved that the efficiency of such an engine, operating reversibly at every stage and returning to its initial state (cyclic process), can be given by the expression

$$\frac{W}{Q_2} = \frac{Q_2 - Q_1}{Q_2} \qquad (3-29)$$

We know that the heat flow in the operation of the engine follows the temperature gradient, so that the heat absorbed and rejected can be related directly to temperatures. Now, Lord Kelvin used the ratios of the two heat quantities Q_2 and Q_1 of the Carnot cycle to establish the Kelvin temperature scale

$$\frac{Q_2}{Q_1} = \frac{T_2}{T_1} \qquad (3-30)$$

We can therefore write, by combining equations (3–28), (3–29), and (3–30),

$$\text{Efficiency} = \frac{Q_2 - Q_1}{Q_2} = \frac{T_2 - T_1}{T_2} \qquad (3-31)$$

It is observed from equation (3–31) that the higher T_2 becomes and the lower T_1 becomes, the greater is the efficiency of the engine. When T_1 reaches absolute zero on the Kelvin scale, the reversible heat engine converts heat completely into work, and its theoretic efficiency becomes unity. This can be seen by setting $T_1 = 0$ in equation (3–31). Since absolute zero is considered unattainable, however, an efficiency of unit is impossible, and heat can never be completely converted to work. We can write this statement using the notation of limits as follows:

$$\lim_{T_1 \to 0} \frac{W}{Q} = 1 \qquad (3-32)$$

If $T_2 = T_1$ in equation (3–31), the cycle is isothermal and the efficiency is zero, confirming the earlier statement that heat is isothermally unavailable for conversion into work.

Example 3–5. A steam engine operates between the temperatures of 373° and 298° K. (*a*) What is the theoretic efficiency of the engine? (*b*) If the engine is supplied with 1000 cal of heat Q_2, what is the theoretic work in ergs?

(*a*)

$$\text{Efficiency} = \frac{W}{Q_2} = \frac{373 - 298}{373}$$

$$= 0.20 \text{ or } 20\%$$

(*b*)

$$W = 1000 \times 0.20 = 200 \text{ cal}$$

$$200 \text{ cal} \times 4.184 \times 10^7 \text{ erg/cal} = 8.36 \times 10^9 \text{ ergs}$$

Entropy. When equation (3–31) is written as

$$\frac{W}{Q_2} = \frac{T_2 - T_1}{T_2} \qquad (3-33)$$

$$W = \frac{Q_2 T_2}{T_2} - \frac{Q_2 T_1}{T_2} \qquad (3-34)$$

$$W = Q_2 - T_1 \frac{Q_2}{T_2} \qquad (3-35)$$

it can be seen that only part of the heat Q_2 is converted to work in the engine. For example, suppose that the energy $T_1 Q_2/T_2 = 800$ cal. This is the heat Q_1 that is returned to the sink at the lower temperature and is unavailable for work. One can easily show that Q_1 is equal to $T_1 Q_2/T_2$ of equation (3–35). The term Q_2/T_2 is known as the *entropy change* of the reversible process at T_2, and Q_1/T_1 is the entropy change at T_1. When the entropy changes at the two temperatures are calculated, they are both found to equal 2.7 cal/deg. The entropy change ΔS_2 during the absorption of heat is positive, however, since Q_2 is positive. At the lower temperature where heat is expelled, Q_1 is negative and the entropy change ΔS_1 is negative. The total entropy change ΔS_{cycle} in the reversible cyclic process is thus zero.

$$\Delta S_2 = \frac{Q_{2\text{rev}}}{T_2} = \frac{1000 \text{ cal}}{373} = 2.7 \text{ cal/deg}$$

$$\Delta S_1 = -\frac{Q_{1\text{rev}}}{T_1} = -\frac{800}{298} = -2.7 \text{ cal/deg}$$

$$\therefore \Delta S_{\text{cycle}} = \Delta S_2 + \Delta S_1 = 0$$

We may also note that if Q_2 is the heat absorbed by an engine at T_2, then $-Q_2$ must be the heat lost by the surroundings (the hot reservoir) at T_2, and the entropy of the surroundings is

$$\Delta S_{\text{surr}} = -\frac{Q_2}{T_2}$$

Hence, for any system and its surroundings, or *universe*

$$\Delta S_{\text{total system}} = \Delta S_{\text{syst}} + \Delta S_{\text{surr}} = 0 \qquad (3-36)$$

Thus we have two cases in which $\Delta S = 0$: (*a*) a system in a reversible cyclic process and (*b*) a system and its surroundings undergoing any reversible proces.

Entropy S may be defined as the molar energy per degree of absolute temperature that is unavailable for work, and, as shown in Table 3–1, it is the capacity factor of thermal energy. For the absorption of heat in any step of a reversible process, the entropy change is written as

$$\Delta S = \frac{Q_{rev}}{T} \qquad (3-37)$$

and for an infinitesimal change

$$dS = \frac{q_{rev}}{T} \qquad (3-38)$$

In an *irreversible process*, the entropy change of the total system or universe (a system and its surroundings) is always positive, because ΔS_{surr} is always less than ΔS_{syst} in an irreversible process. Consider the heat being absorbed irreversibly by an ideal gas at T_2 in the example just given. The entropy of the system depends only on the initial and final states; thus, $\Delta S = 2.7$ cal/deg is the same for an irreversible process as it is for a reversible process. The work done in an irreversible process is less than the maximum work, however, and $\Delta S_{surr} = Q_{surr}/T_2$ is less than -2.7 cal/deg, say -2.5 cal/deg. For this irreversible process

$$\Delta S_{total\ system} = \Delta S_{syst} + \Delta S_{surr} = 2.7 - 2.5 = 0.2$$

Therefore, in an irreversible process, the entropy of the system and its surroundings is increasing. In mathematical symbols, it is written,

$$\Delta S_{total\ system} > 0 \qquad (3-39)$$

and this can serve as a criterion of spontaneity of a process.

Two examples of entropy calculations will now be given, first considering a reversible process and second an irreversible process.

Example 3–6. What is the entropy change accompanying the vaporization of 1 mole of water in equilibrium with its vapor at 25° C? In this reversible isothermal process, the heat of vaporization ΔH_v required to convert the liquid to the vapor state is 10,500 cal/mole.

The process is carried out at a constant pressure so that $Q = \Delta H_v$, and since it is a reversible process, the entropy change can be written as

$$\Delta S = \frac{\Delta H_v}{T} = \frac{10,500}{298} = 35.2 \text{ cal/mole deg}$$

The entropy change involved as the temperature changes is often desired in thermodynamics; this relationship is needed for the next example. The heat absorbed at constant pressure is given by equation (3–22), $q_P = C_P\ dT$, and for a reversible process

$$\frac{C_P\ dT}{T} = \frac{q_{rev}}{T} = dS \qquad (3-40)$$

Integrating between T_1 and T_2 yields

$$\Delta S = C_P \ln \frac{T_2}{T_1} = 2.303 C_P \log \frac{T_2}{T_1} \qquad (3-41)$$

Example 3–7. Compute the entropy change in the (irreversible) transition of a mole of liquid water to crystalline water at $-10°$ C at constant pressure. The entropy is obtained by calculating the entropy changes for several *reversible* steps.

We first reversibly convert supercooled liquid water at $-10°$ to liquid water at 0° C, then change this to ice at 0° C, and finally cool the ice reversibly to $-10°$ C. The sum of the entropy changes of these steps gives ΔS_{water}. To this we add the entropy change undergone by the surroundings so as to obtain the total entropy change. If the process is spontaneous, the result will be a positive value. If the system is at equilibrium, that is, if liquid water is in equilibrium with ice at $-10°$ C, there is no tendency for the transition to occur, and the total entropy change will be zero. Finally, if the process is not spontaneous, the total entropy change will be negative.

The heat capacity of water is 18 cal/deg, and that of ice is 9 cal/deg within this temperature range.

The reversible change of water at $-10°$ C to ice at $-10°$ C is carried out as follows:

$$H_2O_{(l,-10°)} \rightarrow H_2O_{(l,0°)};\ \Delta S = C_P \ln \frac{T_{final}}{T_{initial}} = 0.67$$

$$H_2O_{(l,0°)} \rightarrow H_2O_{(s,0°)};\ \Delta S = \frac{q_{rev}}{T} = \frac{-1437}{273.2} = -5.26$$

$$H_2O_{(s,0°)} \rightarrow H_2O_{(s,-10°)};\ \Delta S = C_P \ln \frac{T_{final}}{T_{initial}} = -0.34$$

$$H_2O_{(l,-10°)} \rightarrow H_2O_{(s,-10°)};\ \Delta S_{H_2O} = -4.93 \text{ cal/mole deg}$$

The entropy of water decreases during the process since ΔS is negative, but we cannot judge the spontaneity of the process until we also calculate ΔS of the surroundings.

For the entropy change of the surroundings, we consider the water to be in equilibrium with a large bath at $-10°$ C, and the heat liberated when the water freezes is absorbed by the bath without a significant temperature increase. Thus, the reversible absorption of heat by the bath is given by

$$\Delta S_{bath} = -\frac{q_{rev}}{T} = \frac{1343}{263.2} = 5.10 \text{ cal/mole deg}$$

where 1343 cal/mole is the heat of fusion of water at $-10°$ C.

$$\therefore \Delta S_{total\ system} = \Delta S_{H_2O} + \Delta S_{bath}$$
$$= -4.91 + 5.10$$
$$= 0.17 \text{ cal/mole deg}$$

The process in *Example 3–7* is spontaneous since $\Delta S > 0$. This criterion of spontaneity is not a convenient one, however, for it requires a calculation of the entropy change both in the system and the surroundings. The free energy functions, to be treated in a later section, do not demand information concerning the surroundings and are more suitable criteria of spontaneity.

Entropy and Disorder. The impossibility of converting all thermal energy into work results from the "disorderliness" of the molecules existing in the system. Every substance at room temperature possesses a certain amount of entropy owing to molecular motion. The large number of molecules of a gas confined in a cylinder (Fig. 3–3) are traveling in all directions, and some of these will not contribute to driving the piston.

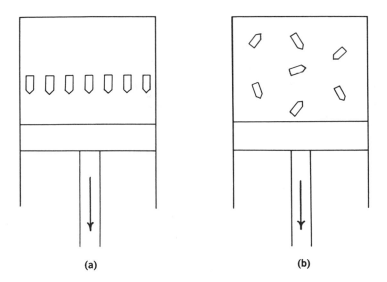

Fig. 3–3. Cylinders containing gas molecules showing (*a*) low entropy, or orderliness, and (*b*) high entropy, or disorderliness. The orderly motion of the molecules in (*a*) could be converted almost entirely into the work of driving the piston; however, nature knows no regimentation of this kind. An actual gas is composed of a large proportion of "wrong-way" molecules with a high degree of freedom or entropy as seen in (*b*). This randomness of motion results in a loss of work, but apparently molecules, like people, are willing to sacrifice some efficiency for greater freedom. (Modified from W. M. Latimer, Chem. Eng. News, **31,** 3366, 1953.)

Latimer[2] states that the entropy of the gas is associated with these "wrong-way molecules," which are manifesting their individual freedom to go in any direction they please. All systems tend to an increased freedom of motion, and the increase in randomness or disorderliness in a natural process is embodied in the second law of thermodynamics. The law may now be stated in the form: *a spontaneous reaction involving a system and its surroundings proceeds in the direction of increased entropy; when the system finally reaches equilibrium, the net entropy change undergone by the system and its surroundings is equal to zero.*

The idea of entropy may become clearer to the student when he or she understands the relationship of entropy and the number of configurations W that a system can assume, as shown by Boltzmann:

$$S = k \ln W \qquad (3\text{-}42)*$$

In this equation k is the Boltzmann constant (the gas constant R divided by Avogadro's number, $R/N = 1.38066 \times 10^{-16}$ erg deg^{-1} molecule^{-1}. When a molecule can assume an increasing number of arrangements, W, as happens when a large flexible protein molecule passes from the solid into the liquid state, the entropy of the system increases, as expressed by equation (3–42). When the protein is bound into a limited number of configurations by the presence of, say, a zinc atom, the entropy of the protein–zinc complex decreases. Thus, the increase in entropy with increasing number of configurations of a molecule, and the de-

crease in entropy with restriction or ordering of the structure, is nicely described by Boltzmann's concept given in equation (3–42).

THE THIRD LAW OF THERMODYNAMICS

The third law of thermodynamics states that the entropy of a pure crystalline substance is zero at absolute zero because the crystal arrangement must show the greatest orderliness at this temperature. The third law cannot be applied to supercooled liquids because their entropy at 0° K is probably not zero.

As a consequence of the third law, it is possible to calculate the absolute entropies of pure substances. The absolute entropy of a perfect crystal at any temperature may be determined from a knowledge of the heat capacity, so long as there is no change of phase during the temperature rise. By integration of equation (3–40),

$$\Delta S = \int_0^T \frac{C_P}{T}\, dT = 2.303 \int_0^T C_P\, d\log T \qquad (3\text{-}43)$$

from $T = 0°$ where $S = 0$ to T where $S = S$. The integral of equation (3–43) is obtained by plotting C_P values against $\log T$ and determining the area under the curve by use of a planimeter.

FREE ENERGY FUNCTIONS AND APPLICATIONS

Two new thermodynamic properties, the *Gibbs free energy* G and the *Helmholtz free energy* or *work function* A are now introduced, and some applications of these important functions to chemistry and pharmacy

---

*His ingenious and renowned formula, $S = k \ln W$, is carved on Ludwig Boltzmann's tombstone in Vienna. As k is named the Boltzmann constant, it has been suggested that R be called the molar Boltzmann constant.

are considered. According to Roseveare,[3] these functions may be related to the other thermodynamic quantities in the following way. Disregarding electric and other forms of energy, we consider PV work as the only useful work or *external energy* that a system can accomplish. The heat content or *total energy* of the system is then divided into *internal* and *external energy*:

$$H = E + PV \qquad (3\text{-}44)$$
$$\text{Total} \quad \text{Internal} \quad \text{External}$$
$$\text{energy} \quad \text{energy} \quad \text{energy}$$

By a second classification, the total heat may be divided into isothermally available or *free energy G* and isothermally unavailable energy, TS:

$$H = G + TS \qquad (3\text{-}45)$$
$$\text{Total} \quad \text{Isothermally} \quad \text{Isothermally}$$
$$\text{energy} \quad \text{available} \quad \text{unavailable}$$
$$\text{energy} \quad \text{energy}$$

Finally, the internal energy can be divided into isothermally available internal energy or work function A and isothermally unavailable energy TS. Thus, for an isothermal process

$$E = A + TS \qquad (3\text{-}46)$$
$$\text{Internal} \quad \text{Isothermally} \quad \text{Isothermally}$$
$$\text{energy} \quad \text{available} \quad \text{unavailable}$$
$$\quad \text{internal} \quad \text{energy}$$
$$\quad \text{energy}$$

A number of relationships may be obtained by rearranging these quantities and placing various restrictions on the processes described. Thus, equation (3–45) is rearranged to

$$G = H - TS \qquad (3\text{-}47)$$

and substituting $E + PV$ for H, we have

$$G = E + PV - TS \qquad (3\text{-}48)$$

Since $A = E - TS$ from equation (3–46), equation (3–48) can be written as

$$G = A + PV \qquad (3\text{-}49)$$

Pressure and Temperature Coefficients of Free Energy. By differentiating equation (3–48), one obtains several useful relationships between free energy and the pressure and temperature. Applying the differential of a product, $d(uv) = u\,dv + V\,du$, to equation (3–48), we obtain the result:

$$dG = dE + P\,dV + V\,dP - T\,dS - S\,dT \qquad (3\text{-}50)$$

Now, in a reversible process in which $q_{rev} = T\,dS$, the first law, restricted to expansion work (i.e., $dE = q_{rev} - P\,dV$), can be written

$$dE = T\,dS - P\,dV \qquad (3\text{-}51)$$

and substituting dE of equation (3–51) into equation (3–50) gives

$$dG = T\,dS - P\,dV + P\,dV + V\,dP - T\,dS - S\,dT$$

or

$$dG = V\,dP - S\,dT \qquad (3\text{-}52)$$

At constant temperature, the last term becomes zero, and equation (3–52) reduces to

$$dG = V\,dP \qquad (3\text{-}53a)$$

or

$$\left(\frac{\partial G}{\partial P}\right)_T = V \qquad (3\text{-}53b)$$

At constant pressure, the first term on the right side of equation (3–52) becomes zero, and

$$dG = -S\,dT \qquad (3\text{-}54)$$

or

$$\left(\frac{\partial G}{\partial T}\right)_P = -S \qquad (3\text{-}55)$$

To obtain the isothermal change of free energy, equation (3–53a) is integrated between states 1 and 2 at constant temperature

$$\int_{G_1}^{G_2} dG = \int_{P_1}^{P_2} V\,dP \qquad (3\text{-}56)$$

For an ideal gas, the volume V is equal to nRT/P, thus allowing the equation to be integrated:

$$\Delta G = (G_2 - G_1) = nRT \int_{P_1}^{P_2} \frac{dP}{P}$$

$$\Delta G = nRT \ln \frac{P_2}{P_1} = 2.303nRT \log \frac{P_2}{P_1} \qquad (3\text{-}57)$$

in which ΔG is the free energy change of an *ideal gas* undergoing an *isothermal* reversible or irreversible alteration.

Example 3–8. What is the free energy change when 1 mole of an ideal gas is compressed from 1 atm to 10 atm at 25° C?

$$\Delta G = 2.303 \times 1.987 \times 298 \times \log \frac{10}{1}$$

$$\Delta G = 1364 \text{ cal}$$

The change in free energy of a solute when the concentration is altered is given by the equation

$$\Delta G = 2.303nRT \log \frac{a_2}{a_1} \qquad (3\text{-}58)$$

in which n is the number of moles of solute and a_1 and a_2 are the initial and final activities of the solute (see pp. 69, 131 for a discussion of activities).

Example 3–9. Borsook and Winegarden[4] roughly computed the free energy change when the kidneys transfer various chemical constituents at body temperature (37° C or 310.2° K) from the blood plasma to the more concentrated urine. The ratio of concentrations was assumed to be equal to the ratio of activities in equation (3–58).

The concentration of urea in the plasma is 0.00500 mole/liter; the concentration in the urine is 0.333 mole/liter. Calculate the free energy change in transporting 0.100 mole of urea from the plasma to the urine.

$$\Delta G = 2.303 \times 0.100 \times 1.987 \times 310.2 \times \log \frac{0.333}{0.00500}$$

$$\Delta G = 259 \text{ cal}$$

This result means that 259 cal of work must be done on the system, or this amount of net work must be performed by the kidneys to bring about the transfer.

Maximum Net Work. The maximum work W_{max} of a reversible process is not all available for accomplishing *useful work* since some must be used as PV work to bring about the expansion or contraction of the system. The net available work is thus $W_{max} - P \Delta V$.

The maximum work W_{max} can be expressed in terms of the work function A as follows. For an isothermal change, equation (3–46) can be written

$$A_2 - A_1 = (E_2 - E_1) - T(S_2 - S_1)$$

or

$$\Delta A = \Delta E - T \Delta S \qquad (3\text{--}59)$$

and from the definition of entropy, assuming the process is reversible, $T \Delta S$ is equal to Q, and

$$\Delta A = \Delta E - Q \qquad (3\text{--}60)$$

or from the first law

$$-\Delta A = W_{max} \qquad (3\text{--}61)$$

The free energy G, like the work function, depends only on the initial and final states of the system so that dG is an exact differential, that is, $\Delta G = G_2 - G_1$. For a reaction involving change in free energy, equation (3–49) becomes

$$G_2 - G_1 = (A_2 + P_2V_2) - (A_1 + P_1V_1)$$

$$= (A_2 - A_1) + (P_2V_2 - P_1V_1)$$

and at constant pressure

$$\Delta G = \Delta A + P(V_2 - V_1)$$

$$\Delta G = \Delta A + P \Delta V \qquad (3\text{--}62)$$

By substituting W_{max} from equation (3–61) into equation (3–62), one obtains

$$-\Delta G = W_{max} - P\Delta V \qquad (3\text{--}63)$$

for an isothermal process at constant pressure. Equation (3–63) expresses the fact that the decrease in free energy is equal to the maximum work exclusive of expansion work, that is, the decrease in free energy at constant temperature and pressure equals ($W_{max} - P \Delta V$), which is the *useful* or *maximum net work* that can be obtained from the process. Under those circumstances in which the $P \Delta V$ term is insignificant (in electrochemical cell and surface tension measurements, for example), the free energy decrease is approximately equal to the maximum work.

Criteria of Equilibrium. When net work can no longer be obtained from a process, G is at a minimum and $\Delta G = 0$. This statement signifies that the system is at equilibrium. Let us prove this by considering a system that is at equilibrium (and hence reversible) at a constant temperature and pressure. Now, for a reversible process restricted to expansion work, we have seen in equation (3–52) that $dG = V \, dP - S \, dT$. When we specify that the temperature and pressure be fixed, equation (3–52) becomes

$$dG = 0 \qquad (3\text{--}64)$$

or for a finite change in G,

$$\Delta G = 0 \qquad (3\text{--}65)$$

Therefore, the criterion for equilibrium at constant temperature and pressure is that ΔG be zero. A negative free energy change, $-\Delta G$, is written sometimes as $\Delta G < 0$, and it signifies that the process is a spontaneous one. If ΔG is positive ($\Delta G > 0$), it indicates that net work must be absorbed for the reaction to proceed, and accordingly it is not spontaneous.

When the process occurs isothermally at constant volume rather than constant pressure, ΔA serves as the criterion for spontaneity and equilibrium. It is negative for a spontaneous process and becomes zero at equilibrium.

These criteria, together with the entropy criterion of equilibrium, are listed in Table 3–4.

It was once thought that at constant pressure, a negative ΔH (evolution of heat) was itself proof of a spontaneous reaction. Many natural reactions do occur with an evolution of heat; the spontaneous melting of ice at 10° C, however, is accompanied by an absorption of heat, and a number of other examples can be cited to prove the error of this assumption. The reason ΔH often serves as a criterion of spontaneity can be seen from the familiar expression,

$$\Delta G = \Delta H - T\Delta S$$

If $T \Delta S$ is small compared with ΔH, a negative ΔH will occur when ΔG is negative (i.e., when the process is spontaneous). When $T \Delta S$ is large, however, ΔG may be negative, and the process may be spontaneous even though ΔH is positive.

The entropy of a system, as previously stated, is a measure of the natural "wrong-way" tendency or, as Gibbs has called it, the "mixed-upness" of molecules. All systems spontaneously tend toward randomness, according to the second law, so that *the more disordered a system becomes, the higher is its probability and the greater its entropy.* Hence, we can write the equation just given as

$$\Delta G = \begin{bmatrix} \text{difference in bond energies or} \\ \text{attractive energies between} \\ \text{products and reactants, } \Delta H \end{bmatrix}$$

$$- \begin{bmatrix} \text{change in probability} \\ \text{during the process,} \\ T \Delta S \end{bmatrix} \qquad (3\text{--}66)$$

TABLE 3–4. *Criteria for Spontaneity and Equilibrium*

Function	Restrictions	Sign of Function		
		Spontaneous	Nonspontaneous	Equilibrium
ΔS	Total system, $\Delta E = 0$, $\Delta V = 0$	+ or > 0	− or < 0	0
ΔG	$\Delta T = 0$, $\Delta P = 0$	− or < 0	+ or > 0	0
ΔA	$\Delta T = 0$, $\Delta V = 0$	− or < 0	+ or > 0	0

We can state that ΔG will become negative and the reaction will be spontaneous either when the heat content decreases or the probability of the system increases at the temperature of the reaction.

Thus, although the conversion of ice into water at 25° C requires an absorption of heat or 1650 cal/mole, the reaction leads to a more probable arrangement of the molecules; that is, an increased freedom of molecular movement. Hence, the entropy increases, and $\Delta S = 6$ cal/mole deg is sufficiently positive to make ΔG negative, despite the positive value of ΔH.

$$\Delta G = 1650 - (298 \times 6) = -138 \text{ cal/mole}$$

Many of the complexes of Chapter 11 form in solution with an absorption of heat, and the processes are spontaneous only because the entropy change is positive. The increase in randomness occurs for the following reason. The dissolution of solutes in water may be accompanied by a *decrease* in entropy, because both the water molecules and the solute molecules lose freedom of movement as hydration occurs. In complexation, this highly ordered arrangement is disrupted as the separate ions or molecules react through coordination, and the constituents thus exhibit more freedom in the final complex than they had in the hydrated condition. The increase in entropy associated with this increased randomness results in a spontaneous reaction as reflected in the negative value of ΔG.

Conversely, some association reactions are accompanied by a decrease in entropy, and they occur in spite of the negative ΔS only because the heat of reaction is sufficiently negative. For example, the Lewis acid–base reaction by which iodine is rendered soluble in aqueous solution,

$$I^-_{(aq)} + I_{2(aq)} = I_3^-_{(aq)}; \quad \Delta H_{25°} = -5100 \text{ cal}$$

is accompanied by a ΔS of -4 cal/mole deg. It is spontaneous because

$$\Delta G = -5100 - [298 \times (-4)]$$
$$= -5100 + 1192 = -3908 \text{ cal/mole}$$

The reader should not be surprised to find a negative entropy associated with a spontaneous reaction. The ΔS values considered here are the changes in entropy of the *substance alone*, and not of the total system, that is, the substance and its immediate surroundings. When ΔS is used as a test of the spontaneity of a reaction, the entropy change of the entire system must be considered. For reactions at constant temperature and pressure, which are the most common types, the change in free energy is ordinarily used as the criterion in place of ΔS. It is more convenient since we need not compute any changes in the surroundings.

By referring back to *Example 3–7*, it will be seen that ΔS was negative for the change from liquid to solid water at $-10°$ C. This is to be expected since the molecules lose some of their freedom when they pass into the crystalline state. The entropy of water plus its surroundings increases during the transition, however; and it is a spontaneous process. The convenience of using ΔG instead of ΔS to obtain the same information is apparent from the following example, which may be compared with the more elaborate analysis required in *Example 3–7*.

Example 3–10. ΔH and ΔS for the transition from liquid water to ice at $-10°$ C and at 1 atm pressure are -1343 cal/mole and -4.91 cal/mole deg, respectively. Compute ΔG for the phase change at this temperature ($-10°$ C $= 263.2°$ K) and indicate whether or not the process is spontaneous.

$$\Delta G = -1343 - [263.2 \times (-4.91)] = -51 \text{ cal/mole} = -213 \text{ J}$$

The process is spontaneous, as reflected in the negative value of ΔG.

Open Systems. The systems considered so far have been closed. They exchange heat and work with their surroundings, but the processes involve no transfer of matter, so that the amount of the components of the system remains constant.

The term *component* should be clarified before we proceed. A phase consisting of w_2 grams of NaCl dissolved in w_1 grams of water is said to contain two independently variable masses or two *components*. Although the phase contains the species Na^+, Cl^-, $(H_2O)_n$, H_3O^+, OH^-, etc., they are not all independently variable. Because H_2O and its various species, H_3O^+, OH^-, $(H_2O)_n$, etc., are in equilibrium, the mass m of water alone is sufficient to specify these species. All forms can be derived from the simple species, H_2O. Similarly, all forms of sodium chloride can be represented by the single species NaCl, and the system therefore consists of just two components, H_2O and NaCl. As stated on p. 37, the *number of components* of a system is the smallest number of independently variable chemical substances that must be specified to describe the phases quantitatively.

In an open system in which the exchange of matter among phases also must be considered, any one of the extensive properties such as volume or free energy becomes a function of temperature, pressure, and the number of moles of the various components.

Chemical Potential. For an infinitesimal reversible change of state, the free energy change in a two-component phase (binary system) is given by

$$dG = \left(\frac{\partial G}{\partial T}\right)_{P,n_1,n_2} dT + \left(\frac{\partial G}{\partial P}\right)_{T,n_1,n_2} dP$$
$$+ \left(\frac{\partial G}{\partial n_1}\right)_{T,P,n_2} dn_1 + \left(\frac{\partial G}{\partial n_2}\right)_{T,P,n_1} dn_2 \quad (3-67)$$

According to Gibbs (who is credited with the development of a great part of chemical thermodynamics), the *chemical potential* of a component, say n_1, is defined as

$$\left(\frac{\partial G}{\partial n_1}\right)_{T,P,n_2} = \mu_1 \quad (3-68)$$

and equation (3-67) is written more conveniently as

$$dG = \left(\frac{\partial G}{\partial T}\right)_{P,n_1,n_2} dT + \left(\frac{\partial G}{\partial P}\right)_{T,n_1,n_2} dP$$
$$+ \mu_1 dn_1 + \mu_2 dn_2 \quad (3-69)$$

Now, from equations (3-55) and (3-53b), $(\partial G/\partial T)_P = -S$ *and* $(\partial G/\partial P)_T = V$ for a closed system. These relationships also apply to an open system, so that equation (3-69) can be written

$$dG = -S\,dT + V\,dP + \mu_1\,dn_1$$
$$+ \mu_2\,dn_2 + \cdots \quad (3-70)$$

The chemical potential, also known as the *partial molar free energy*, can be defined in terms of other extensive properties, the definition given in equation (3-68), however, is the most useful. It states that, at constant temperature and pressure and with the amounts of the other components held constant, the chemical potential of a component i is equal to the change in the free energy brought about by an infinitesimal change in the number of moles n_i of the component. It may be considered as the change in free energy, for example, of an aqueous sodium chloride solution when 1 mole of NaCl is added to a large quantity of the solution, so that the composition does not undergo a measurable change.

At constant temperature and pressure, the first two right-hand terms of equation (3-70) become zero, and

$$dG_{T,P} = \mu_1\,dn_1 + \mu_2\,dn_2 \quad (3-71)$$

or, in abbreviated notation,

$$dG_{T,P} = \Sigma \mu_i\,dn_i \quad (3-72)$$

which, upon integration, gives

$$G_{T,P,N} = \mu_1 n_1 + \mu_2 n_2 + \cdots \quad (3-73)$$

for a system of constant composition, $N = n_1 + n_2 + \ldots$. In equation (3-73), the sum of the right-hand terms equals the total free energy of the system at constant pressure, temperature, and composition. Therefore, μ_1, $\mu_2 \ldots \mu_n$ can be considered as the contributions per mole of each component to the total free energy. The chemical potential, like any other partial molar quantity, is an *intensive* property, in other words, it is independent of the number of moles of the components of the system.

For a closed system at equilibrium and constant temperature and pressure, the free energy change is zero, $dG_{T,P} = 0$, and equation (3-72) becomes

$$\mu_1\,dn_1 + \mu_2\,dn_2 + \cdots = 0 \quad (3-74)$$

for all the phases of the overall system, which is closed.

Equilibrium in a Heterogeneous system. We begin with an example suggested by Klotz.[5] For a two-phase system consisting of, say, iodine distributed between water and an organic phase, the overall system is a closed one, whereas the separate aqueous and organic solutions of iodine are open. The chemical potential of iodine in the aqueous phase is written as μ_{Iw}, and in the organic phase, μ_{Io}. When the two phases are in equilibrium at constant temperature and pressure, the free energy changes dG_w and dG_o of the two phases must be equal since the free energy of the overall system is zero. Therefore, the chemical potentials of iodine in both phases are identical. This can be shown by allowing an infinitesimal amount of iodine to pass from the water to the organic phase in which, at equilibrium, according to equation (3-74),

$$\mu_{Iw}\,dn_{Iw} + \mu_{Io}\,dn_{Io} = 0 \quad (3-75)$$

Now, a decrease of iodine in the water is exactly equal to an increase of iodine in the organic phase:

$$-dn_{Iw} = dn_{Io} \quad (3-76)$$

Substituting (3-76) into (3-75) gives

$$\mu_{Iw}\,dn_{Iw} + \mu_{Io}(-dn_{Iw}) = 0 \quad (3-77)$$

and finally

$$\mu_{Iw} = \mu_{Io} \quad (3-78)$$

This conclusion may be generalized by stating that the chemical potential of a component is identical in all phases of a heterogeneous system when the phases are in equilibrium at a fixed temperature and pressure. Hence, we write

$$\mu_{i_\alpha} = \mu_{i_\beta} = \mu_{i_\gamma} = \cdots \quad (3-79)$$

in which $\alpha, \beta, \gamma \ldots$ are various phases among which the substance i is distributed. For example, in a saturated aqueous solution of sulfadiazine, the chemical potential of the drug in the solid phase is the same as the chemical potential of sulfadiazine in the solution phase.

When two phases are not in equilibrium at constant temperature and pressure, the total free energy of the system tends to decrease, and the substance passes spontaneously from a phase of higher chemical potential to one of lower chemical potential until the potentials are equal. Hence, the chemical potential of a substance can be used as a measure of the *escaping tendency* of the component from its phase. The concept of escaping tendency, defined on page 106, will be used in various chapters throughout the book. The analogy between chemical potential and electric or gravitational potential is evident, the flow in these cases always being from the higher to the lower potential and continuing until all parts of the system are at a uniform potential.

For a phase consisting of a *single pure substance*, the chemical potential is the free energy of the substance per mole. This can be seen by beginning with

$$dG = \left(\frac{\partial G}{\partial n}\right)_{T,P} dn = \mu \, dn \qquad (3-80)$$

for a pure substance at constant pressure and temperature. By integrating equation (3–80), noting that $G = 0$ when $n = 0$, we obtain

$$G = \mu n$$

or

$$\mu = \frac{G}{n} \qquad (3-81)$$

For a two-phase system of a single component, for example, liquid water and water vapor in equilibrium at constant temperature and pressure, the *molar free energy G/n* is identical in all phases. This statement can be verified by combining equations (3–79) and (3–81).

Clausius–Clapeyron Equation. If the temperature and pressure of a two-phase system of one component, for example, of liquid water (*l*) and water vapor (*v*) in equilibrium, are changed by a small amount, the molar free energy changes are equal and

$$dG_l - dG_v \qquad (3-82)$$

In a phase change, the free energy changes for 1 mole of the liquid vapor are given by equation (3–52)

$$dG = V \, dP - S \, dT$$

From equations (3–82) and (3–52)

$$V_l \, dP - S_l \, dT = V_v \, dP - S_v \, dT$$

or

$$\frac{dP}{dT} = \frac{S_v - S_l}{V_v - V_l} = \frac{\Delta S}{\Delta V} \qquad (3-83)$$

Now, at constant pressure, the heat absorbed in the reversible process (equilibrium condition) is equal to the molar latent heat of vaporization, and from the second law we have

$$\Delta S = \frac{\Delta H_v}{T} \qquad (3-84)$$

Substituting (3–84) into (3–83) gives

$$\frac{dP}{dT} = \frac{\Delta H_v}{T \, \Delta V} \qquad (3-85)$$

where $\Delta V = V_v - V_l$, the difference in the molar volumes in the two phases. This is the *Clapeyron equation*, which was introduced in one of its forms on page 31.

The vapor will obey the ideal gas law to a good approximation when the temperature is far enough away from the critical point so that V_v may be replaced by RT/P. Furthermore, V_l is insignificant compared with V_v. In the case of water at 100° C, for example, $V_v = 30.2$ liters and $V_l = 0.0188$ liters.

Under these restrictive circumstances, equation (3–85) becomes

$$\frac{dP}{dT} = \frac{P \, \Delta H_v}{RT^2} \qquad (3-86)$$

which is known as the *Clausius–Clapeyron equation*. It can be integrated between the limits of the vapor pressures P_1 and P_2 and corresponding temperatures T_1 and T_2, assuming ΔH_v is constant over the temperature range considered:

$$\int_{P_1}^{P_2} \frac{dP}{P} = \frac{\Delta H}{R} \int_{T_1}^{T_2} T^{-2} \, dT \qquad (3-87)$$

$$[\ln P]_{P_1}^{P_2} = \frac{\Delta H_v}{R}\left[\left(-\frac{1}{T_2}\right) - \left(-\frac{1}{T_1}\right)\right] \qquad (3-88)$$

$$\ln P_2 - \ln P_1 = \frac{\Delta H_v}{R}\left(\frac{1}{T_1} - \frac{1}{T_2}\right) \qquad (3-89)$$

and finally

$$\ln \frac{P_2}{P_1} = \frac{\Delta H_v(T_2 - T_1)}{RT_1T_2},$$

or,

$$\log \frac{P_2}{P_1} = \frac{\Delta H_v(T_2 - T_1)}{2.303RT_1T_2} \qquad (3-90)$$

This equation is used to calculate the mean heat of vaporization of a liquid if its vapor pressure at two temperatures is available. Conversely, if the mean heat of vaporization and the vapor pressure at one temperature are known, the vapor pressure at another temperature can be obtained.

The Clapeyron and Clausius–Clapeyron equations are important in the study of various phase transitions and in the development of the equations of some of the colligative properties.

Example 3–11. The average heat of vaporization of water can be taken as about 9800 cal/mole within the range of 20° to 100° C. What is the vapor pressure at 95° C? The vapor pressure P_2 at temperature $T_2 = 373°$ K (100° C) is 78 cm Hg, and R is expressed as 1.987 cal/deg mole.

$$\log \frac{78.0}{P_1} = \frac{9800}{2.303 \times 1.987}\left(\frac{373 - 368}{368 \times 373}\right)$$

$$P_1 = 65 \text{ cm Hg}$$

Fugacity. Recall that for a reversible isothermal process restricted to PV work, $(\partial G/\partial P)_T = V$ (equation

[3–53*b*]). The analogous equation relating the change of chemical potential to pressure changes is

$$\left(\frac{\partial \mu_i}{\partial P}\right)_{T, n_1, n_2 \dots} = \overline{V}_i \qquad (3-91)$$

where $\overline{V}_i$ is the partial molar volume of component i and is equal to RT/P_i for an ideal gas, or

$$\int d\mu_i = RT \int \frac{dP}{P_i}$$

$$\mu_i = RT \ln P_i + \mu^\circ \qquad (3-92)$$

in which the integration constant μ° depends only on the temperature and the nature of the gas. It is the chemical potential of component i in the reference state where P_i is equal to 1. When a mixture of real gases does not behave ideally, a function known as the *fugacity f* can be introduced to replace pressure, just as activities are introduced to replace concentration in nonideal solutions. Equation (3–92) becomes

$$\mu_i = \mu^\circ + RT \ln f_i \qquad (3-93)$$

Activities: Activity Coefficients. If the vapor above a solution can be considered to behave ideally, the chemical potential of the solvent in the vapor state in equilibrium with the solution can be written in the form of equation (3–92). If Raoult's law (pp. 106–107) is now introduced for the solvent $P_1 = P_1^\circ X_1$, equation (3–92) becomes

$$\mu_1 = \mu_1^\circ + RT \ln P_1^\circ + RT \ln X_1 \qquad (3-94)$$

Combining the first and second right-hand terms into a single constant gives

$$\mu_1 = \mu^\circ + RT \ln X_1 \qquad (3-95)$$

for an ideal solution. We see that the reference state μ° is equal to the chemical potential μ_1 of the pure solvent (i.e., $X_1 = 1$). For nonideal solutions, equation (3–95) is modified by introducing the "effective concentration" or *activity* of the solvent to replace the mole fraction (see pp. 131–134 for more on activities.):

$$\mu_1 = \mu^\circ + RT \ln a_1 \qquad (3-96)$$

or where

$$a = \gamma X \qquad (3-97)$$

and γ is referred to as the *activity coefficient*:

$$\mu_1 = \mu^\circ + RT \ln \gamma_1 X_1 \qquad (3-98)$$

For the *solute* on the mole fraction scale

$$\mu_2 = \mu^\circ + RT \ln a_2 \qquad (3-99)$$

$$\mu_2 = \mu^\circ + RT \ln \gamma_2 X_2 \qquad (3-100)$$

Based on the practical (molal and molar) scales

$$\mu_2 = \mu^\circ + RT \ln \gamma_m m \qquad (3-101)$$

$$\mu_2 = \mu^\circ + RT \ln \gamma_c c \qquad (3-102)$$

Equations (3–96) and (3–99) are frequently used as definitions of activity.

Gibbs–Helmholtz Equation. For an isothermal process at constant pressure proceeding between the initial and final states 1 and 2, equation (3–47) yields

$$G_2 - G_1 = (H_2 - H_1) - T(S_2 - S_1)$$

$$\Delta G = \Delta H - T \Delta S \qquad (3-103)$$

Now, equation (3–55) may be written as

$$-\Delta S = -(S_2 - S_1) = \left(\frac{\partial G_2}{\partial T}\right)_P - \left(\frac{\partial G_1}{\partial T}\right)_P$$

or

$$-\Delta S = \left[\frac{\partial (G_2 - G_1)}{\partial T}\right]_P = \left[\frac{\partial (\Delta G)}{\partial T}\right]_P \qquad (3-104)$$

Substituting equation (3–104) into (3–103) gives

$$\Delta G = \Delta H + T \left[\frac{\partial (\Delta G)}{\partial T}\right]_P \qquad (3-105)$$

which is one form of the *Gibbs–Helmholtz equation*.

Standard Free Energy and the Equilibrium Constant. Many of the processes of pharmaceutical interest such as complexation, protein binding, the dissociation of a weak electrolyte, or the distribution of a drug between two immiscible phases are reactions at equilibrium and can be described by an equilibrium constant, K. The relationship between the equilibrium constant and the standard free energy change of the reaction, ΔG°, is one of the more important applications of thermodynamics used to solve equilibrium problems.

Consider a closed system at constant pressure and temperature, such as the chemical reaction

$$aA + bB \rightleftharpoons cC + dD \qquad (3-106)$$

The free energy change of the reaction is

$$\Delta G = \Sigma \Delta G_{products} - \Sigma \Delta G_{reactants} \qquad (3-107)$$

Equation (3–106) represents a closed system made up of several components. Therefore, at constant T and P the total free energy change of the products and reactants in equation (3–107) is given as the sum of the chemical potential μ of each component times the number of moles (p. 67). At equilibrium, ΔG is zero and equation (3–107) becomes

$$\Delta G = (a\mu_A + b\mu_B) - (c\mu_C + d\mu_D) = 0 \qquad (3-108)$$

When the reactants and products are ideal gases the chemical potential of each component is expressed in terms of partial pressure (equation (3–92)). For nonideal gases, μ is written in terms of fugacities (equation (3–93)). The corresponding expressions for solutions are given by equations (3–96) to (3–102). Let us use the more general expression that relates the chemical potential to the activity (equation (3–96)). Substituting this equation for each component in equation (3–108) yields

$$c(\mu^\circ_C + RT \ln a_C) + d(\mu^\circ_D + RT \ln a_D) - $$
$$a(\mu^\circ_A + RT \ln a_A) - b(\mu^\circ_B + RT \ln a_B) = 0 \quad (3-109)$$

Rearranging equation (3-109) gives

$$c\,\mu^\circ_C + d\,\mu^\circ_D - a\mu^\circ_A - b\mu^\circ_B + RT(\ln a^c_C + \ln a^d_D) - $$
$$RT(\ln a^a_A + \ln a^b_B) = 0 \quad (3-110)$$

Since μ° is the partial molar free energy change or chemical potential under standard conditions and is multiplied by the number of moles in equation (3-110), the algebraic sum of the terms involving μ° represents the *total standard free energy change of the reaction*, and is called ΔG°:

$$\Delta G^\circ = c\mu^\circ_C + d\mu^\circ_D - a\mu^\circ_A - b\mu^\circ_B \quad (3-111)$$

or, in general,

$$\Delta G^\circ = \Sigma\, n\mu^\circ(\text{products}) - \Sigma\, n\mu^\circ(\text{reactants}) \quad (3-112)$$

Using the rules of logarithms, equation (3-110) is expressed as

$$\Delta G^\circ + RT \ln \frac{a^c_C\, a^d_D}{a^a_A\, a^b_B} = 0 \quad (3-113)$$

or, in general,

$$\Delta G^\circ = -RT \ln \frac{\Sigma a^n(\text{products})}{\Sigma a^n(\text{reactants})} \quad (3-114)$$

Since ΔG° is a constant at constants P and T, and RT is also constant, it follows that the logarithm of the ratio of activities must also be a constant. Equation (3-113) or (3-114) is then written as

$$\Delta G^\circ = -RT \ln K \quad (3-115)$$

Equation (3-115) is a very important expression that relates the standard free energy change of a reaction ΔG° to the equilibrium constant K. This expression allows one to compute K knowing ΔG° and vice versa.

The equilibrium constant has been expressed in terms of activities. Analogously, it can be given as the ratio of partial pressures, fugacities (for gases), and as the ratio of the different concentration expressions used in solutions (mole fraction, molarity, molality). The equilibrium constant is dimensionless, the ratio of activities or concentration canceling the units. However, the numerical value of K differs depending on the units used (activity, mole fraction, fugacity, etc.).

Example 3-12. Derive an expresssion for the free energies, ΔG and ΔG°, of the reaction

$$\text{Fe}_{(s)} + \text{H}_2\text{O}_{(g)} = \text{FeO}_{(s)} + \text{H}_{2(g)}$$

Since the chemical potential of a solid is constant (it does not depend on concentration), the equilibrium constant depends only on the pressures (or fugacities) of the gases. Using pressures

$$\Delta G = \mu^\circ_{\text{FeO}_{(s)}} + \mu^\circ_{\text{H}_{2(g)}} - \mu^\circ_{\text{Fe}(s)} - \mu^\circ_{\text{H}_2\text{O}(g)} + RT\, P_{\text{H}_{2(g)}} - $$
$$RT\, P_{\text{H}_2\text{O}_{(g)}} = 0$$
$$\Delta G = \Delta G^\circ + RT \ln P_{\text{H}_{2(g)}} - RT\, P_{\text{H}_2\text{O}_{(g)}} = 0$$

and

$$\Delta G^\circ = -RT \ln \frac{P_{\text{H}_{2(g)}}}{P_{\text{H}_2\text{O}_{(g)}}}$$

The magnitude and sign of ΔG° indicate whether the reaction is spontaneous but only under *standard conditions* (see pp. 67, 134). When the reaction is not at equilibrium, $\Delta G \neq 0$ and the free energy change is

$$\Delta G = \Delta G^\circ + RT \ln \frac{\Sigma a^n(\text{products})}{\Sigma a^n(\text{reactants})} \neq 0 \quad (3-116)$$

or

$$\Delta G = \Delta G^\circ + RT \ln Q \quad (3-117)$$

where Q, like K, is the ratio of activities (equation [3-116]) fugacities, or concentration units of the products and reactants, but under different conditions than those of equilibrium. Q should not be confused with K (the ratio of activities, fugacities, and so on under *standard conditions at equilibrium* [see p. 134, for definitions of standard state]).

Example 3-13. Sodium cholate is a bile salt that plays an important role in the dissolution or dispersion of cholesterol and other lipids in the body. Sodium cholate may exist either as monomer or dimer (or higher n-mers) in aqueous solution. Let us consider the equilibrium monomer–dimer reaction[6]:

$$2(\text{monomer}) \overset{K}{\rightleftharpoons} \text{dimer}$$

which states that two moles (or molecules) of monomer form one mole (or molecule) of dimer.

(a) If the molar concentration at 25° C of monomeric species is 4×10^{-3} mole/liter and the concentration of dimers is 3.52×10^{-5} mole/liter, what is the equilibrium constant and the standard free energy for the dimerization process?

$$K = \frac{[\text{dimer}]}{[\text{monomer}]^2} = \frac{3.52 \times 10^{-5}}{(4 \times 10^{-3})^2} = 2.20$$

$$\ln K = 0.788$$

$$\Delta G^\circ = -RT \ln K = -(1.9872 \times 298 \times 0.788) = -466.6 \text{ cal/mole}$$

The process is spontaneous under standard conditions.

(b) While keeping the concentration of monomer constant, suppose that one is able to remove part of the dimeric species by physical or chemical means so that its concentration is now four times less than the original dimer concentration. Compute the free energy change. What is the effect on the equilibrium?

The concentration of dimer is now

$$\frac{3.52 \times 10^{-5}}{4} = 8.8 \times 10^{-6} \text{ mole/liter}$$

Since the conditions are not at equilibrium, equation (3-117) should be used. First calculate Q:

$$Q = \frac{[\text{dimer}]}{[\text{monomer}]^2} = \frac{8.8 \times 10^{-6}}{(4 \times 10^{-3})^2} = 0.550; \ln Q = -0.598$$

and from equation (3-117),

$$\Delta G = -466.6 + [1.9872 \times 298 \times (-0.598)] = -820.7 \text{ cal/mole}$$

ΔG is negative, Q is less than K, and the reaction shifts to the right side of the equation with the formation of more dimer.

If we remove monomer from the solution, the reaction is shifted to the left side, forming monomer, and ΔG becomes positive. Suppose that [monomer] is now 1×10^{-3} mole/liter and [dimer] is 3.52×10^{-5} mole/liter:

$$Q = \frac{3.52 \times 10^{-5}}{(1 \times 10^{-3})^2} = 35.2; \ln Q = 3.561$$

$$\Delta G = -466.6 + (1.9872 \times 298 \times 3.561) = +1642 \text{ cal/mole}$$

The positive sign of ΔG indicates that the reaction does not proceed forward spontaneously.

The van't Hoff Equation. The effect of temperature on equilibrium constants is obtained by writing the equation

$$\ln K = -\frac{\Delta G°}{RT} \qquad (3-118)$$

and differentiating with respect to temperature to give

$$\frac{d \ln K}{dT} = -\frac{1}{R}\frac{d(\Delta G°/T)}{dT} \qquad (3-119)$$

The Gibbs–Helmholtz equation may be written in the form (cf. one of the thermodynamics books given in the footnote on p. 53):

$$\frac{d(\Delta G/T)}{dT} = -\frac{\Delta H}{T^2} \qquad (3-120)$$

Expressing equation (3–120) in a form for the reactants and products in their standard states, in which ΔG becomes equal to $\Delta G°$, and substituting into equation (3–119), yields

$$\frac{d \ln K}{dT} = \frac{\Delta H°}{RT^2} \qquad (3-121)$$

in which $\Delta H°$ is the standard heat of reaction. Equation (3–121) is known as the *van't Hoff equation*. It may be integrated, assuming $\Delta H°$ to be constant over the temperature range considered; it thus becomes

$$\ln \frac{K_2}{K_1} = \frac{\Delta H°}{R}\left(\frac{T_2 - T_1}{T_1 T_2}\right) \qquad (3-122)$$

Equation (3–122) allows one to compute the heat of a reaction if the equilibrium constants at T_1 and T_2 are available. Conversely, it can be used to supply the equilibrium constant at a definite temperature if it is known at another temperature. $\Delta H°$ varies with temperature, however, and equation (3–122) gives only an approximate answer; more elaborate equations are required to obtin accurate results. The solubility of a solid in an ideal solution is a special type of equilibrium, and it is not surprising that equation (10–11), p. 221, can be written as

$$\ln \frac{X_2}{X_1} = \frac{\Delta H_f}{R}\left(\frac{T_2 - T_1}{T_1 T_2}\right) \qquad (3-123)$$

which closely resembles equation (3–122). These expressions will be encountered in later chapters.

Combining equations (3–103) and (3–118) yields yet another form of the van't Hoff equation, namely

$$\ln K = -(\Delta H°/R)1/T + \Delta S°/R \qquad (3-124)$$

or

$$\log K = -[\Delta H°/(2.303R)]1/T + \Delta S°/(2.303R) \qquad (3-125)$$

in which $\Delta S°/R$ is the intercept on the $\ln K$ axis of a plot of $\ln K$ versus $1/T$.

Whereas equation (3–122) provides a value of $\Delta H°$ based on the use of two K values at their corresponding absolute temperatures, T_1 and T_2, equations (3–124) and (3–125) give the values of $\Delta H°$ and $\Delta S°$, and therefore the value of $\Delta G° = \Delta H° - T\Delta S°$. In the least-squares linear regression equations (3–124) and (3–125), one uses as many $\ln K$ and corresponding $1/T$ values as are available from experimentation.

Example 3–14. In a study of the transport of pilocarpine across the corneal membrane of the eye, Mitra and Mikkelson[7] presented a van't Hoff plot of the log of the ionization constant, $\log K_a$, of pilocarpine versus the reciprocal of the absolute temperature, $T^{-1} = 1/T$.

Using the data in Table 3–5, regress $\log K_a$ versus T^{-1}. With reference to the van't Hoff equation (equation 3–124), obtain the standard heat (enthalpy), $\Delta H°$, of ionization for pilocarpine and the standard entropy for the ionization process. From $\Delta H°$ and $\Delta S°$ calculate $\Delta G°$ at 25° C. What is the significance of the signs and the magnitudes of $\Delta H°$, $\Delta S°$, and $\Delta G°$?

Answers:

$$\Delta H° = 9784 \text{ cal/mole}$$
$$= 40.94 \text{ kJ/mole}$$
$$\Delta S° = 1.30 \text{ cal/mole deg}$$
$$\Delta G°_{25°} = \Delta H° - T\Delta S° = 9397 \text{ cal/mole}$$

These thermodynamic values have the following significance. $\Delta H°$ is a large positive value that indicates that the ionization of pilocarpine (as its conjugate acid) should increase as the temperature is elevated. The increasing values of K_a in the table show this to be a fact. The standard entropy increase, $\Delta S° = 1.30$ entropy units, although small, provides a force for the reaction of the pilocarpinium ions to form pilocarpine (Fig. 3–4). The positively charged pilocarpine molecules, because of their ionic nature, are probably held in a more orderly arrangement than the predominantly nonionic pilocarpine in the aqueous environment. This increase in disorder in the dissociation process accounts

TABLE 3–5. *Ionization Constants of Pilocarpine at Various Temperatures*

Temperature				
$(t)°$ C	$T(°$ K)	$1/T \times 10^{3*}$	$K_a \times 10^{7*}$	$\log K_a$
15	288	3.47	0.74	−7.13
20	293	3.41	1.07	−6.97
25	298	3.35	1.26	−6.90
30	303	3.30	1.58	−6.80
35	308	3.24	2.14	−6.67
40	313	3.19	2.95	−6.53
45	318	3.14	3.98	−6.40

*When a column is headed $1/T \times 10^3$ it means that the numbers in this column are 1000 (i.e., 10^3) times *larger* than the actual numbers. Thus the first entry in column 3 has the real value 3.47×10^{-3} or 0.00347. Likewise, in the next column $K_a \times 10^7$ signifies that the number 0.74 and the other entries in this column are to be accompanied by the exponential value 10^{-7}, not 10^{+7}. Thus, the first value in the fourth column should be read as 0.74×10^{-7} and the last value 3.98×10^{-7}. (From A. K. Mitra and T. J. Mikkelson, J. Pharm. Sci. 77, 772, 1988, (reproduced with permission of the publishers.)

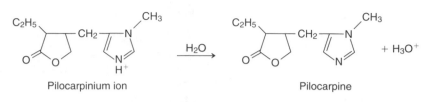

Fig. 3–4. Reaction of pilocarpinium ion to yield pilocarpine base.

for the increased entropy, which, however, is a small value: $\Delta S° = 1.30$ entropy units. Note that a positive $\Delta H°$ does not mean that the ionization will not occur; rather, it signifies that the equilibrium constant for the forward reaction (ionization) will be a small value, say $K_a \cong 1 \times 10^{-7}$, as observed in Table 3–5. A further explanation regarding the sign of $\Delta H°$ is helpful here. Mahan[8] has pointed out that in the first stage of ionization of phosphoric acid (p. 149), for example,

$$H_3PO_4 \rightarrow H^+ + H_2PO_4^-; \quad \Delta H° = -3.1 \text{ kcal/mole}$$

the hydration reaction of the ions being bound to the water molecules is sufficiently exothermic to produce the necessary energy for ionization; that is, enough energy to remove the proton from the acid, H_3PO_4. For this reason, $\Delta H°$ in the first stage of ionization is negative and $K_1 = 7.5 \times 10^{-3}$ at 25° C (see Table 7–1). In the second stage,

$$H_2PO_4^- \rightarrow H^+ + HPO_4^{2-}; \quad \Delta H° = 0.9 \text{ kcal/mole}$$

$\Delta H°$ is now positive, the reaction is *endothermic*, and $K_2 = 6.2 \times 10^{-8}$. Finally, in the third stage,

$$HPO_4^{2-} \rightarrow H^+ + PO_4^{3-}; \quad \Delta H° = 4.5 \text{ kcal/mole}$$

$\Delta H°$ is a relatively large positive value and $K_3 = 2.1 \times 10^{-13}$. These $\Delta H°$ and K_a values show that increasing energy is needed to remove the positively charged proton as the negative charge increases in the acid from the first to the third stage of ionization. Positive $\Delta H°$ (endothermic reaction) values do not signal nonionization of the acid—that is, that the process is nonspontaneous—but rather simply show that the forward reaction, represented by its ionization constant, becomes smaller and smaller.

References and Notes

1. I. M. Klotz and R. M. Rosenberg, *Chemical Thermodynamics*, Benjamin/Cummings, Menlo Park, Calif., 1972, pp. 113–114.
2. W. M. Latimer, Chem. Eng. News **31**, 3366, 1953.
3. W. E. Roseveare, J. Chem. Educ. **15**, 214, 1938.
4. H. Borsook and H. M. Winegarden, Proc. Natl. Acad. Sci. U.S.A. **17**, 3, 1931.
5. J. M. Klotz, *Chemical Thermodynamics*, Prentice-Hall, Englewood Cliffs, N.J., 1950, p. 226.
6. M. Vadnere and S. Lindenbaum, J. Pharm. Sci. **71**, 875, 1982.
7. A. K. Mitra and T. J. Mikkelson, J. Pharm. Sci. **77**, 771, 1988.
8. B. H. Mahan, *Elementary Chemical Thermodynamics*, Benjamin/Cummings, Menlo Park, Calif., 1963, pp. 139–142.
9. H. A. Bent, *The Second Law*, Oxford, 1965, pp. 15, 381; J. Bronowsky, *The Ascent of Man*, Little, Brown, Boston, 1973, pp. 286, 288.
10. S. Glasstone, *Thermodynamics for Chemists*, Van Nostrand, 1947, pp. 53, 503.
11. A. V. Hill, *Adventures in Biophysics*, Oxford University Press, Oxford, 1931.
12. D. D. Wagman et al., *Selected Values of Chemical Thermodynamic Properties*, National Bureau of Standards, Washington, D.C., 1968.
13. J. W. Moncrief and W. H. Jones, *Elements of Physical Chemistry*, Addison-Wesley, Reading, Mass., 1977, pp. 69, 119.
14. A. H. Taylor and R. H. Crist, J. Am. Chem. Soc. **63**, 1377, 1941.
15. S. Glasstone, *Textbook of Physical Chemistry*, Van Nostrand, New York, 1946, p. 834.

Problems*

3–1. Why is alcohol used in thermometers for measuring very low temperatures, whereas mercury is used for high temperatures? *Hint:* Look up in a handbook of chemistry and physics the melting points of alcohol and mercury.

3–2. Calculate the work to vaporize 1.73 moles of water at 0.68 atm pressure and a temperature of 373° K. Assume that the vapor behaves as an ideal gas. *Hint:* The volume may be calculated using the ideal gas equation and the work may be calculated using $W = P\Delta V$. ΔV is the difference in volume between liquid water at 373° K, i.e., 18.795 cm³/mole × 1.73 mole, and its vapor at 373° K.

Answer: The work is 52.96 liter atm or 5366 J (1 liter atm = 101.328 J).

3–3. By the use of thermodynamic calculations, we can relate work done and heat produced in various processes regardless of how seemingly unrelated the processes might be. Consider the following: A 30-year-old man weighing 70 kg (154 lb) produces 3600 kcal of heat per 24 hours working 8 hours as a brick layer and bowling in the evenings. If this heat were used to raise the temperature of 200 kg of water (specific heat of water = 1 cal g⁻¹ deg⁻¹)† that was originally at 25° C, how hot would the water become?

**Problem 3–4 is modified from J. W. Moncrief and W. H. Jones, *Elements of Physical Chemistry*, Addison-Wesley, Reading, Mass., 1977, p. 15, example 7. Problem 3–5 is modified from Moncrief and Jones, ibid, p. 28, example 12. Problem 3–14 is modified from Moncrief and Jones, ibid, p. 96. Problem 3–15 is modified from Moncrief and Jones, ibid, p. 64, example 17. Problem 3–20 is from Moncrief and Jones, ibid, p. 123, problem 6.6. Problem 3–23 is from Moncrief and Jones, ibid, p. 123, problem 6.8. Problem 3–27 is from A. L. Lehninger, *Bioenergetics*, 2nd Edition, Benjamin/Cummins, Menlo Park, Calif., 1971, pp 30, 31; I. M. Klotz, *Introduction to Biomolecular Energetics*, Academic Press, Orlando, Fl., p. 24.*

†The term *heat capacity* is usually expressed in cal or joules mole⁻¹ deg⁻¹. When it is referred to as 1 gram or 1 kilogram of material rather than as 1 mole it is called *specific heat* rather than *heat capacity.*

Answer: The temperature of the mass of water would be raised 18° K ≡ 18° C. The final temperature would be 25° + 18° = 43° C.

3–4. An athlete resting on his back on the floor lifts an 80-lb dumbbell 2 feet above his head. From physics we know that force = mass × acceleration of gravity, and the force multiplied by the distance the mass is lifted yields the work done or energy used.

(a) How much work is done when the dumbbell is lifted 500 times?

(b) If we assume that the energy expended is obtained totally from burning body fat, how many pounds will the athlete lose in this exercise? Approximately 9.0 kilocalories of metabolic energy are obtained per gram of fat burned.

(c) How many lifts of the 80-lb weight would be required to lose 1 lb of fat?

(d) It is agreed that exercise such as weight-lifting is excellent to tone the muscles of the body. From your calculations do you find that it also contributes significantly to weight reduction as part of a diet regimen?

Answers: **(a)** $W = 1.09 \times 10^5$ J or 2.6×10^4 cal = 26 kcal (food calories). **(b)** The person loses 2.9 g or 0.006 lb. **(c)** More than 8000 lifts would be required to lose 1 lb of fat from the body (actually 8333 lifts).

3–5. An active adult woman generates about 3000 kcal of heat per day and it is lost through metabolism. If all the heat is lost by evaporation of moisture from the skin, how much water is lost in a 24-hour day? The heat of vaporization of water is $\Delta H_v \approx 10,000$ cal/mole and the density is 0.997049 g/cm^3 at 25° C.

Answer: 5.4 liters or 5.7 quarts. Of course, water is also eliminated by way of the kidneys, lungs, and feces, and the water loss from these various routes with normal food intake should also be taken into account.

3–6. James Joule found a waterfall in Switzerland that was 920 ft (280.42 m) high. The potential energy of the water at the top of the falls is converted at the bottom into kinetic energy (heat) by friction, as observed in Figure 3–2, and Joule was interested in studying these energy changes. What is the difference in the temperature between the top and the bottom of the falls which Joules would have been expected to find if he had used a very accurate thermometer?

Use SI units in your calculations, then repeat using cgs units. Assume that the velocity of the water at the top of the falls is essentially zero so that we are considering only the potential energy of fall. The specific heat of water is 1 cal/g °K in the cgs system.

Answer: 0.66° K, 0.66° C

3–7. As we learned on page 58, Joule had a bad day. He did not have the attention of his bride on their honeymoon nor was he successful in his study of the thermodynamics of waterfalls. According to Bent,[9] Joule later did estimate—probably from the kind of calculations in *Example 3–4*—that the water at the base of Niagara Falls at the Canadian–U.S. border (Horseshoe Falls) should be approximately 0.2° Fahrenheit warmer than the water at the top of the falls.

Using the calculation given in *Example 3–4*, estimate the height of Horseshoe Falls. Check the height you have calculated with the actual height given in an encyclopedia.

Answer: 154 feet or 46.9 meters

3–8. At the beginning of the nineteenth century, Dulong and Petit determined the heat capacity, C_v, of solid elements to be approximately 6 cal mole^{-1} °K^{-1}.

A bar of iron, atomic weight = 55.847 g, falls accidentally from the top of a building 93 meters high. Taking the molar heat capacity C_v of iron as approximately 6 cal mole^{-1} °K^{-1}, compute the increase in temperature of the bar as it falls from the top of the building to the street. Use SI units in your calculations.

We actually desire the heat capacity per gram (i.e., the specific heat), or, since we are using SI units, we want the heat capacity per kilogram. To convert from calories/mole to calories/gram we divide the molar heat capacity of iron by its "molecular" or atomic weight, 55.847 g. Thus,

$$C_v = \frac{6 \text{ cal mole}^{-1} \text{ °K}^{-1}}{55.847 \text{ g mole}^{-1}} = 0.1074 \text{ cal/g °K} = 107.4 \frac{\text{cal}}{\text{kg °K}}$$

The calculations are analogous to those for the waterfall's temperature change, *Problem 3–6. Hint:* Express C_v in J/(kg °K).

Answer: The increase in temperature of the iron bar as a result of falling 93 meters from the top of the building to the street below is 2.03° C = 2.03° K.

3–9. The molar heat capacity at constant pressure, C_p, varies with temperature. The changes in the heat capacity, ΔC_p, for a reaction at a fixed temperature is given by the expression

$$\Delta C_p = \sum (nC_p)_{products} - \sum (nC_p)_{reactants}$$

where Σ stands for "the sum of" and n is the number of moles of the compound.

C_p can be calculated at different temperatures using the empirical equation

$$C_p = \alpha + \beta T + \gamma T^2 + \ldots$$

where α, β, and γ are constant coefficients. C_p and ΔC_p are given here in cal °K^{-1} mole^{-1}.

Calculate C_p for CO$_{(g)}$, H$_{2(g)}$, and CH$_3$OH$_{(g)}$ at 25° C and compute the change in heat capacity, ΔC_p, for the reaction:

$$CO_{(g)} + H_{2(g)} \rightarrow CH_3OH_{(g)}$$

Data for *Problem 3–9**

	CO$_{(g)}$	H$_{2(g)}$	CH$_3$OH$_{(g)}$
α	6.342	6.947	4.398
$\beta \times 10^3$	1.836	−0.20	24.274
$\gamma \times 10^6$	−0.2801	0.4808	−6.855

*From S. Glasstone, *Thermodynamics for Chemists*, Van Nostrand, New York, 1947, pp. 53, 503.

Answer: C_p(CO) = 6.864 cal °K^{-1} mole^{-1}; C_p(H$_2$) = 6.930 cal °K^{-1} mole^{-1}; C_p(CH$_3$OH) = 11.025 cal °K^{-1} mole^{-1}. For the reaction at 25°C, $\Delta C_p = -9.699$ cal °K^{-1} mole^{-1}

3–10. Equation (3–22b) on page 57, the Kirchhoff equation, demonstrates the effect of temperature on the heat of reaction. Integration of equation (3–22b) between T_1 and T_2 is shown as

$$\Delta H_2 - \Delta H_1 = \int_{T_1}^{T_2} \Delta C_P \, dT$$

Over a small temperature range, ΔC_p may be considered constant, then the above integration simplifies to

$$\Delta H_2 - \Delta H_1 = \Delta C_p(T_2 - T_1)$$

Compute ΔH_2° for the synthesis of methanol at 35° C, using ΔH_1° at 25° C as −21.68 kcal per mole as obtained in *Problem 3–12*, and ΔC_p as the value, −9.699 cal/(deg mole), obtained in *Problem 3–9*, as the value at 25° C. Remember to write ΔC_p as -9.699×10^{-3} kcal/(deg mole) in order to obtain ΔH_2° in kcal/mole.

Answer: ΔH_2° (at 35° C) = −21.78 kcal/mole

3–11. The heat of reaction associated with the preparation of calcium hydroxide is represented as

$$CaO_{(s)} + H_2O_{(liq)} = Ca(OH)_{2(s)}; \quad \Delta H_{25^\circ} = -15.6 \text{ kcal}$$

What is the standard heat of formation ΔH° of Ca(OH)$_2$ at 25° C? The standard heat of formation of water ΔH°(H$_2$O$_{(liq)}$) = −68.3 kcal/mole and the standard heat of formation of calcium oxide ΔH° (CaO$_{(s)}$) = −151.9 kcal/mole.

Answer: ΔH° [Ca(OH)$_{2(s)}$] = −235.8 kcal/mole

3–12. The synthesis of methanol involves the reaction of carbon monoxide and hydrogen gas. The reaction, together with values at 25°

C for S^0 cal deg^{-1} mole^{-1}, ΔH_f° in kcal mole^{-1}, and ΔG_f° in kcal mole^{-1}, is given as follows[10]:

$$CO_{(g)} + 2H_{2(g)} \rightarrow CH_3OH_{(g)}$$

Data for *Problem 3-12*

	$CO_{(g)}$	$H_{2(g)}$	$CH_3OH_{(g)}$
S^0	47.219	31.208	56.63
ΔH_f°	−26.416	0	−48.10
ΔG_f°	−32.78	0	−38.90

(a) Calculate ΔH° for the synthesis of methanol under standard conditions. (b) Calculate ΔG°, using the above data. (c) From ΔG° and ΔH°, compute ΔS° at 25° C. Compare this value with ΔS° obtained directly from S^0 in the above table.

Answers: (a) ΔH° = −21.684 kcal/mole; (b) ΔG° = −6.12 kcal/mole; (c) ΔS° (from ΔG° and ΔH°) = −52.20 cal/mole degree. ΔS° (from S^0 values in the table) = −53.01 cal/mole deg.

3-13. What is the theoretical efficiency of a steam engine operating between the boiler at 20 atm, where the boiling point of water T_2 is 209° C (482° K), and the low temperature reservoir or sink, where the temperature T_1 is 30° C (303° K).*

Answer: Efficiency = 0.37 or 37%

3-14. What is the minimum work in joules that must be done by a refrigerator to freeze 1 avoirdupois pound (453.6 grams) of water at 0° C with the surroundings at 23° C? How much heat is discharged into the room at room temperature (23° C)? The heat of fusion of ice is 1438 cal/mole or 1438/18.016 g/mole = 79.8 cal/g (in the range of 0° to 100°). Thus, 79.8 cal/g × 453.6 g of heat must be removed from the water to form ice (from 0° or 273° K [T_1] to 296° K [T_2]).

The principle of a refrigerator (or air conditioner) is the opposite to that of a heat engine.* The refrigerator fluid takes up heat at the low temperature of the refrigerator and discharges it at the higher temperature of the surroundings (see p. 60 for an explanation of a heat engine).

Since heat is discharged in a refrigerator (or air conditioner) rather than taken up, as in a heat engine, the work has the opposite sign to that given in equation (3-29):

$$-\frac{W}{Q_1} = \frac{T_2 - T_1}{T_1}$$

$$-W = \left(\frac{T_2 - T_1}{T_1}\right) Q_1$$

What is the efficiency $(T_2 - T_1)/T_1$ or, as it is called, the *coefficient of performance* of this refrigerator?

Answer: The work required to remove the heat from 1 pound of water and form ice at 0° C is 1.28×10^4 J in a refrigerator in an environment at 23° C. The coefficient of performance of the refrigerator is 0.084 or 8.4%.

3-15. What is the entropy change involved in the fusion of 1 mole of ice at 0° C? What is the entropy change in the surroundings? The heat of fusion of ice is 79.67 cal/g.

Answer: ΔS_{H_2O} = 5.26 cal/(mole deg); $\Delta S_{surr.}$ = −5.26 cal/(mole deg)

3-16. A Thermos jug, insulated so that no heat enters or leaves the container (adiabatic), contains 2 moles of ice at −10° C and 8.75 moles of liquid water at 20° C. (See *Examples 3-6* and *3-7* on p. 62.)

Calculate the change in entropy, ΔS, accompanying the melting of the ice and elevation of its temperature to 0.496° C in the form of liquid water. Also calculate ΔS for the lowering of the temperature of the water from 20° C to the final temperature of 0.496° C. The molar

---

*From S. Glasstone, *Thermodynamics for Chemists.* Van Nostrand, New York, 1947, pp. 138, 139.

heat of fusion of ice is 1437 cal/mole and C_p for ice is 9 cal/(deg mole); C_p for liquid water is 18 cal/(deg mole).

Obtain the total entropy change ΔS_T and state whether the process is spontaneous or not.

Answers (see *Example 3-7*): The heat needed to raise the temperature of the ice and melt it results from the cooling of the water in the insulated Thermos jug.

In heating 2 moles of ice from −10° C to 0° C, the entropy change in this reversible process at constant pressure is 0.671 cal/deg.

Melting of the 2 mole of ice reversibly at 0° C is accompanied by an entropy change of 10.52 cal/deg.

The 2 moles of ice that have now been melted to liquid water is heated to 0.496° C and this step involves an entropy change of 0.0653 cal/deg.

Finally, the 8.75 moles of liquid water added to the jug at 20° C is cooled reversibly to 0.496° C. The entropy change in this final step is −10.84 cal/deg.

The total entropy change is

$$\Delta S_T = 0.671 + 10.52 + 0.0653 − 10.84 = 0.42 \text{ cal } °K^{-1}$$

It is left for the student to calculate each of these above values and to state whether the process is spontaneous or not.

3-17. At 50° C, a certain protein denatures reversibly with a heat of reaction of 29,288 J mole^{-1}:

$$\text{native protein} \rightleftarrows \text{denatured protein};$$

$$\Delta H_{50^\circ} = 29,288 \text{ J mole}^{-1}$$

The system is at equilibrium and $\Delta G = 0$. Compute the entropy change for the reaction.

Answer: ΔS = 90.6 J °K^{-1} mole^{-1}

3-18. According to Hill,[11] the stomach excretes HCl in the concentration of 0.14 M from the blood where the concentration is 5.0×10^{-8} M. Calculate the work done by the body in the transport (excretion) of 1 mole of HCl at a temperature of 37° C.

Answer: 9150 cal/mole

3-19. Rework *Example 3-11*, page 68, first converting ΔH_V into the units of joules/mole and P_2 into Pascals (Pa = N m^{-2} = kg m^{-1} s^{-2}). Calculate ΔH_V in J/mole and P_1 in units of Pascals.

Answer: ΔH_V = 41003 J/mole; P_1 = 86908 Pa

3-20. For the ionization of acetic acid in aqueous solution,

$$\begin{array}{cccc} & CH_3COOH \text{ (aq)} = & CH_3COO^- \text{ (aq)} + & H^+ \text{ (aq)} \\ \Delta G_f^\circ = & −95.48 & −88.99 & 0.00 \end{array}$$

The *standard free energies of formation* G_f° at 25° C are given immediately under each species in kcal/mole. Calculate the standard free energy change ΔG° for this reaction; and from the thermodynamic equation giving the equilibrium constant (ionization constant), $\Delta G^\circ = -RT \ln K$, calculate K for acetic acid. Compare your result with the value found in Table 7-1.

Answer: ΔG° = 6490 cal/mole; $K = 1.75 \times 10^{-5}$

3-21. Given the standard free energy of formation, ΔG°, and the standard enthalpy of formation, ΔH°, calculate the standard entropy change ΔS° and the equilibrium constant K for the reaction

$$CO_2 \text{ (g)} + H_2O \text{ (liq)} = HCO_3^- \text{ (aq)} + H^+ \text{ (aq)}$$

The values for ΔG° and ΔH° are obtained from tables of standard thermochemical data (Wagman et al.[12]) for 1 mole at 1 atm pressure and 25° C, where (aq) refers to a hypothetical ideal aqueous solution. The values of ΔG° and ΔH° for H$^+$ (aq) are taken as 0.00.

For the various species in solution, the values of ΔG° and ΔH° in kcal/mole are as follows:

	CO_2(g)	H_2O(liq)	HCO_3^-(aq)	H^+(aq)
ΔG° (kcal/mole)	−94.254	−56.687	−140.3	0.0
ΔH° (kcal/mole)	−94.051	−68.315	−164.8	0.0

Answer: ΔS° = −44 e.u.; $K = 1.59 \times 10^{-8}$

3-22. For the reaction of carbon dioxide and molecular hydrogen to form carbon monoxide:

$$CO_2(g) + H_2(g) = CO(g) + H_2O(liq)$$

calculate the standard free energy of the process at 25° C and obtain the equilibrium constant K. The standard heat of formation for $CO_2(g)$ is $\Delta H_f^\circ = -94.051$ kcal/mole and its standard entropy is $S^\circ = 51.06$ cal/deg mole. The standard heat of formation of $CO(g)$ is $\Delta H_f^\circ = -26.416$ kcal/mole and its standard entropy is $S^\circ = 47.2$ cal/deg mole. The standard heat of formation of water (liq) is $\Delta H_f^\circ = -68.315$ kcal/mole and its standard entropy $S^\circ = 18.5$ cal/deg mole. Finally, the standard entropy of $H_2(g)$ is $S^\circ = 31.208$ cal/deg mole. By convention its ΔH_f° is 0.0.

Answer: $\Delta G^\circ = 4260$ cal/mole; $K = 7.54 \times 10^{-4}$

3–23. For one of the steps in the citric acid (Krebs) cycle,[13]

(a)

	oxaloacetate^{2-} +	$H_2O \rightarrow$	pyruvate +	HCO_3^-
ΔG°(kcal/mol)	-190.53	-56.69	-113.32	-140.29

and for another step in this complex series of chemical reactions required for energy production in the body,

(b)

	oxaloacetate^{2-}	+ acetate $\rightarrow$	citrate^{3-}
ΔG°(kcal/mol)	-190.53	-88.99	-273.90

Calculate ΔG° and K at 37° C for these two reactions.

Answer: **(a)** $\Delta G^\circ = -6.39$ kcal/mole, $K = 3.2 \times 10^4$; **(b)** $\Delta G^\circ = 5.62$ kcal/mole, $K = 1.1 \times 10^{-4}$

3–24. Diluted hydriodic acid (HI) is a pharmaceutical product containing 10% of HI and about 0.8% of hypophosphorous acid (H_3PO_2) to prevent discoloration of the aqueous preparation in the presence of light and air.

Hydriodic acid is prepared on a large scale by several processes, principally by the interaction of I_2 and H_2S. Diluted hydriodic may be made into a syrup with dextrose and used for the therapeutic properties of the iodides and as a vehicle for expectorant drugs.

Taylor and Crist[14] investigated the reaction of hydrogen and iodine to form hydrogen iodide at a temperature of 457.6° C (730.75° K),

$$H_2 + I_2 = 2\ HI$$

They obtained the following results in which K is the equilibrium constant,

Data for *Problem 3–24*

$K = \dfrac{[HI]^2}{[H_2][I_2]}$		
H_2 mole/liter	I_2 mole/liter	HI mole/liter
3.841×10^{-3}	1.524×10^{-3}	1.687×10^{-2}
1.696×10^{-3}	1.696×10^{-3}	1.181×10^{-2}
5.617×10^{-3}	0.5936×10^{-3}	1.270×10^{-2}

(a) Calculate the equilibrium constants for the three experiments shown above and obtain the average of these K values at 730.75° K.

(b) At 666.8° K the average equilibrium constant $K_{av.}$ for the reaction of I_2 and H_2 to form hydrogen iodide (hydriodic acid) is 60.80.[15] Calculate the enthalpy change ΔH° for the reaction over the temperature range of 666.8 to 730.75° K.

(c) Does the constant, K, increase or decrease as the temperature is elevated? What does this say about an increased or decreased production of hydrogen iodide from its elements as the temperature is elevated? Do these results suggest that the reaction would be exothermic or endothermic? What quantitative result do you have to answer this last question? How does the van't Hoff equation (equation 3–122) help to answer this question?

Answers: **(a)** $K_{av.} = 48.49$; **(b)** $\Delta H^\circ = -3425$ cal $= -14330$ J; **(c)** this series of questions is left for the student to assure himself or herself of an understanding of chemical equilibria.

3–25. Equation (3–115) allows the student to calculate the free energy change at the three separate temperatures for the reaction of hydrogen and iodine to yield hydrogen iodide. Given the experimentally determined K values and corresponding absolute temperatures,

Data for *Problem 3–25*

K	45.62	48.49	60.80
T (°K)	763.8	730.8	666.8

calculate the standard free energy change at these three temperatures.

Answer: ΔG° at 763.8° K $= -5799$ cal; ΔG° at 730.8° K $= -5637$ cal; ΔG° at 666.8° K $= -5443$ cal

3–26. A student cannot find the heat of vaporization, the heat of sublimation, or the heat of fusion of water in her handbook of chemical properties, but she is able to find a table of vapor pressures (in mm Hg) for liquid water in equilibrium with its vapor at temperatures from $-15°$ C to $+20°$ C, and for ice in equilibrium with its vapor from $-50°$ C to 0° C.

For ice passing directly to water vapor (sublimation), and for the conversion of liquid water to vapor (vaporization), the following values are found (Table 3–6).

(a) Plot the sublimation and vaporization curves in the form of ln(vapor pressure) vs. $1/T$ (°K^{-1}).

(b) Using the indefinite integrated form of the Clausius–Clapeyron equation,

$$\ln P = -\frac{\Delta H}{R}\frac{1}{T} + \text{constant}$$

calculate the heat of vaporization and the heat of sublimation for water within the temperature ranges found in Table 3–6. ΔH is the heat of vaporization or the heat of sublimation. Linear regression on the data in Table 3–6, ln(vapor pressure) vs. $1/T$, yields $(-\Delta H/R)$ as the slope from which ΔH_v or ΔH_s is obtained. An estimate of the slope,

$$\frac{\ln P_2 - \ln P_1}{\left(\dfrac{1}{T_2} - \dfrac{1}{T_1}\right)}$$

may also be obtained from a plot of ln P versus $1/T$ on rectangular coordinate graph paper. Use least-squares linear regression, or the

TABLE 3–6. *Vapor Pressures for the Sublimation and Vaporization of Water, for Problem 3–26*

Ice → vapor (sublimation)		liq. water → vapor (vaporization)	
Vapor press. (mm Hg)	t (° C)	Vapor press. (mm Hg)	t (°C)
0.0296	-50	1.436	-15
0.0966	-40	1.691	-13
0.2859	-30	2.149	-10
0.476	-25	2.715	-7
0.776	-20	3.163	-5
1.241	-15	3.673	-3
1.950	-10	4.579	0
3.013	-5	6.593	5
4.579	0	9.209	10
—	—	12.788	15
—	—	17.535	20

slope of the line obtained from a plot of the data, to calculate ΔH_v and ΔH_s.

(c) For conversion of a solid to a vapor at constant temperature the process should be independent of the path: solid → liquid → vapor; therefore, $\Delta H_s = \Delta H_v + \Delta H_f$, where ΔH_f is the enthalpy change involved in the fusion (melting) process.

Compute ΔH_f (for the transition water → ice) from ΔH_v and ΔH_s obtained in (b).

Answers: (b) For ice to water vapor (sublimation) the least-squares line is expressed by the equation $\ln P_s = -6146.5\,\dfrac{1}{T} + 24.025$; $r^2 = 0.9999$; for sublimation, ice to vapor, $\Delta H_s = 12{,}214$ cal/mol within a range of -50 to $0°$ C. For liquid water to vapor (vaporization), $\ln P_v = -5409\,\dfrac{1}{T} + 21.321$; $r^2 = 0.9999$; $\Delta H_v = 10{,}749$ cal/mol within a range of $-15°$ to $20°$ C. (c) Finally, one calculates $\Delta H_f = 1465$ cal/mole. Experimentally, $\Delta H_f(H_2O) = 1440$ cal/mole.*

(*A satisfactory ΔH of sublimation is not always obtained by this procedure.)

3–27. In the breakdown (metabolism) of glycogen in the muscle of man to form lactate, glucose 1-phosphate is converted to glucose 6-phosphate in the presence of the enzyme phosphoglucomutase:

$$\text{glucose 1-phosphate} \rightleftharpoons \text{glucose 6-phosphate}$$

This biochemical reaction has been studied in some detail in a number of laboratories and the standard free energy change, $\Delta G°$, is found to be about -1727 cal/mole. Calculate the equilibrium constant K at $25°$ C.

$$K = \frac{[\text{glucose 6-phosphate}]}{[\text{glucose 1-phosphate}]}$$

Hint: The application of equation (3–115) allows one to calculate the equilibrium constant.

Answer: K = 18.45

4
Physical Properties of Drug Molecules*

Electromagnetic Radiation
Atomic Spectra
Molecular Spectra
Ultraviolet and Visible Spectrophotometry
Fluorescence and Phosphorescence
Dielectric Constant and Induced Polarization
Permanent Dipole Moment of Polar Molecules

Infrared Spectroscopy
Electron Spin and Nuclear Magnetic Resonance Spectroscopy
Refractive Index and Molar Refraction
Optical Rotation
Circular Dichroism

A study of the physical properties of drug molecules is a prerequisite for product formulation and often leads to a better understanding of the interrelationship between molecular structure and drug action. These properties may be thought of as either *additive* (derived from the sum of the properties of the individual atoms or functional groups within the molecule) or *constitutive* (dependent on the structural arrangement of the atoms within the molecule). Mass is an additive property, whereas optical rotation may be thought of as a constitutive property.

Many physical properties are constitutive and yet have some measure of additivity. Molar refraction of a compound, for example, is the sum of the refraction (p. 95) of the atoms and groups making up the compound. The arrangements of atoms in each group are different, however, and so the refractive index of two molecules will be different; that is, the individual groups in two different molecules contribute different amounts to the overall refraction of the molecules.

A sample calculation will clarify the principle of additivity and constitutivity. The molar refractions of the two compounds,

$$
\begin{array}{c}
O \\
\parallel \\
C_2H_5 - C - CH_3
\end{array}
$$

and

$$CH_3 - CH = CH - CH_2 - OH,$$

having exactly the same number of carbon, hydrogen, and oxygen atoms, are calculated using Table 4–1.

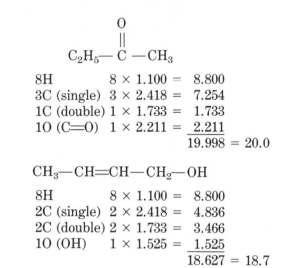

$$
\begin{array}{c}
O \\
\parallel \\
C_2H_5 - C - CH_3
\end{array}
$$

8H	$8 \times 1.100 =$	8.800
3C (single)	$3 \times 2.418 =$	7.254
1C (double)	$1 \times 1.733 =$	1.733
1O (C=O)	$1 \times 2.211 =$	2.211
		19.998 = 20.0

$$CH_3 - CH = CH - CH_2 - OH$$

8H	$8 \times 1.100 =$	8.800
2C (single)	$2 \times 2.418 =$	4.836
2C (double)	$2 \times 1.733 =$	3.466
1O (OH)	$1 \times 1.525 =$	1.525
		18.627 = 18.7

Thus, although these two compounds have the same number of atoms of a definite kind, their molar

TABLE 4–1. *Atomic and Group Contributions to Molar Refraction**

C—(single)	2.418
—C=(double)	1.733
—C≡(triple)	2.398
Phenyl (C_6H_5)	25.463
H	1.100
O (C=O)	2.211
O (O—H)	1.525
O (ether, ester, C—O)	1.643
Cl	5.967
Br	8.865
I	13.900

*These values are reported for the D-line of sodium as the light source. (From *Lange's Handbook,* 12th Edition, J. Dean, Ed., McGraw-Hill, New York, 1979, p. 10–94. See also Bower et al., in *Physical Methods of Organic Chemistry,* 3rd Edition, A. Weissberger, Ed., Vol. 1, Part II, Chapter 28, Wiley-Interscience, New York, 1960.)

*This chapter was prepared by Dr. Allan E. Klein, Director of Quality Assurance and Regulatory Affairs, Oneida Research Services, One Halsey Road, Whitesboro, NY.

refractions are not the same. The molar refractions of the atoms are additive, but the carbon and oxygen atoms are constitutive in refraction. A single-bonded carbon does not add equally as a double-bonded carbon, and a carbonyl oxygen (C=O) is not the same as a hydroxyl oxygen; therefore, the two compounds exhibit additive–constitutive properties and have different molar refractions.

Additive, constitutive, and additive–constitutive properties, the nature of the interaction between these properties, and the attributes of atoms or groups of atoms will be discussed in this chapter and in other sections of the book, including Chapter 10.

Physical properties encompass specific relations between the molecules and well-defined forms of energy or other external "yardsticks" of measurement. For example, the concept of weight uses the force of gravity as an external measure to compare the mass of objects, while that of optical rotation uses plane-polarized light to describe the optical rotation of molecules. Ideally, a physical property should be easily measured or calculated, and such measurements should be reproducible.

By carefully associating specific physical properties with the chemical nature of closely related molecules, conclusions can be drawn that (1) describe the spatial arrangement of drug molecules, (2) provide evidence for the relative chemical or physical behavior of a molecule, and (3) suggest methods for the qualitative and quantitative analysis of a particular pharmaceutical agent. The first and second of these associations often lead to implications about chemical nature and potential action that are necessary for the creation of new molecules with selective pharmacologic activity. The third provides the researcher with tools for drug design and manufacturing and offers the analyst a wide range of methods for assessing the quality of drug products.

This chapter describes some of the important physical properties of molecules that represent well-defined interactions with electromagnetic energy as found in spectroscopy. Quantities have been expressed in Standard International (SI) units (p. 2) in all practical cases.

ELECTROMAGNETIC RADIATION

Electromagnetic energy can be characterized as a continuous waveform of radiation, the nature of which depends on the size and shape of the wave. As with all forms of radiation, electromagnetic radiation can be described in terms of both a wave model and a field vibrating about a point in space. In either case, the radiation has a characteristic frequency, usually a large number. This frequency, ν, is the number of waves passing a fixed point in 1 second. The wavelength, λ, is the extent of a single wave of radiation, that is, the distance between two successive maxima of the wave, and is related to frequency by

$$\lambda \nu = c \qquad (4-1)$$

in which c is the speed of light, 3×10^8 m/sec. Wavenumber, $\bar{\nu}$, can be defined as

$$\bar{\nu} = \nu/c \qquad (4-2)$$

in which the wavenumber (in cm^{-1}) represents the number of wavelengths found in 1 cm of radiation in a vacuum.

The electromagnetic spectrum is classified according to its wavelength, or its corresponding wavenumber, as illustrated in Table 4–2. The wavelength becomes shorter as the corresponding radiant energy increases. According to the elementary quantum theory, the radiant energy absorbed by a chemical species has certain discrete values corresponding to the individual energy transitions that can occur in an atom or molecule. As we shall discuss, the wavelength of the

TABLE 4–2. *Electromagnetic Spectrum*

Region of the Spectrum	Wavelength	Wavenumber	Frequency	Source
	λ (m)*	$\bar{\nu}$ (cm^{-1})†	Hz‡	
	10^{-13}	10^{11}	3×10^{21}	
Gamma rays	3×10^{-10}	3.3×10^7	1×10^{18}	Nuclear transformations
X-rays	3×10^{-8}	3.3×10^5	1×10^{16}	Inner-shell electron transitions
	(= 30 nm)			
Vacuum ultraviolet	2×10^{-7}	5×10^4	1.5×10^{15}	Ionization and valence electron transitions
	(= 200 nm)			
Near ultraviolet	4×10^{-7}	2.5×10^4	7.5×10^{14}	
Visible	7.5×10^{-7}	1.3×10^4	4×10^{14}	Valence electron transitions
	(= 750 nm)			
Near infrared (overtone region)	2.5×10^{-6}	4×10^3	1.2×10^{14}	
Infrared (fundamental region)	2.5×10^{-5}	4×10^2	1.2×10^{13}	Molecular vibrations
Far infrared	10^{-3}	10^1	3×10^{11}	Molecular vibrations or rotations
Microwaves	10^{-1}	10^{-1}	3×10^9	Electron spin transitions
Radiowaves	10^3	10^{-5}	3×10^5	Nuclear spin transitions

*m = meter.
†$\bar{\nu}$ = wavenumber.
‡Hz = hertz = waves/sec.

quantized electromagnetic energy determines the molecular or atomic information we receive from the resulting spectra.

ATOMIC SPECTRA

Spectra can be derived from the interactions between electromagnetic radiation of certain wavelengths and the electrons in orbitals of an atom. These interactions produce emission spectra if large amounts of energy, which can be from a flame or some other energy source, excite electrons in the atoms. In losing their excitation energy, some of these atoms emit discrete radiation while returning to a less energetic state. The interactions produce absorption spectra if radiation of a particular wavelength is passed through a sample and the decrease in the intensity of the radiation due to electronic excitation is measured. The absorption or emission of quantized energy corresponds to an electronic orbital transition in an atom or, as we shall presently discuss, a molecule. According to the Bohr model, the energy of an electron in a definite orbital is

$$E = -\frac{2\pi^2 Z^2 m e^4}{n^2 h^2} \qquad (4\text{-}3)$$

in which Z is the atomic number or effective nuclear charge of the atom, m is the mass of the electron (9.1×10^{-31} kg), n is the principal quantum number of the orbit, e is the charge on the electron (1.602×10^{-19} coulomb or 1.519×10^{-14} $\text{m}^{3/2}$ $\text{kg}^{1/2}$ s^{-1}), and h is Planck's constant, 6.626×10^{-34} joule second. If we represent E as the energy of a photon of electromagnetic radiation and $c\bar{v} = v$, the frequency of the radiation

$$E = hc\bar{v} \qquad (4\text{-}4)$$

as suggested by Planck in 1900 as the basis of the quantum theory of atomic structure. Substituting equation (4-4) in equation (4-3), we obtain

$$\bar{v} = -\frac{2\pi^2 Z^2 m e^4}{n^2 h^3 c}$$

$$= -\frac{2 \times (3.14)^2 \times (1)^2 \times (9.1 \times 10^{-31} \times (1.519 \times 10^{-14})^4}{n^2 \times (6.626 \times 10^{-34})^3 \times (3 \times 10^8)}$$

$$= \frac{-1.097 \times 10^7}{n^2} \text{ m}^{-1} = \frac{-109{,}700}{n^2} \text{ cm}^{-1} \qquad (4\text{-}5)$$

If $n = 1$, corresponding to the ground state of the hydrogen atom, the numerator, $-109{,}700$ cm^{-1}, represents the energy difference in wavenumber between the quantized energy in the ground state and that in the next electronic orbital (in which $n = 2$). This frequency 109,700 cm^{-1}, is known as the *Rydberg constant*, $\boldsymbol{R}_\infty$, and it is related to the quantized energy of the atom by the simple relation

$$\bar{v} = \boldsymbol{R}_\infty \left(\frac{1}{n_1^2} - \frac{1}{n_2^2} \right) \qquad (4\text{-}6)$$

in which n_1 and n_2 are the principal quantum numbers for the orbital states involved in an electronic transition of the atom.

In general, the difference between electron energy levels, $E_2 - E_1$, having respective quantum numbers, n_2 and n_1, is given by the expression

$$E_2 - E_1 = \frac{2\pi^2 Z^2 m e^4}{h^2} \left(\frac{1}{n_1^2} - \frac{1}{n_2^2} \right) \qquad (4\text{-}7)$$

Example 4–1. (a) What is the energy of a quantum of radiation absorbed to promote the electron in the hydrogen atom from its ground state ($n_1 = 1$) to the second orbital, $n_2 = 2$?

$$E_2 - E_1 = \frac{2 \times (3.14)^2 \times (1)^2 \times (9.1 \times 10^{-31}) \times (1.519 \times 10^{-14})^4}{(6.626 \times 10^{-34})^2}$$

$$\times \left(\frac{1}{(1)^2} - \frac{1}{(2)^2} \right)$$

$$= 1.63 \times 10^{-18} \text{ joule}$$

Note that the joule $= \text{kg} \times \text{m}^2 \times \text{s}^{-2}$ (SI units; see Table 1–3).

(b) If we substitute equation (4-6) into equation (4-7), we can obtain

$$E_2 - E_1 = \frac{2\pi^2 Z^2 m e^4}{h^2} \left(\frac{\bar{v}}{\boldsymbol{R}_\infty} \right) \qquad (4\text{-}8)$$

Using this equation, what is the wavelength of the spectral line when an electron passes from the $n = 1$ orbital to the $n = 2$ orbital, where $E_2 - E_1 = 1.63 \times 10^{-18}$ joule?

$$E_2 - E_1 = 1.63 \times 10^{-18} =$$

$$= \frac{2 \times (3.14)^2 \times (1)^2 \times (9.1 \times 10^{-31}) \times (1.519 \times 10^{-14})^4}{(6.626 \times 10^{-34})^2}$$

$$\times \left(\frac{\bar{v}}{109{,}700} \right)$$

$$\bar{v} = \frac{(1.63 \times 10^{-18}) \times (1.097 \times 10^5) \times (6.626 \times 10^{-34})^2}{2 \times (3.14)^2 \times (1)^2 \times (9.1 \times 10^{-31}) \times (1.519 \times 10^{-14})^4}$$

$$= 82{,}091 \text{ cm}^{-1}$$

and therefore, from equations (4-1) and (4-2),

$$\lambda = \frac{1}{\bar{v}} = \frac{1}{82{,}091} = 1.21 \times 10^{-5} \text{ cm} = 121 \text{ nm}$$

This is the first line of the Lyman ultraviolet series of the atomic spectra for hydrogen. Note that, from equation (4-3), the electron of the hydrogen atom in the ground state, $n = 1$, has a lower energy (-2.18×10^{-18} joules) than in the next highest electron state, $n = 2 (-0.55 \times 10^{-18}$ joules).

When the electron acquires sufficient energy to leave the atom, it is regarded as infinitely distant from the nucleus, and the nucleus is considered no longer to affect the electron. The energy required for this process, which results in the ionization of the nucleus, is known as the *ionization potential*. If we consider this process as occurring when $n = \infty$, then the ionization potential from the ground state ($n = 1$) to $n = \infty$ is

$$E_2 - E_1 = \frac{2\pi^2 Z^2 m e^4}{h^2} \left(\frac{1}{1} - \frac{1}{\infty} \right)$$

TABLE 4–3. *Spectral Wavelengths Associated with Electronic Transitions Used in the Detection of Particular Elements*

Element	Wavelength (nm)
As	193.7
Ca	422.7
Na	589.0
Cu	324.8
Hg	253.7
Li	670.8
Pb	405.8
Zn	213.9
K	766.5

since $1/\infty \cong 0$, then

$$E_2 - E_1 = \frac{2\pi^2 Z^2 m e^4}{h^2}$$

This is equivalent to $-E$ for $n = 1$, according to equation (4–3). Thus, the ionization potential exactly equals the negative energy of the electron in the ground state. This is correct according to the definition of ground state energy, which may be thought of as the difference in energy between the $n = 1$ orbital and a distance infinitely far away.

Each element of the periodic table has a characteristic atomic spectrum that can be associated with its electronic transition states. Atomic spectra can be used to identify and quantify specific elements. Some of the more sensitive spectral wavelengths associated with particular atoms are given in Table 4–3.

Atomic spectroscopy has pharmaceutical applications in analyzing for metal ions from drug products and in the quality control of parenteral electrolyte solutions. For example, blood levels of lithium, used to treat bipolar disorder (manic-depression), can be analyzed by atomic spectroscopy to determine overdosing of lithium salts.

MOLECULAR SPECTRA

The absorption of electromagnetic radiation by molecules includes vibrational and rotational transitions, as well as the electronic transitions just described for atoms. These additional transitions make the spectra of molecules more complex than those of atoms. The additional transitions result from energy interactions that produce either vibrations within the molecule associated with the stretching or bending of bonds between the atoms, or the rotation of the molecule about its center of gravity. In the case of vibration, the interatomic bonds may be thought of as springs between atoms (see Fig. 4–10), which can vibrate in various stretching or bending configurations depending on their energy levels, while in rotation, the motion is similar to that of a top spinning according to its energy level. In addition, the molecule may have some kinetic energy associated with its translational (straight-line) motion in a particular direction.

The energy levels associated with these various transitions differ greatly from one another. The energy associated with movement of an electron from one orbital to another (electronic transitions) is typically about 10^{-18} joule, while the energy involved in vibrational changes is about 10^{-19} to 10^{-20} joule depending on the atoms involved, and the energy for rotational change is about 10^{-21} joule. The energy associated with translational change is even smaller, about 10^{-35} joule. The precise energies associated with these individual transitions depend on the atoms and bonds that compose the molecule. Each electronic energy state of a molecule normally has several possible vibrational states, and each of these has several rotational states, as shown in Figure 4–1. The translational states are so numerous and the energy levels between translational states so small that they are normally considered as a continuous form of energy and are not treated as quantized. The total energy of a molecule is the sum of its electronic, vibrational, rotational, and translational energies.

When a molecule absorbs electromagnetic radiation, it can undergo certain transitions that depend on the quantized amount of energy absorbed. In Figure 4–1, the absorption of radiation (line a) equivalent to the energy transition ΔE_1 results in the electronic transition from the lowest level of the ground state (S_0) to an excited electronic state (S_1) with a somewhat different rotational energy. Electronic transitions of molecules involve energies corresponding to ultraviolet or visible radiation, whereas purely vibrational transitions (line b) involve near-infrared radiation, and rotational transitions (line c) are associated with low-energy radiation over the entire infrared wavelength region. The relatively large energy associated with an electronic tran-

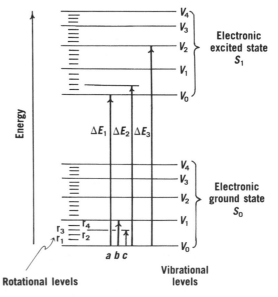

Fig. 4–1. Molecular energy levels and (a) electronic, (b) vibrational, and (c) rotational transitions. Vibrational and rotational energy levels have been exaggerated compared with electronic energy levels in this figure. (Modified from H. H. Bauer, G. D. Christian, and J. E. Reilly, *Instrumental Analysis*, Allyn and Bacon, Boston, 1978.)

sition usually leads to a variety of different vibrational and rotational changes. Slight differences in the vibrational and rotational nature of the excited electronic state complicate the spectrum. These differences lead to broad bands, characteristic of the ultraviolet and visible regions, rather than the sharp, narrow lines characteristic of individual vibrational or rotational changes in the infrared region.

The energy absorbed by a molecule may be found only at a few discrete wavelengths in the ultraviolet, visible, and infrared regions, or the absorptions may be numerous and at longer wavelengths than originally expected. The latter case, involving longer wavelength radiation, is normally found for molecules that have resonance structures, such as benzene, in which the bonds are elongated by the resonance and have lower energy transitions than would be expected otherwise. Electromagnetic energy may also be absorbed by a molecule from the microwave and radiowave regions (see Table 4–2). Low-energy transitions involve the spin of electrons in the microwave region and the spin of nuclei in the radiowave region. The study of these transitions constitutes the fields of electron spin resonance (ESR) and nuclear magnetic resonance (NMR) spectroscopy. These various forms of molecular spectroscopy are discussed in the following sections.

ULTRAVIOLET AND VISIBLE SPECTROPHOTOMETRY

When organic molecules in solution, or as a liquid, are exposed to light in the visible and ultraviolet regions of the spectrum (see Table 4–2), they absorb light of particular wavelengths depending on the type of electronic transition that is associated with the absorption. Such electronic transitions depend on the electron bonding within the molecule.[1] For example, paraffins that contain σ-type bonds can undergo only $\sigma \rightarrow \sigma^*$ electronic transitions from their lowest energy, or ground, state. The * indicates the excited state of the electron after absorption of a quantized amount of energy. These σ electronic transitions occur exclusively from the relatively high energy available from short-wavelength radiation in the vacuum ultraviolet region (wavelengths typically between 100 and 150 nm). If a carbonyl group is present in a molecule, however, the oxygen atom of this functional group possesses a pair of nonbonding (n) electrons that can undergo $n \rightarrow \pi^*$ or $n \rightarrow \sigma^*$ electronic orbital transitions. These transitions require a lower energy than do $\sigma \rightarrow \sigma^*$ transitions and therefore occur from the absorption of longer wavelengths of radiation. For acetone, these $n \rightarrow \pi^*$ or $n \rightarrow \sigma^*$ transitions occur at 280 and 190 nm, respectively. For aldehydes and ketones, the region of the ultraviolet spectrum between 270 and 290 nm is associated with their carbonyl $n \rightarrow \pi^*$ electronic transitions, and this fact can be used for identification. Thus, the types of electronic orbitals present in the ground state of the molecule dictate the region of the spectrum in which absorption can take place. Those parts of a molecule that can be directly associated with an absorption of ultraviolet or visible light, such as the carbonyl group, are called *chromophores*.

The magnitude of the absorption of light at a fixed wavelength can be calculated by using *Beer's law*. This equation relates the amount of light absorbed (A) to the concentration of absorbing substance (c in g/liter) and the length of the path of radiation passing through the sample (b in cm) as

$$A = abc \qquad (4-9)$$

in which a is a constant known as *absorptivity* for a particular absorbing species (in units of liter $g^{-1} cm^{-1}$). If the units of c are moles/liter, then the constant is termed ϵ, the *molar absorptivity* (in units of liter $mole^{-1} cm^{-1}$). The absorptivity depends not only on the molecule whose absorbance is being determined, but also on the type of solvent being used, as well as on the temperature and the wavelength of light used for the analysis. The quantity A is termed the *absorbance* and is related to the *transmittance* of light (T) by

$$A = \log \frac{I_o}{I} = -\log T \qquad (4-10)$$

in which I_o is the intensity of the incident light beam and I is in the intensity of light after it emerges from the sample.

Example 4–2. (a) A solution of $c = 2 \times 10^{-5}$ moles/liter of chlordiazepoxide dissolved in 0.1 N sodium hydroxide was placed in a fused silica cell having an optical path of 1 cm. The absorbance A was found to be 0.648 at a wavelength of 260 nm. What is the molar absorptivity? (b) If a solution of chlordiazepoxide had an absorbance of 0.298 in a 1-cm cell at 260 nm, what is its concentration?

(a)

$$\epsilon = \frac{A}{bc} = \frac{6.48 \times 10^{-1}}{1 \times (2 \times 10^{-5})}$$
$$= 3.24 \times 10^4 \text{ liter mole}^{-1} \text{ cm}^{-1}$$

(b)

$$c = \frac{A}{b\epsilon} = \frac{2.98 \times 10^{-1}}{1 \times (3.24 \times 10^4)} = 9.20 \times 10^{-6} \text{ moles/liter}$$

The large value of ϵ indicates that chlordiazepoxide absorbs strongly at this wavelength. This molar absorptivity is characteristic of the drug dissolved in 0.1 N NaOH at this wavelength, and is not the same in 0.1 N HCl. A lactam is formed from the drug under an acid condition that has an absorbance maximum at 245 rather than 260 nm, and a correspondingly different ϵ value.

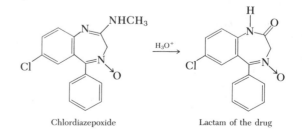

Chlordiazepoxide   Lactam of the drug

Example 4–3. Aminacrine is an antiinfective agent with the following molecular structure:

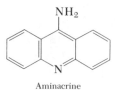

Aminacrine

Its highly conjugated acridine ring produces a complex ultraviolet spectrum in dilute sulfuric acid that includes absorption maxima at 260, 313, 326, 381, 400, and 422 nm. The molar absorptivities of the absorbances at 260 and 313 nm are 63,900 and 1130 liter mole^{-1} cm^{-1} respectively. What is the minimum amount of aminacrine that can be detected at each of these two wavelengths?

If we assume an absorbance level of $A = 0.002$ corresponding to a minimum detectable concentration of the drug, then, at 260 nm,

$$c = \frac{A}{b \times \epsilon} = \frac{0.002}{1 \times 63900} = 3.13 \times 10^{-8} \text{ mole/liter}$$

while at 381 nm

$$c = \frac{0.002}{1 \times 1130} = 1.77 \times 10^{-6} \text{ mole/liter}$$

Nearly 100 times greater sensitivity in detecting the drug is possible with the 260-nm absorption band. The absorbance level of 0.002 was chosen by judging this value to be a significant signal above instrumental noise (i.e., interference generated by the spectrophotometer in the absence of the drug). For a particular analysis, this minimum absorbance level for detection of a compound will depend on both the instrumental conditions and the sample state, for example, the solvent chosen for dissolution of the sample.

Characteristic ϵ values for selected drugs together with their wavelength of maximum absorbance (at which the ϵ values were calculated) are given in Table 4–4. Sometimes the absorbance found in the literature is expressed as $E^{1\%}_{1cm}$. This is the absorbance through a 1-cm path length of a solution containing 1 g of solute per 100 mL of solution. The $E^{1\%}_{1cm}$ term is being discontinued and replaced by the ϵ value for molar absorptivity.

A molecule may have more than one characteristic absorption wavelength band, and the complete spectrum in the ultraviolet and visible wavelength regions can provide information for the positive identification of a compound. A recording spectrophotometer is usually used to obtain such a spectrum. A schematic diagram of a typical double-beam spectrophotometer is shown in Figure 4–2. The beam of light from the source, usually a deuterium lamp, passes through a prism or grating monochromator to sort the light according to wavelength and spread the wavelengths over a wide range. This permits a particular wavelength region to be easily selected by passing it through the appropriate slits. The selected light is then split into two separate beams by a rotating mirror, or "chopper"—one beam for the reference, which is typically the blank solvent used to dissolve the sample, and the other for the sample cell. After each beam passes through its respective cell, it is reflected onto a second mirror in another chopper assembly, which alternatively selects either the reference or the combined beams to focus onto the photomultiplier detector. The rapidly changing current signal from the detector is proportional to the intensity of the particular beam, and this is fed into an amplifier, which electronically separates the signals of the reference beam from those of the sample beam. The final difference in beam signals is automatically recorded on a strip-chart recorder. The recording obtained is a plot of the intensity, usually as absorbance, against the wavelength, as shown in Figure 4–3. Standard solutions of known but varying concentration are used in quantitative analysis as the samples in the spectrophotometer. The absorbance of each solution is determined at one selected wavelength (typically an absorption maximum). The absorbance is plotted against the concentration, as shown in Figure 4–4, to obtain what is known as a Beer's law plot. The concentration of an "unknown" sample can then be determined by interpolation from such a graph.

Spectrophotometry is a useful tool for studying chemical equilibria or determining the rate of chemical reactions. The chemical species participating in the equilibria must have different absorption spectra, and one simply observes the variation in absorption at a representative wavelength for each species while the pH or other equilibrium variable is changed. If one determines the concentrations of the species from Beer's law and knows the pH of the solution, one can

TABLE 4–4.   *Molar Absorptivity of Some Drugs Measured in a 1-cm Cell*

Drug	ϵ (liter mole^{-1} cm^{-1})	Wavelength (nm)	Solvent
Codeine phosphate	1,570	284	Water
Colchicine	29,200	243	Ethanol
(+)-3-Hydroxy-*N*-methylmorphinan (Dextrorphan)	2,360	279	0.1 *N* Sulfuric acid
Reserpine	14,500	267	Chloroform
Riboflavine	35,500	222	Water
Tetracycline hydrochloride	16,200	380	Water
Tolazoline	24	257	Ethanol
Prednisolone	17,500	263	Ethanol

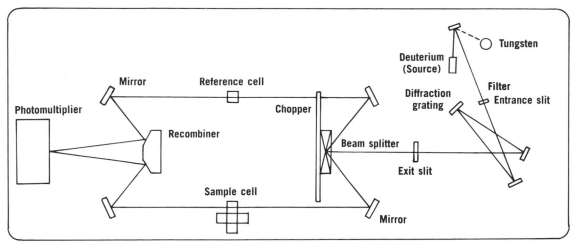

Fig. 4-2. Schematic diagram of a double-beam spectrophotometer, Bausch and Lomb Spectronic 2000. (From J. P. Malone, L. E. DeLong, and J. C. Defendorf, Am. Lab. **12,** 78, 1980. Copyright 1980 by International Scientific Communications, Inc.)

calculate an approximate pK_a for a drug. For example, if the drug is a free acid (HA) in equilibrium with its base (A^-), then

$$pK_a = pH + \log [HA]/[A^-] \qquad (4-11)$$

When $[HA] = [A^-]$, as determined by their respective absorbances in the spectrophotometric determination, $pK_a \cong pH$.

Example 4-4. Phenobarbital shows a maximum absorption of 240 nm as the monosodium salt (A^-), while the free acid (HA) shows no absorption maxima in the wavelength region from 230 to 290 nm. If the free acid in water is slowly titrated with known volumes of dilute NaOH, measuring the pH of the solution and the absorbance at 240

nm after each titration, one reaches a maximum absorbance value at pH 10 after the addition of 10 mL of titrant. How can pK_a be determined from this titration?

By plotting the absorbance against the pH over the titration range to pH = 10, one may obtain the midpoint in absorbance, where half the free acid has been titrated, and $[HA] = [A^-]$ (Fig. 4-5). The pH corresponding to this absorbance midpoint is approximately equal to the pK_a, namely, pK_{a_1} for the first ionization stage of phenobarbital. This midpoint occurs at a pH of 7.3; therefore, the $pK_a \cong 7.3$. For more accurate pK_a determinations, refer to the discussion beginning on page 204.

Reaction rates can be measured easily if a particular reaction species has an absorption spectrum that is noticeably different from the spectra of other reactants or products. One can follow the rate of appearance or disappearance of the selected species by recording its absorbance at specific times during the reaction process. If no other reaction species absorbs at the

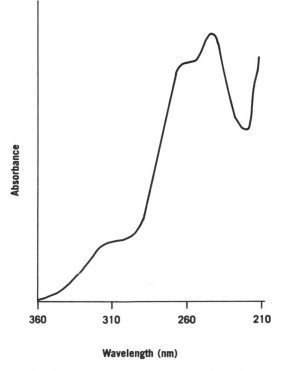

Fig. 4-3. The absorbance of light by a solution of chlordiazepoxide as a function of the wavelength in nanometers.

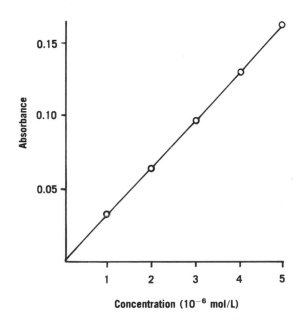

Fig. 4-4. A Beer's law plot of absorbance against the concentration of chlordiazepoxide.

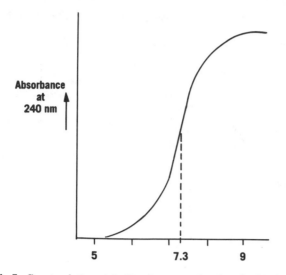

Fig. 4–5. Spectrophotometric titration curve for phenobarbital. The absorbance of the monosodium salt at 240 nm is plotted against the pH of the solution.

particular wavelength chosen for this determination, the reaction rate will simply be proportional to the rate of change of absorbance with reaction time.

An example of the use of spectrophotometry for the determination of reaction rates in pharmaceutics is given in the work of Jivani and Stella,[2] where the disappearance of *para*-aminosalicylic acid from solution was used to determine its rate of decarboxylation.

Spectrophotometry can be used to study enzyme reactions and to evaluate the effects of drugs on enzymes. For example, the analysis of clavulanic acid can be accomplished by measuring the ultraviolet absorption of penicillin G at 240 nm, as described by Gutman et al.[3] Clavulanic acid inhibits the activity of β-lactamase enzymes, which are capable of degrading penicillin G to penicilloic acid: where R is $C_6H_5CH_2—$. The method first requires that the rate of absorbance change at 240 nm be measured with a solution containing penicillin G and a β-lactamase enzyme. Duplicate experiments are then performed with increasing standard concentrations of clavulanic acid. These show a decrease in absorbance change, equivalent to the enzyme inhibition from the drug, as the concentration of the drug increases. The concentration of an unknown amount of clavulanic acid is measured by comparing its rate of enzyme inhibition with that of the standards.

Although these applications are often helpful in pharmaceutical calculations, the major use of spectro-

photometry today is in the field of quantitative analysis, in which the absorbance of chromophors is determined. Various applications of spectrophotometry are discussed by Schulman and Vogt.[4]

FLUORESCENCE AND PHOSPHORESCENCE

A molecule that initially absorbs ultraviolet light to reach an excited state and then emits ultraviolet or visible light in returning to the ground state is said to undergo *photoluminescence*. This emission of light may be described as either fluorescence or phosphorescence, depending on the mechanism by which the electron finally returns to the ground state.

The overall mechanism can be described as

$$S_0 + UV \rightarrow S^* \rightarrow S_0 + \text{Fluorescence}$$
(Ground state) (Singlet)

$$T^* \rightarrow S_0 + \text{Phosphorescence}$$
(Triplet)

in which, in addition to the singlet excited state (S*) discussed previously, we have a triplet (T*) state, associated with the production of phosphorescence. The triplet state of the excited electron occurs when the excited singlet electron changes spin so that it is now of the same spin as its originally paired electron in the ground-state orbital. The triplet state usually cannot be achieved by excitation from the ground state, this being termed a "forbidden" transition according to the quantum theory. It is usually reached through the process of *intersystem crossing*, in which the excited singlet (S*) converts spontaneously to a triplet by a change in electron spin, usually with some energy loss. These changes, together with the energies involved, are represented schematically in Figure 4–6.

The triplet state (T*) is usually considered more stable (i.e., having a longer lifetime) than the excited singlet state (S*). The length of time during which light will be emitted after the molecule has become excited depends on the lifetime of the electronic transition. Therefore, we can expect phosphorescence to occur for a longer period after excitation than fluorescence. Ordinarily, fluorescence occurs between 10^{-6} to 10^{-9} second after excitation. Because of this short lifetime, fluorescence is usually measured while the molecule is being excited. A typical filter fluorometer is shown in Figure 4–7. Fluorescence intensity is measured in this

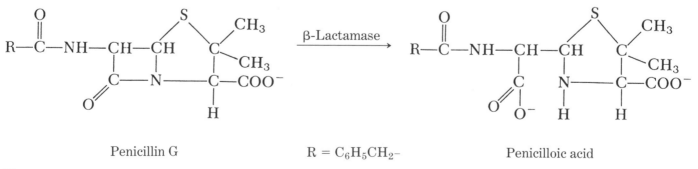

Penicillin G $R = C_6H_5CH_2-$ Penicilloic acid

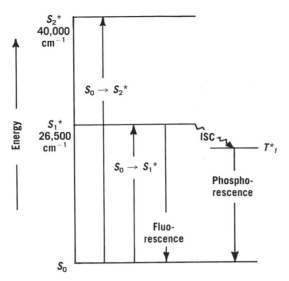

Fig. 4–6. Schematic energy-level diagram for a molecule that fluoresces or phosphoresces. ISC stands for intersystem crossing; S_0, S^*, and T are described in the text.

system by placing the photomultiplier detector at right angles to the light beam that is producing the excitation. The signal intensity is recorded as relative fluorescence against a standard solution. Since photoluminescence can occur in any direction from the sample, the detector will sense a part of the total emission at a characteristic wavelength and will not be capable of detecting radiation from the light beam used for excitation. Fluorescence normally has a longer wavelength than the radiation used for the excitation, principally because of internal energy losses within the excited molecule before the fluorescent emission occurs. Phosphorescence typically has still longer wavelengths than fluorescence, owing to the energy difference that occurs in intersystem crossing as well as the loss of energy due to internal conversion over a longer lifetime.

Photoluminescence occurs only in those molecules that can undergo the specified photon emissions after excitation with consequent return to the ground state. Many molecules do not possess any photoluminescence, although they can absorb ultraviolet light. In these cases, the return to the ground state from the singlet excited state occurs through the internal conversion of excitation energy into vibrational energy or through collisions with other molecules resulting in energy transfer. These energy conversions result finally in the production of heat rather than photoluminescence. Most often, a molecule that fluoresces or phosphoresces contains at least one aromatic ring. Examples of drugs that fluoresce are given in Table 4–5 along with their characteristic excitation and emission wavelengths, which can be used for qualitative or quantitative analyses. Photoluminescent analysis is normally more sensitive and selective than absorption spectrophotometry.

A thorough review of the applications of photoluminescence to the analysis of pharmaceuticals is given by Schulman and Sturgeon.[5]

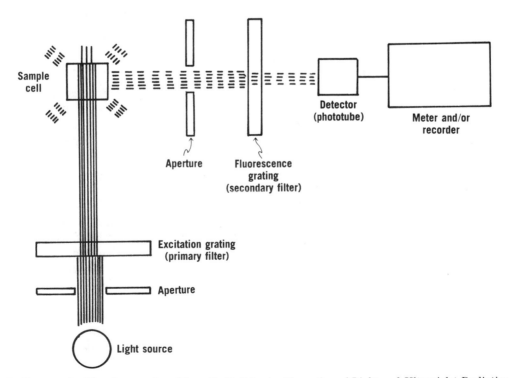

Fig. 4–7. Schematic diagram of a filter fluorometer. (From G. H. Schenk, *Absorption of Light and Ultraviolet Radiation*, Allyn and Bacon, Boston, 1973, p. 260.)

TABLE 4–5. *Fluorescence of Some Drugs*

Drug	Excitation Wavelength (nm)	Emission Wavelength (nm)	Solvent
Phenobarbital	255	410–420	0.1 *N* NaOH
Hydroflumethiazide	333	393	1 *N* HCl
Quinine	350	~450	0.1 *N* H_2SO_4
Thiamine	365	~440	Isobutanol, after oxidation with ferricyanide
Aspirin	280	335	1% Acetic acid in chloroform
Tetracycline hydrochloride	330	450	0.05 *N* NaOH(aq)
Fluorescein	493.5	514	pH-2 (aq.)
Riboflavine	455	520	Ethanol
Hydralazine	320	353	Conc. H_2SO_4

DIELECTRIC CONSTANT AND INDUCED POLARIZATION

A molecule can maintain a separation of electric charge either through induction by an external electric field or by a permanent charge separation within a polar molecule. To fully understand the concepts of charge separation, it is necessary to understand the concept of the dielectric constant.

Consider two parallel conducting plates, such as the plates of an electric condenser, which are separated by some medium across a distance r, as shown in Figure 4–8, and apply a potential across the plates. Electricity will flow from the left plate to the right plate through the battery until the potential difference of the plates equals that of the battery supplying the initial potential difference. The *capacitance*, C (in farads), is equal to the quantity of electric charge, q (in coulombs), stored on the plates, divided by the potential difference, V (in volts), between the plates:

$$C = q/V \qquad (4-12)$$

The capacitance of the condenser in Figure 4–8 depends on the type of medium separating the plates as well as on the thickness r. When a vacuum fills the space between the plates, the capacitance is C_0. This value is used as a reference to compare capacitances when other substances fill the space. If water fills the space, the capacitance is increased, since the water molecule can orientate itself so that its negative end lies nearest the positive condenser plate and its positive end lies nearest the negative plate. This alignment provides additional movement of charge because of the increased ease with which electrons can flow between the plates. Thus, additional charge can be placed on the plates per unit of applied voltage.

The capacitance of the condenser filled with some material, C_x, divided by the reference standard C_0, is referred to as the *dielectric constant*, ϵ:

$$\epsilon = C_x/C_0 \qquad (4-13)$$

The dielectric constant ordinarily has no dimensions, since it is the ratio of two capacitances. Dielectric constants of some liquids are listed in Table 4–6. By

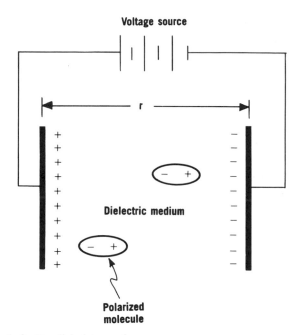

Fig. 4–8. Parallel plate condenser.

definition, the dielectric constant of a vacuum is unity. Dielectric constants can be determined by oscillometry, in which the frequency of a signal is kept constant by electrically changing the capacitance between the two parallel plates. The liquid whose dielectric constant is being measured is placed in a glass container between the two plates during the experiment. The dielectric constants of solvent mixtures can be related to drug solubility as described by Gorman and Hall[6] and ϵ for drug vehicles can be related to drug plasma concentration as reported by Pagay et al.[7]

If nonpolar molecules in a suitable solvent are placed between the plates of a charged capacitor, an *induced polarization* of the molecules can occur. This *induced dipole* occurs because of the separation of electric charge within the molecule when it is placed in the electric field between the plates. The electrons and nuclei are displaced from their original positions in this induction process. This temporary induced dipole moment is proportional to the field strength of the

TABLE 4–6. *Dielectric Constants of Some Liquids at 25° C*

Substance	Dielectric Constant, ϵ	
N-Methylformamide	182	
Hydrogen cyanide	114	
Formamide	110	
Water	78.5	
Glycerol	42.5	
Methanol	32.6	
Tetramethylurea	23.1	
Acetone	20.7	
n-Propanol	20.1	
Isopropanol	18.3	
Isopentanol	14.7	
1-Pentanol	13.9	
Benzyl alcohol	13.1	
Phenol	9.8	(60° C)
Ethyl acetate	6.02	
Chloroform	4.80	
Hydrochloric acid	4.60	
Diethyl ether	4.34	(20° C)
Acetonitrile	3.92	
Carbon disulfide	2.64	
Triethylamine	2.42	
Toulene	2.38	
Beeswax (solid)	2.8	
Benzene	2.27	
Carbon tetrachloride	2.23	
1,4-Dioxane	2.21	
Pentane	1.84	(20° C)
Furfural	41	(20° C)
Pyridine	12.3	
Methyl salicylate	9.41	(30° C)

capacitor and the *induced polarizability*, α_p, which is a characteristic property of the particular molecule. Polarizability is defined as the ease with which an ion or molecule can be polarized by any external force, whether it be an electric field, light energy, or another molecule. Large-size anions have large polarizabilities because of their loosely held outer electrons. Polarizabilities for molecules are found in Table 4–7. The units on α_p are $Å^3$ or 10^{-24} cm^3.

From electromagnetic theory, it is possible to obtain the relationship

$$\frac{\epsilon - 1}{\epsilon + 2} = \frac{4}{3} \pi n \alpha_p \qquad (4-14)$$

in which n is the number of molecules per unit volume. Equation (4–14) is known as the *Clausius–Mossotti equation.* Multiplying both sides by the molecular weight of the substance, M, and dividing both sides by the density, ρ, we obtain

TABLE 4–7. *Polarizabilities*

Molecule	$\alpha_p \times 10^{24}$ cm^3
H_2O	1.68
N_2	1.79
HCl	3.01
HBr	3.5
HI	5.6
HCN	5.9

$$\left(\frac{\epsilon - 1}{\epsilon + 2}\right) \frac{M}{\rho} = \frac{4}{3} \frac{\pi n M \alpha_p}{\rho} = \frac{4}{3} \pi N \alpha_p = P_i \qquad (4-15)$$

in which N is Avogadro's number, 6.023×10^{23} mole^{-1}, and P_i is known as the *induced molar polarization*. P_i represents the induced dipole moment per mole of nonpolar substance when the electric field strength of the condenser, V/m in volts per meter, is unity.

Example 4–5. Chloroform has a molecular weight of 119 g/mol and a density of 1.43 g/cm³ at 25° C. What is the induced molar polarizability of chloroform?

$$P_i = \frac{(\epsilon - 1)}{(\epsilon + 2)} \times \frac{M}{\rho} = \frac{(4.8 - 1)}{(4.8 + 2)} \times \frac{119}{1.43} = 46.5 \text{ cm}^3/\text{mole}$$

The concept of induced dipole moments can be extended from the condenser model just discussed to the model of a nonpolar molecule in solution surrounded by ions. In this case, an anion would repel molecular electrons while a cation would attract them. This would cause an interaction of the molecule in relation to the ions in solution and produce an induced dipole. The distribution and ease of attraction or repulsion of electrons in the nonpolar molecule will affect the magnitude of this induced dipole, as would the applied external electric field strength.

PERMANENT DIPOLE MOMENT OF POLAR MOLECULES

In a polar molecule, the separation of positively and negatively charged regions can be permanent, and the molecule will possess a *permanent dipole moment*, μ. This is a nonionic phenomenon, and although regions of the molecule may possess charges, these charges should balance each other so the molecule as a whole will have no net charge. The water molecule, for example, possesses a permanent dipole. The magnitude of the permanent dipole, μ, is independent of any induced dipole from an electric field. It is defined as the vector sum of the individual charge moments within the molecule, including those from bonds and lone-pair electrons. The vectors depend on the distance of separation between the charges. The unit of μ is the *debye*, with 1 debye equal to 10^{-18} esu cm.* This is derived from the charge on the electron (about 10^{-10} esu) multiplied by the average distance between charged centers on a molecule (about 10^{-8} cm).

In an electric field, molecules with permanent dipole moments can also have induced dipoles. The polar molecule, however, tends to orient itself with its negatively charged centers closest to positively charged centers on other molecules *before* the electric field is applied, so that when the applied field is present, the orientation is in the direction of the field. Maximum

---

*The esu (electrostatic unit) is the measure of electrostatic charge, defined as a charge in a vacuum that repels a like charge 1 centimeter away with a force of 1 dyne. In SI units, 1 debye = 3.34×10^{-30} coulomb-meter.

dipole moment occurs when the molecules are oriented most perfectly. Absolutely perfect orientation can never occur owing to the thermal energy of the molecules, which contributes to agitation against the molecular alignment. The *total* molar polarization, P, is the sum of induction and permanent dipole effects:

$$P = P_i + P_0 = \left(\frac{\epsilon - 1}{\epsilon + 2}\right) \frac{M}{\rho} \quad (4-16)$$

in which P_0 is the orientation polarization of the permanent dipoles. P_0 is equal to $4\pi N\mu^2/9\,kT$, in which k is the Boltzmann constant, 1.38×10^{-23} J° K^{-1}. Since P_0 depends on the temperature, T, equation (4–16) can be rewritten in a linear form as

$$P = P_i + A\,\frac{1}{T} \quad (4-17)$$

in which the slope A is $4\pi N\mu^2/9k$, and P_i is the y intercept. If P is obtained at several temperatures and plotted against $1/T$, the slope of the graph can be used to calculate μ, and the intercept can be applied to

compute α_p. The values of P can be obtained from equation (4–16) by measuring the dielectric constant and the density of the polar compound at various temperatures. The dipole moments of several compounds are listed in Table 4–8.

In solution, the permanent dipole of a solvent such as water can strongly interact with the solute molecules. This interaction contributes to solvent effect and is associated, in the case of water, with the hydration of ions and molecules. The symmetry of the molecule can also be associated with its dipole moment. For example, benzene and *p*-dichlorobenzene are symmetric planar molecules and have dipole moments of zero. Meta and ortho derivatives of benzene, however, are not symmetric and have significant dipole moments, as listed in Table 4–8.

Permanent dipole moments can be correlated with biologic activities of certain molecules to obtain valuable information about the relationship of physical properties and charge separation in a class of compounds. For example, the insecticidal activity of the three isomers of DDT, shown in the following structures, can be associated with their permanent dipole moments. The para isomer, *p,p'*-DDT, has the smallest dipole moment and the greatest activity. This may be due to the fact that greater solubility in a nonpolar solvent may be related to a small dipole moment for a solute. The more soluble molecule most readily penetrates the lipoidal membranes of the insect and attacks the enzymes of the insect's nervous system. Hence, the lower the dipole moment of the isomer, the greater its insecticidal action.

TABLE 4–8. *Dipole Moments of Some Compounds*

Compound	Dipole Moment (Debye units)
p-Dichlorobenzene	0
H$_2$	0
Carbon dioxide	0
Benzene	0
1,4-Dioxane	0
Carbon monoxide	0.12
Hydrogen iodide	0.38
Hydrogen bromide	0.78
Hydrogen chloride	1.03
Dimethylamine	1.03
Barbital	1.10
Phenobarbital	1.16
Ethylamine	1.22
Formic acid	1.4
Acetic acid	1.4
Phenol	1.45
Ammonia	1.46
m-Dichlorobenzene	1.5
Tetrahydrofuran	1.63
n-Propanol	1.68
Chlorobenzene	1.69
Ethanol	1.69
Methanol	1.70
Dehydrocholesterol	1.81
Water	1.84
Chloroform	1.86
Cholesterol	1.99
Ethylenediamine	1.99
Acetylsalicylic acid	2.07
o-Dichlorobenzene	2.3
Acetone	2.88
Hydrogen cyanide	2.93
Nitromethane	3.46
Acetanilide	3.55
Androsterone	3.70
Acetonitrile	3.92
Methyltestosterone	4.17
Testosterone	4.32
Urea	4.56
Sulfanilamide	5.37

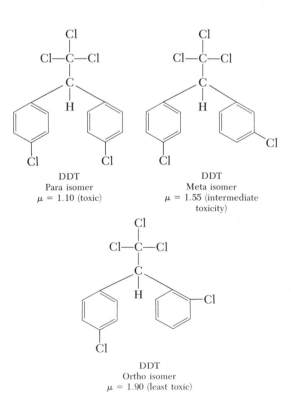

DDT
Para isomer
$\mu = 1.10$ (toxic)

DDT
Meta isomer
$\mu = 1.55$ (intermediate toxicity)

DDT
Ortho isomer
$\mu = 1.90$ (least toxic)

The importance of dipole interactions should not be underestimated. For ionic solutes and nonpolar solvents, ion-induced dipole interactions have an essential role in solubility phenomena. For drug-receptor bonding, dipole forces are believed to contribute to this essentially noncovalent interaction, as described by Kollman.[8] For solids composed of molecules with permanent dipole moments, the dipole force contributes to the crystalline arrangement and overall structural nature of the solid. Ice crystals are organized through their dipole forces. Additional interpretations of the significance of dipole moments are given by Minkin et al.[9]

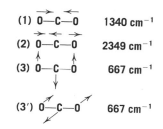

Fig. 4–9. The normal vibrational modes of CO_2 and their respective wavenumbers, showing the directions of motion in reaching the extreme of the harmonic cycle. (Modified from W. S. Brey, *Physical Chemistry and Its Biological Applications*, Academic Press, New York, 1978, p. 316.)

INFRARED SPECTROSCOPY

The study of the interaction of electromagnetic radiation with vibrational or rotational resonances within a molecular structure is termed *infrared spectroscopy*. Normally, infrared radiation in the region from about 2.5 to 50 μm, equivalent to 4000 to 200 cm^{-1} in wavenumber, is used in commercial spectrometers to determine most of the important vibration or vibration–rotation transitions. The individual masses of the vibrating or rotating atoms or functional groups, as well as the bond strength and molecular symmetry, determine the frequency (and, therefore, also the wavelength) of the infrared absorption. The absorption of infrared radiation occurs only if the permanent dipole moment of the molecule changes with a vibrational or rotational resonance. The molecular symmetry relates directly to the permanent dipole moment, as already discussed. Bond stretching or bending *resonances* (i.e., the harmonic oscillations associated with the stretching or bending of the bond) may affect this symmetry, thereby shifting the dipole moment as found for (2), (3), and (3′) in Figure 4–9. Other resonances, such as (1) for CO_2 in Figure 4–9, do not affect the dipole moment and do not produce infrared absorption. Resonances that *shift* the dipole moments can give rise to infrared absorption by molecules, even those considered to have no permanent dipole moment, such as benzene or CO_2. The frequencies of infrared absorption bands correspond closely to vibrations from particular parts of the molecule. The bending and stretching vibrations for acetaldehyde, together with the associated infrared frequencies of absorption, are shown in Figure 4–10. In addition to the fundamental absorption bands, shown in this figure, each of which corresponds to a vibration or vibration–rotation resonance and a change in the dipole moment, weaker overtone bands may be observed for multiples of each of these frequencies (in wavenumbers). For example, an overtone band may appear for acetaldehyde at 3460 cm^{-1}, which corresponds to twice the frequency (2 × 1730 cm^{-1}) for the carbonyl stretching band. Since the frequencies are simply associated with harmonic motion of the radiant energy, the overtones may be thought of as simple multiples that are exactly in phase with the fundamental frequency and can therefore "fit" into the same resonant vibration within the molecule.

Since the vibrational resonances of a complex molecule often can be attributed to particular bonds or groups, they behave as though they resulted from vibrations in a diatomic molecule. This means that vibrations produced by similar bonds and atoms are associated with infrared bands over a small frequency range, even though these vibrations may occur in completely different molecules. Some characteristic infrared stretching vibrations are listed according to bond and atomic group in Table 4–9. The infrared spectrum of a molecule can be used for structural identification by applying tables such as Table 4–9. This qualitative use is the principal application of infrared spectroscopy in pharmacy. A typical infrared spectrum of theophylline is shown in Figure 4–11. The spectrum "fingerprints" the drug and provides one method of verifying compounds. The individual bands can be associated with particular groups. For example, the band at 1660 cm^{-1}, (*a*) in Figure 4–11, is due to a carbonyl stretching vibration for theophylline.

Infrared spectra can be complex, and characteristic frequencies vary depending on the physical state of the molecule being examined. For example, hydrogen bonding between sample molecules may change the spectra. For alcohols in dilute carbon tetrachloride solution, there is little intermolecular hydrogen bonding, and the hydroxyl stretching vibration occurs at about 3600 cm^{-1}. The precise position and shape of the infrared band associated with the hydroxyl group depends on the concentration of the alcohol and the degree of hydrogen bonding. Steric effects, the size and relative charge of neighboring groups, and phase changes can effect similar frequency shifts.

The use of infrared spectroscopy in pharmacy has centered on its applications for drug identification, as described by Chapman and Moss.[10] The development of Fourier Transform-Infrared (FT-IR) spectrometry, as described by Durig,[11] has enhanced infrared applica-

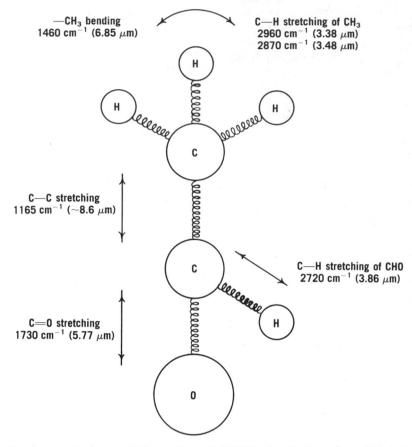

—CH₃ bending
1460 cm⁻¹ (6.85 μm)

C—H stretching of CH₃
2960 cm⁻¹ (3.38 μm)
2870 cm⁻¹ (3.48 μm)

C—C stretching
1165 cm⁻¹ (~8.6 μm)

C—H stretching of CHO
2720 cm⁻¹ (3.86 μm)

C=O stretching
1730 cm⁻¹ (5.77 μm)

Fig. 4—10. Bending and stretching frequencies for acetaldehyde. (From H. H. Willard et al., *Instrumental Methods of Analysis*, 4th Edition, Van Nostrand, New York, 1965.)

TABLE 4—9. *Characteristic Infrared Stretching Vibrations of Some Functional or Atomic Groups*

Group	Characteristic Wavenumber Range (cm⁻¹)
C—F (monofluoro)	1110–1000
C—Cl (monochloro)	730– 650
C—Br (monobromo)	680– 515
C—I (monoiodo)	600– 500
C=N	1620–1690
C≡N	2100–2300
N=N	1500–1560
N—H	3200–3600
C—C	600–1500
C=C (olefin)	1620–1700
C=C (aromatic)	1430–1650
C≡C	2100–2300
C—O (alcohol)	1075–1400
C=O	1600–1900
C—H (alkane)	2850–3000
C—H (alkene)	3000–3100
C—H (aromatic)	3000–3100
O—H	3200–3700

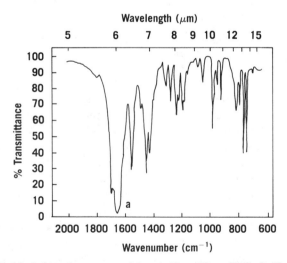

Fig. 4—11. Infrared spectrum of theophylline. (From E. G. C. Clarke, Ed., *Isolation and Identification of Drugs*, Pharmaceutical Press, London, 1969.)

tions for both qualitative and quantitative analysis of drugs owing to the greater sensitivity and the enhanced ability to analyze aqueous samples with FT-IR instrumentation. A thorough survey of the techniques and applications of infrared spectroscopy is provided by Smith[12] and by Willard et al.[13]

ELECTRON SPIN AND NUCLEAR MAGNETIC RESONANCE SPECTROSCOPY

Electromagnetic radiation is characterized as waves that have both an electric vector and a magnetic vector at 90° to each other, as shown in Figure 4–12. Certain forms of spectroscopy measure differences in magnetic

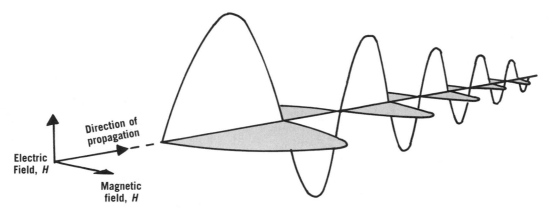

Fig. 4–12. Wave model of electromagnetic radiation showing electrical and magnetic vectors.

energy levels of electrons or nuclei through their relationship to certain frequencies of electromagnetic radiation. A species with an odd number of (or unpaired) electrons placed in an external magnetic field can produce resonance between energy levels of the unpaired electron's magnetic moment at a frequency in the microwave region of the electromagnetic spectrum (see Table 4–2). This resonance is associated with the spin of the unpaired electron, and the study of this effect is termed electron spin resonance (ESR) or, alternatively, electron paramagnetic resonance (EPR) spectroscopy. The microwave frequency at which resonance occurs depends upon the external magnetic field. For example, a frequency at 10 Hz* typically will be found for resonances produced with a magnetic field H of 0.35 T.[†] Resonance of the unpaired electron is specifically associated with the energy difference, ΔE, between the two spin states that an electron can have according to the quantum theory. When the electron is an external magnetic field,

$$\Delta E = h\nu = g\beta_e H \qquad (4-18)$$

in which ν is the resonance frequency in the microwave region, β_e is a constant known as the *Bohr magneton* with a value of 9.27×10^{-24} joule/tesla, H is the applied magnetic field, and g is termed the spectroscopic *splitting factor*. The g *factor* is characteristic for certain metal complexes with unpaired electrons. For organic free radicals, g is nearly equal to its value for a free electron, 2.0023, which is the ratio of the electron's *spin* magnetic moment to its *orbital* magnetic moment.

Electron spin resonance spectroscopy has been applied to the study of free radical processes, including pathways of photosynthesis, and to the structure of metal complexes. It is useful only for species that possess unpaired electrons. The addition of substances with unpaired electrons to systems such as lipids or enzymes that do not contain odd electrons, however,

affords the lipids or enzymes a *spin label*. This permits studies of the structural environment near the spin label through changes in the pattern of the ESR spectrum. Applications of ESR are described by Swartz et al.[14]

The interaction of electromagnetic radiation from the radiowave region of the spectrum (see Table 4–2) with the spin of *nuclei* in a magnetic field is studied by nuclear magnetic resonance (NMR) spectroscopy. All atomic nuclei have a charge attributed to their protons and, in addition, may have a spin about their nuclear axis. Spinning charges, whether they be nuclei or electric currents in closed circuits, generate magnetic fields, that is, they have magnetic moments. The total angular momentum of the spinning charges from the particles of a particular nucleus is characterized by the spin quantum number, I. A nucleus in the ground state, which is the only state we shall discuss here since we are dealing with low-energy transitions, can have a value of I from 0, which denotes no nuclear spin, increasing to $\frac{1}{2}$, 1, $\frac{3}{2}$, etc. This value of I is directly related to the atomic number and mass number of the nucleus so that nuclei with even atomic and mass numbers have $I = 0$ and no spin and no magnetic moment. Such nuclei include ^{12}C and ^{16}O. Nuclei with odd mass numbers have I of half-integral value, while nuclei with odd atomic numbers but even mass numbers have I of integral value. Both of these last cases give rise to nuclei with magnetic moments and, consequently, NMR signals. Examples include ^{1}H, ^{13}C, ^{15}N, and ^{19}F, which have $I = \frac{1}{2}$, and ^{2}H and ^{14}N, which have $I = 1$.

The concept of NMR is based on the fact that nuclei with magnetic moments, μ, *precess*, that is, rotate like a gyroscope, about the axis of an applied magnetic field. This precession occurs only through certain orientations, or nuclear *spin states*, with their own I values, as shown in Figure 4–13. The nuclear spin states are separated by the energy difference ΔE, so that

$$\Delta E = h\nu = \mu H(1 - \sigma)/I \qquad (4-19)$$

in which σ is the shielding constant for a particular atom (i.e., a measure of its susceptibility to induction from a

---

*Hertz, Hz., is frequency in waves per second.

[†]The tesla, T, is the unit of magnetic flux density: One T induces a voltage of 1 volt in a 1-m long conductor that is moving at 1 m/sec. The tesla is equivalent to 10^4 gauss, the unit that the tesla replaced.

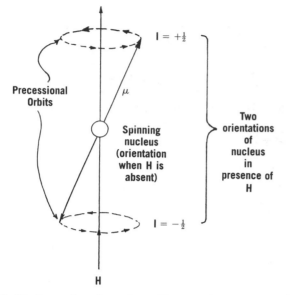

Fig. 4–13. Precession of a nucleus with magnetic moment, μ, about the axis of an applied magnetic field, H. (Modified from D. Betteridge and H. E. Hallam, *Modern Analytical Methods*, The Chemical Society, London, 1972, p. 201.)

magnetic field), H is the external magnetic field strength, μ is the nuclear magnetic moment, and ν is some radio frequency. In actual practice, equation (4–19) can be applied to spectroscopy by gradually varying the magnetic field strength, H, while keeping the radio frequency, ν, constant. At some particular H value, a nuclear spin transition will take place that flips the nuclei from one spin state to another (for example, from $I = -\frac{1}{2}$ to $+\frac{1}{2}$, as in Fig. 4–13). In some spectrometers, the experiment can be done in the reverse fashion: keeping H constant and varying ν. In either case, equation (4–19) applies, and the particular value of ν depends on H.

Example 4–6. (*a*) What is the energy change associated with the ^1H nuclear spin of chloroform, which has a shielding constant, σ, of -7.25×10^{-6} and a nuclear magnetic moment, μ, of 1.410620×10^{-26} J/T in a magnetic field H of 1 tesla? The spin quantum number I for ^1H is 0.5.

From equation (4–19):

$\Delta E = \mu H (1 - \sigma)/I = (1.410620 \times 10^{-26}) \times 1 \times (1.00000725)/(0.5)$

$= 2.821260 \times 10^{-26}$ J*

(*b*) What is the radio frequency at which resonance will occur for this nuclear spin transition under the stated conditions? From equation (4–19):

$$\nu = \frac{\Delta E}{h} = \frac{2.821260 \times 10^{-26}}{6.626196 \times 10^{-34}} = 4.257738 \times 10^7 \text{ Hz}$$

Tetramethylsilane (TMS) is often used as a reference compound in proton NMR because the resonance frequency of its one proton signal, from its four identical methyl groups, is below that for most other compounds. In addition, TMS is relatively stable and inert.

---

*We have assumed an exaggerated level of significance for this value, i.e., six significant digits after the decimal point, to show a subsequent relationship.

$$\begin{array}{c} CH_3 \\ | \\ CH_3-Si-CH_3 \\ | \\ CH_3 \end{array}$$

Tetramethylsilane

Example 4–7. What is the radio frequency at which resonance occurs for TMS in a magnetic field of 1 tesla?

The shielding constant is 0.000, and $\Delta E = 2.821240 \times 10^{-26}$ J for TMS, so

$$\nu = \frac{\Delta E}{h} = \frac{2.821240 \times 10^{-26}}{6.626196 \times 10^{-34}} = 4.257707 \times 10^7 \text{ Hz}$$

From the examples just given, it is important to note that the difference in the resonance frequency between chloroform and TMS at a constant magnetic field strength is only $(4.257738 \times 10^7) - (4.257707 \times 10^7) = 310$ Hz or waves/sec. This small radio frequency difference is equivalent to more than half the total range within which ^1H NMR signals are detected. Consequently, the instrument needs to scan only a relatively narrow range of radio frequencies with a constant magnetic field strength for what is termed *frequency-swept NMR*. Alternatively, the instrument may sweep a narrow region of magnetic field strength while the radio frequency is constant, for *field-swept NMR*.

The value of the shielding constant, σ, for a particular nucleus will depend on local magnetic fields, including those produced by nearby electrons within the molecule. This effect is promoted by placing the molecule within a large external magnetic field, H. Greater shielding will occur with higher electron density near a particular nucleus, and this reduces the frequency (assuming frequency-swept NMR) at which resonance takes place. Thus, for TMS, the high electron density from the Si atom produces enhanced shielding and, therefore, a lower resonance frequency. The relative difference between a particular NMR signal and a reference signal (usually from TMS for proton NMR) is termed the *chemical shift*, δ, given in parts per million (ppm). It is defined as

$$\delta = (\sigma_r - \sigma_s) \times 10^6 \qquad (4-20)$$

in which σ_r and σ_s are the shielding constants for the reference and sample nucleus, respectively.

If the separation between the sample and reference resonance is ΔH or $\Delta\nu$, then

$$\delta = \frac{\Delta H}{H_R} \times 10^6 = \frac{\Delta\nu}{\nu_R} \times 10^6 \qquad (4-21)$$

in which H_R or ν_R are the magnetic field strength or radio frequency for the nuclei* depending on whether field-swept or frequency-swept NMR is used.

---

*In our example, the proton ^1_1H resonates at 42.57×10^6 Hz at a field strength of 1 tesla.

Example 4-8. What is the chemical shift of the chloroform proton using TMS as a reference?

Substituting the frequencies obtained from *Examples 4-6b* and *4-7* into equation (4-21), we obtain the chemical shift:

$$\delta = \frac{\Delta\nu}{\nu_R} \times 10^6$$

$$= \frac{(4.257738 \times 10^7) - (4.257707 \times 10^7)}{42.57 \times 10^6} \times 10^6$$

$$= \frac{310 \times 10^6}{42.57 \times 10^6} = 7.28 \text{ ppm}$$

This is an approximate value owing to the relative accuracy used to determine each frequency in the example. The accepted experimental value for this chemical shift is 7.25 ppm. Identical chemical shifts are obtained using either frequency or field sweeping as the experimental measurement, since the relative changes (i.e., ΔH or $\Delta\nu$) to the reference value are directly proportional by either NMR method. The chemical shift of a nucleus provides information about its local magnetic environment and therefore can "type'" a nuclear species. Table 4-10 lists some representative proton chemical shifts. Figure 4-14 shows a proton NMR spectrum for benzyl acetate, $CH_3COOCH_2C_6H_5$, using TMS as a reference. Notice that each signal band represents a particular type of proton, that is, the proton at $\delta = 2.0$ is from the CH_3 group, while that at 5.0 is due to CH_2, and the protons at about 7.3 are from the aromatic protons. The *integral* curve above the spectrum is the sum of the respective band areas, and its stepwise height is proportional to the number of protons represented by each band.

An example of the application of NMR to the direct analysis of a pharmaceutical is given by Hanna and Lau-Cam[15] for succinylcholine chloride injections. This NMR assay involves the addition of a known amount of acetamide, as an internal standard, to a freeze-dried sample of the succinylcholine injection. The mixture is dissolved in deuterium oxide (D_2O) and the NMR spectrum obtained. The integral of the band at 3.27 ppm, from the 18 protons in CH_3 groups attached to N atoms in succinylcholine chloride, that is,

TABLE 4-10. *Proton Chemical Shifts for Representative Chemical Groups or Compounds*

Compound or Group	ppm
TMS $(CH_3)_4Si$	0.00
CH_4	0.23
Cyclohexane	1.44
Acetone	2.08
CH_3Cl	3.06
$CHCl_3$	7.25
Benzene	7.27
Ethylene	5.28
Acetylene	1.80
R—OH (hydrogen-bonded)	0.5–5.0
R_2—NH	1.2–2.1
Carboxylic acids (R—COOH)	10–13
H_2O	~4.7

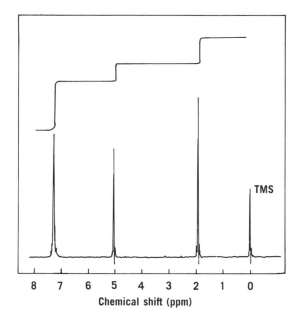

Fig. 4-14. Proton NMR spectrum of benzyl acetate with TMS as a reference. The TMS band appears at the far right. The upper curve is an integration of the spectral bands, the height of the step at each being proportional to the area under that band. (From W. S. Brey, *Physical Chemistry and Its Biological Applications*, Academic Press, New York, 1978, p. 498.)

$$\left[\begin{array}{c} CH_2COOCH_2CH_2\overset{+}{N}(CH_3)_3 \\ | \\ CH_2COOCH_2CH_2\underset{+}{N}(CH_3)_3 \end{array}\right] 2Cl^-$$

Succinylcholine Chloride

and the integral from the band at 2.01 ppm, due to the three methyl protons of acetamide (CH_3CONH_2), are determined. The amount of succinylcholine chloride in an injection sample is then calculated from

$$C = W/V \times Iu/Is \times EWu/EWs \qquad (4-22)$$

in which C is the concentration, in mg/mL, of the succinylcholine chloride, W is the weight, in mg, of acetamide taken as the internal standard, V is the volume, in mL, of succinylcholine chloride injection being tested, Iu and Is are the average integrals of the 3.27-ppm band from succinylcholine chloride and the 2.01-ppm band from acetamide, respectively, EWu is the formula weight (molecular weight) of succinylcholine chloride divided by the number of protons producing the signal band (i.e., 361.31/18), and EWs is the formula weight of the internal standard divided by its signal protons (i.e., 59.07/3).

Example 4-9. What is the concentration (in mg/mL) of succinylcholine chloride in a 1-mL injection sample to which 93 mg of acetamide internal standard is added, and which produces average integral signals at 3.27 ppm and 2.01 ppm of 2158 and 2045 units, respectively?

$$C = W/V \times Iu/Is \times EWu/EWs = 93/1 \times 2158/2045 \times \frac{361.31/18}{59.07/3}$$

$$= 93 \times 1.06 \times 20.07/19.69$$

$$= 100 \text{ mg/mL}$$

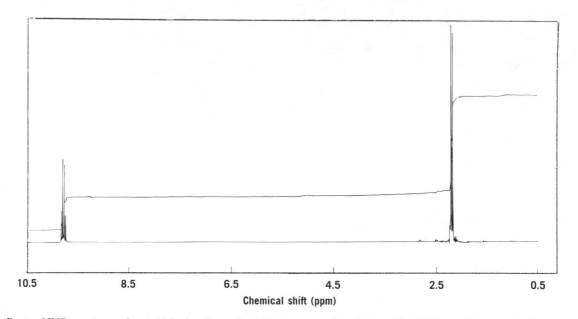

Fig. 4–15. Proton NMR spectrum of acetaldehyde. (From A. S. V. Burgen and J. C. Metcalfe, J. Pharm. Pharmacol. **22**, 156, 1970.)

In Figure 4–14, the signal bands are of simple shape, with little apparent complexity. Such sharp single bands are known as *singlets* in NMR terminology. In most NMR spectra, the bands are not as simple, since each particular nucleus can be coupled by spin interactions to neighboring nuclei. If these neighboring nuclei are in different local magnetic environments, owing primarily to differences in electron densities, splitting of the bands can occur. This leads to *multiplet* patterns, with several lines for a single resonant nucleus. The pattern of splitting in the multiplet can provide valuable information concerning the nature of the neighboring nuclei.

Figure 4–15 shows the proton NMR spectrum of acetaldehyde, CH_3CHO, in which the doublet of the CH_3 group (right side of the figure) is produced from coupling to the neighboring single proton, and the quartet of the lone proton in the CHO group (left side of the figure) is produced from coupling to the three methyl protons. In any molecule, if the representative coupled nuclei are in proportion as A_X:A_Y on neighboring groups, then the resonance band for A_X will be split into $(2_Y \times I + 1)$ lines, in which I is the spin quantum number for the nuclei, while that for A_Y will be split into $(2_X \times I + 1)$ lines, assuming the nuclei are in different local environments. For example, with acetaldehyde, A_X:A_Y is CH_3:CH, and the resulting proton splitting pattern is A_X (CH_3) as two lines and A_Y (CH) as four lines. This splitting produces *first-order* spectra when the difference in ppm between all the lines of a multiplet (known as the *coupling constant*, J) is small compared with the difference in the chemical shift, δ, between the coupled nuclei. First-order spectra produce simple multiplets with intensities determined by the coefficients of the binomial expansion: a doublet of intensity 1:1; a triplet, 1:2:1; a quartet, 1:3:3:1. Further details of multiplicity and the interpretation of NMR spectra can be found in the book by Bauer et al.[16]

The typical range for NMR chemical shifts depends on the nucleus being observed: for protons, it is about 15 ppm with organic compounds, while it is about 400 ppm for ^{13}C or ^{19}F spectra. Table 4–11 gives the basic NMR resonance for certain pure isotopes, together with their natural abundances. As the natural abundance of the isotope decreases, the relative sensitivity of NMR gets proportionally smaller.

TABLE 4–11. *Basic NMR Resonances and Natural Abundance of Selected Isotopes**

Isotope	NMR Frequency (MHz) at Field Strength (T)		Natural Abundance (%)
	1.0000 T	2.3487 T	
^1_1H	42.57	100.00	99.985
$^{13}_6C$	10.71	25.14	1.108
$^{15}_7N$	4.31	10.13	0.365
$^{19}_9F$	40.05	94.08	100

*From A. J. Gordon and R. A. Ford, *The Chemist's Companion*, Wiley, New York, 1972, p. 314.

The development of ^{13}C NMR spectroscopy in recent years has been influenced by the application of *spin decoupling* to intensify and simplify the otherwise complex ^{13}C NMR spectra. Decoupling of the proton spins is produced by continuously irradiating the entire proton spectral range with broad-band radiofrequency radiation. This decoupling produces the collapse of multiplet signals into simpler and more intense signals. It also produces an effect known as the *nuclear Overhauser effect* (NOE), in which decoupling of the protons produces a dipole–dipole interaction and energy transfer to the carbon nuclei, resulting in greater relaxation (i.e., rate of loss of energy from nuclei in the higher spin state to the lower spin state), and, consequently, a greater population of carbon nuclei in the lower spin state (see Fig. 4–13). Since this greater population in the lower spin state permits a greater absorption signal in NMR, the NOE can increase the carbon nuclei signal by as much as a factor of three. These factors—proton spin decoupling and the NOE—have enhanced the sensitivity of ^{13}C NMR and, therefore, compensate for the low natural abundance of ^{13}C as well as the smaller magnetic moment, μ, of ^{13}C compared with that for hydrogen.

A powerful extension of this enhancement of ^{13}C spectra involves systematically decoupling only specific protons by irradiating at particular radiofrequencies rather than by broad-band irradiation. Such systematic decoupling permits individual carbon atoms to show multiplet collapse and signal intensification, as mentioned above, when protons coupled to the particular carbon atom are irradiated. These signal changes allow particular carbon nuclei in a molecular structure to be associated with particular protons, and produce what is termed *two-dimensional NMR spectrometry*. The techniques involved in these experiments are described by Farrar.[17]

Nuclear magnetic resonance is a versatile tool in pharmaceutical research. Spectra can provide powerful evidence for a particular molecular conformation of a drug, including the distinction between closely related isomeric structures. This identification is normally based on the relative position of chemical shifts as well a peak multiplicity and other parameters associated with spin coupling. Drug–receptor interactions can be distinguished and characterized through specific changes in the NMR spectrum of the unbound drug after the addition of a suitable protein binder. These changes are due to restrictions in drug orientation. Burgen and Metcalfe[18] describe applications of NMR to problems involving drug-membrane and drug–protein interactions. An illustration of these interactions analyzed by both ESR and NMR spectroscopy is given by Lawrence and Gill[19] using ESR, and by Tamir and Lichtenberg[20] using proton-NMR techniques. The ESR and proton-NMR results show that the psychotropic tetrahydrocannabinols reduce the molecular ordering in the bilayer of liposomes used as simple models of biologic membranes. These results suggest that the cannabinoids exert their psychotropic effects by way of a nonspecific interaction of the cannabinoid with lipid constituents, principally cholesterol, of nerve cell membranes. The use of NMR in pharmaceutical research, with particular reference to analytical problems, has been reviewed by Rackham.[21]

REFRACTIVE INDEX AND MOLAR REFRACTION

Light passes more slowly through a substance than through a vacuum. As light enters a denser substance, the advancing waves at the interface are modified by being closer together owing to their slower speed and shorter wavelength, as shown in Figure 4–16. If the light enters the denser substance at an angle, as shown, one part of the wave slows down more quickly as it passes the interface, and this produces a bending of the wave toward the interface. This phenomenon is called *refraction*. If light enters a less dense substance, it is refracted away from the interface rather than toward it. The relative value of this effect between two substances is given by the *refractive index*, n:

$$n = \frac{\sin i}{\sin r}$$

$$= \frac{\text{velocity of light in first substance}}{\text{velocity of light in second substance}} \quad (4-23)$$

in which $\sin i$ is the sine of the angle of the incident ray of light and $\sin r$ is the sine of the angle of the refracted ray. Normally, the numerator is taken as the velocity of light in air, and the denominator is the material being investigated. The refractive index, by this convention, is greater than 1 for substances denser than air. Theoretically, the reference state where $n = 1$ should be for light passing through a vacuum; however, the use of air as a reference produces a difference in n of only

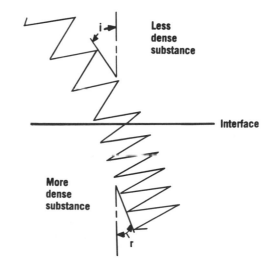

Fig. 4–16. Waves of light passing an interface between two substances of different density.

0.03% from that in a vacuum and is more commonly used.

Refractive index varies with the wavelength of light and the temperature. Normally, these values are identified when a refractive index is listed; for example, n_D^{20} signifies the refractive index using the D-line emission of sodium, at 589 nm, at a temperature of 20° C. Pressure must also be held constant in measuring the refractive index of gases. Refractive index can be used to identify a substance, to measure its purity, and to determine the concentration of one substance dissolved in another. Typically, a refractometer is used to determine refractive index.

The *molar refraction*, R_m, is related to both the refractive index and the molecular properties of a compound being tested. It is expressed as

$$R_m = \frac{n^2 - 1}{n^2 + 2} \left(\frac{M}{\rho} \right) \qquad (4\text{-}24)$$

in which M is the molecular weight and ρ is the density of the compound. The R_m value of a compound can often be predicted from the structural features of the molecule. Each constituent atom or group contributes a portion to the final R_m value, as discussed earlier in connection with additive-constitutive properties (see Table 4–1). For example, acetone has an R_m produced from three carbons ($R_m = 7.254$), six hydrogens (6.6), and a carbonyl oxygen (2.21) to give a total R_m of 16.1 cm³/mol. Because R_m is independent of the physical state of the molecule, this value can often be used to distinguish between structurally different compounds, such as keto and enol tautomers.

Light incident upon a molecule induces vibrating dipoles, and the greater the refractive index at a particular wavelength, the greater is the dipolar induction. The interaction of light photons with the polarizable electrons of a dielectric causes a reduction in the velocity of light. The dielectric constant, being a measure of polarizability, is greatest when dipolar interactions with light are proportionally large. The refractive index for light of long wavelengths, n_∞, is related to the dielectric constant for a nonpolar molecule, ϵ, by the expression:

$$\epsilon = n_\infty^2 \qquad (4\text{-}25)$$

Molar polarization, P_i, equation (4–15), can be considered roughly equivalent to molar refraction, R_n, and can be written as

$$P_i = \left(\frac{n_\infty^2 - 1}{n_\infty^2 + 2} \right) \frac{M}{\rho} = \frac{4}{3} \pi N \alpha_p \qquad (4\text{-}26)$$

From this equation, the polarizability α_p of a nonpolar molecule may be obtained from a measurement of refractive index. For practical purposes, the refractive index at a finite wavelength is used. This introduces only a relatively small error, approximately 5%, in the calculation.

OPTICAL ROTATION

By passing light through a polarizing prism, such as a Nicol prism, the randomly distributed vibrations of radiation are sorted so that only those vibrations occurring in a single plane are emitted. The velocity of this *plane-polarized* light can become slower or faster as it passes through a substance, in a manner similar to that discussed for refraction. This change in velocity results in refraction of the polarized light in a particular direction for an *optically active* substance. A clockwise rotation, looking into the beam of polarized light, defines a substance that is *dextrorotatory*, whereas a counterclockwise rotation defines a *levorotatory* substance. The dextrorotatory substance, which may be thought of as rotating the beam to the right, produces an *angle of rotation*, α, that is defined as positive (+); while the levorotatory substance, which would rotate the beam to the left, has an α that is defined as negative (−). Molecules that have an asymmetric center and therefore lack symmetry about a single plane are optically active, whereas symmetric molecules are optically inactive and consequently do not rotate the plane of polarized light. Optical activity can be considered as the interaction of a plane-polarized radiation with electrons in a molecule to produce electronic polarization. This interaction rotates the direction of vibration of the radiation by altering the electric field. A *polarimeter* is used to measure optical activity.

Optical rotation, α, depends on the density of an optically active substance, since each molecule provides an equal but small contribution to the rotation. The *specific rotation*, $\{\alpha\}_\lambda^t$, at a specified temperature t and wavelength λ (usually the D-line of sodium), is characteristic for a pure, optically active substance. It is expressed by the equation

$$\{\alpha\}_\lambda^t = \frac{\alpha v}{lg} \qquad (4\text{-}27)$$

in which l is the length in decimeters (dm*) of the light path through the sample, and g is the number of grams of optically active substance in v mL of volume. If the substance is dissolved in a solution, the solvent as well as the concentration should be reported with the specific rotation. The specific rotations of some drugs are found in Table 4–12. The subscript D on [α] indicates that the measurement of specific rotation is made at a wavelength (λ) of 589 nm for sodium light. When the concentration is not specified, as in Table 4–12, the concentration is assumed to be 1 gram per milliliter of solvent. The specific rotation of steroids, carbohydrates, aminoacids, and other compounds of biologic importance are found in the *CRC Handbook of Chemistry and Physics*, CRC Press, Boca Raton, Fl.

---

*Decimeters was the unit chosen because of the long sample cells normally used in polarimeters. The decimeter = 10 cm = 1/10 m.

TABLE 4-12. *Specific Rotations*

Drug	$[\alpha]_D$	Temperature (°C)	Solvent
Ampicillin	+283°	20	Water
Aureomycin	+296°	23	Water
Benzylpenicillin	+305°	25	Water
Camphor	+41° to +43°	25	Ethanol
Colchicine	−121°	17	Chloroform
Cyanocobalamin	−60°	23	Water
Ergonovine	−16°	20	Pyridine
Nicotine	−162°	20	Pure liquid
Propoxyphene	+67°	25	Chloroform
Quinidine	+230°	15	Chloroform
Reserpine	−120°	25	Chloroform
Tetracycline hydrochloride	−253	24	Methanol
d-Tubocurarine chloride	+190°	22	Water
Yohimbine	+51° to +62°	20	Ethanol

Optical Rotatory Dispersion. Optical rotation changes as a function of the wavelength of light, and *optical rotatory dispersion* (ORD) is the measurement of the angle of rotation as a function of the wavelength. By varying the wavelength of light, the specific rotation for an optically active substance will change. A graph of specific rotation versus wavelength shows an inflection and then passes through zero at the wavelength of maximum absorption of polarized light as shown in Figure 4–17. This change in specific rotation is known as the *Cotton effect*. By convention, compounds whose specific rotations show a maximum *before* passing through zero as the wavelength of polarized light becomes smaller are said to show a *positive Cotton effect*, whereas if {α} shows a maximum *after* passing through zero (under the same conditions of approaching shorter wavelengths), the compound shows a *negative Cotton effect*. Enantiomers can be characterized by the Cotton effect, as shown in Figure 4–18. In addition, ORD is often useful for the structural examination of organic compounds. For example, one can readily distinguish between two steroids with keto groups at positions 3 and 17 by examination of rotatory dispersion curves.

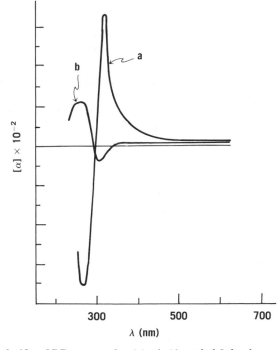

Fig. 4–18. ORD curves for (*a*) *cis*-10-methyl-2-decalone and (*b*) trans-10-methyl-2-decalone. Note that (*a*) has a positive cotton effect, while (*b*) has a negative cotton effect. (From *Optical Rotatory Dispersion*, by C. Djerassi. Copyright © 1960, McGraw-Hill Book Company, New York. Used with the permission of McGraw-Hill Book Company.)

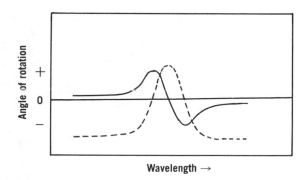

Fig. 4–17. The Cotton effect. Variation of the angle of rotation (solid line) in the vicinity of an absorption band of polarized light (dashed line). (Modified from W. S. Brey, *Physical Chemistry and Its Biological Applications*, Academic Press, New York, 1978, p. 330.)

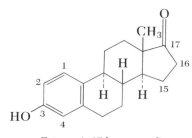

Estrone (a 17-keto steroid)

Detailed discussion of ORD is given by Crabbe.[22]

CIRCULAR DICHROISM

Plane-polarized light is described as the vector sum of two circularly polarized components. Circularly polarized light has an electric vector that spirals around the direction of propagation. In plane-polarized light, there can be two such vectors, each spiraling in the opposite direction. For an optically active substance, the values of the index of refraction n of the two vectors cannot be the same. This difference changes the relative rate at which the polarized light spirals about its direction of propagation.

Likewise, the speeds of the two components of polarized light become unequal as they pass through an optically active substance that is capable of absorbing light over a selected wavelength range. This is the same as saying that the two components of polarized light have different absorptivities at a particular wavelength of light. This effect causes circularly polarized light to become elliptically polarized, and this is termed *circular dichroism* (CD). The Cotton effect is the unequal absorption of light by the two components of circularly polarized light in the wavelength region near an absorption band. Circular dichroism spectra are plots of molar ellipticity, ([θ]), which is proportional to the difference in absorptivities between the two components of circularly polarized light, against the wavelength of light. Molar ellipticity is given by

$$[\theta] = \frac{[\psi]M}{100} = 3300 \, (\epsilon_L - \epsilon_R) \text{ deg liter mole}^{-1} \text{ dm}^{-1}$$

$$(4-28)$$

where 1 dm is written for 10 cm, and [ψ] is the specific ellipticity analogous to specific rotation, M is the molecular weight, and ϵ_L and ϵ_R are the molar absorptivities for the left and right components of circularly polarized light at a selected wavelength. The applications of CD to interactions between small molecules and macromolecules are reviewed by Perrin and Hart.[23] Its application to the determination of the activity of penicillin was described by Rasmussen and Higuchi.[24] The activity is measured as the change in the CD spectra of penicillin after addition of penicillinase, which enzymatically cleaves the β-lactam ring to form the penicilloate ion, as shown for penicillin G on p. 84. Typical CD spectra for benzylpenicillin and its hydrolysis product are shown in Figure 4–19. The direct determination of penicillins by CD and the distinction of penicillins from cephalosporins by their CD spectra has been described by Purdie and Swallows.[25] The penicillins all have single positive CD bands with maxima at 230 nm, while the cephalosporins have two CD bands, a positive one with a maximum at 260 nm and a negative one with maximum at 230 nm (wavelengths for maxima are given to within ±2 nm). This permits easy differentiation between penicillins and cephalosporins by CD spectropolarimetry.

References and Notes

1. W. S. Brey, *Physical Chemistry and Its Biological Applications*, Academic Press, New York, 1978, Chapter 9.
2. S. G. Jivani and V. J. Stella, J. Pharm. Sci. **74**, 1274, 1985.
3. A. L. Gutman, V. Ribon, and J. P. Leblanc, Anal. Chem. **57**, 2344, 1985.
4. S. G. Schulman and B. S. Vogt, in J. W. Munson, Ed., *Pharmaceutical Analysis: Modern Methods, Part B*, Marcel Dekker, New York, 1984, Chapter 8.
5. S. G. Schulman and R. J. Sturgeon, in J. W. Munson, ed. *Pharmaceutical Analysis: Modern Methods, Part A*, Marcel Dekker, New York, 1984, Chapter 4.
6. W. G. Gorman and G. D. Hall, J. Pharm. Sci. **53**, 1017, 1964.
7. S. N. Pagay, R. I. Poust and J. L. Colaizzi, J. Pharm. Sci. **63**, 44, 1974.
8. P. A. Kollman, in M. E. Wolff, Ed., *The Basis of Medicinal Chemistry, Burger's Medicinal Chemistry, Part I*, Wiley, New York, 1980, Chapter 7.
9. V. I. Minkin, O. A. Osipov and Y. A. Zhadanov, *Dipole Moments in Organic Chemistry*, Plenum Press, New York, 1970.
10. D. I. Chapman and M. S. Moss, in E. G. C. Clarke, Ed., *Isolation and Identification of Drugs*, Pharmaceutical Press, London, 1969, pp. 103–122.
11. J. R. Durig, Ed., *Chemical, Biological, and Industrial Applications of Infrared Spectroscopy*, Wiley, New York, 1985. R. A. Hoult, *Development of the Model 1600 FT-IR Spectrophotometer*, Perkin Elmer Corp., Norwalk, Conn. R. J. Bell, *Introductory Fourier Transform Spectroscopy*, Academic Press, New York, 1972. P. R. Griffith, *Chemical Infrared Fourier Transform Spectroscopy*, Wiley, New York, 1975. R. J. Markovich and C. Pidgeon, Pharm. Res. **8**, 663, 1991.
12. A. L. Smith, *Applied Infrared Spectroscopy*, Wiley, New York, 1979.
13. H. H. Willard, L. L. Merritt, J. A. Dean and F. A. Settle, *Instrumental Methods of Analysis*, 6th Edition, Van Nostrand, New York, 1981, Chapter 7.
14. H. M. Swartz, J. R. Bolton and D. C. Borg, Eds., *Biological Applications of Electron Spin Resonance*, Wiley, New York, 1972.
15. G. M. Hanna and C. A. Lau-Cam, Anal. Let. **18**, 2183, 1985.
16. H. H. Bauer, G. D. Christian and J. E. O'Reilly, *Instrumental Analysis*, Allyn and Bacon, Boston, 1978, Chapter 12.

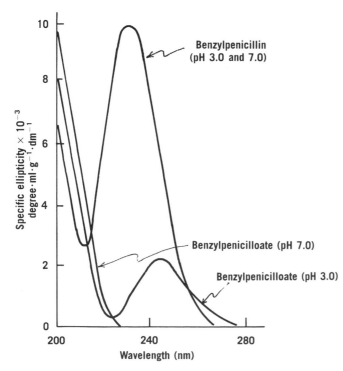

Fig. 4–19. CD spectra of benzylpenicillin and its penicilloic acid derivative at pH 7.0. (From C. E. Rassmussen and T. Higuchi, J. Pharm. Sci. **60**, 1616, 1971, reproduced with permission of the copyright owner.)

17. T. C. Farrar, Anal. Chem. **59**, 749A, 1987.
18. A. S. V. Burgen and J. C. Metcalfe, J. Pharm. Pharmacol. **22**, 153, 1970.
19. D. K. Lawrence and E. W. Gill, Mol. Pharmacol. **11**, 595, 1975.
20. J. Tamir and D. Lichtenberg, J. Pharm. Sci. **72**, 458, 1983.
21. D. M. Rackham, Talanta **23**, 269, 1976.
22. P. Crabbe, *ORD and CD in Chemistry and Biochemistry*, Academic Press, New York, 1972.
23. J. H. Perin and P. A. Hart, J. Pharm. Sci. **59**, 431, 1970.
24. C. E. Rasmussen and T. Higuchi, J. Pharm. Sci. **60**, 1608, 1971.
25. N. Purdie and K. A. Swallows, Anal. Chem. **59**, 1349, 1987.
26. G. M. Hanna and C. Lav-Cam, Pharmazie **39**, 816, 1984.

Problems

4-1. The wavelength for the detection of lithium by its atomic emission spectra is 670.8 nm. What is the energy of the photon of radiation that corresponds to this emission line for lithium?

Answer: 2.93×10^{-19} J

4-2. Describe at least one limitation to the usefulness of atomic emission methods for the detection of trace metals (for example, selenium) dissolved in blood. (J. A. Dean, Editor, *Lange's Handbook of Chemistry*, McGraw-Hill, New York, 1979, contains tables of emission lines.)

4-3. A urine sample is being analyzed for trace levels of copper by atomic emission. The following flame emission intensities (EI) were obtained at a wavelength of 324.8 nm for the 24-hour urine sample, which had a total volume of 980 mL. A set of copper samples (CS) yielded EI values as shown in the table.

Data for *Problem 4-3*

Copper samples (CS)	Emission intensity (EI)
Cu standard, 0.5 µg/mL	20
Cu standard, 1.0 µg/mL	38
Cu standard, 1.5 µg/mL	61
Cu standard, 2.0 µg/mL	80
Urine sample	32

What is the concentration of copper in the 24-hour urine sample? If the normal copper level in urine is approximately 20 µg per 24-hour sample, does this calculated copper concentration indicate an unusually high pathologic condition?

Hint: Regress CS in µg/mL against EI: $CS = a + b$ EI. From the equation, if the relationship is linear, obtain µg/mL for copper in the urine sample having an EI of 32. This is the result per milliliter; but the volume of the 24-hour urine sample is 980 mL. Calculate the micrograms of copper in the urine over a 24-hour period.

Answer: 797 µg per 24-hour sample. This is an unusually high copper level in urine and indicates a pathologic condition.

4-4. A single tablet of colchicine is dissolved in 100 mL of ethanol and its absorbance maximum at 243 nm is measured as 0.438 in a 1-cm path-length cell. Using the molar absorptivity for colchicine given in Table 4-4, what is the amount, in mg, of colchicine in the tablet? The molecular weight of colchicine is 399.4 g/mole.

Answer: 0.60 mg per tablet.

4-5. The ultraviolet spectrum of saccharin has absorption maxima in methanol at 285, 276, and 226 nm and corresponding molar absorptivities (ϵ) of 775, 951, and 8570 liter mole^{-1} cm^{-1}, respectively. Assuming a minimum absorbance level of $A = 0.002$, what is the minimum detectable concentration of saccharin at each of its absorption maxima wavelengths? Which of these wavelengths would be suitable for the analysis of the amount of saccharin in a tablet with a label claim of 1/4 grain sodium saccharin when the tablet is dissolved in 50 mL of methanol? The molecular weight of sodium saccharin is 205.16 g/mole. Assume that the pathlength of the cell is 1 cm.

Answer: At 285 nm, $c = 2.6 \times 10^{-6}$ mole/liter; at 276 nm, $c = 2.1 \times 10^{-6}$ mole/liter; and at 226 nm, $c = 2.3 \times 10^{-7}$ mole/liter. The

1/4 grain sodium saccharin tablet in a 50-mL solution provides a concentration of 1.58×10^{-3} mole/liter, which is larger than the minimum detectable concentrations at 285, 276, and 226 nm. Any of these three wavelengths is suitable for the analysis.

4-6. A sample of 20 acetaminophen tablets is selected to determine the average amount of active ingredient. The weight of a tablet is 400 mg. Acetaminophen tablets are finely powdered and a portion of the powder (400 mg) is transferred to a 250-mL volumetric flask, diluted with ethanol to volume, mixed, and filtered. One milliliter of the filtrate is transferred to a second 250-mL volumetric flask and diluted with ethanol to volume. The absorbance of this solution, A, is 0.340 at 250 nm, in a 1-cm cell. The molar absorptivity, ϵ, of acetaminophen is 13,500, and its molecular weight is 151.2 g/mole. Calculate the deviation from the labeled amount (250 mg per tablet) in the sample of tablets assayed. The quantity of acetaminophen must be within the limits of 90 and 110 per cent.

Answer: The amount of acetaminophen per tablet is 237.5 mg. The deviation from the labeled claim is 5 per cent, which is within the limits established.

4-7. The Beer's law plot, as shown in Figure 4-4, is a straight line relating absorbance to concentration. Describe an experimental condition in which the Beer's law plot might be a curved line, with the slope of the curve decreasing at higher concentrations. From a molecular point of view, what is the cause of deviations from ideal solution behavior at high concentrations?

4-8. The molecular weight of diethyl ether is 74.12 g/mole and its density is 0.7134 g/cm^3 at 20° C. What is the induced molar polarization, P_i, of diethyl ether? See Table 4-6 for the dielectric constant of diethyl ether. What is the calculated induced polarizability, α_p, for diethyl ether at 20° C?

Answer: $P_i = 54.73$ cm^3/mole; $\alpha_p = 2.17 \times 10^{-23}$ cm^3

4-9. The following table of concentrations and absorbance values, A, was produced for solutions of nitrazepam in 0.1-N sulfuric acid. The absorbance A was measured at 277.5 nm. What is the average molar absorptivity, ϵ, of nitrazepam in 0.1-N sulfuric acid calculated from the three sets of data in the table? A 1-cm path-length cell was used for the experiment. Draw the Beer's law plot associated with the data given in the table. The molecular weight of nitrazepam is 281.3 g/mole.

Data for *Problem 4-9*

Concentration (C) (mg/L)	Absorbance (A)
0.394	0.06
0.844	0.13
1.160	0.25

Answer: Average molar absorptivity, $\epsilon = 4.29 \times 10^4$ liter mole^{-1} cm^{-1}.

4-10. The $E_{1cm}^{1\%}$ value for the ultraviolet absorbance of indomethacin at 318 nm is 182 per 100 mL g^{-1} cm^{-1}. (See page 82 for $E_{1\,cm}^{1\%}$.) What is the molar absorptivity, ϵ, corresponding to this $E_{1\,cm}^{1\%}$ value? The molecular weight of indomethacin is 357.81 g/mole.

Answer: $\epsilon = 6512$ liter mole^{-1} cm^{-1}

4-11.* The methyl group protons of nicotine have a shielding constant σ of -2.2×10^{-6} and the nuclear magnetic moment, μ_H, is 1.41062×10^{-26} J/T for the proton in NMR spectroscopy. The spin quantum number, I, is equal to 1/2. **(a)** What is the frequency ν_R at which resonance will occur for the methyl group of nicotine at a magnetic field strength H of 1 tesla? **(b)** What is the chemical shift, δ, in ppm of the methyl protons of nicotine under the same conditions

---

*Both an H and a lower case h appear in this problem and they must not be confused. H is the magnetic field given in the units of *teslas* and h is the Planck's constant, 6.6262×10^{-27} erg sec.

using TMS as a reference? TMS has a resonance frequency ν_R of 4.257707×10^7 Hz under the stated conditions. See *Examples 4–6, 4–7,* and *4–8.*

Answer: **(a)** $\nu_R = 4.257716 \times 10^7$ Hz. **(b)** Chemical shift, $\delta = 2.11$ ppm. (*Note:* δ may equal 2.16 if ν is carried out to several more decimal places.)

4–12. A blood serum sample is being analyzed for isoniazid by fluorescence induced with salicylaldehyde. The following relative fluorescence emission intensities are obtained for a blank sample with no drug, a standard of 0.80 µg/mL, and the serum sample: 1.2, 60.5, and 38.4, respectively. Assuming that the emission intensity is proportional to the isoniazid concentration, determine the isoniazid concentration in µg/mL in the serum.

Answer: The standard isoniazid sample of 0.80 µg/mL yields a fluorescence emission intensity of 60.5–1.2, or 59.3 where 1.2 is a correction for the blank. The isoniazid in the serum sample produces a fluorescence intensity of 38.4–1.2. Thus, by the method of proportions, one directly obtains the isoniazid concentration, 0.50 µg/mL.

4–13. An aqueous solution of maltose containing 15.3 g per 100 mL was observed in a polarimeter to have a rotation of 20° at 25° C using the sodium D-line. The polarimeter cell was 10 cm long. What is the specific rotation, $\{\alpha\}_D^{25°}$, of maltose? *Note:* cell length must be expressed in decimeters.

Answer: $\{\alpha\}_D^{25°} = 131°$

4–14. Calculate the total molar polarization for water, using the dielectric constant at 25° C given in Table 4–6 and equation (4–16).

Answer: $P = 17.4$ cm^3/mole

4–15. A forensic scientist is attempting to identify a sample as either a codeine or cocaine salt by infrared spectroscopy. The infrared spectrum shows no strong bands between 1600 and 2000 cm^{-1}, some strong bands in the region of 1400 to 1500 cm^{-1}, and some broad bands in the region 3200 to 3700 cm^{-1}. Based on this data, which compound is associated with the spectrum? Use Table 4–9 as a guide.

4–16. The diphenhydramine hydrochloride content of a capsule formulation can be determined by proton NMR using t-butyl alcohol as an internal standard.[26] The integral I_u of the 6 N-methyl protons in the diphenhydramine band at 2.85 ppm is divided by the integral I_s of the nine methyl protons of t-butyl alcohol in the band at 1.27 ppm using equation (4–22). If a single capsule's contents v is assayed, using $W = 25$ mg of t-butyl alcohol as the internal standard, and the

average integrals of the bands at 2.85 and 1.27 ppm are 1200 and 7059 units, respectively, what is the amount C (in mg per capsule) of diphenhydramine hydrochloride in the capsule? The formula weights (molecular weights) for diphenhydramine hydrochloride EW_u and t-butyl alcohol EW_s are 291.9 g/mole and 74.1 g/mole, respectively.

Answer: 25 mg of diphenhydramine hydrochloride per capsule

4–17. Explain why deuterium oxide rather than water is used to dissolve the sample of succinylcholine chloride for NMR analysis, as described in *Example 4–9.* Give examples of other solvents that are suitable for proton NMR analysis. (*Hint:* See references to books at the end of this chapter for examples of suitable solvents for NMR spectroscopy.)

4–18. (a) Calculate the molar refraction, R_m, of methanol using Table 4–1 for the molar refraction of contributing atoms and groups. Compare the result with that obtained by using equation (4–24). The refractive index n of methanol is 1.326, its molecular weight is 32.04 g/mole, and its density is 0.7866 g/cm^3 at 25° C.

(b) What are the units on R_m?

Answer: The values in Table 4–1 yield R_m for methanol as 8.343 cm^3/mole; and with the density of methanol as 0.7866 g/cm^3 at 25° C, equation (4–24) yields the value $R_m = 8.218$. The student should readily be able to attach the proper units to R_m.

4–19. What is the molar ellipticity $[\Theta]$ for a penicillin V solution with a specific ellipticity, $[\Psi]$, of 1.04×10^5 deg mL/g dm at 230 nm? Penicillin has a molecular weight of 350 g/mole.

Answer: From equation (4–28), the molar ellipticity $[\Theta]$ is 364 deg liter mole^{-1} dm^{-1}.

4–20. The refractive index n for quinoline, an antimalarial drug, is 1.627 at 20° C using light from the D-line emission of sodium. If the incident light, passing through air, is at an angle of 45° from the perpendicular to the surface of the quinoline liquid, what is the angle of its direction inside the quinoline?

Answer: 25°45′

4–21. The specific rotation of digoxin at 20° C using light from the D-line of sodium, $\{\alpha\}_D^{20}$, is $+30.4°$. If an optical rotation, α, of $+15.2°$ is obtained at the same temperature and wavelength of light for a 10-mL solution in a 1-dm length cell, wavelength of light for a 10-mL solution in a 1-dm length cell, what is the concentration, g, of digoxin (in g/mL) in the solution?

Answer: $g = 5$ grams in 10 mL or a concentration of 0.5 g/mL.

5

Solutions of Nonelectrolytes

Concentration Expressions
Equivalent Weights
Solutions of Nonelectrolytes

Ideal and Real Solutions
Colligative Properties
Molecular Weight Determination

Materials may be mixed together to form a true solution, a colloidal solution, or a coarse dispersion. A *true solution* is defined as a mixture of two or more components that form a homogeneous molecular dispersion, in other words, a one-phase system, the composition of which can vary over a wide range. The terms in this definition warrant further comment, and an attempt at clarification is made in the following paragraphs.

A *system* is a bounded space or a definite quantity of substance that is under observation and experimentation. Under some circumstances, the system may consist only of radiant energy or an electric field, containing no material substances. The term *phase* has already been defined in Chapter 2 as a distinct homogeneous part of a system separated by definite boundaries from other parts of the system. Each phase may be consolidated into a contiguous mass or region, such as a single piece of ice floating in water, or it may be distributed as small particles throughout the system, such as oil droplets in an emulsion or solid particles in a pharmaceutical suspension.

These latter two are examples of *coarse dispersions*, the diameter of the particles in emulsions and suspensions for the most part being larger than 0.1 μm (100 Å or 10^{-5} cm). A *colloidal dispersion* represents a system having a particle size intermediate between that of a true solution and a coarse dispersion, roughly 10 to 5000 Å. A colloidal dispersion may be considered as a two-phase system (heterogeneous) under certain circumstances and as a one-phase system (homogeneous) under others. A colloidal dispersion of silver proteinate in water is heterogeneous since it consists of distinct particles constituting a separate phase. A colloidal dispersion of acacia or sodium carboxymethylcellulose in water, on the other hand, is homogeneous. It does not differ significantly from a solution of sucrose and

may be considered as a single-phase system or true solution.[1]

A solution composed of only two substances is known as a *binary solution*, and the components or constituents are referred to as the *solvent* and the *solute*. We use the terms *component* and *constituent* interchangeably here, as do other authors, to represent the pure chemical substances that make up a solution. The *number of components* has a definite significance in the phase rule, as explained on p. 37. The constituent present in the greater amount in a binary solution is arbitrarily designated as the solvent and the constituent in the lesser amount as the solute. When a solid is dissolved in a liquid, however, the liquid is usually taken as the solvent and the solid as the solute, irrespective of the relative amounts of the constituents.

When water is one of the constituents of a liquid mixture, it is usually considered the solvent. When dealing with mixtures of liquids that are miscible in all proportions, such as alcohol and water, it is less meaningful to classify the constituents as solute and solvent.

Properties of Solutions. The physical properties of substances may be classified as *colligative, additive,* and *constitutive*. Some of the constitutive and additive properties of molecules were considered in Chapter 4. In the field of thermodynamics, physical properties of systems are classified as *extensive* properties, depending on the quantity of the matter in the system (e.g., mass and volume) and *intensive* properties, which are independent of the amount of the substances in the system (e.g., temperature, pressure, density, surface tension, and viscosity of a pure liquid).

Colligative properties depend mainly on the number of particles in a solution. The colligative properties of solutions are osmotic pressure, vapor pressure lowering, freezing point depression, and boiling point elevation. The values of the colligative properties are approximately the same for equal concentrations of different nonelectrolytes in solution regardless of the species or chemical nature of the constituents. In considering the colligative properties of solid-in-liquid solutions, it is assumed that the solute is nonvolatile and that the pressure of the vapor above the solution is provided entirely by the solvent.

Additive properties depend on the total contribution of the atoms in the molecules or on the sum of the properties of the constituents in a solution. An example of an additive property of a compound is the molecular weight, that is, the sum of the masses of the constituent atoms.

The masses of the components of a solution are also additive, the total mass of the solution being the sum of the masses of the individual components.

Constitutive properties depend on the arrangement and to a lesser extent on the number and kind of atoms within a molecule. These properties give clues to the constitution of individual compounds and groups of molecules in a system. Many physical properties may be partly additive and partly constitutive. The refraction of light, electric properties, surface and interfacial characteristics, and the solubility of drugs are at least in part constitutive and in part additive properties; these are considered in other sections of the book.

Types of Solutions. A solution may be classified according to the states in which the solute and solvent occur, and since three states of matter (gas, liquid, and crystalline solid) exist, nine types of homogeneous mixtures of solute and solvent are possible. These types, together with some examples, are given in Table 5–1.

When solids or liquids dissolve in a gas to form a gaseous solution, the molecules of the solute can be treated thermodynamically like a gas; similarly, when gases or solids dissolve in liquids, the gases and the solids can be considered to exist in the liquid state. In the formation of solid solutions, the atoms of the gas or liquid take up positions in the crystal lattice and behave like atoms or molecules of solids.

The solutes (whether gases, liquids, or solids) are divided into two main classes: *nonelectrolytes* and *electrolytes*. Nonelectrolytes are substances that do not yield ions when dissolved in water and therefore do not conduct an electric current through the solution. Examples of nonelectrolytes are sucrose, glycerin, naphthalene, and urea. The colligative properties of solutions of nonelectrolytes are fairly regular. A 0.1-molar solution of a nonelectrolyte produces approximately the same colligative effect as any other nonelectrolytic solution of equal concentration. Electrolytes are substances that form ions in solution, conduct the electric current, and show apparent "anomalous" colligative properties, that is, they produce a considerably greater freezing point depression and boiling point elevation than do nonelectrolytes of the same concentration. Examples of electrolytes are hydrochloric acid, sodium sulfate, ephedrine, and phenobarbital.

Electrolytes may be subdivided further into *strong electrolytes* and *weak electrolytes* depending on whether the substance is completely or only partly ionized in water. Hydrochloric acid and sodium sulfate are strong electrolytes, whereas ephedrine and phenobarbital are weak electrolytes. The classification of electrolytes according to Arrhenius and the discussion of the modern theories of electrolytes are found in Chapter 6.

CONCENTRATION EXPRESSIONS

The concentration of a solution may be expressed either in terms of the quantity of solute in a definite *volume of solution* or as the quantity of solute in a definite *mass of solvent or solution*. The various expressions are summarized in Table 5–2.

Molarity and Normality.[2] Molarity and normality are the expressions commonly used in analytical work. All solutions of the same molarity contain the same number of solute molecules in a definite volume of solution. When a solution contains more than one solute, it may have different molar concentrations with respect to the various solutes. For example, a solution can be 0.001 molar (0.001 M) with respect to phenobarbital and 0.1 M with respect to sodium chloride. One liter of such a solution is prepared by adding 0.001 mole of phenobarbital (0.001 mole × 232.32 g/mole = 0.2323 g) and 0.1 mole of sodium chloride (0.1 mole × 58.45 g/mole = 5.845 g) to enough water to make 1000 mL of solution.

Difficulties are sometimes encountered when one desires to express the molarity of an ion or radical in a solution. A molar solution of sodium chloride is 1 M with respect to both the sodium and the chloride ion, whereas a molar solution of Na_2CO_3 is 1 M with respect to the carbonate ion and 2 M with respect to the sodium ion, since each mole of this salt contains 2 moles of sodium ions. A molar solution of sodium chloride is also 1 normal (1 N) with respect to both its ions; however, a molar solution of sodium carbonate is 2 N with respect to both the sodium and the carbonate ion.

Molar and normal solutions are popular in chemistry since they may be brought to a convenient volume; a

TABLE 5–1. *Types of Solutions*

Solute	Solvent	Example
Gas	Gas	Air
Liquid	Gas	Water in oxygen
Solid	Gas	Iodine vapor in air
Gas	Liquid	Carbonated water
Liquid	Liquid	Alcohol in water
Solid	Liquid	Aqueous sodium chloride solution
Gas	Solid	Hydrogen in palladium
Liquid	Solid	Mineral oil in paraffin
Solid	Solid	Gold—silver mixture, mixture of alums

TABLE 5–2. *Concentration Expressions*

Expression	Symbol	Definition
Molarity	M, c	Moles (gram molecular weights) of solute in 1 liter of solution
Normality	N	Gram equivalent weights of solute in 1 liter of solution
Molality	m	Moles of solute in 1000 g of solvent
Mole fraction	X, N	Ratio of the moles of one constituent (e.g., the solute) of a solution to the total moles of all constituents (solute and solvent)
Mole percent		Moles of one constituent in 100 moles of the solution. Mole percent is obtained by multiplying mole fraction by 100.
Percent by weight	% *w/w*	Grams of solute in 100 g of solution
Percent by volume	% *v/v*	Milliliters of solute in 100 mL of solution
Percent weight-in-volume	% *w/v*	Grams of solute in 100 mL of solution
Milligram percent	—	Milligrams of solute in 100 mL of solution

volume aliquot of the solution, representing a known weight of solute, is easily obtained by the use of the burette or pipette.

Both molarity and normality have the disadvantage of changing value with temperature because of the expansion or contraction of liquids, and should not be used when one wishes to study the properties of solutions at various temperatures. Another difficulty arises in the use of molar and normal solutions for the study of properties such as vapor pressure and osmotic pressure, which are related to the concentration of the solvent. The volume of the solvent in a molar or a normal solution is not usually known, and it varies for different solutions of the same concentration, depending upon the solute and solvent involved.

Molality. A molal solution is prepared in terms of weight units and does not have the disadvantages just discussed; therefore, molal concentration appears more frequently than molarity and normality in theoretic studies. It is possible to convert molality into molarity or normality if the final volume of the solution is observed or if the density is determined. In aqueous solutions more dilute than 0.1 *M*, it usually may be assumed for practical purposes that molality and molarity are equivalent. For example, a 1% solution by weight of sodium chloride with a specific gravity of 1.0053 is 0.170 *M* and 0.173 molal (0.173 *m*). The following difference between molar and molal solutions should also be noted. If another solute, containing neither sodium nor chloride ions, is added to a certain volume of a molal solution of sodium chloride, the solution remains 1 *m* in sodium chloride, although the total volume and the weight of the solution increase. Molarity, of course, *decreases* when another solute is added because of the increase in volume of the solution.

Molal solutions are prepared by adding the proper weight of solvent to the carefully weighed quantity of the solute. The volume of the solvent can be calculated from the specific gravity, and the solvent may then be measured from a burette rather than weighed.

Mole Fraction. Mole fraction is used frequently in experimentation involving theoretical considerations since it gives a measure of the relative proportion

of moles of each constituent in a solution. It is expressed as

$$X_1 = \frac{n_1}{n_1 + n_2} \qquad (5-1)$$

$$X_2 = \frac{n_2}{n_1 + n_2} \qquad (5-2)$$

for a system of two constituents.

X_1 is the mole fraction of constituent 1 (the subscript 1 is ordinarily used as the designation for the solvent), X_2 is the mole fraction of constituent 2 (usually the solute), and n_1 and n_2 are the number of moles of the constituents in the solution. The sum of the mole fractions of solute and solvent must equal unity. Mole fraction is also expressed in percentage terms by multiplying X_1 or X_2 by 100. In a solution containing 0.01 mole of solute and 0.04 mole of solvent, the mole fraction of the solute $X_2 = 0.01/(0.04 + 0.01) = 0.20$. Since the mole fractions of the two constituents must equal 1, the mole fraction of the solvent is 0.8. The mole percent of the solute is 20%; the mole percent of the solvent is 80%.

The manner in which mole fraction is defined allows one to express the relationship between the number of solute and solvent molecules in a simple, direct way. In the example just given, it is readily seen that two out of every 10 molecules in the solution are solute molecules, and it will be observed later that many of the properties of solutes and solvents are directly related to their mole fraction in the solution. For example, the partial vapor pressure above a solution brought about by the presence of a volatile solute is equal to the vapor pressure of the pure solute multiplied by the mole fraction of the solute in the solution.

Percent Expressions. The percentage method of expressing the concentration of pharmaceutical solutions is quite common. Percent by weight signifies the number of grams of solute per 100 grams of solution. A 10% by weight (% *w/w*) aqueous solution of glycerin contains 10 g of glycerin dissolved in enough water (90 g) to make 100 g of solution. Percent by volume is expressed as the volume of solute in milliliters contained in 100 mL of the solution. Alcohol (USP) contains 92.3% by weight and 94.9% by volume of C_2H_5OH at 15.56°, that is, it contains 92.3 g of C_2H_5OH in 100 g of solution or 94.9 mL of C_2H_5OH in 100 mL of solution.

Calculations Involving Concentration Expressions. The calculations involving the various concentration expressions are illustrated in the following example.

Example 5–1. An aqueous solution of exsiccated ferrous sulfate was prepared by adding 41.50 g of $FeSO_4$ to enough water to make 1000 mL of solution at 18° C. The density of the solution is 1.0375, and the molecular weight of $FeSO_4$ is 151.9. Calculate (a) the molarity; (b) the molality; (c) the mole fraction of $FeSO_4$, the mole fraction of water, and the mole percent of the two constituents; and (d) the percent by weight of $FeSO_4$.

(a) Molarity

$$\text{Moles of } FeSO_4 = \frac{\text{g of } FeSO_4}{\text{molecular weight}}$$

$$= \frac{41.50}{151.9} = 0.2732$$

$$\text{Molarity} = \frac{\text{moles of } FeSO_4}{\text{liters of solution}} = \frac{0.2732}{1 \text{ liter}} = 0.2732 \, M$$

(b) Molality

$$\text{Grams of solution} = \text{volume} \times \text{density};$$
$$1000 \times 1.0375 = 1037.5 \text{ g}$$

Grams of solvent = grams of solution − grams of $FeSO_4$ = 1037.5 − 41.5 = 996.0 g

$$\text{Molality} = \frac{\text{moles of } FeSO_4}{\text{kg of solvent}} = \frac{0.2732}{0.996} = 0.2743 \, m$$

(c) Mole fraction and mole percent

$$\text{Moles of water} = \frac{996}{18.02} = 55.27 \text{ moles}$$

Mole fraction of $FeSO_4$,

$$X_2 = \frac{\text{moles of } FeSO_4}{\frac{\text{moles}}{\text{water}} + \frac{\text{moles}}{FeSO_4}} = \frac{0.2732}{55.27 + 0.2732} = 0.0049$$

Mole fraction of water,

$$X_1 = \frac{55.27}{55.27 + 0.2732} = 0.9951$$

Notice that $X_1 + X_2 = 0.9951 + 0.0049 = 1.0000$

Mole percent of $FeSO_4 = 0.0049 \times 100 = 0.49\%$

Mole percent of water $= 0.9951 \times 100 = 99.51\%$

(d) Percent by weight

Percent by weight of $FeSO_4$

$$= \frac{\text{g of } FeSO_4}{\text{g of solution}} \times 100$$

$$= \frac{41.50}{1037.5} \times 100 = 4.00\%$$

One may use the table of conversion equations, Table 5–3, to convert concentration expressions, say molality, into its value in molarity or mole fraction. Or, knowing the weight w_1 of a solvent, the weight w_2 of the solute, and the molecular weight M_2 of the solute, one can calculate the molarity c or the molality m of the solution. As an exercise, the reader should derive an expression relating X_1 to X_2 to the weights w_1 and w_2 and the solute's molecular weight M_2. The data in

TABLE 5–3. *Conversion Equations for Concentration Terms*

A. Molality (moles of solute/kg of solvent, *m*) and mole fraction of solute (X_2).

$$X_2 = \frac{m}{m + \dfrac{1000}{M_1}}$$

$$m = \frac{1000 \, X_2}{M_1(1 - X_2)}$$

$$= \frac{1000 \, (1 - X_1)}{M_1 X_1}$$

B. Molarity (moles of solute/liter of solution, c) and mole fraction of solute (X_2).

$$X_2 = \frac{c}{c + \dfrac{1000\rho - cM_2}{M_1}}$$

$$c = \frac{1000 \, \rho X_2}{M_1(1 - X_2) + M_2 X_2}$$

C. Molality (*m*) and molarity (*c*).

$$m = \frac{1000 \, c}{1000\rho - M_2 \, c}$$

$$c = \frac{1000\rho}{\dfrac{1000}{m} + M_2}$$

D. Molality (*m*) and molarity (*c*) in terms of weight of solute, w_2, weight of solvent, w_1, and molecular weight, M_2, of solute.

$$m = \frac{w_2/M_2}{w_1/1000} = \frac{1000 \, w_2}{w_1 M_2}$$

$$c = \frac{1000 \, \rho w_2}{M_2(w_1 + w_2)}$$

Definition of terms:
ρ = density of the solution (g/cm³)
M_1 = molecular weight of the solvent
M_2 = molecular weight of the solute
X_1 = mole fraction of the solvent
X_2 = mole fraction of the solute
w_1 = weight of the solvent (g, mg, kg, etc.)
w_2 = weight of the solute (g, mg, kg, etc.)

Example 5–1 are useful to determine whether your derived equation is correct.

EQUIVALENT WEIGHTS[2]

A gram atom of hydrogen weighs 1.008 g and consists of 6.02×10^{23} atoms (Avogadro's number) of hydrogen. This gram atomic weight of hydrogen combines with 6.02×10^{23} atoms of fluorine and with half of 6.02×10^{23} atoms of oxygen. One gram atom of fluorine weighs 19 g and one gram atom of oxygen weighs 16 g. Therefore, 1.008 g of hydrogen combines with 19 grams of fluorine and with half of 16 or 8 grams of oxygen. The quantities of fluorine and oxygen combining with 1.008 g of hydrogen are referred to as the equivalent weight of the combining atoms. One equivalent (Eq) of fluorine (19 g) combines with 1.008 g of hydrogen. One equivalent of oxygen (8 g) also combines with 1.008 g of hydrogen.

We observe that 1 equivalent weight (19 g) of fluorine is identical with its atomic weight. Not so with oxygen; its gram equivalent weight (8 g) is equal to half its atomic weight. Stated otherwise, the atomic weight of fluorine contains 1 equivalent of fluorine, while the atomic weight of oxygen contains two equivalents. The equation relating these atomic quantities is as follows (the equation for molecules is quite similar to that for atoms, as seen in the next paragraph):

$$\text{Equivalent weight} = \frac{\text{Atomic weight}}{\begin{array}{c}\text{Number of equivalents}\\\text{per atomic weight (valence)}\end{array}} \quad (5\text{--}3)$$

The number of equivalents per atomic weight, namely 1 for fluorine and 2 for oxygen, are the common *valences* of these elements. (Many elements may have more than one valence and hence several equivalent weights, depending on the reaction under consideration.) Magnesium will combine with two atoms of fluorine, and each fluorine can combine with one atom of hydrogen. Therefore, the valence of magnesium is 2, and its equivalent weight, according to equation (5–3), is one half its atomic weight (24/2 = 12 g/equivalent). Aluminum will combine with three atoms of fluorine; the valence of aluminum is therefore 3 and its equivalent weight is one third its atomic weight, or 27/3 = 9 g/equivalent.

The concept of equivalent weights not only applies to atoms but also extends to molecules. The equivalent weight of sodium chloride is identical to its molecular weight, 58.5 g/Eq, that is, the equivalent weight of sodium chloride is the sum of the equivalent weights of sodium (23 g) and chlorine (35.5 g), or 58.5 g/Eq. The equivalent weight of sodium chloride is identical to its molecular weight, 58.5 g, since the valence of sodium and chlorine are each 1 in the compound. The equivalent weight of Na_2CO_3 is numerically half of its molecular weight. The valence of the carbonate ion, CO_3^{2-}, is 2, and its equivalent weight is 60/2 = 30 g/Eq. Although the valence of sodium is unity, two atoms are present in Na_2CO_3, providing a weight of 2 × 23 g = 46 g; its equivalent weight is one half of this, or 23 g/Eq. The equivalent weight of Na_2CO_3 is therefore 30 + 23 = 53 g, which is one half the molecular weight. The relationship of equivalent weight to molecular weight for molecules such as NaCl and Na_2CO_3 is (compare equations [5–3] for atoms):

Equivalent weight (g/Eq)

$$= \frac{\text{molecular weight (g/mole)}}{\text{equivalent/mole}} \quad (5\text{--}4)$$

Example 5–2. (a) What is the number of equivalents per mole of K_3PO_4, and what is the equivalent weight of this salt? (b) What is the equivalent weight of KNO_3? (c) What is the number of equivalents per mole of $Ca_3(PO_4)_2$, and what is the equivalent weight of this salt?

(a) K_3PO_4 represents 3 equivalents per mole, and its equivalent weight is numerically equal to one third its molecular weight— namely, 212 g/mole ÷ 3 Eq/mole = 70.7 g/Eq.

(b) The equivalent weight of KNO_3 is also equal to its molecular weight, or 101 g/Eq.

(c) The number of equivalents per mole for $Ca_3(PO_4)_2$ is 6 (i.e., three calcium ions each with a valence of 2 or two phosphate ions each with a valence of 3). The equivalent weight of $Ca_3(PO_4)_2$ is therefore one sixth its molecular weight, or 310/6 = 51.7 g/Eq.

For a complex salt such as monobasic potassium phosphate (potassium acid phosphate), KH_2PO_4 (molecular weight, 136 g), the equivalent weight depends on how the compound is used. If it is used for its potassium content, the equivalent weight is identical to its molecular weight, or 136 g. When used as a buffer for its hydrogen content, the equivalent weight is one half the molecular weight, 136/2 = 68 g, since two hydrogen atoms are present. When used for its phosphate content, the equivalent weight of KH_2PO_4 is one third the molecular weight, 136/3 = 45.3 g, since the valence of phosphate is 3.

As defined in Table 5–2, the normality of a solution is the equivalent weight of the solute in 1 liter of solution. For NaF, KNO_3, and HCl, the number of equivalent weights equals the number of molecular weights, and normality is identical with molarity. For H_3PO_4, the equivalent weight is one third the molecular weight, 98 g/3 = 32.67 g/Eq, assuming complete reaction, and a 1-*N* solution of H_3PO_4 is prepared by weighing 32.67 g of H_3PO_4 and bringing it to a volume of 1 liter with water. For a 1-*N* solution of sodium bisulfate (sodium acid sulfate), $NaHSO_4$ (molecular weight 120 g), the weight of salt needed depends on the species for which the salt is used. If used for sodium or hydrogen, the equivalent weight would equal the molecular weight, or 120 g/Eq. If the solution were used for its sulfate content, 120/2 = 60 g of $NaHSO_4$ would be weighed out and sufficient water added to make a liter of solution.

In electrolyte replacement therapy in the hospital, solutions containing various electrolytes are injected into the body to correct serious electrolytes imbalances. The concentrations are usually expressed as equivalents per liter or milliequivalents per liter. For example, the normal plasma concentration of sodium ions in humans is about 142 mEq/liter; the normal plasma concentration of bicarbonate ions, HCO_3^-, is 27 mEq/liter. Equation (5–4) is useful for calculating the quantity of salts needed to prepare electrolyte solutions in hospital practice. The moles in the numerator and denominator of equation (5–4) may be replaced with, say, liters, to give

$$\text{Equivalent weight (in g/Eq)} = \frac{\text{grams/liter}}{\text{equivalents/liter}} \quad (5\text{--}5)$$

or

Equivalent weight (in mg/mEq)

$$= \frac{\text{milligrams/liter}}{\text{milliequivalents/liter}} \quad (5\text{--}6)$$

Equivalent weight (analogous to molecular weight) is expressed in grams/Eq, or what amounts to the same units, mg/mEq.

Example 5-3. Human plasma contains about 5 mEq/liter of calcium ions. How many milligrams of calcium chloride dihydrate, $CaCl_2 \cdot 2H_2O$ (molecular weight 147 g/mole), are required to prepare 750 mL of a solution equal in Ca^{2+} to human plasma? The equivalent weight of the dihydrate salt $CaCl_2 \cdot 2H_2O$ is half its molecular weight, $147/2 = 73.5$ g/Eq, or 73.5 mg/mEq. Using equation (5-6),

$$73.5 \text{ mg/mEq} = \frac{\text{mg/liter}}{5 \text{ mEq/liter}}$$

$$73.5 \text{ mg/mEq} \times 5 \text{ mEq/liter} = 367.5 \text{ mg/liter}$$

For 750 cm³, $367.5 \times \dfrac{750 \text{ mL}}{1000 \text{ mL}} = 275.6$ mg of $CaCl_2 \cdot 2H_2O$

Example 5-4. Calculate the number of equivalents per liter of potassium chloride, molecular weight 74.55 g/mole, present in a 1.15% w/v solution of KCl.

Using equation (5-5) and noting that the equivalent weight of KCl is identical to its molecular weight,

$$74.55 \text{ g/Eq} = \frac{11.5 \text{ g/liter}}{\text{Eq/liter}}$$

$(11.5 \text{ g/liter})/(74.55 \text{ g/Eq}) = 0.154$ Eq/liter (or 154 mEq/liter)

Example 5-5. What is the Na^+ content in mEq/liter of a solution containing 5.00 g of NaCl per liter of solution? The molecular weight and therefore the equivalent weight of NaCl is 58.5 g/Eq or 58.5 mg/mEq.

$$\text{mEq/liter} = \frac{\text{mg/liter}}{\text{Eq. wt.}} = \frac{5000 \text{ mg/liter}}{58.5 \text{ mg/mEq}} = 85.47 \text{ mEq of } Na^+ \text{ per liter}$$

SOLUTIONS OF NONELECTROLYTES

As stated earlier, the colligative properties of nonelectrolytes are ordinarily regular; on the other hand, solutions of electrolytes show apparent deviations. The remainder of this chapter relates to solutions of nonelectrolytes, except where comparison with an electrolyte system is desirable for clarity. Solutions of electrolytes are dealt with in Chapter 6.

IDEAL AND REAL SOLUTIONS

An ideal gas is defined in Chapter 2 as one in which there is no attraction between the molecules, and it is found desirable to establish an ideal gas equation to which the properties of real gases tend as the pressure approaches zero. Consequently, the ideal gas law is referred to as a *limiting law*. It is convenient to define an *ideal solution* as one in which there is no change in the properties of the components, other than dilution, when they are mixed to form the solution. No heat is evolved or absorbed during the mixing process, and the final volume of the solution represents an additive property of the individual constituents. Stated another way, no shrinkage or expansion occurs when the substances are mixed. The constitutive properties, for example, the vapor pressure, refractive index, surface tension, and viscosity of the solution, are the weighted averages of the properties of the pure individual constituents.

Ideal solutions are formed by mixing substances with similar properties. For example, when 100 mL of methanol is mixed with 100 mL of ethanol, the final volume of the solution is 200 mL, and no heat is evolved or absorbed. The solution is nearly *ideal*.

When 100 mL of sulfuric acid is combined with 100 mL of water, however, the volume of the solution is about 180 mL at room temperature, and the mixing is attended by a considerable evolution of heat; the solution is said to be *nonideal*, or real. As with gases, some solutions are quite ideal in moderate concentrations, while others approach ideality only under extreme dilution.

To summarize, whereas ideality in a gas implies the *complete absence* of attractive forces, ideality in a solution means *complete uniformity* of attractive forces. Since a liquid is a highly condensed state, it cannot be expected to be devoid of attractive forces; nevertheless, if, in a mixture of A and B molecules, the forces between A and A, B and B, and A and B are all of the same order, the solution is considered to be ideal according to the definition just given.

Escaping Tendency.[3] It is common knowledge that two bodies are in thermal equilibrium when their temperatures are the same. If one body is heated to a higher temperature than the other, heat will flow "downhill" from the hotter to the colder body until both bodies are again in thermal equilibrium. We can describe this process in another way by using the concept of *escaping tendency*, and say that the heat in the hotter body has a greater escaping tendency that in the colder one. Temperature is a quantitative measure of the escaping tendency of heat, and at thermal equilibrium, when both bodies finally have the same temperature, the escaping tendency of each constituent is the same in all parts of the system.

A quantitative measure of the escaping tendencies of material substances undergoing physical and chemical transformations is *free energy*. For a pure substance, the free energy per mole, or the *molar free energy*, provides a measure of escaping tendency; for the constituent of a solution it is the *partial molar free energy* or *chemical potential* that is used as an expression of escaping tendency. Chemical potential is discussed in Chapter 3. The free energy of a mole of ice is greater than that of liquid water at 1 atm above 0° C and is spontaneously converted into water, since

$$\Delta G = G_{liq} - G_{ice} < 0$$

At 0° C, at which temperature the system is in equilibrium, the molar free energies of ice and water are identical and $\Delta G = 0$. In terms of escaping tendencies, we can say that above 0° C, the escaping tendency of ice is greater than the escaping tendency of liquid water, whereas at equilibrium, the escaping tendencies of water in both phases are identical.

Ideal Solutions and Raoult's Law. The vapor pressure of a solution is a particularly important property since it serves as a quantitative expression of escaping tendency. In 1887, Raoult recognized that, in an ideal solution, the partial vapor pressure of each volatile constituent is equal to the vapor pressure of the pure constituent multiplied by its mole fraction in the solution. Thus, for two constituents A and B:

$$p_A = p_A°X_A \qquad (5-7)$$

$$p_B = p_B°X_B \qquad (5-8)$$

in which p_A and p_B are the partial vapor pressures of the constituents over the solution when the mole fraction concentrations are X_A and X_B respectively. The vapor pressures of the pure components are $p_A°$ and $p_B°$. For example, if the vapor pressure of ethylene chloride in the pure state is 236 mm Hg at 50° C, then in a solution consisting of a mole fraction of 0.4 ethylene chloride and 0.6 benzene, the partial vapor pressure of ethylene chloride is 40% of 236 or 94.4 mm. Thus, in an ideal solution, when liquid A is mixed with liquid B, the vapor pressure of A is reduced by dilution with B in a manner depending on the mole fractions of A and B present in the final solution. This will diminish the escaping tendency of each constituent, leading to a reduction in the rate of escape of the molecules of A and B from the surface of the liquid.

Example 5-6. What is the partial vapor pressure of benzene and of ethylene chloride in a solution at a mole fraction of benzene of 0.6? The vapor pressure of pure benzene at 50° C is 268 mm, and the corresponding $p_A°$ for ethylene chloride is 236 mm.

$$p_B = 268 \times 0.6 = 160.8 \text{ mm}$$

$$p_A = 236 \times 0.4 = 94.4 \text{ mm}$$

If additional volatile components are present in the solution, each will produce a partial pressure above the solution, which can be calculated from Raoult's law. The total pressure is the sum of the partial pressures of all the constituents. In *Example 5-6*, the total vapor pressure P is calculated as follows:

$$P = p_A + p_B = 160.8 + 94.4 = 255.2 \text{ mm}$$

The vapor pressure–composition curve for the binary system benzene and ethylene chloride at 50° C is shown in Figure 5–1. The three lines represent the partial pressure of ethylene chloride, the partial pressure of benzene, and the total pressure of the solution as a function of the mole fraction of the constituents.

Aerosols and Raoult's Law. Aerosol dispensers have been used to package some drugs since the early 1950s. An aerosol contains the drug concentrated in a solvent or carrier liquid and a propellant mixture of the proper vapor characteristics. Trichloromonofluoromethane (designated as propellant 11) and dichlorodifluoromethane (designated as propellant 12) were used in various proportions to yield the proper vapor pressure and density at room temperature. Although still used with drugs, these halogenated hydrocarbons are no longer used in cosmetic aerosols and have been replaced

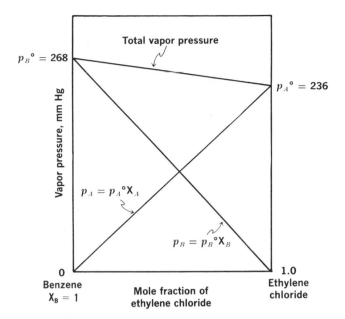

Fig. 5–1. Vapor pressure–composition curve for an ideal binary system.

by nitrogen and unsubstituted hydrocarbons (see *Problem 5–9*).

Example 5–7. The vapor pressure of pure propellant 11 (MW 137.4) at 21° C is $p_{11}° = 13.4$ pounds/square inch (psi) and that of propellant 12 (MW 120.9) is $p_{12}° = 84.9$ psi. A 50:50 mixture by gram weight of the two propellants consists of 50 g : 137.4 g mole^{-1} = 0.364 mole of propellant 11, and 50 g/120.9 g mole^{-1} = 0.414 mole of propellant 12. What is the partial pressure of propellants 11 and 12 in the 50:50 mixture, and what is the total vapor pressure of this mixture?

$$p_{11} = \frac{n_{11}}{n_{11} + n_{12}} p_{11}° = \frac{0.364}{0.364 + 0.414}(13.4) = 6.27 \text{ psi}$$

$$p_{12} = \frac{n_{12}}{n_{11} + n_{12}} p_{12}° = \frac{0.414}{0.364 + 0.414}(84.9) = 45.2 \text{ psi}$$

The total vapor pressure of the mixture is

$$6.27 + 45.2 = 51.5 \text{ psi}$$

To convert to gauge pressure (psig), one subtracts the atmospheric pressure of 14.7 psi:

$$51.5 - 14.7 = 36.8 \text{ psig}$$

The psi values just given are measured with respect to zero pressure rather than with respect to the atmosphere, and are sometimes written psia to signify *absolute* pressure.

Real Solutions. Ideality in solutions presupposes complete uniformity of attractive forces (p. 106). Many examples of solution pairs are known, however, in which the "cohesive" attraction of A for A exceeds the "adhesive" attraction existing between A and B. Similarly, the attractive forces between A and B may be greater than those between A and A or B and B. This may occur even though the liquids are miscible in all proportions. Such mixtures are *real* or *nonideal;* that is, they do not adhere to Raoult's law throughout the entire range of composition. Two types of deviation from Raoult's law are recognized; *negative deviation* and *positive deviation*.

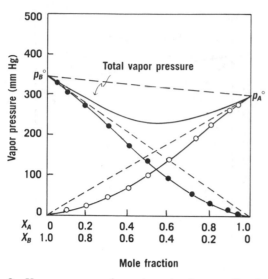

Fig. 5-2. Vapor pressure of a system showing negative deviation from Raoult's law.

When the "adhesive" attractions between molecules of different species exceed the "cohesive" attractions between like molecules, the vapor pressure of the solution is less than that expected from Raoult's ideal solution law, and *negative deviation* occurs. If the deviation is sufficiently great, the total vapor pressure curve shows a minimum, as observed in Figure 5–2, where *A* is chloroform and *B* is acetone.

The dilution of constituent *A* by additions of *B* normally would be expected to reduce the partial vapor pressure of *A*; this is the simple dilution effect embodied in Raoult's law. In the case of liquid pairs that show negative deviation from the law, however, the addition of *B* to *A* tends to reduce the vapor pressure of *A* to a greater extent than can be accounted for by the simple dilution effect. Chloroform and acetone manifest such an attraction for one another through the formation of a hydrogen bond, thus further reducing the escaping tendency of each constituent. This pair forms a weak compound,

$$Cl_3C\text{—}H \cdots O\text{=}C(CH_3)_2$$

which may be isolated and identified. Reactions between dipolar molecules, or between a dipolar and a nonpolar molecule, may also lead to negative deviations. The interaction in these cases, however, is usually so weak that no definite compound can be isolated.

When the interaction between *A* and *B* molecules is less than that between molecules of the pure constituents, the presence of *B* molecules reduces the interaction of the *A* molecules, and *A* molecules correspondingly reduce the *B–B* interaction. Accordingly, the dissimilarity of polarities or internal pressures of the constituents results in a greater escaping tendency of both the *A* and the *B* molecules. The partial vapor pressure of the constituents is greater than that expected from Raoult's law, and the system is said to

exhibit *positive deviation*. The total vapor pressure often shows a maximum at one particular composition if the deviation is sufficiently large. An example of positive deviation is shown in Figure 5–3. Liquid pairs that demonstrate positive deviation are benzene and ethyl alcohol, carbon disulfide and acetone, and chloroform and ethyl alcohol.

Raoult's law does not apply over the entire concentration range in a nonideal solution. It describes the behavior of either component of a real liquid pair only when that substance is present in high concentration and thus is considered to be the solvent. Raoult's law may be expressed as

$$p_{solvent} = p°_{solvent}X_{solvent} \qquad (5\text{–}9)$$

in such a situation, and it is valid only for the solvent of a nonideal solution that is sufficiently dilute with respect to the solute. It cannot hold for the component in low concentration, that is, the solute, in a dilute nonideal solution.

These statements will become clearer when one observes, in Figure 5–2, that the actual vapor pressure curve of chloroform (component *A*) approaches the ideal curve defined by Raoult's law as the solution composition approaches pure chloroform. Raoult's law can be used to describe the behavior of chloroform when it is present in high concentration (i.e., when it is the solvent). The ideal equation is not applicable to acetone (component *B*), however, which is present in low concentration in this region of the diagram, since the actual curve for acetone does not coincide with the ideal

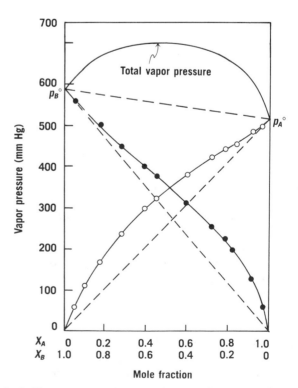

Fig. 5-3. Vapor pressure of a system showing positive deviation from Raoult's law.

line. When one studies the left side of Figure 5–2, one observes that the conditions are reversed: acetone is considered to be the solvent here, and its vapor pressure curve tends to coincide with the ideal curve. Chloroform is the solute in this range, and its curve does not approach the ideal line. Similar considerations apply to Figure 5–3.

Henry's Law. The vapor pressure curves for both acetone and chloroform as *solutes* are observed to lie considerably below the vapor pressure of an ideal mixture of this pair. The molecules of solute, being in relatively small number in the two regions of the diagram, are completely surrounded by molecules of solvent and so reside in a uniform environment. Therefore, the partial pressure or escaping tendency of chloroform at low concentration is in some way proportional to its mole fraction, but, as observed in Figure 5–2, the proportionality constant is not equal to the vapor pressure of the pure substance. The vapor pressure–composition relationship of the solute cannot be expressed by Raoult's law, but instead by an equation known as *Henry's law:*

$$p_{\text{solute}} = k_{\text{solute}} X_{\text{solute}} \qquad (5\text{–}10)$$

in which k for chloroform is less than $p^{\circ}_{\text{CHCl}_3}$. Henry's law applies to the solute and Raoult's applies to the solvent in dilute solutions of real liquid pairs. Of course, Raoult's law also applies over the entire concentration range (to both solvent and solute) when the constituents are sufficiently similar to form an ideal solution. Under any circumstance, when the partial vapor pressures of both of the constituents are directly proportional to the mole fractions over the entire range, the solution is said to be ideal; Henry's law becomes identical with Raoult's law, and k becomes equal to p°. Henry's law is used for the study of gas solubilities and will be discussed in Chapter 10.

Distillation of Binary Mixtures. The relationship between vapor pressure (and hence boiling point) and composition of binary liquid phases is the underlying principle in distillation. In the case of miscible liquids, instead of plotting vapor pressure versus composition, it is more useful to plot the boiling points of the various mixtures, determined at atmospheric pressure, against composition.

The higher the vapor pressure of a liquid—that is, the more volatile it is—the lower the boiling point. Since the vapor of a binary mixture is always richer in the more volatile constituent, the process of distillation can be used to separate the more volatile from the less volatile constituent. Figure 5–4 shows a mixture of a high-boiling liquid *A* and a low-boiling liquid *B*. A mixture of these substances having the composition *a* is distilled at the boiling point *b*. The composition of the vapor v_1 in equilibrium with the liquid at this temperature is *c*; this is also the composition of the distillate when it is condensed. The vapor is therefore richer in *B* than the liquid from which it was distilled. If a

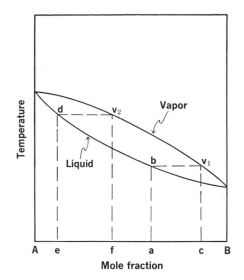

Fig. 5–4. Boiling point diagram of an ideal binary mixture.

fractionating column is used, *A* and *B* can be completely separated. The vapor rising in the column is met by the condensed vapor or downward-flowing liquid. As the rising vapor is cooled by contact with the liquid, some of the lower-boiling fraction condenses, and the vapor contains more of the volatile component than it did when it left the retort. Therefore, as the vapor proceeds up the fractionating column, it becomes progressively richer in the more volatile component *B*, and the liquid returning to the distilling retort becomes richer in the less volatile component *A*.

Figure 5–4 shows the situation for a pair of miscible liquids exhibiting ideal behavior. Since vapor pressure curves can show maxima and minima (see Figs. 5–2 and 5–3), it follows that boiling point curves will show corresponding minima and maxima, respectively. With these mixtures, distillation produces either pure *A* or pure *B* plus a mixture of constant composition and constant boiling point. This latter is known as an *azeotrope* (Greek: boil unchanged) or *azeotropic mixture*. It is not possible to separate such a mixture completely into two pure components by simple fractionation. If the vapor pressure curves show a minimum (i.e., negative deviation from Raoult's law), the azeotrope has the highest boiling point of all the mixtures possible; it is therefore least volatile and remains in the flask, while either pure *A* or pure *B* is distilled off. If the vapor pressure curve exhibits a maximum (showing a positive deviation from Raoult's law), the azeotrope has the lowest boiling point and forms the distillate. Either pure *A* or pure *B* then remains in the flask.

When a mixture of HCl and water is distilled at atmospheric pressure, an azeotrope is obtained that contains 20.22% by weight of HCl and that boils at 108.58° C. The composition of this mixture is accurate and reproducible enough that the solution can be used as a standard in analytic chemistry. Mixtures of water and acetic acid and of chloroform and acetone yield azeotropic mixtures with maxima in their boiling point curves and minima in their vapor pressure curves. Mixtures of ethanol and water and of methanol and benzene both show the reverse behavior, namely minima in the boiling point curves and maxima in the vapor pressure curves.

When a mixture of two practically *immiscible* liquids is heated, while being agitated to expose the surfaces of both liquids to the vapor phase, each constituent independently exerts its own vapor pressure as a function of temperature as though the other constituent were not present. Boiling begins and distillation may be effected when the sum of the partial pressures of the two immiscible liquids just exceeds the atmospheric pressure. This principle is applied in *steam distillation*, whereby many organic compounds insoluble in water can be purified at a temperature well below the point at which decomposition occurs. Thus bromobenzene alone boils at 156.2° C, while water boils at 100° C at a pressure of 760 mm Hg. A mixture of the two, however, in any proportion, boils at 95° C. Bromobenzene may thus be distilled at a temperature 61° C below its normal boiling point. Steam distillation is particularly useful for obtaining volatile oils from plant tissues without decomposing the oils.

COLLIGATIVE PROPERTIES

When a *nonvolatile solute* is combined with a *volatile solvent*, the vapor above the solution is provided solely by the solvent. The solute reduces the escaping tendency of the solvent, and, on the basis of Raoult's law, the vapor pressure of a solution containing a nonvolatile solute is lowered proportional to the relative number (rather than the weight concentration) of the solute molecules. The freezing point, boiling point, and osmotic pressure of a solution also depend on the relative proportion of the molecules of the solute and the solvent. These are called *colligative properties* (Greek: collected together) since they depend chiefly on the number rather than on the nature of the constituents.

Lowering of the Vapor Pressure. According to Raoult's law, the vapor pressure, p_1, of a solvent over a dilute solution is equal to the vapor pressure of the pure solvent, $p_1°$, times the mole fraction of solvent in the solution, X_1. Since the solute under discussion here is considered to be nonvolatile, the vapor pressure of the solvent p_1 is identical to the total pressure of the solution p.

It is more convenient to express the vapor pressure of the solution in terms of the concentration of the solute, rather than the mole fraction of the solvent, and this may be accomplished in the following way. The sum of the mole fractions of the constituents in a solution is unity:

$$X_1 + X_2 = 1 \qquad (5\text{--}11)$$

Therefore,

$$X_1 = 1 - X_2 \qquad (5\text{--}12)$$

in which X_1 is the mole fraction of the solvent and X_2 is the mole fraction of the solute. Raoult's equation may be modified by substituting equation (5–12) for X_1 to give

$$p = p_1°(1 - X_2) \qquad (5\text{--}13)$$

$$p_1° - p = p_1°X_2 \qquad (5\text{--}14)$$

$$\frac{p_1° - p}{p_1°} = \frac{\Delta p}{p_1°} = X_2 = \frac{n_2}{n_1 + n_2} \qquad (5\text{--}15)$$

In equation (5–15), $\Delta p = p_1° - p$ is the lowering of the vapor pressure and $\Delta p/p_1°$ is the *relative vapor pressure lowering*. The relative vapor pressure lowering depends only on the mole fraction of the solute X_2, that is, on the number of solute particles in a definite volume of solution. Therefore, the relative vapor pressure lowering is a *colligative property*.

Example 5–8. Calculate the relative vapor pressure lowering at 20° C for a solution containing 171.2 g of sucrose (w_2) in 1000 g (w_1) of water. The molecular weight of sucrose (M_2) is 342.3 and the molecular weight of water (M_1) is 18.02 g/mole.

$$\text{Moles of sucrose} = n_2 = \frac{w_2}{M_2} = \frac{171.2}{342.3} = 0.500$$

$$\text{Moles of water} = n_1 = \frac{w_1}{M_1} = 1000/18.02 = 55.5$$

$$\frac{\Delta p}{p_1°} = X_2 = \frac{n_2}{n_1 + n_2}$$

$$\frac{\Delta p}{p_1°} = \frac{0.50}{55.5 + 0.50} = 0.0089$$

Notice that in *Example 5–8*, the relative vapor pressure lowering is a dimensionless number, as would be expected from its definition. The result may also be stated as a percentage; the vapor pressure of the solution has been lowered 0.89% by the 0.5 mole of sucrose.

The mole fraction, $n_2/(n_1 + n_2)$, is nearly equal to, and may be replaced by, the mole ratio n_2/n_1 in a dilute solution such as this one. Then, the relative vapor pressure lowering can be expressed in terms of molal concentration of the solute by setting the weight of solvent w_1 equal to 1000 grams. For an aqueous solution,

$$X_2 = \frac{\Delta p}{p_1°} \cong \frac{n_2}{n_1} = \frac{w_2/M_2}{1000/M_1} = \frac{m}{55.5} = 0.018\ m \qquad (5\text{--}16)$$

Example 5–9. Calculate the vapor pressure when 0.5 mole of sucrose is added to 1000 g of water at 20° C. The vapor pressure of water at 20° C is 17.54 mm Hg. The vapor pressure lowering of the solution is

$$\Delta p = p_1°X_2 \cong p_1° \times 0.018 \times m$$

$$= 17.54 \times 0.018 \times 0.5$$

$$= 0.158\ \text{mm} \cong 0.16\ \text{mm}$$

The final vapor pressure is

$$17.54 - 0.16 = 17.38\ \text{mm}$$

Determination of the Vapor Pressure of Solutions. The vapor pressure of a solution may be determined directly by means of a manometer, and the vapor pressure lowering is then obtained by subtracting the vapor pressure of the solution from the vapor pressure of the pure solvent. For dilute aqueous solutions, however, the vapor pressure lowering, as seen in *Example 5–9*, is so slight as to produce a serious error in the measurement. Accurate differential manometers have been developed and are available for measuring small differences in vapor pressure.[4]

The *isopiestic method* is used frequently for the precise determination of vapor pressures. The solution whose vapor pressure is to be determined and a solution containing a standard solute, for example, potassium chloride, are placed in separate dishes in a closed container, as shown in Figure 5–5. The vapor of the solution with the higher pressure passes to the one with the lower pressure until the vapor pressures of the two solutions are the same, that is, *isopiestic* (Greek: equal pressure). When there is no further change in weight, the solutions are analyzed to determine their concentrations. The vapor pressures of potassium chloride solutions of various concentrations have been determined accurately, and tables of these values are available in the literature. The vapor pressure of the test solution, which is isopiestic with the potassium chloride solution, is thus readily obtained. Knowing the vapor pressure of water at this temperature, it is a simple matter to calculate the vapor pressure lowering of the solution. Robinson and Sinclair and Scatchard et al.[5] discuss the details of the method.

Hill and Baldes[6] described an apparatus consisting essentially of a combination of various wires of different alloys formed into two loops and connected to a galvanometer, as shown in Figure 5–6, for determining the relative vapor pressures of small amounts of liquids. This thermoelectric method depends on measuring the change in potential as a solution of known vapor pressure and an unknown evaporate in a chamber

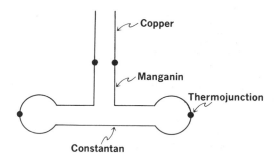

Fig. 5–6. Hill–Baldes apparatus for the thermoelectric determination of vapor pressure. (After E. J. Baldes, J. Sci. Instr. **11**, 223, 1934.)

maintained at a constant humidity. The vapor pressure lowering of the solution is then obtained from a standard curve of vapor pressure versus galvanometer readings of potential. This method has been used to study the colligative properties of ophthalmic solutions.[7]

A modern variation of the thermoelectric method for determining vapor pressure lowering is embodied in the Wescor vapor pressure "osmometer" shown in Figure 5–7. In this instrument, the test solution, which is typically on the order of less than 10 microliters, is absorbed onto a filter paper disk. The disk is placed in a sealed chamber near the thermocouple, which is cooled below the dew point of the solution. The thermocouple is then equilibrated to the dew point of the solution, whereupon its potential is recorded. By electronically zeroing the instrument at the ambient temperature before the dew point reading, the potential determined is proportional to the vapor pressure lowering. Reference standard solutions are used to calibrate the potential readings against known vapor pressures at the ambient temperature. This instrument has been applied to monitoring diuretic therapy,[8] quantitating sodium in isotonic solutions,[9] and studying the colligative properties of parenteral solutions.[10]

Describing this instrument as an "osmometer" is inappropriate. Various thermoelectric vapor pressure and freezing point instruments have been termed "osmometers," even though no membrane diffusion is involved in their operation. It would perhaps be more appropriate to call these instruments "vapor pressure differentiometers." UIC, Inc., of Joliet, Ill., manufactures vapor pressure osmometers, membrane osmometers, and a colloidal/oncotic osmometer for the automatic analysis of blood and biologic fluids.

Thermoelectric vapor pressure instruments have also been described that use separate chambers for the reference and sample and use thermistors instead of thermocouples as detectors.[11] The thermistor "osmometers" measure changes in resistance and are reported to have a sensitivity of 1×10^{-4} molal concentration, based on a sucrose solution standard. Studies of the colligative properties of nucleosides have been reported using such an instrument.[12]

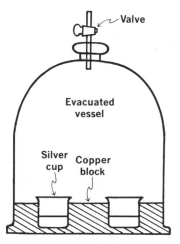

Fig. 5–5. Apparatus for the isopiestic method.

Fig. 5–7. Vapor pressure osmometer (Wescor Inc., Logan, Utah). Dial A is used to calibrate the instrument within the range of 200 to 2000 milliosmolality (mOsm/kg) using a standard solution of known osmolality (see p. 137 for a discussion on milliosmolality). The control B is used to calibrate the instrument in the range of 0 to 200 mOsm/kg. C is the off-on power switch, D the sample holder, and E the sample slide. F is a chamber-sealing knob that is tightened after the sample slide is pushed fully in to center the sample holder in the chamber under F. A drop of sample solution placed in the holder comes to equilibrium in the chamber, and a thermocouple hygrometer provides an accurate readout of mOsm/kg in the display window.

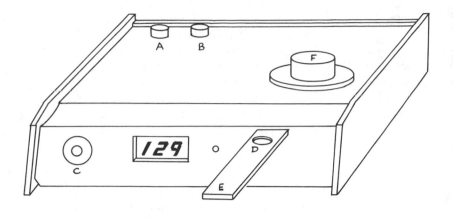

Elevation of the Boiling Point. As stated in Chapter 2, the normal boiling point is the temperature at which the vapor pressure of the liquid becomes equal to an external pressure of 760 mm Hg. The boiling point of a solution of a nonvolatile solute is higher than that of the pure solvent, owing to the fact that the solute lowers the vapor pressure of the solvent. This may be seen by referring to the curves in Figure 5–8. The vapor pressure curve for the solution lies below that of the pure solvent, and the temperature of the solution must be elevated to a value above that of the solvent in order to reach the normal boiling point. The elevation of the boiling point is shown in the figure as $T - T_o = \Delta T_b$. The ratio of the elevation of the boiling point, ΔT_b, to the vapor pressure lowering, $\Delta p = p° - p$, at 100° C is approximately a constant at this temperature; it is written as

$$\frac{\Delta T_b}{\Delta p} = k' \qquad (5-17)$$

or

$$\Delta T_b = k' \, \Delta p \qquad (5-18)$$

Moreover, since $p°$ is a constant, the boiling point elevation may be considered proportional to $\Delta p/p°$, the relative lowering of vapor pressure. By Raoult's law, however, the relative vapor pressure lowering is equal to the mole fraction of the solute; therefore,

$$\Delta T_b = kX_2 \qquad (5-19)$$

Since the boiling point elevation depends only on the mole fraction of the solute, it is a colligative property.

In dilute solutions, X_2 is equal approximately to $m/(1000/M_1)$ (equation [5–16]), and equation (5–19) may be written as

$$\Delta T_b = \frac{kM_1}{1000} \, m \qquad (5-20)$$

or

$$\Delta T_b = K_b m \qquad (5-21)$$

in which ΔT_b is known as the *boiling point elevation* and K_b is called the *molal elevation constant* or the *ebullioscopic constant*. K_b has a characteristic value for each solvent, as seen in Table 5–4. It may be considered as the boiling point elevation for an ideal 1 m solution. Stated another way, K_b is the ratio of the boiling point elevation to the molal concentration in an extremely dilute solution in which the system is approximately ideal.

The preceding discussion constitutes a plausible argument leading to the equation for boiling point elevation. A more satisfactory derivation of equation (5–21), however, involves the application of the Clapeyron equation (pp. 31, 68), which is written as

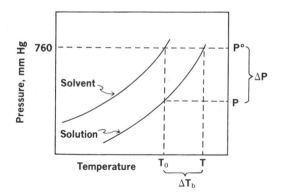

Fig. 5–8. Boiling point elevation of the solvent due to addition of a solute (not to scale).

TABLE 5–4. *Ebullioscopic and Cryoscopic Constants for Various Solvents*

Substance	Boiling Point (°C)	K_b	Freezing Point (°C)	K_f
Acetic acid	118.0	2.93	16.7	3.9
Acetone	56.0	1.71	−94.82*	2.40*
Benzene	80.1	2.53	5.5	5.12
Camphor	208.3	5.95	178.4	37.7
Chloroform	61.2	3.54	−63.5	4.96
Ethyl alcohol	78.4	1.22	−114.49*	3*
Ethyl ether	34.6	2.02	−116.3	1.79*
Phenol	181.4	3.56	42.0	7.27
Water	100.0	0.51	0.00	1.86

*From G. Kortum and J. O'M. Bockris, *Textbook of Electrochemistry*, Vol. II, Elsevier, New York 1951, pp. 618, 620.

$$\frac{\Delta T_b}{\Delta p} = T_b \frac{V_v - V_l}{\Delta H_v} \qquad (5\text{-}22)$$

V_v and V_l are the molar volume of the gas and the molar volume of the liquid, respectively. T_b is the boiling point of the solvent and ΔH_v the molar heat of vaporization. Since V_l is negligible compared to V_v, the equation becomes

$$\frac{\Delta T_b}{\Delta p} = T_b \frac{V_v}{\Delta H_v} \qquad (5\text{-}23)$$

and V_v, the volume of 1 mole of gas, is replaced by $RT_b/p°$ to give

$$\frac{\Delta T_b}{\Delta p} = \frac{RT_b^2}{p°\Delta H_v} \qquad (5\text{-}24)$$

or

$$\Delta T_b = \frac{RT_b^2}{\Delta H_v} \frac{\Delta p}{p°} \qquad (5\text{-}25)$$

From equation (5–16), $\Delta p/p_1° = X_2$, and equation (5–25) may be written

$$\Delta T_b = \frac{RT_b^2}{\Delta H_v} X_2 = kX_2 \qquad (5\text{-}26)$$

which provides a more exact equation with which to calculate ΔT_b.

Replacing the relative vapor pressure lowering $\Delta p/p_1°$ by $m/(1000/M_1)$ according to the approximate expression (equation [5–16]), in which $w_2/M_2 = m$ and $w_1 = 1000$, the formula becomes

$$\Delta T_b = \frac{RT_b^2 M_1}{1000\ \Delta H_v} m = K_b m \qquad (5\text{-}27)$$

Equation (5–27) provides a less exact expression to calculate ΔT_b.

For water at 100° C, $T_b = 373.2°$ K, $\Delta H_v = 9720$ cal/mole, $M_1 = 18.02$ g/mole, and $R = 1.987$ cal/mole deg.

$$K_b = \frac{1.987 \times (373.2)^2 \times 18.02}{1000 \times 9720} = 0.513 \text{ deg kg/mole}$$

Example 5–10. A 0.200 *m* aqueous solution of a drug gave a boiling point elevation of 0.103° C. Calculate the approximate molal elevation constant for the solvent, water. Substituting into equation (5–21) yields

$$K_b = \frac{\Delta T_b}{m} = \frac{0.103}{0.200} = 0.515 \text{ deg kg/mole}$$

The proportionality between ΔT_b and the molality is exact only at infinite dilution, at which the properties of real and ideal solutions coincide. The ebullioscopic constant K_b of a solvent can be obtained experimentally by measuring ΔT_b at various molal concentrations and extrapolating to infinite dilution ($m = 0$), as seen in Figure 5–9.

Determination of Boiling Point Elevation. Boiling point elevation is determined experimentally by placing a

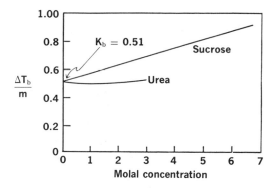

Fig. 5–9. The influence of concentration on the ebullioscopic constant.

weighed amount of the solute and the solvent in a glass vessel provided with a thermometer and a reflux condenser. In the *Cottrell boiling point apparatus*, the vapor and the boiling solvent are pumped by the force of ebullition through a glass tube and sprayed over the thermometer bulb to obtain an invariant equilibrium temperature. The boiling point of the pure solvent is determined in the same apparatus.

Depression of the Freezing Point. The normal freezing point or melting point of a pure compound is the temperature at which the solid and the liquid phases are in equilibrium under a pressure of 1 atm. Equilibrium here means that the tendency for the solid to pass into the liquid state is the same as the tendency for the reverse process to occur, since both the liquid and the solid have the same escaping tendency. The value T_o, observed in Figure 5–10, for water saturated with air at this pressure is arbitrarily assigned a temperature of 0° C. The *triple point* of air-free water, at which solid, liquid, and vapor are in equilibrium, lies at a pressure of 4.58 mm Hg and a temperature of 0.0098° C. It is not identical with the ordinary freezing point of water at atmospheric pressure, as explained on page 38, but is rather the freezing point of water under the pressure of its own vapor. We shall use the triple point in the following argument, since the depression ΔT_f here does

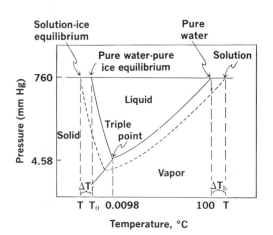

Fig. 5–10. Depression of the freezing point of the solvent, water, by a solute (not to scale).

not differ significantly from ΔT_f at a pressure of 1 atm. The two freezing point depressions referred to are illustrated in Figure 5–10. ΔT_b of Figure 5–8 is also shown in the diagram.

If a solute is dissolved in the liquid at the triple point, the escaping tendency or vapor pressure of the liquid solvent is lowered below that of the pure solid solvent. The temperature must drop in order to reestablish equilibrium between the liquid and the solid. Because of this fact, the freezing point of a solution is always lower than that of the pure solvent. It is assumed that the solvent freezes out in the pure state rather than as a *solid solution* containing some of the solute. When such a complication does arise, special calculations, not considered here, must be used.

The more concentrated the solution, the farther apart are the solvent and the solution curves in the diagram (see Fig. 5–10) and the greater is the freezing point depression. Accordingly, a situation exists analogous to that described for the boiling point elevation, and the freezing point depression is proportional to the molal concentration of the solute. The equation is

$$\Delta T_f = K_f m \qquad (5\text{–}28)$$

or

$$\Delta T_f = K_f \frac{1000\, w_2}{w_1 M_2} \qquad (5\text{–}29)$$

ΔT_f is the *freezing point depression*, and K_f is the *molal depression constant* or the *cryoscopic constant*, which depends on the physical and chemical properties of the solvent.

The freezing point depression of a solvent is a function only of the number of particles in the solution, and for this reason it is referred to as a *colligative* property. The depression of the freezing point, like the boiling point elevation, is a direct result of the lowering of the vapor pressure of the solvent. The value of K_f for water is 1.86. It may be determined experimentally by measuring $\Delta T_f/m$ at several molal concentrations and extrapolating to zero concentration. As seen in Figure 5–11, K_f approaches the value of 1.86 for water

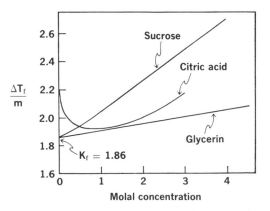

Fig. 5–11. The influence of concentration on the cryoscopic constant for water.

solutions of sucrose and glycerin as the concentrations tend toward zero, and equation (5–28) is valid only in very dilute solutions. The apparent cryoscopic constant for higher concentrations may be obtained from Figure 5–11. For work in pharmacy and biology, the K_f value 1.86 may be rounded off to 1.9, which is good approximation for practical use with aqueous solutions where concentrations are usually lower than 0.1 M. The value K_f for the solvent in a solution of citric acid is observed not to approach 1.86. This abnormal behavior is to be expected when dealing with solutions of electrolytes. Their irrationality will be explained in Chapter 6, and proper steps will be taken to correct the difficulty.

K_f may also be derived from Raoult's law and the Clapeyron equation. For water at its freezing point, $T_f = 273.2°$ K, ΔH_f is 1437 cal/mole, and

$$K_f = \frac{1.987 \times (273.2)^2 \times 18.02}{1000 \times 1437} = 1.86 \text{ deg kg/mole}$$

The cryoscopic constants, together with the ebullioscopic constants, for some solvents at infinite dilution are given in Table 5–4.

Example 5–11. What is the freezing point of a solution containing 3.42 g of sucrose and 500 g of water? The molecular weight of sucrose is 342. In this relatively dilute solution, K_f is approximately equal to 1.86.

$$\Delta T_f = K_f m = K_f \frac{1000\, w_2}{w_1 M_2}$$

$$\Delta T_f = 1.86 \times \frac{1000 \times 3.42}{500 \times 342}$$

$$\Delta T_f = 0.037° \text{ C}$$

Therefore, the freezing point of the aqueous solution is $-0.037°$ C.

Example 5–12. What is the freezing point depression of a 1.3-m solution of sucrose in water?

From the graph (see Fig. 5–11), one observes that the cryoscopic constant at this concentration is about 2.1 rather than 1.86. Thus, the calculation becomes

$$\Delta T_f = K_f \times m = 2.1 \times 1.3 = 2.73° \text{ C}$$

Determination of Freezing Point Lowering. Several methods are available for the determination of freezing point lowering. They include (*a*) the Beckmann method and (*b*) the equilibrium method.

The apparatus for the determination of the freezing point of a solution using the Beckmann method is seen in Figure 5–12. It consists of a jacketed tube with a sidearm through which the test material may be introduced. A Beckmann thermometer* is supported in the tube and extends into the test solution. A glass stirrer passes through a tube in the stopper and is operated manually or by means of a motor as shown in Figure 5–12. The tube and jacket are supported in a vessel containing a cooling mixture of salt and ice.

---

*The Beckmann thermometer is of the differential type that may be set arbitrarily to function within a 5° temperature range between $-10°$ and $+140°$ C and is graduated in 0.01° divisions. The temperature can be estimated to within about $\pm0.005°$ C.

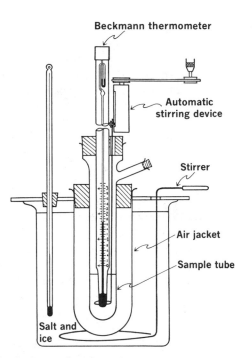

Fig. 5–12. Beckmann freezing point apparatus.

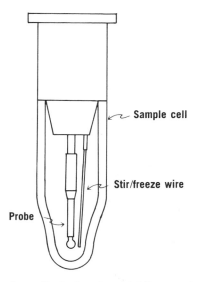

Fig. 5–13. Sensing unit of a freezing point "osmometer." The other parts of the osmometer, not shown, include a stirring motor, refrigeration unit, calibration dials, on-off switch, and a window that displays the freezing point value at equilibrium. The solution in the sample cell is supercooled several degrees below its freezing point; the tip of the stir/freeze wire then vibrates to form ice crystals. The temperature of the sample solution rises to its freezing point with the liberation of heat of fusion. The probe senses the equilibrium temperature, and it is read out in the display window (Advanced Digimatic osmometer, Model 3DII, Advanced Instruments, Inc., Needham Heights, MA).

In carrying out a determination, the temperature is read on the Beckmann differential thermometer at the freezing point of the pure solvent, water. A known weight of the solute is introduced into the apparatus, containing a given weight of solvent, and the freezing point of the solution is read and recorded.

Example 5–13. The freezing point of water on the scale of the Beckmann thermometer is 1.112° C and the value for an aqueous solution of the solute is 0.120° C. What is the apparent K_f value if the concentration of the solution is 0.50 m?

$$K_f = \frac{\Delta T_f}{m} = \frac{(1.112 - 0.120)}{0.50} = \frac{0.992}{0.50}$$

$$= 1.98$$

Johlin[13] described a semimicro apparatus for the determination of the freezing point of small quantities of physiologic solutions. Results may be obtained with as little as 1 mL of solution. The apparatus is now available commercially as the Osmette S, Model 400Z, from Precision Systems, Waltham, Mass., and the Advanced Digimatic Osmometer, Model 3DII, Advanced Instruments, Inc., Needham Heights, Mass. A schematic of the freezing point osmometer is shown in Figure 5–13.

The equilibrium method[14] is the most accurate procedure for obtaining freezing point data. The freezing point of the pure solvent is determined accurately by intimately mixing the solid and liquid solvent (ice and water) in a jacketed tube or Dewar flask. When equilibrium is established, the temperature of the mixture is read with a Beckmann thermometer or with a multijunction thermocouple and a potentiometer. According to Ballard and Goyan,[15] a thermistor may be used instead of a thermocouple. The solution, mixed with ice frozen from the pure solvent, is then placed in the flask, and when equilibrium is again attained, the temperature is recorded. A sample of the liquid phase is removed and analyzed at the time of measurement to determine accurately the concentration of the solution. The accuracy of the method can be improved by simultaneously placing the two ends of the thermocouple into two vacuum jacketed flasks, one containing the pure liquid in equilibrium with solid solvent and the other containing the solution in equilibrium with solid solvent. The difference in freezing points of the two systems can be determined to within ±0.00002° C.

Ethylene glycol is the common antifreeze used in automobile cooling systems, air conditioners, freeze-drying apparatus, and so on. It has a high boiling point and may be retained in a car's radiator for as long as a year or more. It is therefore known as a *permanent* antifreeze. The same freezing point depression equation (5–28) that we have already used—namely, $\Delta T_f = K_f m$—is used to estimate the effectiveness of an antifreeze to lower the freezing point of water in a car's cooling system. We see from the equation that the property of reducing the freezing point of water varies only with the molality of an antifreeze and not with the chemical characteristic of the agent. Methanol, denatured ethanol, propylene glycol, glycerol, and even sugars and honey have been used as antifreezes. However, ethylene glycol's high boiling point makes it particularly attractive. An automobile antifreeze is now used year-round; it raises the boiling point of water, just as it lowers the freezing point, and thus prevents the loss of fluid through evaporation in the summer.

A more exact expression for freezing point depression is

$$\Delta T_f = \frac{RT_f\, T}{\Delta H_f}\ln X_1 \qquad (5\text{--}30)$$

For a very dilute solution we can make the approximation that

$$\ln X_1 = \ln(1 - X_2) \simeq X_2 \qquad (5\text{--}31)$$

Therefore, equation (5–30) becomes

$$\Delta T_f = \frac{RT_f T}{\Delta H_f}X_2 \qquad (5\text{--}32)$$

in which T_f is the freezing point of the solvent, T is the freezing point of the solution, and ΔH_f is the heat of fusion of the solvent.

Example 5–14. How many liters of ethylene glycol (Caution, Poisonous!) must be added to a car's cooling system, which holds 12 kg of fluid, to protect the car from freezing at a temperature of $+10°$ F? The molecular weight of ethylene glycol is 62.07 g/mole and its density $d_4^0 = 1.1274$ g/cm³. The heat of fusion of water is 1436 cal/mole. Use equation (5–32) and compare your result with that obtained from equation (5–28) on page 114.

We use the equation on the front leaf of the book to convert $10°$ F to $-12.22°$ C, which is a lowering of the freezing point of water, $0°$ C, to $-12.22°$ C, or $\Delta T_f = +12.22$

From equation (5–32),

$$X_2 - \frac{\Delta T_f \cdot \Delta H_f}{RT_f T} = \frac{(12.22)(1436)}{(1.9872)(273.2)(260.8)} = 0.1239$$

The quantity $X_2 = 0.1239$ is now expressed in molality; that is, in moles/kg water, and from moles/kg water to grams/kg water, then to mL/kg water, and finally to liters per 12 kg of fluid in the car's cooling system.

$$\text{molality,}^*\; m, = \frac{1000\,X_2}{M_1(1 - X_2)} = \frac{1000 \times 0.1239}{18.015(1 - 0.1239)}$$

$$= 7.850 \text{ moles/kg water}$$

7.850 moles/kg water $\times$ 62.07 g/mole $= 487.25$ g/kg water

487.25 g/kg water $\div$ 1.1274 g/mL $= 432.19$ mL/kg water

432.19 mL/kg water $\times$ 12 kg fluid $= 5186.3$ mL $= 5.19$ liters

Using the more approximate equation (5–28), $\Delta T_f = K_f m$ in which $K_f = 1.86$ deg kg/mole, $\Delta T_f = 12.22$ deg, and molality, m, is

$$m = \Delta T_f/K_f = 12.22°/1.86 = 6.570 \text{ mole/kg water}$$

$$\frac{6.570 \times 62.07}{1.1274} \times 12 \text{ kg fluid} = 4340.5 \text{ mL} = 4.34 \text{ liters}$$

A fair comparison—5.19 liters versus 4.34 liters—is obtained using the more exact equation (5–32) and the less exact equation (5–28).

Osmotic Pressure. If cobalt chloride is placed in a parchment sac and suspended in a beaker of water, the water gradually becomes red as the solute diffuses

---

*See Table 5–3, page 104 for conversion equations used to change from one concentration unit to another. Note that in this example, an excess number of significant figures are retained until the final step, when they are rounded off. This is an acceptable procedure, particularly when using a hand calculator or computer.

throughout the vessel. In this process of *diffusion*, both the solvent and the solute molecules migrate freely. On the other hand, if the solution is confined in a membrane permeable only to the solvent molecules, the phenomenon known as *osmosis* (Greek: a push or impulse)[16] occurs, and the barrier that permits only the molecules of one of the components (usually water) to pass through is known as a *semipermeable membrane*. A thistle tube, over the wide opening of which is stretched a piece of untreated cellophane, can be used to demonstrate the principle, as shown in Figure 5–14. The tube is partly filled with a concentrated solution of sucrose and the apparatus is lowered into a beaker of water. The passage of water through the semipermeable membrane into the solution eventually creates enough pressure to drive the sugar solution up the tube until the hydrostatic pressure of the column of liquid equals the pressure causing the water to pass through the membrane and enter the thistle tube. When this occurs, the solution ceases to rise in the tube. Osmosis is therefore defined as the passage of the solvent into a solution through a semipermeable membrane. This process tends to equalize the escaping tendency (p. 106) of the solvent on both sides of the membrane. Escaping tendency can be measured in terms of vapor pressure or the closely related colligative property, *osmotic pressure*. It should be evident that osmosis can also take place when a concentrated solution is separated from a less concentrated solution by a semipermeable membrane.

Osmosis in some cases is believed to involve the passage of solvent through the membrane by a distillation process, or by dissolving in the material of the membrane in which the solute is insoluble. In other cases, the membrane may act as a sieve, having a pore size sufficiently large to allow passage of solvent but not of solute molecules.

In either case, the phenomenon of osmosis really depends on the fact that the chemical potential (a thermodynamic expression of escaping tendency, discussed on page 106), of a solvent molecule in solution is less than exists in the pure solvent. Solvent therefore

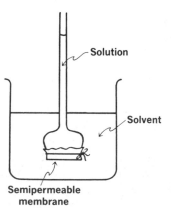

Fig. 5–14. Apparatus for demonstrating osmosis.

passes spontaneously into the solution until the chemical potentials of solvent and solution are equal. The system is then at equilibrium. It may be advantageous for the student to consider osmosis in terms of the following sequence of events. (1) The addition of a nonvolatile solute to the solvent forms a solution in which the vapor pressure of the solvent is reduced (see Raoult's law). (2) If pure solvent is now placed adjacent to the solution but separated from it by a semipermeable membrane, solvent molecules will pass through the membrane into the solution in an attempt to dilute out the solute and raise the vapor pressure back to its original value (namely, that of the original solvent). (3) The osmotic pressure that is set up as a result of this passage of solvent molecules may be determined either by measuring the hydrostatic head appearing in the solution or by applying a known pressure that just balances the osmotic pressure and prevents any net movement of solvent molecules into the solution. The latter is the preferred technique. The osmotic pressure thus obtained is proportional to the reduction in vapor pressure brought about by the concentration of solute present. Since this is a function of the molecular weight of the solute, osmotic pressure is a colligative property and may be used to determine molecule weights.

As contrasted to the *freezing point* osmometer (Fig. 5–13), an *osmotic pressure* osmometer (Fig. 5–15) is based on the same principle as the thistle tube apparatus shown in Figure 5–14. Once equilibrium has been attained, the height of the solution in the capillary tube on the solution side of the membrane is greater by the amount h than the height in the capillary tube on the solvent (water) side. The hydrostatic head, h, is related to the osmotic pressure through the expression, osmotic pressure π (atm) = height h × solution density ρ × gravity acceleration. The two tubes of large bore are for filling and discharging the liquids from the compartments of the apparatus. The height of liquid in these two large tubes does not enter into the calculation of osmotic pressure. The determination of osmotic pressure is discussed in some detail in the next section.

Measurement of Osmotic Pressure. The osmotic pressure of the sucrose solution referred to in the last section is not measured conveniently by observing the height that the solution attains in the tube at equilibrium. The concentration of the final solution is not known since the passage of water into the solution dilutes it and alters the concentration. A more exact measure of the osmotic pressure of the undiluted solution is obtained by determining the excess pressure on the solution side that just prevents the passage of solvent through the membrane. Osmotic pressure is defined as the excess pressure, or pressure greater than that above the pure solvent, that must be applied to the solution to prevent the passage of the solvent through a perfect semipermeable membrane. In this definition, it is assumed that a semipermeable sac containing the solution is immersed in the *pure* solvent.

In 1877, the botanist Pfeffer measured the osmotic pressure of sugar solutions, using a porous cup impreg-

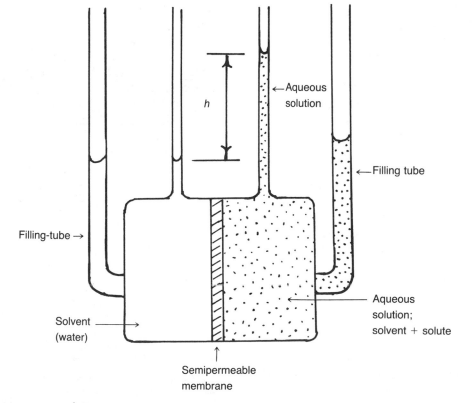

Fig. 5–15. Osmotic pressure osmometer.

nated with a deposit of cupric ferrocyanide $(Cu_2Fe(CN)_6)$ as the semipermeable membrane. The apparatus was provided with a manometer to measure the pressure. Although many improvements have been made through the years, including the attachment of sensitive pressure transducers to the membrane that can be electronically amplified to produce a signal[17] the direct measurement of osmotic pressure remains difficult and inconvenient. Nevertheless, osmotic pressure is the colligative property best suited to the determination of the molecular weight of polymers such as proteins.

Van't Hoff and Morse Equations for Osmotic Pressure. In 1886, van't Hoff recognized in Pfeffer's data a proportionality between osmotic pressure, concentration, and temperature and suggested a relationship that corresponded to the equation for an ideal gas. Van't Hoff concluded that there was an apparent analogy between solutions and gases and that the osmotic pressure in a dilute solution was equal to the pressure that the solute would exert if it were a gas occupying the same volume. The equation is

$$\pi V = nRT \qquad (5-33)$$

in which π is the osmotic pressure in atm, V is the volume of the solution in liters, n is the number of moles of solute, R is the gas constant equal to 0.082 liter atm/mole deg, and T is the absolute temperature.

The student should be cautioned not to take van't Hoff's analogy too literally, for it leads to the belief that the solute molecules "produce" the osmotic pressure by exerting pressure on the membrane, just as gas molecules create a pressure by striking the walls of a vessel. It is more correct, however, to consider the osmotic pressure as resulting from the relative escaping tendencies of the *solvent* molecules on the two sides of the membrane. Actually, equation (5–33) is a limiting law applying to dilute solutions, and it simplifies into this form from a more exact expression (equation [5–39]) only after introducing a number of assumptions that are not valid for real solutions.

Example 5–15. One gram of sucrose, molecular weight 342, is dissolved in 100 mL of solution at 25° C. What is the osmotic pressure of the solution?

$$\text{Moles of sucrose} = \frac{1.0}{342} = 0.0029$$

$$\pi \times 0.10 = 0.0029 \times 0.082 \times 298$$

$$\pi = 0.71 \text{ atm}$$

Equation (5–33), the van't Hoff equation, can be expressed as

$$\pi = \frac{n}{V} RT = cRT \qquad (5-34)$$

in which c is the concentration of the solute in moles per liter (molarity). Morse and others have shown that when the concentration is expressed in molality rather than molarity, the results compare more nearly with the experimental findings. The Morse equation is

$$\pi = RTm \qquad (5-35)$$

Thermodynamics of Osmotic Pressure and Vapor Pressure Lowering. Osmotic pressure and the lowering of vapor pressure, both colligative properties, are inextricably related, and this relationship may be obtained from certain thermodynamic considerations.

We begin by considering a sucrose solution in the right-hand compartment of the apparatus shown in Figure 5–16, and the pure solvent—water—in the left-hand compartment. The two compartments are separated by a semipermeable membrane through which water molecules, but not sucrose molecules, can pass. It is assumed that the gate in the air space connecting the solutions can be shut during osmosis. The external pressure, say 1 atmosphere, above the pure solvent is P_o, while the pressure on the solution, provided by the piston in Figure 5–16 and needed to maintain equilbrium, is P. The difference between the two pressures at equilibrium, $P - P_o$, or the excess pressure on the solution, just required to prevent passage of water into the solution, is the osmotic pressure π.

Let us now consider the alternative transport of water through the air space above the liquids. Should the membrane be closed off and the gate in the air space opened, water molecules pass from the pure solvent to the solution by way of the vapor state by a distillation process. The space above the liquids actually serves as a "semipermeable membrane," just as does the real membrane at the lower part of the apparatus. The vapor pressure $p°$ of water in the pure solvent under the influence of the atmospheric pressure P_o is greater than the vapor pressure p of water in the solution by an amount $p° - p = \Delta p$. To bring about equilibrium, a pressure P must be exerted by the piston on the solution to increase the vapor pressure of the solution until it is equal to that of the pure solvent, $p°$. The

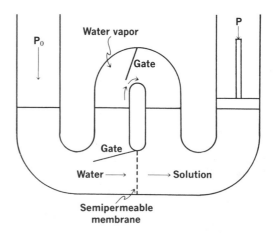

Fig. 5–16. Apparatus for demonstrating the relationship between osmotic pressure and vapor pressure lowering.

excess pressure that must be applied, $P - P_o$, is again the osmotic pressure π. The operation of such an apparatus thus demonstrates the relationship between osmotic pressure and vapor pressure lowering.

By following this analysis further, it should be possible to obtain an equation relating osmotic pressure and vapor pressure. Observe that both osmosis and the distillation process are based on the principle that the escaping tendency of water in the pure solvent is greater than that in the solution. By application of an excess pressure, $P - P_o = \pi$, on the solution side of the apparatus, it is possible to make the escaping tendencies of water in the solvent and solution identical. A state of equilibrium is produced; thus, the free energy of solvent on both sides of the membrane or on both sides of the air space is made equal, and $\Delta G = 0$.

To relate vapor pressure lowering and osmotic pressure, we must obtain the free energy changes involved in (a) transferring a mole of solvent from solvent to solution by a distillation process through the vapor phase and (b) transferring a mole of solvent from solvent to solution by osmosis.

$$(a) \qquad \Delta G = RT \ln \frac{p}{p^\circ} \qquad (5\text{--}36)$$

is the increase in free energy at a definite temperature for the passage of 1 mole of water to the solution through the vapor phase;

$$(b) \qquad \Delta G = -V_1(P - P_o) = -V_1\pi \qquad (5\text{--}37)$$

is the increase in free energy at constant temperature for the passage of 1 mole of water into the solution by osmosis. In equation (5–37), V_1 is the volume of 1 mole of solvent, or more correctly, it is the *partial molar volume*, that is, the change in volume of the solution on the addition of 1 mole of solvent to a large quantity of solution.

Equating equations (5–36) and (5–37) gives

$$-\pi V_1 = RT \ln \frac{p}{p^\circ} \qquad (5\text{--}38)$$

and eliminating the minus sign by inverting the logarithmic term yields

$$\pi = \frac{RT}{V_1} \ln \frac{p^\circ}{p} \qquad (5\text{--}39)$$

Equation (5–39) is a more exact expression for osmotic pressure than are equations (5–34) and (5–35), and it applies to concentrated as well as dilute solutions, provided that the vapor follows the ideal gas laws.

The simpler equation (5–35) for osmotic pressure may be obtained from equation (5–39), assuming that the solution obeys Raoult's law,

$$p = p^\circ X_1 \qquad (5\text{--}40)$$

$$\frac{p}{p^\circ} = X_1 = 1 - X_2 \qquad (5\text{--}41)$$

Equation (5–39) can thus be written

$$\pi V_1 = -RT \ln (1 - X_2) \qquad (5\text{--}42)$$

and $\ln (1 - X_2)$ can be expanded into a series

$$\ln (1 - X)_2 = -X_2 - \frac{X_2^2}{2} - \frac{X_2^3}{3} \cdots - \frac{X_2^n}{n} \qquad (5\text{--}43)$$

When X_2 is small, that is, when the solution is dilute, all terms in the expansion beyond the first may be neglected, and

$$\ln (1 - X_2) \cong -X_2 \qquad (5\text{--}44)$$

so that

$$\pi V_1 = RT X_2 \qquad (5\text{--}45)$$

For a dilute solution, X_2 equals approximately the mole ratio n_2/n_1, and equation (5–45) becomes

$$\pi \cong \frac{n_2}{n_1 V_1} RT \qquad (5\text{--}46)$$

in which $n_1 V_1$, the number of moles of solvent multiplied by the volume of 1 mole, is equal to the total volume of solvent V in liters. For a dilute aqueous solution, the equation becomes

$$\pi = \frac{n_2}{V} RT = RTm \qquad (5\text{--}47)$$

which is Morse's expression, equation (5–35).

Example 5–16. Compute π for a 1-m aqueous solution of sucrose using both equation (5–35) and the more exact thermodynamic equation (5–39). The vapor pressure of the solution is 31.207 mm Hg and the vapor pressure of water is 31.824 mm Hg at 30.0° C. The molar volume of water at this temperature is 18.1 cm³/mole, or 0.0181 liter/mole.

(a) By the Morse equation,

$$\pi = RTm = 0.082 \times 303 \times 1$$

$$\pi = 24.8 \text{ atm}$$

(b) By the thermodynamic equation,

$$\pi = \frac{RT}{V_1} \ln \frac{p^\circ}{p}$$

$$\pi = \frac{0.082 \times 303}{0.0181} \times 2.303 \log \frac{31.824}{31.207}$$

$$= 27.0 \text{ atm}$$

The experimental value for the osmotic pressure of a 1-m solution of sucrose at 30° C is 27.2 atm.

MOLECULAR WEIGHT DETERMINATION

The four colligative properties that have been discussed in this chapter—vapor pressure lowering, freezing point lowering, boiling point elevation, and osmotic pressure—may be used to calculate the molecular weights of nonelectrolytes present as solutes. Thus, the lowering of the vapor pressure of a solution containing a nonvolatile solute depends only on the mole fraction of the solute. This allows the molecular weight of the solute to be calculated in the following manner.

Since the mole fraction of solvent, $n_1 = w_1/M_1$, and the mole fraction of solute, $n_2 = w_2/M_2$, in which w_1 and w_2 are the weights of solvent and solute of molecular weight M_1 and M_2 respectively, equation (5–15) can be expressed as

$$\frac{p_1{}^\circ - p_1}{p_1{}^\circ} = \frac{n_2}{n_1 + n_2} = \frac{w_2/M_2}{w_1/M_1 + w_2/M_2} \quad (5\text{–}48)$$

In dilute solutions in which w_2/M_2 is negligible compared with w_1/M_1, the former term may be omitted from the denominator, and the equation simplifies to

$$\frac{\Delta p}{p_1{}^\circ} = \frac{w_2/M_2}{w_1/M_1} \quad (5\text{–}49)$$

The molecular weight of the solute M_2 is obtained by rearranging equation (5–49) to

$$M_2 = \frac{w_2 M_1 p_1{}^\circ}{w_1 \Delta p} \quad (5\text{–}50)$$

Mason and Gardner[18] have used the isopiestic method, outlined previously (p. 111), for the determination of molecular weights by vapor pressure lowering.

The molecular weight of a nonvolatile solute can similarly be determined from the boiling point elevation of the solution. Knowing K_b, the molal elevation constant, for the solvent and determining T_b, the boiling point elevation, one can calculate the molecular weight of a nonelectrolyte. Since $1000\, w_2/w_1$ is the weight of solute per kilogram of solvent, molality (moles/kilogram of solvent) can be expressed as

$$m = \frac{w_2/M_2}{w_1} \times 1000 = \frac{1000 w_2}{w_1 M_2} \quad (5\text{–}51)$$

and

$$\Delta T_b = K_b m \quad (5\text{–}52)$$

then

$$\Delta T_b = K_b \frac{1000 w_2}{w_1 M_2} \quad (5\text{–}53)$$

or

$$M_2 = K_b \frac{1000 w_2}{w_1 \Delta T_b} \quad (5\text{–}54)$$

Example 5–17. A solution containing 10.0 g of sucrose dissolved in 100 g of water has a boiling point of 100.149° C. What is the molecular weight of sucrose?

$$M_2 = 0.51 \times \frac{1000 \times 10.0}{100 \times 0.149}$$

$$= 342 \text{ g/mole}$$

As was shown in Figure (5–10), the lowering of vapor pressure arising from the addition of a nonvola-tile solute to a solvent results in a depression of the freezing point. By rearranging equation (5–29).

$$M_2 = K_f \frac{1000 w_2}{\Delta T_f\, w_1} \quad (5\text{–}55)$$

in which w_2 is the number of grams of solute dissolved in w_1 grams of solvent. It is thus possible to calculate the molecular weight of the solute from cryoscopic data of this type.

Example 5–18. The freezing point depression of a solution of 2.000 g of 1,3-dinitrobenzene in 100.0 g of benzene was determined by the equilibrium method and was found to be 0.6095° C. Calculate the molecular weight of 1,3-dinitrobenzene.

$$M_2 = 5.12 \times \frac{1000 \times 2.000}{0.6095 \times 100.0} = 168.0 \text{ g/mole}$$

The van't Hoff and Morse equations may be used to calculate the molecular weight of solutes from osmotic pressure data provided the solution is sufficiently dilute and ideal. The manner in which osmotic pressure is used to calculate the molecular weight of colloidal materials is discussed in Chapter 15.

Example 5–19. Fifteen grams of a new drug dissolved in water to yield 1000 mL of solution at 25° C was found to produce an osmotic pressure of 0.6 atm. What is the molecular weight of the solute?

$$\pi = cRT = \frac{c_g RT}{M_2} \quad (5\text{–}56)$$

in which c_g is in g/liter of solution. Thus,

$$\pi = \frac{15 \times 0.0821 \times 298}{M_2}$$

or

$$M_2 = \frac{15 \times 24.45}{0.6} = 612 \text{ g/mole}$$

Choice of Colligative Properties. Each of the colligative properties seems to have certain advantages and disadvantages for the determination of molecular weights. The boiling point method can be used only when the solute is nonvolatile and when the substance is not decomposed at boiling temperatures. The freezing point method is satisfactory for solutions containing volatile solutes, such as alcohol, since the freezing point of a solution depends on the vapor pressure of the solvent alone. The freezing point method is easily executed and yields results of high accuracy for solutions of small molecules. It is sometimes inconvenient to use freezing point or boiling point methods, however, since they must be carried out at definite temperatures. Osmotic pressure measurements do not have this disadvantage, and yet the difficulties inherent in this method preclude its wide use. In summary, it may be said that the cryoscopic and newer vapor pressure techniques are the methods of choice, except for high polymers, in which instance the osmotic pressure method is used (pp. 401–402).

Since the colligative properties are interrelated, it should be possible to determine the value of one property from a knowledge of any other. The relationship between vapor pressure lowering and osmotic pressure has already been shown. Freezing point depression and osmotic pressure can be related approximately as follows. The molality from the equation $m = \Delta T_f/K_f$ is substituted in the osmotic pressure equation, $\pi = RTm$, to give, at $0°$ C,

$$\pi = RT \frac{\Delta T_f}{K_f} = \frac{22.4}{1.86} \Delta T_f \qquad (5\text{-}57)$$

or

$$\pi \cong 12\Delta T_f \qquad (5\text{-}58)$$

Lewis[19] suggested an equation:

$$\pi = 12.06 \, \Delta T_f - 0.021 \, \Delta T_f^2 \qquad (5\text{-}59)$$

which gives accurate results.

Example 5–20. A sample of human blood serum has a freezing point of $-0.53°$ C. What is the approximate osmotic pressure of this sample at $0°$ C? What is its more accurate value as given by the Lewis equation?

$$\pi = 12 \times 0.53 = 6.36 \text{ atm}$$
$$\pi = 12.06 \times 0.53 - 0.021(0.53)^2 = 6.39 \text{ atm}$$

Table 5–5 presents the equations and their constants in summary form. All equations are approximate and are useful only for dilute solutions in which the volume occupied by the solute is negligible with respect to that of the solvent.

Example 5–21. In your laboratory you wish to study the applicability of various colligative property methods for determining the molecular weights of small and large molecules. You begin by comparing the freezing point depression method and the osmotic pressure method. To obtain freezing point depressions and osmotic pressures, you decide to use the following hypothetical data for both large and small drug molecules, and then compare the relative precision of the two methods. Let $M_2 = 250$ g/mole (small drug); $M_2 = 1,000,000$ g/mole (macromolecule). The concentration is 1% (w/v) or 10 g/1000 cm^3 for both macromolecular and small-drug aqueous solutions. The density of both aqueous solutions is 1.010 g/cm^3 and the temperature is 298° K.

Use the equations on page 120 for freezing point depression and osmotic pressure with $K_f = 1.86$ and $R = 0.0821$ liter atm deg^{-1} mol^{-1}.

The weight of the solutions is

$$1000 \text{ cm}^3 \times 1.010 \text{ g/cm}^3 = 1010 \text{ g solution}$$

For the small-drug solution, equation (5–55),

$$\Delta T_f = K_f \frac{1000 \, w_2}{w_1 M_2} = 1.86 \times \frac{1000 \times 10}{(1010 - 10)250} = 0.0744 \text{ deg}$$

Osmotic pressure may be calculated using either the van't Hoff (equation [5–33]) or the Morse (equation [5–35]) expression. Beginning with the van't Hoff equation (5–33), we have equation (5–56):

$$\pi = c_g \, RT/M_2 = (10 \times 0.0821 \times 298)/250 = 0.979 \text{ atm}$$
$$0.979 \text{ atm} \times 760 \text{ mm Hg/atm} = 744 \text{ mm Hg}$$

Use of the Morse equation (5–35) proceeds as follows for the small drug:

$$\pi = RTm$$

where $m = 1000 \, w_2/w_1 M_2$ (equation [5–51]).
Therefore,

$$\pi = (RT) \frac{1000 \, w_2}{w_1} \frac{1}{M_2}$$
$$= (0.0821 \times 298) \frac{1000 \times 10}{(1010 - 10)} \frac{1}{250} = 0.979 \text{ atm}$$

Changing to mm Hg,

$$0.979 \text{ atm} \times 760 \text{ mm Hg/atm} = 743.8 \text{ mm Hg}$$

In actual experimental work, the capillary tube of the osmometer contains an aqueous solution and not mercury (see Fig. 5–15). Therefore, the height in the capillary calculated as mm Hg is converted into millimeters of solution. This is done using the conversion factor:

$$\text{mm aqueous solution} = \text{mm Hg} \times \frac{13.534 \text{ g/cm}^3 \text{ for Hg at } 25° \text{ C}}{\text{density of solution (g/cm}^3) \text{ at } 25° \text{ C}}$$

The van't Hoff and the Morse equations yielded an osmotic pressure of 743.8 mm Hg as seen above. This value is then changed to mm aqueous solution:

$$743.8 \text{ mm Hg} \times \frac{13.534}{1.010} = 9967 \text{ mm solution}$$

for the small-drug molecule of molecular weight 250 g/mole.
For the freezing point depression of the macromolecular solution, $M_2 = 10^6$ g/mole,

$$\Delta T_f = (1.86) \frac{1000 \times 10}{(1010 - 10)} \frac{1}{10^6} = 1.860 \times 10^{-5} \text{ deg}$$

Applying the Morse equation to obtain the osmotic pressure of the large molecule gives

$$\pi = (0.0821 \times 298) \frac{1000 \times 10}{(1010 - 10)} \frac{1}{10^6} = 2.45 \times 10^{-4} \text{ atm}$$

Changing to mm Hg and then to mm aqueous solution:

$$2.45 \times 10^{-4} \text{ atm} \times 760 \text{ mm Hg/atm} = 0.186 \text{ mm Hg}$$
$$0.186 \text{ mm Hg} \times \frac{13.534}{1.010} = 2.492 \text{ mm solution}$$

This analysis shows that the freezing point depression method *(cryoscopic method)* is quite adequate for small-molecular-weight determinations, a 1% solution giving $\Delta T_f \cong 0.07$ deg, which is easily read on a Beckmann thermometer. Not so for a large polymeric

TABLE 5–5. *Approximate Expressions for the Colligative Properties*

Colligative Property	Expression	Proportionality Constant in Aqueous Solution
Vapor pressure lowering	$\Delta p = 0.018 p_1° \, m$	$0.018 p_1° = 0.43$ at 25° C
		$= 0.083$ at 0° C
Boiling point elevation	$\Delta T_b = K_b m$	$K_b = 0.51$
Freezing point depression	$\Delta T_f = K_f m$	$K_f = 1.86$
Osmotic pressure	$\pi = RTm$	$RT = 24.4$ at 25° C
		$= 22.4$ at 0° C

drug molecule. The cryoscopic method yields $\Delta T_f = 1.8 \times 10^{-5}$ deg, which cannot be read accurately by any thermometric device readily available in the laboratory. The values given above are differences in degrees and may be expressed as either Kelvin or centigrade degrees. When we turn to osmometry, the situation brightens for the large-molecule analysis. Although it is slower and more tedious than freezing point depression work, and need not be used for small molecules, which are easily analyzed by cryoscopy, osmometry provides values that are easily read on the millimeter scale for polymeric molecules of molecular weights as large as several millions.

A summary of the comparative results is as follows:

Cryoscopy		
Molecular Size	Molecular Weight	ΔT_f
Small molecule, 1% (*w/v*)	250 g/mole	0.074 deg
Large molecule, 1% (*w/v*)	10^6 g/mole	1.860×10^{-5} deg

Osmometry		
Molecular Size	Molecular Weight	π
		van't Hoff / Morse
Small molecule, 1% (*w/v*)	250 g/mole	9967 mm sol. / 9967 mm sol.
Large molecule, 1% (*w/v*)	10^6 g/mole	2.492 mm sol. / 2.492 mm sol.

References and Notes

1. H. R. Kruyt, *Colloid Science*, Vol. II, Elsevier, New York, 1949, Chapter 1.
2. W. H. Chapin and L. E. Steiner, *Second Year College Chemistry*, Wiley, New York, 1943, Chapter 13; M. J. Sienko, *Stoichiometry and Structure*, Benjamin, New York, 1964.
3. G. N. Lewis and M. Randall, *Thermodynamics*, McGraw-Hill, New York, 1923, Chapter 16.
4. S. Glasstone, *Textbook of Physical Chemistry*, 2nd Ed., Van Nostrand, New York, 1946, p. 628.
5. R. A. Robinson and D. A. Sinclair, J. Am. Chem. Soc. **56**, 1830, 1934; G. Scatchard, W. J. Hamer and S. E. Wood, J. Am. Chem. Soc. **60**, 3061, 1938.
6. A. V. Hill, Proc. R. Soc. London, **A127**, 9, 1930; E. J. Baldes, J. Sci. Instr. **11**, 223, 1934; R. R. Roepke, J. Phys. Chem. **46**, 359, 1942.
7. C. G. Lund et al., Acta Pharm. Intern. **1**, 3, 1950; Science, **109**, 149, 1949.
8. W. K. Barlow, P. G. Schneider, S. L. Schult and M. Viebell, Medical Electronics, April, 1978.
9. P. K. Ng and J. L. Lundblad, J. Pharm. Sci. **68**, 239, 1979.
10. W. H. Streng, H. E. Huber and J. T. Carstensen, J. Pharm. Sci. **67**, 384, 1978; H. E. Huber, W. H. Streng and H. G. H. Tan, J. Pharm. Sci. **68**, 1028, 1979.
11. R. D. Johnson and F. M. Goyan, J. Pharm. Sci. **56**, 757, 1967; F. M. Goyan, R. D. Johnson and H. N. Borazan, J. Pharm. Sci. **60**, 117, 1971.
12. H. N. Borazan, J. Pharm. Sci. **62**, 923, 1973.
13. J. M. Johlin, J. Biol. Chem. **91**, 551, 1931.
14. L. H. Adam, J. Am. Chem. Soc. **37**, 481, 1915; G. Scatchard, P. T. Jones, and S. S. Prentiss, J. Am. Chem. Soc. **54**, 2676, 1932.
15. B. E. Ballard and F. M. Goyan, J. Am. Pharm. Assoc., Sci. Ed. **47**, 40, 1958; **47**, 783, 1958.
16. M. P. Tombs and A. R. Peacock, *The Osmotic Pressure of Biological Macromolecules*, Clarendon, Oxford, 1974, p. 1.
17. W. K. Barlow and P. G. Schneider, *Colloid Osmometry*, Logan, Utah, Wescor, Inc., 1978.
18. C. M. Mason and H. M. Gardner, J. Chem. Educ. **13**, 188, 1939.
19. G. N. Lewis, J. Am. Chem. Soc. **30**, 668, 1908.

Problems

5–1. A solution of sucrose (molecular weight 342) is prepared by dissolving 0.5 g in 100 g of water. Compute (**a**) the weight percent, (**b**) the molal concentration, and (**c**) the mole fraction of sucrose and of water in the solution.

Answers: (**a**) 0.498% by weight; (**b**) 0.0146 m; (**c**) 0.00026 mole fraction of sucrose; 0.99974 mole fraction of water

5–2. An aqueous solution of glycerin, 7.00% by weight, is prepared. The solution is found to have a density of 1.0149 g/cm³ at 20° C. The molecular weight of glycerin is 92.0473 and its density is 1.2609 g/cm³ at 20° C. What is the molarity, molality, and percent by volume?

Answer: 0.7718 M, 0.8177 m, 5.63% v/v

5–3. What is the normality of a 25.0-mL solution of hydrochloric acid, that neutralizes 20.0-mL of a 0.50-N sodium hydroxide solution?

Answer: 0.40 N

5–4. How many grams of Na_2SO_4 (molecular weight 142) are required to make 1.2 liters of a 0.5-N solution?

Answer: 42.6 g

5–5. (**a**) Give the number of equivalents per mole of HCl, H_3PO_4, and $Ba(OH)_2$. (**b**) What is the equivalent weight of each of these compounds?

Answers: (**a**) The number of equivalents is 1, 3, and 2, respectively. (**b**) The equivalent weights of these compounds are 36.5 g/Eq, 32.7 g/Eq, and 85.7 g/Eq, respectively.

5–6. What is the equivalent weight of anhydrous $NaAl(SO_4)_2$ (molecular weight 242) when used for its sodium, aluminum, and sulfate content, respectively?

Answer: 242 g/Eq, 80.7 g/Eq, and 60.5 g/Eq, respectively

5–7. If normal human plasma contains about 3 mEq/liter of the hydrogen phosphate ion HPO_4^{2-}, how many milligrams of dibasic potassium phosphate, K_2HPO_4 (molecular weight 174), are required to supply the needed HPO_4^{2-} for an electrolyte replacement in the hospital?

Answer: 261 mg/liter

5–8. How many grams of $Ca_3(PO_4)_2$ are required to prepare 170 mL of a 0.67-N solution? The molecular weight of $Ca_3(PO_4)_2$ is 310.

Answer: 5.88 g

5–9. The vapor pressure p_B^0 of pure butane is 2.3966 atm at 25° C and that of n-pentane p_p° is 0.6999 atm at 25° C. Using Raoult's law, calculate the partial vapor pressure of n-butane (molecular weight 58.12) and n-pentane (molecular weight 72.15) in a mixture of 50 g of each of these two vapors at 25° C in atm and in pounds/in.².

Answer: 1.327 atm and 0.312 atm. To convert atm to pounds/in.², multiply by 14.70.

5–10. The vapor pressures of pure "Freon 11" and pure "Freon 12" at 25° C are 15 lb/in.² and 85 lb/in.² respectively. In the preparation of a pharmaceutical aerosol these two propellants were mixed together in the mole ratio of 0.6 to 0.4.

(**a**) What are the partial vapor pressures of "Freon 11" and "Freon

12" in a mixture having a mole ratio of 0.6 to 0.4, assuming that the mixture follows Raoult's law?

(b) What is the total vapor pressure of this mixture at 25° C?

(c) An aerosol can safely be packaged in a glass container protected with a plastic coating as long as the pressure does not exceed about 35 lb/in.^{2} (20 lb/in.^{2} in gauge pressure) at room temperature. Can such a container be used for the preparation described in this example? Can freons be used today in pharmaceutical areosols?

Answers: **(a)** p_{11} = 9 lb/in.^{2}; p_{12} = 34 lb/in.^{2}; **(b)** P = 43 lb/in.^{2}

5–11. (a) State Henry's law and discuss its relationship to Raoult's law. **(b)** How is Henry's law used in the study of gases in solution?

Answers: **(a)** See the sections on Raoult's law and Henry's law (pp. 107–109). **(b)** See *Problems 5–12* and *5–13* in this chapter, and *Problems 10–3* through *10–6* in Chapter 10.

5–12.* One may wonder how a fish breathes oxygen when the oxygen is dissolved in water. It is the peculiar gill system of a fish that allows it to take up the oxygen into its body directly from water. The solubility of oxygen in the air dissolved in water is calculated using Henry's law, $p_{O_2} = kX_{O_2}$. The partial pressure p_{O_2} of O_2 in the air at 25° C is 0.20 atm and that of N_2 is 0.80 atm. The Henry law constants at 25° C are given in the table.

Data for *Problem 5–12*

Gas	mm Hg per mole fraction of gas	atmospheres per mole fraction of gas
O_2	3.30×10^7	4.34×10^4
N_2	6.51×10^7	8.57×10^4

(a) Calculate X_{O_2}, the mole fraction of oxygen and X_{N_2}, the mole fraction of nitrogen gas in air at 25° C.

(b) What is the total mole fraction concentration of these two gases in water at 25° C?

(c) In air, oxygen constitutes 20% or one fifth of the total pressure (see above). What fractional contribution does oxygen make to the concentration of the two gases *in water?*

(d) Is the dissolved air a fish breathes in water proportionately greater in oxygen than the air we land animals breathe?

Answers: **(a)** X_{O_2} = 4.61 × 10^{-6}; X_{N_2} = 9.33 × 10^{-6}; **(b)** total mole fraction concentration = 13.94 × 10^{-6}; **(c)** in water, oxygen constitutes one third of the pressure; **(d)** yes: one third is greater than one fifth

5–13. The partial vapor pressure of oxygen dissolved in water in equilibrium with the atmosphere at 25° C is 200 mm, and the Henry's law constant k is 3.3 × 10^7 mm Hg/mole fraction of O_2. What is the concentration of oxygen in water expressed in mole fraction?

Answer: 6.06 × 10^{-6}

5–14. The freezing point lowering of a solution containing 1.00 gram of a new drug and 100 grams of water is 0.573° C at 25° C. **(a)** What is the molecular weight of the compound? **(b)** What is the boiling point of the solution? **(c)** What is the osmotic pressure of the solution?

Answers: **(a)** 32.46 g/mole; **(b)** b.p. 100.157° C; **(c)** 7.54 atm. Using equation (5–35), π = 6.87 atm.

5–15. (a) Derive an equation relating osmotic pressure and the lowering of the vapor pressure of a solution at 25° C. Refer to Table 5–5 for equations relating π to Δp.

(b) Give an explanation for the manner in which an osmotic membrane functions. Use a diagram of the cell and membrane to show the flow of the component liquids and the production of osmotic pressure.

Partial Answer: **(a)** At 25° C, π = 56.93 Δp.

5–16. A 105-g sample of polyethylene glycol 400 (PEG 400) was dissolved in 500 g of water, and the vapor pressure of the solution was found to be 122.6 torr at 56.0° C. The boiling point elevation of this solution over that of pure water (100° C at 1 atm) was determined to be 0.271° C. The vapor pressure of pure water, p_1^0, at 56° C is 123.80 torr. Calculate the molecular weight of this sample of PEG 400 using vapor pressure lowering, boiling point elevation, and osmotic pressure. The "400" of PEG means that the molecular weight of this polymer is approximately 400 g/mole. The density of water at 56° C is 0.985 g/cm^3. Experimentally, π was obtained as 0.0138 atm.

Answers: From vapor pressure lowering, M_2 = 390 g/mole. From boiling point elevation, M_2 = 395 g/mole. From osmotic pressure, M_2 = 411 g/mole.

5–17. Determine the boiling point elevation constant K_b for carbon tetrachloride. You can obtain the molecular weight and boiling point of CCl_4 from the *Merck Index*. To obtain the heat of vaporization ΔH_v at the boiling point, you will need to consult the *CRC Handbook of Chemistry and Physics* or other sources that give ΔH_v for CCl_4 at various temperatures. CRC gives ΔH_v values in units of BTU/lb or cal/g and temperatures in Fahrenheit or Celsius degrees, up to 120° F (48.89° C).

(a) Plot the ΔH_v values versus temperature and extrapolate the line (by eye) to 76.7° C, the boiling point of CCl_4. The molecular weight of CCl_4 is 153.84 g/mole. Convert ΔH_v in cal/g to cal/mole and degrees C to degrees Kelvin, then square the temperature for use in the cryoscopic constant equation, $K_b = RT_b^2 M_1/(1000 \cdot \Delta H_v)$ (p. 113).

(b) You may care to use linear, quadratic, or cubic regression of ΔH_v against temperature on a hand calculator or personal computer to obtain the best fit of the data and the most satisfactory extrapolation to give ΔH_v at the boiling point of carbon tetrachloride.

Answers: **(a)** K_b = 5.0 to 5.2 depending on the method of extrapolation used. **(b)** Using cubic regression, K_b = 5.13.

5–18. A solution of drug is prepared by dissolving 15.0 g in 100 g of water, and is subjected to ebullioscopic analysis. The boiling point elevation is 0.28° C. Compute the molecular weight of the drug.

Answer: 275 g/mole

5–19. In the summer the vaporization of the cooling fluid of a car is retarded by the presence of ethylene glycol, which acts by increasing the boiling point of water. **(a)** For the ethylene glycol-in-water solution discussed in *Example 5–14* calculate the boiling point elevation of water in degrees Fahrenheit using equation (5–26). The heat of vaporization of water is 9720 cal/mole. The mole fraction X_2 of ethylene glycol in the aqueous solution is 0.1239. **(b)** Compare the result with that obtained by using the less exact expression, $\Delta T_b = K_b m$.

Answers: **(a)** Using the mole fraction equation one obtains the boiling point elevation of water, ΔT_b, in Fahrenheit degrees as 6.35° F. **(b)** ΔT_b = 7.20° F

5–20. (a) What is the boiling point rise for a 0.437 molal solution of anthracene in chloroform? Use equation 5–52, page 120. **(b)** The molecular weight of anthracene is 178.2 g/mole. Using equation (5–53), page 120, check your result in (a); i.e., calculate ΔT_b.

Answers: **(a)** ΔT_b = 1.586° C; **(b)** ΔT_b = 1.586° C

5–21. A solution containing 0.2223 grams of benzanthine penicillin G in 1000 grams of benzene has a freezing point of 0.00124° below that of the pure solvent (5.5° C for benzene). What is the molecular weight of benzanthine penicillin G?

Answer: 918 g/mole (actual mol. wt. = 909 g/mole)

5–22. Five grams of a new drug (a nonelectrolyte) are dissolved in 250 g of water, and the solution is subjected to a cryoscopic analysis to obtain the molecular weight. The freezing point depression is found to be 0.120° C. Compute the molecular weight.

Answer: 310 g/mole

5–23. (a) Compute the freezing point depression of 1 g of methylcellulose (molecular weight 26,000 g/mole) dissolved in 100 g of water.

(b) Using the Morse equation, compute the osmotic pressure of this solution at 20° C. Express the result in cm of solution. To convert mm

---

*Problem 5–12 is modified from J. W. Moncrief and W. H. Jones, *Elements of Physical Chemistry*, Addison-Wesley, Reading, Mass., 1977, p. 115.

of mercury to mm solution, mm solution = mm Hg $\times \dfrac{\rho_{Hg}}{\rho_{solution}}$. The density of mercury at 20° C is 13.5462 g/mL. Assume that the density of the solution is 1 g/mL.

(c) Assume that you have a thermometer in which you are able to accurately read 0.05° C and estimate the value to 0.005° C. Can you use freezing point depression of the methylcellulose solution to determine the molecular weight of this polymer? Can you use osmotic pressure to obtain the molecular weight?

Answers: (a) $\Delta T_f = 0.0007°$ C; (b) $\pi = 9.9$ cm; (c) the freezing point depression is too small to read on most thermometers. You should use osmotic pressure to determine the molecular weight of methylcellulose.

5-24. (a) Calculate the cryoscopic constant of benzene. The heat of fusion, ΔH_f, is 2360 cal/mole, and the melting point of benzene is 5.5° C. Its molecular weight is 78.11 g/mole.

(b) Calculate the ebullioscopic constant of phenol. Its heat of vaporization is 9730 cal/mole and its boiling temperature is 181.4° C. The molecular weight of phenol is 94.11 g/mole. Compare your results with those found in Table 5-4.

Answers: (a) K_f (benzene) = 5.10 deg kg/mole; (b) K_b (phenol) = 3.97 deg kg/mole

5-25. Compute the freezing point depression of a 0.20% w/v glucose solution. The molecular weight of glucose is 180 gram/mole.

Answer: $\Delta T_f = 0.02°$

5-26. What concentration of ethylene glycol is required to protect a car's cooling system from freezing down to −20° F? Express the concentration in grams of antifreeze per 100 grams of fluid in the system. The molecular weight of ethylene glycol is 62.07 g/mole.

Answer: 96.6 grams of ethylene glycol per 100 grams of fluid

5-27. It is winter and you are caught in your home at night in a severe winter storm of snow and ice; the temperature is −20° F. Your child is sick and you must get to the village pharmacy 10 miles away in the morning to have the child's prescription filled. You just brought home a new car but you forgot to have it serviced with antifreeze. You have a 5-pound bag of sucrose in the house and you know that the volume of the car's coolant system is 9 quarts (1 quart = 0.9463 liters).

(a) How far can the temperature drop overnight in your driveway (no garage) before the coolant system would freeze if you added 5 pounds of sugar to the water in the radiator and were sure that it dissolved completely? The molecular weight of sucrose is 342 g/mole and 1 lb (avoirdupois) = 0.4536 kg.

(b) All means of transportation, including taxis, buses, and emergency vehicles, are tied up because of the storm. The demands on the pharmacy, grocery and other stores are such that they cannot deliver. What other solutions might you arrive at to handle this emergency, should the addition of sucrose not protect the car's coolant system?

Answers: (a) $\Delta T_f = 1.09°$ C or 1.96° F. These results show that the use of sucrose will be of little help. (b) Discuss with your classmates other possibilities to deal with this emergency.

5-28. What is the osmotic pressure of a solution of urea (molecular weight 60) containing 0.30 g of the drug in 50 mL of water at 20° C? Use the van't Hoff equation.

Answer: 2.4 atm

5-29. Compute the osmotic pressure of a 0.60-m aqueous mannitol solution using (a) equation (5-35) and (b) equation (5-39). The vapor pressure of the solution p at 20° C is 17.349 mm Hg and the vapor pressure of water $p°$ at the same temperature is 17.535 mm Hg. The molar volume of water at 20° C is 0.0181 liter/mole.

Answers: (a) 14.4 atm; (b) 14.3 atm

5-30. If the freezing point of blood is −0.52° C, what is its osmotic pressure at 25° C? What is the vapor pressure lowering of blood at this temperature?

Answer: $\pi = 6.84$ atm; $\Delta p = 0.12$ mm Hg

5-31. A new alkaloid, guayusine, was isolated from a South American plant, *Guayusa multiflora*. A solution containing 0.473 g of the alkaloid per 500 mL of aqueous solution produced an osmotic pressure of 0.060 atm (i.e., 45.6 mm of Hg or 619 mm of solution) at 25° C. The drug does not associate or dissociate in aqueous solution. Calculate the approximate molecular weight of guayusine.

Answer: 386 g/mole

5-32. The freezing point depression of 2.0 grams of antigesic, a new antipyretic and analgesic, in 100 mL of aqueous solution was found to be 0.198° C. (a) Compute the osmotic pressure of the solution. (b) Compute the molecular weight of antigesic from its osmotic pressure. ΔT_f and π are related through the equations $\Delta T_f = K_f c_g$ and $\pi = RT c_g$ where RT is taken as 22.43 at 0° C and c_g is concentration in g/liter. The drug behaves almost ideally in dilute aqueous solution. It does not dissociate or associate in water; therefore, equation (5-57) is adequate to yield an approximate molecular weight.

Answer: (a) $\pi = 2.39$ atm; (b) $M_2 = 188$ g/mole

5-33. A new polypeptide drug has been synthesized and its molecular weight is estimated to be in the range of 10,000 daltons (1 dalton = 1 g/mole). Which colligative property method would be best for accurately determining its molecular weight? The question is answered by calculating ΔT_b, ΔT_f, Δp, and π at 20° C for a 1% solution of the drug in water. The vapor pressure $p_1°$ of water at 20° C is 17.54 mm Hg. The density of the solution is 1.015 g/mL, and the density of mercury needed to convert mm Hg to mm solution is 13.5462 g/mL at 20° C.

Answer: $\pi = 243$ mm of solution; $\Delta T_b = 5.07 \times 10^{-4}$ deg; $\Delta T_f = 1.85 \times 10^{-3}$ deg; $\Delta p = 3.14 \times 10^{-3}$ mm Hg. The best colligative property to determine the molecular weight of this macromolecule is osmotic pressure, for the easiest to measure is $\pi = 243$ mm solution. The other values are too small to measure accurately. The determination of the molecular weights of macromolecules is discussed in Chapter 15.

6

Solutions of Electrolytes

Properties of Solutions of Electrolytes
Arrhenius Theory of Electrolytic Dissociation
Theory of Strong Electrolytes

Coefficients for Expressing Colligative
Properties

The first satisfactory theory of ionic solutions was that proposed by Arrhenius in 1887. The theory was based largely on studies of electric conductance by Kohlrausch, colligative properties by van't Hoff, and chemical properties such as heats of neutralization by Thomsen. Arrhenius[1] was able to bring together the results of these diverse investigations into a broad generalization known as the theory of electrolytic dissociation.

Although the theory proved quite useful for describing weak electrolytes, it was soon found unsatisfactory for strong and moderately strong electrolytes. Accordingly, many attempts were made to modify or replace Arrhenius's ideas with better ones, and finally, in 1923, Debye and Hückel put forth a new theory. It is based on the principles that *strong electrolytes* are completely dissociated into ions in solutions of moderate concentration and that any deviation from complete dissociation is due to interionic attractions. Debye and Hückel expressed the deviations in terms of activities, activity coefficients, and ionic strengths of electrolytic solutions. These quantities, which had been introduced earlier by Lewis, are discussed in this chapter together with the theory of interionic attraction. Other aspects of modern ionic theory and the relationships between electricity and chemical phenomena are considered in following chapters.

We begin with a discussion of some of the properties of ionic solutions that led to Arrhenius theory of electrolytic dissociation.

PROPERTIES OF SOLUTIONS OF ELECTROLYTES

Electrolysis. When, under a potential of several volts, a direct electric current (dc) flows through an electrolytic cell (Figure 6–1), a chemical reaction occurs. The process is known as *electrolysis*. Electrons enter the cell from the battery or generator at the *cathode* (road down); they combine with positive ions or *cations*, in the solution, and the cations are accordingly reduced. The negative ions, or *anions*, carry electrons through the solution and discharge them at the *anode* (road up), and the anions are accordingly oxidized. *Reduction* is the addition of electrons to a chemical species, and *oxidation* is removal of electrons from a species. The current in a solution consists of a flow of positive and negative ions toward the electrodes, whereas the current in a metallic conductor consists of a flow of free electrons migrating through a crystal lattice of fixed positive ions. Reduction occurs at the cathode, where electrons enter from the external circuit and are added to a chemical species in solution. Oxidation occurs at the anode where the electrons are removed from a chemical species in solution and go into the external circuit.

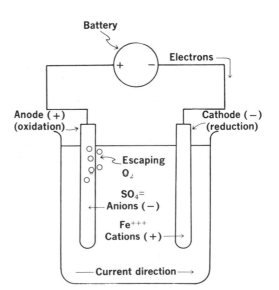

Fig. 6–1. Electrolysis in an electrolytic cell.

125

In the electrolysis of a solution of ferric sulfate in a cell containing platinum electrodes, a ferric ion migrates to the cathode where it picks up an electron and is reduced:

$$Fe^{3+} + e = Fe^{2+} \qquad (6-1)$$

The sulfate ion carries the current through the solution to the anode, but it is not easily oxidized; therefore, hydroxyl ions of the water are converted into molecular oxygen, which escapes at the anode, and sulfuric acid is found in the solution around the electrode. The oxidation reaction at the anode is

$$OH^- = \tfrac{1}{4}O_2 + \tfrac{1}{2}H_2O + e \qquad (6-2)$$

Platinum electrodes are used here since they do not pass into solution to any extent. When *attackable* metals, such as copper or zinc, are used as the anode, their atoms tend to lose electrons, and the metal passes into solution as the positively charged ion.

In the electrolysis of cupric chloride between platinum electrodes, the reaction at the cathode is

$$\tfrac{1}{2}Cu^{2+} + e = \tfrac{1}{2}Cu \qquad (6-3)$$

while at the anode, chloride and hydroxyl ions are converted respectively into gaseous molecules of chlorine and oxygen, which then escape. In each of these two examples, the net result is the transfer of one electron from the cathode to the anode.

Transference Numbers. It should be noted that the flow of electrons through the solution from right to left in Figure 6–1 is accomplished by the movement of cations to the right as well as anions to the left. The fraction of total current carried by the cations or by the anions is known as the *transport* or *transference number* t_+ or t_-.

$$t_+ = \frac{\text{current carried by cations}}{\text{total current}} \qquad (6-4)$$

$$t_- = \frac{\text{current carried by anions}}{\text{total current}} \qquad (6-5)$$

The sum of the two transference numbers is obviously equal to unity:

$$t_+ + t_- = 1 \qquad (6-6)$$

The transference numbers are related to the velocities of the ions, the faster-moving ion carrying the greater fraction of current. The velocities of the ions in turn depend on hydration as well as ion size and charge. Hence, the speed and the transference numbers are not necessarily the same for positive and for negative ions. For example, the transference number of the sodium ion in a 0.10-*M* solution of NaCl is 0.385. Because it is greatly hydrated, the lithium ion in a 0.10-*M* solution of LiCl moves slower than the sodium ion and hence has a lower transference number, viz., 0.317.

Electrical Units. According to Ohm's law, the strength of an electric current *I* in amperes flowing through a metallic conductor is related to the difference in applied potential or voltage *E* and the resistance *R* in ohms, as follows:

$$I = \frac{E}{R} \qquad (6-7)$$

The current strength *I* is the rate of flow of current or the quantity *Q* of electricity (electronic charge) in coulombs flowing per unit time:

$$I = \frac{Q}{t} \qquad (6-8)$$

and

Quantity of electric charge, *Q*
$$= \text{current, } I \times \text{time, } t \qquad (6-9)$$

The quantity of electric charge is expressed in coulombs (1 coul = 3×10^9 electrostatic units of charge, or esu), the current in amperes, and the electric potential in volts.

Electric energy consists of an intensity factor, electromotive force or voltage, and a quantity factor, coulombs.

$$\text{Electric energy} = E \times Q \qquad (6-10)$$

Faraday's Laws. In 1833 and 1834, Michael Faraday announced his famous laws of electricity, which may be summarized in the statement, *the passage of 96,500 coulombs of electricity through a conductivity cell produces a chemical change of 1 gram equivalent weight of any substance.* The quantity 96,500 is known as the faraday, *F*. The best estimate of the value today is 9.648456×10^4 coulombs per gram equivalent.

A univalent negative ion is an atom to which a valence electron has been added; a univalent positive ion is an atom from which an electron has been removed. Each gram equivalent of ions of any electrolyte carries Avogadro's number (6.02×10^{23}) of positive or negative charges. Hence, from Faraday's laws, the passage of 96,500 coulombs of electricity results in the transport of 6.02×10^{23} electrons in the cell. A faraday is an Avogadro's number of electrons, corresponding to the mole, which is an Avogadro's number of molecules. The passage of 1 faraday of electricity causes the electrolytic deposition of the following number of gram atoms or "moles" of various ions: $1Ag^+$, $1Cu^+$, $\tfrac{1}{2}Cu^{2+}$, $\tfrac{1}{2}Fe^{2+}$, $\tfrac{1}{3}Fe^{3+}$. Thus, the number of positive charges carried by 1 gram equivalent of Fe^{3+} is 6.02×10^{23}, but the number of positive charges carried by 1 gram atom or 1 mole of ferric ions is $3 \times 6.02 \times 10^{23}$.

Faraday's laws can be used to compute the charge on an electron in the following way. Since 6.02×10^{23} electrons are associated with 96,500 coulombs of electricity, each electron has a charge *e* of

$$e = \frac{96,500 \text{ coulombs}}{6.02 \times 10^{23} \text{ electrons}}$$

$$= 1.6 \times 10^{-19} \text{ coulombs/electron} \qquad (6-11)$$

and since 1 coulomb $= 3 \times 10^9$ esu

$$e = 4.8 \times 10^{-10} \text{ electrostatic units}$$
$$\text{of charge/electron} \quad (6\text{-}12)$$

Electrolytic Conductance. The resistance R in ohms of any uniform metallic or electrolytic conductor is directly proportional to its length l in cm and inversely proportional to its cross-sectional area A in cm^2,

$$R = \rho \frac{l}{A} \quad (6\text{-}13)$$

in which ρ is the resistance between opposite faces of a 1-cm cube of the conductor and is known as the *specific resistance.*

The *conductance* C is the reciprocal of resistance,

$$C = \frac{1}{R} \quad (6\text{-}14)$$

and hence can be considered as a measure of the ease with which current can pass through the conductor. It is expressed in reciprocal ohms or *mhos*. From equation (6–13),

$$C = \frac{1}{R} = \frac{1}{\rho}\frac{A}{l} \quad (6\text{-}15)$$

The *specific conductance* κ is the reciprocal of specific resistance and is expressed in mhos/cm.

$$\kappa = \frac{1}{\rho} \quad (6\text{-}16)$$

It is the conductance of a solution confined in a cube 1 cm on an edge as seen in Figure 6–2. The relationship between specific conductance and conductance or resistance is obtained by combining equations (6–15) and (6–16).

$$\kappa = C\frac{l}{A} = \frac{1}{R}\frac{l}{A} \quad (6\text{-}17)$$

Measuring the Conductance of Solutions. The Wheatstone bridge assembly for measuring the conductance of a solution is shown in Figure 6–3. The solution of unknown resistance R_x is placed in the cell and

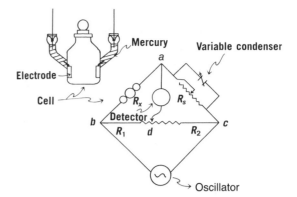

Fig. 6–3. Wheatstone bridge for conductance measurements.

connected in the circuit. The contact point is moved along the slide wire bc until at some point, say d, no current from the source of alternating current (oscillator) flows through the detector (earphones or oscilloscope). When the bridge is balanced the potential at a is equal to that at d, the sound in the earphones or the oscillating pattern on the oscilloscope is at a minimum, and the resistances R_s, R_1, and R_2 are read. In the balanced state, the resistance of the solution R_x is obtained from the equation

$$R_x = R_s \frac{R_1}{R_2} \quad (6\text{-}18)$$

The variable condenser across resistance R_s is used to produce a sharper balance. Some conductivity bridges are calibrated in conductance as well as resistance values. The electrodes in the cell are platinized with platinum black by electrolytic deposition so that catalysis of the reaction will occur at the platinum surfaces, and formation of a nonconducting gaseous film will not occur on the electrodes.

Water that is carefully purified by redistillation in the presence of a little permanganate is used to prepare the solutions. Conductivity water, as it is called, has a specific conductance of about 0.05×10^{-6} mho/cm at 18° C, whereas ordinary distilled water has a value somewhat over 1×10^{-6} mho/cm. For most conductivity studies, "equilibrium water" containing CO_2 from the atmosphere is satisfactory. It has a specific conductance of about 0.8×10^{-6} mho/cm.

The specific conductance κ is computed from the resistance R_x or conductance C by use of equation (6–17). The quantity l/A, the ratio of distance between electrodes to the area of the electrode, has a definite value for each conductance cell; it is known as the *cell constant*, K. Equation (6–17) thus can be written

$$\kappa = KC = K/R \quad (6\text{-}19)$$

(The subscript x is no longer needed on R and is therefore dropped.) It would be difficult to measure l and A, but it is a simple matter to determine the cell constant experimentally. The specific conductance of several standard solutions has been determined in carefully calibrated cells. For example, a solution

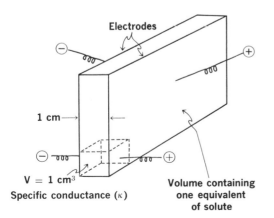

Fig. 6–2. Relationship between specific conductance and equivalent conductance.

containing 7.45263 g of potassium chloride in 1000 g of water has a specific conductance of 0.012856 mho/cm at 25° C. A solution of this concentration contains 0.1 mole of salt per cubic decimeter (100 cm^3) of water and is known as a 0.1 *demal* solution. When such a solution is placed in a cell and the resistance is measured, the cell constant can be determined by use of equation (6–19).

Example 6–1. A 0.1-demal solution of KCl was placed in a cell whose constant K was desired. The resistance R was found to be 34.69 ohms at 25° C.

$$K = \kappa R = 0.012856 \text{ mho/cm} \times 34.69 \text{ ohms}$$
$$= 0.4460 \text{ cm}^{-1}$$

Example 6–2. When the cell described in *Example 6–1* was filled with a 0.01-N Na$_2$SO$_4$ solution, it had a resistance of 397 ohms. What is the specific conductance?

$$\kappa = \frac{K}{R} = \frac{0.4460}{397} = 1.1234 \times 10^{-3} \text{ mho/cm}$$

Equivalent Conductance. To study the dissociation of molecules into ions, independent of the concentration of the electrolyte, it is convenient to use equivalent conductance rather than specific conductance. All solutes of equal normality produce the same number of ions when completely dissociated, and equivalent conductance measures the current-carrying capacity of this given number of ions. Specific conductance, on the other hand, measures the current-carrying capacity of all ions in a unit volume of solution and accordingly varies with concentration.

Equivalent conductance Λ is defined as the conductance of a solution of sufficient volume to contain 1 gram equivalent of the solute when measured in a cell in which the electrodes are spaced 1 cm apart. The equivalent conductance Λ_c at a concentration of c gram equivalents per liter is calculated from the product of the specific conductance κ and the volume V in cm^3 that contains 1 gram equivalent of solute. The cell may be imagined as having electrodes 1 cm apart and to be of sufficient area so that it can contain the solution. The cell is shown in Figure 6–2.

$$V = \frac{1000 \text{ cm}^3/\text{liter}}{c \text{ Eq/liter}} = \frac{1000}{c} \text{ cm}^3/\text{Eq} \quad (6–20)$$

The equivalent conductance is obtained when κ, the conductance per cm^3 of solution (i.e., the specific conductance), is multiplied by V, the volume in cm^3 that contains 1 gram equivalent weight of solute. Hence, the equivalent conductance Λ_c, expressed in units of mho cm^2/Eq, is given by the expression

$$\Lambda_c = \kappa \times V \quad (6–21)$$
$$= \frac{1000 \, \kappa}{c} \text{ mho cm}^2/\text{Eq}$$

If the solution is 0.1 N in concentration, then the volume containing 1 gram equivalent of the solute will be 10,000 cm^3, and, according to equation (6–21), the equivalent conductance will be 10,000 times as great as the specific conductance. This is seen in *Example 6–3.*

Example 6–3. The measured conductance of a 0.1-N solution of a drug is 0.0563 mho at 25° C. The cell constant at 25° C is 0.520 cm^{-1}. What is the specific conductance and what is the equivalent conductance of the solution at this concentration?

$$\kappa = 0.0563 \times 0.520 = 0.0293 \text{ mho/cm}$$
$$\Lambda_c = 0.0293 \times 1000/0.1$$
$$= 293 \text{ mho cm}^2/\text{Eq}$$

Equivalent Conductance of Strong and Weak Electrolytes. As the solution of a strong electrolyte is diluted, the *specific conductance* κ *decreases* because the number of ions per unit volume of solution is reduced. (It sometimes goes through a maximum before decreasing.) Conversely, the *equivalent conductance* Λ of a solution of a strong electrolyte steadily *increases* on dilution. The increase in Λ with dilution is explained as follows. The quantity of electrolyte remains constant at 1 gram equivalent according to the definition of equivalent conductance; however, the ions are hindered less by their neighbors in the more dilute solution and hence can move faster. The equivalent conductance of a weak electrolyte also increases on dilution, but not as rapidly at first.

Kohlrausch was one of the first investigators to study this phenomenon. He found that the equivalent conductance was a linear function of the square root of the concentration for strong electrolytes in dilute solutions, as illustrated in Figure 6–4. The expression for Λ_c, the equivalent conductance at a concentration c (Eq/L), is

$$\Lambda_c = \Lambda_0 - b\sqrt{c} \quad (6–22)$$

in which Λ_0 is the intercept on the vertical axis and is known as the *equivalent conductance at infinite dilution*. The constant b is the slope of the line for the strong electrolytes shown in Figure 6–4.

When the equivalent conductance of a weak electrolyte is plotted against the square root of the concentra-

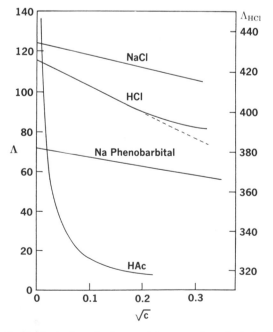

Fig. 6–4. Equivalent conductance of strong and weak electrolytes.

tion, as shown for acetic acid in Figure 6–4, the curve cannot be extrapolated to a limiting value, and Λ_o must be obtained by a method such as is described in the following paragraph. The steeply rising curve for acetic acid results from the fact that the dissociation of weak electrolytes increases on dilution, with a large increase in the number of ions capable of carrying the current.

Kohlrausch concluded that the ions of all electrolytes begin to migrate independently as the solution is diluted; the ions in dilute solutions are so far apart that they do not interact in any way. Under these conditions, Λ_o is the sum of the equivalent conductances of the cations $l_c{}^o$ and the anions $l_a{}^o$ at infinite dilution

$$\Lambda_o = l_c{}^o + l_a{}^o \qquad (6\text{–}23)$$

Based on this law, the known Λ_o values for certain electrolytes can be added and subtracted to yield Λ_o for the desired weak electrolyte. The method is illustrated in the following example.

Example 6–4. What is the equivalent conductance at infinite dilution of the weak acid phenobarbital? The Λ_o of the strong electrolytes, HCl, sodium phenobarbital (NaP), and NaCl are obtained from the experimental results shown in Figure 6–4. The values are $\Lambda_{oHCl} = 426.2$, $\Lambda_{oNaP} = 73.5$, and $\Lambda_{oNaCl} = 126.5$ mho cm²/Eq.

Now, by Kohlrausch's law of the independent migration of ions,

$$\Lambda_{oHP} = l_{H+}^o + l_{P-}^o$$

and

$$\Lambda_{oHCl} + \Lambda_{oNaP} - \Lambda_{oNaCl} = l_{H+}^o + l_{Cl-}^o + l_{Na+}^o + l_{P-}^o - l_{Na+}^o - l_{Cl-}^o$$

which, on simplifying the right-hand side of the equation, becomes

$$\Lambda_{oHCl} + \Lambda_{oNaP} - \Lambda_{oNaCl} = l_{H+}^o + l_{P-}^o$$

Therefore,

$$\Lambda_{oHP} = \Lambda_{oHCl} + \Lambda_{oNaP} - \Lambda_{oNaCl}$$

and

$$\Lambda_{oHP} = 426.2 + 73.5 - 126.5$$
$$= 373.2 \text{ mho cm}^2/\text{Eq}$$

Colligative Properties of Electrolytic Solutions and Concentrated Solutions of Nonelectrolytes. As stated in the previous chapter, van't Hoff observed that the osmotic pressure of dilute solutions of nonelectrolytes, such as sucrose and urea, could be expressed satisfactorily by the equation, $\pi = RTc$, equation (5–34), page 118, in which R is the gas constant, T is the absolute temperature, and c is the concentration in moles per liter. Van't Hoff found, however, that solutions of electrolytes gave osmotic pressures approximately two, three, and more times larger than expected from this equation, depending on the electrolyte investigated. By introducing a correction factor i to account for the irrational behavior of ionic solutions, he wrote

$$\pi = iRTc \qquad (6\text{–}24)$$

By the use of this equation, van't Hoff was able to obtain calculated values that compared favorably with the experimental results of osmotic pressure. Van't Hoff recognized that i approached the number of ions into which the molecule dissociated as the solution was made increasingly dilute.

The factor i may also be considered to express the departure of concentrated solutions of nonelectrolytes from the laws of ideal solutions. The deviations of concentrated solutions of nonelectrolytes can be explained on the same basis as deviations of real solutions from Raoult's law, considered in the preceding chapter. They included differences of internal pressures of the solute and solvent, polarity, compound formation or complexation, and association of either the solute or solvent. The departure of electrolytic solutions from the colligative effects in ideal solutions of nonelectrolytes may be attributed—in addition to the factors just enumerated—to dissociation of weak electrolytes and to interaction of the ions of strong electrolytes. Hence, the van't Hoff factor i accounts for the deviations of real solutions of nonelectrolytes and electrolytes, regardless of the reason for the discrepancies.

The i factor is plotted against the molal concentration of both electrolytes and nonelectrolytes in Figure 6–5. For nonelectrolytes, it is seen to approach unity, and for strong electrolytes, it tends toward a value equal to the number of ions formed upon dissociation. For example, i approaches the value of 2 for solutes such as NaCl and CaSO₄, 3 for K₂SO₄ and CaCl₂, and 4 for K₃Fe(C)₆ and FeCl₃.

The van't Hoff factor can also be expressed as the ratio of any colligative property of a real solution to that of an ideal solution of a nonelectrolyte, since i represents the number of times greater that the colligative effect is for a real solution (electrolyte or nonelectrolyte) than for an ideal nonelectrolyte.

The colligative properties in dilute solutions of electrolytes are expressed on the molal scale by the equations

$$\Delta p = 0.018 i p_1{}^\circ m \qquad (6\text{–}25)$$
$$\pi = iRTm \qquad (6\text{–}26)$$
$$\Delta T_f = iK_f m \qquad (6\text{–}27)$$
$$\Delta T_b = iK_b m \qquad (6\text{–}28)$$

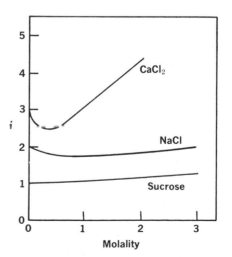

Fig. 6–5. Van't Hoff i factor of representative compounds.

Equation (6–25) applies only to aqueous solutions, whereas (6–26), (6–27), and (6–28) are independent of the solvent used.

Example 6–5. What is the osmotic pressure of a 2.0-*m* solution of sodium chloride at 20° C?

The *i* factor for a 2.0-*m* solution of sodium chloride as observed in Figure 6–5 is about 1.9.

$$\pi = 1.9 \times 0.082 \times 293 \times 2.0 = 91.3 \text{ atm}$$

ARRHENIUS THEORY OF ELECTROLYTIC DISSOCIATION

During the period in which van't Hoff was developing the solution laws, the Swedish chemist Svante Arrhenius was preparing his doctoral thesis on the properties of electrolytes at the University of Uppsala in Sweden. In 1887, he published the results of his investigations and proposed the now classic theory of dissociation.[1] The new theory resolved many of the anomalies encountered in the earlier interpretations of electrolytic solutions. Although the theory was viewed with disfavor by some influential scientists of the nineteenth century, Arrhenius's basic principles of electrolytic dissociation were gradually accepted and are still considered valid today. The theory of the existence of ions in solutions of electrolytes even at ordinary temperatures remains intact, aside from some modifications and elaborations that have been made through the years to bring it into line with certain stubborn experimental facts.

The original Arrhenius theory, together with the alterations that have come about as a result of the intensive research on electrolytes, is summarized as follows. When electrolytes are dissolved in water, the solute exists in the form of ions in the solution, as seen in the following equations

$$H_2O + \underset{\text{[Ionic compound]}}{Na^+Cl^-} \rightarrow Na^+ + Cl^- + H_2O$$

[Strong electrolyte] (6–29)

$$H_2O + \underset{\substack{\text{[Covalent} \\ \text{compound]}}}{HCl} \rightarrow H_3O^+ + Cl^-$$

[Strong electrolyte] (6–30)

$$H_2O + \underset{\substack{\text{[Covalent} \\ \text{compound]}}}{CH_3COOH} \rightleftharpoons H_3O^+ + CH_3COO^-$$

[Weak electrolyte] (6–31)

The solid form of sodium chloride is marked with + and − signs in reaction (6–29) to indicate that sodium chloride exists as ions even in the crystalline state. If electrodes are connected to a source of current and are placed in a mass of fused sodium chloride, the molten compound will conduct the electric current, since the crystal lattice of the pure salt consists of ions. The addition of water to the solid dissolves the crystal and separates the ions in solution.

Hydrogen chloride exists essentially as neutral molecules rather than as ions in the pure form, and does not conduct electricity. When it reacts with water, however, it ionizes according to reaction (6–30). H_3O^+ is the modern representation of the hydrogen ion in water and is known as the *hydronium* or *oxonium* ion. In addition to H_3O^+, other hydrated species of the proton probably exist in solution, but they need not be considered here.[2]

Sodium chloride and hydrochloric acid are *strong electrolytes* because they exist almost completely in the ionic form in moderately concentrated aqueous solutions. Inorganic acids such as HCl, HNO_3, H_2SO_4, and HI; inorganic bases as NaOH and KOH of the alkali metal family and $Ba(OH)_2$ and $Ca(OH)_2$ of the alkaline earth group; and most inorganic and organic salts are highly ionized and belong to the class of strong electrolytes.

Acetic acid is a *weak electrolyte*, the oppositely directed arrows in equation (6–31) indicating that an equilibrium between the molecules and ions is established. Most organic acids and bases and some inorganic compounds, such as H_3BO_3, H_2CO_3, and NH_4OH, belong to the class of weak electrolytes. Even some salts (lead acetate, $HgCl_2$, HgI, and HgBr) and the complex ions $Hg(NH_3)_2^+$, $Cu(NH_3)_4^{2+}$, and $Fe(CN)_6^{3-}$ are weak electrolytes.

Faraday applied the term *ion* (Greek: wanderer) to these species of electrolytes and recognized that the cations (positively charged ions) and anions (negatively charged ions) were responsible for conducting the electric current. Before the time of Arrhenius's publications, it was believed that a solute was not spontaneously decomposed in water, but rather dissociated appreciably into ions only when an electric current was passed through the solution.

Drugs and Ionization. Some drugs, such as anionic and cationic antibacterial and antiprotozoal agents, are more active when in the ionic state. Other compounds, such as the hydroxybenzoate esters (parabens) and many general anesthetics, bring about their biologic effects as nonelectrolytes. Still other compounds, such as the sulfonamides, are thought to exert their drug action both as ions and as neutral molecules.[3]

Degree of Dissociation. Arrhenius did not originally consider strong electrolytes to be ionized completely except in extremely dilute solutions. He differentiated between strong and weak electrolytes by the fraction of the molecules ionized: the *degree of dissociation* α. A strong electrolyte was one that dissociated into ions to a high degree and a weak electrolyte one that dissociated into ions to a low degree.

Arrhenius determined the degree of dissociation directly from conductance measurements. He recognized that the equivalent conductance at infinite dilution Λ_o was a measure of the complete dissociation of the solute into its ions and that Λ_c represented the number of solute particles present as ions at a concentration *c*. Hence, the fraction of solute molecules ionized, or the degree of dissociation, was expressed by the equation[4]

$$\alpha = \frac{\Lambda_c}{\Lambda_o} \qquad (6-32)$$

in which Λ_c/Λ_o is known as the *conductance ratio*.

Example 6–6. The equivalent conductance of acetic acid at 25° C and at infinite dilution is 390.7 mho cm²/Eq. The equivalent conductance of a 5.9×10^{-3} M solution of acetic acid is 14.4 mho cm²/Eq. What is the degree of dissociation of acetic acid at this concentration?

$$\alpha = \frac{14.4}{390.7} = 0.037 \text{ or } 3.7\%$$

The van't Hoff factor i can be connected with the degree of dissociation α in the following way. The i factor equals unity for an ideal solution of a nonelectrolyte; however, a term must be added to account for the particles produced when a molecule of an electrolyte dissociates. For 1 mole of calcium chloride, which yields 3 ions per molecule, the van't Hoff factor is given by

$$i = 1 + \alpha(3 - 1) \qquad (6-33)$$

or, in general, for an electrolyte yielding v ions,

$$i = 1 + \alpha(v - 1) \qquad (6-34)$$

from which is obtained an expression for the degree of dissociation,

$$\alpha = \frac{i - 1}{v - 1} \qquad (6-35)$$

The cryoscopic method is used to determine i from the expression

$$\Delta T_f = iK_f m \qquad (6-36)$$

or

$$i = \frac{\Delta T_f}{K_f m} \qquad (6-37)$$

Example 6–7. The freezing point of a 0.10-m solution of acetic acid is −0.188° C. Calculate the degree of ionization of acetic acid at this concentration. Acetic acid dissociates into two ions, that is, $v = 2$.

$$i = \frac{0.188}{1.86 \times 0.10} = 1.011$$

$$\alpha = \frac{i - 1}{v - 1} = \frac{1.011 - 1}{2 - 1} = 0.011$$

In other words, according to the result of *Example 6–7* the fraction of acetic acid present as free ions in a 0.10-m solution is 0.011. Stated in percentage terms, acetic acid in 0.1 m concentration is ionized to the extent of about 1%.

THEORY OF STRONG ELECTROLYTES

Arrhenius used α to express the degree of dissociation of both strong and weak electrolytes, and van't Hoff introduced the factor i to account for the deviation of strong and weak electrolytes and nonelectrolytes

from the ideal laws of the colligative properties, regardless of the nature of these discrepancies. According to the early ionic theory, the degree of dissociation of ammonium chloride, a strong electrolyte, was calculated in the same manner as that of a weak electrolyte.

Example 6–8. The freezing point depression for a 0.01-m solution of ammonium chloride is 0.0367° C. Calculate the "degree of dissociation" of this electrolyte.

$$i = \frac{\Delta T_f}{K_f m} = \frac{0.0367°}{1.86 \times 0.010} = 1.97$$

$$\alpha = \frac{1.97 - 1}{2 - 1} = 0.97$$

The Arrhenius theory is now accepted for describing the behavior only of weak electrolytes. The degree of dissociation of a weak electrolyte can be calculated satisfactorily from the conductance ratio Λ_c/Λ_o or obtained from the van't Hoff i factor.

Many inconsistencies arise, however, when an attempt is made to apply the theory to solutions of strong electrolytes. In dilute and moderately concentrated solutions, they dissociate almost completely into ions, and it is not satisfactory to write an equilibrium expression relating the concentration of the ions and the minute amount of undissociated molecules, as is done for weak electrolytes (Chapter 7). Moreover, a discrepancy exists between α calculated from the i value and α calculated from the conductivity ratio for strong electrolytes in aqueous solutions having concentrations greater than about 0.5 M.

For these reasons, one does not account for the deviation of a strong electrolyte from ideal nonelectrolyte behavior by calculating a degree of dissociation. It is more convenient to consider a strong electrolyte as completely ionized and to introduce a factor that expresses the deviation of the solute from 100% ionization. The *activity* and *osmotic coefficient*, discussed in subsequent paragraphs, are used for this purpose.

Activity and Activity Coefficients. An approach that conforms well to the facts and that has evolved from a large number of studies on solutions of strong electrolytes ascribes the behavior of strong electrolytes to an electrostatic attraction between the ions.

The large number of oppositely charged ions in solutions of electrolytes influence one another through *interionic attractive forces*. Although this interference is negligible in dilute solutions, it becomes appreciable at moderate concentrations. In solutions of weak electrolytes, regardless of concentration, the number of ions is small and the interionic attraction correspondingly insignificant. Hence, the Arrhenius theory and the concept of the degree of dissociation are valid for solutions of weak electrolytes but not for strong electrolytes.

Not only are the ions interfered with in their movement by the "atmosphere" of oppositely charged ions surrounding them; they also can associate at high concentration into groups known as *ion pairs*, for example, Na^+Cl^-, and ion triplets, $Na^+Cl^-Na^+$. Associations of still higher orders may exist in solvents of low dielectric constant, in which the force of attraction of oppositely charged ions is large.

Because of the electrostatic attraction and ion association in moderately concentrated solutions of strong electrolytes, the values of the freezing point depression and the other colligative properties are less than expected for solutions of unhindered ions. Consequently, a strong electrolyte may be *completely ionized*, yet *incompletely dissociated* into free ions.

One may think of the solution as having an "effective concentration'" or, as it is called, an *activity*. The activity, in general, is less than the actual or stoichiometric concentration of the solute, not because the strong electrolyte is only partly ionized, but rather because some of the ions are effectively "taken out of play" by the electrostatic forces of interaction.

At infinite dilution in which the ions are so widely separated that they do not interact with one another, the activity a of an ion is equal to its concentration, expressed as molality or molarity. It is written on a molal basis at infinite dilution as

$$a = m \qquad (6\text{–}38)$$

or

$$\frac{a}{m} = 1 \qquad (6\text{–}39)$$

As the concentration of the solution is increased, the ratio becomes less than unity because the effective concentration or activity of the ions becomes less than the stoichiometric or molal concentration. This ratio is known as the *practical activity coefficient* γ_m on the molal scale, and the formula is written, for a particular ionic species, as

$$\frac{a}{m} = \gamma_m \qquad (6\text{–}40)$$

or

$$a = \gamma_m m \qquad (6\text{–}41)$$

On the molarity scale, another *practical activity coefficient* γ_c is defined as

$$a = \gamma_c c \qquad (6\text{–}42)$$

and on the mole fraction scale, a *rational activity coefficient* is defined as

$$a = \gamma_x X \qquad (6\text{–}43)$$

One sees from equations (6–41), (6–42), and (6–43) that these coefficients are proportionality constants relating activity to molality, molarity, and mole fraction, respectively, for an ion. The activity coefficients take on a value of unity and are thus identical in infinitely dilute solutions. The three coefficients usually decrease and assume different values as the concentration is increased; however, the differences among the three activity coefficients may be disregarded in dilute

solutions in which $c \cong m < 0.01$. The concept of activity and activity coefficient was first introduced by Lewis and Randall[5] and may be applied to solutions of nonelectrolytes and weak electrolytes as well as to the ions of strong electrolytes.

A cation and an anion in an aqueous solution may each have a different ionic activity. This is recognized by using the symbol a_+ when speaking of the activity of a cation and the symbol a_- when speaking of the activity of an anion. An electrolyte in solution contains each of these ions, however, so it is convenient to define a relationship between the activity of the electrolyte $a_\pm$ and the activities of the individual ions. The activity of an electrolyte is defined by its *mean ionic activity*, which is given by the relation

$$a_\pm = (a_+{}^m a_-{}^n)^{1/(m+n)} \qquad (6\text{–}44)$$

in which the exponents m and n give the stoichiometric number of given ions that are in solution. Thus, an NaCl solution has a mean ionic activity of

$$a_\pm = (a_{Na^+} a_{Cl^-})^{1/2}$$

whereas an $FeCl_3$ solution has a mean ionic activity of

$$a_\pm = (a_{Fe^{+3}} a_{Cl^-}{}^3)^{1/4}$$

The ionic activities of equation (6–44) may be expressed in terms of concentrations using any of equations (6–41) to (6–43). Using equation (6–42) one obtains from equation (6–44) the expression

$$a_\pm = [(\gamma_+ c_+)^m (\gamma_- c_-)^n]^{1/(m+n)} \qquad (6\text{–}45)$$

or

$$a_\pm = (\gamma_+{}^m \gamma_-{}^n)^{1/(m+n)} (c_+{}^m c_-{}^n)^{1/(m+n)} \qquad (6\text{–}46)$$

The *mean ionic activity coefficient* for the electrolyte can be defined by

$$\gamma_\pm = (\gamma_+{}^m \gamma_-{}^n)^{1/(m+n)} \qquad (6\text{–}47)$$

and

$$\gamma_\pm^{m+n} = \gamma_+{}^m \gamma_-{}^n \qquad (6\text{–}48)$$

Substitution of equation (6–47) into equation (6–46) yields

$$a_\pm = \gamma_\pm (c_+{}^m c_-{}^n)^{1/(m+n)} \qquad (6\text{–}49)$$

In using equation (6–49), it should be noted that the concentration of the electrolyte c is related to the concentration of its ions by

$$c_+ = mc \qquad (6\text{–}50)$$

and

$$c_- = nc \qquad (6\text{–}51)$$

Example 6–9. What is the mean ionic activity of a 0.01 *M* solution of $FeCl_3$?

$$a_\pm = \gamma_\pm (c_+ c_-{}^3)^{1/4} = \gamma_\pm[(0.01)(3 \times 0.01)^3]^{1/4}$$
$$= 2.3 \times 10^{-2} \gamma_\pm$$

It is possible to obtain the *mean ionic activity coefficient* $\gamma_{\pm}$ of an electrolyte by several experimental methods as well as by a theoretic approach. The experimental methods include distribution coefficient studies, electromotive force measurement, colligative property methods, and solubility determinations. (These results may then be used to obtain approximate activity coefficients for individual ions, where this is desired.[6])

Debye and Hückel have developed a theoretic method by which it is possible to calculate the activity coefficient of a single ion as well as the mean ionic activity coefficient of a solute without recourse to experimental data. Although the theoretic equation agrees with experimental findings only in dilute solutions (so dilute, in fact, that some chemists have referred jokingly to such solutions as "slightly contaminated water"), it has certain practical value in solution calculations. Furthermore, the Debye-Hückel equation provides a remarkable confirmation of modern solution theory.

The mean ionic activity coefficients of a number of strong electrolytes are found in Table 6–1. The results of various investigators vary in the third decimal place; therefore, most of the entries in the table have been recorded only to two places, providing sufficient precision for the calculations in this book. Although the values in the table are given at various molalities, we may accept these activity coefficients for problems involving molar concentrations (in which $m < 0.1$) since, in dilute solutions, the difference between molality and molarity is not great.

The mean values of Table 6–1 for NaCl, $CaCl_2$, and $ZnSO_4$ are plotted in Figure 6–6 against the square root of the molality. The reason for plotting the square root of the concentration is due to the form that the Debye–Hückel equation takes (p. 135). The activity coefficient approaches unity with increasing dilution. As the concentrations of some of the electrolytes are increased, their curves pass through minima and rise again to values greater than unity. Although the curves for different electrolytes of the same ionic class coincide at lower concentrations, they differ widely at higher values. The initial decrease in the activity coefficient

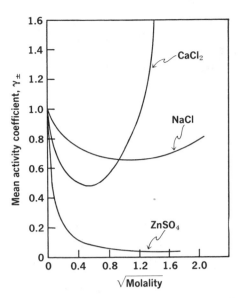

Fig. 6–6. Mean ionic activity coefficients of representative electrolytes plotted against the square root of concentration.

with increasing concentration is due to the interionic attraction, which causes the activity to be less than the stoichiometric concentration. The rise in the activity coefficient following the minimum in the curve of an electrolyte, such as HCl and $CaCl_2$, can be attributed to the attraction of the water molecules for the ions in concentrated aqueous solution. This *solvation* reduces the interionic attractions and increases the activity coefficient of the solute. It is the same effect that results in the salting out of nonelectrolytes from aqueous solutions to which electrolytes have been added.

Activity of the Solvent. Thus far, the discussion of activity and activity coefficients has centered on the solute and particularly on electrolytes. It is customary to define the activity of the solvent on the mole fraction scale. When a solution is made infinitely dilute, it can be considered to consist essentially of pure solvent. Therefore, $X_1 \cong 1$, and the solvent behaves ideally in conformity with Raoult's law. Under this condition, the mole fraction can be set equal to the activity of the solvent, or

$$a = X_1 = 1 \qquad (6-52)$$

TABLE 6–1. *Mean Ionic Activity Coefficients of Some Strong Electrolytes at 25° C on the Molal Scale*

Molality (m)	HCl	NaCl	KCl	NaOH	CaCl₂	H₂SO₄	Na₂SO₄	CuSO₄	ZnSO₄
0.000	1.00	1.00	1.00	1.00	1.00	1.00	1.00	1.00	1.00
0.005	0.93	0.93	0.93	—	0.79	0.64	0.78	0.53	0.48
0.01	0.91	0.90	0.90	0.90	0.72	0.55	0.72	0.40	0.39
0.05	0.83	0.82	0.82	0.81	0.58	0.34	0.51	0.21	0.20
0.10	0.80	0.79	0.77	0.76	0.52	0.27	0.44	0.15	0.15
0.50	0.77	0.68	0.65	0.68	0.51	0.16	0.27	0.067	0.063
1.00	0.81	0.66	0.61	0.67	0.73	0.13	0.21	0.042	0.044
2.00	1.01	0.67	0.58	0.69	1.55	0.13	0.15	—	0.035
4.00	1.74	0.79	0.58	0.90	2.93	0.17	0.14	—	—

As the solution becomes more concentrated in solute, the activity of the solvent ordinarily becomes less than the mole fraction concentration, and the ratio can be given, as for the solute, by the rational activity coefficient

$$\frac{a}{X_1} = \gamma_x \qquad (6-53)$$

or

$$a = \gamma_x X_1 \qquad (6-54)$$

The activity of a volatile solvent can be determined rather simply. The ratio of the vapor pressure p_1 of the solvent in a solution to the vapor pressure of pure solvent $p_1°$ is approximately equal to the *activity* of the solvent at ordinary pressures: $a_1 = p_1/p°$.

Example 6-10. The vapor pressure of water in a solution containing 0.5 mole of sucrose in 1000 g of water is 17.38 mm, and the vapor pressure of pure water at 20° C is 17.54 mm. What is the activity (or escaping tendency) of water in the solution?

$$a = \frac{17.38}{17.54} = 0.991$$

Reference State. The assignment of activities to the components of solutions provides a measure of the extent of departure from ideal solution behavior. For this purpose, a *reference state* must be established in which each component behaves ideally. The reference state may be defined as the solution in which the concentration (mole fraction, molal or molar) of the component is equal to the activity:

$$\text{activity} = \text{concentration}$$

or, what amounts to the same thing, the activity coefficient is unity,

$$\gamma_i = \frac{\text{activity}}{\text{concentration}} = 1$$

The reference state for a solvent on the mole fraction scale was shown in equation (6-52) to be the pure solvent.

The reference state for the solute may be chosen from one of several possibilities. If a liquid solute is miscible with the solvent (e.g., in a solution of alcohol in water), the concentration may be expressed in mole fraction, and the pure liquid may be taken as the reference state, as was done for the solvent. For a liquid or solid solute having a limited solubility in the solvent, the reference state is ordinarily taken as the infinitely dilute solution in which the concentration of the solute and the ionic strength (see the following) of the solution are small. Under these conditions, the activity is equal to the concentration, and the activity coefficient is unity.

Standard State. The activities ordinarily used in chemistry are relative activities. It is not possible to know the absolute value of the activity of a component; therefore, a standard must be established just as was done in Chapter 1 for the fundamental measurable properties.

The *standard state* of a component in a solution is the state of the component at unit activity. The relative activity in any solution is then the ratio of the activity in that state relative to the value in the standard state. When defined in these terms, activity is a dimensionless number.

The pure liquid at 1 atm and at a definite temperature is chosen as the standard state of a solvent or of a liquid solute miscible with the solvent, since, for the pure liquid, $a = 1$. Because the mole fraction of a pure solvent is also unity, mole fraction is equal to activity, and the reference state is identical with the standard state.

The standard state of the solvent in a solid solution is the pure solid at 1 atm and at a definite temperature. The assignment of $a = 1$ to pure liquids and pure solids will be found to be convenient in later discussions on equilibria and electromotive force.

The standard state for a solute of limited solubility is more difficult to define. The activity of the solute in an infinitely dilute solution, although equal to the concentration, is not unity, and the standard state is thus not the same as the reference state. The standard state of the solute is defined as a hypothetic solution of unit concentration (mole fraction, molal or molar) having, at the same time, the characteristics of an infinitely dilute or ideal solution. For complete understanding, this definition requires careful development, as carried out by Klotz and Rosenberg.[7]

Ionic Strength. In dilute solutions of nonelectrolytes, activities and concentrations are considered to be practically identical, since electrostatic forces do not bring about deviations from ideal behavior in these solutions. Likewise, for weak electrolytes that are present alone in solution, the differences between the ionic concentration terms and activities are usually disregarded in ordinary calculations, since the number of ions present is small, and the electrostatic forces are negligible.

However, for strong electrolytes and for solutions of weak electrolytes together with salts and other electrolytes, such as exist in buffer systems, it is important to use activities instead of concentrations. The activity coefficient, and hence the activity, may be obtained by using one of the forms of the Debye–Hückel equation (considered below) if one knows the ionic strength of the solution. Lewis and Randall[8] introduced the concept of *ionic strength* μ to relate interionic attractions and activity coefficients. The ionic strength is defined on the molar scale as

$$\mu = \tfrac{1}{2}(c_1 z_1^2 + c_2 z_2^2 + c_3 z_3^2 + \cdots + c_j z_j^2) \quad (6-55)$$

or, in abbreviated notation

$$\mu = \tfrac{1}{2} \sum_1^j c_i z_i^2 \qquad (6-56)$$

in which the summation symbol $\sum_{1}^{j}$ indicates that the product of cz^2 terms for all the ionic species in the solution, from the first one to the jth species, are to be added together. The term c_i is the concentration in moles per liter of any of the ions and z_i is its valence. Ionic strength represents the contribution to the electrostatic forces of the ions of all types. It depends on the total number of ionic charges and not on the specific properties of the salts present in the solution. It was found that bivalent ions are equivalent not to two but to four univalent ions; hence, by introducing the square of the valence, proper weight is given to the ions of higher charge. The sum is divided by two because positive ion–negative ion pairs contribute to the total electrostatic interaction, whereas we are interested in the effect of each ion separately.

Example 6–11. What is the ionic strength of (a) 0.010 M KCl, (b) 0.010 M $BaSO_4$, and (c) 0.010 M Na_2SO_4, and (d) what is the ionic strength of a solution containing all three electrolytes together with salicylic acid in 0.010 M concentration in aqueous solution?

(a) KCl
$$\mu = \tfrac{1}{2}[(0.01 \times 1^2) + (0.01 \times 1^2)]$$
$$= 0.010$$

(b) $BaSO_4$
$$\mu = \tfrac{1}{2}[(0.01 \times 2^2) + (0.01 \times 2^2)]$$
$$= 0.040$$

(c) Na_2SO_4
$$\mu = \tfrac{1}{2}[(0.02 \times 1^2) + (0.01 \times 2^2)]$$
$$= 0.030$$

(d) The ionic strength of a 0.010-M solution of salicylic acid is 0.003 as calculated from a knowledge of the ionization of the acid at this concentration (using the equation $[H_3O^+] = \sqrt{K_a c}$ of pp. 145, 155). Unionized salicyclic acid does not contribute to the ionic strength.

The ionic strength of the mixture of electrolytes is the sum of the ionic strengths of the individual salts. Thus,

$$\mu_{\text{total}} = \mu_{\text{KCl}} + \mu_{\text{BaSO}_4} + \mu_{\text{Na}_2\text{SO}_4} + \mu_{\text{HSal}}$$
$$= 0.010 + 0.040 + 0.030 + 0.003$$
$$= 0.083$$

Example 6–12. A buffer contains 0.3 mole of K_2HPO_4 and 0.1 mole of KH_2PO_4 per liter of solution. Calculate the ionic strength of the solution.

The concentrations of the ions of K_2HPO_4 are $[K^+] = 0.3 \times 2$ and $[HPO_4^{2-}] = 0.3$. The values for KH_2PO_4 are $[K^+] = 0.1$ and $[H_2PO_4^-] = 0.1$. Any contributions to μ by further dissociation of $[HPO_4^{2-}]$ and $[H_2PO_4^-]$ are neglected.

$$\mu = \tfrac{1}{2}(0.3 \times 2 \times 1^2) + (0.3 \times 2^2) + (0.1 \times 1^2) + (0.1 \times 1^2)]$$
$$\mu = 1.0$$

It will be observed in *Example 6–11* that the ionic strength of a 1:1 electrolyte such as KCl is the same as the molar concentration; μ of a 1:2 electrolyte such as Na_2SO_4 is three times the concentration; and μ for a 2:2 electrolyte is four times the concentration.

The mean ionic activity coefficients of electrolytes should be expressed at various ionic strengths instead of concentrations. Lewis has shown the uniformity in activity coefficients when they are related to ionic strength:

(a) The activity coefficient of a strong electrolyte is roughly constant in all dilute solutions of the same ionic strength, irrespective of the type of salts that are used to provide the additional ionic strength.

(b) The activity coefficients of all strong electrolytes of a single class, for example, all uni-univalent electrolytes, are approximately the same at a definite ionic strength, provided the solutions are dilute.

The results in Table 6–1 illustrate the similarity of the mean ionic activity coefficients for 1:1 electrolytes at low concentrations (below 0.1 m) and the differences that become marked at higher concentrations.

Bull[9] pointed out the importance of the principle of ionic strength in biochemistry. In the study of the influence of pH on biologic action, the effect of the variable salt concentration in the buffer may obscure the results unless the buffer is adjusted to a constant ionic strength in each experiment. If the biochemical action is affected by the specific salts used, however, even this precaution may fail to yield satisfactory results. Further use will be made of ionic strength in the chapters on ionic equilibria, solubility, and kinetics.

The Debye–Hückel Theory. Debye and Hückel derived an equation based on the principles that strong electrolytes are completely ionized in dilute solution and that the deviations of electrolytic solutions from ideal behavior are due to the electrostatic effects of the oppositely charged ions. The equation relates the activity coefficient of a particular ion or the mean ionic activity coefficient of an electrolyte to the valence of the ions, the ionic strength of the solution, and the characteristics of the solvent. The mathematical derivation of the equation is not attempted here but can be found in Lewis and Randall's *Thermodynamics* as revised by Pitzer and Brewer.[10] The equation may be used to calculate the activity coefficients of drugs, the values of which have not been obtained experimentally and are not available in the literature.

According to the theory of Debye and Hückel, the activity coefficient γ_i of an ion of valence z_i is given by the expression

$$\log \gamma_i = -Az_i^2\sqrt{\mu} \tag{6–57}$$

Equation (6–57) yields a satisfactory measure of the activity coefficient of an ion species up to an ionic strength μ of about 0.02. For water at 25° C, A, a factor that depends only on the temperature and the dielectric constant of the medium, is approximately equal to 0.51. The values of A for various solvents of pharmaceutical importance are found in Table 6–2.

The form of the Debye–Hückel equation for a binary electrolyte, consisting of ions with valences of z_+ and z_- and present in a dilute solution ($\mu < 0.02$), is

$$\log \gamma_\pm = -Az_+z_-\sqrt{\mu} \tag{6–58}$$

TABLE 6–2. *Values of A for Solvents at 25° C*

Solvent	Dielectric Constant ϵ	A^*_{calc}
Acetone	20.70	3.76
Ethanol	24.30	2.96
Water	78.54	0.509

$^*A_{(calc)} = \dfrac{1.824 \times 10^6}{(\epsilon \times T)^{3/2}}$ in which ϵ is the dielectric constant and T is the absolute temperature on the Kelvin scale.

The symbols z_+ and z_- stand for the valences or charges, ignoring algebraic signs, on the ions of the electrolyte whose mean ionic activity coefficient is sought. The coefficient in equation (6–58) is γ_x, the rational activity coefficient (i.e., $\gamma_\pm$ on the mole fraction scale), but in dilute solutions for which the Debye–Hückel equation is applicable, γ_x can be assumed without serious error to be equal also to the practical coefficients, γ_m and γ_c, on the molal and molar scales.

Example 6–13. Calculate the mean ionic activity coefficient for $0.005\ M$ atropine sulfate (1:2 electrolyte) in an aqueous solution containing $0.01\ M$ NaCl at 25° C. Since the drug is a uni-bivalent electrolyte, $z_1 z_2 = 1 \times 2 = 2$. A for water at 25° C is 0.51.

μ for atropine sulfate $= \frac{1}{2}[(0.005 \times 2 \times 1^2) + (0.005 \times 2^2)] = 0.015$

μ for NaCl $\qquad = \frac{1}{2}[(0.01 \times 1^2) + (0.01 \times 1^2)] = \underline{\ 0.01\ }$

$\qquad$ Total $\mu \qquad\qquad\qquad\qquad\qquad\qquad = 0.025$

$$\log \gamma_\pm = -0.51 \times 2 \times \sqrt{0.025}$$
$$\log \gamma_\pm = -1.00 + 0.839 = -0.161$$
$$\gamma_\pm = 0.690$$

With the present-day accessibility of the hand calculator, the intermediate step in this calculation (needed only when log tables are used) may be deleted.

Thus one observes that the activity coefficient of a strong electrolyte in dilute solution depends on the total ionic strength of the solution, the valence of the ions of the drug involved, the nature of the solvent, and the temperature of the solution. Notice that although the ionic strength term results from the contribution of all ionic species in solution, the $z_1 z_2$ terms apply only to the drug, the activity coefficient of which is being determined.

Extension of the Debye–Hückel Equation to Higher Concentrations. The limiting expressions, equations (6–57) and (6–58), are not satisfactory above an ionic strength of about 0.02, and (6–58) is not completely satisfactory for use in *Example 6–13*. A formula that applies up to an ionic strength of perhaps 0.1 is

$$\log \gamma_\pm = -\frac{Az_+z_-\sqrt{\mu}}{1 + a_i B\sqrt{\mu}} \qquad (6\text{–}59)$$

The term a_i is the mean distance of approach of the ions and is called the *mean effective ionic diameter* or the *ion size parameter*. Its exact significance is not known; however, it is somewhat analogous to the b

term in the van der Waals gas equation. The term B, like A, is a constant influenced only by the nature of the solvent and the temperature. The values of a_i for several electrolytes at 25° C are given in Table 6–3, and the values of B and A for water at various temperatures are shown in Table 6–4. The values of A for various solvents, as previously mentioned, are listed in Table 6–2.

Since a_i for most electrolytes equals 3 to 4×10^{-8} and B for water at 25° C equals 0.33×10^8, the product of a_i and B is approximately unity. Equation (6–59) then simplifies to

$$\log \gamma_\pm = -\frac{Az_+z_-\sqrt{\mu}}{1 + \sqrt{\mu}} \qquad (6\text{–}60)$$

Example 6–14. Calculate the activity coefficient of a $0.004M$ aqueous solution of sodium phenobarbital at 25° C, which has been brought to an ionic strength of 0.09 by the addition of sodium chloride. Use equations (6–58), (6–59), and (6–60) and compare the results.

Equation (6–58): $\log \gamma_\pm = -0.51\sqrt{0.09}$; $\gamma_\pm = 0.70$

Equation (6–59): $\log \gamma_\pm =$

$$-\frac{0.51\sqrt{0.09}}{1 + [(2 \times 10^{-8}) \times (0.33 \times 10^8) \times \sqrt{0.09}]}; \gamma_\pm = 0.75$$

Equation (6–60): $\log \gamma_\pm = -\dfrac{0.51\sqrt{0.09}}{1 + \sqrt{0.09}}$; $\gamma_\pm = 0.76$

These results may be compared with the experimental values for some uni-univalent electrolytes in Table 6–1 at a molal concentration of about 0.1.

For still higher concentrations, that is, at ionic strengths above 0.1, the observed activity coefficients for some electrolytes pass through minima and then

TABLE 6–3. *Mean Effective Ionic Diameter for Some Electrolytes at 25° C*

Electrolyte	a_i (cm)
HCl	5.3×10^{-8}
NaCl	4.4×10^{-8}
KCl	4.1×10^{-8}
Methapyrilene HCl	3.9×10^{-8}
MgSO$_4$	3.4×10^{-8}
K$_2$SO$_4$	3.0×10^{-8}
AgNO$_3$	2.3×10^{-8}
Sodium phenobarbital	2.0×10^{-8}

TABLE 6–4. *Values of A and B for Water at Various Temperatures*

Temperature (°C)	A	B
0	0.488	0.325×10^8
15	0.500	0.328×10^8
25	0.509	0.330×10^8
40	0.524	0.333×10^8
70	0.560	0.339×10^8
100	0.606	0.348×10^8

increase with concentration; in some cases they become greater than unity, as seen in Figure 6–6. To account for the increase in $\gamma_\pm$ at higher concentrations, an empirical term $C\mu$ can be added to the Debye–Hückel equation, resulting in the expression

$$\log \gamma_\pm = -\frac{Az_+z_-\sqrt{\mu}}{1 + a_iB\sqrt{\mu}} + C\mu \qquad (6-61)$$

This equation gives satisfactory results in solutions of concentrations as high as 1 M. The mean ionic activity coefficient obtained from equation (6–61) is γ_x; however, it is not significantly different from γ_m and γ_c even at this concentration. Zografi et al.[11] have used the extended Debye–Hückel equation (equation (6–61)) in a study of the interaction between the dye orange II and quarternary ammonium salts.

Investigations have resulted in equations that extend the concentration to about 5 moles/liter.[12]

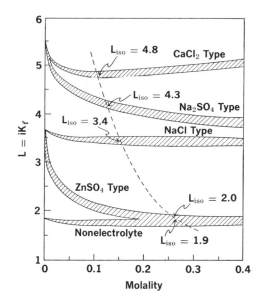

Fig. 6–7. L_{iso} values of various ionic classes.

COEFFICIENTS FOR EXPRESSING COLLIGATIVE PROPERTIES

Although activities may be used to bring the colligative properties of strong electrolytes into line with experimental results, the equations are complicated and are not treated in this book. Activities are more valuable in connection with equilibria expressions and electrochemical calculations. The use of activities for calculating the colligative properties of weak electrolytes is particularly inconvenient, for it also requires a knowledge of the degree of dissociation.

The L Value. The van't Hoff expression $\Delta T_f = iK_f m$ probably provides the best single equation for computing the colligative properties of nonelectrolytes, weak electrolytes, and strong electrolytes. It can be modified slightly for convenience in dilute solutions by substituting molar concentration c and by writing iK_f as L, so that

$$\Delta T_f = Lc \qquad (6-62)$$

L has been computed from experimental data for a number of drugs by Goyan et al.[13] It varies with the concentration of the solution. At a concentrtion of drug that is isotonic with body fluids, $L = iK_f$ is designated here as L_{iso}. It has a value equal to about 1.9 (actually 1.86) for nonelectrolytes, 2.0 for weak electrolytes, 3.4 for uni-univalent electrolytes, and larger values for electrolytes of high valences. A plot of iK_f against the concentration of some drugs is presented in Figure 6–7, in which each curve is represented as a band to show the variability of the L values within each ionic class. The approximate L_{iso} for each of the ionic classes may be obtained from the dashed line running vertically through the figure. The application of L_{iso} to the preparation of isotonic drug solutions is described in Chapter 8.

Osmotic Coefficient. Other methods of correcting for the deviations of electrolytes from ideal colligative behavior have been suggested. One of these is based on the fact that as the solution becomes more dilute, i approaches ν, the number of ions into which an electrolyte dissociates, and at infinite dilution, $i = \nu$, or $i/\nu = 1$. Proceeding in the direction of more concentrated solutions, i/ν becomes less (and sometimes greater) than unity.

The ratio i/ν is designated as g and is known as the *practical osmotic coefficient* when expressed on a molal basis. In the case of a weak electrolyte, it provides a measure of the degree of dissociation. For strong electrolytes g is equal to unity for complete dissociation, and the depature of g from unity, that is, $1 - g$, in moderately concentrated solutions is an indication of the interionic attraction. Osmotic coefficients, g, for electrolytes and nonelectrolytes are plotted against ionic concentration, νm, in Figure 6–8. Since $g = 1/\nu$ or $i = g\nu$ in a dilute solution, the cryoscopic equation may be written

$$\Delta T_f = g\nu K_f m \qquad (6-63)$$

The molal osmotic coefficients of some salts are listed in Table 6–5.

Example 6–15. The osmotic coefficient of LiBr at 0.2 m is 0.944 and the L_{iso} value is 3.4. Compute ΔT_f for this compound using g and L_{iso}. Disregard the difference between molality and molarity.

$$\Delta T_f = g\nu K_f m = 0.944 \times 2 \times 1.86 \times 0.2$$
$$= 0.70°$$
$$\Delta T_f = L_{iso}c = 3.4 \times 0.2 = 0.68°$$

Osmolality. Although osmotic pressure (pp. 117–119) classically is given in atmospheres, in clinical practice it is expressed in terms of osmols (Osm) or milliosmols (mOsm). A solution containing 1 mole (1 gram molecular weight) of a nonionizable substance in 1 kg of water (a

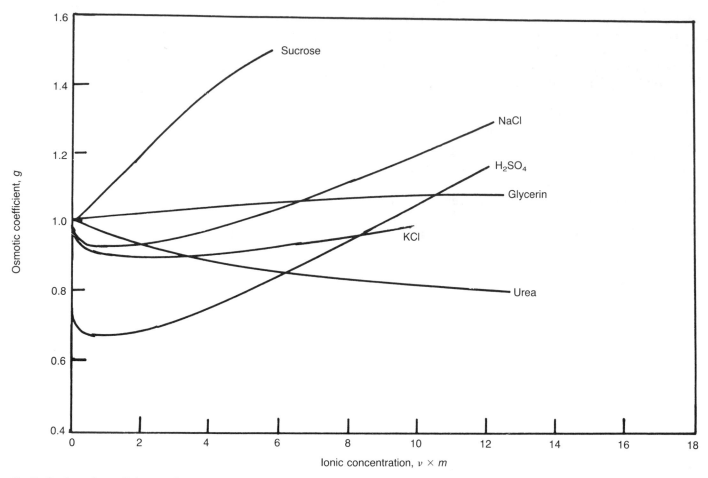

Fig. 6—8. Osmotic coefficient, *g*, for some common solutes. (From G. Scatchard, W. Hamer and S. Wood, J. Am. Chem. Soc. **60**, 3061, 1938. Reproduced with permission of the copyright owner.)

1-*m* solution) is referred to as a 1-osmolal solution. It contains 1 osmol (Osm) or 1000 milliosmols (mOsm) of solute per kilogram of solvent. Osmolality measures the total number of particles dissolved in a kilogram of water, that is, the osmols per kilogram of water, and depends on the electrolytic nature of the solute. An ionic species dissolved in water will dissociate to form ions or "particles." These ions tend to associate somewhat, however, owing to their ionic interactions. The apparent number of "particles" in solution, as measured

by osmometry or one of the other colligtive methods, will depend on the extent of these interactions. An un-ionized material (i.e., a nonelectrolyte) is used as the reference solute for osmolality measurements, ionic interactions being insignificant for a nonelectrolyte. For an electrolyte that dissociates into ions in a dilute solution, osmolality or milliosmolality can be calculated from

$$\text{Milliosmolality (mOsm/kg)} = i \cdot mm \quad (6\text{--}64)$$

TABLE 6—5. *Osmotic Coefficients, g, at 25° C**

m	NaCl	KCl	H_2SO_4	Sucrose	Urea	Glycerin
0.1	0.9342	0.9264	0.6784	1.0073	0.9959	1.0014
0.2	0.9255	0.9131	0.6675	1.0151	0.9918	1.0028
0.4	0.9217	0.9023	0.6723	1.0319	0.9841	1.0055
0.6	0.9242	0.8987	0.6824	1.0497	0.9768	1.0081
0.8	0.9295	0.8980	0.6980	1.0684	0.9698	1.0105
1.0	0.9363	0.8985	0.7176	1.0878	0.9631	1.0128
1.6	0.9589	0.9024	0.7888	1.1484	0.9496	1.0192
2.0	0.9786	0.9081	0.8431	1.1884	0.9346	1.0230
3.0	1.0421	0.9330	0.9922	1.2817	0.9087	1.0316
4.0	1.1168	0.9635	1.1606	1.3691	0.8877	1.0393
5.0	1.2000	0.9900	—	1.4477	0.8700	1.0462

*From G. Scatchard, W. G. Hamer and S. E. Wood, J. Am. Chem. Soc. **60**, 3061, 1938. Reproduced with permission of the copyright owner.

in which i (see p. 129) is approximately the number of ions formed per molecule and mm is the millimolal concentration. If no ionic interactions occurred in a solution of sodium chloride, i would equal 2.0. In a typical case, for a 1:1 electrolyte in dilute solution, i is approximately 1.86 rather than 2.0, owing to ionic interaction between the positively and negatively charged ions.

Example 6–16. What is the milliosmolality of a 0.120-m solution of potassium bromide? What is its osmotic pressure in atmospheres?

For a 120 millimolal solution of KBr:

Milliosmolality = $1.86 \times 120 = 223$ mOsm/kg

A 1-osmolal solution raises the boiling point 0.52° C, lowers the freezing point 1.86° C, and produces an osmotic pressure of 24.4 atm at 25° C. Therefore, a 0.223 Osm/kg solution yields an osmotic pressure of $24.4 \times 0.223 = 5.44$ atm.

Refer to the reports by Streng et al.[14] and Murty et al.[15] for discussions on the use of osmolality and osmolarity in clinical pharmacy. Molarity (moles of solute per liter of solution) is used in clinical practice more frequently than molality (moles of solute per kilogram of solvent). Also, osmolarity is used more frequently than osmolality in labeling parenteral solutions in the hospital. Yet osmolarity cannot be measured and must be calculated from the experimentally determined osmolality of a solution. As shown by Murty et al.,[15] the conversion is made using the relation:

Osmolarity = (measured osmolality)

$\times$ (solution density in g/mL

$-$ anhydrous solute concentration in g/mL) (6–65)

According to Streng et al.,[14] osmolality is converted to osmolarity using the equation

mOsm/liter solution = mOsm/(kg H_2O)

$\times [d_1°(1 - 0.001 \bar{v}_2°)]$ (6–66)

where $d_1°$ is the density of the solvent and $\bar{v}_2°$ is the partial molal volume of the solute at infinite dilution.

Example 6–17. A 30-g/L solution of sodium bicarbonate contains 0.030 g/mL of anhydrous sodium bicarbonate. The density of this solution was found to be 1.0192 g/mL at 20° C, and its measured milliosmolality was 614.9 mOsm/kg. Convert milliosmolality to milliosmolarity.

Milliosmolarity = 614.9 mOsm/kg H_2O

$\times$ (1.0192 g/mL $-$ 0.030 g/mL)

= 608.3 mOsm/L solution

Example 6–18. A 0.154-molal sodium chloride solution has a milliosmolality of 286.4 mOsm/kg (see *Example* (6–19)). Calculate the milliosmolarity, mOsm/L solution, using equation (6–66). The density of the solvent—water—at 25° C is $d_1° = 0.9971$ g/cm³, and the partial molal volume of the solute—sodium chloride—is $\bar{v}_2° = 16.63$ mL/mole.

Milliosmolality = (286.4 mOsm/kg H_2O)

$\times [0.9971(1 - 0.001(16.63))]$

= 280.8 mOsm/L solution

As noted here, osmolarity differs from osmolality by only 1 or 2%. However, in more concentrated solutions of polyvalent electrolytes together with buffers, preservatives, and other ions, the difference may become significant. For accuracy in the preparation and labeling of parenteral solutions, osmolality should be measured carefully with a vapor pressure or freezing point osmometer (rather than calculated) and the results converted to osmolarity using equation (6–65) or (6–66). UIC, Inc., of Joliet, Ill. manufactures a cryoscopic osmometer for automatic osmolality determinations.

Whole blood, plasma, and serum are complex liquids consisting of proteins, glucose, nonprotein nitrogenous materials, sodium, potassium, calcium, magnesium, chloride, and bicarbonate ions. The serum electrolytes, constituting less than 1% of the blood's weight, determine the osmolality of the blood. Sodium chloride contributes a milliosmolality of 275, while glucose and the other constituents together provide about 10 mOsm/kg to the blood.

Colligative properties such as freezing point depression are related to osmolality through equations (6–27) and (6–63).

$$\Delta T_f \cong K_f i m \qquad (6–67)$$

in which $i = gv$ and $im = gvm$ is osmolality.

Example 6–19. Calculate the freezing point depression of (a) a 0.154-m solution of NaCl and (b) a 0.154-m solution of glucose. What are the milliosmolalities of these two solutions?

(a) From Table 6–5, g for NaCl at 25° C is about 0.93, and since NaCl ionizes into two ions, $i = v \cdot g = 2 \times 0.93 = 1.86$. From equation (6–64), the osmolality of a 0.154-m solution is $i \cdot m = 1.86 \times 0.154 = 0.2864$. The milliosmolality of this solution is therefore 286.4 mOsm/kg. Using equation (6–67), with K_f also equal to 1.86, we obtain for the freezing point depression of a 0.154-m solution—or its equivalent, a 0.2864-Osm/kg solution—of NaCl

$$\Delta T_f = (1.86)(1.86)(0.154)$$

$$= (1.86)(0.2864) = 0.53° C$$

(b) Glucose is a nonelectrolyte, producing only one particle for each of its molecules in solution, and for a nonelectrolyte, $i = v = 1$ and $g = i/v = 1$. Therefore, the freezing point depression of a 0.154-m solution of glucose is approximately

$$\Delta T_f = K_f i m = (1.86)(1.00)(0.154)$$

$$= 0.286° C$$

which is nearly one half of the freezing point depression provided by sodium chloride, a 1:1 electrolyte that provides two particles rather than one particle in solution.

The osmolality of a nonelectrolyte such as glucose is identical to its molal concentration since osmolality = $i \times$ molality, and i for a nonelectrolyte is 1.00. The milliosmolality of a solution is 1000 times its osmolality or, in this case, 154 mOsm/kg.

Ohwaki et al.[16] studied the effect of osmolality on the nasal absorption of secretin, a hormone used in the treatment of duodenal ulcers. They found that maximum absorption through the nasal mucosa occurred at a sodium chloride milliosmolarity of about 860 mOsm/L (0.462 M), possibly owing to structural changes in the epithelial cells of the nasal mucosa at this high mOsm/L value.

Although the osmolality of blood and other body fluids is contributed mainly by the content of sodium chloride, the osmolality and milliosmolality of these complex solutions by convention are calculated based on i or nonelectrolytes, that is, i is taken as unity, and osmolality becomes equal to molality. This principle is best described by an example.

Example 6–20. Freezing points were determined using the blood of 20 normal subjects and were averaged to $-0.5712°$ C. This value of course is equivalent to a freezing point depression of $+0.5712°$ C below the freezing point of water because the freezing point of water is taken as $0.000°$ C at atmospheric pressure. What is the average milliosmolality, x, of the blood of these subjects?

Using equation (6–67) with the arbitrary choice of $i = 1$ for body fluids, we obtain

$$0.5712 = (1.86)(1.00)\, x$$

$$x = 0.3071 \text{ Osm/kg}$$

$$= 307.1 \text{ mOsm/kg}$$

It is noted in *Example 20* that although the osmolality of blood and its freezing point depression are contributed mainly by NaCl, an i value of 1 was used for blood rather than $gv = 1.86$ for an NaCl solution.

The milliosmolality for blood obtained by various workers using osmometry, vapor pressure, and freezing point depression apparatus (Chapter 5) ranges from about 250 to 350 mOsm/kg.[17] The normal osmolality of body fluids is given in medical handbooks[18] as 275 to 295 mOsm/kg, but normal values are likely to fall in an even narrower range of 286 ± 4 mOsm/kg.[19] Freezing point and vapor pressure osmometers are now used routinely in the hospital. A difference of 50 mOsm/kg or more from the accepted values of a body fluid suggests an abnormality such as liver failure, hemorrhagic shock, uremia, or other toxic manifestations. Body water and electrolyte balance are also monitored by measurement of milliosmolality. Colligative property measurements and apparatus are describe in Chapter 5.

References and Notes

1. S. Arrhenius, Z. Physik, Chem. **1**, 631, 1887.
2. H. L. Clever, J. Chem. Educ. **40**, 637, 1963; P. A. Giguère, J. Chem. Educ. **56**, 571, 1979; R. P. Bell, *The Proton in Chemistry*, 2nd Edition, Chapman and Hall, London, 1973, pp. 13–25.
3. A. Albert, *Selective Toxicity*, Chapman and Hall, London, 1979, pp. 344, 373–384.
4. S. Arrhenius, J. Am. Chem. Soc. **34**, 361, 1912.
5. G. N. Lewis and M. Randall, *Thermodynamics*, McGraw-Hill, New York, 1923, p. 255.
6. S. Glasstone, *An Introduction to Electrochemistry*, Van Nostrand, New York, 1942, pp. 137–139.
7. I. M. Klotz and R. M. Rosenberg, *Chemical Thermodynamics*, 3rd Edition, W. A. Benjamin, Menlo Park, Calif., 1973, Chapter 19.
8. G. N. Lewis and M. Randall, *Thermodynamics*, McGraw-Hill, New York, 1923, p. 373.
9. H. B. Bull, *Physical Biochemistry*, 2nd Edition, Wiley, New York, 1951, p. 79.
10. G. N. Lewis and M. Randall, *Thermodynamics*. Revised by K. S. Pitzer and L. Brewer, 2nd Edition, McGraw-Hill, New York, 1961, Chapter 23.
11. G. Zografi, P. Patel and N. Weiner, J. Pharm. Sci. **53**, 545, 1964.
12. R. H. Stokes and R. A. Robinson, J. Am. Chem. Soc. **70**, 1870, 1948; Eigen and Wicke, J. Phys. Chem. **58**, 702, 1954.
13. F. M. Goyan, J. M. Enright and J. M. Wells, J. Am. Pharm. Assoc., Sci. Ed. **33**, 74, 1944.
14. W. H. Streng, H. E. Huber and J. T. Carstensen, J. Pharm. Sci. **67**, 384, 1978; H. E. Huber, W. H. Streng, and H. G. H. Tan, J. Pharm. Sci. **68**, 1028, 1979.
15. B. S. R. Murty, J. N. Kapoor and P. O. DeLuca, Am. J. Hosp. Pharm. **33**, 546, 1976.
16. T. Ohwaki, H. Ando, F. Kakimoto, K. Uesugi, S. Watanabe, Y. Miyake and M. Kayano, J. Pharm. Sci. **76**, 695, 1987.
17. C. Waymouth, In Vitro **6**, 109, 1970.
18. M. A. Kaupp, et al., Eds., *Current Medical Diagnosis & Treatment*, Lange, Los Altos, Calif., 1986, pp. 27, 1113.
19. L. Glasser, et al., Am. J. Clin. Pathol. **60**, 695–699, 1973.
20. L. Barcza and L. Lenner, J. Pharm. Sci. **77**, 622, 1988.
21. S.-Y.P. King, A. M. Basista and G. Torosian, J. Pharm. Sci. **78**, 95, 1989.

Problems

6–1. The equivalent conductance Λ_0 of the sodium salt of a sulfonamide at infinite dilution was found by experiment to be 100.3 mho cm^2/Eq. The Λ_0 for HCl is 426.16; for NaCl, 126.45. What is Λ_0 for the free acid (the free sulfonamide)?

Answer: 400 mho cm^2/Eq

6–2. The equivalent conductance at infinite dilution for the following strong electrolytes are given: $\Lambda_0(\text{HCl}) = 426.16$, $\Lambda_0(\text{NaAc}) = 91.0$, and $\Lambda_0(\text{NaCl}) = 126.45$ mho cm^2/Eq. Compute the equivalent conductance at infinite dilution for acetic acid.

Answer: 390.7 mho cm^2/Eq

6–3. The equivalent conductances Λ_c (mho cm^2/Eq) of NaCl at several molar concentrations, c, are

Data for *Problem 6–3*

c	0.09	0.04	0.01
Λ_c	113.34	117.70	122.08

(a) Plot Λ_c against $\sqrt{c}$ as in Figure 6–4. Compute Λ_0 and the equation of the line (use least squares).

(b) The transference number, t_c, of Na$^+$ at infinite dilution is 0.396. Compute the ionic equivalent conductance of Na$^+$, Cl$^-$, and the transference number of Cl$^-$ at infinite dilution.

Answers: (a) The equation of the line is $\Lambda_c = 126.45 - 43.70\sqrt{c}$; $r^2 = 0.9999$. The intercept $\Lambda_0 = 126.45$ ohm^{-1} cm^2/Eq.

(b) From the definition of transference number and the Kohlrausch law, equation 6–23, we can use the transference numbers to calculate the ionic equivalent conductances $\ell_c°$ and $\ell_a°$ in which $\ell_a° = \Lambda_0\, t_{a-}°$; $\ell_c° = \Lambda_0\, t_{c+}°$; and $\Lambda_0 = \ell_a° + \ell_c°$; $t_{a-}° = 0.604$.

In the literature we find $\ell_a° = 76.34$, $\ell_c° = 50.07$ mho cm^2/Eq.

6–4. Chloral hydrate is one of the oldest hypnotic drugs. It was synthesized in 1832 and is still of some importance in general anesthesia and in some types of neurosis. The conductance Λ_c of a 1-molar solution of NaCl in water at 25° C decreases with the addition of increasing amounts of chloral hydrate. The measured conductances Λ_c of the 1-M aqueous solution of NaCl in the presence of various amounts of chloral hydrate are

Data for *Problem 6–4*

Chloral hydrate, c (molar conc., M)	0.2	0.4	0.6	0.8
Λ_c (mho cm^2/Eq)	78.92	74.30	69.68	65.06

Barcza and Lenner[20] found a direct relationship between Λ_c and the chloral hydrate concentration, c.

(a) Plot c on he x-axis against Λ_c and extrapolate to zero concentration of chloral hydrate to get Λ_c for the 1-M aqueous solution of NaCl.

(b) Compute Λ_c for the 1-M aqueous solution of NaCl using the equation obtained in *Problem 6–3*. Do your results correlate with those obtained in *Problem 6–3*?

(c) Why does the conductivity of the 1-M aqueous solution of NaCl decrease as chloral hydrate is added?

Answers: (a) Extrapolating by eye, using a ruler, one obtains $\Lambda_c = 83$ mho cm²/Eq. By least-squares regression we obtain the linear equation, $\Lambda_c = 83.54 - 23.1c$; $r^2 = 1.000$. The intercept, 83.54 mho cm²/Eq, is the value of Λ_c for 1-M NaCl in the absence of chloral hydrate.

(b) From the equation obtained in *Problem 6–3*, $\Lambda_c(1 \text{ M}) = 126.45 - 43.70\sqrt{1.0} = 82.75$ mho cm²/Eq. That value compares well with the intercept value found above in (a).

(c) *Hint:* Consider the size and therefore the velocity of the large anionic complex relative to the small Cl^- ion,

$$CCl_3-CH{\overset{\displaystyle OH \,.}{\underset{\displaystyle OH \,.}{\diagup \atop \diagdown}}} \!\!: Cl^-$$

6–5. A 1.0 m solution of sucrose had an observed osmotic pressure of 24.8 atm at 0° C. Calculate the van't Hoff i factor for sucrose at this concentration.

Answer: i = 1.11 (a dimensionless number).

6–6.* Calcium chloride may be used to melt the ice from sidewalks. How many pounds (avoirdupois) of $CaCl_2$ are required to melt a layer of ice 0.5 inch thick on a sidewalk 50 ft long and 4 ft wide if the temperature of ice is 10° F? The molecular weight of $CaCl_2$ is 110.99 g/mole. The density of the ice at 10° F is 0.9973 g/mL, and the degree of ionization α of $CaCl_2$ is 0.8.

Answer: 145 lb (66 kg). Some ice will sublime and pass directly from the solid into the vapor state. This and other factors such as heating by the sun will render the answer given here a rough approximation. However, the calculation will give the city winter emergency crews an estimate of the amount of $CaCl_2$ needed for clearing sidewalks and streets. (*Note:* Some cities are no longer using "salt" on streets and sidewalks because of its pollution problems.)

6–7. Some cooks add salt to a kettle of water in which they are boiling peeled corn or unpeeled potatoes. In addition to improving the flavor, this practice is reputed to cook and soften the food better. (a) Is there any scientific justification for this? Explain. (b) What is the concentration of NaCl in grams of salt per kg of water needed to obtain a significant rise in the boiling point, say 5° C? (c) Would this concentration of NaCl render the food too salty to the taste?

Partial Answer: (b) Concentration of NaCl solution = 4.9 molal or 286 g salt/kg water. (c) Check with a good cook about the saltiness of the food in this concentration of salt solution.

6–8. The data for an isotonic solution of aureomycin hydrochloride is found in Table 8–4, page 183. The freezing point depression ΔT_f for a 1% solution (1 g/dL) is listed as 0.06°. (a) What is the van't Hoff factor i and the degree of dissociation α for this antibiotic in the 1% w/v solution? At this low concentration, one may assume molarity is approximately equal to molality. (b) Repeat the calculation for atropine sulfate and physostigmine salicylate, and find the i and α values for these additional two solutions.

Answers: (a) $i = 1.753$; $\alpha = 0.753$. Aureomycin is dissociated to the extent of 75.3%. (b) For the salt, $(atropine)_2 SO_4$, $i = 2.614$; $\alpha =$

0.807. For physostigmine salicylate, $i = 1.999$; $\alpha = 0.999$. Atropine sulfate is 81% dissociated and physostigmine salicylate is 99.9% dissociated.

6–9. Using the data and the value of Λ_0 given in *Problem 6–3*, compute the degree of ionization α of a 0.09-m solution of NaCl, the i value, and the freezing point depression.

Answer: You will need equation (6–27), page 129, and equations (6–32) and (6–34), page 131. $\alpha = 0.896$; $i = 1.896$; $\Delta T_f = 0.32$ deg

6–10. The equivalent conductance of a sulfonamide at 0.01 M concentration was found by experiment to be 1.104. The equivalent conductance of the drug at infinite dilution is 400.0. What is the degree of dissociation of the weak electrolyte at this concentration?

Answer: 0.00276 or 0.28%

6–11. (a) The vapor pressure of water over an aqueous solution of a drug is 721 mm Hg at 100° C. What is the activity of water in this solution? (b) Methanol has a boiling point of 64.7° C. The vapor pressure of methanol in a methanolic solution of a sulfonamide is 703 mm Hg. What is the activity of methanol in this solution at 64.7° C? (c) Chlorine has a vapor pressure of 10.0 atm at 35.6° C. In a mixture of chlorine and carbon tetrachloride the vapor pressure of chlorine is 9.30 atm at 35.6° C. What is the activity of chlorine in the mixture?

(d) Formic acid has a vapor pressure of 40.0 mm Hg at 24° C. In a mixture of formic acid and acetic acid, formic acid has a vapor pressure of 32.2 mm at 24° C. What is the activity of formic acid in the mixture?

Answer: (a) $a = 0.949$; (b) $a = 0.925$; (c) $a = 0.930$; (d) $a = 0.805$.

6–12.* The vapor pressure $p_1°$ of water at 25° C is 23.8 torr. (a) Compute the lowering of the vapor pressure of water when 25 g of $CaCl_2$ is added to 100 g of water. The molecular weight of $CaCl_2$ is 110.99 g/mole. (b) Compute the activity and the activity coefficient of water in the solution.

Answers: (a) The vapor pressure is lowered from 23.8 torr to 20.91 torr or $\Delta p_1 = 2.89$ torr. (b) $a_1 - 0.879$; $\gamma_1 = 0.915$ (you will need to calculate X_1 the mole fraction of water, to obtain this activity coefficient, 0.915, for water).

6–13. If 15 g of a strong electrolyte, NaOH, molecular weight 40.01 g/mole, is added to 100 g of water at 25° C, the vapor pressure of pure water, viz. 23.8 mm Hg, is lowered. (a) Calculate the vapor pressure of the solution. (b) The activity coefficient γ_1 of the water in the solution is given using the equation $\gamma_1 = p_1/X_1 p_1°$. This we are assured of because $\gamma_1 X_1 = a_1 = p_1/p_1°$, which we know to be the equation to obtain activities for gases and vapors. Calculate the activity coefficient and the activity of water in this solution.

Answers: (a) 20.59 torr; (b) $\gamma_1 = 0.934$; $a_1 = 0.865$

6–14. The vapor pressure of pure water (23.8 torr) at 25° C is lowered when 100 g of the nonelectrolyte, glucose, is added to 1000 g of the water. The molecular weight of glucose is 180.16 g/mole. What is the activity and the activity coefficient of water at this temperature and concentration of glucose?

Answer: $a_1 = 0.990$; $\gamma_1 = 1.000$. Thus in a 100·g/kg H_2O solution of glucose (fairly concentrated, 0.56 molal), both the activity and the activity coefficient of water may be taken as approximately equal to 1.0. This is not so for a solution of an electrolyte, as seen in *Problems 6–12* and *6–13*.

6–15. Compute the mean ionic activity coefficient of a 0.01-M aqueous solution of diphenylhydantoin sodium containing 0.01 M KCl at 25° C. Use the limiting Debye-Hückel equation.

Answer: $\gamma_\pm = 0.85$

6–16. Using the extended Debye–Hückel equation, compute the mean ionic activity coefficient of a 0.05-M solution of epinephrine hydrochloride containing a 0.05 M potassium chloride.

Answer: $\gamma_\pm = 0.75$

6–17. (a) What amount of $CaCl_2$ (in moles/liter) should be added to a 0.02-M solution of neomycin sulfate to produce an ionic strength of 0.09?

(b) Calculate the mean ionic activity and the mean ionic activity coefficient for the 0.02-M solution of neomycin sulfate at an ionic strength of 0.09 and 25° C. Use both equations (6–58) and (6–60) (pp. 135, 136) and compare the results.

---

*Problems 6–6 and 6–12 are modified from J. W. Moncrief and W. H. Jones, *Elements of Physical Chemistry*, Addison-Wesley, Reading, Mass., 1977, pp. 146 and 124, respectively.

Answers: (a) 0.01 M $CaCl_2$. (b) From equation (6–58), $\gamma_\pm = 0.494$ and $a_\pm = 0.0157$. From equation (6–60), $\gamma_\pm = 0.582$ and $a_\pm = 0.0185$. The results from the two equations are different. The ionic strength of the solution is 0.02 M, so equation (6–60) is required.

6–18. King and associates[21] investigated the properties of a new anticancer agent, brequinar sodium. The solubility in water at room temperature ($\approx 23°$ C) was found to be 0.274 M. The compound is a 1:1 electrolyte.

(a) Compute the mean ionic activity and the mean ionic activity coefficient in the saturated solution (0.274 M) at 23° C.

(b) After adding a 0.01-M solution of NaCl the solubility decreased because of the common ion effect, Na^+ being the common ion (see p. 231). The new solubility value was 0.245 M. Compute new values for the mean ionic activity and the mean ionic activity coefficient. Choose the proper equation to obtain the most accurate value for $\gamma_\pm$.

Answers: (a) The ionic strength is 0.274; $\gamma_\pm = 0.668$ (equation 6–60) and $a_\pm = 0.183$. (b) The ionic strength is 0.245 for the drug and 0.01 for NaCl; $\gamma_\pm = 0.674$ and $a_\pm = 0.165$.

6–19. A solution contains 0.003 M of sodium phenobarbital together with a buffer consisting of 0.20 M sodium acetate and 0.30 M acetic acid. Acetic acid is a weak electrolyte; its degree, or fraction, of dissociation α at this concentration is 0.008 and the undissociated species do not contribute to the ionic strength. What is the ionic strength of the solution?

Answer: $\mu = 0.205$

6–20. A solution contains 0.05 M $AlCl_3$ and 0.2 M Na_2HPO_4. What is the ionic strength of this solution?

Answer: 0.90

6–21. Ringer's solution USP has been designed to have approximately the same ionic strength as that of normal blood. Calculate the ionic strength of blood from the concentration of the constituents of Ringer's solution.

Answer: $\mu = 0.16$

6–22. The freezing point depression of a solution containing 4 g of methapyrilene hydrochloride in 100 mL of solution was 0.423°. Methapyrilene hydrochloride dissociates into two ions and has a molecular weight of 297.85. Calculate (a) the van't Hoff factor i, (b) the osmotic coefficient g, and (c) the L value for the drug at this concentration.

Answer: (a) $i = 1.69$; (b) $g = 0.85$; (c) $L = 3.16$

6–23. The equivalent conductance of acetic acid is 48.15 mho cm²/Eq at a concentration of 1×10^{-3} mole/liter. The value at infinite dilution as calculated in *Problem 6–2* is 390.7. Compute α, i, and L at this concentration.

Answer: $\alpha = 0.12$; $i = 1.12$; $L = 2.1$

6–24. The L_{iso} value of an aqueous solution of ascorbic acid is 1.90 and its osmotic pressure at 37° is $\pi = 1182$ mm Hg. Compute i, ΔT_f, and the degree of dissociation α.

Answer: $i = 1.02$; $\Delta T_f = 0.11°$; $\alpha = 0.02$ or 2% dissociated

6–25. Calculate the freezing point depression and the milliosmolality of 0.25-M solutions of sodium iodide, sodium bicarbonate, and calcium chloride, and of 340 millimolal solutions of griseofulvin and pentobarbital. What is the osmotic pressure in atmospheres of the sodium bicarbonate solution; of the pentobarbital solution at 25° C?

(*Hint:* Sodium bicarbonate, like sodium iodide, provides two particles in solution. Pentobarbital and grisseofulvin can be assumed to be nonelectrolytes, and the i value for their solutions is taken as unity. For $CaCl_2$, $i = 2.6$.)

Partial Answer: Milliosmolality of sodium iodide is 465 mOsm/kg and its freezing point depression is 0.86° C. The osmotic pressure of the pentobarbital solution is 8.3 atm.

6–26. A 0.120-molal solution of potassium bromide has a milliosmolality of 1.86×120 millimolal $= 223$ mOsm/kg (see *Example 6–16*, p. 139). The density of water at 25° C is 0.997 g/cm³, and the partial molar volume of KBr is $\bar{v}_2^° = 33.97$ cm³/mole. Calculate the milliosmolarity, mOsm/(liter solution), of this KBr solution using equation (6–66).

Answer: 214.8 mOsm/(liter solution).

6–27. Partial pressures (in mm Hg), p_1, of acetone at various mole fractions, X_1, are given in the following table for a mixture of acetone and chloroform.

Data for *Problem 6–27*

X_1	1.000	0.950	0.925	0.878	0.710	0.575
p_1(mm)	344.5	327.5*	317.0*	299.7	230.7	173.7

*These points have been added to the data.
Source: Data from J. von Zawidzki as reported by I. M. Klotz and R. M. Rosenberg, *Chemical Thermodynamics*, W. A. Benjamin, Menlo Park, Cal., 1972, pp. 355, 356. Some points are omitted and two points have been added near $X_1 = 1.000$.

(a) Compute the activity and activity coefficient for acetone at various X_1 values in these solutions.

(b) Plot both the experimental p_1 values and the Raoult law pressures versus X_1. Discuss the deviations from Raoult's law and its implications regarding possible intermolecular interaction between chloroform and acetone.

Partial Answer: (a) X_1 1.0   0.878   0.575
             a_1 1.0   0.870   0.504
             γ_1 1.0   0.991   0.877
This tabular answer states that when $X_1 = 1.0$, $a_1 = 1.0$ and $\gamma_1 = 1.0$, and so on

6–28. The mole fraction concentrations and vapor pressures in mm Hg (torr) for a new general anesthetic, theasotrate, in ethanol at 45° C are given in the table below. Calculate the activities and activity coefficients for the new drug.

Data for *Problem 6–28*

X_1	1.000	0.942	0.740	0.497
p_1(mm)	402	377	277	174

Partial Answer: For $X_1 = 0.942$, $a_1 = 0.938$, $\gamma_1 = 0.996$

7
Ionic Equilibria

Modern Theories of Acids, Bases, and Salts
Acid–Base Equilibria
Sörensen's pH Scale

Species Concentration as a Function of pH
Calculation of pH
Acidity Constants

MODERN THEORIES OF ACIDS, BASES, AND SALTS

As pointed out in the previous chapter, Arrhenius defined an acid as a substance that liberates hydrogen ions and a base as a substance that supplies hydroxyl ions on dissociation. Because of a need for a broader concept, Brönsted in Copenhagen and Lowry in London independently proposed parallel theories in 1923.[1] The *Brönsted–Lowry theory*, as it has come to be known, is more useful than the Arrhenius theory for the representation of ionization in both aqueous and nonaqueous systems.

Brönsted–Lowry Theory. According to the Brönsted–Lowry theory, an acid is a substance, charged or uncharged, that is capable of donating a proton; and a base is a substance, charged or uncharged, that is capable of accepting a proton from an acid. The relative strengths of acids and bases are measured by the tendencies of these substances to give up and take on protons. Hydrochloric acid is a strong acid in water since it gives up its proton readily, whereas acetic acid is a weak acid because it gives up its proton only to a small extent. The strength of an acid or base varies with the solvent. Hydrochloric acid is a weak acid in glacial acetic acid and acetic acid is a strong acid in liquid ammonia. Consequently, the strength of an acid depends not only on its ability to give up a proton, but also on the ability of the solvent to accept the proton from the acid. This is called the *basic strength* of the solvent.

Solvents may be classified as protophilic, protogenic, amphiprotic, and aprotic. A *protophilic* or basic solvent is one that is capable of accepting protons from the solute. Such solvents as acetone, ether, and liquid ammonia fall into this group. A *protogenic* solvent is a proton-donating compound and is represented by acids such as formic acid, acetic acid, sulfuric acid, liquid HCl, and liquid HF. *Amphiprotic* solvents act as both

proton acceptors and proton donors, and this class includes water and the alcohols. *Aprotic* solvents, such as the hydrocarbons, neither accept nor donate protons, and, being neutral in this sense, they are useful for studying the reactions of acids and bases free of solvent effects.

In the Brönsted–Lowry classification, acids and bases may be anions such as HSO_4^- and CH_3COO^-, cations such as NH_4^+ and H_3O^+, or neutral molecules such as HCl and NH_3. Water can act as either an acid or a base and thus is amphiprotic. Acid–base reactions occur when an acid reacts with a base to form a new acid and a new base. Since the reactions involve a transfer of a proton, they are known as *protolytic reactions* or *protolysis*.

In the reaction between HCl and water, HCl is the acid and water the base.

$$HCl + H_2O \rightarrow H_3O^+ + Cl^- \qquad (7-1)$$
$$\text{Acid}_1 \quad \text{Base}_2 \quad \text{Acid}_2 \quad \text{Base}_1$$

Acid_1 and base_1 stand for an *acid–base pair* or *conjugate pair*, as do acid_2 and base_2. Since the bare proton, H^+, is practically nonexistent in aqueous solution, what is normally referred to as the hydrogen ion consists of the hydrated proton, H_3O^+, known as the *hydronium ion*. Higher solvated forms may also exist in solution.[*] In an ethanolic solution, the "hydrogen ion" is the proton attached to a molecule of solvent, represented as $C_2H_5OH_2^+$. In equation (7-1), hydrogen chloride, the acid, has donated a proton to water, the base, to form the corresponding acid, H_3O^+, and the base, Cl^-.

---

*Reports have appeared in the literature[2] describing the discovery of a polymer of the hydrogen ion consisting of 21 molecules of water surrounding one hydrogen ion, namely

$$H^+ \cdot (H_2O)_{21}$$

The reaction of HCl with water is one of ionization. Neutralization and hydrolysis are also considered as acid–base reactions or protolysis following the broad definitions of the Brönsted–Lowry concept. Several examples illustrate these types of reactions, as shown in Table 7–1. The displacement reaction, a special type of neutralization, involves the displacement of a weaker acid, acetic, from its salt in the reaction shown below.

Lewis Electronic Theory. Other theories have been suggested for describing acid–base reactions, the most familiar of which is the *electronic theory* of Lewis.[3]

According to the Lewis theory, an acid is a molecule or ion that accepts an electron pair to form a covalent bond. A base is a substance that provides the pair of unshared electrons by which the base coordinates with an acid. Certain compounds, such as boron trifluoride and aluminum chloride, although not containing hydrogen and consequently not serving as proton donors, are nevertheless acids in this scheme. Many substances that do not contain hydroxyl ions, including amines, ethers, and carboxylic acid anhydrides, are classified as bases according to the Lewis definition. Two Lewis acid-base reactions follow:

$$
\text{H}^+ \text{ (solvated)} + \underset{\text{Base}}{:\overset{\overset{\displaystyle H}{|}}{\underset{\underset{\displaystyle H}{|}}{N}}-H} = \left[\text{H}\!:\!\overset{\overset{\displaystyle \cdot\cdot}{N}}{\underset{\underset{\displaystyle \cdot\cdot}{H}}{}}\!:\!\text{H} \right]^+ \quad (7\text{--}2)
$$

$$
\underset{\text{Acid}}{\overset{\overset{\displaystyle Cl}{|}}{\underset{\underset{\displaystyle Cl}{|}}{Cl-B}}} + \underset{\text{Base}}{:O\!\!\begin{matrix} \diagup CH_3 \\ \diagdown CH_3 \end{matrix}} = \overset{\overset{\displaystyle Cl}{|}}{\underset{\underset{\displaystyle Cl}{|}}{Cl-B\!:\!O}}\begin{matrix} \diagup CH_3 \\ \diagdown CH_3 \end{matrix} \quad (7\text{--}3)
$$

The Lewis system is probably too broad for convenient application to ordinary acid–base reactions, and those processes that are most conveniently expressed in terms of this electronic classification should be referred to simply as a form of electron sharing rather than as acid–base reactions.[4] The Lewis theory is finding increasing use for describing the mechanism of many organic and inorganic reactions. It will be mentioned again in the chapters on solubility and complexation. The Brönsted–Lowry nomenclature is particularly useful for describing ionic equilibria and is used extensively in this chapter.

TABLE 7–1. *Examples of Acid–Base Reactions*

	Acid$_1$		Base$_2$		Acid$_2$		Base$_1$
Neutralization	NH_4^+	+	OH^-	=	H_2O	+	NH_3
Neutralization	H_3O^+	+	OH^-	=	H_2O	+	H_2O
Neutralization	HCl	+	NH_3	=	NH_4^+	+	Cl^-
Hydrolysis	H_2O	+	CH_3COO^-	=	CH_3COOH	+	OH^-
Hydrolysis	NH_4^+	+	H_2O	=	H_3O^+	+	NH_3
Displacement	HCl	+	CH_3COO^-	=	CH_3COOH	+	Cl^-

ACID–BASE EQUILIBRIA

Equilibrium may be defined as a balance between two opposing forces or actions. This statement does not imply cesssation of the opposing reactions, suggesting rather a dynamic equality between the velocities of the two. Chemical equilibrium maintains the concentrations of the reactants and products constant.

Most chemical reactions proceed in both a forward and reverse direction if the products of the reaction are not removed as they form. Some reactions, however, proceed nearly to completion and, for practical purposes, may be regarded as irreversible. The topic, chemical equilibria, is concerned with truly reversible systems and includes reactions such as the ionization of weak electrolytes.

The ionization or protolysis of a weak electrolyte, acetic acid, in water may be written in the Brönsted–Lowry manner as

$$\underset{\text{Acid}_1}{\text{HAc}} + \underset{\text{Base}_2}{\text{H}_2\text{O}} \rightleftharpoons \underset{\text{Acid}_2}{\text{H}_3\text{O}^+} + \underset{\text{Base}_1}{\text{Ac}^-} \quad (7\text{--}4)$$

The arrows pointing in the forward and reverse directions indicate that the reaction is proceeding to the right and left simultaneously. According to the law of mass action, the velocity or rate of the forward reaction R_f is proportion to the concentration of the reactants:

$$R_f = k_1 \times [\text{HAc}]^1 \times [\text{H}_2\text{O}]^1 \quad (7\text{--}5)$$

The speed of the reaction is usually expressed in terms of the decrease in the concentration of either of the reactants per unit time. The terms, rate, speed, and velocity, have the same meaning here. The reverse reaction

$$R_r = k_2 \times [\text{H}_3\text{O}^+]^1 \times [\text{Ac}^-]^1 \quad (7\text{--}6)$$

expresses the rate R_r of reformation of un-ionized acetic acid. Since only one mole of each constituent appears in the reaction, each term is raised to the first power, and the exponents need not appear in subsequent expressions for the dissociation of acetic acid and similar acids and bases. The symbols k_1 and k_2 are proportionality constants commonly known as *specific reaction rates* for the forward and the reverse reactions, respectively, and the brackets [ ] indicate concentrations. A better representation of the facts would be had by replacing concentrations with activities, but for the present discussion, the approximate equations are adequate.

Ionization of Weak Acids. According to the concept of equilibrium, the rate of the forward reaction decreases with time as acetic acid is depleted, whereas the rate of the reverse reaction begins at zero and increases as larger quantities of hydrogen ions and acetate ions are formed. Finally, a balance is attained when the two rates are equal, that is, when

$$R_f = R_r \quad (7\text{--}7)$$

The *concentrations* of products and reactants are not necessarily equal at equilibrium; it is the *speeds* of the forward and reverse reactions that are the same. Since equation (7–7) applies at equilibrium, equations (7–5) and (7–6) may be set equal:

$$k_1 \times [HAc] \times [H_2O] = k_2 \times [H_3O^+] \times [Ac^-] \qquad (7-8)$$

and solving for the ratio, k_1/k_1, one obtains

$$k = \frac{k_1}{k_2} = \frac{[H_3O^+][Ac^-]}{[HAc][H_2O]} \qquad (7-9)$$

In dilute solutions of acetic acid, water is in sufficient excess to be regarded as constant at about 55.3 moles per liter (1 liter H_2O at 25° C weights 997.07 g, and 997.07/18.02 = 55.3). It is thus combined with k_1/k_2 to yield a new constant K_a, the *ionization constant* or the *dissociation constant* of acetic acid.

$$K_a = 55.3\, k = \frac{[H_3O^+][Ac^-]}{[HAc]} \qquad (7-10)$$

Equation (7–10) is the equilibrium expression for the dissociation of acetic acid, and the dissociation constant K_a is an equilibrium constant in which the essentially constant concentration of the solvent is incorporated. In the discussion of equilibria involving charged as well as uncharged acids, according to the Brönsted–Lowry nomenclature, the term *ionization constant K_a* is not satisfactory and is replaced by the name *acidity constant*. Similarly, for charged and uncharged bases, the term *basicity constant* is now often used for K_b, to be discussed in the next section.

In general, the acidity constant for an uncharged weak acid, HB, may be expressed by the following:

$$HB + H_2O \rightleftharpoons H_3O^+ + B^- \qquad (7-11)$$

$$K_a = \frac{[H_3O^+][B^-]}{[HB]} \qquad (7-12)$$

Equation (7–10) may be presented in a more general form using the symbol c to represent the initial molar concentration of acetic acid and x to represent the concentration $[H_3O^+]$. The latter quantity is also equal to $[Ac^-]$ since both ions are formed in equimolar concentration. The concentration of acetic acid remaining at equilibrium $[HAc]$ can be expressed as $c - x$. The reaction, equation (7–4), is

$$\begin{array}{ccc} HAc + H_2O \rightleftharpoons & H_3O^+ + & Ac^- \\ (c - x) & x & x \end{array} \qquad (7-13)$$

and the equilibrium expression (7–10) becomes

$$K_a = \frac{x^2}{c - x} \qquad (7-14)$$

in which c is large in comparison with x. The term $c - x$ may be replaced by c without appreciable error, giving the equation

$$K_a \cong \frac{x^2}{c} \qquad (7-15)$$

which may be rearranged as follows for the calculation of the hydrogen ion concentration of weak acids:

$$x^2 = K_a c$$

$$x = [H_3O^+] = \sqrt{K_a c} \qquad (7-16)$$

Example 7–1. In a liter of a 0.1-*M* solution, acetic acid was found by conductivity analysis to dissociate into 1.32×10^{-3} gram ions ("moles") each of hydrogen and acetate ion at 25° C. What is the acidity or dissociation constant K_a for acetic acid?

According to equation (7–4), at equilibrium, 1 mole of acetic acid has dissociated into 1 mole each of hydrogen ion and acetate ion. The concentration of ions is expressed as moles per liter and less frequently as molality. A solution containing 1.0078 g of hydrogen ions in a liter represents 1 gram ion or 1 mole of hydrogen ions. The molar concentration of each of these ions is expressed as x. If the original amount of acetic acid was 0.1 mole per liter, then at equilibrium the undissociated acid would equal $0.1 - x$, since x is the amount of acid that has dissociated. The calculations according to equation (7–12) are:

$$K_a = \frac{(1.32 \times 10^{-3})^2}{0.1 - (1.32 \times 10^{-3})}$$

It is of little significance to retain the small number, 1.32×10^{-3}, in the denominator, and the calculations become

$$K_a = \frac{(1.32 \times 10^{-3})^2}{0.1}$$

$$K_a = \frac{1.74 \times 10^{-6}}{1 \times 10^{-1}} = 1.74 \times 10^{-5}$$

The value of K_a in *Example 7–1* means that, at equilibrium, the ratio of the product of the ionic concentrations to that of the undissociated acid is 1.74×10^{-5}; that is to say, the dissociation of acetic acid into its ions is small, and acetic acid may be considered as a weak electrolyte.

When a salt formed from a strong acid and a weak base, ammonium chloride, is dissolved in water, it dissociates completely as follows:

$$NH_4^+Cl^- \xrightarrow{H_2O} NH_4^+ + Cl^- \qquad (7-17)$$

The Cl^- is the conjugate base of a strong acid, HCl, which is 100% ionized in water. Thus, the Cl^- cannot react any further. In the Brönsted–Lowry system, NH_4^+ is considered to be a cationic acid that can form its conjugate base, NH_3, by donating a proton to water as follows:

$$NH_4^+ + H_2O \rightleftharpoons H_3O^+ + NH_3 \qquad (7-18)$$

$$K_a = \frac{[H_3O^+][NH_3]}{[NH_4^+]} \qquad (7-19)$$

In general, for charged acids, BH^+, the reaction is written

$$BH^+ + H_2O \rightleftharpoons H_3O^+ + B \qquad (7-20)$$

and the acidity constant is

$$K_a = \frac{[H_3O^+][B]}{[BH^+]} \qquad (7-21)$$

Ionization of Weak Bases. Nonionized weak bases, B, exemplified by NH_3, react with water as follows:

$$B + H_2O \rightleftharpoons OH^- + BH^+ \qquad (7-22)$$

$$K_b = \frac{[OH^-][BH^+]}{[B]} \qquad (7-23)$$

which, by a procedure like that used to obtain equation (7-16), leads to:

$$[OH^-] = \sqrt{K_b c} \qquad (7-24)$$

Example 7-2. The basicity or ionization constant K_b for morphine base is 7.4×10^{-7} at 25° C. What is the hydroxyl ion concentration of a 0.0005-M aqueous solution of morphine?

$$[OH^-] = \sqrt{7.4 \times 10^{-7} \times 5.0 \times 10^{-4}}$$
$$[OH^-] = \sqrt{37.0 \times 10^{-11}} = \sqrt{3.7 \times 10^{-10}}$$
$$x = [OH^-] = 1.92 \times 10^{-5} \text{ moles/liter}$$

Salts of strong bases and weak acids, such as sodium acetate, dissociate completely in acqueous solution to given ions:

$$Na^+CH_3COO^- \xrightarrow{H_2O} Na^+ + CH_3COO^- \qquad (7-25)$$

The sodium ion cannot react with water, since it would form NaOH, which is a strong electrolyte and would dissociate completely into its ions. The acetate anion is a Brönsted–Lowry weak base, and

$$CH_3COO^- + H_2O \rightleftharpoons OH^- + CH_3COOH$$

$$K_b = \frac{[OH^-][CH_3COOH]}{[CH_3COO^-]} \qquad (7-26)$$

In general, for an anionic base, B^-

$$B^- + H_2O \rightleftharpoons OH^- + HB$$

$$K_b = \frac{[OH^-][HB]}{[B^-]} \qquad (7-27)$$

The acidity and basicity constants for a number of pharmaceutically important acids and bases are listed in Tables 7-2 and 7-3. The last column gives the *dissociation exponent* or pK value, which is discussed on pages 152 and 162.

The Ionization of Water. The concentration of hydrogen or hydroxyl ions in solutions of acids or bases may be expressed as gram ions per liter or as moles per liter. A solution containing 17.008 g of hydroxyl ions or 1.008 g of hydrogen ions per liter is said to contain 1 gram ion or 1 mole of hydroxyl or hydrogen ions per liter. Owing to the ionization of water, it is possible to establish a quantitative relationship between the hydrogen and hydroxyl ion concentration of any aqueous solution.

The concentration of either the hydrogen or the hydroxyl ion in acidic, neutral, or basic solutions is usually expressed in terms of the hydrogen ion concentration or, more conveniently, in pH units.

In a manner corresponding to the dissociation of weak acids and bases, water ionizes slightly to yield hydrogen and hydroxyl ions. As previously observed, a weak electrolyte requires the presence of water or some other polar solvent for ionization. Accordingly, one molecule of water may be thought of as a weak electrolytic solute that reacts with another molecule of water as the solvent. This *autoprotolytic* reaction is represented as

$$H_2O + H_2O \rightleftharpoons H_3O^+ + OH^- \qquad (7-28)$$

The law of mass action is then applied to give the equilibrium expression

$$\frac{[H_3O^+][OH^-]}{[H_2O]^2} = k \qquad (7-29)$$

The term for molecular water in the denominator is squared since the reactant is raised to a power equal to the number of molecules appearing in the equation, as required by the law of mass action. Because molecular water exists in great excess relative to the concentrations of hydrogen and hydroxyl ions, $[H_2O]^2$ is considered as a constant and is combined with k to give a new constant, K_w, known as the *dissociation constant*, the *autoprotolysis constant*, or the *ion product* of water:

$$K_w = k \times [H_2O]^2 \qquad (7-30)$$

The value of the ion product is approximately 1×10^{-14} at 25° C; it depends strongly upon temperature, as shown in Table 7-4. In any calculations involving the ion product, one must be certain to use the proper value of K_w for the temperature at which the data are obtained.

Substituting equation (7-30) into (7-29) gives the common expression for the ionization of water:

$$[H_3O^+] \times [OH^-] = K_w \cong 1 \times 10^{-14} \text{ at 25° C} \qquad (7-31)$$

In *pure* water, the hydrogen and hydroxyl ion concentrations are equal, and each has the value of approximately 1×10^{-7} mole per liter at 25° C.*

$$[H_3O^+] = [OH^-] \cong \sqrt{1 \times 10^{-14}} \qquad (7-32)$$
$$\cong 1 \times 10^{-7}$$

When an acid is added to pure water, some hydroxyl ions, provided by the ionization of water, must always remain. The increase in hydrogen ions is offset by a decrease in the hydroxyl ions, so that K_w remains constant at about 1×10^{-14} at 25° C.

Example 7-3. A quantity of HCl (1.5×10^{-3} M) is added to water at 25° C to increase the hydrogen ion concentration from 1×10^{-7} to 1.5×10^{-3} moles per liter. What is the new hydroxyl ion concentration?

From equation (7-31),

$$[OH^-] = \frac{1 \times 10^{-14}}{1.5 \times 10^{-3}}$$
$$= 6.7 \times 10^{-12} \text{ moles/liter}$$

Relationship Between K_a and K_b. A simple relationship exists between the dissociation constant of a weak acid, HB, and that of its conjugate base, B^-, or between

---

*Under laboratory conditions, distilled water in equilibrium with air contains about 0.03% by volume of CO_2, corresponding to a hydrogen ion concentration of about 2×10^{-6} (pH $\cong$ 5.7).

TABLE 7–2. *Ionization or Acidity Constants for Weak Acids at 25° C*

Weak Acids	MW	K_a		pK_a
Acetaminophen	151.16		1.20×10^{-10}	9.92
Acetic	60.05		1.75×10^{-5}	4.76
Acetylsalicylic	180.15		3.27×10^{-4}	3.49
p-Aminobenzoic acid	137.13	K_1	2.24×10^{-5}	4.65
		K_2	1.58×10^{-5}	4.80
Amobarbital	226.27		1.15×10^{-8}	7.94
Ascorbic	176.12	K_1	5.0×10^{-5}	4.3
		K_2	1.6×10^{-12}	11.8
Barbital	184.19		1.23×10^{-8}	7.91
Barbituric	128.09		1.05×10^{-4}	3.98
Benzoic	122.12		6.30×10^{-5}	4.20
Benzyl penicillin	334.38		1.74×10^{-3}	2.76
Boric	61.84	K_1	5.8×10^{-10}	9.24
Butylparaben	194.22		4.0×10^{-9}	8.4
Caffeine	194.19		1×10^{-14}	14.0
Carbonic	44.01	K_1	4.31×10^{-7}	6.37
		K_2	4.7×10^{-11}	10.33
Citric (1 H₂O)	210.14	K_1	7.0×10^{-4}	3.15
		K_2	1.66×10^{-5}	4.78
		K_3	4.0×10^{-7}	6.40
Dichloroacetic	128.95		5×10^{-2}	1.3
Formic	48.02		1.77×10^{-4}	3.75
Fumaric	116.07	K_1	9.3×10^{-4}	3.03
		K_2	4.2×10^{-5}	4.38
Gallic	170.1		4×10^{-5}	4.4
α-D-Glucose	180.16		8.6×10^{-13}	12.1
Glycerophosphoric	172.08	K_1	3.4×10^{-2}	1.47
		K_2	6.4×10^{-7}	6.19
Glycine (protonated cation)	75.07	K_1	4.5×10^{-3}	2.35
		K_2	1.7×10^{-10}	9.78
Hydroquinone	110.11		1.1×10^{-10} (18°)	9.96
Lactic	90.08		1.39×10^{-4}	3.86
Maleic	116.07	K_1	1.0×10^{2}	2.00
		K_2	5.5×10^{-7}	6.26
Malic	134.09	K_1	4×10^{-4}	3.4
		K_3	9×10^{-6}	5.1
Malonic	104.06	K_1	1.40×10^{-3}	2.85
		K_2	2.0×10^{-6}	5.70
Mandelic	152.14		4.29×10^{-4}	3.37
Methylparaben	152.14		4.0×10^{-9}	8.4
Monochloroacetic	94.50		1.40×10^{-3}	2.86
Oxalic (2 H₂O)	126.07	K_1	5.5×10^{-2}	1.26
		K_2	5.3×10^{-5}	4.28
Penicillin V	350.38		1.86×10^{-3}	2.73
Pentobarbital	226.28		1.0×10^{-8}	8.0
Phenobarbital	232.23		3.9×10^{-8}	7.41
Phenol	95.12		1×10^{-10}	10.0
Phenytoin (Dilantin)	252.26		7.9×10^{-9}	8.1
Phosphoric	98.00	K_1	7.5×10^{-3}	2.12
		K_2	6.2×10^{-8}	7.21
		K_3	2.1×10^{-13}	12.67
Picric	229.11		4.2×10^{-1}	0.38
Propionic	74.08		1.34×10^{-5}	4.87
Propylparaben	180.20		4.0×10^{-9}	8.4
Saccharin	183.18		2.1×10^{-12}	11.7
Salicylic	138.12		1.06×10^{-3}	2.97
Succinic	118.09	K_1	6.4×10^{-5}	4.19
		K_2	2.3×10^{-6}	5.63
Sucrose	342.30		2.4×10^{-13} (19° C)	12.62
Sulfacetamide	214.24		1.35×10^{-6}	5.87
Sulfadiazine	250.28		3.3×10^{-7}	6.48
Sulfamerazine	264.30		8.7×10^{-8}	7.06
Sulfapyridine	249.29		3.6×10^{-9}	8.44
Sulfathiazole	255.32		7.6×10^{-8}	7.12
Sulfisomidine	278.34		3.4×10^{-8}	7.47
Sulfisoxazole	267.30		1.0×10^{-5}	5.0
Tartaric	150.09	K_1	9.6×10^{-4}	3.02
		K_2	4.4×10^{-5}	4.36
Tetracycline	444.43	K_1	5.01×10^{-4}	3.30
		K_2	2.09×10^{-8}	7.68
		K_3	2.04×10^{-10}	9.69
Trichloroacetic	163.40		1.3×10^{-1}	0.89
Valeric	102.13		1.56×10^{-5}	4.81

TABLE 7-3. *Ionization or Basicity Constants for Weak Bases at 25° C**

Weak Bases	MW	K_b		pK_b	pK_a (conjugate acid)
Acetanilide	135.16		4.1×10^{-14} (40°)	13.39	0.61
Ammonia	35.05		1.74×10^{-5}	4.76	9.24
Apomorphine	267.31		1.0×10^{-7}	7.00	7.00
Atropine	289.4		4.5×10^{-5}	4.35	9.65
Benzocaine	165.19		6.0×10^{-12}	11.22	2.78
Caffeine	194.19	K_1	3.98×10^{-11}	10.4	3.6
		K_2	4.07×10^{-14}	13.4	0.6
Cocaine	303.35		2.6×10^{-6}	5.59	8.41
Codeine	299.36		1.6×10^{-6}	5.8	8.2
Ephedrine	165.23		2.3×10^{-5}	4.64	9.36
Epinephrine	183.20	K_1	7.9×10^{-5}	4.1	9.9
		K_2	3.2×10^{-6}	5.5	8.5
Erythromycin	733.92		6.3×10^{-6}	5.2	8.8
Ethylenediamine	60.10		7.1×10^{-8}	7.15	6.85
Glycine	75.07		2.3×10^{-12}	11.65	2.35
Hydroquinone	110.11		4.7×10^{-6}	5.33	8.67
Morphine	285.33		7.4×10^{-7}	6.13	7.87
Nalorphine	311.37		6.3×10^{-7}	6.2	7.8
Papaverine	339.39		8×10^{-9}	8.1	5.9
Physostigmine	275.34	K_1	7.6×10^{-7}	6.12	7.88
		K_2	5.7×10^{-13}	12.24	1.76
Pilocarpine	208.25	K_1	7×10^{-8}	7.2	6.8
		K_2	2×10^{-13}	12.7	1.3
Procaine	236.30		7×10^{-6}	5.2	8.8
Pyridine	79.10		1.4×10^{-9}	8.85	5.15
Quinacrine (dihydrochloride)	472.88		1.0×10^{-6}	6.0	8.0
Quinine	324.41	K_1	1.0×10^{-6}	6.00	8.00
		K_2	1.3×10^{-10}	9.89	4.11
Reserpine	608		4×10^{-8}	7.4	6.6
Scopolamine	303.35		1.6×10^{-6}	5.8	8.2
Strychnine	334.40	K_1	1×10^{-6}	6.0	8.0
		K_2	2×10^{-12}	11.7	2.3
Theobromine	180.17	K_1	7.76×10^{-7}	6.11	7.89
		K_2	4.8×10^{-14}	13.3	0.7
Theophylline	180.17	K_1	1.58×10^{-9}	8.80	5.20
		K_2	5.0×10^{-14}	13.3	0.7
Thiourea	76.12		1.25×10^{-12}	11.90	2.1
Tolbutamide	270.34		2.0×10^{-9}	8.7	5.3
Urea	60.06		1.5×10^{-14}	13.82	0.18

*Additional pKs for acids and bases of pharmaceutical interest are found in R. F. Doerge, Ed., *Wilson and Gisvold's Textbook of Organic Medicinal and Pharmaceutical Chemistry*, 8th Ed., Lippincott, Philadelphia, 1982, pp. 841–847; D. W. Newton and R. B. Kluza. Drug Intel. Clin. Pharm. **12,** 546, 1978.

TABLE 7-4. *Ion Product of Water at Various Temperatures**

Temperature (°C)	$K_w \times 10^{14}$	pK_w
0	0.1139	14.944
10	0.2920	14.535
20	0.6809	14.167
24	1.000	14.000
25	1.008	13.997
30	1.469	13.833
37	2.57	13.59
40	2.919	13.535
50	5.474	13.262
60	9.614	13.017
70	15.1	12.82
80	23.4	12.63
90	35.5	12.45
100	51.3	12.29
300	400	11.40

*From Harned and Robinson, Trans. Far. Soc. **36,** 973, 1940, and other sources.

BH^+ and B, when the solvent is amphiprotic. This can be obtained by multiplying equation (7–12) by equation (7–27):

$$K_a K_b = \frac{[H_3O^+][B^-]}{[HB]} \cdot \frac{[OH^-][HB]}{[B^-]} \qquad (7\text{–}33)$$

$$= [H_3O^+][OH^-] = K_w$$

and

$$K_b = \frac{K_w}{K_a} \qquad (7\text{–}34)$$

or

$$K_a = \frac{K_w}{K_b} \qquad (7\text{–}35)$$

Example 7–4. Ammonia has a K_b of 1.74×10^{-5} at 25° C. Calculate K_a for its conjugate acid, NH_4^+.

$$K_a = \frac{K_w}{K_b} = \frac{1.00 \times 10^{-14}}{1.74 \times 10^{-5}}$$

$$= 5.75 \times 10^{-10}$$

Ionization of Polyprotic Electrolytes. Acids that donate a single proton and bases that accept a single proton are called *monoprotic electrolytes*. A polyprotic (polybasic) acid is one that is capable of donating two or more protons, and a polyprotic base is capable of accepting two or more protons. A diprotic (dibasic) acid, such as carbonic acid, ionizes in two stages, and a triprotic (tribasic) acid, such as phosphoric acid, ionizes in three stages. The equilibria involved in the protolysis or ionization of phosphoric acid, together with the equilibrium expressions, are

$$H_3PO_4 + H_2O = H_3O^+ + H_2PO_4^- \qquad (7\text{--}36)$$

$$\frac{[H_3O^+][H_2PO_4^-]}{[H_3PO_4]} = K_1 = 7.5 \times 10^{-3} \qquad (7\text{--}37)$$

$$H_2PO_4^- + H_2O = H_3O^+ + HPO_4^{2-}$$

$$\frac{[H_3O^+][HPO_4^{2-}]}{[H_2PO_4^-]} = K_2 = 6.2 \times 10^{-8} \qquad (7\text{--}38)$$

$$HPO_4^{2-} + H_2O = H_3O^+ + PO_4^{3-}$$

$$\frac{[H_3O^+][PO_4^{3-}]}{[HPO_4^{2-}]} = K_3 = 2.1 \times 10^{-13} \qquad (7\text{--}39)$$

In any polyprotic electrolyte, the primary protolysis is greatest, and succeeding stages become less complete at any given acid concentration.

The negative charges on the ion HPO_4^{2-} make it difficult for water to remove the proton from the phosphate ion, as reflected in the small value of K_3. Thus, phosphoric acid is weak in the third stage of ionization, and a solution of this acid contains practically no PO_4^{3-} ions.

Each of the species formed by the ionization of a polyprotic acid can also act as a base. Thus, for the phosphoric acid system:

$$PO_4^{3-} + H_2O \rightleftharpoons HPO_4^{2-} + OH^- \qquad (7\text{--}40)$$

$$K_{b1} = \frac{[HPO_4^{2-}][OH^-]}{[PO_4^{3-}]} = 4.8 \times 10^{-2} \qquad (7\text{--}41)$$

$$HPO_4^{2-} + H_2O \rightleftharpoons H_2PO_4^- + OH^- \qquad (7\text{--}42)$$

$$K_{b2} = \frac{[H_2PO_4^-][OH^-]}{[HPO_4^{2-}]} = 1.6 \times 10^{-7} \qquad (7\text{--}43)$$

$$H_2PO_4^- + H_2O \rightleftharpoons H_3PO_4 + OH^- \qquad (7\text{--}44)$$

$$K_{b3} = \frac{[H_3PO_4][OH^-]}{[H_2PO_4^-]} = 1.3 \times 10^{-12} \qquad (7\text{--}45)$$

In general, for a polyprotic acid system for which the parent acid is H_nA, there are $n + 1$ possible species in solution:

$$H_nA + H_{n-j}A^{-j} + \cdots + HA^{-(n-1)} + A^{n-} \qquad (7\text{--}46)$$

in which j represents the number of protons dissociated from the parent acid and goes from 0 to n. The total concentration of all species must be equal to C_a, or

$$[H_nA] + [H_{n-j}A^{-j}] + \cdots$$

$$+ [HA^{-(n-1)}] + [A^{n-}] = C_a \qquad (7\text{--}47)$$

Each of the species pairs in which j differs by 1 constitutes a conjugate acid–base pair, and in general

$$K_j K_{b(n+1-j)} = K_w \qquad (7\text{--}48)$$

in which K_j represents the various acidity constants for the system. Thus, for the phosphoric acid system described by equations (7–37) to (7–45):

$$K_1 K_{b3} = K_2 K_{b2} = K_3 K_{b1} = K_w \qquad (7\text{--}45)$$

Ampholytes. In the preceding section, equations (7–37), (7–38), (7–41) and (7–43) demonstrated that in the phosphoric acid system, the species $H_2PO_4^-$ and HPO_4^{2-} can function either as acids or bases. A species that can function either as an acid or as a base is called an *ampholyte* and is said to be *amphoteric* in nature. In general, for a polyprotic acid system, all the species, with the exception of H_nA and A^{n-}, are amphoteric.

Amino acids and proteins are ampholytes of particular interest in pharmacy. If glycine hydrochloride is dissolved in water, it ionizes as follows:

$$^+NH_3CH_2COOH + H_2O \rightleftharpoons$$

$$^+NH_3CH_2COO^- + H_3O^+ \qquad (7\text{--}50)$$

$$^+NH_3CH_2COO^- + H_2O \rightleftharpoons$$

$$NH_2CH_2COO^- + H_3O^+ \qquad (7\text{--}51)$$

The species $^+NH_3CH_2COO^-$ is amphoteric in that, in addition to reacting as an acid as shown in equation (7–51), it can react as a base with water as follows:

$$^+NH_3CH_2COO^- + H_2O \rightleftharpoons$$

$$^+NH_3CH_2COOH + OH^- \qquad (7\text{--}52)$$

The amphoteric species $^+NH_3CH_2COO^-$ is called a *zwitterion* and differs from the amphoteric species formed from phosphoric acid in that it carries both a positive and a negative charge, and the whole molecule is electrically neutral. The pH at which the zwitterion concentration is a maximum is known as the *isoelectric point*. At the isoelectric point the net movement of the solute molecules in an electric field is negligible.

SÖRENSEN'S pH SCALE

The hydrogen ion concentration of a solution varies from approximately 1 in a 1-*M* solution of a strong acid to about 1×10^{-14} in a 1-*M* solution of a strong base, and the calculations often become unwieldly. To alleviate this difficulty, Sörensen[5] suggested a simplified method of expressing hydrogen ion concentration. He established the term *pH*, which was originally written as p_H^+, to represent the hydrogen ion potential, and he defined it as the common logarithm of the reciprocal of the hydrogen ion concentration:

$$pH = \log \frac{1}{[H_3O^+]} \quad (7-53)$$

According to the rules of logarithms, this equation can be written as

$$pH = \log 1 - \log [H_3O^+] \quad (7-54)$$

and since the logarithm of 1 is zero,

$$pH = -\log [H_3O^+] \quad (7-55)$$

equations (7–53) and (7–55) are identical; they are acceptable for approximate calculations involving pH.

The pH of a solution may be considered in terms of a numeric scale having values from 0 to 14, which expresses in a quantitative way the degree of acidity (7 to 0) and alkalinity (7 to 14). The value 7 at which the hydrogen and hydroxyl ion concentrations are about equal at room temperature is referred to as the *neutral point*, or neutrality. The neutral pH at 0° C is 7.47, and at 100° C it is 6.15 (cf. Table 7–4). The scale relating pH to the hydrogen and hydroxyl ion concentration of a solution is given in Table 7–5, and the pH of a number of pharmaceutical vehicles and solutions frequently used as vehicles are found in Table 7–6.

Conversion of Hydrogen Ion Concentration to pH. The student should practice converting from hydrogen ion concentration to pH, and vice versa, until he or she is proficient in these logarithmic operations. The following examples are given to afford a review of the mathematical operations involving logarithms. Equation (7–55) is more convenient for these calculations than equation (7–53).

Example 7–5. The hydronium ion concentration of a 0.05-*M* solution of HCl is 0.05 *M*. What is the pH of this solution?

TABLE 7–5. *The pH Scale and Corresponding Hydrogen and Hydroxyl Ion Concentrations*

pH	$[H_3O^+]$ (moles/liter)	$[OH^-]$ (moles/liter)	
0	$10^0 = 1$	10^{-14}	↑
1	10^{-1}	10^{-13}	
2	10^{-2}	10^{-12}	
3	10^{-3}	10^{-11}	Acidic
4	10^{-4}	10^{-10}	
5	10^{-5}	10^{-9}	
6	10^{-6}	10^{-8}	
7	10^{-7}	10^{-7}	Neutral
8	10^{-8}	10^{-6}	
9	10^{-9}	10^{-5}	
10	10^{-10}	10^{-4}	
11	10^{-11}	10^{-3}	Basic
12	10^{-12}	10^{-2}	
13	10^{-13}	10^{-1}	
14	10^{-14}	$10^0 = 1$	↓

$$pH = -\log (5.0 \times 10^{-2}) = -\log 10^{-2} - \log 5.0$$
$$= 2 - 0.70 = 1.30$$

The hand calculator permits one to obtain pH simply by use of the log function followed by a change of sign.

A better definition of pH involves the activity rather than the concentration of the ions:

$$pH = -\log a_{H^+} \quad (7-56)$$

and since the activity of an ion is equal to the activity coefficient multiplied by the molal or molar concentration (equation (6–42),

hydronium ion concentration × activity coefficient

= hydronium ion activity

the pH may be computed more accurately from the formula

$$pH = -\log (\gamma_\pm \times c) \quad (7-57)$$

Example 7–6. The mean molar ionic activity coefficient of a 0.05-*M* solution of HCl is 0.83 at 25° C. What is the pH of the solution?

$$pH = -\log (0.83 \times 0.05) = 1.38$$

If sufficient NaCl is added to the HCl solution to produce a total ionic strength of 0.5 for this mixture of uni-univalent electrolytes, the activity coefficient is 0.77. What is the pH of this solution?

$$pH = -\log (0.77 \times 0.05) = 1.41$$

Hence, the addition of a neutral salt affects the hydrogen ion activity of a solution, and activity coefficients should be used for the accurate calculations of pH.

Example 7–6 dealt with the pH of a strong acid. For a weak electrolyte (*Example 7–7*), pH is calculated in the same manner from the hydrogen ion concentration.

Example 7–7. The hydronium ion concentration of a 0.1-*M* solution of barbituric acid was found to be 3.24×10^{-3} *M*. What is the pH of the solution?

$$pH = -\log (3.24 \times 10^{-3})$$
$$pH = 3 - \log 3.24 = 2.49$$

For practical purposes, activities and concentrations are equal in solutions of weak electrolytes to which no salts are added, since the ionic strength is small.

Conversion of pH to Hydrogen Ion Concentration. The following example illustrates the method of converting pH to $[H_3O^+]$.

Example 7–8. If the pH of a solution is 4.72, what is the hydronium ion concentration?

$$pH = -\log [H_3O^+] = 4.72$$
$$\log [H_3O^+] = -4.72 = -5 + 0.28$$
$$[H_3O^+] = \text{antilog } 0.28 \times \text{antilog } (-5)$$
$$[H_3O^+] = 1.91 \times 10^{-5} \text{ moles/liter}$$

The use of a hand calculator bypasses this two-step procedure. One simply enters −4.72 into the calculator and presses the key for antilog or 10^x in order to obtain $[H_3O^+]$.

p*K* and pOH. The use of pH to designate the negative logarithm of hydronium ion concentration has proved to be so convenient that expressing numbers less than

TABLE 7—6. *Approximate pH Numbers of Some Pharmaceutical Specialties and Vehicles**

Product	pH	Manufacturer
Acacia syrup	5.0	
Acromycin-V syrup	4.0—5.0	Lederle
Actifed syrup	5.0—7.2	Burroughs Wellcome
Ambenyl	5.5—6.0	Marion
Anspor for oral suspension	3.5—6.0	SmithKline Beecham
Antepar syrup	5.7—6.3	Burroughs Wellcome
Aromatic Eriodictyon syrup	7.0—8.0	
Artane	2.0—3.0	Lederle
Aventyl liquid	2.5—4.0	Lilly
Bactrium suspension	5.0—6.0	Roche
Benadryl elixir	7.0	Parke—Davis
Bentyl HCl	5.0—5.5	Merrell—National
Benzaldehyde compound elixir	6.0	
Bromides syrup	4.5	
Butisol sodium elixir	9.7	Wallace Laboratories
Calcidrin syrup	4.0—5.0	Abbott
Catnip and fennel elixir	8.0	
Cerose	5.0—5.2	Ives
Cerose-DM	5.0—5.2	Ives
Cetro-Cirose	5.3	Ives
Cheracol	4.0	Upjohn
Cherry syrup	3.5—4.0	
Chlor-Trimeton maleate syrup	4.4—5.6	Schering
Cibalith-S	4.0—5.0	Ciba
Compound cardamom elixir	7.5	
Comtrex Cough Formula	4.5—5.5	Bristol—Meyers
Comtrex Multi-Symptom Liquid	4.3	Bristol—Meyers
Contac Cough and Congestion Formula	4.3	SmithKline Beecham
Contac Cough, Chest Congestion and Sore Throat Formula	4.5	SmithKline Beecham
Contac Jr. Nondrowsy Cold Liquid	4.5	SmithKline Beecham
Contac Nighttime Cold Medicine	5.6	SmithKline Beecham
Cosanyl	3.0	Health Care Industries
Darvon-N suspension	4.0—6.0	Lilly
Decadron elixir	3.0—3.4	Merck Sharp & Dohme
Demazin syrup	4.5—6.0	Schering
Dimetapp elixir	2.2—3.2	Robins
Diuril oral suspension	3.5—4.0	Merck Sharp & Dohme
Donnagel suspension	4.0—5.5	Robins
Donnatal elixir	4.0—5.5	Robins
Elixir Alurate Verdum	2.5	Hoffmann—La Roche
Excedrin PM liquid	4.6	Bristol—Myers
Feosol elixir	2.0—2.4	SmithKline Beecham
Gantanol suspension	4.7—5.0	Roche
Gantrisin syrup	4.5—5.0	Roche
Glycyrrhiza syrup	6.0—6.5	
Haldol	2.8—3.8	McNeil
Homicebrin	3.5—4.0	Lilly
Hydriodic acid syrup	1.0	Lilly
Ilosone suspension	4.5—6.0	Lilly
Iso-alcoholic elixir	5.0	
Kaopectate	4.2	Upjohn
Lanoxin pediatric elixir	6.8—7.2	Burroughs Wellcome
Lipo Gantrisin	4.3—4.8	Roche
Lipomul oral	5.0	Upjohn
Mestinon syrup	4.2—4.8	Roche
Naldecon adult syrup	4.0—5.0	Bristol Laboratories
Naldecon CX solution	4.5—5.5	Bristol Laboratories
Naldecon DX adult liquid	4.5—5.5	Bristol Laboratories
Naldecon DX pediatric drops	3.7—4.7	Bristol Laboratories
Naldecon DX pediatric syrup	2.7—3.7	Bristol Laboratories
Naldecon EX pediatric Drops	3.5—4.5	Bristol Laboratories
Naldecon EX pediatric syrup	3.0—4.0	Bristol Laboratories
Naldecon pediatric drops	4.0—5.0	Bristol Laboratories
Naldecon pediatric syrup	4.0—5.0	Bristol Laboratories
Naldecon senior DX syrup	4.5—5.5	Bristol Laboratories
Neldecon senior EX syrup	4.5—5.5	Bristol Laboratories
Naprosyn (naproxin) suspension	2.2—3.7	Syntex
Nasalide (flunisolidate) nasal solution	4.5—6.0	Syntex
Nembutal elixir	3.2—4.0	Abbott
Noctec	4.8—5.2	Squibb
Novafed liquid	2.5—4.5	Dow
Novahistine DH	2.5—4.0	Dow
Novahistine elixir	2.5—4.0	Dow
Novahistine expectorant	2.5—4.0	Dow
Orange syrup	2.5—3.0	
Orthoxicol	2.5—3.0	Upjohn
Pepsin, lactated	4.0—5.0	
Periactin syrup	3.5—4.5	Merck Sharp & Dohme

TABLE 7-6. *(continued)*

Phenobarbital elixir	6.0	
Prolixin elixir	5.3–5.8	Squibb
Pyribenzamine elixir	4.5	Ciba
Raspberry syrup	3.0	
Robitussin	2.3–3.0	Robins
Romilar CF	4.9	Block
Roniacol elixir	4.0–5.0	Roche
Sarsaparilla, compound syrup	5.0	
Stelazine concentrate	2.2–3.2	SmithKline Beecham
Sudafed syrup	2.5–3.5	Burroughs Wellcome
Sudafed Plus syrup	2.5–4.0	Burroughs Wellcome
Sumycin syrup	3.5–6.0	Squibb
Suptra suspension	5.0–6.0	Burroughs Wellcome
Surbex	3.7–3.9	Abbott
Synarel (nafarelin acetate) nasal solution	5.2±0.5	Syntex
Syrup	6.5–7.0	
Tagamet liquid	5.0–6.5	SmithKline Beecham
Taka-Diastase	6.0	Parke–Davis
Taractan concentrate	3.5–4.5	Roche
Tegretol suspension	3.0–5.0	Geigy
Terpin hydrate elixir	6.0	
Terpin hydrate elixir and codeine	8.0	
Theragran liquid	4.7–5.2	Squibb
Thiamine HCl elixir	4.0–5.0	
Thorazine concentrate, 30 mg	3.0–4.0	SmithKline Beecham
Thorazine concentrate, 100 mg	2.4–3.4	SmithKline Beecham
Thorazine syrup	4.0–5.0	SmithKline Beecham
Toradol IM (ketorolac tromethamine) injection	7.4±0.5	Syntex
Tuss-Ornade liquid	4.0–4.4	SmithKline Beecham
Tussend expectorant	2.5–4.5	Dow
Tussend liquid	2.0–4.0	Dow
Tylenol with codeine elixir	4.0–6.1	McNeil
Valadol liquid	3.8–6.1	Squibb
Vitamin B complex elixir	4.0–5.0	
White Pine compound syrup	6.5	
Wild Cherry syrup	4.5	

*Results are correct to about ±0.3 pH unit. Some of the products are suspensions, whereas others contain nonaqueous vehicles. The pH values in the table therefore are not necessarily the same as those obtained in aqueous systems and are accordingly called pH numbers (p. 201). These pH ranges are used by the pharmaceutical manufacturers as quality control specifications and are kindly supplied by the companies.

unity in "p" notation has become a standard procedure. The mathematician would say that "p" is a *mathematical operator* that acts on the quantity, $[H^+]$, K_a, K_b, K_w, etc., to convert the value into the negative of its common logarithm. In other words, the term "p" is used to express the negative logarithm of the term following the "p". For example, pOH expresses $-\log [OH^-]$, pK_a is used for $-\log K_a$, and pK_w is $-\log K_w$. Thus, equations (7–31) and (7–33) can be expressed as

$$pH + pOH = pK_w \qquad (7–58)$$

$$pK_a + pK_b = pK_w \qquad (7–59)$$

in which pK is often called the *dissociation exponent.*

The pK of weak acidic and basic drugs are ordinarily determined by ultraviolet spectrophometry (p. 81) and potentiometric titration (p. 204). They may also be obtained by solubility analysis[6–8] (p. 233) and by a partition coefficient method.[8]

SPECIES CONCENTRATION AS A FUNCTION OF pH

As was shown in the preceding sections, polyprotic acids, H_nA, can ionize in successive stages to yield $n + 1$ possible species in solution. In many studies of pharmaceutical interest, it is important to be able to calculate the concentration of all acidic and basic species in solution.

The concentrations of all species involved in successive acid–base equilibria change with pH and can be represented solely in terms of equilibrium constants and the hydronium ion concentration. These relationships can be obtained by defining all species in solution as fractions, α, of total acid, C_a, added to the system (see equation (7–47) for C_a).

$$\alpha_0 = [H_nA]/C_a \qquad (7–60a)$$

$$\alpha_1 = [H_{n-1}A^{-1}]/C_a \qquad (7–60b)$$

and in general.

$$\alpha_j = [H_{n-j}A^{-j}]/C_a \qquad (7–61a)$$

and

$$\alpha_n = [A^{-n}]/C_a \qquad (7–61b)$$

in which j represents the number of protons that have ionized from the parent acid. Thus, dividing equation (7–47) by C_a and using equations (7–60a) to (7–61b) gives

$$\alpha_0 + \alpha_j + \cdots + \alpha_{n-1} + \alpha_n = 1 \qquad (7–62)$$

All of the α values can be defined in terms of equilibrium constants, α_0, and H_3O^+ as follows:

$$K_1 = \frac{[H_{n-1}A^-][H_3O^+]}{[H_nA]} = \frac{\alpha_1 C_a[H_3O^+]}{\alpha_0 C_a} \quad (7\text{--}63)$$

therefore

$$\alpha_1 = K_1\alpha_0/[H_3O^+] \quad (7\text{--}64)$$

$$K_2 = \frac{[H_{n-2}A^{2-}][H_3O^+]}{[H_{n-1}A^-]} = \frac{[H_{n-2}A^{2-}][H_3O^+]^2}{K_1[H_nA]}$$

$$= \frac{\alpha_2 C_a[H_3O^+]^2}{\alpha_0 C_a K_1} \quad (7\text{--}65)$$

or

$$\alpha_2 = \frac{K_1 K_2 \alpha_0}{[H_3O^+]^2} \quad (7\text{--}66)$$

and, in general

$$\alpha_j = (K_1 K_2 \ldots K_j)\alpha_0/[H_3O^+]^j \quad (7\text{--}67)$$

Inserting the appropriate forms of equation (7–67) into equation (7–62) gives

$$\alpha_0 + \frac{K_1\alpha_0}{[H_3O^+]} + \frac{K_1 K_2 \alpha_0}{[H_3O^+]^2}$$

$$+ \cdots + \frac{K_1 K_2 \ldots K_n \alpha_0}{[H_3O^+]^n} = 1 \quad (7\text{--}68)$$

Solving for α_0 yields

$$\alpha_0 = [H_3O^+]^n/\{[H_3O^+]^n + K_1[H_3O]^{n-1}$$

$$+ K_1 K_2[H_3O^+]^{n-2} + \cdots + K_1 K_2 \ldots K_n\} \quad (7\text{--}69)$$

or

$$\alpha_0 = \frac{[H_3O^+]^n}{D} \quad (7\text{--}70)$$

in which D represents the denominator of equation (7–69). Thus, the concentration of H_nA as a function of $[H_3O^+]$ can be obtained by substituting equation (7–60a) into equation (7–70) to give

$$[H_nA] = \frac{[H_3O^+]^n C_a}{D} \quad (7\text{--}71)$$

Substituting equation (7–60b) into equation (7–64) and the resulting equation into equation (7–70) gives

$$[H_{n-1}A^{-1}] = \frac{K_1[H_3O^+]^{n-1}C_a}{D} \quad (7\text{--}72)$$

In general,

$$[H_{n-j}A^{-j}] = \frac{K_1 \ldots K_j[H_3O^+]^{n-j}C_a}{D} \quad (7\text{--}73)$$

and

$$[A^{-n}] = \frac{K_1 K_2 \ldots K_n C_a}{D} \quad (7\text{--}74)$$

Although these equations appear complicated, they are in reality quite simple. The term D in equations (7–70) to (7–74) is a power series in $[H_3O^+]$, each term multiplied by equilibrium constants. The series starts with $[H_3O^+]$ raised to the power representing n, the total number of dissociable hydrogens in the parent acid, H_nA. The last term is the product of all the acidity constants. The intermediate terms can be obtained from the last term by substituting $[H_3O^+]$ for K_n to obtain the next-to-last term, then substituting $[H_3O^+]$ for K_{n-1} to obtain the next term, and so on, until the first term is reached. The following equations show the denominators D to be used in equation (7–70) to (7–74) for various types of polyprotic acids:

H_4A: $D = [H_3O^+]^4 + K_1[H_3O^+]^3 + K_1K_2[H_3O^+]^2$

$$\qquad + K_1K_2K_3[H_3O^+] + K_1K_2K_3K_4 \quad (7\text{--}75)$$

H_3A: $D = [H_3O^+]^3 + K_1[H_3O^+]^2$

$$\qquad + K_1K_2[H_3O^+] + K_1K_2K_3 \quad (7\text{--}76)$$

H_2A: $D = [H_3O^+]^2 + K_1[H_3O^+] + K_1K_2 \quad (7\text{--}77)$

HA: $D = [H_3O^+] + K_a \quad (7\text{--}78)$

In all instances, for a species in which j protons have ionized, the numerator in equations (7–70) to (7–74) is C_a multiplied by the term from the denominator D that has $[H_3O^+]$ raised to the $n - j$ power. Thus, for the parent acid H_2A, the appropriate equation for D would be equation (7–77). The molar concentrations of the species $H_nA(j = 0)$, $HA^-(j = 1)$, and $A^{2-}(j = 2)$ can be given as

$$[H_2A] = \frac{[H_3O^+]^2 C_a}{[H_3O^+]^2 + K_1[H_3O^+] + K_1K_2} \quad (7\text{--}79)$$

$$[HA^-] = \frac{K_1[H_3O^+]C_a}{[H_3O^+]^2 + K_1[H_3O^+] + K_1K_2} \quad (7\text{--}80)$$

$$[A^{2-}] = \frac{K_1K_2 C_a}{[H_3O^+]^2 + K_1[H_3O^+] + K_1K_2} \quad (7\text{--}81)$$

These equations can be used directly to solve for molar concentrations. It should be obvious, however, that lengthy calculations are needed for substances such as citric acid or ethylenediaminetetraacetic acid, requiring the use of a digital computer to obtain solutions in a reasonable time. Graphic methods have been used to simplify the procedure.[9]

CALCULATION OF pH

Proton Balance Equations. According to the Brönsted–Lowry theory, every proton donated by an acid must be accepted by a base. Thus, an equation accounting for the total proton transfers occurring in a system should be of fundamental importance in describing any acid–base equilibria in that system. This can be accomplished by establishing a proton balance equation (PBE) for each system. In the PBE, the sum of the concentration terms for species that form by proton consumption is equated to the sum of the concentration terms for species that are formed by the release of a proton.

For example, when HCl is added to water, it dissociates completely into H_3O^+ and Cl^- ions. The H_3O^+ is a species that is formed by the consumption of a proton (by water acting as a base), and the Cl^- is formed by the release of a proton from HCl. In all aqueous solutions, H_3O^+ and OH^- result from the dissociation of two water molecules according to equation (7–28). Thus, OH^- is a species formed from the release of a proton. The PBE for the system of HCl in water is

$$[H_3O^+] = [OH^-] + [Cl^-]$$

Although H_3O^+ is formed from two reactions, it is included only once in the PBE. The same would be true for OH^- if it came from more than one source.

The general method for obtaining the PBE is as follows:

(a) Always start with the species added to water.

(b) On the left side of the equation, place all species that can form when protons are consumed by the starting species.

(c) On the right side of the equation, place all species that can form when protons are released from the starting species.

(d) Each species in the PBE should be multiplied by the number of protons lost or gained when it is formed from the starting species.

(e) Add $[H_3O^+]$ to the left side of the equation, and $[OH^-]$ to the right side of the equation. These result from the interaction of two molecules of water, as shown previously.

Example 7–9. What is the PBE when H_3PO_4 is added to water?
The species $H_2PO_4^-$ forms with the release of one proton.
The species HPO_4^{2-} forms with the release of two protons.
The species PO_4^{3-} forms with the release of three protons.

$$[H_3O^+] = [OH^-] + [H_2PO_4^-] + 2[HPO_4^{2-}] + 3[PO_4^{3-}]$$

Example 7–10. What is the PBE when Na_2HPO_4 is added to water?
The salt dissociates into $2Na^+$ and $1\ HPO_4^{2-}$; Na^+ is neglected in the PBE since it is not formed from the release or consumption of a proton; HPO_4^{2-}, however, does react with water and is considered to be the starting species.
The species $H_2PO_4^-$ results with the consumption of one proton.
The species of H_3PO_4 can form with the consumption of two protons.
The species PO_4^{3-} can form with the release of one proton.

$$[H_3O^+] + [H_2PO_4^-] + 2[H_3PO_4] = [OH^-] + [PO_4^{3-}]$$

Example 7–11. What is the PBE when sodium acetate is added to water?
The salt dissociates into one Na^+ and one CH_3COO^- ion. The CH_3COO^- is considered to be the starting species. The CH_3COOH can form when CH_3COO^- consumes one proton.

$$[H_3O^+] + [CH_3COOH] = [OH^-]$$

The PBE allows the pH of any solution to be calculated readily, as follows:

(a) Obtain the PBE for the solution in question.

(b) Express the concentration of all species as a function of equilibrium constants and $[H_3O^+]$ using equations (7–71) to (7–74).

(c) Solve the resulting expression for $[H_3O^+]$ using any assumptions that appear valid for the system.

(d) Check all assumptions.

(e) If all assumptions prove valid, convert $[H_3O^+]$ to pH.

If the solution contains a base, it is sometimes more convenient to solve the expression obtained in part *(b)* for $[OH^-]$, then convert this to pOH, and finally to pH by use of equation (7–58)

Solutions of Strong Acids and Bases. Strong acids and bases are those that have acidity or basicity constants greater than about 10^{-2}. Thus, they are considered to ionize 100% when placed in water. When HCl is placed in water, the PBE for the system is given by

$$[H_3O^+] = [OH^-] + [Cl^-] = \frac{K_w}{[H_3O^+]} + C_a \qquad (7–82a)$$

which can be rearranged to give

$$[H_3O^+]^2 - C_a[H_3O^+] - K_w = 0 \qquad (7–82b)$$

in which C_a is the total acid concentration. This is a quadratic equation of the general form

$$aX^2 + bX + c = 0 \qquad (7–83)$$

which has the solution

$$X = \frac{-b \pm \sqrt{b^2 - 4ac}}{2a} \qquad (7–84)$$

Thus, equation (7–82b) becomes

$$[H_3O^+] = \frac{C_a + \sqrt{C_a^2 + 4K_w}}{2} \qquad (7–85)$$

in which only the positive root is used, since $[H_3O^+]$ can never be negative.

When the concentration of acid is $1 \times 10^{-6}\ M$ or greater, $[Cl^-]$ becomes much greater than* $[OH^-]$ in equation (7–82a), and C_a^2 becomes much greater than $4K_w$ in equation (7–85). Thus, both equations simplify to

$$[H_3O^+] \cong C_a \qquad (7–86)$$

A similar treatment for a solution of a strong base such as NaOH gives

$$[OH^-] = \frac{C_b + \sqrt{C_b^2 + 4K_w}}{2} \qquad (7–87)$$

and

$$[OH^-] \cong C_b \qquad (7–88)$$

if the concentration of base is 1×10^6 molar or greater.

Conjugate Acid–Base Pairs. Use of the PBE enables us to develop one master equation that can be used to solve for the pH of solutions composed of weak acids,

---

*To adopt a definite and consistent method of making approximations throughout this chapter, the expression "much greater than" means that the larger term is at least 20 times greater than the smaller term.

weak bases, or a mixture of a conjugate acid–base pair. To do this, consider a solution made by dissolving both a weak acid, HB, and a salt of its conjugate base, B^-, in water. The acid–base equilibria involved are

$$HB + H_2O \rightleftharpoons H_3O^+ + B^- \qquad (7-89)$$

$$B^- + H_2O \rightleftharpoons OH^- + HB \qquad (7-90)$$

$$H_2O + H_2O \rightleftharpoons H_3O^+ + OH^- \qquad (7-91)$$

The PBE for this system is

$$[H_3O^+] + [HB] = [OH^-] + [B^-] \qquad (7-92)$$

The concentrations of the acid and the conjugate base may be expressed as

$$[HB] = \frac{[H_3O^+]C_b}{[H_3O^+] + K_a} \qquad (7-93)$$

$$[B^-] = \frac{K_aC_a}{[H_3O^+] + K_a} \qquad (7-94)$$

Equation (7–93) contains C_b (concentration of base added as the salt) rather than C_a, since in terms of the PBE, the species HB was generated from the species B^- added in the form of the salt. Equation (7–94) contains C_a (concentration of HB added), since the species B^- in the PBE came from the HB added. Inserting equations (7–93) and (7–94) into equation (7–92) gives

$$[H_3O^+] + \frac{[H_3O^+]C_b}{[H_3O^+] + K_a}$$
$$= [OH^-] + \frac{K_aC_a}{[H_3O^+] + K_a} \qquad (7-95)$$

which can be rearranged to yield

$$[H_3O^+] = K_a \frac{(C_a - [H_3O^+] + [OH^-])}{(C_b + [H_3O^+] - [OH^-])} \qquad (7-96)$$

This equation is exact and was developed using no assumptions.[†] It is, however, quite difficult to solve. Fortunately, for real systems, the equation may be simplified.

Solutions Containing Only a Weak Acid. If the solution contains only a weak acid, C_b is zero, and $[H_3O^+]$ is generally much greater than $[OH^-]$. Thus, equation (7–96) simplifies to

$$[H_3O^+]^2 + K_a[H_3O^+] - K_aC_a = 0 \qquad (7-97)$$

which is a quadratic equation with the solution

$$[H_3O^+] = \frac{-K_a + \sqrt{K_a^2 + 4K_aC_a}}{2} \qquad (7-98)$$

In many instances, $C_a \gg [H_3O^+]$, and equation (7–97) simplifies to (p. 145)

$$[H_3O^+] = \sqrt{K_aC_a} \qquad (7-99)$$

Example 7–12. Calculate the pH of a 0.01-M solution of salicylic acid, which has a $K_a = 1.06 \times 10^{-3}$ at 25° C.

(a) Using equation (7–99),

$$[H_3O^+] = \sqrt{(1.06 \times 10^{-3}) \times (1.0 \times 10^{-2})}$$
$$= 3.26 \times 10^{-3}\ M$$

The approximation that $C_a \gg H_3O^+$ is not valid.

(b) Using equation (7–98),

$$[H_3O^+] = -\frac{(1.06 \times 10^{-3})}{2}$$
$$+ \frac{\sqrt{(1.06 \times 10^{-3})^2 + 4(1.06 \times 10^{-3})(1.0 \times 10^{-2})}}{2}$$

$$= 2.77 \times 10^{-3}\ M$$

$$pH = -\log (2.77 \times 10^{-3}) = 2.56$$

The example just given illustrates the importance of checking the validity of all assumptions made in deriving the equation used for calculating $[H_3O^+]$. The simplified equation (7–99) gives an answer for $[H_3O^+]$ with a relative error of 18% as compared with the correct answer given by equation (7–98).

Example 7–13. Calculate the pH of a 1 g/100 mL solution of ephedrine sulfate. The molecular weight of the salt is 428.5, and K_b for ephedrine base is 2.3×10^{-5}.

(a) The ephedrine sulfate, $(BH^+)_2SO_4$, dissociates completely into two BH^+ cations and one SO_4^{2-} anion. Thus, the concentration of the weak acid (ephedrine cation) is twice the concentration, C_s, of the salt added.

$$C_a = 2C_s = \frac{2 \times 10\ \text{g/liter}}{428.5\ \text{g/mole}} = 4.67 \times 10^{-2}\ M$$

(b)

$$K_a = \frac{1.00 \times 10^{-14}}{2.3 \times 10^{-5}} = 4.35 \times 10^{-10}$$

(c)

$$[H_3O^+] = \sqrt{(4.35 \times 10^{-10}) \times (4.67 \times 10^{-2})}$$
$$= 4.51 \times 10^{-6}\ M$$

All assumptions are valid.

$$pH = -\log (4.51 \times 10^{-6}) = 5.35$$

Solutions Containing Only a Weak Base. If the solution contains only a weak base, C_a is zero, and $[OH^-]$ is generally much greater than $[H_3O^+]$. Thus, equation (7–96) simplifies to

$$[H_3O^+] = \frac{K_a[OH^-]}{C_b - [OH^-]} = \frac{K_aK_w}{[H_3O^+]C_b - K_w} \qquad (7-100)$$

This equation can be solved for either $[H_3O^+]$ or $[OH^-]$. Solving for $[H_3O^+]$ using the left and far-right parts of equation (7–100) gives

$$C_b[H_3O^+]^2 - K_w[H_3O^+] - K_aK_w = 0 \qquad (7-101)$$

which has the solution

$$[H_3O^+] = \frac{K_w + \sqrt{K_w^2 + 4C_bK_aK_w}}{2C_b} \qquad (7-102)$$

[†]Except that, in this and all subsequent developments for pH equations, it is assumed that concentration may be used in place of activity.

If $K_a \gg [H_3O^+]$, which is generally true for solutions of weak bases, equation (7–100) gives

$$[H_3O^+] = \sqrt{\frac{K_a K_w}{C_b}} \qquad (7\text{--}103)$$

Equation (7–100) can be solved for $[OH^-]$ by using the left and middle portions and converting K_a to K_b to give

$$[OH^-] = \frac{-K_b + \sqrt{K_b^2 + 4K_b C_b}}{2} \qquad (7\text{--}104)$$

and if $C_b \gg [OH^-]$, which generally obtains for solutions of weak bases,

$$[OH^-] = \sqrt{K_b C_b} \qquad (7\text{--}105)$$

A good exercise for the student would be to prove that equation (7–103) is equal to equation (7–105). The applicability of both these equations will be shown in the following examples.

Example 7–14. What is the pH of a 0.0033-*M* solution of cocaine base, which has a basicity constant of 2.6×10^{-6}?

$$[OH^-] = \sqrt{(2.6 \times 10^{-6}) \times (3.3 \times 10^{-3})}$$
$$= 9.26 \times 10^{-5} \ M$$

All assumptions are valid.

$$pOH = -\log (9.26 \times 10^{-5}) = 4.03$$
$$pH = 14.00 - 4.03 = 9.97$$

Example 7–15. Calculate the pH of a 0.165-*M* solution of sodium sulfathiazole. The acidity constant for sulfathiazole is 7.6×10^{-8}.

(a) The salt $Na^+ B^-$ dissociates into one Na^+ and one B^- as described by equations (7–24) to (7–27). Thus, $C_b = C_s = 0.165 \ M$. Since K_a for a weak acid such as sulfathiazole is usually given, rather than K_b for its conjugate base, equation (7–103) is preferred over equation (7–105).

$$[H_3O^+] = \sqrt{\frac{(7.6 \times 10^{-8}) \times (1.00 \times 10^{-14})}{0.165}}$$
$$= 6.79 \times 10^{-11} \ M$$

All assumptions are valid.

$$pH = -\log (6.79 \times 10^{-11}) = 10.17$$

Solutions Containing a Single Conjugate Acid–Base Pair. In a solution composed of a weak acid and a salt of that acid, for example, acetic acid and sodium acetate; or a weak base and a salt of that base, for example, ephedrine and ephedrine hydrochloride, C_a and C_b are generally much greater than either $[H_3O^+]$ or $[OH^-]$. Thus, equation (7–96) simplifies to

$$[H_3O^+] = \frac{K_a C_a}{C_b} \qquad (7\text{--}106)$$

Example 7–16. What is the pH of a solution containing acetic acid 0.3 *M* and sodium acetate 0.05 *M*?

$$[H_3O^+] = \frac{(1.75 \times 10^{-5}) \times (0.3)}{5.0 \times 10^{-2}}$$
$$= 1.05 \times 10^{-4} \ M$$

All assumptions are valid.

$$pH = -\log (1.05 \times 10^{-4}) = 3.98$$

Example 7–17. What is the pH of a solution containing ephedrine 0.1 *M* and ephedrine hydrochloride 0.01 *M*? Ephedrine has a basicity constant of 2.3×10^{-5}; thus, the acidity constant for its conjugate acid is 4.35×10^{-10}.

$$[H_3O^+] = \frac{(4.35 \times 10^{-10}) \times (1.0 \times 10^{-2})}{1.0 \times 10^{-1}}$$
$$= 4.35 \times 10^{-11} \ M$$

All assumptions are valid.

$$pH = -\log (4.35 \times 10^{-11}) = 10.36$$

Solutions made by dissolving in water both an acid and its conjugate base, or a base and its conjugate acid, are examples of buffer solutions. These solutions are of great importance in pharmacy and are covered in greater detail in the next two chapters.

Two Conjugate Acid–Base Pairs. The Brönsted–Lowry theory and the PBE enable a single equation to be developed that is valid for solutions containing an ampholyte, which forms a part of two dependent acid–base pairs. An amphoteric species can be added directly to water, or it can be formed by the reaction of a diprotic weak acid, H_2A, or a diprotic weak base, A^{2-}. Thus, it is convenient to consider a solution containing a diprotic weak acid, H_2A, a salt of its ampholyte, HA^-, and a salt of its diprotic base, A^{2-}, in concentrations C_a, C_{ab}, and C_b, respectively. The total PBE for this system is

$$[H_3O^+] + [H_2A]_{ab} + [HA^-]_b + 2[H_2A]_b$$
$$= [OH^-] + [HA^-]_a + 2[A^{2-}]_a$$
$$+ [A^{2-}]_{ab} \qquad (7\text{--}107)$$

in which the subscripts refer to the source of the species in the PBE, that is, $[H_2A]_{ab}$ refers to H_2A generated from the ampholyte, and $[H_2A]_b$ refers to the H_2A generated from the diprotic base. Replacing these species concentrations as a function of $[H_3O^+]$ gives

$$[H_3O^+] + \frac{[H_3O^+]^2 C_{ab}}{D} + \frac{K_1 [H_3O^+] C_b}{D}$$
$$+ \frac{2[H_3O^+]^2 C_b}{D} = \frac{K_w}{[H_3O^+]}$$
$$+ \frac{K_1 [H_3O^+] C_a}{D} + \frac{2K_1 K_2 C_a}{D}$$
$$+ \frac{K_1 K_2 C_{ab}}{D} \qquad (7\text{--}108)$$

Multiplying through by $[H_3O^+]$ and D, which is given by equation (7–77), gives

$$[H_3O^+]^4 + [H_3O^+]^3 (K_1 + 2C_b + C_{ab})$$
$$+ [H_3O^+]^2 [K_1(C_b - C_a) + K_1 K_2 - K_w]$$
$$- [H_3O^+][K_1 K_2 (2C_a + C_{ab}) + K_1 K_w]$$
$$- K_1 K_2 K_w = 0 \qquad (7\text{--}109)$$

This is a general equation that has been developed using no assumptions and that can be used for solutions made by adding a diprotic acid to water, adding an ampholyte to water, adding a diprotic base to water, and by combinations of these substances added to water. It is also useful for tri- and quadriprotic acid systems, because K_3 and K_4 are much smaller than K_1 and K_2 for all acids of pharmaceutical interest. Thus, these polyprotic acid systems may be handled in the same manner as a diprotic acid system.

Solutions Containing Only a Diprotic Acid. If a solution is made by adding a diprotic acid, H_2A, to water to give a concentration, C_a, the terms C_{ab} and C_b in equation (7–109) are zero. In almost all instances, the terms containing K_w can be dropped, and after dividing through by $[H_3O^+]$, equation (7–109) becomes

$$[H_3O^+]^3 + [H_3O^+]^2 K_1 - [H_3O^+](K_1 C_a - K_1 K_2)$$
$$- 2K_1 K_2 C_a = 0 \quad (7\text{–}110)$$

If $C_a \gg K_2$, as is usually true,

$$[H_3O^+]^3 + [H_3O^+]^2 K_1 - [H_3O^+]K_1 C_a$$
$$- 2K_1 K_2 C_a = 0 \quad (7\text{–}111)$$

If $[H_3O^+] \gg 2K_2$, the term $2K_1 K_2 C_a$ can be dropped, and dividing through by $[H_3O^+]$ yields the quadratic equation

$$[H_3O^+]^2 + [H_3O^+]K_1 - KC_a = 0 \quad (7\text{–}112)$$

The assumptions $C_a \gg K_2$ and $[H_3O^+] \gg 2K_2$ will be valid whenever $K_2 \ll K_1$. Equation (7–112) is identical to equation (7–97), which was obtained for a solution containing a monoprotic weak acid. Thus, if $C_a \gg [H_3O^+]$, equation (7–112) simplifies to equation (7–99).

Example 7–18. Calculate the pH of a 1.0×10^{-3}-M solution of succinic acid. $K_1 = 6.4 \times 10^{-5}$ and $K_2 = 2.3 \times 10^{-6}$.
(a) Use equation (7–99), since K_1 is approximately 30 times K_2.
$$[H_3O^+] = \sqrt{(6.4 \times 10^{-5}) \times (1.0 \times 10^{-3})}$$
$$= 2.53 \times 10^{-4} \, M$$
The assumption that $C_a \gg [H_3O^+]$ is not valid.
(b) Use the quadratic equation (7–112):
$$[H_3O^+] = -(6.4 \times 10^{-5})/2$$
$$+ \frac{\sqrt{(6.4 \times 10^{-5})^2 + 4(6.4 \times 10^{-5})(1.0 \times 10^{-3})}}{2}$$
$$= 2.23 \times 10^{-4} \, M$$
Note that C_a is much greater than K_2, and $[H_3O^+]$ is much greater than $2K_2$.
$$pH = -\log (2.23 \times 10^{-4}) = 3.65$$

Solutions Containing Only an Ampholyte. If an ampholyte, HA^-, is dissolved in water to give a solution with concentration, C_{ab}, the terms C_a and C_b in equation (7–109) are zero. For most systems of practical importance, the first, third, and fifth terms of equation (7–109) are negligible when compared with the second and fourth terms, and the equation becomes

$$[H_3O^+] = \sqrt{\frac{K_1 K_2 C_{ab} + K_1 K_w}{K_1 + C_{ab}}} \quad (7\text{–}113)$$

The term $K_2 C_{ab}$ is generally much greater than K_w, and

$$[H_3O^+] = \sqrt{\frac{K_1 K_2 C_{ab}}{K_1 + C_{ab}}} \quad (7\text{–}114)$$

If the solution is concentrated enough that $C_{ab} \gg K_1$,

$$[H_3O^+] = \sqrt{K_1 K_2} \quad (7\text{–}115)$$

Example 7–19. Calculate the pH of a 5.0×10^{-3}-M solution of sodium bicarbonate at 25° C. The acidity constants for carbonic acid are $K_1 = 4.3 \times 10^{-7}$ and $K_2 = 4.7 \times 10^{-11}$.
Since $K_2 C_{ab} (23.5 \times 10^{-14})$ is much greater than K_w, and $C_{ab} \gg K_1$, equation (7–115) can be used.
$$[H_3O^+] = \sqrt{(4.3 \times 10^{-7}) \times (4.7 \times 10^{-11})}$$
$$= 4.5 \times 10^{-9} \, M$$
$$pH = -\log (4.5 \times 10^{-9}) = 8.35$$

Solutions Containing Only a Diacidic Base. In general, the calculations for solutions containing weak bases are easier to handle by solving for $[OH^-]$ rather than $[H_3O^+]$. Any equation in terms of $[H_3O^+]$ and acidity constants can be converted into terms of $[OH^-]$ and basicity constants by substituting $[OH^-]$ for $[H_3O^+]$, K_{b1} for K_1, K_{b2} for K_2, and C_b for C_a. These substitutions are made into equation (7–109). Furthermore, for a solution containing only a diacidic base, C_a and C_{ab} are zero; all terms containing K_w can be dropped; $C_b \gg K_{b2}$; and $[OH^-] \gg 2K_{b2}$. The following expression results:

$$[OH^-]^2 + [OH^-]K_{b1} - K_{b1} C_b = 0 \quad (7\text{–}116)$$

If $C_b \gg [OH^-]$, the equation simplifies to

$$[OH^-] = \sqrt{K_{b1} C_b} \quad (7\text{–}117)$$

Example 7–20. Calculate the pH of a 1.0×10^{-3}-M solution of Na_2CO_3. The acidity constants for carbonic acid are $K_1 = 4.31 \times 10^{-7}$ and $K_2 = 4.7 \times 10^{-11}$.
(a) using equation (7–48),
$$K_{b1} = \frac{K_w}{K_2} = \frac{1.00 \times 10^{-14}}{4.7 \times 10^{-11}} = 2.1 \times 10^{-4}$$
$$K_{b2} = \frac{K_w}{K_1} = \frac{1.00 \times 10^{-14}}{4.31 \times 10^{-7}} = 2.32 \times 10^{-8}$$
(b) Since $K_{b2} \ll K_{b1}$, one uses equation (7–117):
$$[OH^-] = \sqrt{(2.1 \times 10^{-4}) \times (1.0 \times 10^{-3})}$$
$$= 4.6 \times 10^{-4} \, M$$
The assumption that $C_b \gg [OH^-]$ is not valid, and equation (7–116) must be used. (See equations (7–83) and (7–84) for the solution of a quadratic equation.)
$$[OH^-] = -(2.1 \times 10^{-4})/2$$
$$+ \frac{\sqrt{(2.1 \times 10^{-4})^2 + 4(2.1 \times 10^{-4})(1.0 \times 10^{-3})}}{2}$$
$$= 3.7 \times 10^{-4} \, M$$
$$pOH = -\log (3.7 \times 10^{-4}) = 3.4$$
$$pH = 14.00 - 3.4 = 10.6$$

Use of the simplified equation (7–117) gives an answer for $[OH^-]$ that has a relative error of 24% as compared with the correct answer given by equation (7–116). It is absolutely essential that all assumptions made in the calculation of $[H_3O^+]$ or $[OH^-]$ be verified!

Two Independent Acid–Base Pairs. Consider a solution containing two independent acid–base pairs:

$$HB_1 + H_2O \rightleftharpoons H_3O^+ + B_1^-$$

$$K_1 = \frac{[H_3O^+][B_1^-]}{[HB_1]} \qquad (7\text{–}118)$$

$$HB_2 + H_2O \rightleftharpoons H_3O^+ + B_2^-$$

$$K_2 = \frac{[H_3O^+][B_2^-]}{[HB_2]} \qquad (7\text{–}119)$$

A general equation for calculating the pH of this type of solution can be developed by considering a solution made by adding to water the acids HB_1 and HB_2 in concentrations C_{a1} and C_{a2}, and the bases B_1^- and B_2^- in concentrations C_{b1} and C_{b2}. The PBE for this system would be

$$[H_3O^+] + [HB_1]_{B1} + [HB_2]_{B2}$$
$$= [OH^-] + [B_1^-]_{A1} + [B_2^-]_{A2} \qquad (7\text{–}105)$$

in which the subscripts refer to the source of the species in the PBE. Replacing these species concentrations as a function of $[H_3O^+]$ gives

$$[H_3O^+] + \frac{[H_3O^+]C_{b1}}{[H_3O^+] + K_1} + \frac{[H_3O^+]C_{b2}}{[H_3O^+] + K_2}$$
$$= \frac{K_w}{[H_3O^+]} + \frac{K_1 C_{a1}}{[H_3O^+] + K_1}$$
$$+ \frac{K_2 C_{a2}}{[H_3O^+] + K_2} \qquad (7\text{–}121)$$

which can be rearranged to:

$$[H_3O^+]^4 + [H_3O^+]^3(K_1 + K_2 + C_{b1} + C_{b2})$$
$$+ [H_3O^+]^2[K_1(C_{b2} - C_{a1}) + K_2(C_{b1} - C_{a2}) + K_1 K_2 - K_w]$$
$$- [H_3O^+][K_1 K_2(C_{a1} + C_{a2}) + K_w(K_1 + K_2)] - K_1 K_2 K_w = 0$$
$$\qquad (7\text{–}122)$$

Although this equation is extremely complex, it simplifies readily when applied to specific systems.

Solutions Containing Two Weak Acids. In systems containing two weak acids, C_{b1} and C_{b2} are zero, and all terms in K_w can be ignored in equation (7–122). For all systems of practical importance, C_{a1} and C_{a2} are much greater than K_1 and K_2, so the equation simplifies to

$$[H_3O^+]^2 + [H_3O^+](K_1 + K_2)$$
$$- (K_1 C_{a1} + K_2 C_{a2}) = 0 \qquad (7\text{–}123)$$

If C_{a1} and C_{a2} are both greater than $[H_3O^+]$, the equation simplifies to

$$[H_3O^+] = \sqrt{K_1 C_{a1} + K_2 C_{a2}} \qquad (7\text{–}124)$$

Example 7–21. What is the pH of a solution containing acetic acid, 0.01 mole/liter, and formic acid, 0.001 mole/liter?

$$[H_3O^+]$$
$$= \sqrt{(1.75 \times 10^{-5})(1.0 \times 10^{-2}) + (1.77 \times 10^{-4})(1.0 \times 10^{-3})}$$
$$= 5.93 \times 10^{-4}\ M$$
$$pH = -\log(5.93 \times 10^{-4}) = 3.23$$

Solutions Containing a Salt of a Weak Acid and a Weak Base. The salt of a weak acid and a weak base, such as ammonium acetate, dissociates almost completely in aqueous solution to yield NH_4^+ and Ac^-. the NH_4^+ is an acid and can be designated as HB_1, and the base Ac^- can be designated as B_2^- in equations (7–118) and (7–119). Since only a single acid, HB_1, and a single base, B_2^-, were added to water in concentrations C_{a1} and C_{b2} respectively, all other stoichiometric concentration terms in equation (7–112) are zero. In addition, all terms containing K_w are negligibly small and may be dropped, simplifying the equation to

$$[H_3O^+]^2(K_1 + K_2 + C_{b2})$$
$$+ [H_3O^+][K_1(C_{b2} - C_{a1}) + K_1 K_2]$$
$$- K_1 K_2 C_{a1} = 0 \qquad (7\text{–}125)$$

In solutions containing a salt such as ammonium acetate, $C_{a1} = C_{b2} = C_s$. C_s is the concentration of salt added. In all systems of practical importance, $C_s \gg K_1$ or K_2, and equation (7–125) simplifies to:

$$[H_3O^+]^2 C_s + [H_3O^+]K_1 K_2 - K_1 K_2 C_s = 0 \qquad (7\text{–}126)$$

which is a quadratic equation that can be solved in the usual manner. In most instances, however, $C_s \gg [H_3O^+]$, and the quadratic equation reduces to

$$[H_3O^+] = \sqrt{K_1 K_2} \qquad (7\text{–}127)$$

Equations (7–118) and (7–119) illustrate the fact that K_1 and K_2 are not the successive acidity constants for a single diprotic acid system, and equation (7–127) is not the same as equation (7–115); instead, K_1 is the acidity constant for HB_1 ($Acid_1$) and K_2 is the acidity constant for the conjugate acid, HB_2 ($Acid_2$) of the base B_2^-. The determination of $Acid_1$ and $Acid_2$ can be illustrated using ammonium acetate, and considering the acid and base added to the system interacting as follows:

$$\underset{Acid_1}{NH_4^+} + \underset{Base_2}{Ac^-} \rightleftharpoons \underset{Acid_2}{HAc} + \underset{Base_1}{NH_3} \qquad (7\text{–}128)$$

Thus, for this system, K_1 is the acidity constant for the ammonium ion, and K_2 is the acidity constant for acetic acid.

Example 7–22. Calculate the pH of a 0.01-*M* solution of ammonium acetate. The acidity constant for acetic acid is $K_2 = K_a = 1.75 \times 10^{-5}$, and the basicity constant for ammonia is $K_b = 1.74 \times 10^{-5}$.

(a) K_1 can be found by dividing K_b for ammonia into K_w:

$$K_1 = \frac{1.00 \times 10^{-14}}{1.74 \times 10^{-5}} = 5.75 \times 10^{-10}$$

$$[H_3O^+] = \sqrt{(5.75 \times 10^{-10}) \times (1.75 \times 10^{-5})}$$

$$= 1.00 \times 10^{-7} \, M$$

Note that all of the assumptions are valid.

$$\text{pH} = -\log (1.00 \times 10^{-7}) = 7.00$$

When ammonium succinate is dissolved in water, it dissociates to yield two NH_4^+ cations and 1 succinate (S^{2-}) anion. These ions can enter into the following acid-base equilibrium:

$$\underset{\text{Acid}_1}{NH_4^+} + \underset{\text{Base}_2}{S^{2-}} \; \rightleftharpoons \; \underset{\text{Acid}_2}{HS^-} + \underset{\text{Base}_1}{NH_3} \qquad (7-129)$$

In this system, $C_{b2} = C_s$ and $C_{a1} = 2C_s$, the concentration of salt added. If C_s is much greater than either K_1 or K_2, equation (7–125) simplifies to

$$[H_3O^+]^2 - [H_3O^+]K_1 - 2K_1K_2 = 0 \qquad (7-130)$$

and if $2K_2 \gg [H_3O^+]$,

$$[H_3O^+] = \sqrt{2K_1K_2} \qquad (7-131)$$

In this example, equation (7–129) shows that K_1 is the acidity constant for the ammonium cation, and K_2, referring to Acid$_2$, must be the acidity constant for the bisuccinate species HS^-, or the second acidity constant for succinic acid.

In general, when Acid$_2$ comes from a polyprotic acid H_nA, equation (7–125) simplifies to

$$[H_3O^+]^2 - [H_3O^+]K_1(n - 1) - nK_1K_2 = 0 \qquad (7-132)$$

and

$$[H_3O^+] = \sqrt{nK_1K_2} \qquad (7-133)$$

using the same assumptions that were used in developing equations (7–129) and (7–130).

It should be pointed out that in deriving equations (7–129) to (7–133), the base was assumed to be monoprotic. Thus, it would appear that these equations should not be valid for salts such as ammonium succinate or ammonium phosphate. For all systems of practical importance, however, the solution to these equations yields a pH value above the final pK_a for the system. Therefore, the concentrations of all species formed by the addition of more than one proton to a polyacidic base will be negligibly small, and the assumption of only a one-proton addition becomes quite valid.

Example 7–23. Calculate the pH of a 0.01-M solution of ammonium succinate. As shown in equation (7–129), K_1 is the acidity constant for the ammonium cation, which was found in the previous example to be 5.75×10^{-10}, and K_2 refers to the acid succinate (HS^-) or the second acidity constant for the succinic acid system. Thus, $K_2 = 2.3 \times 10^{-6}$.

$$[H_3O^+] = \sqrt{2(5.75 \times 10^{-10}) \times (2.3 \times 10^{-6})}$$

$$= 5.14 \times 10^{-8}$$

$$\text{pH} = -\log (5.14 \times 10^{-8}) = 7.29$$

Solutions Containing a Weak Acid and a Weak Base. In the preceding section, the acid and base were added in the form of a single salt. They can be added as two separate salts or an acid and a salt, however, forming buffer solutions (see Chapter 8) whose pH is given by equation (7–127). For example, consider a solution made by dissolving equimolar amounts of sodium acid phosphate, NaH_2PO_4, and disodium citrate, $Na_2HC_6H_5O_7$, in water. Both salts dissociate to give the amphoteric species $H_2PO_4^-$ and $HC_6H_5O_7^{2-}$, causing a problem in deciding which species to designate as HB_1 and which to designate as B_2^- in equations (7–118) and (7–119). This problem can be resolved by considering the acidity constants for the two species in question. The acidity constant for $H_2PO_4^-$ is 7.2 and that for the species $HC_6H_5O_7^{2-}$ is 6.4. The citrate species, being more acidic, acts as the acid in the following equilibrium:

$$\underset{\text{Acid}_1}{HC_6H_5O_7^{2-}} + \underset{\text{Base}_2}{H_2PO_4^-} \rightleftharpoons$$

$$\underset{\text{Acid}_2}{H_3PO_4} + \underset{\text{Base}_1}{C_6H_5O_7^{3-}} \qquad (7-134)$$

Thus, K_1 in equation (7–127) is K_3 for the citric acid system, and K_2 in equation (7–127) is K_1 for the phosphoric acid system.

Example 7–24. What is the pH of a solution containing NaH_2PO_4 and disodium citrate (disodium hydrogen citrate) $Na_2HC_6H_5O_7$, both in a concentration of 0.01 M? The third acidity constant for $HC_6H_5O_7^{2-}$ is 4.0×10^{-7}, while the first acidity constant for phosphoric acid is 7.5×10^{-3}.

$$[H_3O^+] = \sqrt{(4.0 \times 10^{-7}) \times (7.5 \times 10^{-3})}$$

$$= 5.48 \times 10^{-5} \, M$$

All assumptions are valid.

$$\text{pH} = -\log (5.48 \times 10^{-5}) = 4.26$$

The equilibrium shown in equation (7–134) illustrates the fact that the system made by dissolving NaH_2PO_4 and $Na_2HC_6H_5O_7$ in water is identical to that made by dissolving H_3PO_4 and $Na_3C_6H_5O_7$ in water. In the latter case, H_3PO_4 is HB_1, and the tricitrate is B_2^-, and if the two substances are dissolved in equimolar amounts, equation (7–127) is valid for the system.

A slightly different situation arises for equimolar combinations of substances such as succinic acid, $H_2C_4H_4O_4$, and tribasic sodium phosphate, Na_3PO_4. In this case it is obvious that succinic acid is the acid that can protonate the base to yield the species $HC_4H_4O_4^-$ and HPO_4^{2-}. The acid succinate (pK_a 5.63) is a stronger acid than HPO_4^{2-} (pK_a 12.0), however, and an equilibrium cannot be established between these species and the species originally added to water. Instead, the HPO_4^{2-} is protonated by the acid succinate to give $C_4H_4O_4^{2-}$ and $H_2PO_4^-$. This is illustrated in the following:

$$H_2C_4H_4O_4 + PO_4^{3-} \rightarrow$$

$$HC_4H_4O_4^- + HPO_4^{2-} \qquad (7-135)$$

$$HC_4H_4O_4^- + HPO_4^{2-} \rightleftharpoons$$
Acid$_1$ Base$_2$

$$C_4H_4O_4^{2-} + H_2PO_4^- \qquad (7-136)$$
Base$_1$ Acid$_2$

Thus, K_1 in equation (7–136) is K_2 for the succinic acid system, and K_2 in equation (7–127) is actually K_2 from the phosphoric acid system.

Example 7–25. Calculate the pH of a solution containing succinic acid and tribasic sodium phosphate, each at a concentration of 0.01 M. The second acidity constant for the succinic acid system is 2.3×10^{-6}. The second acidity constant for the phosphoric acid system is 6.2×10^{-8}.

(a)

$$[H_3O^+] = \sqrt{(2.3 \times 10^{-6})(6.2 \times 10^{-8})}$$
$$= 3.78 \times 10^{-7} \, M$$

All assumptions are valid.

$$pH = -\log(3.78 \times 10^{-7}) = 6.42$$

(b) Equation (7–127) can also be solved by taking logarithms of both sides to yield

$$pH = \tfrac{1}{2}(pK_1 + pK_2)$$
$$= \tfrac{1}{2}(5.63 + 7.21) = 6.42 \qquad (7-137)$$

Equations (7–135) and (7–136) illustrate the fact that solutions made by dissolving equimolar amounts of $H_2C_4H_4O_4$ and Na_3PO_4, $NaHC_4H_4O_4$ and Na_2HPO_4, or $Na_2C_4H_4O_4$ and NaH_2PO_4 in water all equilibrate to the same pH and are identical.

ACIDITY CONSTANTS

One of the most important properties of a drug molecule is its acidity constant, which for many drugs can be related to physiologic and pharmacologic activity,[10-12] solubility (see Chapter 10), rate of solution,[13] extent of binding,[14] and rate of absorption.[15]

Effect of Ionic Strength Upon Acidity Constants. In the preceding sections, the solutions were considered dilute enough that the effect of ionic strength upon the acid–base equilibria could be ignored. A more exact treatment for the ionization of a weak acid, for example, would be

$$HB + H_2O \rightleftharpoons H_3O^+ + B$$

$$K = \frac{a_{H_3O^+} a_B}{a_{HB}} = \frac{[H_3O^+][B]}{[HB]} \cdot \frac{\gamma_{H_3O^+} \gamma_B}{\gamma_{HB}} \qquad (7-138)$$

in which K is the thermodynamic acidity constant, and the charges on the species have been omitted to make the equations more general. Equation (7–138) illustrates the fact that in solving equations involving acidity constants, both the concentration and activity coefficient of each species must be considered. One way to simplify the problem would be to define the acidity constant as an apparent constant in terms of the hydronium ion activity and species concentrations and activity coefficients, as follows:

$$K = a_{H_3O^+} \frac{[B]}{[HB]} \frac{\gamma_B}{\gamma_{HB}} = K' \frac{\gamma_B}{\gamma_{HB}} \qquad (7-139)$$

and

$$pK' = pK + \log \frac{\gamma_B}{\gamma_{HB}} \qquad (7-140)$$

The following form of the Debye–Hückel equation[16] can be used for ionic strengths up to about 0.3 M:

$$-\log \gamma_i = \frac{0.51 Z_i^2 \sqrt{\mu}}{1 + aB\sqrt{\mu}} - K_s \mu \qquad (7-141)$$

in which Z_i is the charge on the species i. The value of the constants $a \cdot B$ can be taken to be approximately 1 at 25° C, and K_s is a "salting out" constant. At moderate ionic strengths, K_s can be assumed to be approximately the same for both the acid and its conjugate base.[16] Thus, for an acid with charge Z, going to a base with charge $Z - 1$:

$$pK' = pK + \frac{0.51(2Z - 1)\sqrt{\mu}}{1 + \sqrt{\mu}} \qquad (7-142)$$

Example 7–26. Calculate pK_2' for citric acid at an ionic strength of 0.01 M. Assume that $pK_2 = 4.78$. The charge on the acidic species is -1.

$$pK_2' = 4.78 + \frac{0.51(-3)\sqrt{0.01}}{1 + \sqrt{0.01}}$$
$$= 4.78 - 1.53(0.091) = 4.64$$

If either the acid or its conjugate base is a zwitterion, it will have a large dipole moment, and the expression for its activity coefficient must contain a term K_r, the "salting in" constant.[17] Thus, for the zwitterion [+ −]:

$$-\log \gamma_{+-} = (K_r - K_s)\mu \qquad (7-143)$$

The first ionization of an amino acid such as glycine hydrochloride involves an acid with a charge of +1 going to the zwitterion, [+−]. Combining equations (7–143) and (7–141) with equation (7–140) gives

$$pK_1' = pK_1 + \frac{0.51\sqrt{\mu}}{1 + \sqrt{\mu}} - K_r\mu \qquad (7-144)$$

The second ionization step involves the zwitterion going to a species with a charge of -1. Thus, using equations (7–143), (7–141), and (7–140) gives

$$pK_2' = pK_2 - \frac{0.51\sqrt{\mu}}{1 + \sqrt{\mu}} + K_r\mu \qquad (7-145)$$

The "salting in" constant, K_r, is approximately 0.32 for alpha-amino acids in water, and approximately 0.6 for dipeptides.[17] Use of these values for K_r enables equations (7–144) and (7–145) to be used for solutions with ionic strengths up to about 0.3 M.

The procedure to be used in solving pH problems in which the ionic strength of the solution must be considered would be as follows:

(*a*) Convert all pK values needed for the problem into pK' values.

(*b*) Solve the appropriate equation in the usual manner.

Example 7–27. Calculate the pH of 0.01-M solution of acetic acid to which enough KCl had been added to give an ionic strength of 0.01 M at 25° C. The pK_a for acetic acid is 4.76.

(*a*)

$$pK'_a = 4.76 - \frac{0.51\sqrt{0.10}}{1 + \sqrt{0.10}}$$

$$= 4.76 - 0.12 = 4.64$$

(*b*) Taking logarithms of equation (7–99) gives

$$pH = \tfrac{1}{2}(pK'_a - \log C_a)$$

in which we now write pK_a as pK'_a

$$pH = \tfrac{1}{2}(4.64 + 2.00) = 3.32$$

Example 7–28. Calculate the pH of 10^{-3}-M solution of glycine at an ionic strength of 0.10 at 25° C. The pK_a values for glycine are p$K_1 = 2.35$ and p$K_2 = 9.78$.

(*a*)

$$pK'_1 = 2.35 + \frac{0.51\sqrt{0.10}}{1 + \sqrt{0.10}} - 0.32(0.10)$$

$$= 2.35 + 0.12 - 0.03 = 2.44$$

(*b*)

$$pK'_2 = 9.78 - \frac{0.51\sqrt{0.10}}{1 + \sqrt{0.10}} + 0.32(0.10)$$

$$= 9.78 - 0.12 + 0.03 = 9.69$$

(*c*) Taking logarithms of equation (7–115) gives

$$pH = \tfrac{1}{2}(pK_1 + pK_2)$$

$$= \tfrac{1}{2}(2.44 + 9.69) = 6.07$$

The pH value that is calculated using the apparent acidity constants, designated K', in place of the thermodynamic acidity constants K, is defined as the negative logarithm of the *hydronium ion activity*. Taking antilogarithms, therefore, would give the hydronium ion activity, *not* the hydronium ion *concentration*. If the hydronium ion concentration is desired, it can be obtained by dividing the hydronium ion activity by the mean ionic activity coefficient for the electrolyte (p. 150).

Free Energy of Ionization and the Effect of Temperature Upon Ionic Equilibria. Recall from Chapter 3 that the standard free energy change $\Delta G°$ of a reaction is related to the equilibrium constant. Therefore, the standard free energy change of an ionization reaction can be computed from the ionization constant, K_a:

$$\Delta G° = -RT \ln K_a \qquad (7\text{–}146)$$

Using the pK_a, equation (7–146) can be written as

$$\Delta G° = 2.303\, RT\, pK_a \qquad (7\text{–}147)$$

Example 7–29. The pK_a value for the weak acid amobarbital at 25° C is 7.96 (Table 7–7). Compute the standard free energy change for the ionization of this barbituric acid derivative.

$$\Delta G° = 2.303 \times 1.9872 \times 298 \times 7.96$$

$$= 10,855.9 \text{ cal/mole}$$

$$= 10.86 \text{ kcal/mole}$$

Notice that although $\Delta G°$ is positive, it is not $\Delta G°$ but rather ΔG that determines whether or not a process is spontaneous, according to Chapter 3, equation (3–117)

$$\Delta G = \Delta G° + RT \ln Q \qquad (7\text{–}148)$$

Example 7–30. An organic acid dissociates according to the reaction

$$HA + H_2O = H_3O^+ + A^-$$

The dissociation exponent pK_a of the acid at 25° C is 5.0. Assume that the reaction proceeds at a rate slow enough that the concentration of the products may be determined at any time. Disregard the difference between activities and concentrations. Compute (*a*) the standard free energy $\Delta G°$ and (*b*) the free energy change ΔG accompanying the reaction when 0.1 mole per liter of the acid has dissociated sufficiently to form 10^{-4} mole per liter of ions. (*c*) In terms of the sign of $\Delta G°$ state whether or not the reaction is spontaneous.

(*a*)

$$\Delta G° = 2.303 \times 1.987 \times 298 \times 5.0$$

$$= 6818 \text{ cal/mole}$$

(*b*) The reaction quotient Q, expressed in concentrations, is

$$Q = \frac{[H_3O^+][A]}{[H\Lambda]} = \frac{10^{-4} \times 10^{-4}}{10^{-1} - 10^{-4}} \cong 10^{-7}$$

The concentration of water, being great, is not altered significantly by the reaction and thus does not appear in the quotient. Alternatively, it may be stated that the $[H_2O]$ term does not appear because water is present essentially at unit activity, pure water at 1 atm and 25° C being taken as the standard state of H_2O. Q must not be confused with the equilibrium constant K, the latter being the ratio of the concentrations of the reactant and products as the forward and reverse reactions proceed under the conditions of dynamic equilibrium.

$$\Delta G = \Delta G° + 2.303\, RT \log \frac{a_{\text{prod}}}{a_{\text{react}}} = 2.303\, RT\, pK + 2.303\, RT \log Q$$

$$\Delta G = 6818 + (2.303 \times 1.987 \times 298 \times \log 10^{-7})$$

$$= 6818 - 9546 = -2728 \text{ cal/mole}$$

(*c*) The conversion of 0.1 mole per liter of acid into 10^{-4} mole per liter of its ions is a spontaneous reaction since ΔG is negative at constant pressure and temperature.

By writing equation (7–148) as

$$\Delta G = RT \ln \frac{Q}{K}$$

it can be seen that the sign and hence the spontaneity of the reaction depends on the relative values of the quantities Q and K. If Q is smaller than K, signifying that the concentrations (activities) of the products are yet below the values at equilibrium, ΔG will have a negative sign, and the process will move spontaneously toward a state of equilibrium. If Q is larger than K, the concentrations of the products are greater than the equilibrium values, ΔG will have a positive sign, and the process will be nonspontaneous. If $K = Q$, then $\Delta G = 0$, and the system is at equilibrium.

The positive value of $\Delta G°$ signifies that the electrolyte in its standard state of unit activity cannot dissociate spontaneously into ions of unit activity. Ionization does occur, nevertheless, its possibility being shown by the sign of ΔG and not by the sign of $\Delta G°$. This fact was brought out in *Example 7–30*, in which neither the reactant nor the products were in their standard states.

The *CRC Handbook of Physics and Chemistry*, 63rd ed., p. D-62 gives the following standard thermodynamic values, where *f* stands for free energy or enthalpy of *formation* (see p. 59 for an explanation of the standard enthalpy [heat] of formation; standard free energy of formation is defined in an analogous way). $S°$ is a standard thermodynamic property, as designated by the superscript "o." It is not a *difference* in entropies, ΔS, as in the case of enthalpy and free energy, but is rather absolute entropy of a substance based on its entropy value above zero degrees Kelvin.

Now, the change in enthalpy, entropy, or free energy in a reaction may be characterized by the standard enthalpy, entropy, and free energy changes, $\Delta H°$, $\Delta S°$, and $\Delta G°$. These are obtained by taking the differences between the $\Delta H_f°$, $S°$, and $\Delta G_f°$ of the product and reactant.

Example 7–31. In the case of the ionization of acetic acid in aqueous solution at 25° C (298.15° K), we can use these thermodynamic properties to calculate the dissociation (ionization) constant, K_a, and the dissociation exponent, pK_a.

Standard Thermodynamic Values For Ionization Of Acetic Acid*

	CH₃COOH ⟶	CH₃COO⁻ ⟶	H⁺
$\Delta H_f°$ (kcal/mole)	−116.10	−116.16	0
$\Delta G_f°$ (kcal/mole)	− 94.8	− 88.29	0
$S°$ (cal/deg mole)	42.7	20.7	0

*Standard thermodynamic values vary somewhat from one literature source to another.

In its standard state of 1 molar aqueous solution, the value of the hydrogen ion for these thermodynamic properties is zero, as seen in the table.

The standard enthalpy and standard entropy changes, $\Delta H°$ and $\Delta S°$, for the ionization reaction are the values for the product, CH_3COO^-, minus the values for the reactant at 25° C:

$$\Delta H° = (-116.16) - (-116.10) = -0.060 \text{ kcal/mole}$$
$$= -60.0 \text{ cal/mole}$$
$$\Delta S° = \quad 20.7 - \quad 42.7 \quad = -22.0 \text{ cal/deg mole}$$

Now, from equation (7–147),

$$pK_a = +\Delta G°/(2.303\,RT) \tag{7–149}$$

Since

$$\Delta G° = \Delta H° - T\Delta S° \tag{7–150}$$

we also have

$$2.303 \cdot \log K_a = \frac{\Delta S°}{R} - \frac{\Delta H°}{RT} \tag{7–151}$$

Therefore, knowing $\Delta H_f°$ and $S°$ or simply having $\Delta G_f°$ (as found in *Problem 3–20*) for both reactants and products, we can obtain K_a and pK_a for the ionization of weak acids and weak bases. This procedure may also be used to calculate equilibria constants for nonionic chemical reactions (*Problem 3–22*).

Continuing with the case of acetic acid and using equation (7–151),

$$2.303 \log K_a = \frac{-22.0}{1.9872} - \frac{-60.0}{(1.9872)(298.15)} = -10.96958$$
$$\log K_a = 4.763; \quad K_a = 1.73 \times 10^{-5}$$
$$pK_a = 4.76$$

Example 7–32. Calculate the K_a and pK_a for the first and second ionization stages of H_2CO_3 at 25° C in aqueous solution. The data are as follows*:

	$\Delta H_f°$	$S°$	$\Delta G_f°$
H_2CO_3 aq	−167.22	44.8	−148.94
HCO_3^- aq	−165.39	21.8	−140.26
CO_3^{2-} aq	−161.84	−13.6	−126.17

*CRC Handbook of Chemistry and Physics, 63rd ed. CRC Press, Boca Raton, Fla., p. D–60.

$\Delta H_f°$ and $\Delta G_f°$ are the heat and free energy of formation at 25° C (298.15° K), respectively. $S°$ is the absolute entropy at 25° C. The "o" indicates that these thermodynamic quantities are for each species in its standard state of 1 molal aqueous solution at 1 atmosphere pressure and ordinary temperature.

The reaction for the first stage is

$$H_2CO_3 \rightarrow HCO_3^- + H^+$$

and the standard enthalpy, entropy, and free energies are

$$\Delta H° = \Delta H_f°(HCO_3^- \text{ aq}) - \Delta H_f°(H_2CO_3)$$
$$(-165.39) \quad - \quad (-167.22) = 1.830 \text{ kcal/mole}$$
$$= 1830 \text{ cal/mole}$$
$$\Delta S° = S°(HCO_3^- \text{ aq}) - S°(H_2CO_3)$$
$$(21.8) \quad - \quad (44.8) \quad = -23.0 \text{ cal/deg mole}$$
$$\Delta G° = \Delta G_f°(HCO_3^- \text{ aq}) - \Delta G_f°(H_2CO_3)$$
$$(-140.26) \quad - \quad (-148.94) \quad = 8.680 \text{ kcal/mole}$$
$$= 8680 \text{ cal/mole}$$

The ionization constant for the first stage of ionization of H_2CO_3 is obtained from the equation, $\Delta G° = \Delta H° - T\Delta S° = -RT \ln K_1$, or

$$\ln K_1 = \frac{\Delta S_{12}°}{R} - \frac{\Delta H_{12}°}{RT} = -\frac{\Delta G_{12}°}{RT}$$

TABLE 7–7. pK_a and $\Delta G°$ Values for Substituted Barbituric Acids, 25° C*

Compound	pK_a	$\Delta G°$ (kcal/mol)
5-Allyl-5-isopropylbarbituric acid (Aprobarbital)‡	8.02	10.96
5-5-Diallylbarbituric acid (Dial)	7.81	10.66
5,5-Dibromobarbituric acid‡	5.68	7.75
5,5-Dichlorobarbituric acid‡	5.55	7.57
5,5-Diethylbarbituric acid (Barbital)†,‡	7.98	10.89
5,5-Dimethylbarbituric acid‡	8.51	11.61
5-Ethyl-5-butylbarbituric acid (Butethal)§	7.98	10.89
5-Ethyl-5-isopropylbarbituric acid (Probarbital)‡	8.14	11.11
5-Ethyl-5-(l-methylbutyl)barbituric acid (Pentobarbital)§, ‖	8.13	11.09
5-Ethyl-5-(3-methylbutyl)barbituric acid (Amobarbital)§	7.96	10.86
5-Ethyl-5-phenylbarbituric acid (Phenobarbital)¶	7.48	10.20
5-Methyl-5-phenylbarbituric acid (Rutonal)‡	7.78	10.61

*This table was provided by R. J. Prankerd, College of Pharmacy, University of Florida, Gainesville, Fla.
†From G. G. Manov, K. E. Schuette and F. S. Kirk, J. Res. Nat. Bur. Stand. **48**, 84–91, 1952.
‡From R. H. McKeown, J. Chem. Soc., Perk. II, 506–514, 1980.
§From A. I. Biggs, J. Chem. Soc. 2485–2488, 1956.
‖From R. J. Prankerd, Ph.D. Thesis, University of Otago, New Zealand, 1985.
¶From D. R. Baird, R. H. McKeown and R. J. Prankerd, School of Pharmacy, University of Otago, New Zealand. Unpublished data.

TABLE 7–8. *Thermodynamic Constants of Ionization**

Electrolyte	A	C	D	$T_{max}°$ K	pK_{Tmax}	$\Delta G°_{25° C}$ cal/mole	$\Delta H°_{25° C}$ cal/mole	$\Delta S°_{25° C}$ cal/deg mole
Formic acid	1342.85	0.015168	5.2743	297.5	3.7519	5117	−23	−17.6
Acetic acid	1170.48	0.013399	3.1649	295.6	4.7555	6486	−92	−22.1
Propionic acid	1213.26	0.014055	3.3860	293.8	4.8729	6647	−163	−22.8
Boric acid	2193.55	0.016499	3.0395	364.6	8.9923	12596	3328	−31.1
Barbital	2324.47	0.011856	3.3491	†	†	†	†	†
Lactic acid	1304.72	0.014926	4.9639	‡	‡	‡	‡	‡

*From H. S. Harned and B. B. Owen, Physical Chemistry of Electrolytic Solutions, Reinhold, New York, 1958.
†See *Problem 7–42* on page 168.
‡See *Problem 7–43* on page 168.

Substituting the values from the table for the first stage, $H_2CO_3 \rightarrow HCO_3^- + H^+$, we obtain

$$\ln K_1 = \frac{-23.0}{1.9872} - \frac{1830}{(1.9872)(298.15)} = -14.663; \log K_1 = \ln K_1/2.303$$

$$-\log K_1 = pK_1 = 6.37$$

(The value in Table 7–1 is 6.37.)

One can also obtain the dissociation constant using $\Delta G_{12}°$, where $_{1,2}$ refers to the values for the species H_2CO_3 and HCO_3^-, respectively. From the table we obtain $\Delta G_{12}° = 8.68$ kcal/mole or 868.0 cal/mole:

$$\ln K_1 = -\frac{8680}{(1.9872)(298.15)} = -14.650; \log K_1 = \ln K_1/2.303$$

$$pK_1 = -\log K_1 = 6.36$$

As an exercise, the student should calculate K_2 and pK_2, the values for the second stages of the ionization of H_2CO_3. Compare your values with those found in Table 7–1. The pK_a and $\Delta G°$ values for some substituted barbituric acids at 25° C are found in Table 7–7.

Harned and Owen[18] suggest the following empiric equation by which to relate the ionization constants and temperature:

$$\log K = -\frac{A}{T} - CT + D \qquad (7–152)$$

in which A, C, and D are constants obtained by careful experimentation. Ionization constants of many of the weak electrolytes pass through a maximum value between 0° and 60° C, and the temperature at which maximum ionization occurs is given by the expression

$$T_{max} = \sqrt{\frac{A}{C}} \qquad (7–153)$$

The dissociation exponent at this temperature is

$$pK_{Tmax} = 2\sqrt{AC} - D \qquad (7–154)$$

The thermodynamic quantities for ionization are also obtained by use of the constants A, C, and D.

$$\Delta G° = 2.3026R(A - DT + CT^2) \qquad (7–155)$$

$$\Delta H° = 2.3026R(A - CT^2) \qquad (7–156)$$

$$\Delta S° = 2.3026R(D - 2CT) \qquad (7–157)$$

The results of Harned and Owen[18] for some representative weak electrolytes are listed in Table 7–8.

References and Notes

1. J. N. Brönsted, Rec. Trav. Chim. **42**, 718, 1923; Chem. Revs. **5**, 231, 1928; T. M. Lowry, J. Chem. Soc. **123**, 848, 1923.
2. A. W. Castleman, Jr., J. Chem. Phys. **94**, 3268, 1991; Chem. Eng. News **69** [14], 47, April 8, 1991.
3. W. F. Luder and S. Zuffanti, *Electronic Theory of Acids and Bases*, Wiley, New York, 1947; G. N. Lewis, *Valency and the Structure of Atoms and Molecules*, Reinhold, New York, 1923.
4. R. P. Bell, *Acids and Bases*, Methuen, London, 1952, Chapter 7.
5. S. P. L. Sörensen, Biochem. Z. **21**, 201, 1909.
6. S. F. Kramer and G. L. Flynn, J. Pharm. Sci. **61**, 1896, 1972.
7. P. A. Schwartz, C. T. Rhodes and J. W. Cooper, Jr., J. Pharm. Sci. **66**, 994, 1977.
8. J. Blanchard, J. O. Boyle and S. Van Wagenen, J. Pharm. Sci. **77**, 548, 1988.
9. T. S. Lee and L. Gunnar Sillen, *Chemical Equilibrium in Analytical Chemistry*, Interscience, New York, 1959; J. N. Butler, *Solubility and pH Calculations*, Addison-Wesley, Reading, Mass., 1964; A. J. Bard, *Chemical Equilibrium*, Harper & Row, New York, 1966.
10. P. B. Marshall, Br. J. Pharmacol. **10**, 270, 1955.
11. P. Bell and R. O. Roblin, J. Am. Chem. Soc. **64**, 2905, 1942.
12. I. M. Klotz, J. Am. Chem. Soc. **66**, 459, 1944.
13. W. E. Hamlin and W. I. Higuchi, J. Pharm. Sci. **55**, 205, 1966.
14. M. C. Meyer and D. E. Guttman, J. Pharm. Sci. **57**, 245, 1968.
15. B. B. Brodie, "Physico-Chemical Factors in Drug Absorption" in T. B. Binns, *Absorption and Distribution of Drugs*, Williams & Wilkins, Baltimore, 1964, pp. 16–48.
16. J. T. Edsall and J. Wyman, *Biophysical Chemistry*, Vol. 1, Academic Press, New York, 1958, p. 442.
17. J. T. Edsall and J. Wyman, ibid., p. 443.
18. H. S. Harned and B. B. Owen, *Physical Chemistry of Electrolytic Solutions*, Reinhold, New York, 1958, pp. 665, 667, 758.
19. M. J. Nieto, J. L. Gonzalez, A. Dominguez-Gil and J. M. Lanao, J. Pharm. Sci. **76**, 228, 1987.
20. B. H. Mahon, *Elementary Chemical Thermodynamics*, W. A. Benjamin, Menlo Park, CA., 1963 p. 140.
21. H. A. Bent, *The Second Law*, Oxford University Press, Oxford, 1965, pp. 397–415.
22. Y. K. Agrawal, R. Giridhar and S. K. Menon, J. Pharm. Sci. **76**, 903, 1987.
23. H. A. Bent, *The Second Law*, Oxford University Press, Oxford, 1965, p. 402.
24. A. P. Kurtz and T. D. J. D'Silva, J. Pharm. Sci. **76**, 599, 1987.

Problems

7–1. Practice calculations involving pH, pOH, and ionic concentration in aqueous solutions.

(a) Convert pH = 2.54 to hydrogen ion concentration, $[H^+]$.

(b) What is the pH of a 7.93×10^{-4} molar solution of a strong acid?

(c) If the pH of a solution of a strong base is 8.75, what is its hydroxyl ion concentration? What is its hydrogen ion concentration?

(d) What is the pH of a 0.00379-M solution of HNO_3? What is its pOH?

(e) Convert the hydroxyl ion concentration, 0.00915 M to pH.

(f) Calculate the pH of a 2.37×10^{-3} M solution of sulfuric acid. H_2SO_4 dissociates completely as a strong electrolyte in a dilute solution, as found in the present problem.

(g) A 0.017-M solution of HCl is mixed with a 0.017-M solution of NaOH. What is the pH of the final mixture?

(h) What is the pH of a 0.034-M solution of NaCl?

(i) The solubility of phenobarbital in water at 25° C is 0.14% (w/v). What is the pH of the saturated solution?

(j) If 15 mL of 0.02 M NaOH is added to 15 mL of 0.02 M acetic acid, what is the pH of the solution? Convert the pH to hydrogen ion concentration.

(k) The pOH of a drug solution is 6.82; what is the pH of the solution? What is the hydroxyl ion concentration if the solution is a strong base?

(l) What is the pH and pOH of a 5×10^{-8} M solution of HCl at 25° C?

(m) Calculate the pH of a 0.06-M solution of formic acid.

Answers: **(a)** $[H_3O^+] = 2.88 \times 10^{-3}$; **(b)** pH = 3.10; **(c)** $[OH^-] = 5.62 \times 10^{-6}$, $[H_3O^+] = 1.78 \times 10^{-9}$; **(d)** pH = 2.42, pOH = 11.58; **(e)** pH = 11.96; **(f)** pH = 2.32; **(g)** pH = 7.07; **(h)** pH = 7.08; **(i)** pH = 4.81; **(j)** pH = 8.53, $[H_3O^+] = 2.95 \times 10^{-9}$; **(k)** pH = 7.18, $[OH^-] = 1.51 \times 10^{-7}$; **(l)** pH = 6.89, pOH = 7.11; **(m)** pH = 2.49.

7-2. If 100 mL of 0.005 M sulfathiazole is mixed with 57 mL of 0.003 M sodium hydroxide, what is the pH of the mixture? What is the pOH of the solution? Sulfathiazole reacts in part with NaOH to give sodium sulfathiazole. *Hint:* Use the Henderson–Hasselbalch equation (8–8) in the form

$$pH = pK_a + \log \frac{[\text{sodium sulfathiazole}]}{[\text{sulfathiazole}]}$$

The pK_a of sulfathiazole is 7.12.

Answer: pH = 6.84, pOH = 7.16

7-3.(a) What is the mole percent of free phenobarbital in solution at pH 8.00? **(b)** What is the mole percent of free cocaine in solution at pH 8.00? (The fraction of nonionized drug in the form of a weak acid is obtained using equation (13–95), and as a weak base, equation (13–96)). (Also see equations (13–77) and (13–78) for the ionized rather than the nonionized case.)

Answers: **(a)** 23%; **(b)** 28%

7-4. **(a)** What is the pH of a 5 g per 100 mL solution of phenol? **(b)** What is the hydroxyl ion concentration of the solution?

Answers: **(a)** pH = 5.14; **(b)** $[OH^-] = 1.38 \times 10^{-9}$

7-5. Compute the hydronium ion concentration and pH of a 0.001-M solution of acetic acid using both the approximate and the more exact quadratic equations.

Answer: approximate $[H_3O^+] = 1.32 \times 10^{-4}$ M, pH = 3.88; exact $[H_3O^+] = 1.24 \times 10^{-4}$ M, pH = 3.91

7-6. Calculate the pH of a 1% (w/v) solution of morphine sulfate. The molecular weight of this salt is 668.76.

Answer: pH = 4.70

7-7. What is the pH of a 1:200 aqueous solution of ephedrine at 25°?

Answer: pH = 10.92

7-8. Calculate the pH of a 0.01-M solution of tartaric acid.

Answer: pH = 2.58

7-9. Calculate the pH of a 0.01-M solution of physostigmine at 25° C.

Answer: pH = 9.94

7-10. Calculate the pH of a solution containing 0.1 M acetic acid and 0.1 M formic acid.

Answer: pH = 2.36

7-11. What is the hydronium ion concentration and the pH of a solution at 25° C containing 0.01 mole/liter of sulfadiazine and 0.05

mole/liter of sulfisoxazole? The necessary data are found in Table 7–2.

Answer: $[H_3O^+] = 7.094 \times 10^{-4}$ mole/liter; pH = 3.15

7-12. **(a)** What is the PBE for a solution of ammonium chloride? **(b)** What is the PBE for a solution containing equimolecular amounts of Na_2HPO_4 and ammonium chloride?

Answers: **(a)** $[H_3O^+] = [OH^-] + [NH_3]$; **(b)** $[H_3O^+] + 2[H_3PO_4] + [H_2PO_4^-] = [OH^-] + [NH_3] + [PO_4^{3-}]$

7-13. What is the isoionic pH of the ampholyte *p*-aminobenzoic acid ($^+NH_3C_6H_4COO^-$), which has the two acidity constants, $pK_1 = 2.3$ and $pK_2 = 4.9$?

Answer: pH = 3.6

7-14. The sulfonamides can exist in the form of an ampholyte $^+NH_3C_6H_4SO_2NR^-$ in aqueous solution. The two acidity constants of sulfadiazine are $pK_1 = 2.1$ and $pK_2 = 6.5$. Calculate the isoionic point for this drug.

Answer: pH = 4.3

7-15. Cefroxadine, a β-lactam antibiotic, has two ionizable groups, $-COOH$ and NH_2 (Nieto et al.[19]). The equilibrium for this ampholyte may be represented as

$$^+NH_3\text{—R—COOH} \underset{K_1}{\overset{-H^+}{\rightleftharpoons}} {}^+NH_3\text{—R—COO}^- \underset{K_2}{\overset{-H^+}{\rightleftharpoons}} NH_2\text{—R—COO}^-$$

Calculate the pH of a 4.7×10^{-3} M solution of cefroxadine at 25° C. The dissociation constants are $K_1 = 6.92 \times 10^{-4}$ M and $K_2 = 1.17 \times 10^{-7}$ M. Use equation (7–115) and the more exact equation (7–114) to obtain the pH of this ampholyte.

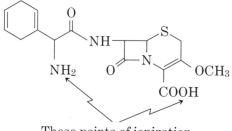

These points of ionization become NH_3^+ and COO^-

Cefroxadine

Answer: More exact result, pH = 5.08; less exact result, pH = 5.05. At this pH the zwitterionic form of cefroxadine, $^+NH_3$–R–COO^-, predominates.

7-16. What is the pH of a solution containing acetic acid 0.1 M and sodium acetate 0.02 M?

Answer: pH = 4.06

7-17.(a) Calculate the pH of a 0.1-M solution of ammonium borate. **(b)** Calculate the pH of a 0.1-M solution of ammonium propionate.

Answers: **(a)** pH = 9.24; **(b)** pH = 7.06

7-18. What is the pH of a 0.01-M solution of $(NH_4)_3PO_4$?

Answer: pH = 10.72

7-19. What is the pH of a solution containing equimolar amounts of succinic acid and tribasic sodium citrate?

Answer: pH = 5.20

7-20. Aminophylline is a complex of theophylline ($C_7H_8N_4O_2$) and ethylenediamine $C_2H_4(NH_2)_2 \cdot 2H_2O$ and belongs to the therapeutic category of smooth muscle relaxant. It behaves as a weak base with a $pK_b = 5.0$.

(a) Compute the concentration in mole/liter of ionized aminophylline (BH^+) in aqueous solution at 25° C when the reaction, $B + H_2O \rightleftharpoons BH^+ + OH^-$, is at equilibrium. The total concentration of aminophylline is 0.003 mole/liter.

(b) What is the pH of the solution at 25° C?

Answers: **(a)** The concentration of the conjugate acid species (BH^+) at equilibrium is 1.68×10^{-4} mole/liter; **(b)** pH = 10.23

7-21. What is the pH of a sulfadiazine sodium solution containing 0.5 mole of drug in 1000 mL of solution?

Answer: pH = 10.09

7–22.* An aspirin tablet (acetylsalicylic acid, pK_a 3.49, molecular weight 180.15 g/mole), was taken orally with cold water to make a solution of aspirin in the stomach fluids of 0.00167 mole/liter. The cold water produced a temperature in the stomach temporarily of 25° C.

(a) What is the percentage of aspirin in the ionic form, $C_6H_4(OOCCH_3)COO^-$, in the stomach in which the pH of the fluid is 3.20? See equation (13–77).

(b) Determine $\Delta G°$ for the ionization of aspirin at 25° C.

(c) compute ΔG for the ionization of aspirin at a molar concentration of 0.00167 in the stomach, assuming that the fluids are at a temperature of 25° C. Is the ionization of aspirin under these conditions a spontaneous process?

Answers: **(a)** % of ionization = 33.9; **(b)** $\Delta G° = 4762$ cal/mole; **(c)** $\Delta G = -65$ cal/mole. ΔG being negative, the reaction is spontaneous.

7–23.* **(a)** Calculate K_a and pK_a for the ionization of formic acid.

Data for *Problem 7–23*

	HCOOH	→ HCOO⁻	+ H⁺
$\Delta H_f°$ (kcal/mole)	−101.68	−101.71	0
$S°$ (cal/deg mole)	39.0	22.0	0

Source: Data from CRC *Handbook of Chemistry and Physics*, 63rd ed. p. D-60

(b) Calculate K_a and pK_a for formic acid using the free energies of formation, in which $\Delta G°_f(HCOO^-)$ is −83.9 kcal/mole and $\Delta G°_f(HCOOH)$ is −89.0 kcal/mole.

Answers: **(a)** $K_a = 2.03 \times 10^{-4}$, p$K_a = 3.69$; **(b)** $K_a = 1.83 \times 10^{-4}$; p$K_a = 3.74$. Compare your results with the K_a and pK_a values found in Table 7–2.

7–24. The ionization of sulfisomidine, pK_a – 7.47, is shown as

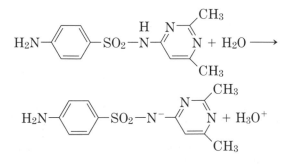

When taken orally the drug exists as a 0.073-M aqueous solution in the upper intestinal tract where the pH is 5.83.

(a) Calculate the percent of sulfisomidine in the ionic form in the solution in the intestinal tract (use equation (13–77)).

(b) Obtain the standard free energy change, $\Delta G°$, for the ionization reaction at 25° C, and explain the meaning of this result.

(c) What is the value of ΔG for the ionization in the intestinal tract, and what is the interpretation of this result?

Answers: **(a)** the percent ionization, 2.24%, is small in the intestinal tract where the pH of the environment is 5.83. **(b)** The standard free energy change is $\Delta G° = 10,191$ cal/mole. This large positive value for $\Delta G°$ suggests that the ionization reaction does not proceed far to the right in the above equation. Sulfisomidine is therefore a weak acid, which corroborates the ionization constant of 3.39×10^{-8}, the pK_a of 7.47, and the percentage ionization of 2.24%. **(c)** The free energy change, ΔG, for the reaction is 4156 cal/mole. Because of the positive value of ΔG the ionization reaction is not

---

*Problems 7–22 and 7–23 are modified from J. W. Moncrief and W. H. Jones *Elements of Physical Chemistry*, Addison-Wesley, Reading, MA., 1977, p. 123.

spontaneous. This predominantly nonionic antibacterial compound will probably be well absorbed through the intestinal mucosa. If the pH is raised, the drug will not be 50% or more ionized until the pH becomes 7.47 in the GI tract.

If the pK_a of the drug were, say, 3.0, it would be largely ionized (99.9%) at pH 5.83 in the GI tract. It would then not be significantly absorbed by passive diffusion, except at special places along the gut where ionic species are absorbed by facilitated transport mechanisms.

7–25. Phosphoric acid ionizes in three stages, as shown on page 149, and the species $H_2PO_4^-$ and HPO_4^{2-} in the body help to maintain the pH at a value of about 7.4. Calculate the K_a and pK_a for the first, second, and third stages of ionization of phosphoric acid. The required data, $\Delta H°_f$ and $S°$, are given in the table.[20]

Data for *Problem 7–25*

	$\Delta H°_f$ kcal/mole	$S°$ cal/deg mole
H_3PO_4(aq)	−308.2	42.1
$H_2PO_4^-$(aq)	−311.3	21.3
HPO_4^{2-}(aq)	−310.4	−8.6
PO_4^{3-}(aq)	−306.9	−52.0
H^+(aq)	0	0

The ionization for the first stage is often written for thermodynamic calculations as

$$H_3PO_4(aq) \rightleftharpoons H_2PO_4^-(aq) + H^+(aq)$$

It is shown on page 149 as

$$H_3PO_4 + H_2O = H_2PO_4^- + [H_3O^+]$$

Liquid water is written H_2O(liq) and the hydronium ion, $[H_3O^+]$, in aqueous solution as $[H_3O^+]$(aq). The $\Delta H°_f$ and $S°$ values for H_2O(liq) and $[H_3O^+]$(aq) are identical (Bent[21]) and may be eliminated. The values for H^+(aq) are by convention set equal to zero and may also be dropped.

Partial Answer: $K_1 = 5.3 \times 10^{-3}$, p$K_1 = 2.27$

7–26. The equation for the first stage of ionization of phosphoric acid and the standard free energies of formation $\Delta G°_f$ of the reactants and products are

$$H_3PO_4(aq) + H_2O(liq) \rightleftharpoons H_2PO_4^-(aq) + H_3O^+(aq)$$

$\Delta G°_f$ (kcal/mole) −274.2   −52.69   −271.3   −56.69

(a) Compute the first ionization constant K_1 from standard free energies of formation (Bent[21]). Compare your result with the K_1 in Table 7–2 and with the value obtained in *Problem 7–25*, using $\Delta H°_f$ and $S°$.

(b) Compute the standard free energy of formation of HPO_4^{2-}, knowing that pK_2, the "dissociation exponent" for the second stage of ionization of phosphoric acid, is 7.21.

Answers: **(a)** $K_1 = 7.49 \times 10^{-3}$, p$K_1 = 2.13$; **(b)** $\Delta G° = +9.84$ kcal/mole

7–27. Magnesium carbonate is the active ingredient in some over-the-counter antacid products. It reacts with HCl in the stomach, neutralizing some of the acid and releasing CO_2 according to the reaction

$$MgCO_3(s) + 2HCl(aq) \overset{K}{\rightleftharpoons} MgCl_2(aq) + CO_2(g) + H_2O(liq)$$

$\Delta G_f°$ (25° C) −241.9   2(−31.372)   −171.444   −94.254   −56.687
(kcal/mole)

In the equation s stands for solid, g for gas, liq for liquid, and aq for aqueous solution. Below each term of the equation is given the standard free energy of formation.

You have just ingested a newly formulated 100-mg magnesium carbonate tablet. **(a)** If you follow this with a second tablet, how will it affect the equilibrium established following the first tablet, as shown in the equation? **(b)** How will the equilibrium be affected if instead of taking another tablet you burp and expel some of the CO_2 formed in the reaction? **(c)** Compute the standard free energy change $\Delta G°$ of this reaction, and use $\Delta G°$ to obtain the equilibrium constant for the reaction.

Answers: **(a)** The reaction proceeds to the right, maintaining the value of the equilibrium constant, K. **(b)** Following a burp, the reaction also proceeds to the right so as to maintain the value of K. **(c)** $\Delta G° = -17.741$ kcal/mole, $K = 1.01 \times 10^{13}$

7–28. Some nonprescription antacid tablets contain magnesium oxide as the active ingredient to react with HCl of the stomach. The equation for the reaction, together with the standard heat of formation, standard free energy of formation, and the standard absolute entropy, is

$$MgO(s) \quad + \quad 2HCl(aq) \quad \rightleftharpoons \quad MgCl_2(aq) \quad + \quad H_2O(liq)$$

	MgO(s)	2HCl(aq)	MgCl$_2$(aq)	H$_2$O(liq)
$\Delta H_f° \left(\dfrac{\text{kcal}}{\text{mole}}\right)$	-143.81	$2(-39.952)$	-191.48	-68.315
$\Delta G_f° \left(\dfrac{\text{kcal}}{\text{mole}}\right)$	-136.10	$2(-31.372)$	-171.444	-56.687
$S° \left(\dfrac{\text{cal}}{\text{deg} \cdot \text{mole}}\right)$	6.380	$2(13.5)$	-6.117	16.71

Notice that the standard thermodynamic values for HCl(aq) have each been shown multiplied by 2 since 2 molecules of HCl appear in the equation. Tables of the standard thermodynamic properties are obtained from the National Bureau of Standards and are found in the appendixes of some thermodynamic books. The CRC *Handbook of Chemistry and Physics* contains a number of these values.

(a) Using the $\Delta G°_f$ values of the magnesium oxide reaction, calculate the standard free energy change $\Delta G°$ accompanying the reaction when an MgO antacid tablet interacts with the acid in the stomach.

(b) Having obtained $\Delta G°$ for the reaction, and assuming a temperature of 25° C, determine the constant, K, for the reaction.

(c) Use $\Delta H°_f$ and $S°$ values to obtain $\Delta G°$ and K for the reaction. Do you get the same results as under (a) and (b)?

(d) In terms of the chemical species in the reaction, describe what occurs when the first magnesium oxide antacid tablet is followed by a second or third tablet. In what way are $\Delta G°$ and K changed? What happens to the pH of the stomach fluid?

Partial Answer: **(a)** $\Delta G° = -29.287$ kcal/mole; **(b)** $K = 2.93 \times 10^{21}$. the large value for K demonstrates that the reaction goes essentially to completion (from left to right in the equation).

7–29. pK_a values of sulfacetamide have been determined by Agrawal et al.[22] in mixtures of dioxane and water at 25° C as given in the table.

Data (a) for *Problem 7–29*

Mole fraction of dioxane:	0.083	0.123	0.147	0.175
Temp (°C)		pK_a		
25	6.75	7.24	7.46	7.75
35	6.50	7.00	7.23	7.51

(a) Compute the standard free energy, standard enthalpy, and standard entropy for the ionization reaction $HA \rightleftharpoons H^+ + A^-$ in the four mixtures of dioxane and water at the two temperatures. Prepare a table of results as shown in data table (b). From the thermodynamic result obtained, is it possible to decide whether or not the reaction is a spontaneous process? If not spontaneous, would it be impossible for this reaction to occur? (*Hint:* The value of $\Delta H°$ may be obtained using the van't Hoff equation (equation 3–124, p. 71). Once $\Delta G°$ and $\Delta H°$ are known, $\Delta S°$ is readily calculated.

(b) Plot the pK_a values (vertical axis) against the mole fraction of dioxane and extrapolate the lines to zero concentration of dioxane (100% water, 0% dioxane). Read off the pK_a values in water at 25° C and 35° C.

(c) Using least-squares regression analysis, regress pK_a versus mole fraction of dioxane both at 25° C and 35° C. Compare these results with pK_a (25° C) and pK_a (35° C) obtained by extrapolation in (b).

Answers: **(a)** The values of $\Delta G°$, $\Delta H°$, and $\Delta S°$ for 0.175 mole fraction of dioxane have been given you in data table (b). Complete the table. **(b)** By extrapolation: $pK_a = 5.87$ at 25° C and 5.58 at 35° C in 100% water. **(c)** By least-squares regression analysis: $pK_a = 5.87$ at 25° C and 5.61 at 35° C in 100% water.

Data (b) for *Problem 7–29*

Mole fraction of dioxane:	0.083		0.123		0.147		0.175	
Temperature (°C)	25°	35°	25°	35°	25°	35°	25°	35°
$\Delta G° \dfrac{\text{kcal}}{\text{mole}}$							10.6	10.6
$\Delta H° \dfrac{\text{kcal}}{\text{mole}}$							10.1	
$\Delta S° \dfrac{\text{cal}}{\text{deg} \cdot \text{mole}}$							-1.61	

7–30. (a) The pK_a of amobarbital at 20° C is 8.06. What is the standard free energy change for the dissociation of this barbiturate at 20° C? **(b)** If the standard entropy change $\Delta S°$ for this reaction is -3.1 cal/(deg mole), what is the enthalpy change $\Delta H°$ at this temperature?

Answers: **(a)** 10,813 cal/mole; **(b)** 9904 cal/mole

7–31. From the dissociation constant K_a of acetic acid at 25° C, compute the standard free energy change using the equation $\Delta G° = -RT \ln K$. If $\Delta H°$ for this dissociation at 25° C is -92 cal/mole, what is the value for $\Delta S°$? (*Hint:* $\Delta G° = \Delta H° - T \Delta S°$.)

Answer: $\Delta G° = 6490$ cal/mole; $\Delta S° = -22$ cal/(deg mole)

7–32. Mercurous chloride (calomel) is a white powder, used in the past as an antiseptic and a cathartic. Mercurous chloride, mixed with mercuric chloride, is permitted by the Environmental Protection Agency as a fungicide to prevent fungus infections in certain trees, grasses, grains, and textiles.

The formation of mercurous chloride from its elements—liquid mercury and gaseous chlorine—is written, together with the standard enthalpy and free energy of formation and the standard absolute entropy, as

$$Hg(liq) + \tfrac{1}{2}Cl_2(g) = \tfrac{1}{2}Hg_2Cl_2(s)$$

	Hg(liq)	$\tfrac{1}{2}$Cl$_2$(g)	$\tfrac{1}{2}$Hg$_2$Cl$_2$(s)
$\Delta H°_f$ values (kcal/mole)	0.0	0.0	$\tfrac{1}{2}(-63.32)$
$\Delta G°_f$ values (kcal/mole)	0.0	0.0	$\tfrac{1}{2}(-50.35)$
$S°$ values (cal/[deg mole])	18.5	$\tfrac{1}{2}(53.286)$	$\tfrac{1}{2}(46.8)$

(a) Calculate $\Delta G°$ from the $\Delta G°_f$ values for the reaction of mercury and chlorine to form calomel. (Notice that the heat and free energy of formation of the elements Hg(liq) and Cl$_2$(g) are zero, therefore the value for the formation of Hg$_2$Cl$_2$ (-63.32 kcal/mole) is the *heat of formation* and -50.35 kcal/mole is the *free energy of formation* obtained by calorimetry. These are values for the heat and the free energy of formation found in a table of $\Delta H°_f$ and $\Delta G°_f$. The superscript ° indicates that the values are for the elements in their standard states.

(b) Using the $\Delta H°_f$ and $S°$ values, calculate $\Delta G°$ for the reaction and compare its value with that obtained in (a).

(c) Using $\Delta G°$ from (a) or (b), calculate the equilibrium constant for the reaction at 25° C.

Data for *Problem 7–33*

	$CH_3COOH(liq)$	$+$	$C_2H_5OH(liq)$	$=$	$CH_3COOC_2H_5(liq)$	$+$	$H_2O(liq)$
$\Delta H°_f$ (kcal/mole)	-116.4		$-66.20*$		$-114.49*$		-68.317
$\Delta G°_f$ (kcal/mole)	-93.8		-41.77		$-79.70**$		-56.690
$S°$ (cal/[deg mole])	38.2		38.4		62.0		16.716

(Below the equation are listed the standard heat of formation, the standard free energy of formation, and the standard absolute entropy.

Source: The values not designated with asterisks are from H. A. Bent, *The Second Law*, Oxford University Press, Oxford, 1965, pp. 398, 402.

*From J. A. Dean, Editor, *Lange's Handbook of Chemistry*, McGraw-Hill, New York, 1979, Table 9–2.

**Modified from the Lange Handbook value.

(d) Does the value obtained for $\Delta G°$ allow one to determine whether this process is spontaneous or not?

Answers: **(a)** $\Delta G° = -25.175$ kcal/mole; **(b)** $\Delta G°$ (from $\Delta H°$ and $\Delta S°$) $= -25.177$ kcal/mole; **(c)** $K_{(298° K)} = 2.84 \times 10^{18}$; **(d)** refer to page 161 for the relationship of $\Delta G°$ to spontaneity of a reaction.

7–33. In order to prepare the ester, ethyl acetate, acetic acid is reacted with ethyl alcohol at 25° C as shown in the table above.

(a) Using the $\Delta G°_f$ values, calculate $\Delta G°$ for the reaction at 25° C and the equilibrium constant, K.

(b) Using the $\Delta H°_f$, and $S°$ values, calculate $\Delta G°$ and K at 25° C and compare the results with those obtained in (a).

(c) According to the equation, if the reaction proceeded completely to the right, 1 mole each of acetic acid and ethyl alcohol would yield 1 mole each of ethyl acetate and water. However, the equilibrium constant K found in (a) or (b) shows that the reaction does not proceed completely to the right, for if that were the case, K would have the value of infinity. Let us suppose that 0.0027 M each of acetic acid and ethyl alcohol react together at 25° C to form the products, ethyl acetate and water. The amounts of acetic acid and ethyl alcohol are of course used up at the same rate to form ethyl acetate and water in equal amounts. What will be the concentration of the ester, ethyl acetate, at equilibrium? The following procedure is suggested. Having calculated the value of K in (a) and (b), and assigning x as the concentration of both ethyl acetate and water, one obtains the expression

$$\frac{x \cdot x}{(0.0027 \quad x)(0.0027 \quad x)} = K \cong 4.0$$

Note that at equilibrium, the original concentration 0.0027 M each for acetic acid and ethyl alcohol is reduced by the equilibrium concentration, x, for both ethyl acetate and water.

The equation for the reaction and the associated thermodynamic quantities are found in the table above. The value designated with a double asterisk was modified from the *Lange's Handbook* value of -79.52 to -79.70 to bring the $\Delta G°$ values into agreement by the two methods of calculation required for answers (a) and (b).

Answers: **(a)** $K = 3.99$ (if -79.52 kcal/mole had been used for $\Delta G°_f$ of ethyl acetate, as mentioned above, K would have been obtained as 2.95). **(b)** Using $\Delta H°_f$ and $S°$ values, $\Delta G° = -837.9$ cal/mole; $K = 4.11$. The value of K obtained experimentally from the concentrations of the reactants and the products at equilibrium, rather than the thermodynamic approach used here, is $K = 4.00$. **(c)** The concentration of ethyl acetate at equilibrium by experimentation is 0.0018 mole/liter. An equal concentration, 0.0018 M of water is formed. The concentration of acetic acid and ethyl alcohol is therefore each 0.0027 $- 0.0018$, or 0.0009 M, and the equilibrium expression appears as

$$K = \frac{(0.0018)(0.0018)}{(0.0027 - 0.0018)(0.0027 - 0.0018)} = 4.00$$

7–34. Once $\Delta H°$, the standard heat of reaction, is found at 25° C and the constant K for the reaction is known, also at 25° C, the van't Hoff equation (equation 3–124), may be employed to obtain K, the reaction constant for ionization over a range of temperatures from roughly 0° C to 50° C. The ionization of acetic acid and the standard heat of formation for the species involved in the reaction are:

$$CH_3COOH(aq) \rightarrow CH_3COO^-(aq) + H^+$$

$\Delta H°_f$ (kcal/mole)	-116.743^{23}	-116.843	0

(a) Calculate $\Delta H°$ at 25° C and using K_a for acetic acid at 25° C, substitute these values into the van't Hoff equation to obtain K_a at 0° C and 37° C. **(b)** If a curved line of K_a versus temperature occurs for an acid such as acetic, is it possible to obtain K_a values at say, 0° and 37° C, knowing the K_a value at 25° C? *Hint:* Plot on the same graph the values of ln K_a against 1/T given in CRC, p. D-174, and the values of ln K_a against 1/T you obtained under (a) and compare the results.

Partial Answer: **(a)** The ionization constant K_a for acetic acid at 0° C is 1.777×10^{-5}. The CRC *Handbook of Chemistry and Physics*, 63rd ed., p. D-174 gives K_a (acetic acid) as 1.657×10^{-5} at 0° C, 1.754 $\times 10^{-5}$ at 25° C; by extrapolation we obtain $K_a = 1.739 \times 10^{-5}$ at 37° C. The K_a value for acetic acid is greater at 25° C than at 0° C or 37° C (CRC, p. D-174). This is not true for all acids in water.

7–35. The standard free energy $\Delta G°$ is 10.26 kcal/mole and the standard heat content or enthalpy $\Delta H°$ is 19.32 kcal/mole for the dissociation of sulfathiazole at 35° C. (The term *standard* in thermodynamics refers to the value of the thermodynamic property, $\Delta G°$, $\Delta H°$, or $\Delta S°$ at ordinary temperatures [usually 25° C] and at 1 atm pressure).

(a) Compute the dissociation exponent, pK_a, at 35° C.

(b) The $\Delta G°$ and $\Delta S°$ values at a temperature T_1, say 35° C, can be used to compute pK_a at another temperature T_2, say 20° C, according to the equation

$$pK_a = \frac{\Delta G°_{T_1} - \Delta S°_{T_1} (T_2 - T_1)}{2.303 R T_2}$$

where $\Delta S°$ at the temperature T_1 (35° C) is calculated from the $\Delta G°$ and $\Delta H°$ values given above at 35° C. Compute the pK_a of sulfathiazole at 20° C.

Answers: **(a)** pK_a (35° C) = 7.28; **(b)** pK_a (20° C) = 7.32

7–36. The pH of a 1:500 aqueous solution of ephedrine was determined with a pH meter and was found to be 10.70. Calculate the pK_b for ephedrine.

Answer: $pK_b = 4.68$ (cf. Table 7–3, p. 148)

7–37. Calculate α, the degree of dissociation of 0.01 molar physostigmine, disregarding the secondary ionization. α is the concentration of the ionized form, [physostigmine$^+$] = [OH$^-$]/C_b, where C_b is the concentration of the compound. The student may use the relationship, [OH$^-$]/C_b or equation (13–78), p. 342.

Answer: 0.0087 or 0.87%

7–38. The weak acid, corresponding to the salt benzylpenicillin sodium, molecular weight 356.38, has a pK_a of 2.76. the drug is dissolved in isotonic sodium chloride solution (0.9 g NaCl per 100 mL) to make a 3% w/v solution of the antibiotic. **(a)** What is the pH of this solution, disregarding activity coefficients? **(b)** What is the result using ionic activity coefficients? (Use the Debye–Hückel equation.)

Answer: **(a)** pH = 7.84; **(b)** pH = 7.68

7–39. What is the hydroxyl ion concentration of an aqueous solution containing 0.1 g per 1000 mL of reserpine and 9 g per 1000 mL of sodium chloride? The molecular weight of reserpine is 608. Calculate the results **(a)** without activity coefficients, and **(b)** with activity coefficients, using the Debye–Hückel equation.

Answer: **(a)** [OH$^-$] = 2.56×10^{-6} M; **(b)** [OH$^-$] = 1.84×10^{-6} M

7–40. In a study of insecticidal oximes ($R_2C\!\!=\!\!NOH$) Kurtz and D'Silva[24] postulated a relationship between the pK_a value of an oxime and its proton chemical shift, δ_{OH} (see pp. 92 and 93 for a description of chemical shift). To learn whether pK_a values could be obtained from NMR data, the authors determined chemical shifts of the hydroxyl proton, δ_{OH}, of selected oximes with known pK_a values. pK_a and δ_{OH} values are listed in the table.

(a) Plot pK_a on the vertical axis versus the experimentally determined δ_{OH} values on the horizontal axis.

(b) Use least-squares linear regression analysis, regressing pK_a versus δ_{OH} to obtain an equation relating these two variables. How well do the coefficients of your equation correspond to those of Kurtz and D'Silva?

(c) Use your equation of the least-squares regression line to calculate the pK_a from $\delta_{OH} = 11.15$ for acetophenone oxime. Compare your calculated pK_a with the literature value, $pK_a = 11.41$, for acetophenone oxime.

Data for *Problem 7–40*

Known pK_a and Experimental δ_{OH} Values		
Compound	δ_{OH}	pK_a
2-Propanone oxime	10.12	12.42
2-Butanone oxime	10.14	12.45
3-Pentanone oxime	10.18	12.60
Acetophenone oxime	11.15	11.41
Benzaldehyde oxime	11.19	10.78
4-Nitrobenzaldehyde oxime	11.84	9.88
2,3-Butanedione monooxime	12.27	9.34
3-Oximinopentane-2,4-dione	12.92	7.38
2-Oximino-1,3-dithiolane	11.15	10.70

Partial Answer: (b) The equation obtained using the nine oximes from the work of Kurtz and D'Silva is

$$pK_a = 29.92 - 1.71\,\delta_{OH}; \quad r^2 = 0.967, \quad n = 9$$

(n stands for the number of compounds involved in the regression as independent variables)

(c) The pK_a of acetophenone oxime calculated from the equation under (b) above is 10.85. The literature value is 11.41.

7–41. Kurtz and D'Silva[24] used NMR chemical shift data to obtain the pK_a of a number of oximes, as described in *Problem 7–40*. Furthermore, these workers observed that the sensitivity of phenol pK_a values was similar to that of oxime pK_a values for changes in proton chemical shift, δ_{OH}. That is, the slope of the plot of pK_a versus δ_{OH} for oximes was nearly the same as that for phenols. Thus, it should be possible to use a single equation to express the pK_a vs. δ_{OH} values for both oximes and phenols. To test this possibility the authors used 20 oxime pK_a values and 51 phenol pK_a values and regressed these against measured δ_{OH} values. Kurtz and D'Silva added an *indicator variable** to account for the difference in these two classes of chemicals. The indicator variable I is taken as equal to unity for each phenol in the equation and as zero for each compound which is an oxime, giving the expression

$$pK_a = a + b(\delta_{OH}) + c(I)$$

The 20 pK_a and δ_{OH} values for the oximes and the 51 pK_a and δ_{OH} values for the phenols are entered into a computer program designed to handle linear regression with indicator variables. As the oxime and phenol data are entered, I is given a value of 0 for each oxime and a value of 1 for each phenol. The computer-generated results (see the statistical package, SPSS, 1975, pp. 373–375) provide values for a, b, and c in the above equation.

In essence, the indicator variable produces different intercepts and thus divides the results into two separate lines having the same slope. The lines in this case represent the two classes of compounds, oximes and phenols; and the single equation relating pK_a and δ_{OH} for these two classes is, according to Kurtz and D'Silva,

$$pK_a = 28.15 - 1.55\,\delta_{OH} - 3.96I, \quad r^2 = 0.97$$

Plot the two lines on a graph of pK_a against δ_{OH}. Locate the points for benzaldehyde oxime and 2-3 butanedione monooxime on the one line, and phenol and 2-nitrophenol on the other line. Use the observed (measured) δ_{OH} values for these four compounds:

Data for *Problem 7–41*

Compound	Measured δ_{OH}
Benzaldehyde oxime	11.19
2,3-Butanedione monooxime	12.27
Phenol	9.23*
2-Nitrophenol	10.82*

*From G. Socrates, Trans. Faraday Soc. **66**, 1052, 1966.

and the above equation, to calculate the pK_a values.

Answer:

	pK_a	
Compound	Calculated	Literature
Benzaldehyde oxime	10.81	10.78
2,3-Butanedione monooxime	9.13	9.34
Phenol	9.88	9.97
2-Nitrophenol	7.42	7.14

7–42. The constants, A, C, and D for barbital found in Table 7–8 were obtained from a precision e.m.f. study of the pK_a–temperature dependence. Compute T_{max}, pK_{Tmax}, $\Delta G°$, $\Delta H°$, and $\Delta S°$ at physiologic temperature using equation (7–152) through (7–157) on page 163, and introduce them into the squares[†] of Table 7–8.

Partial Answer: $T_{max} = 443°$ C; $\Delta G° = 11.1$ kcal/mole

7–43. The constants A, C, and D for lactic acid in Table 7–8 are obtained using equations (7–152) through (7–157) on page 163. Calculate the values for T_{max}, pK_{Tmax}, $\Delta G°$, $\Delta H°$, and $S°$ at 25° C and introduce them into the squares, [‡], of Table 7–8.

Partial Answer: $pK_{Tmax} = 3.86$; $\Delta H° = -101$ cal/mole

---

*Indicator variables, also called *dummy variables*, are described in SPSS, McGraw-Hill, 1975, p. 373

8
Buffered and Isotonic Solutions

The Buffer Equation
Buffer Capacity
Buffers in Pharmaceutical and Biologic
   Systems

Buffered Isotonic Solutions
Methods of Adjusting Tonicity and pH

Buffers are compounds or mixtures of compounds that, by their presence in solution, resist changes in pH upon the addition of small quantities of acid or alkali. The resistance to a change in pH is known as *buffer action*. According to Roos and Borm,[1] Koppel and Spiro published the first paper on buffer action in 1914 and suggested a number of applications, which were later elaborated by Van Slyke.[2]

If, to water or a solution of sodium chloride, a small amount of a strong acid or base is added, the pH is altered considerably; such systems have no buffer action.

A combination of a weak acid and its conjugate base (i.e., its salt), or a weak base and its conjugate acid act as buffers. If 1 mL of a 0.1-N HCl solution is added to 100 mL of pure water, the pH is reduced from 7 to 3. If the strong acid is added to a 0.01-M solution containing equal quantities of acetic acid and sodium acetate, the pH is changed only 0.09 pH units, because the base Ac^- ties up the hydrogen ions according to the reaction

$$Ac^- + H_3O^+ \rightleftharpoons HAc + H_2O \qquad (8-1)$$

If a strong base, sodium hydroxide, is added to the buffer mixture, acetic acid neutralizes the hydroxyl ions as follows:

$$HAc + OH^- \rightleftharpoons H_2O + Ac^- \qquad (8-2)$$

THE BUFFER EQUATION

Common Ion Effect and the Buffer Equation for a Weak Acid and Its Salt. The pH of a buffer solution and the change in pH upon the addition of an acid or base may be calculated by use of the *buffer equation*. This expression is developed by considering the effect of a salt on the ionization of a weak acid when the salt and the acid have an ion in common.

For example, when sodium acetate is added to acetic acid, the dissociation constant for the weak acid,

$$K_a = \frac{[H_3O^+][Ac^-]}{[HAc]} = 1.75 \times 10^{-5} \qquad (8-3)$$

is momentarily disturbed since the acetate ion supplied by the salt increases the $[Ac^-]$ term in the numerator. To reestablish the constant K_a at 1.75×10^{-5}, the hydrogen ion term in the numerator $[H_3O^+]$ is instantaneously decreased, with a corresponding increase in $[HAc]$. Therefore, the constant K_a remains unaltered, and the equilibrium is shifted in the direction of the reactants. Consequently, the ionization of acetic acid,

$$HAc + H_2O \rightleftharpoons H_3O^+ + Ac^- \qquad (8-4)$$

is *repressed* upon the addition of the common ion $[Ac^-]$. This is an example of the *common ion effect*. The pH of the final solution is obtained by rearranging the equilibrium expression for acetic acid:

$$[H_3O^+] = K_a \frac{[HAc]}{[Ac^-]} \qquad (8-5)$$

If the acid is weak and ionizes only slightly, the expression $[HAc]$ may be considered to represent the total concentration of acid, and it is written simply as [acid]. In the slightly ionized acidic solution, the acetate concentration $[Ac^-]$ may be considered as having come entirely from the salt, sodium acetate. Since 1 mole of sodium acetate yields 1 mole of acetate ion, $[Ac^-]$ is equal to the total salt concentration and is replaced by the term [salt]. Hence, equation (8-5) is written,

$$[H_3O^+] = K_a \frac{[acid]}{[salt]} \qquad (8-6)$$

Equation (8–6) may be expressed in logarithmic form, with the signs reversed, as

$$-\log[H_3O^+] = -\log K_a - \log[acid] + \log[salt] \quad (8\text{–}7)$$

from which is obtained an expression, known as the *buffer equation* or the *Henderson–Hasselbalch equation*, for a weak acid and its salt:

$$pH = pK_a + \log \frac{[salt]}{[acid]} \quad (8\text{–}8)$$

The ratio [acid]/[salt] in equation (8–6) has been inverted by undergoing the logarithmic operations in (8–7) and it appears in (8–8) as [salt]/[acid]. pK_a, the negative logarithm of K_a, is called the *dissociation exponent* (p. 152).

The buffer equation is important in the preparation of buffered pharmaceutical solutions; it is satisfactory for calculations within the pH range of 4 to 10.

Example 8–1. What is the pH of 0.1-*M* acetic acid solution, $pK_a = 4.76$? What is the pH after enough sodium acetate has been added to make the solution 0.1 *M* with respect to this salt?

The pH of the acetic acid solution is calculated by use of the logarithmic form of equation (7–99) on p. 155.

$$pH = \tfrac{1}{2}pK_a - \tfrac{1}{2}\log c$$

$$pH = 2.38 + 0.50 = 2.88$$

The pH of the buffer solution containing acetic acid and sodium acetate is determined by use of the buffer equation (8–8):

$$pH = 4.76 + \log \frac{0.1}{0.1} = 4.76$$

It is seen from *Example 8–1* that the pH of the acetic acid solution has been *increased* almost 2 pH units; that is, the acidity has been *reduced* to about one hundredth of its original value by the addition of an equal concentration of a salt with a common ion. This example bears out the statement regarding the repression of ionization upon the addition of a common ion.

Sometimes it is desired to know the ratio of salt to acid in order to prepare a buffer of a definite pH. *Example 8–2* demonstrates the calculation involved in such a problem.

Example 8–2. What is the molar ratio, [salt]/[acid], required to prepare an acetate buffer of pH 5.0? Also express the result in mole percent.

$$5.0 = 4.76 + \log \frac{[salt]}{[acid]}$$

$$\log \frac{[salt]}{[acid]} = 5.0 - 4.76 = 0.24$$

$$\frac{[salt]}{[acid]} = \text{antilog } 0.24 = 1.74$$

Therefore, the mole ratio of salt to acid is 1.74/1. Mole percent is mole fraction multiplied by 100. The mole fraction of salt in the salt–acid mixture is 1.74/(1 + 1.74) = 0.635, and in mole percent, the result is 63.5%.

The Buffer Equation for a Weak Base and Its Salt. Buffer solutions are not ordinarily prepared from weak bases and their salts because of the volatility and instability of the bases and because of the dependence of their pH on

pK_w, which is often affected by temperature changes. Pharmaceutical solutions—for example, a solution of ephedrine base and ephedrine hydrochloride—however, often contain combinations of weak bases and their salts.

The buffer equation for solutions of weak bases and the corresponding salts may be derived in a manner analogous to that for the weak acid buffers. Accordingly,

$$[OH^-] = K_b \frac{[base]}{[salt]} \quad (8\text{–}9)$$

and using the relationship, $[OH^-] = K_w/[H_3O^+]$, the buffer equation becomes

$$pH = pK_w - pK_b + \log \frac{[base]}{[salt]} \quad (8\text{–}10)$$

Example 8–3. What is the pH of a solution containing 0.10 mole of ephedrine and 0.01 mole of ephedrine hydrochloride per liter of solution? The pK_b of ephedrine is 4.64.

$$pH = 14.00 - 4.64 + \log \frac{0.10}{0.01}$$

$$pH = 9.36 + \log 10 = 10.36$$

Activity Coefficients and the Buffer Equation. A more exact treatment of buffers begins with the replacement of concentrations by activities in the equilibrium of a weak acid:

$$K_a = \frac{a_{H_3O^+} a_{Ac^-}}{a_{HAc}} = \frac{(\gamma_{H_3O^+} c_{H_3O^+}) \times (\gamma_{Ac^-} c_{Ac^-})}{\gamma_{HAc} c_{HAc}} \quad (8\text{–}11)$$

The activity of each species is written as the activity coefficient multiplied by the molar concentration. The activity coefficient of the undissociated acid γ_{HAc} is essentially 1 and may be dropped. Solving for the hydrogen ion activity and pH, defined as $-\log a_{H_3O^+}$, yields the equations

$$a_{H_3O^+} = \gamma_{H_3O^+} \times c_{H_3O^+} = K_a \frac{c_{HAc}}{\gamma_{Ac^-} c_{Ac^-}} \quad (8\text{–}12)$$

$$pH = pK_a + \log \frac{[salt]}{[acid]} + \log \gamma_{Ac^-} \quad (8\text{–}13)$$

From the Debye–Hückel expression (equation (6–59), p. 136) for an aqueous solution of a univalent ion at 25° C having an ionic strength not greater than about 0.1 or 0.2, we write

$$\log \gamma_{Ac^-} = \frac{-0.5\sqrt{\mu}}{1 + \sqrt{\mu}}$$

and equation (8–13) then becomes

$$pH = pK_a + \log \frac{[salt]}{[acid]} - \frac{0.5\sqrt{\mu}}{1 + \sqrt{\mu}} \quad (8\text{–}14)$$

The general equation for buffers of polybasic acids is

$$pH = pK_n + \log \frac{[salt]}{[acid]} - \frac{A(2n-1)\sqrt{\mu}}{1 + \sqrt{\mu}} \quad (8\text{–}15)$$

in which n is the stage of the ionization. (See *Problem 8–3*, p. 187).

Example 8–4. A buffer contains 0.05 mole per liter of formic acid and 0.10 mole per liter of sodium formate. The pK_a of formic acid is 3.75. The ionic strength of the solution is 0.10. Compute the pH (*a*) with and (*b*) without consideration of the activity coefficient correction.

(*a*)

$$pH = 3.75 + \log \frac{0.10}{0.05} - \frac{0.5\sqrt{0.10}}{1 + \sqrt{0.10}}$$

$$= 3.93$$

(*b*)

$$pH = 3.75 + \log \frac{0.10}{0.05} = 4.05$$

Some Factors Influencing the pH of Buffer Solutions. The addition of neutral salts to buffers changes the pH of the solution by altering the ionic strength, as shown in equation (8–13). Changes in ionic strength and hence in the pH of a buffer solution may also be brought about by dilution. The addition of water in moderate amounts, while not changing the pH, may cause a small positive or negative deviation because it alters activity coefficients and because water itself can act as a weak acid or base. Bates[3] has expressed this quantitatively in terms of a *dilution value*, which is the change in pH on diluting the buffer solution to one half its original strength. Some dilution values for National Bureau of Standards buffers are found in Table 9–2, p. 199. A positive dilution value signifies that the pH rises with dilution, and a negative value signifies that the pH decreases with dilution of the buffer.

Temperature also influences buffers. Kolthoff and Tekelenburg[4] determined the *temperature coefficient of pH*, that is, the change in pH with temperature, for a large number of buffers. The pH of acetate buffers was found to increase with temperature, whereas the pH of boric acid–sodium borate buffers decreased with temperature. Although the temperature coefficient of acid buffers was relatively small, the pH of most basic buffers was found to change more markedly with temperature, owing to K_w, which appears in the equation of basic buffers and which changes significantly with temperature. Bates[3] refers to several basic buffers that show only a small change of pH with temperature and can be used in the pH range of 7 to 9. The temperature coefficients for the calomel electrode are given in Bates,[3] Table 10–10.

Drugs as Buffers. It is important to recognize that solutions of drugs that are weak electrolytes also manifest buffer action. Salicylic acid solution in a soft glass bottle is influenced by the alkalinity of the glass. It might be thought at first that the reaction would result in an appreciable increase in pH; however, the sodium ions of the soft glass combine with the salicylate ions to form sodium salicylate. Thus, there arises a solution of salicylic acid and sodium salicylate—a buffer solution that resists the change in pH. Similarly, a solution of ephedrine base manifests a natural buffer protection against reductions in pH. Should hydrochloric acid be added to the solution, ephedrine hydrochloride is formed, and the buffer system—ephedrine plus ephedrine hydrochloride—will resist large changes in pH until the ephedrine is depleted by reaction with the acid. Therefore, a drug in solution may often act as its own buffer over a definite pH range. Such buffer action, however, is often too weak to counteract pH changes brought about by the carbon dioxide of the air and the alkalinity of the bottle. Additional buffers are therefore frequently added to drug solutions to maintain the system within a certain pH range. A quantitative measure of the efficiency or capacity of a buffer to resist pH changes will be discussed in a later section.

pH Indicators. Indicators may be considered as weak acids or weak bases that act like buffers and also exhibit color changes as their degree of dissociation varies with pH. For example, methyl red shows its full alkaline color, yellow, at a pH of about 6 and its full acid color, red, at about pH 4. Indicators therefore offer a convenient alternative method to electrometric techniques (Chapter 9) for determining the pH of a solution.

The dissociation of an acid indicator is given here in simplified form:

$$\underset{\substack{\text{Acid}_1 \\ \text{(acid color)}}}{\text{HIn}} + \underset{\text{Base}_2}{\text{H}_2\text{O}} \rightleftharpoons \underset{\text{Acid}_2}{\text{H}_3\text{O}^+} + \underset{\substack{\text{Base}_1 \\ \text{(alkaline color)}}}{\text{In}^-} \qquad (8\text{–}16)$$

The equilibrium expression is

$$\frac{[\text{H}_3\text{O}^+][\text{In}^-]}{[\text{HIn}]} = K_{\text{In}} \qquad (8\text{–}17)$$

HIn is the un-ionized form of the indicator, which gives the acid color, and In^- is the ionized form, which produces the basic color. K_{In} is referred to as the *indicator constant*. If an acid is added to a solution of the indicator, the hydrogen ion concentration term on the right-hand side of equation (8–16) is increased, and the ionization is repressed by the common ion effect. The indicator is then predominantly in the form of HIn, the acid color. If base is added, $[\text{H}_3\text{O}^+]$ is reduced by reaction of the acid with the base, reaction (8–16) proceeds to the right, yielding more ionized indicator In^-, and the base color predominates. Thus, the color of an indicator is a function of the pH of the solution. A number of indicators with their useful pH ranges are listed in Table 8–1.

The equilibrium expression (8–16) may be treated in a manner similar to that for a buffer consisting of a weak acid and its salt or conjugate base. Hence

$$[\text{H}_3\text{O}^+] = K_{\text{In}} \frac{[\text{HIn}]}{[\text{In}^-]} \qquad (8\text{–}18)$$

and since [HIn] represents the acid color of the indicator and the conjugate base $[\text{In}^-]$ represents the

TABLE 8–1. *Color, pH and pKin, the Indicator Constant, of Some Common Indicators*

	Color			
Indicator	Acid	Base	pH Range	pK_{In}
Thymol blue (acid range)	red	yellow	1.2– 2.8	1.5
Methyl violet	blue	violet	1.5– 3.2	—
Methyl orange	red	yellow	3.1– 4.4	3.7
Bromcresol green	yellow	blue	3.8– 5.4	4.7
Methyl red	red	yellow	4.2– 6.2	5.1
Bromcresol purple	yellow	purple	5.2– 6.8	6.3
Bromthymol blue	yellow	blue	6.0– 7.6	7.0
Phenol red	yellow	red	6.8– 8.4	7.9
Cresol red	yellow	red	7.2– 8.8	8.3
Thymol blue (alkaline range)	yellow	blue	8.0– 9.6	8.9
Phenolphthalein	colorless	red	8.3–10.0	9.4
Alizarin yellow	yellow	lilac	10.0–12.0	—
Indigo carmine	blue	yellow	11.6–14	—

basic color, these terms may be replaced by the concentration expressions, [acid] and [base]. The formula for pH as derived from equation (8–18) becomes

$$pH = pK_{In} + \log \frac{[\text{base}]}{[\text{acid}]} \qquad (8\text{–}19)$$

Example 8–5.* An indicator, methyl red, is present in its ionic form *In⁻*, in a concentration of 3.20×10^{-3} M and in its molecular form, *HIn*, in an aqueous solution at 25° C in a concentration of 6.78×10^{-3} M. From Table 8–1 we observe a pK_{In} of 5.1 for methyl red. What is the pH of this solution?

$$pH = 5.1 + \log \frac{3.20 \times 10^{-3}}{6.78 \times 10^{-3}} = 4.77$$

Just as a buffer shows its greatest efficiency when pH = pK_a, an indicator exhibits its *middle tint* when [base]/[acid] = 1 and pH = pK_{In}. The most efficient indicator range, corresponding to the effective buffer interval, is about 2 pH units, that is, $pK_{In} \pm 1$. The reason for the width of this color range may be explained as follows. It is known from experience that one cannot discern a change from the acid color to the salt or conjugate base color until the ratio of [base] to [acid] is about 1 to 10. That is, there must be at least 1 part of the basic color to 10 parts of the acid color before the eye can discern a change in color from acid to alkaline. The pH value at which this change is perceived is given by the equation

$$pH = pK_{In} + \log \frac{1}{10} = pK_{In} - 1 \qquad (8\text{–}20)$$

Conversely, the eye cannot discern a change from the alkaline to the acid color until the ratio of [base] to [acid] is about 10 to 1, or

$$pH = pK_{In} + \log \frac{10}{1} = pK_{In} + 1 \qquad (8\text{–}21)$$

Therefore, when base is added to a solution of a buffer in its acid form, the eye first visualizes a change in color at $pK_{In} - 1$, and the color ceases to change any further at $pK_{In} + 1$. The effective range of the indicator between its full acid and full basic color may thus be expressed as

$$pH = pK_{In} \pm 1 \qquad (8\text{–}22)$$

As buffers may be mixed to cover a wide pH range, so also can several indicators be combined to yield so-called *universal indicators*. The *Merck Index* suggests one such universal indicator consisting of a mixture of methyl yellow, methyl red, bromthymol blue, thymol blue, and phenolphthalein, which covers the range from pH 1 to 11.

The colorimetric method for the determination of pH is probably less accurate and less convenient but also less expensive than the electrometric method. It may be used in the determination of the pH of aqueous solutions that are not colored or turbid, and it is particularly useful for the study of acid–base reactions in nonaqueous solutions. The details of the method are given in the treatise of Kolthoff and Rosenblum.[5] Wyss[6] has discussed the determination of the pH of solutions in the prescription laboratory. In general, the colorimetric determination of pH involves the following steps.

(a) Determine the approximate pH of the solution by the addition of several drops of a universal indicator. Wide-range pH papers, prepared by applying a universal indicator solution to paper strips, may be used.

(b) A series of Clark–Lubs buffer solutions as modified by Bower and Bates,[7] differing by 0.2 pH unit and within the pH range of the unknown solution, are chosen. Several drops of an indicator solution, having a pK_{In} approximately equal to the pH of the unknown solution so that it changes color within the pH range

---

*In dealing with indicators, one is concerned only with the color changes and not with the concentrations of the colored species of the indicator. Example (8–5) simply shows that if the concentrations of the colored species were known, the same equation could be used in principle for indicator solutions as for buffer systems to calculate the pH of a solution.

under consideration, are added to each buffer sample and to the unknown solution contained in suitable test tubes.

(c) The colors of the buffers of known pH are matched with the color of the unknown solution; accordingly, the pH of the unknown solution can be determined to within 0.1 pH unit.

Narrow-range pH papers may be used in the same way as the indicator solution by comparing the color when a drop of buffer and a drop of the unknown solution are applied to adjacent strips.

Goyan and Coutsouris[8] concluded that it was possible to cover the pH range from 4 to 8 by the use of only three indicators, bromcresol green, bromthymol blue, and thymol blue. For details of this method, refer to the original article.

A final note of caution should be added regarding the colorimetric method. Since indicators themselves are acids (or bases), their addition to unbuffered solutions whose pH is to be determined will change the pH of the solution. The colorimetric method is therefore not applicable to the determination of the pH of sodium chloride solution or similar unbuffered pharmaceutical preparations unless special precautions are taken in the measurement. Some medicinal solutions and pharmaceutical vehicles, however, to which no buffers have been added, are buffered by the presence of the drug itself (p. 171) and can withstand the addition of an indicator without a significant change in pH. Errors in the result may also be introduced by the presence of salts and proteins, and these errors must be determined for each indicator over the range involved.

BUFFER CAPACITY

Thus far it has been stated that a buffer counteracts the change in pH of a solution upon the addition of a strong acid, a strong base, or other agents that tend to alter the hydrogen ion concentration. Furthermore, it has been shown in a rather qualitative manner how this buffer action is manifested by combinations of weak acids and weak bases together with their salts. The resistance to changes of pH now remains to be discussed in a more quantitative way.

The magnitude of the resistance of a buffer to pH changes is referred to as the buffer capacity β. It is also known as *buffer efficiency, buffer index,* and *buffer value.* Koppel and Spiro[1] and Van Slyke[2] introduced the concept of buffer capacity and defined it as the ratio of the increment of strong base (or acid) to the small change in pH brought about by this addition. For the present discussion, the approximate formula,

$$\beta = \frac{\Delta B}{\Delta \mathrm{pH}} \qquad (8-23)$$

may be used, in which delta, Δ, has its usual meaning,

a *finite change*, and ΔB is the small increment in gram equivalents per liter of strong base added to the buffer solution to produce a pH change of ΔpH. According to equation (8–23), the buffer capacity of a solution has a value of 1 when the addition of 1 gram Eq of strong base (or acid) to 1 liter of the buffer solution results in a change of 1 pH unit. The significance of this index will be appreciated better when it is applied to the calculation of the capacity of a buffer solution.

Approximate Calculation of Buffer Capacity. Consider an acetate buffer containing 0.1 mole each of acetic acid and sodium acetate in 1 liter of solution. To this are added 0.01-mole portions of sodium hydroxide. When the first increment of sodium hydroxide is added, the concentration of sodium acetate, the [salt] term in the buffer equation, increases by 0.01 mole/liter, and the acetic acid concentration [acid] decreases proportionately, because each increment of base converts 0.01 mole of acetic acid into 0.01 mole of sodium acetate according to the reaction

$$\mathrm{HAc} + \mathrm{NaOH} \rightleftharpoons \mathrm{NaAc} + \mathrm{H_2O} \qquad (8-24)$$
$$(0.1 - 0.01) \quad (0.01) \quad (0.1 + 0.01)$$

The changes in concentration of the salt and the acid by the addition of a base are represented in the buffer equation (8–8) by using the modified form:

$$\mathrm{pH} = \mathrm{p}K_a + \log \frac{[\text{salt}] + [\text{base}]}{[\text{acid}] - [\text{base}]} \qquad (8-25)$$

Before the addition of the first portion of sodium hydroxide, the pH of the buffer solution is

$$\mathrm{pH} = 4.76 + \log \frac{(0.1 + 0)}{(0.1 - 0)} = 4.76 \qquad (8-26)$$

The results of the continual addition of sodium hydroxide are shown in Table 8–2. The student should verify the pH values and buffer capacities by the use of equations (8–25) and (8–23) respectively.

As may be seen from Table 8–2, the buffer capacity is not a fixed value for a given buffer system, but rather depends on the amount of base added. The buffer capacity changes as the ratio log [salt]/[acid] increases with added base. With the addition of more sodium hydroxide, the buffer capacity decreases rapidly, and,

TABLE 8–2. *Buffer Capacity of Solutions Containing Equimolar Amounts (0.1 M) of Acetic Acid and Sodium Acetate*

Moles of NaOH Added	pH of Solution	Buffer Capacity, β
0	4.76	
0.01	4.85	0.11
0.02	4.94	0.11
0.03	5.03	0.11
0.04	5.13	0.10
0.05	5.24	0.09
0.06	5.36	0.08

when sufficient base has been added to convert the acid completely into sodium ions and acetate ions, the solution no longer possesses an acid reserve. The buffer has its greatest capacity before any base is added where [salt]/[acid] = 1, and, therefore, according to equation (8–8), pH = pK_a. The buffer capacity is also influenced by an increase in the total concentration of the buffer constituents since, obviously, a great concentration of salt and acid provides a greater alkaline and acid reserve. The influence of concentration on buffer capacity is treated following the discussion of Van Slyke's equation.

A More Exact Equation for Buffer Capacity. The buffer capacity calculated from equation (8–23) is only approximate. It gives the average buffer capacity over the increment of base added. Koppel and Spiro[1] and Van Slyke[2] developed a more exact equation,

$$\beta = 2.3C \frac{K_a[H_3O^+]}{(K_a + [H_3O^+])^2} \qquad (8-27)$$

where C is the total buffer concentration, that is, the sum of the molar concentrations of the acid and the salt. Equation (8–27) permits one to compute the buffer capacity at any hydrogen ion concentration—for example, at the point where no acid or base has been added to the buffer.

Example 8–6. At a hydrogen ion concentration of 1.75×10^{-5} (pH = 4.76), what is the capacity of a buffer containing 0.10 mole each of acetic acid and sodium acetate per liter of solution? The total concentration, $C = $ [acid] + [salt], is 0.20 mole per liter, and the dissociation constant is 1.75×10^{-5}.

$$\beta = \frac{2.3 \times 0.20 \times (1.75 \times 10^{-5}) \times (1.75 \times 10^{-5})}{[(1.75 \times 10^{-5}) + (1.75 \times 10^{-5})]^2}$$

$$= 0.115$$

Example 8–7. Prepare a buffer solution of pH 5.00 having a capacity of 0.02. The steps in the solution of the problem are:

(a) One chooses a weak acid having a pK_a close to the pH desired. Acetic acid, $pK_a = 4.76$, is suitable in this case.

(b) The ratio of salt and acid required to produce a pH of 5.00 was found in *Example 8–2* to be [salt]/[acid] = 1.74/1.

(c) The buffer capacity equation (8–27) is used to obtain the total buffer concentration, $C = $ [salt] + [acid]

$$0.02 = 2.3C \frac{(1.75 \times 10^{-5}) \times (1 \times 10^{-5})}{[(1.75 \times 10^{-5}) + (1 \times 10^{-5})]^2}$$

$$C = 3.75 \times 10^{-2} \text{ mole/liter}$$

(d) Finally from (b), [salt] = 1.74 × [acid], and from (c):

$$C = (1.74 \times \text{[acid]}) + \text{[acid]}$$

$$= 3.75 \times 10^{-2} \text{ mole/liter}$$

Therefore

$$\text{[acid]} = 1.37 \times 10^{-2} \text{ mole/liter}$$

and

$$\text{[salt]} = 1.74 \times \text{[acid]}$$

$$= 2.38 \times 10^{-2} \text{ mole/liter}$$

The Influence of Concentration on Buffer Capacity. The buffer capacity is affected not only by the [salt]/[acid] ratio but also by the total concentrations of acid and salt. As shown in Table 8–2, when 0.01 mole of base was added to a 0.1 molar acetate buffer, the pH increased from 4.76 to 4.85 or a ΔpH of 0.09.

If the concentration of acetic acid and sodium acetate is raised to 1 molar, the pH of the original buffer solution remains at about 4.76, but now, upon the addition of 0.01 mole of base, it becomes 4.77, a ΔpH of only 0.01. The calculation, disregarding activity coefficients, is

$$\text{pH} = 4.76 + \log \frac{(1.0 + 0.01)}{(1.0 - 0.01)} = 4.77 \quad (8-28)$$

Therefore, an increase in the concentration of the buffer components results in a greater buffer capacity or efficiency. This conclusion is also evident in equation (8–27), where an increase in the total buffer concentration, $C = $ [salt] + [acid], obviously results in a greater value of β.

In summary, the buffer capacity depends on (a) the value of the ratio [salt]/[acid], increasing as the ratio approaches unity; and (b) the magnitude of the individual concentrations of the buffer components, the buffer becoming more efficient as the salt and acid concentrations are increased.

Maximum Buffer Capacity. An equation expressing the maximum buffer capacity may be derived from the buffer capacity formula of Koppel and Spiro[1] and Van Slyke[2] (equation (8–27)). The maximum buffer capacity occurs where pH = pK_a, or, in equivalent terms, where $[H_3O^+] = K_a$. Substituting $[H_3O^+]$ for K_a in both the numerator and denominator of equation (8–27) gives

$$\beta_{max} = 2.303C \frac{[H_3O^+]^2}{(2[H_3O^+])^2} = \frac{2.303}{4} C$$

$$\beta_{max} = 0.576C \qquad (8-29)$$

in which C is the total buffer concentration.

Example 8–8. What is the maximum buffer capacity of an acetate buffer with a total concentration of 0.020 mole per liter?

$$\beta_{max} = 0.576 \times 0.020$$

$$= 0.01152 \text{ or } 0.012$$

Neutralization Curves and Buffer Capacity. A further understanding of buffer capacity can be obtained by considering the titration curves of strong and weak acids when they are mixed with increasing quantities of alkali. The reaction of an equivalent of an acid with an equivalent of a base is called neutralization; it may be expressed according to the method of Brönsted and Lowry. The neutralization of a strong acid by a strong base and weak acid by a strong base are written, as explained on pp. 143–145, in the form

| Acid₁ | Base₂ | Acid₂ | Base₁ |

$$H_3O^+(Cl^-) + (Na^+)OH^- = H_2O + H_2O + Na^+ + Cl^-$$

$$HAc + (Na^+)OH^- = H_2O + (Na^+)Ac^-$$

in which $(H_3O^+)(Cl^-)$ is the hydrated form of HCl in water. The neutralization of a strong acid by a strong base simply involves a reaction between hydronium and hydroxyl ions and is usually written

$$H_3O^+ + OH^- = 2H_2O \qquad (8\text{--}30)$$

Since (Cl^-) and (Na^+) appear on both sides of the equation just given, they may be disregarded without influencing the result. The reaction between the strong acid and strong base proceeds almost to completion; however, the weak acid–strong base reaction is incomplete, since Ac^- reacts in part with water, that is, it hydrolyzes to regenerate the free acid.

The neutralization of 10 mL of 0.1 N HCl (curve I) and 10 mL of 0.1 N acetic acid (curve II) by 0.1 N NaOH is shown in Figure 8–1. The plot of pH versus milliliters of NaOH added produces the titration curve. It is computed as follows for HCl. Before the first increment of NaOH is added, the hydrogen ion concentration of the 0.1-N solution of HCl is 10^{-1} mole/liter and the pH = 1, disregarding activities and assuming HCl to be completely ionized. The addition of 5 mL of 0.1 N NaOH neutralizes 5 mL of 0.1 N HCl, leaving 5 mL of the original HCl in 10 + 5 = 15 mL of solution, or $[H_3O^+] = \frac{5}{15} \times 0.1 = 3.3 \times 10^{-2}$ mole per liter and pH = 1.48. When 10 mL of base has been added, all the HCl is converted to NaCl, and the pH, disregarding the difference between activity and concentration resulting from the ionic strength of the NaCl solution, is 7. This is known as the equivalence point of the titration. Curve I in Figure 8–1 results from plotting such data. It is seen that the pH does not change markedly until nearly all the HCl is neutralized. Hence, a solution of a strong acid has a high buffer capacity below a pH of 2. Likewise, a strong base has a high buffer capacity above a pH of 12.

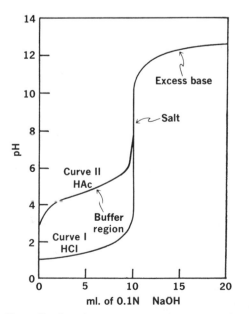

Fig. 8–1. Neutralization of a strong acid and a weak acid by a strong base.

The buffer capacity equations considered thus far have pertained exclusively to mixtures of weak electrolytes and their salts. The buffer capacity of a solution of a strong acid was shown by Van Slyke to be directly proportional to the hydrogen ion concentration, or

$$\beta = 2.303\,[H_3O^+] \qquad (8\text{--}31)$$

The buffer capacity of a solution of a strong base is similarly proportional to the hydroxyl ion concentration,

$$\beta = 2.303\,[OH^-] \qquad (8\text{--}32)$$

The total buffer capacity of a water solution of a strong acid or base at any pH is the sum of the separate capacities just given, equations (8–31) and (8–32), or

$$\beta = 2.303([H_3O^+] + [OH^-]) \qquad (8\text{--}33)$$

Example 8–9. What is the buffer capacity of a solution of hydrochloric acid having a hydrogen ion concentration of 10^{-2} mole per liter?

The hydroxyl ion concentration of such a solution is 10^{-12}, and the total buffer capacity is

$$\beta = 2.303(10^{-2} + 10^{-12})$$
$$\beta = 0.023$$

The OH^- concentration is obviously so low in this case that it may be neglected in the calculation.

Three equations are normally used to obtain the data for the titration curve of a weak acid (curve II of Figure 8–1), although a single equation that is somewhat complicated can be used. Suppose that increments of 0.1 N NaOH are added to 10 mL of a 0.1-N HAc solution.

(*a*) The pH of the solution, before any NaOH has been added, is obtained from the equation for a weak acid (p. 155, equation (7–99)).

$$pH = \tfrac{1}{2}pK_a - \tfrac{1}{2}\log c$$
$$= 2.38 - \tfrac{1}{2}\log 10^{-1} = 2.88$$

(*b*) At the equivalence point, where the acid has been converted completely into sodium ions and acetate ions, the pH is computed from the equation for a salt of a weak acid and strong base (p. 156, equation (7–103)) in log form:

$$pH = \tfrac{1}{2}\,pK_w + \tfrac{1}{2}\,pK_a + \tfrac{1}{2}\log c$$
$$= 7.00 + 2.38 + \tfrac{1}{2}\log(5 \times 10^{-2})$$
$$= 8.73$$

The concentration of the acid is given in the last term of this equation as 0.05, because the solution has been reduced to half its original value by mixing it with an equal volume of base at the equivalence point.

(*c*) Between these points on the neutralization curve, the increments of NaOH convert some of the acid to its conjugate base Ac^- to form a buffer mixture, and the pH of the system is calculated from the buffer equation. When 5 mL of base is added, the equivalent of 5 mL of 0.1 N acid remains and 5 mL of 0.1 N Ac$^-$ is formed, and using the Henderson–Hasselbalch equation,

$$pH = pK_a + \log \frac{[salt]}{[acid]}$$

$$= 4.76 + \log \frac{5}{5} = 4.76$$

The slope of the curve is a minimum and the buffer capacity is greatest at this point, where the solution shows the smallest pH change per gram equivalent of base added. The buffer capacity of a solution is the reciprocal of the slope of the curve at a point corresponding to the composition of the buffer solution. As seen in Figure 8–1, the slope of the line is a minimum, and the buffer capacity is greatest at half-neutralization, where pH = pK_a.

The titration curve for a tribasic acid such as H_3PO_4 consists of three stages, as shown in Figure 8–2. These may be considered as being produced by three separate acids (H_3PO_4, $pK_1 = 2.21$; $H_2PO_4^-$, $pK_2 = 7.21$; and HPO_4^{2-}, $pK_3 = 12.67$) whose strengths are sufficiently different so that their curves do not overlap. The curves may be plotted by using the buffer equation and their ends joined by smooth lines to produce the continuous curve of Figure 8–2.

A mixture of weak acids, whose pK_a values are sufficiently alike (differing by no more than about 2 pH units) so that their buffer regions overlap, can be used as a *universal buffer* over a wide range of pH values. A buffer of this type was introduced by Britton and Robinson.[9] The three stages of citric acid—$pK_1 = 3.15$, $pK_2 = 4.78$, $pK_3 = 6.40$—are sufficiently close to provide overlapping of neutralization curves and efficient buffering over this range. Adding Na_2HPO_4, whose conjugate acid $H_2PO_4^-$ has a pK_2 of 7.2,

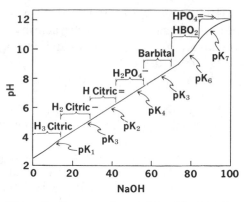

Fig. 8–3. Neutralization curve for a universal buffer. The horizontal axis is marked off in milliliters of 0.2 N NaOH. (After H. T. Britton, *Hydrogen Ions*, Vol. I, D. Van Nostrand, New York, 1956, p. 368.)

diethylbarbituric acid, $pK_1 = 7.91$, and boric acid, $pK_1 = 9.24$, provides a universal buffer that covers the pH range of about 2.4 to 12. The neutralization curve for the universal buffer mixture is linear between pH 4 and 8, as seen in Figure 8–3, because the successive dissociation constants differ by only a small value.

A titration curve depends on the ratio of the successive dissociation constants. Theoretically, when one K is equal to or less than 16 times the previous K, that is, when successive pKs do not differ by greater than 1.2 units, the second ionization begins well before the first is completed, and the titration curve is a straight line with no inflection points. Actually the inflection is not noticeable until one K is about 50 to 100 times that of the previous K value.

The buffer capacity of several acid–salt mixtures is plotted against pH in Figure 8–4. A buffer solution is useful within a range of about ±1 pH unit about the pK_a of its acid, where the buffer capacity is roughly greater than 0.01 or 0.02, as observed in Figure 8–4. Accordingly, the acetate buffer should be effective over a pH range of about 3.8 to 5.8, and the borate buffer should be effective over a range of 8.2 to 10.2. In each case, the greatest capacity occurs where [salt]/[acid] = 1 and pH = pK_a. Because of interionic effects, buffer capacities do not in general exceed a value of 0.2. The buf-

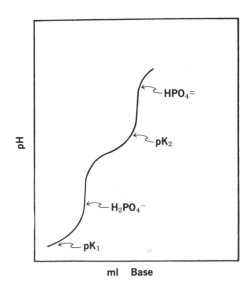

Fig. 8–2. Neutralization of a tribasic acid.

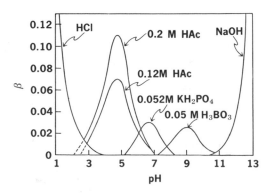

Fig. 8–4. The buffer capacity of several buffer systems as a function of pH. (Modified from R. G. Bates, *Electrometric pH Determinations*, Wiley, New York, 1954.)

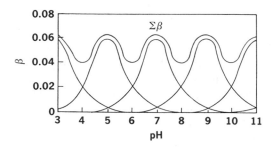

Fig. 8–5. The total buffer capacity of a universal buffer as a function of pH. From I. M. Kolthoff and C. Rosenblum, *Acid–Base Indicators*, Macmillan, New York, 1937, p. 29.)

fer capacity of a solution of the strong acid HCl becomes marked below a pH of 2, and the buffer capacity of a strong base NaOH becomes significant above a pH of 12.

The buffer capacity of a combination of buffers, the pK_a values of which overlap to produce a universal buffer, is plotted in Figure 8–5. It is seen that the total buffer capacity $\Sigma\beta$ is the sum of the β values of the individual buffers. In this figure, it is assumed that the maximum β's of all buffers in the series are identical.

BUFFERS IN PHARMACEUTICAL AND BIOLOGIC SYSTEMS

In Vivo Biologic Buffer Systems. *Blood* is maintained at a pH of about 7.4 by the so-called primary buffers in the plasma and the secondary buffers in the erythrocytes. The plasma contains carbonic acid/bicarbonate and acid/alkali sodium salts of phosphoric acid as buffers. Plasma proteins, which behave as acids in blood, can combine with bases and so act as buffers. In the erythrocytes, the two buffer systems consist of hemoglobin/oxyhemoglobin and acid/alkali potassium salts of phosphoric acid.

The dissociation exponent pK_1 for the first ionization stage of carbonic acid in the plasma at body temperature and an ionic strength of 0.16 is about 6.1. The buffer equation for the carbonic acid/bicarbonate buffer of the blood is

$$pH = 6.1 + \log \frac{[HCO_3^-]}{[H_2CO_3]} \quad (8-34)$$

in which $[H_2CO_3]$ represents the concentration of CO_2 present as H_2CO_3 dissolved in the blood. At a pH of 7.4, the ratio of bicarbonate to carbonic acid in normal blood plasma is

$$\log \frac{[HCO_3^-]}{[H_2CO_3]} = 7.4 - 6.1 = 1.3$$

or

$$[HCO_3^-]/[H_2CO_3] = 20/1 \quad (8-35)$$

This result checks with experimental findings, since the actual concentrations of bicarbonate and carbonic

acid in the plasma are about 0.025 *M* and 0.00125 *M* respectively.

The buffer capacity of the blood in the physiologic range pH 7.0 to 7.8 is obtained as follows. According to Peters and Van Slyke,[10] the buffer capacity of the blood owing to hemoglobin and other constituents, exclusive of bicarbonate, is about 0.025 gram equivalents per liter per pH unit. The pH of the bicarbonate buffer in the blood (i.e. pH 7.4) is rather far removed from the pH (6.1) where it exhibits maximum buffer capacity; therefore, the bicarbonate's buffer action is relatively small with respect to that of the other blood constituents. According to the calculation just given, the ratio $[NaHCO_3]/[H_2CO_3]$ is 20:1 at pH 7.4. Using equation (8–27), the buffer capacity for the bicarbonate system ($K_1 = 4 \times 10^{-7}$) at a pH of 7.4 ($[H_3O^+] = 4 \times 10^{-8}$) is found to be roughly 0.003. Therefore, the total buffer capacity of the blood in the physiologic range, the sum of the capacities of the various constituents, is 0.025 + 0.003 = 0.028. Salenius[11] reported a value of 0.0318 ± 0.0035 for whole blood, whereas Ellison et al.[12] obtained a buffer capacity of about 0.039 gram equivalents per liter per pH unit for whole blood, of which 0.031 was contributed by the cells and 0.008 by the plasma.

Usually when the pH of the blood goes below 6.9 or above 7.8, life is in serious danger. The pH of the blood in diabetic coma is alleged to drop as low as about 6.8.

Lacrimal fluid, or tears, have been found to have a great degree of buffer capacity, allowing a dilution of 1:15 with neutral distilled water before an alteration of pH is noticed.[13] In the terminology of Bates,[14] this would be referred to today as *dilution value* rather than buffer capacity (p. 171). The pH of tears is about 7.4, with a range of 7 to 8 or slightly higher. Pure conjunctival fluid is probably more acidic than the tear fluid commonly used in pH measurements. This is because pH increases rapidly when the sample is removed for analysis because of the loss of CO_2 from the tear fluid.

Urine. The 24-hour urine collection of a normal adult has a pH averaging about 6.0 units; it may be as low as 4.5 or as high as 7.8. When the pH of the urine is below normal values, hydrogen ions are excreted by the kidneys. Conversely, when the urine is above pH 7.4, hydrogen ions are retained by action of the kidneys in order to return the pH to its normal range of values.

Pharmaceutical Buffers. Buffer solutions are used frequently in pharmaceutical practice, particularly in the formulation of ophthalmic solutions. They also find application in the colorimetric determination of pH and for those research studies in which pH must be held constant.

Gifford[15] suggested two stock solutions, one containing boric acid and the other monohydrated sodium carbonate, which, when mixed in various proportions, yield buffer solutions with pH values from about 5 to 9.

Sörensen[16] proposed a mixture of the salts of sodium phosphate for buffer solutions of pH 6 to 8. Sodium chloride is added to each buffer mixture to make it isotonic with body fluids.

A buffer system suggested by Palitzsch[17] and modified by Hind and Goyan[18] consists of boric acid, sodium borate, and sufficient sodium chloride to make the mixtures isotonic. It is used for ophthalmic solutions in the pH range of 7 to 9.

The buffers of Clark and Lubs,[19] based on the original pH scale of Sörensen, have been redetermined at 25° C by Bower and Bates[7] so as to conform to the present definition of pH (p. 200). Between pH 3 and 11, the older values were about 0.04 unit lower than the values now assigned, and at the ends of the scale, the differences were greater. The original values were determined at 20° C, whereas most experiments today are performed at 25° C.

The Clark–Lubs mixtures and their corresponding pH ranges are:

(a) HCl and KCl, pH 1.2 to 2.2

(b) HCl and potassium hydrogen phthalate, pH 2.2 to 4.0

(c) NaOH and potassium hydrogen phthalate, pH 4.2 to 5.8

(d) NaOH and KH_2PO_4, pH 5.8 to 8.0

(e) H_3BO_3, NaOH and KCl, pH 8.0 to 10.0

With regard to mixture (a), consisting of HCl and KCl and used for the pH range from 1.0 to 2.2, it will be recalled from the discussion of the neutralization curve (I), Figure 8–1, that HCl alone has considerable buffer efficiency below pH 2. KCl is a neutral salt and is added to adjust the ionic strength of the buffer solutions to a constant value of 0.10; the pH calculated from the equation, $-\log a_{H^+} = -\log (\gamma_\pm c)$, corresponds closely to the experimentally determined pH. The role of the KCl in the Clark–Lubs buffer is sometimes erroneously interpreted as that of a salt of the buffer acid, HCl, corresponding to the part played by sodium acetate as the salt of the weak buffer acid, HAc. Potassium chloride is added to (e), the borate buffer, to produce an ionic strength comparable to that of (d), the phosphate buffer, where the pH of the two buffer series overlap.

Buffer solutions are discussed in the USP XXII on pp. 1598, 1599, 1784, and 1785. A buffer commonly used in biologic research (pH 7 to 9) and reported in the *Merck Index* is TRIS, aminohydroxymethyl propanediol.

Preparation of Pharmaceutical Buffer Solutions. The pharmacist may be called upon at times to prepare buffer systems, the formulas for which do not appear in the literature. The following steps should be helpful in the development of a new buffer.

(a) Select a weak acid having a pK_a approximately equal to the pH at which the buffer is to be used. This will ensure maximum buffer capacity.

(b) From the buffer equation, calculate the ratio of salt and weak acid required to obtain the desired pH. The buffer equation is satisfactory for approximate calculations within the pH range of 4 to 10.

(c) Consider the individual concentrations of the buffer salt and acid needed to obtain a suitable buffer capacity. A *concentration* of 0.05 to 0.5 *M* is usually sufficient; and a *buffer capacity* of 0.01 to 0.1 is generally adequate.

(d) Other factors of some importance in the choice of a pharmaceutical buffer include availability of chemicals, sterility of the final solution, stability of the drug and buffer on aging, cost of materials, and freedom from toxicity. For example, a borate buffer, because of its toxic effects, certainly cannot be used to stabilize a solution to be administered orally or parenterally.

(e) Finally, one should determine the pH and buffer capacity of the completed buffered solution using a reliable pH meter. In some cases, sufficient accuracy is obtained by the use of pH papers. Particularly when the electrolyte concentration is high, it may be found that the pH calculated by use of the buffer equation is somewhat different from the experimental value. This is to be expected when activity coefficients are not taken into account, and it emphasizes the necessity for carrying out the actual determination.

Influence of Buffer Capacity and pH on Tissue Irritation. Solutions to be applied to tissues or administered parenterally are liable to cause irritation if their pH is greatly removed from the normal pH of the relevant body fluid. Consequently, the pharmacist must consider this point when formulating ophthalmic solutions, parenteral products, and fluids to be applied to abraded surfaces. Of possible greater significance than the actual pH of the solution is its buffer capacity and the volume to be used in relation to the volume of body fluid with which the buffered solution will come in contact. The buffer, capacity of the body fluid should also be considered. Tissue irritation, due to large pH differences between the solution being administered and the physiologic environment in which it is used, will be minimal (a) the lower the buffer capacity of the solution, (b) the smaller the volume used, for a given concentration, and (c) the larger the volume and buffer capacity of the physiologic fluid.

Friedenwald et al.[20] claimed that the pH of solutions for introduction into the eye may vary from 4.5 to 11.5 without marked pain or damage. This statement evidently would be true only if the buffer capacity were kept low. Martin and Mims[21] found that Sörensen's phosphate buffer produced irritation in the eyes of a number of subjects when used outside the narrow pH range of 6.5 to 8, whereas a boric acid solution of pH 5 produced no discomfort in the eyes of the same subjects. Martin and Mims concluded that a pH range of nonirritation cannot be established absolutely but rather depends upon the buffer employed. In light of the previous discussion, this apparent anomaly can be explained partly in terms of the low buffer capacity of boric acid as compared with that of the phosphate buffer (cf. *Problems 8–12* and *8–13*, p. 188) and partly to the difference of the physiologic response to various ion species.

Riegelman and Vaughn[22] assumed that the acid-neutralizing power of the tears when 0.1 mL of a 1% solution of a drug is instilled into the eye is roughly equivalent to 10 microliters of a 0.01-N strong base. They point out that while in a few cases irritation of the eye may result from the presence of the free base form of a drug at the physiologic pH, it is more often due to the acidity of the eye solution. For example, since only one carboxyl group of tartaric acid is neutralized by epinephrine base in epinephrine bitartrate, a 0.06-M solution of the drug has a pH of about 3.5. The prolonged pain resulting from instilling two drops of this solution into the eye is presumably due to the unneutralized acid of the bitartrate, which requires ten times the amount of tears to restore the normal pH of the eye as compared with the result following two drops of epinephrine hydrochloride. Solutions of pilocarpine salts also possess sufficient buffer capacity to cause pain or irritation owing to their acid reaction when instilled into the eye.

Parenteral solutions for injection into the blood are usually not buffered, or they are buffered to a low capacity so that the buffers of the blood may readily bring them within the physiologic pH range. If the drugs are to be injected only in small quantities and at a slow rate, their solutions can be buffered weakly to maintain approximate neutrality.

Following oral administration, aspirin is absorbed more rapidly in systems buffered at low buffer capacity than in systems containing no buffer or in highly buffered preparations, according to Mason.[23] Thus, the buffer capacity of the buffer should be optimized to produce rapid absorption and minimal gastric irritation of orally administered aspirin.

In addition to the adjustment of tonicity and pH for ophthalmic preparations, similar requirements are demanded for nasal delivery of drugs. This has become all the more important in recent years since the nasal passage is now used for the administration of systemic drugs (see pp. 525–527 for nasal dosage forms). Insulin, for example, is more effective by nasal administration than by other nonparenteral routes.[24]

Stability vs. Optimum Therapeutic Response. For the sake of completeness, some mention must be made at this point of the effect of buffer capacity and pH on the stability and therapeutic response of the drug being used in solution.

As will be discussed later (Chapter 10), the undissociated form of a weakly acidic or basic drug often has a higher therapeutic activity than the dissociated salt form. This is because the former is lipid soluble and can penetrate body membranes readily, whereas the ionic form, not being lipid soluble, can penetrate membranes only with greater difficulty. Thus Swan and White[25] and Cogan and Kinsey[26] observed an increase in therapeutic response of weakly basic alkaloids (used as ophthalmic drugs) as the pH of the solution, and hence concentration of the undissociated base, was increased. At a pH of about 4, these drugs are predominantly in the ionic form, and penetration is slow or insignificant. When the tears bring the pH to about 7.4, the drugs may exist to a significant degree in the form of the free base, depending on the dissociation constant of the drug.

Example 8–10. The pK_b of pilocarpine is 7.15 at 25° C. Compute the mole percent of free base present on 25° C and at a pH of 7.4.

$$C_{11}H_{16}N_2O_2 + H_2O \rightleftharpoons C_{11}H_{16}N_2O_2H^+ + OH^-$$

Pilocarpine base   Pilocarpine ion

$$pH = pK_w - pK_b + \log \frac{[\text{base}]}{[\text{salt}]}$$

$$7.4 = 14.00 - 7.15 + \log \frac{[\text{base}]}{[\text{salt}]}$$

$$\log \frac{[\text{base}]}{[\text{salt}]} = 7.40 - 14.00 + 7.15 = 0.55$$

$$\frac{[\text{base}]}{[\text{salt}]} = \frac{3.56}{1}$$

$$\text{mole percent of base} = \frac{[\text{base}]}{[\text{salt}] + [\text{base}]} \times 100$$

$$= [3.56/(1 + 3.56)] \times 100 = 78\%$$

Hind and Goyan[27] pointed out that the pH for maximum stability of a drug for ophthalmic use may be far below that of the optimum physiologic effect. Under such conditions, the solution of the drug can be buffered at a low buffer capacity and at a pH that is a compromise between that of optimum stability and the pH for maximum therapeutic action. The buffer is adequate to prevent changes in pH due to the alkalinity of the glass or acidity of CO_2 from dissolved air. Yet, when the solution is instilled in the eye, the tears participate in the gradual neutralization of the solution; conversion of the drug occurs from the physiologically inactive form to the undissociated base. The base can then readily penetrate the lipoidal membrane. As the base is absorbed at the pH of the eye, more of the salt is converted into base to preserve the constancy of pK_b; hence, the alkaloidal drug is gradually absorbed.

pH and Solubility. The relationship of pH and the solubility of weak electrolytes will be treated in some detail in Chapter 10. At this point it is necessary only to point out briefly the influence of buffering on the solubility of an alkaloidal base. At a low pH, a base is predominantly in the ionic form, which is usually very soluble in aqueous media. As the pH is raised, more undissociated base is formed as calculated by the method illustrated in *Example 8–10*. When the amount of base exceeds the limited water solubility of this form, free base precipitates from solution. Therefore, the solution should be buffered at a sufficiently low pH so that the concentration of alkaloidal base in equilibrium with its salt is calculated to be less than the solubility of the free base at the storage temperature. Stabilization against precipitation can thus be maintained.

BUFFERED ISOTONIC SOLUTIONS

Reference has already been made to the in vivo buffer systems, such as blood and lacrimal fluid, and the desirability for buffering pharmaceutical solutions under certain conditions. In addition to carrying out pH adjustment, pharmaceutical solutions that are meant for application to delicate membranes of the body should also be adjusted to approximately the same osmotic pressure (Chapter 5) as that of the body fluids. Isotonic solutions cause no swelling or contraction of the tissues with which they come in contact, and produce no discomfort when instilled in the eye, nasal tract, blood, or other body tissues. Isotonic sodium chloride is a familiar pharmaceutical example of such a preparation.

The need to achieve isotonic conditions with solutions to be applied to delicate membranes is dramatically illustrated by mixing a small quantity of blood with aqueous sodium chloride solutions of varying tonicity. For example, if a small quantity of blood, defibrinated to prevent clotting, is mixed with a solution containing 0.9 g NaCl per 100 mL, the cells retain their normal size. The solution has essentially the same salt concentration and hence the same osmotic pressure as the red blood cell contents, and is said to be *isotonic* with blood. If the red blood cells are suspended in a 2.0% NaCl solution, the water within the cells passes through the cell membrane in an attempt to dilute the surrounding salt solution until the salt concentrations on both sides of the erythrocyte membrane are identical. This outward passage of water causes the cells to shrink and become wrinkled or *crenated*. The salt solution in this instance is said to be *hypertonic* with respect to the blood cell contents. Finally, if the blood is mixed with 0.2% NaCl solution or with distilled water, water enters the blood cells, causing them to swell and finally burst, with the liberation of hemoglobin. This phenomenon is known as *hemolysis*, and the weak salt solution or water is said to be *hypotonic* with respect to the blood.

The student should appreciate that the red blood cell membrane is not impermeable to all drugs; that is, it is not a perfect semipermeable membrane. Thus, it will permit the passage of not only water molecules, but also solutes such as urea, ammonium chloride, alcohol, and boric acid.[28] A 2.0% solution of boric acid has the same osmotic pressure as the blood cell contents when determined by the freezing point method and is therefore said to be *isosmotic* with blood. The molecules of boric acid pass freely through the erythrocyte membrane, however, regardless of concentration. As a result, this solution acts essentially as water when in contact with blood cells. Being extremely hypotonic

with respect to the blood, boric acid solution brings about rapid hemolysis. Therefore, a solution containing a quantity of drug calculated to be isosmotic with blood is isotonic *only* when the blood cells are impermeable to the solute molecules and permeable to the solvent, water. It is interesting to note that the mucous lining of the eye acts as a true semipermeable membrane to boric acid in solution. Accordingly, a 2.0% boric acid solution serves as an isotonic ophthalmic preparation.

To overcome this difficulty, Husa[29] has suggested that the term *isotonic* should be restricted to solutions having equal osmotic pressures with respect to a particular membrane. Goyan and Reck[30] felt that, rather than restricting the use of the term in this manner, a new term should be introduced that is defined on the basis of the sodium chloride concentration. These workers defined the term *isotonicity value* as the concentration of an aqueous NaCl solution having the same colligative properties as the solution in question. Although all solutions having an isotonicity value of 0.9 g NaCl per 100 mL of solution need not *necessarily* be isotonic with respect to the living membranes concerned. Nevertheless, many of them are roughly isotonic in this sense, and all may be considered isotonic across an ideal membrane. Accordingly, the term *isotonic* is used with this meaning throughout the present chapter. Only a few substances—those that penetrate animal membranes at a sufficient rate—will show exception to this classification.

The remainder of this chapter is concerned with a discussion of isotonic solutions and the means by which they may be buffered.

Measurement of Tonicity. The tonicity of solutions may be determined by one of two methods. First, in the *hemolytic* method, the effect of various solutions of the drug is observed on the appearance of red blood cells suspended in the solutions. The various effects produced have been described in the previous section. Husa and his associates[29] have used this method. In their later work, a quantitative method developed by Hunter[31] was used based on the fact that a hypotonic solution liberates oxyhemoglobin in direct proportion to the number of cells hemolyzed. By such means, the van't Hoff i factor (p. 129) can be determined and the value compared with that computed from cryoscopic data, osmotic coefficient, and activity coefficient.[32]

Husa has found that a drug having the proper i value as measured by freezing point depression or computed from theoretic equations nevertheless may hemolyze human red blood cells; it was on this basis that he suggested restriction of the term *isotonic* to solutions having equal osmotic pressures with respect to a particular membrane.

The second approach used to measure tonicity is based on any of the methods that determine colligative properties, as discussed in Chapter 5. Goyan and Reck[30] investigated various modifications of the Hill–Baldes technique[33] (p. 111) for measuring tonicity. This method is based on a measurement of the slight temperature differences arising from differences in the vapor pressure of thermally insulated samples contained in constant-humidity chambers.

One of the first references to the determination of the freezing point of blood and tears (as was necessary to make solutions isotonic with these fluids) was that of Lumiere and Chevrotier,[34] in which the values of $-0.56°$ and $-0.80°$ C were given respectively for the two fluids. Following work by Pedersen-Bjergaard and co-workers,[35,36] however, it is now well established that $-0.52°$ is the freezing point of both human blood and lacrimal fluid. This temperature corresponds to the freezing point of a 0.90% NaCl solution, which is therefore considered to be isotonic with both blood and lacrimal fluid.

Calculating Tonicity Using L_{iso} Values. Since the freezing point depressions for solutions of electrolytes of both the weak and strong types are always greater than those calculated from the equation, $\Delta T_f = K_f c$, a new factor, $L = iK_f$, is introduced to overcome this difficulty.[37] The equation already discussed in Chapter 6, p. 137, is

$$\Delta T_f = Lc \qquad (8-36)$$

The L value may be obtained from the freezing point lowering of solutions of representative compounds of a given ionic type at a concentration c that is isotonic with body fluids. This specific value of L is symbolized as L_{iso} (p. 137).

The L_{iso} value for a 0.90% (0.154-M) solution of sodium chloride, which has a freezing point depression of 0.52° and is thus isotonic with body fluids, is 3.4:

$$L_{iso} = \frac{\Delta T_f}{c} \qquad (8-37)$$

$$L_{iso} = \frac{0.52°}{0.154} = 3.4$$

The interionic attraction in solutions that are not too concentrated is roughly the same for all uni-univalent electrolytes regardless of the chemical nature of the various compounds of this class, and all have about the

same value for L_{iso}, namely 3.4. As a result of this similarity between compounds of a given ionic type, a table can be arranged listing the L value for each class of electrolytes at a concentration that is isotonic with body fluids. The L_{iso} values obtained in this way are found in Table 8–3.

It will be observed that for dilute solutions of nonelectrolytes, L_{iso} is approximately equal to K_f. Table 8–3 is used to obtain the approximate ΔT_f for a solution of a drug, if the ionic type can be correctly ascertained. A plot of iK_f against molar concentration of various types of electrolytes, from which the values of L_{iso} can be read, is shown in Figure 6–7, p. 137.

Example 8–11. What is the freezing point lowering of a 1% solution of sodium propionate (molecular weight 96)? Since sodium propionate is a uni-univalent electrolyte, its L_{iso} value is 3.4. The molar concentration of a 1% solution of this compound is 0.104.

$$\Delta T_f = 3.4 \times 0.104 = 0.35° \qquad (8-38)$$

Although 1 g per 100 mL of sodium propionate is not the isotonic concentration, it is still proper to use L_{iso} as a simple average that agrees with the concentration range expected for the finished solution. The selection of L values in this concentration region is not sensitive to minor changes in concentration; no pretense to an accuracy greater than about 10% is implied or needed in these calculations.

The calculation of *Example 8–11* may be simplified by expressing molarity c as grams of drug contained in a definite volume of solution. Thus

$$\text{Molarity} = \frac{\text{moles}}{\text{liter}}$$

$$= \frac{\text{weight in grams}}{\substack{\text{molecular weight} \\ \text{in g/mole}}} \div \frac{\text{volume in mL}}{1000 \text{ mL/liter}} \qquad (8-39)$$

or

$$c = \frac{w}{MW} \times \frac{1000}{v} \qquad (8-40)$$

in which w is the grams of solute, MW is the molecular weight of the solute, and v is the volume of solution in milliliters. Substituting in equation (8–36)

TABLE 8–3. *Average L_{iso} Values for Various Ionic Types**

Type	L_{iso}	Examples
Nonelectrolytes	1.9	Sucrose, glycerin, urea, camphor
Weak electrolytes	2.0	Boric acid, cocaine, phenobarbital
Di-divalent electrolytes	2.0	Magnesium sulfate, zinc sulfate
Uni-univalent electrolytes	3.4	Sodium chloride, cocaine hydrochloride, sodium phenobarbital
Uni-divalent electrolytes	4.3	Sodium sulfate, atropine sulfate
Di-univalent electrolytes	4.8	Zinc chloride, calcium bromide
Uni-trivalent electrolytes	5.2	Sodium citrate, sodium phosphate
Tri-univalent electrolytes	6.0	Aluminum chloride, ferric iodide
Tetraborate electrolytes	7.6	Sodium borate, potassium borate

*From J. M. Wells, J. Am. Pharm. Assoc., Pract. Ed. **5**, 99, 1944.

$$\Delta T_f = L_{iso} \times \frac{w \times 1000}{MW \times v} \qquad (8\text{-}41)$$

The problem in *Example (8–11)* can be solved in one operation by the use of equation (8–41) without the added calculation needed to obtain the molar concentration.

$$\Delta T_f = 3.4 \times \frac{1 \times 1000}{96 \times 100} = 3.4 \times 0.104$$

$$= 0.35°$$

The student is encouraged to derive expressions of this type; certainly equations (8–40) and (8–41) should not be memorized, for they are not remembered long. The L_{iso} values may also be used for calculating sodium chloride equivalents and Sprowls' V values, as discussed in subsequent sections of this chapter.

METHODS OF ADJUSTING TONICITY AND pH

One of several methods may be used to calculate the quantity of sodium chloride, dextrose, and other substances that may be added to solutions of drugs to render them isotonic.

For discussion purposes, the methods are divided into two classes. In the Class I methods, sodium chloride or some other substance is added to the solution of the drug to lower the freezing point of the solution to −0.52° and thus make it isotonic with body fluids. Under this class are included the *Cryoscopic* method and the *Sodium Chloride Equivalent* method. In the Class II methods, water is added to the drug in a sufficient amount to form an isotonic solution. The preparation is then brought to its final volume with an isotonic or a buffered isotonic dilution solution. Included in this class are the *White–Vincent* method and the *Sprowls* method.

Class I Methods

Cryoscopic Method. The freezing point depressions of a number of drug solutions, determined experimentally or theoretically, are found in Table 8–4. According to the previous section, the freezing point depressions of drug solutions that have not been determined experimentally can be estimated from theoretic considerations, knowing only the molecular weight of the drug and the L_{iso} value of the ionic class.

The calculations involved in the cryoscopic method are explained best by an example.

Example 8–12. How much sodium chloride is required to render 100 mL of a 1% solution of apomorphine hydrochloride isotonic with blood serum?

From Table 8–4 it is found that a 1% solution of the drug has a freezing point lowering of 0.08°. To make this solution isotonic with blood, sufficient sodium chloride must be added to reduce the freezing point by an additional 0.44° (0.52 − 0.08). In the freezing point table,

it is also observed that a 1% solution of sodium chloride has a freezing point lowering of 0.58°. By the method of proportion,

$$\frac{1\%}{X} = \frac{0.58°}{0.44°} \ ; \ X = 0.76\%$$

Thus, 0.76% sodium chloride will lower the freezing point the required 0.44° and will render the solution isotonic. The solution is prepared by dissolving 1.0 g of apomorphine hydrochloride and 0.76 g of sodium chloride in sufficient water to make 100 mL of solution.

Sodium Chloride Equivalent Method. A second method for adjusting the tonicity of pharmaceutical solutions was developed by Mellen and Seltzer.[38] The *sodium chloride equivalent* or, as referred to by these workers, the "tonicic equivalent" of a drug is the amount of sodium chloride that is equivalent to (i.e., has the same osmotic effect as) 1 gram, or other weight unit, of the drug. The sodium chloride equivalents E for a number of drugs are listed in Table 8–4.

When the E value for a new drug is desired for inclusion in Table 8–4, it can be calculated from the L_{iso} value or freezing point depression of the drug according to the formulas derived by Goyan et al.[39] For a solution containing 1 g of drug in 1000 mL of solution, the concentration c expressed in moles per liter may be written as

$$c = \frac{1\ g}{molecular\ weight} \qquad (8\text{-}42)$$

and from equation (8–36)

$$\Delta T_f = L_{iso} \frac{1\ g}{MW}$$

Now E is the weight of NaCl with the same freezing point depression as 1 g of the drug, and for a NaCl solution containing E grams of drug per 1000 mL,

$$\Delta T_f = 3.4 \frac{E}{58.45} \qquad (8\text{-}43)$$

in which 3.4 is the L_{iso} value for sodium chloride and 58.45 is its molecular weight. Equating these two values of ΔT_f yields

$$\frac{L_{iso}}{MW} = 3.4 \frac{E}{58.45} \qquad (8\text{-}44)$$

$$E \cong 17 \frac{L_{iso}}{MW} \qquad (8\text{-}45)$$

Example 8–13. Calculate the approximate E value for a new amphetamine hydrochloride derivative (molecular weight 187).

Since this drug is a uni-univalent salt, it has an L_{iso} value of 3.4. Its E value is calculated from equation (8–45):

$$E = 17 \frac{3.4}{187} = 0.31$$

Calculations for determining the amount of sodium chloride or other inert substance to render a solution isotonic (across an ideal membrane) simply involve multiplying the quantity of each drug in the prescription by its sodium chloride equivalent and subtracting

TABLE 8–4. *Isotonic Values**

Substance	MW	E	V	$\Delta T_f^{1\%}$	L_{iso}
Alcohol, dehydrated	46.07	0.70	23.3	0.41	1.9
Aminophylline	456.46	0.17	5.7	0.10	4.6
Ammonium chloride	53.50	1.08	36	0.64	3.4
Amphetamine sulfate (benzedrine sulfate)	368.49	0.22	7.3	0.13	4.8
Antipyrine	188.22	0.17	5.7	0.10	1.9
Antistine hydrochloride (antazoline hydrochloride)	301.81	0.18	6.0	0.11	3.2
Apomorphine hydrochloride	312.79	0.14	4.7	0.08	2.6
Ascorbic acid	176.12	0.18	6.0	0.11	1.9
Atropine sulfate	694.82	0.13	4.3	0.07	5.3
Aureomycin hydrochloride	544	0.11	3.7	0.06	3.5
Barbital sodium	206.18	0.29	10.0	0.29	3.5
Benadryl hydrochloride (diphenhydramine hydrochloride)	291.81	0.20	6.6	0.34	3.4
Boric acid	61.84	0.50	16.7	0.29	1.8
Butacaine sulfate (butyn sulfate)	710.95	0.20	6.7	0.12	8.4
Caffeine	194.19	0.08	2.7	0.05	0.9
Caffeine and sodium benzoate	—	0.25	8.7	0.28	—
Calcium chloride · $2H_2O$	147.03	0.51	17.0	0.30	4.4
Calcium gluconate	448.39	0.16	5.3	0.09	4.2
Calcium lactate	308.30	0.23	7.7	0.14	4.2
Camphor	152.23	0.20	6.7	0.12	1.8
Chloramphenicol (chloromycetin)	323.14	0.10	3.3	0.06	1.9
Chlorobutanol (chloretone)	177.47	0.24	8.0	0.14	2.5
Cocaine hydrochloride	339.81	0.16	5.3	0.09	3.2
Cupric sulfate · $5H_2O$	249.69	0.18	6.0	0.11	2.6
Dextrose · H_2O	198.17	0.16	5.3	0.09	1.9
Dibucaine hydrochloride (nupercaine hydrochloride)	379.92	0.13	4.3	0.08	2.9
Emetine hydrochloride	553.56	0.10	3.3	0.06	3.3
Ephedrine hydrochloride	201.69	0.30	10.0	0.18	3.6
Ephedrine sulfate	428.54	0.23	7.7	0.14	5.8
Epinephrine bitartrate	333.29	0.18	6.0	0.11	3.5
Epinephrine hydrochloride	219.66	0.29	9.7	0.17	3.7
Ethylhydrocupreine hydrochloride (optochin)	376.92	0.17	5.7	0.10	3.8
Ethylmorphine hydrochloride (dionin)	385.88	0.16	5.3	0.09	3.6
Eucatropine hydrochloride (euphthalmine hydrochloride)	327.84	0.18	6.0	0.11	3.5
Fluorescein sodium	376	0.31	10.3	0.18	6.9
Glycerin	92.09	0.34	11.3	0.20	1.8
Homatropine hydrobromide	356.26	0.17	5.7	0.10	3.6
Lactose	360.31	0.07	2.3	0.04	1.7
Magnesium sulfate · $7H_2O$	246.50	0.17	5.7	0.10	2.5
Menthol	156.26	0.20	6.7	0.12	1.8
Meperidine hydrochloride (demerol hydrochloride)	283.79	0.22	7.3	0.12	3.7
Mercuric chloride (mercury bichloride)	271.52	0.13	4.3	0.08	2.1
Mercuric cyanide	252.65	0.15	5.0	0.09	2.2
Mercuric succinimide	396.77	0.14	4.8	0.08	3.3
Methacholine chloride (mecholyl chloride)	195.69	0.32	10.7	0.19	3.7
Methamphetamine hydrochloride (desoxyephedrine hydrochloride)	185.69	0.37	12.3	0.22	4.0
Metycaine hydrochloride	292.82	0.20	6.7	0.12	3.4
Mild silver protein	—	0.18	6.0	0.11	—
Morphine hydrochloride	375.84	0.15	5.0	0.09	3.3
Morphine sulfate	758.82	0.14	4.8	0.08	6.2
Naphazoline hydrochloride (privine hydrochloride)	246.73	0.27	7.7	0.16	3.3
Neomycin sulfate	—	0.11	3.7	0.06	—
Neostigmine bromide (prostigmine bromide)	303.20	0.22	6.0	0.11	3.2
Nicotinamide	122.13	0.26	8.7	0.15	1.9
Penicillin G potassium	372.47	0.18	6.0	0.11	3.9
Penicillin G Procaine	588.71	0.10	3.3	0.06	3.5
Penicillin G sodium	356.38	0.18	6.0	0.11	3.8
Phenacaine hydrochloride (holocaine hydrochloride)	352.85	0.20	5.3	0.11	3.3

TABLE 8–4.   (continued)

Substance	MW	E	V	$\Delta T_f^{1\%}$	L_{iso}
Phenobarbital sodium	254.22	0.24	8.0	0.14	3.6
Phenol	94.11	0.35	11.7	0.20	1.9
Phenylephrine hydrochloride (neosynephrine hydrochloride)	203.67	0.32	9.7	0.18	3.5
Physostigmine salicylate	413.46	0.16	5.3	0.09	3.9
Physostigmine sulfate	648.45	0.13	4.3	0.08	5.0
Pilocarpine nitrate	271.27	0.23	7.7	0.14	3.7
Potassium acid phosphate (KH_2PO_4)	136.13	0.43	14.2	0.25	3.4
Potassium chloride	74.55	0.76	25.3	0.45	3.3
Potassium iodide	166.02	0.34	11.3	0.20	3.3
Procaine hydrochloride	272.77	0.21	7.0	0.12	3.4
Quinine hydrochloride	396.91	0.14	4.7	0.08	3.3
Quinine and urea hydrochloride	547.48	0.23	7.7	0.14	7.4
Scopolamine hydrobromide (hyoscine hydrobromide)	438.32	0.12	4.0	0.07	3.1
Silver nitrate	169.89	0.33	11.0	0.19	3.3
Sodium acid phosphate ($NaH_2PO_4 \cdot H_2O$)	138.00	0.40	13.3	0.24	3.2
Sodium benzoate	144.11	0.40	13.3	0.24	3.4
Sodium bicarbonate	84.00	0.65	21.7	0.38	3.2
Sodium bisulfite	104.07	0.61	20.3	0.36	3.7
Sodium borate·$10H_2O$	381.43	0.42	14.0	0.25	9.4
Sodium chloride	58.45	1.00	33.3	0.58	3.4
Sodium iodide	149.92	0.39	13.0	0.23	3.4
Sodium nitrate	85.01	0.68	22.7	0.39	3.4
Sodium phosphate, anhydrous	141.98	0.53	17.7	0.31	4.4
Sodium phosphate·$2H_2O$	178.05	0.42	14.0	0.25	4.4
Sodium phosphate·$7H_2O$	268.08	0.29	9.7	0.17	4.6
Sodium phosphate·$12H_2O$	358.21	0.22	7.3	0.13	4.6
Sodium propionate	96.07	0.61	20.3	0.36	3.4
Sodium sulfite, exsiccated	126.06	0.65	21.7	0.38	4.8
Streptomycin sulfate	1457.44	0.07	2.3	0.04	6.0
Strong silver protein	—	0.08	2.7	0.05	—
Sucrose	342.30	0.08	2.7	0.05	1.6
Sulfacetamide sodium	254.25	0.23	7.7	0.14	3.4
Sulfadiazine sodium	272.27	0.24	8.0	0.14	3.8
Sulfamerazine sodium	286.29	0.23	7.7	0.14	3.9
Sulfanilamide	172.21	0.22	7.3	0.13	2.2
Sulfathiazole sodium	304.33	0.22	7.3	0.13	3.9
Tannic acid	—	0.03	1.0	0.02	—
Tetracaine hydrochloride (pontocaine hydrochloride)	300.82	0.18	6.0	0.11	3.2
Tetracycline hydrochloride	480.92	0.14	4.7	0.08	4.0
Tripelennamine hydrochloride (pyribenzamine hydrochloride)	291.83	0.30	7.3	0.17	3.8
Urea	60.06	0.59	19.7	0.35	2.1
Zinc chloride	139.29	0.62	20.3	0.37	5.1
Zinc phenolsulfonate	555.84	0.18	6.0	0.11	5.9
Zinc sulfate·$7H_2O$	287.56	0.15	5.0	0.09	2.5

*The values in Table 8–4 have been obtained from the data of E. R. Hammarlund and K. Pedersen-Bjergaard, J. Am. Pharm. Assoc., Pract. Ed. **19**, 39, 1958; ibid., Sci. Ed. **47**, 107, 1958, and other sources. The values vary somewhat with concentration, and those in the table are for 1 to 3% solutions of the drugs in most instances. A complete table of E and ΔT_f values is found in the *Merck Index*, 11th Edition, Merck, Rahway, NJ, 1989, pp. MISC-79 to MISC-103. For the most recent results of Hammarlund, see J. Pharm. Sci. **70**, 1161, 1981; ibid. **78**, 519, 1989.

Key: MW is the molecular weight of the drug; E is the sodium chloride equivalent of the drug; V is the volume in mL of isotonic solution that can be prepared by adding water to 0.3 g of the drug (the weight of drug in 1 fluid ounce of a 1% solution); $\Delta T_f^{1\%}$ is the freezing point depression of a 1% solution of the drug; and L_{iso} is the molar freezing point depression of the drug at a concentration approximately isotonic with blood and lacrimal fluid.

this value from the concentration of sodium chloride that is isotonic with body fluids, namely, 0.9 g/100 mL.

Example 8–14. A solution contains 1.0 g ephedrine sulfate in a volume of 100 mL. What quantity of sodium chloride must be added to make the solution isotonic? How much dextrose would be required for this purpose?

The quantity of the drug is multiplied by its sodium chloride equivalent E, giving the weight of sodium chloride to which the quantity of drug is equivalent in osmotic pressure

Ephedrine sulfate: 1.0 g × 0.23 = 0.23 g

The ephedrine sulfate has contributed a weight of material osmotically equivalent to 0.23 g of sodium chloride. Since a total of 0.9 g of sodium chloride is required for isotonicity, 0.67 g (0.90 − 0.23) of NaCl must be added.

If one desired to use dextrose instead of sodium chloride to adjust the tonicity, the quantity would be estimated by setting up the following proportion. Since the sodium chloride equivalent of dextrose is 0.16,

$$\frac{1 \text{ g dextrose}}{0.16 \text{ g NaCl}} = \frac{X}{0.67 \text{ g NaCl}}$$

$$X = 4.2 \text{ g of dextrose}$$

Other agents than dextrose may of course be used to replace NaCl. It is recognized that thimerosal becomes less stable in eye drops when a halogen salt is used as an "isotonic agent" (i.e., an agent like NaCl ordinarily used to adjust the tonicity of a drug solution). Reader[40] found that mannitol, propylene glycol, or glycerin—isotonic agents that did not have a detrimental effect on the stability of thimerosal—could serve as alternatives to sodium chloride. The concentration of these agents for isotonicity is readily calculated by use of the equation (see *Example 8–14*):

$$X = \frac{Y \text{ (additional amount of NaCl for isotonicity)}}{E \text{ (grams of NaCl equivalent to 1 g of the isotonic agent)}} \quad (8\text{–}46)$$

where X is the grams of isotonic agent required to adjust the tonicity; Y is the additional amount of NaCl for isotonicity, over and above the osmotic equivalence of NaCl provided by the drugs in the solution; and E is the sodium chloride equivalence of the isotonic agent.

Example 8–15. Let us prepare 200 mL of an isotonic aqueous solution of thimerosal, molecular weight 404.84 g/mole. The concentration of this antiinfective drug is 1:5000, or 0.2 g/1000 mL. The L_{iso} for such a compound, a salt of a weak acid and a strong base (a 1:1 electrolyte), is 3.4 and the sodium chloride equivalent E is

$$E = 17 \frac{L_{iso}}{MW} = 17 \frac{3.4}{404.84} = 0.143$$

The quantity of thimerosal, 0.04 gram for the 200-mL solution, multiplied by its E value, gives the weight of NaCl to which the drug is osmotically equivalent:

$$0.04 \text{ g thimerosal} \times 0.143 = 0.0057 \text{ g NaCl}$$

Since the total amount of NaCl needed for isotonicity is 0.9 g/100 mL, or 1.8 g for the 200-mL solution, and since an equivalent of 0.0057 g of NaCl has been provided by the thimerosal, the additional amount of NaCl needed for isotonicity, Y, is

$$Y = 1.80 \text{ g NaCl needed} - 0.0057 \text{ g NaCl supplied by the drug}$$
$$= 1.794 \text{ g}$$

This is the additional amount of NaCl needed for isotonicity. The result, ~1.8 g NaCl, shows that the concentration of thimerosal is so small that it contributes almost nothing to the isotonicity of the solution. Thus, a concentration of 0.9% NaCl or 1.8 g/200 mL is required.

However, from the work of Reader[40] we know that sodium chloride interacts with mercury compounds such as thimerosal to reduce the stability and effectiveness of this preparation. Therefore, we have decided to replace NaCl with propylene glycol as the isotonic agent.

From equation (8–45) we calculate the E value of propylene glycol, a nonelectrolyte with an L_{iso} value of 1.9 and a molecular weight of 76.09 g/mole.

$$E = 17 \frac{1.9}{76.09} = 0.42$$

Using equation (8–46), $X = Y/E$,

$$X = 1.794/0.42 = 4.3 \text{ g}$$

in which $X = 4.3$ g is the amount of propylene glycol required to adjust the 200-mL solution of thimerosal to isotonicity.

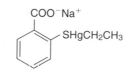

Thimerosal (merthiolate, sodium)

Class II Methods

White–Vincent Method. The Class II methods of computing tonicity involve the addition of water to the drugs to make an isotonic solution, followed by the addition of an isotonic or isotonic-buffered diluting vehicle to bring the solution to the final volume. Stimulated by the need to adjust the pH in addition to the tonicity of ophthalmic solutions, White and Vincent[41] developed a simplified method for such calculations. The derivation of the equation is best shown as follows.

Suppose that one wishes to make 30 mL of a 1% solution of procaine hydrochloride isotonic with body fluid. First, the weight of the drug w is multiplied by the sodium chloride equivalent E.

$$0.3 \text{ g} \times 0.21 = 0.063 \text{ g} \quad (8\text{–}47)$$

This is the quantity of sodium chloride osmotically equivalent to 0.3 g of procaine hydrochloride.

Second, it is known that 0.9 g of sodium chloride, when dissolved in enough water to make 100 mL, yields a solution that is isotonic. The volume V of isotonic solution that can be prepared from 0.063 g of sodium chloride (equivalent to 0.3 g of procaine hydrochloride) is obtained by solving the proportion

$$\frac{0.9 \text{ g}}{100 \text{ mL}} = \frac{0.063 \text{ g}}{V} \quad (8\text{–}48)$$

$$V = 0.063 \times \frac{100}{0.9} \quad (8\text{–}49)$$

$$V = 7.0 \text{ mL} \quad (8\text{–}50)$$

In equation (8–49), the quantity 0.063 is equal to the weight of drug w multiplied by the sodium chloride equivalent E as seen in equation (8–47). The value of the ratio 100/0.9 is 111.1. Accordingly, equation (8–49) may be written

$$V = w \times E \times 111.1 \quad (8\text{–}51)$$

in which V is the volume in milliliters of isotonic solution that may be prepared by mixing the drug with water, w the weight in grams of the drug given in the problem, and E the sodium chloride equivalent obtained from Table 8–4. The constant, 111.1, represents the volume in milliliters of isotonic solution obtained by dissolving 1 g of sodium chloride in water.

The problem may be solved in one step using equation (8–51):

$$V = 0.3 \times 0.21 \times 111.1$$
$$V = 7.0 \text{ mL}$$

TABLE 8–5.   *Isotonic and Isotonic-Buffered Diluting Solutions**

Isotonic Diluting Solutions
Isotonic sodium chloride solution	USP
Dextrose solution	5.6%
Sodium nitrate solution.	1.3%
Ringer's solution.	USP

Isotonic-Buffered Diluting Solutions

Diluting Solution I, pH 4.7

Used for salts such as those of epinephrine, cocaine, dionin, metycaine, nupercaine, optochin, phenacaine, pontocaine, procaine, physostigmine, syntropan, and zinc. For dispensing salts of physostigmine and epinephrine, 2g of sodium bisulfite may be added to the solution to minimize discoloration.
Boric acid, c.p. (H_3BO_3)	20.0 g
Suitable preservative, q.s.	
Sterile distilled water, q.s. ad	1000 mL

Diluting Solution II, pH 6.8

Primarily used for salts of pilocarpine, which are stable for about a month in this buffer.
Sodium acid phosphate ($NaH_2PO_4 \cdot H_2O$) monohydrate	4.60 g
Disodium phosphate (Na_2HPO_4) anhydrous.	4.73 g
Sodium chloride, c.p.	4.80 g
Suitable preservative, q.s.	
Sterile distilled water, q.s. ad	1000 mL

Diluting Solution III, pH 7.4

May be used as a neutral collyrium or as a solvent for drugs that are stable in a neutral solution.
Potassium acid phosphate (KH_2PO_4) anhydrous	1.90 g
Disodium phosphate (Na_2HPO_4) anhydrous.	8.10 g
Sodium chloride, c.p.	4.11 g
Suitable preservative, q.s.	
Sterile distilled water q.s. ad	1000 mL

Diluting Solution IV, pH 9

Used where an alkaline buffer is desired for ophthalmic drugs.
Boric acid	0.43 g
Sodium borate	4.20 g
Suitable preservative, q.s.	
Sterile distilled water, q.s. ad	1000 mL

*From H. W. Hind and F. M. Goyan, J. Am. Pharm. Assoc., Sci. Ed. **36**, 33, 413, 1947; H. W. Hind and I. J. Szekely, J. Am. Pharm. Assoc., Pract. Ed. **14**, 644, 1953; H. B. Kostenbauder, F. B. Gable and A. Martin, J. Am. Pharm. Assoc., Sci. Ed. **42**, 210, 1953.

In order to complete the isotonic solution, enough isotonic sodium chloride solution, another isotonic solution, or an isotonic-buffered diluting solution is added to make 30 mL of the finished product. Several isotonic and isotonic-buffered diluting solutions are found in Table 8–5. These solutions all have isotonicity values of 0.9% NaCl.

When more than one ingredient is contained in an isotonic preparation, the volumes of isotonic solution, obtained by mixing each drug with water, are additive.

Example 8–16. Make the following solution isotonic with respect to an ideal membrane.

Phenacaine hydrochloride . . . . .0.06 g
Boric acid . . . . .0.30 g
Sterilized distilled water, enough to make . . . . .100.0 mL

$$V = [(0.06 \times 0.20) + (0.3 \times 0.50)] \times 111.1$$

$$V = 18 \text{ mL}$$

The drugs are mixed with water to make 18 mL of an isotonic solution, and the preparation is brought to a volume of 100 mL by adding an isotonic diluting solution.

Sprowls Method. A further simplification of the method of White and Vincent was introduced by Sprowls.[42] He recognized that equation (8–51) could be used to construct a table of values of V when the weight

of the drug w was arbitrarily fixed. Sprowls chose as the weight of drug 0.3 g, the quantity for 1 fluid ounce of a 1% solution. The volume V of isotonic solution that can be prepared by mixing 0.3 g of a drug with sufficient water may be computed for drugs commonly used in ophthalmic and parenteral solutions. The method as described by Sprowls[42] is further discussed in several reports by Martin and Sprowls[43] It is now found in the U.S. Pharmacopeia, XXI, p. 1339. A modification of the original table has been made by Hammarlund and Pedersen-Bjergaard[44] and is given in column 4 of Table 8–4, where the volume in milliliters of isotonic solution for 0.3 g of the drug, the quantity for 1 fluid ounce of a 1% solution, is listed. (The volume of isotonic solution in milliliters for 1 g of the drug can also be listed in tabular form if desired by multiplying the values in column 4 by 3.3). The primary quantity of isotonic solution is finally brought to the specified volume with the desired isotonic or isotonic-buffered diluting solutions.

References and Notes

1. A. Roos and W. F. Borm, *Resp. Physiol.* **40**, 1–32, 1980; M. Koppel and K. Spiro, Biochem. Z. **65**, 409–439, 1914.
2. D. D. Van Slyke, J. Biol Chem. **52**, 525, 1922.
3. R. G. Bates, *Electrometric pH Determinations*, Wiley, New York, 1954, pp. 97–104; pp. 116, 338.

4. I. M. Kolthoff and F. Tekelenburg, Rec. Trav. Chim. **46**, 33, 1925.
5. I. M. Kolthoff and C. Rosenblum, *Acid Base Indicators*, Macmillan, New York, 1937.
6. A. P. Wyss, J. Am. Pharm. Assoc., Pract. Ed. **6**, 6, 1945.
7. V. E. Bower and R. G. Bates, J. Research Nat. Bur. Standards **55**, 197, 1955.
8. F. M. Goyan and H. C. Coutsouris, J. Am. Pharm. Assoc., Pract. Ed. **10**, 146, 1949.
9. H. T. S. Britton and R. A. Robinson, J. Chem. Soc., **1931**, 458.
10. J. P. Peters and D. D. Van Slyke, *Quantitative Clinical Chemistry*, Vol. 1, Williams & Wilkins, Baltimore, 1931, Chapter 18.
11. P. Salenius, Scand. J. Clin. Lab. Invest. **9**, 160, 1957.
12. G. Ellison et al., Clin. Chem. **4**, 453, 1958.
13. G. N. Hosford and A. M. Hicks, Arch. Ophthalmol. **13**, 14, 1935; **17**, 797, 1937.
14. R. G. Bates, *Electrometric pH Determinations*, Wiley, New York, 1954, pp. 97–108.
15. S. R. Gifford, Arch. Ophthalmol. **13**, 78, 1935.
16. S. L. P. Sörensen, Biochem. Z. **21**, 131, 1909; **22**, 352, 1909.
17. S. Palitzsch, Biochem. Z. **70**, 333, 1915.
18. H. W. Hind and F. M. Goyan, J. Am. Pharm. Assoc., Sci. Ed. **36**, 413, 1947.
19. W. M. Clark and H. A. Lubs, J. Bacteriol. **2**, 1, 109, 191, 1917.
20. J. S. Friedenwald, W. F. Hughes and H. Herrman, Arch. Ophthalmol. **31**, 279, 1944.
21. F. N. Martin and J. L. Mims, Arch. Ophthalmol. **44**, 561, 1950; J. L. Mims, ibid. **46**, 644, 1951.
22. S. Riegelman and D. G. Vaughn, J. Am. Pharm. Assoc., Pract. Ed. **19**, 474, 1958.
23. W. D. Mason, J. Pharm. Sci. **73**, 1258, 1984.
24. S. Hirai, T. Ikenaga and T. Matsuzawa, Diabetes, **27**, 296, 1977; T. Ohwaki et al., J. Pharm. Sci. **74**, 550, 1985; C. H. Huang, R. Kimura, R. B. Nassar and A. Hussain, J. Pharm. Sci. **74**, 608, 1985.
25. K. C. Swan and N. G. White, Am. J. Ophthalmol. **25**, 1043, 1942.
26. D. G. Cogan and V. E. Kinsey, Arch. Ophthalmol. **27**, 466, 661, 696, 1942.
27. H. W. Hind and F. M. Goyan, J. Am. Pharm. Assoc., Sci. Ed. **36**, 33, 1947.
28. Y. Takeuchi, Y. Yamaoka, Y. Morimoto, I. Kaneko, Y. Fukumori and T. Fukuda, J. Pharm. Sci. **78**, 3, 1989.
29. T. S. Grosicki and W. J. Husa, J. Am. Pharm. Assoc., Sci. Ed. **43**, 632, 1954; W. J. Husa and J. R. Adams, ibid. **33**, 329, 1944, W. D. Easterly and W. J. Husa, ibid. **43**, 750, 1954; W. J. Husa and O. A. Rossi, ibid. **31**, 270, 1942.
30. F. M. Goyan and D. Reck, J. Am. Pharm. Assoc., Sci. Ed. **44**, 43, 1955.
31. F. R. Hunter, J. Clin. Invest. **19**, 691, 1940.
32. C. W. Hartman and W. J. Husa, J. Am. Pharm. Assoc., Sci. Ed. **46**, 430, 1957.
33. A. V. Hill, Proc. R. Soc., London, A **127**, 9, 1930; E. J. Baldes, J. Sci. Instruments **11**, 223, 1934; A. Weissberger, *Physical Methods of Organic Chemistry*, Vol. 1, Part 1, Interscience, New York, 2nd Edition, 1949, p. 546.
34. A. Lumiere and J. Chevrotier, Bull. Sci. Pharmacol. **20**, 711, 1913.
35. C. G. Lund, P. Nielsen and K. Pedersen-Bjergaard, *The Preparation of Solutions Isosmotic with Blood, Tears, and Tissue*, Danish Pharmacopeia Commission, Vol. 2, Einar Munksgaard, Copenhagen, 1947.
36. A. Krogh, C. G. Lund and K. Pedersen-Bjergaard, Acta Physiol. Scand. **10**, 88, 1945.
37. F. M. Goyan, J. M. Enright and J. M. Wells, J. Am. Pharm. Assoc., Sci. Ed. **33**, 74, 1944.
38. M. Mellen and L. A. Seltzer, J. Am. Pharm. Assoc., Sci. Ed. **25**, 759, 1936.
39. F. M. Goyan, J. M. Enright and J. M. Wells, J. Am. Pharm. Assoc., Sci. Ed. **33**, 78, 1944.
40. M. J. Reader, J. Pharm. Sci. **73**, 840, 1984.
41. A. I. White and H. C. Vincent, J. Am. Pharm. Assoc., Pract. Ed. **8**, 406, 1947.
42. J. B. Sprowls, J. Am. Pharm. Assoc., Pract. Ed. **10**, 348, 1949.
43. A. Martin and J. B. Sprowls, Am. Profess. Pharmacist **17**, 540, 1951; Pennsylvania Pharmacist **32**, 8, 1951.
44. E. R. Hammarlund and K. Pedersen-Bjergaard, J. Am. Pharm. Assoc., Pract. Ed. **19**, 38, 1958.
45. E. J. Cohen, F. F. Heyroth, and M. F. Menkin, J. Am. Chem. Soc. **49**, 173, 1927; **50**, 696, 1928.
46. D. D. Van Slyke, A. B. Hastings, C. D. Murray, and J. Sendroy, J. Biol. Chem. **65**, 701, 1925.

Problems

8–1. One desires to adjust a solution to pH 8.8 by the use of a boric acid–sodium borate buffer. What approximate ratio of acid and salt is required?

Answer: The acid:salt ratio is 1:0.36

8–2. What is the pH of a solution containing 0.1 mole of ephedrine and 0.01 mole of ephedrine hydrochloride per liter of solution?

Answer: pH = 10.36

8–3. (a) What is the pH of a buffer consisting of 0.12 M NaH_2PO_4 and 0.08 M Na_2HPO_4, the former acting as the acid and the latter as the salt or conjugate base (see Cohen et al.[45])? (b) What is the value when the ionic strength corrections are made using the Debye–Hückel law? *Hint:* Use equation (8–15). The value for n in the terms pK_n and $(2n - 1)$ is 2 in this problem since the second stage of ionization of phosphoric acid is involved. Thus the equation becomes

$$pH = 7.21 + \log \frac{[Na_2HPO_4]}{[NaH_2PO_4]} - \frac{0.51 \times 3\sqrt{\mu}}{1 + \sqrt{\mu}}$$

Answers: (a) pH = 7.03; (b) pH = 6.46

8–4. What is the pH of an elixir containing 0.002 mole/liter of the free acid sulfisoxazole, and 0.20 mole/liter of the 1:1 salt sulfisoxazole diethanolamine? The pK_a of the acid is 5.30. The activity coefficient γ_{sulf} can be obtained from the appropriate Debye–Hückel equation for this ionic strength. The effect of any alcohol in the elixir on the value of the dissociation constant may be neglected.

Answer: pH = 7.14

8–5. Ascorbic acid (molecular weight 176.12) is too acidic to administer by the parenteral route. The acidity of ascorbic acid is partially neutralized by adding a basic compound, usually sodium carbonate or sodium bicarbonate. Thus, the injectable product contains sodium ascorbate, ascorbic acid, and the neutralizing agent. The molecular weight of ascorbic acid, together with its pK_a, is found in Table 7–2.

(a) What is the pH of an injectable solution containing only ascorbic acid in the concentration of 55 g per liter of solution? $K_1 = 5 \times 10^{-5}$ and $K_2 = 1.6 \times 10^{-12}$.

(b) What is the molar ratio of sodium ascorbate to ascorbic acid, and the percentage of each compound required to prepare an injectable solution with a pH of 5.7?

Answers: (a) pH = 2.40; (b) a 25.1:1 ratio of sodium ascorbate to ascorbic acid, or 96.2 mole percent sodium ascorbate and 3.8 percent of ascorbic acid

8–6. Physostigmine salicylate is used in ophthalmic solutions as a mydriatic and to decrease the intraocular pressure in glaucoma.

(a) What is the pH of a 0.5 percent aqueous solution of physostigmine salicylate, molecular weight 413.5? This compound is the salt of a weak acid, and the pH of the solution may be obtained using equation (7–127) as long as the concentration of the salt, C_s, is much greater than $[H_3O^+]$. The *acidity* constant for the physostigmine cation, K_1, is $10^{-14}/(7.6 \times 10^{-7})$, and the acidity constant for salicylic acid, K_2, is 1.06×10^{-3}. The calculation of the pH of a salt of a weak base and a weak acid is demonstrated in *Example 7–22*. We can disregard the second step in the ionization of physostigmine.

(b) How much is the pH increased by addition to the solution of 0.1% physostigmine base, molecular weight 275.34? See the Henderson–Hasselbalch equation (8–10) for the pH of a solution of a weak base and its corresponding salt.

Answers: (a) pH = 5.43; (b) an increase of 1.93 pH units

8–7. The thermodynamic dissociation exponent pK_1 for carbonic acid at 30° C is 6.33. According to Van Slyke et al.[46] the ionic strength of the blood is roughly 0.16. Compute the apparent dissociation exponent pK'_1 to be used for the carbonic acid of blood at 30° C. Notice that the pH or $-\log a_{H^+}$ is given by the expression

$$pH = pK_1' + \log \frac{[HCO_3^-]}{[H_2CO_3]}$$

$$= pK_1 + \log \frac{[HCO_3^-]}{[H_2CO_3]} + \log \gamma_{HCO_3^-}$$

Therefore,

$$pK_1' = pK_1 + \log \gamma_{(HCO_3^-)} \cong pK_1 - 0.5\sqrt{\gamma}$$

Answer: $pK_1' = 6.13$

8–8. Plot the buffer capacity–pH curve for a barbituric acid–sodium barbiturate buffer of total concentration 0.2 M over the range of pH 1 to 7. What is the maximum buffer capacity and at what pH does β_{max} occur?

Answer: $\beta_{max} = 0.115$ and it occurs at pH 3.98

8–9. What is the buffer capacity of a solution containing 0.20 M acetic acid and 0.10 M sodium acetate?

Answer: $\beta = 0.15$

8–10. Your product research director asks you to prepare a buffer solution of pH 6.5 having a buffer capacity of 0.10. Choose a suitable combination of buffer species and compute the concentrations needed.

One possible answer: Na_2HPO_4 (salt) = 0.052 M
NaH_2PO_4 (acid) = 0.265 M

8–11. To a buffer containing 0.1 mole/liter each of sodium formate and formic acid, 0.01 gram equivalent/liter of sodium hydroxide was added. What is the average buffer capacity of the solution over this pH range?

Answer: $\beta = 0.111$ (if pH is not rounded to 3.84 one may get $\beta = 0.115$ instead of 0.111)

8–12. What is the buffer capacity of a solution containing 0.36 M boric acid at a pH of 7.0? What is the buffer capacity at pH 9.24, i.e., where pH = pK_a? At what pH is β a maximum and what is the value of β_{max}? What is the buffer capacity at pH 10.8? Using the calculated values of β, plot the buffer capacity versus pH. If the student wishes to smooth the buffer curve a little better, he or she may also calculate β at pH 8.20 and at 10.0. When these six points are plotted on the graph and a smooth line is drawn through them, a bell-shaped buffer curve is obtained. See Figure 8–4 for the shapes of several buffer curves.

Partial Answer: β at pH 7.0 = 0.0048; β at pH 8.2 = 0.064; β at pH 9.24 = 0.21; β at pH 10.8 = 0.021, β_{max} is found at pH 9.24 where pH = pK_a; $\beta_{max} = 0.576C = 0.21$.

8–13. What is the buffer capacity for a Sörensen phosphate buffer (a) at pH 5.0 and (b) at pH 7.2? The total buffer concentration is 0.067 M, and the dissociation constant is $K_2 = 6.2 \times 10^{-8}$.

Answers: (a) $\beta = 0.001$; (b) $\beta = 0.04$

8–14. A borate buffer contains 2.5 g of sodium chloride (molecular weight 58.5 g/mole); 2.8 g of sodium borate, decahydrate (molecular weight 381.43); 10.5 g of boric acid (molecular weight 61.84); and sufficient water to make 1000 mL of solution. Compute the pH of the solution (a) disregarding the ionic strength, and (b) taking into account the ionic strength.

Answers: (a) pH disregarding ionic strength is 7.87; (b) including ionic strength, pH = 7.79

8–15. Calculate the buffer capacity of an aqueous solution of the strong base sodium hydroxide having a hydroxyl ion concentration of 3.0×10^{-3} molar.

Answer: $\beta = 0.0069$

8–16. (a) What is the final pH of a solution after mixing 10 mL of a 0.10-M HCl solution with 20 mL of a 0.10-M procaine solution? The pK_b for procaine is found in Table 7–2. (b) Does the solution exhibit buffer capacity?

Answers: (a) pH = 8.8; (b) $\beta_{max} = 0.039$; it shows a weak buffer capacity.

8–17. Assuming that the total bicarbonate buffer concentration in normal blood is about 0.026 mole/liter, what would be the maximum buffer capacity of this buffer and at what pH would β_{max} occur?

Answer: $\beta_{max} = 0.015$ at pH 6.1 (see pp. 177, 178)

8–18. Describe in detail how you would formulate a buffer having approximately the same pH, ionic strength, and buffer capacity as that of blood. The ionic strength of the blood plasma is about 0.16 and the buffer capacity in the physiologic pH range is approximately 0.03 (p. 177). Use the Na_2HPO_4/NaH_2PO_4 buffer and pK_2 of phosphoric acid. Activity coefficients must be considered, and the thermodynamic pK_2 of phosphoric acid must be used to obtain the answer.

Answer: A mixture of 0.044 Na_2HPO_4 and 0.0105 NaH_2PO_4 has a buffer capacity of 0.03 and provides a pH of 7.4. The ionic strength of this mixture is 0.14. The ionic strength may be raised to 0.16 by the addition of 0.02 M NaCl or KCl.

8–19. A titration is conducted beginning with 50 mL of 0.2 N acetic acid and adding (a) 10 mL; (b) 25 mL; (c) 50 mL; and (d) 50.1 mL of 0.2 N NaOH. What is the pH after each increment of base has been added?

Answers: (a) 4.16; (b) 4.76; (c) 8.88; (d) 10.3

8–20. Plot the pH titration curve for the neutralization of 0.1 N barbituric acid by 0.1 N NaOH. What is the pH of the solution at the equivalence point?

Answer: pH = 8.34

8–21. A 1 fluid ounce (29.573 mL) solution contains 4.5 grains (291.60 mg) of silver nitrate. How much sodium nitrate must be added to this solution to make it isotonic with nasal fluid? Assume that nasal fluid has an isotonicity value of 0.9% NaCl.

Answer: 3.83 grains = 248 mg

8–22. Compute the Sprowls V value, the E value, and the freezing point depression of a 1% solution of diphenhydramine hydrochloride.

Answer: $V \div 6.7$ mL, $E \div 0.20$, $\Delta T_f = 0.12$

8–23. A 25% solution of phenylpropanolamine hydrochloride is prepared. The physician desires that 0.25 fluid ounce (7.393 mL) of this solution be made isotonic and adjusted to a pH of 6.8. The Sprowls V value is 12.7. Discuss the difficulties that are encountered in filling the physician's request. How might these difficulties be overcome?

8–24. (a) Compute the isotonic concentration (molarity) from the L_{iso} values given in Table 8–4 for the following substances: sodium borate·$10H_2O$ (sodium tetraborate), phenylephrine hydrochloride, physostigmine sulfate, and calcium gluconate.

(b) What is the volume of water that should be added to 0.3 gram of these substances to produce an isotonic solution?

Partial Answer: (a) 0.0553, 0.149, 0.104, 0.124 mole/liter; (b) check your results against Table 8–4—they may differ from the table values.

8–25. Compute the freezing point depression of 1% solutions of the following drugs: (a) ascorbic acid, (b) calcium chloride, (c) ephedrine sulfate, and (d) methacholine chloride. The percentages of sodium chloride required to make 100 mL of 1% solutions of these drugs isotonic are 0.81%, 0.48%, 0.76%, and 0.67%, respectively. *Hint:* Refer to *Example 8–11.*

Answers: Check your results against Table 8–4.

8–26. (a) Compute the approximate sodium chloride equivalent of MgO (molecular weight = 40.3 g/mole), $ZnCl_2$ (molecular weight = 136.3 g/mole), $Al(OH)_3$ (molecular weight = 77.98 g/mole), and isoniazid (a tuberculostatic drug, weak electrolyte, molecular weight = 137.2 g/mole), using the average L_{iso} values given in Table 8–3. (b) From the E value you calculated in (a), compute the freezing point depression of a 1% solution of these drugs. (c) Can one actually obtain a 1% aqueous solution of MgO or $Al(OH)_3$?

Answers: (a) $E = 0.84, 0.60, 1.31,$ and 0.25; (b) $\Delta T_f^{1\%} = 0.49°$ C, $0.35°$ C, $0.76°$ C, and $0.15°$ C

8–27. Using the sodium chloride equivalent method, make the following solutions isotonic with respect to the mucous lining of the eye (ocular membrane).

(a) Tetracaine hydrochloride   10 grams
    NaCl   x grams
    Sterilize distilled water, enough to make 1000 mL
(b) Tetracaine hydrochloride   0.10 gram
    Boric acid   x grams
    Sterile distilled water, enough to make 10 mL

Answers: **(a)** add 7.2 grams of NaCl; **(b)** add 0.14 gram of boric acid.

8–28. Make the following solution isotonic with respect to blood:

Chlorpromazine hydrochloride	2.5 grams
Ascorbic acid	0.2 gram
Sodium bisulfite	0.1 gram
Sodium sulfate, anhydrous	0.1 gram
Sterile distilled water, enough to make	100 mL

Hint: First, compute the E values of chlorpromazine HCl and sodium sulfate, not given in Table 8–4, from the approximate L_{iso} values given in Table 8–3. The molecular weight of chlorpromazine hydrochloride is 318.9 daltons* and the molecular weight of sodium sulfate is 142.06 daltons.

Answer: Dissolve the drugs in 66.44 mL of water. This solution is isotonic. Add 0.3 gram of NaCl and bring to a volume of 100 mL.

8–29. A new drug having a molecular weight of 300 g/mole produced a freezing point depression of 0.52° C in a 0.145-M solution. What are the calculated L_{iso} value, the E value, and the V value for this drug?

Answer: $L_{iso} = 3.6$, $E = 0.20$, $V = 6.7$ mL

8–30. Using the sodium chloride method, calculate the grams of sodium chloride needed to make 30 mL of a 2% isotonic physostigmine salicylate solution.

Answer: 0.174 gram

8–31. Compute the percent nonionized aminophylline ($pK_b = 5.0$ and molecular weight 421.2 daltons) and its molar concentration after intravenous injection of 10 mL of an aqueous 2.5 w/v solution of aminophylline at 25° C. The normal pH of blood is about 7.4 and the total blood volume is approximately 5 liters. Use the Henderson–Hasselbalch equation in the form

$$pH = pK_w - pK_b - \log \frac{[BH^+]}{[B]}$$

where $\dfrac{[BH^+]}{[B]}$ is the ratio of ionized to nonionized drug.

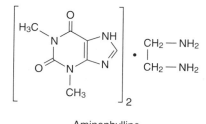

Aminophylline

Answer: Percent of nonionized aminophylline = 2.5%, corresponding to 3.0×10^{-6} mole/liter.

---

*The word *dalton* is used in connection with molecular weight: 1 dalton = 1 g/mole.

9
Electromotive Force and Oxidation—Reduction

Electrochemical Cells

Electrometric Determination of pH, Specific Ions, and Redox Potentials

In Chapter 6, an electrolytic cell was described in which chemical reactions were produced by passing an electric current through an electrolyte solution. In this chapter, we consider the reverse process, in which an electric current is produced by allowing a chemical reaction to occur. Such an electrochemical reaction depends on the relative abilities of species in solution to be oxidized or reduced, and this in turn will be related to processes occurring at the electrodes, which connect the species in solution to any external circuit. The electrochemical reactions may be used to determine pH, activity coefficients, or the quantity of a specific ion in solution. These determinations involve *potentiometry*, in which there is no significant current flow through the system. The application of this technique to pharmacy will be discussed.

ELECTROCHEMICAL CELLS

Electromotive Force of a Cell. An electrochemical cell normally consists of two *electrodes* immersed in an electrolyte solution, or solutions, that are in contact with each other. The Daniell cell, shown in Figure 9–1, is a typical electrochemical cell. It consists of a zinc electrode in a solution of zinc sulfate in one compartment and a copper electrode in a solution of copper sulfate in the other compartment. The compartments are known as the *half-cells* of the electrochemical cell and are separated by a porous diaphragm that allows electric contact between the solutions but does not permit excessive mixing of the two solutions.

Zinc has a greater tendency to ionize, that is, to lose electrons, than does copper. Therefore, a spontaneous reaction can occur when the two half-cells are connected by an external wire; atoms of the zinc electrode go into solution as Zn^{2+} ions and leave electrons behind on the

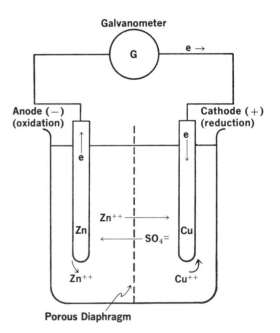

Fig. 9–1. Daniell cell showing oxidation at the anode, reduction at the cathode, and the flow of electrons (e^-) in the external circuit. The Zn^{2+} and SO_4^{2-} ions diffuse through the porous diaphragm in opposite directions to maintain electroneutrality in each half-cell as the reaction proceeds.

electrode. The electrons pass from this negatively charged electrode or *anode* through the external wire to the copper electrode. Here, at the *cathode*, copper ions from the solution take on electrons and deposit copper atoms on the electrode surface. The cathode thus loses electrons to the solution, so that it is considered to be positively charged. This spontaneous reaction corresponds to the oxidation of zinc metal at the zinc electrode while copper ions are being reduced at the copper electrode, which can be expressed in the following *half-reactions:*

Anode reaction (oxidation)

$$Zn = Zn^{2+} + 2e^- \qquad E_{left} \qquad (9-1)$$

Cathode reaction (reduction)

$$Cu^{2+} + 2e^- = Cu \qquad E_{right} \qquad (9-2)$$

Each half-reaction represents the change occurring at a single electrode, and the two half-reactions can be added together to express the overall cell reaction:

$$Zn + Cu^{2+} = Zn^{2+} + Cu$$

$$E_{cell} = E_{left} + E_{right} \qquad (9-3)$$

The individual *electrode potentials* (E_{left} and E_{right}) occur at the junction between each electrode and its surrounding solution. The sum of the two electrode potentials corresponds to E_{cell}, which is the *electromotive force* (emf) or *voltage* of the cell. Note that the term *emf* refers to the voltage of the complete cell, whereas *potential* refers to voltage from an electrode. In accordance with convention, the electrodes of the cell are always written so that *electrons are given up to the external circuit at the left electrode (anode) and accepted from the external circuit at the right electrode (cathode).* A schematic depiction of the Daniell cell therefore is written as

$$Zn|Zn^{2+}(c_{Zn^{2+}}) \parallel Cu^{2+}(c_{Cu^{2+}})|Cu$$

in which a single vertical line represents the junction between two different phases, and the double vertical line indicates a liquid junction, that is, an electric contact between two electrolyte solutions. The concentrations of the different ions in the half-cells (c_{ion}) are also given in the diagram.

The Daniell cell is *reversible;* that is, by applying an external current opposite to and infinitesimally greater than that of the cell, zinc will deposit at the zinc electrode, and copper will go into solution at the copper electrode. An irreversible cell, such as one in which an escape of hydrogen accompanies the chemical reaction, cannot be reversed completely by an infinitesimally greater applied potential. Irreversible cells are not ordinarily used in electrochemical studies, since their operation is not susceptible to thermodynamic treatment. An electrochemical cell, such as the Daniell cell, in which a spontaneous reaction occurs at the electrode surfaces and that can be used to provide electric energy from the chemical reaction occurring within it, is known as a *galvanic cell.*

Types of Electrodes. A number of electrodes of differing types can be constructed, and by combining any two of the electrodes, a variety of cells is obtained. Only a few of the possible types of electrodes that can be made are described here.

Metal–Metal Ion Electrodes. The Daniell cell consists of electrodes of this type. Each electrode is made simply by immersing a metal strip into a solution containing ions of the metal. For example, a nickel electrode can be represented by

$$Ni|Ni^{2+} (c, \text{moles/liter})$$

Amalgam Electrodes. A variation of the metal-metal ion electrode replaces the metal strip by a metal amalgam, and this is immersed in a solution containing the metal ion. An advantage of this type of electrode is that active metals such as sodium or potassium that otherwise would react with aqueous solutions can be used as electrodes. A sodium–amalgam electrode is represented by

$$Na (\text{in Hg at } c_1, \text{moles/liter})|Na^+ (c_2, \text{moles/liter})$$

Metal–Insoluble Salt Electrodes. The calomel (mercurous chloride) electrode and the silver–silver chloride electrode are the most frequently used reference electrodes. Reference electrodes produce an invariant potential that is not affected by changes in solution concentration. They are used with another electrode, usually called the *indicator electrode*, under an infinitesimally small amount of current flow, as described for reversible cells. The measurement of cell potential with a reference electrode will be discussed in a subsequent section.

The calomel electrode (Fig. 9–2) consists of mercury, a paste of mercurous chloride, and a solution of KCl, which provides chloride ions. The electrode is represented by

$$Hg|Hg_2Cl_2|Cl^- (c, \text{moles/liter})$$

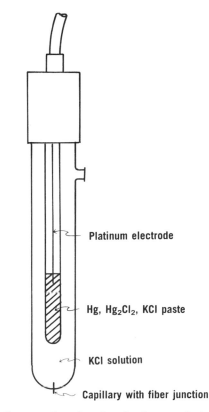

Platinum electrode

Hg, Hg₂Cl₂, KCl paste

KCl solution

Capillary with fiber junction

Fig. 9–2. Cross-section of a calomel reference electrode.

The electrode reaction is

$$Hg = Hg^+ + e^-$$
$$Hg^+ + Cl^- = \tfrac{1}{2}Hg_2Cl_2$$
$$\text{(overall)} \quad Hg + Cl^- = \tfrac{1}{2}Hg_2Cl_2 + e^- \qquad (9\text{--}4)$$

A silver chloride electrode consists of a layer of silver chloride on a silver wire that is immersed in a solution containing chloride ions. This electrode is represented by

$$Ag|AgCl|Cl^- \ (c, \text{ moles/liter})$$

and the electrode process is

$$Ag = Ag^+ + e^-$$
$$Ag^+ + Cl^- = AgCl$$
$$\text{(overall)} \quad Ag + Cl^- = AgCl + e^- \qquad (9\text{--}5)$$

Oxidation–Reduction Electrodes. Although every electrochemical half-cell fundamentally involves an oxidation-reduction reaction, only half-cells containing an inert electrode immersed in a solution consisting of both the oxidized and reduced forms of a substance are called oxidation–reduction electrodes. An advantage of this type of electrode is its ability to function as either a cathode or an anode in a cell. The direction taken by the electrode reaction depends on the potential of the other electrode in the cell.

Platinum is the metal most frequently used for inert electrodes. Gold and silver have limited usefulness as inert electrodes since both are soft and since silver, in addition, is prone to oxidation. A platinum wire immersed in a solution containing ferrous and ferric ions is typical of an electrode in this category. The electrode may be abbreviated as

$$Pt|Fe^{2+} \ (c_1, \text{ moles/liter}), \ Fe^{3+} \ (c_2, \text{ moles/liter})$$

in which the comma designates that both chemical species are in the same solution. The electrode reaction for this half-cell is

$$Fe^{2+} = Fe^{3+} + e^- \qquad (9\text{--}6)$$

Oxidation–reduction electrodes can also be made using organic substances that exist in two different oxidation states. Quinhydrone, an equimolar mixture of benzoquinone, Q, and hydroquinone, H_2Q, which is only slightly soluble in water, are involved in the reversible oxidation–reduction reaction,

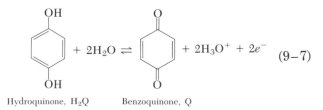

$$\qquad (9\text{--}7)$$

Hydroquinone, H_2Q Benzoquinone, Q

Introducing an inert platinum wire produces an oxidation–reduction electrode. The electrode can be written as

$$Pt|H_2Q, \ Q, \ H_3O^+ \ (c, \text{ moles/liter})$$

The potential of the quinhydrone electrode varies with the H_3O^+ concentration according to the electrode reaction just given. Therefore, hydrogen ion activity (i.e., pH), can be monitored with this electrode.

Gas Electrodes. Bubbling a gas over an inert metal wire immersed in a solution containing ions that can be derived from the gas produces a gas electrode. A platinum electrode, normally coated with colloidal platinum black to increase the effective electric surface area and thereby to facilitate the electrode reaction, can be used. For example, the hydrogen electrode,

$$Pt|H_2 \text{ (known pressure)}|H^+ \ (c, \text{ moles/liter})$$

may have its electrode reaction represented by

$$Pt + H_2 = Pt \cdot H_2$$
$$Pt \cdot H_2 = Pt + \tfrac{1}{2}H^+ + e^-$$
$$\text{(overall)} \qquad H_2 = \tfrac{1}{2}H^+ + e^- \qquad (9\text{--}8)$$

Membrane Electrodes. The use of a thin, ion-sensitive glass membrane enclosing an electrolyte solution has produced electrodes that can detect potentials arising at the glass/solution interface. By carefully controlling the composition of the glass or crystalline membrane, the electrode can become particularly sensitive to certain ions in solution. These ion-selective electrodes are discussed more fully in a subsequent section of this chapter. The pH glass electrode is the most common type of membrane electrode. It consists of a platinum wire dipping into a solution of hydrochloric acid. The wire is in contact with an internal reference electrode, usually either a silver–silver chloride or a calomel electrode, which is sealed within the same high-resistance body, as shown in Figure 9–3. The glass membrane in this electrode is responsive to protons and other monovalent ions but relatively unresponsive to divalent cations. By carefully adjusting the three-dimensional arrangement of cations (including Na^+, Ca^{2+}, Li^+, and Ba^{2+}) located in the silicate structure of the glass membrane, the responsiveness of the electrode to monovalent cations other than hydrogen can be controlled. For example, the usual glass pH electrode produces a "sodium error" caused by the responsiveness of most glass membranes to sodium ions at high pH values. This error can be reduced by employing a glass membrane with a high concentration of lithium ions incorporated in the silicate matrix. The glass membrane pH electrode is represented as

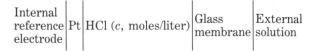

| Internal reference electrode | Pt | HCl (*c*, moles/liter) | Glass membrane | External solution |

In practice, the glass pH electrode must be attached to an external reference electrode to complete the cell. If two glass electrodes are immersed in the same solution and connected to a pH meter, a small potential

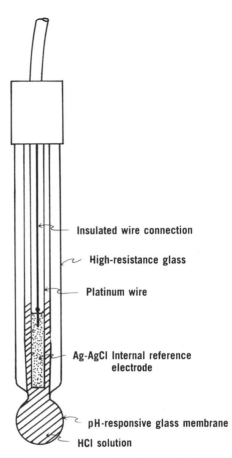

Fig. 9–3. Schematic representation of a typical glass pH electrode.

- Insulated wire connection
- High-resistance glass
- Platinum wire
- Ag-AgCl Internal reference electrode
- pH-responsive glass membrane
- HCl solution

difference can be noticed between the two electrodes. This is due to slight differences in the properties of the individual glass membranes, and for pH measurement, this individual electrode variation requires standardization of each cell containing a glass electrode against a buffer of known pH.

Membrane electrodes may also be fabricated from cellulose, polyethylene, collodion, or liquid ion-exchange resins that are insoluble in water. Salt crystals may also be used in place of glass as ion-selective membrane electrodes.

Microelectrodes. Recent developments in manufacturing have provided electrodes that are small enough to contact a single cell or neural unit in an intact animal. These microelectrodes typically have metal or glass tips, shaped like tapered needles, with electrode diameters on the order of 1 μm or less. The electrodes are composed of the same electrolyte solutions and materials as previously described in this section; however, the entire electrode is usually about the size of a small hypodermic needle or a micropipette, and normally it can be sterilized and implanted in an animal for pharmacologic studies. The use and properties of microelectrodes are described by Ferris.[1]

Measuring the Electromotive Force of Cells. A *voltmeter* draws a measurable amount of current from a circuit; therefore, the voltage determined becomes dependent

on the resistance of the cell to current flow, according to Ohm's law (p. 126), in which $E = IR$. A *potentiometer* measures voltage by opposing the emf of a cell with an applied potential while no current is being drawn through the external circuit. This absence of current flow through the sample cell makes *potentiometry* a useful method for determining the emf of a reversible electrochemical cell. It simply balances one current flow against another without producing changes in potential due to cell resistance. A potentiometer circuit is shown schematically in Figure 9–4. When the key is pressed, an applied current is allowed to flow from the battery (B) through a variable resistor (R) to a galvanometer (G). The variable resistor (R), which is also called a voltage divider, can be adjusted so that the galvanometer, G, shows no current deflection. When this is done, the voltage read on the voltmeter, V, from the applied potential must be equal and exactly opposed to the potential of the cell whose emf is being determined. Thus the potential differences across the points $O–X$ on the resistor (R) must be equal but opposite in sign to the potential of the cell, E_x, when the galvanometer shows no deflection. As long as the galvanometer is balanced quickly by tapping the key (K), current does not flow for an appreciable time while there is a deflection of G, and the emf measured for the cell can be considered a true equilibrium value. This method is sometimes referred to as *null-point potentiometry*.

Thermodynamics of Electrochemical Cells. The work done by an electrochemical cell operating reversibly, $-\Delta G$, equals the electromotive force E multiplied by

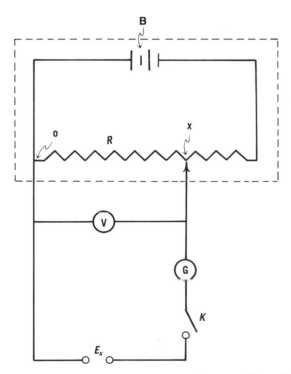

Fig. 9–4. Schematic diagram of a potentiometer. (From R. N. Adams, J. Pharm. Sci. **58** (10), 1172, 1969, reproduced with permission of the copyright owner.)

the number of faradays, nF coulombs, of electricity that pass through the cell

$$-\Delta G = nFE \qquad (9-9)$$

When the electromotive force is positive, the process is spontaneous, which accounts for the negative sign. For the reactants and products under standard conditions, one writes

$$\Delta G° = -nFE° \qquad (9-10)$$

The faraday, F, is approximately 96,500 coulomb/Eq of ions, and n is the number of equivalents of ions reacting or the number of electrons transferred. $E°$ is the cell emf determined by potentiometry under reversible electrochemical conditions at a fixed temperature and pressure.

Example 9–1. What is the free energy change for the cell reaction
$$Cd + Cu^{2+} = Cd^{2+} + Cu$$
in which $E_{cell} = +0.750$ volt?

$\Delta G = -nFE = -$ 2Eq/mole $\times$ 96,500 coulomb/Eq $\times$ 0.750 volt

$\Delta G = -144{,}750$ joule/mole

Equilibrium constants, K, can be obtained from the standard potential using equation (9–10) together with equation (3–115) on page 70.

$$RT \ln K = nFE°$$

or

$$\log K = \frac{nFE°}{2.303RT} \qquad (9-11)$$

Example 9–2. The Daniell cell has a standard potential $E°$ of 1.100 volts. What is the value of K at 25° C for the reaction, $Zn + Cu^{2+} = Zn^{2+} + Cu$, in which the activities of the solid phases, Zn and Cu, are taken as unity?

$$\log K = \frac{2 \times 96{,}500 \text{ coulombs/Eq} \times 1.100 \text{ volt}}{2.303 \times 8.314 JK^{-1} \text{ mole}^{-1} \times 298° K}$$

$$\log K = 37.2$$

$$K = \frac{a_{Zn^{2+}}}{a_{Cu^{2+}}} = 1.6 \times 10^{37}$$

This large value for the equilibrium constant signifies that the chemical reaction in the Daniell cell proceeds essentially to completion.

The Nernst Equation. By convention, any half-cell reaction is written as a reduction, that is, an acceptance of electrons by the reactants to form the products:

$$\underset{\text{(Reactants)}}{\alpha(Ox)} + ne- \rightleftharpoons \underset{\text{(Products)}}{\beta(Rd)} \qquad (9-12)$$

in which α moles of the oxidized species (Ox) in the half-cell is reduced by a reaction involving n electrons to β moles of the reduced species (Rd) in the half-cell. The change is free energy for such a half-cell reduction can be expressed, according to equation (3–116) (p. 70), as

$$\Delta G = \Delta G° + RT \ln \frac{a(Rd)^\beta}{a(Ox)^\alpha} \qquad (9-13)$$

in which $a(Rd)$ signifies some arbitrary activity of the products and $a(Ox)$ some arbitrary activity of the reactants. Following the law of mass action (p. 144), each term is raised to a power equal to the number of moles β of products or α of reactants. Now, $-nFE$ and $-nFE°$ can be substituted into equation (9–13) for ΔG and $\Delta G°$ giving

$$-nFE = -nFE° + RT \ln \frac{a(Rd)^\beta}{a(Ox)^\alpha}$$

and

$$E = E° - \frac{RT}{nF} \ln \frac{a(Rd)^\beta}{a(Ox)^\alpha} \qquad (9-14)$$

Equation (9–14) is known as the *Nernst equation*. $E°$ is the standard potential, that is, the emf when the activities of all reactants and products are unity, and is normally expressed for reductions, as in Table 9–1. The Nernst equation is used to compute either an individual electrode potential or a cell emf from a known $E°$ at a specified temperature, T, for a reaction involving n electrons at specified activities of the reactants and products. At 25° C, equation (9–14) becomes

$$E = E° - \frac{0.0592}{n} \log \frac{a_{products}}{a_{reactants}} \qquad (9-15)$$

The individual *electrode potentials* are calculated from the Nernst equation as shown in *Example 9–3*. The emf of the entire cell obtained using the Nernst equation is discussed in the next section.

Example 9–3. What is the reduction potential at 25° C of platinum wire electrodes immersed in an acidic solution of ferrous ions, at a concentration of 0.50 molal (m), and of ferric ions, at a concentration of 0.25 m? The activity coefficient, γ, for the ferrous ion is 0.435 and that for the ferric ion is 0.390 under the experimental conditions. $E°_{Fe^{3+}\rightarrow Fe^{2+}} = 0.771$ volts from Table 9–1. The electrode reaction, at the inert platinum electrode, is

$$Fe^{3+} + e^- \rightleftharpoons Fe^{2+}$$

The activity of each ion in the electrode reaction is given by $a = \gamma(m)$, so $a = 0.435 \times 0.50 = 0.218$ for the ferrous ion, and $a = 0.390 \times 0.25 = 0.0975$ for the ferric ion. From equation (9–15), with $n = 1$,

$$E_{electrode} = E°_{Fe^{3+}\rightarrow Fe^{2+}} - \frac{0.0592}{1} \log \frac{a_{Fe^{2+}}}{a_{Fe^{3+}}}$$

$$E_{electrode} = 0.771 - 0.0592 \log \frac{0.218}{0.0975}$$

$$= 0.771 - 0.021$$

$$E_{electrode} = 0.750 \text{ volt}$$

In the example just given, the electrode is acting as the cathode, and a reduction is observed. If an electrode reaction is expressed as an oxidation rather than a reduction, that is, the electrode is acting as the anode, then the sign of $E°$ as given in Table 9–1 must be changed, since by convention it is a reduction potential, and equation (9–15) becomes

TABLE 9-1. *Standard Half-cell Reduction Potentials at 25° C*

Reduction Reaction	Reduction Electrode*	$E°$ (volts)
$\frac{1}{2}Cl_2 + e^- = Cl^-$	$Cl^-|Cl_2, Pt$	+1.360
$\frac{1}{4}O_2 + H^+ + e^- = \frac{1}{2}H_2O$	$H^+|O_2, Pt$	+1.229
$Hg^{2+} + e^- = \frac{1}{2}Hg_2^{2+}$	$Hg^{2+}, Hg_2^{2+}|Pt$	+0.907
$Ag^+ + e^- = Ag$	$Ag^+|Ag$	+0.799
$\frac{1}{2}Hg^{2+} + e^- = Hg$	$Hg_2^{2+}|Hg$	+0.854
$Fe^{3+} + e^- = Fe^{2+}$	$Fe^{3+}, Fe^{2+}|Pt$	+0.771
$\frac{1}{2}I_2 + e^- = I^-$	$I^-|I_2$	+0.536
$Fe(CN)_6^{3-} + e^- = Fe(CN)_6^{4-}$	$Fe(CN)_6^{3-}, Fe(CN)_6^{4-}|Pt$	+0.356
$\frac{1}{2}Cu^{2+} + e^- = \frac{1}{2}Cu$	$Cu^{2+}|Cu$	+0.337
$\frac{1}{2}Hg_2Cl_2 + e^- = Hg + Cl^-$	$Cl^-|Hg_2Cl_2, Hg$	+0.268
$AgCl + e^- = Ag + Cl^-$	$Cl^-|AgCl, Ag$	+0.223
$AgBr + e^- = Ag + Br^-$	$Br^-|AgBr, Ag$	+0.071
$H^+ + e^- = \frac{1}{2}H_2$	$H^+|H_2, Pt$	0.000
$\frac{1}{2}Pb^{2+} + e^- = \frac{1}{2}Pb$	$Pb^{2+}|Pb$	-0.126
$AgI + e^- = Ag + I^-$	$I^-|AgI, Ag$	-0.156
$\frac{1}{2}Ni^{2+} + e^- = \frac{1}{2}Ni$	$Ni^{2+}|Ni$	-0.250
$\frac{1}{2}Cd^{2+} + e^- = \frac{1}{2}Cd$	$Cd^{2+}|Cd$	-0.403
$\frac{1}{2}Fe^{2+} + e^- = \frac{1}{2}Fe$	$Fe^{2+}|Fe$	-0.440
$\frac{1}{2}Zn^{2+} + e^- = \frac{1}{2}Zn$	$Zn^{2+}|Zn$	-0.763
$Na + e^- = Na$	$Na^+|Na$	-2.714
$K^+ + e^- = K$	$K^+|K$	-2.925
$Li^+ + e^- = Li$	$Li^+|Li$	-3.045

*A single line represents the boundary between an electrode and its solution. A comma is used to separate two species that are present together in the same phase.

$$E = -E° - \frac{0.0592}{n} \log \frac{a_{products}}{a_{reactants}} \quad (9-16)$$

The reaction in *Example 9-3* expressed as an oxidation becomes

$$Fe^{2+} \rightleftharpoons Fe^{3+} + e^-$$

and the oxidation potential at the anode is

$$E_{electrode} = E_{Fe^{3+} \to Fe^{2+}} - \frac{0.0592}{1} \log \frac{a_{Fe^{3+}}}{a_{Fe^{2+}}}$$

$$E_{electrode} = -0.771 - 0.0592 \log \frac{0.0975}{0.218}$$

$$E_{electrode} = -0.771 + 0.021 = -0.750 \text{ volt}$$

Standard EMF of Cells. The term $E°$ in the Nernst expression, equation (9-14), is defined as the measured emf of a cell, E, when all the reactants and products have unit activity. In the following example, an experimental method to measure $E°$ will be described. This method uses the Debye–Hückel limiting law (Chapter 6) to describe the reactants and products with unit activity.

Consider a cell that consists of a hydrogen gas electrode as the anode and a silver–silver chloride electrode as the cathode immersed in an aqueous solution of hydrochloric acid:

$$Pt|H_2 (P_{atm})|HCl (c, \text{moles/liter})|AgCl|Ag$$

The overall cell reaction is determined by summing the half-reactions at each electrode:

$$\frac{1}{2}H_2 = H^+ + e^-$$
$$\underline{AgCl + e^- = Ag + Cl^-}$$
$$AgCl + \frac{1}{2}H_2 = H^+ + Ag + Cl^- \quad (9-17)$$

At 25° C, the emf of this cell is given by equation (9-15):

$$E = E° - \frac{0.0592}{1} \log \frac{a_{H^+}a_{Ag}a_{Cl^-}}{a_{AgCl}a_{H_2}^{1/2}} \quad (9-18)$$

Since the solid phases are assigned an activity of 1, as mentioned on p. 134, and the pressure of hydrogen gas can be adjusted to 1 atm, at which it behaves ideally and has an activity of 1, equation (9-18) can be simplified to

$$E = E° - 0.0592 \log a_{H^+}a_{Cl^-} \quad (9-19)$$

The individual ionic activities can be expressed in terms of *mean ionic* activities, as described on p. 132 of Chapter 6. This substitution leads to

$$E = E° - 0.0592 \log \gamma_{\pm}^2 c_{H^+}c_{Cl^-} \quad (9-20)$$

in which $\gamma_{\pm}$ is the mean ionic activity coefficient for a solution of hydrochloric acid whose ion concentrations (molality, that is, moles per kilogram of solvent) are c_{H^+} and c_{Cl^-}, respectively. According to the overall reaction for the cell, the concentrations of H^+ and Cl^- must be equal, so equation (9-20) can be expressed as

$$E = E° - 0.0592 \log \gamma_{\pm}^2 c^2 \quad (9-21)$$

in which c is the molar concentration of HCl in the solution. Equation (9-21) can be rearrangd to obtain

$$E + 0.0592 \log c^2 = E° - 0.0592 \log \gamma_{\pm}^2$$

or

$$E + 0.1184 \log c = E° - 0.1184 \log \gamma_{\pm} \quad (9-22)$$

Using the Debye–Hückel limiting law (p. 135), the $\log \gamma_{\pm}$ term in equation (9-22) can be replaced by $-Az^2\sqrt{\mu}$, in which A is a constant for a particular medium (0.509 for water at 25° C), z is the valence of the ions (1 in this example), and μ is the ionic strength of the solution. This gives the equation

$$E + 0.1184 \log c = E° + 0.1184(0.509)\sqrt{\mu}$$

or

$$E + 0.1184 \log c = E° + 0.0603\sqrt{\mu} \quad (9-23)$$

Since $\mu = \frac{1}{2}\Sigma c_i z_i^2$, for i ionic species in solution, according to equation (6-56), then for the cell with only HCl in solution,

$$E + 0.1184 \log c = E° + 0.0603\sqrt{c} \quad (9-24)$$

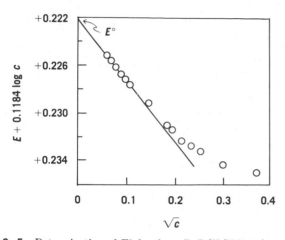

Fig. 9-5. Determination of $E°$ for the cell, $Pt|H_2|HCl$ (c)$|AgCl|Ag$. Notice that the values on the vertical axis decrease in the upward direction, so the negative slope of the line corresponds to a positive value, +0.0603, in equation (9-24).

The Debye-Hückel limiting law is satisfactory only for dilute solutions. Therefore, when we apply equation (9-24) to the actual determination of the standard emf of the cell, we find that a linear relationship between the left-hand side of the equation and the square root of the concentration of HCl, that is, $c^{1/2}$, is obtained only for small values of c. This is shown in Figure 9-5. Extrapolating the line so that it intersects the vertical axis yields a value for $E°$ that corresponds to the emf of the cell at infinite dilution. This is the desired standard emf for the cell in the example, namely, +0.222 volt.

Example 9-4. What is the standard potential, $E°$, for a cell consisting of a hydrogen gas electrode (P = 1 atm) as the anode and a silver-silver bromide electrode as the cathode immersed in a solution of 0.0004 m hydrobromic acid? The cell emf, E, is determined by potentiometry to be 0.4745 volts. The cell can be depicted as

$$Pt|H_2 \text{ (1 atm)}|HBr \text{ (0.0004 } \dot{M})|AgBr|Ag$$

The overall cell reaction is

$$AgBr + \tfrac{1}{2}H_2 = H^+ + Ag + Br^-$$

The equations used for the AgCl cell in our previous example hold also for this cell, so equation (9-24) can be applied:

$$E + 0.1184 \log c = E° + 0.0603\sqrt{c}$$

Therefore,

$$E° = E + 0.1184 \log c - 0.0603\sqrt{c}$$
$$E° = 0.4745 - 0.4023 - 0.0012 = 0.071 \text{ volt}$$

Reference Electrodes and Standard Potentials. The absolute potential of a single electrode cannot be measured but as a relative potential can be assigned by combining the electrode with a *reference electrode* to form a cell and then measuring the cell emf. The potential of the reference electrode is known, so the potential of the unknown electrode can be obtained as a difference. To compare a series of emf's determined in this way for a variety of electrodes, it is necessary to specify whether oxidation or reduction is occurring at

the electrode. According to the Gibbs-Stockholm agreement or convention,* the measured emf should be designated as a *reduction potential*. That is, the unknown electrode is the cathode in the cell, and the relative ability of the electrode to accept electrons is measured against a reference electrode. The cell may thus be written as

$$E_{cell} = E_{reference} + E_{unknown\ electrode} \quad (9-25)$$

in which the unknown electrode is the right electrode in the cell schematic (i.e., the cathode). If the potentials are determined under standard conditions, that is, 25°C, 1 atm pressure, and unit activity of all species, then, for the standard reduction potential,

$$E°_{cell} = E°_{reference} + E°_{unknown\ electrode} \quad (9-26)$$

If the electrodes were switched so that the reference electrode became the cathode and the unknown electrode became the anode, an *oxidation potential* would be determined for the unknown electrode. Oxidation potentials are not normally used for comparing cell potentials, according to convention. It is important to note that oxidation potentials differ from reduction potentials only by having the reverse sign, as demonstrated in *Example 9-3.* Thus, if the standard reduction potential for the silver-silver chloride electrode is +0.223 volt, its oxidation potential must be -0.223 volt.

Consider a cell that consists of a reference hydrogen electrode and a second electrode whose potential is being determined. The cell, according to convention, is represented as

$$E°_{cell} = E°_{H_2(anode)} + E°\ unknown\ electrode_{(cathode)} \quad (9-27)$$

Under unit hydrogen ion activity and standard conditions, the reference hydrogen electrode, which is a primary reference electrode, is arbitrarily assigned a potential of 0.000 volt,

$$E_{H_2}° = 0 \quad (9-28)$$

Thus, according to this definition, the measured standard cell emf corresponds to a standard electrode reduction potential:

$$E°_{cell} = E°\ unknown\ electrode_{(cathode)} \quad (9-29)$$

In addition to the hydrogen electrode, secondary reference electrodes, with which other electrodes can be combined, include the 0.1-N calomel electrode, the 1-N calomel electrode, the saturated calomel electrode (in which the concentration terms refer to the chloride ion concentration), and the silver-silver chloride electrode. These electrodes can be standardized by combining them with the hydrogen electrode, as

---

*This convention was adopted in 1953 at the 17th Conference of the International Union of Pure and Applied Chemistry in Stockholm.

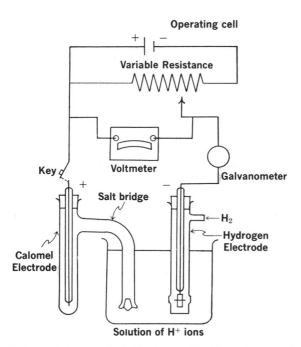

Operating cell

Variable Resistance

Voltmeter

Galvanometer

Key

Salt bridge

H_2

Hydrogen Electrode

Calomel Electrode

Solution of H⁺ ions

Fig. 9–6. Hydrogen electrode in combination with a calomel electrode. (After F. Daniels and R. A. Alberty, *Physical Chemistry*, Wiley, New York, 1955, p. 418.)

shown in Figure 9–6. These secondary reference electrodes are most often used for laboratory measurement since they are rugged and require practically no adjustment before use. In contrast, a hydrogen electrode, in which the hydrogen gas pressure must be carefully controlled, requires careful handling and frequent adjustment.

A KCl solution acts as the electrolyte solution in all of the mentioned secondary reference electrodes. It also acts as a *salt bridge* to make electric contact between the electrode and the rest of the cell. The salt bridge (represented by double lines, ‖, in cell schematic diagrams) minimizes the potential difference that occurs across the liquid boundary between two solutions. The KCl solution in the salt bridge is prevented from mixing to any significant extent with the external solution by introducing a porous ceramic plug or permeable membrane at the boundary between the solutions. The potential difference at this boundary is known as the *liquid junction potential*. In cells that contain such a liquid junction potential, which comes about owing to unequal diffusion of ions across the barrier between the solutions, it is correct to write the overall cell emf as

$$E_{cell} = E_{anode} + E_{junction} + E_{cathode} \quad (9\text{–}30)$$

It is possible to design electrodes with liquid junctions that have minimum junction potential, as described by Durst[2] and by Connors.[2]

Standard and Formal Reduction Potentials. Copper ions accept electrons and are reduced more easily to the corresponding metal than lead ions, and lead ions in

turn are more easily reduced than zinc ions. Therefore, the elements and their respective ions may be arranged in an electromotive series with those ions that accept electrons most readily, that is, those that are reduced most easily under standard conditions at the top of the list in Table 9–1. The standard reduction potentials, $E°$, are the potentials of the reduction reaction, occurring at the cathode, at *unit activity* of reactants and products.

By comparison, the *formal potential* of an electrode is obtained using specified concentrations of all species with equal concentrations of the oxidized and reduced species in the half-cell reaction. The formal potential is an experimentally observable value that takes into account liquid junction potentials, ionic strength, complexation, and other cell variations that will affect the cell emf. For example, the standard reduction potential $E°$ of the calomel electrode, at unit activity of all species, is +0.268 volt, whereas the formal reduction potential of the 0.1-N calomel electrode is +0.334 volt; of the 1-N calomel electrode, +0.280 volt; and of the saturated calomel electrode, +0.242 volt at 25° C. In some cases, the standard reduction potential, $E°$, of an electrode cannot be measured since limited solubility of a species involved in the half-cell reaction prevents obtaining a solution with unit activity. In these cases, only formal potentials can be obtained.

In Table 9–1, the potentials are all standard reduction potentials using the standard hydrogen electrode, with an assigned $E°$ of 0.000 volt as a reference. For an *oxidation* reaction, the sign of the potential in Table 9–1 is reversed. In oxidations, the electrode with a larger positive potential would be oxidized more easily than that with a smaller potential. For example, the $Li|Li^+$ electrode would by oxidized more easily than the $Zn|Zn^{2+}$ electrode.

Example 9–5. Calculate $E°_{cell}$ for an electrochemical cell consisting of a zinc electrode and a copper electrode, each immersed in a solution of its ions at an activity of 1.00.

The cell is written as

$$Zn|Zn^{2+} \ (a = 1) \ \| \ Cu^{2+} \ (a = 1)|Cu$$

in which oxidation takes place at the left electrode and reduction at the right electrode, and electrons flow through the external circuit from left to right. How do we know that oxidation will occur at the zinc electrode and not at the copper electrode?

The standard reduction potentials for the zinc and copper electrodes are −0.763 volt and +0.337 volt, respectively, from Table 9–1. These $E°$ values indicate that copper is reduced more easily than zinc, because of the larger positive $E°$ potential of the copper electrode. It follows, from what has been said previously about oxidation potentials, that zinc must be oxidized more easily, that is, it has a greater standard *oxidation* potential. Therefore, in this particular cell, oxidation must occur at the zinc electrode and reduction at the copper electrode. The overall cell reaction is

$$Zn + Cu^{2+} = Zn^{2+} + Cu$$

The emf of the cell is the sum of the *oxidation* potential of the left electrode and the *reduction* potential of the right electrode. The standard oxidation potential for the zinc half-cell is +0.763, that is, the E° value listed in Table 9–1, but with the *opposite sign*. Equation (9–3), under standard conditions is written as

$$E^\circ_{\text{cell}} = \underset{\text{(oxidation)}}{E^\circ_{\text{left}}} + \underset{\text{(reduction)}}{E^\circ_{\text{right}}}$$

$$= \underset{\text{(oxidation)}}{E^\circ_{\text{Zn}\to\text{Zn}^{2+}}} + \underset{\text{(reduction)}}{E^\circ_{\text{Cu}^{2+}\to\text{Cu}}}$$

$$= \underset{\text{(reduction)}}{-E^\circ_{\text{Zn}^{2+}\to\text{Zn}}} + \underset{\text{(reduction)}}{E^\circ_{\text{Cu}^{2+}\to\text{Cu}}}$$

$$E^\circ_{\text{cell}} = +0.763 + (+0.337) = 1.100 \text{ volts}$$

Example 9–6. Will a silver electrode reduce a lead electrode at 25° C when both half-cells are at unit activity?

The two reduction reactions and their corresponding standard potentials from Table 9–1 are

$$\text{Ag}^+ + e^- = \text{Ag} \qquad E^\circ = +0.799$$
$$\tfrac{1}{2}\text{Pb}^{2+} + e^- = \tfrac{1}{2}\text{Pb} \qquad E^\circ = -0.126$$

The silver potential is more positive than that for lead; therefore, silver is reduced more easily than lead. A silver electrode cannot reduce a lead electrode, and if the cell is written with the mistaken belief that silver is the oxidation electrode and lead is the reduction electrode, the cell emf, when calculated, will be found to have a negative value. The emf of any cell must be positive to provide a flow of electrons in the external circuit from the anode to the cathode, and this can be used as a guide to indicate whether the cell has been written properly. It is useful to remember that *the cell emf must always be positive, whereas the potentials of the individual electrodes can be either positive or negative.*

Suppose the cell is written as

$$\text{Ag}|\text{Ag}^+ \, (a = 1) \, \| \, \text{Pb}^{2+} \, (a = 1)|\text{Pb}$$

and the overall reaction as

$$\text{Ag} + \tfrac{1}{2}\text{Pb}^{2+} = \text{Ag}^+ + \tfrac{1}{2}\text{Pb}$$

$$E^\circ_{\text{cell}} = E^\circ_{\text{Ag}\to\text{Ag}^+} + E^\circ_{\text{Pb}^{2+}\to\text{Pb}} = -0.799 + (-0.126) = -0.925 \text{ volt}$$

This result is wrong since E°_{cell} is negative; the mistake can be corrected by reversing the electrodes:

$$\text{Pb}|\text{Pb}^{2+} \, (a = 1) \, \| \, \text{Ag}^+ \, (a = 1)|\text{Ag}$$

$$\text{Ag}^+ + \tfrac{1}{2}\text{Pb} = \text{Ag} + \tfrac{1}{2}\text{Pb}^{2+}$$

$$E^\circ_{\text{cell}} = E^\circ_{\text{Pb}\to\text{Pb}^{2+}} + E^\circ_{\text{Ag}^+\to\text{Ag}} = +0.126 + (+0.799) = +0.925 \text{ volt}$$

Example 9–7. What is the correct configuration for a cell composed of a ferrocyanide–ferricyanide electrode and a mercurous–mercuric electrode when both half-cells are at unit activity at 25° C? This type of cell is known as an oxidation–reduction system.

The two electrode reactions, when written as reductions, along with their E° values from Table 9–1, are

$$\text{Fe(CN)}_6^{3-} + e^- = \text{Fe(CN)}_6^{4-} \qquad E^\circ = +0.356$$
$$\text{Hg}^{2+} + e^- = \tfrac{1}{2}\text{Hg}_2^{2+} \qquad E^\circ = +0.907$$

The mercurous–mercuric electrode has a larger reduction potential and therefore will oxidize the ferrocyanide to ferricyanide. The cell is correctly written as

$$\text{Pt}|\text{Fe(CN)}_6^{3-}, \text{Fe(CN)}_6^{4-} \, (a = 1) \, \| \, \text{Hg}^{2+}, \text{Hg}_2^{2+} \, (a = 1)|\text{Pt}$$

and the overall reaction is

$$\text{Fe(CN)}_6^{4-} + \text{Hg}^{2+} = \text{Fe(CN)}_6^{3-} + \tfrac{1}{2}\text{Hg}_2^{2+}$$

The calculated E°_{cell} is

$$E^\circ_{\text{cell}} = E^\circ_{\text{Fe(CN)}_6^{4-}\to\text{Fe(CN)}_6^{3-}} + E^\circ_{\text{Hg}^{2+}\to\tfrac{1}{2}\text{Hg}_2^{2+}} =$$
$$-0.356 + (+0.907) = +0.551 \text{ volt}$$

Example 9–8. Compute the emf of the following cell at 25° C:

$$\text{Ag, AgI}|\text{I}^- \, (a = 0.4) \, \| \, \text{Cl}^- \, (a = 0.8)|\text{AgCl, Ag}$$

The cell reaction is

$$\text{I}^- + \text{AgCl} = \text{AgI} + \text{Cl}^-$$

Applying equation (9–15) in which $n = 1$ for this reaction,

$$E_{\text{cell}} = E^\circ_{\text{cell}} - \frac{0.0592}{1} \log \frac{a_{\text{AgI}} a_{\text{Cl}^-}}{a_{\text{I}^-} a_{\text{AgCl}}}$$

The activities of the two solids, AgI and AgCl, are 1 and may be eliminated from the last term of the equation. The standard potential of the cell is the sum of the two standard half-cell potentials:

$$E^\circ_{\text{cell}} - E^\circ_{\text{I}^-\to\text{AgI}} + E^\circ_{\text{AgCl}\to\text{Cl}^-}$$
$$= +0.156 + (+0.223) = +0.379 \text{ volt}$$

and the emf of the cell is

$$E_{\text{cell}} = 0.379 - 0.0592 \log \frac{0.8}{0.4}$$

$$E_{\text{cell}} = 0.379 - 0.018 = +0.361 \text{ volt}$$

Concentration Cells. Thus, far, this chapter has discussed *chemical cells* in which an emf is produced by an oxidation–reduction reaction occurring with two different electrodes. In a concentration cell, the emf results from the differences in *activities* of solutions of the same material constituting the two half-cells.

Suppose that a cell consists of two copper electrodes immersed in copper sulfate solutions at 25° C having activities of 0.01 and 0.05. The cell is represented by

$$\text{Cu}|\text{Cu}^{2+} \, (a_1 = 0.01) \, \| \, \text{Cu}^{2+} \, (a_2 = 0.05)|\text{Cu}$$

The reactions at the anode and the cathode are

$$\text{(Anode)} \qquad \text{Cu} = \text{Cu}^{2+} \, (a_1 = 0.01) + 2e^-$$

$$\text{(Cathode)} \quad \text{Cu}^{2+} \, (a_2 = 0.05) + 2e^- = \text{Cu}$$

and the overall reaction is

$$\text{Cu}^{2+} \, (a_2 = 0.05) = \text{Cu}^{2+} \, (a_1 = 0.01)$$

The corresponding Nernst equations for the individual electrodes are

$$E_{\text{left}} = \underset{\text{(oxidation)}}{E^\circ_{\text{Cu}\to\text{Cu}^{2+}}} - \frac{0.0592}{2} \log a_1$$

$$E_{\text{right}} = \underset{\text{(reduction)}}{E^\circ_{\text{Cu}^{2+}\to\text{Cu}}} - \frac{0.0592}{2} \log \frac{1}{a_2}$$

The equation for the cell emf is

$$E_{\text{cell}} = E_{\text{left}} + E_{\text{right}}$$

$$= \left(E^\circ_{\text{Cu}\to\text{Cu}^{2+}} - \frac{0.0592}{2} \log a_1 \right)$$

$$+ \left(E^\circ_{\text{Cu}^{2+}\to\text{Cu}} - \frac{0.0592}{2} \log \frac{1}{a_2} \right)$$

$$= (E^\circ_{\text{Cu}\to\text{Cu}^{2+}} + E^\circ_{\text{Cu}^{2+}\to\text{Cu}}) - \frac{0.0592}{2} \log \frac{a_1}{a_2}$$

Since $E^\circ_{\text{Cu}\to\text{Cu}^{2+}} = -0.337$ and $E^\circ_{\text{Cu}^{2+}\to\text{Cu}} = +0.337$, $E^\circ_{\text{cell}} = 0$, and the general equation for a concentration cell at 25° C is

$$E_{\text{cell}} = -\frac{0.0592}{n} \log \frac{a_1}{a_2} \qquad (9\text{–}31)$$

The electrolyte at the higher activity a_2 tends to diffuse spontaneously into the solution of lower activity

a_1, and the cell emf arises from this difference in effective concentrations.

Example 9–9. Calculate the cell emf of the concentration cell just discussed.

$$E_{cell} = -\frac{0.0592}{2} \log \frac{0.01}{0.05} = 0.021 \text{ volt}$$

Example 9–10. Calculate the emf at 25° C arising from the cell

$$\text{Ag; AgCl}|\text{Cl}^- \ (a_2 = 0.10) \ \| \ \text{Cl}^- \ (a_1 = 0.01)|\text{Hg}_2\text{Cl}_2, \text{Hg}$$

In this case, we have two different electrodes but a common ion in the electrolyte solutions, so that the cell acts as a chemical cell with some cell emf arising out of the difference in electrolyte activities. The overall reaction is

$$\text{Ag} + \text{Cl}^- \ (a_2 = 0.10) + \tfrac{1}{2}\text{Hg}_2\text{Cl}_2 = \text{AgCl} + \text{Hg} + \text{Cl}^- \ (a_1 = 0.01)$$

The corresponding Nernst equations for the individual electrodes are:

$$E_{left} = E^o_{\substack{\text{Cl}^-\rightarrow\text{AgCl} \\ \text{(oxidation)}}} - \frac{0.0592}{1} \log \frac{a_{AgCl}}{a_{Ag}a_{Cl^-(a_2)}}$$

$$E_{right} = E^o_{1/2\text{Hg}_2\text{Cl}_2\rightarrow\text{Cl}^-} - \frac{0.0592}{1} \log \frac{a_{Hg}a_{Cl^-(a_1)}}{a_{Hg_2Cl_2}}$$

The equation for the cell emf is

$$E_{cell} = E_{left} + E_{right}$$

and since the activity of all solids in the overall reaction is unity, the cell emf becomes

$$E_{cell} = E^o_{Cl^-\rightarrow AgCl} - 0.0592 \log \frac{1}{a_2} + E^o_{1/2Hg_2Cl_2\rightarrow Cl^-} - 0.0592 \log a_1$$

With values from Table 9–1, this becomes

$$E_{cell} = \left(-0.223 - 0.0592 \log \frac{1}{0.10}\right) + \left(+0.268 - 0.0592 \log 0.01\right)$$

$$= -0.282 + 0.386 = +0.104 \text{ volt}$$

It is interesting to note that this cell would be represented incorrectly if the concentrations of chloride in the half-cells were reversed, that is, if $a_2 = 0.01$ and $a_1 = 0.10$. In that case, a negative E_{cell} of -0.014 volt would be calculated, and it would be necessary to represent the calomel as the oxidation electrode on the left and the silver–silver chloride electrode as the reduction electrode on the right to achieve a positive E_{cell}.

ELECTROMETRIC DETERMINATION OF pH, SPECIFIC IONS, AND REDOX POTENTIALS

The determination of pH can be made by means of any electrode whose potential depends on the hydrogen ion activity.[3] The hydrogen and glass electrodes are discussed here as typical pH electrodes. Two hydrogen electrodes may be combined to measure pH, one serving as the indicating electrode and the other as the reference electrode, although this arrangement is not generally used in practice. The calomel and the silver chloride electrode are more convenient as reference electrodes and are typically used with commercial pH meters. The National Bureau of Standards (NBS) determines the pH of its standard buffers in a cell composed of a hydrogen-indicating electrode and a silver–silver chloride reference electrode. Some of the NBS buffers available to laboratories for standardizing pH meters are listed in Table 9–2.

The Hydrogen Electrode. The chemical cell using a hydrogen and a saturated calomel electrode is shown in Figure 9–6. The half-cell reactions together with the overall cell reactions are

Left (oxidation):
$$\text{H}_2 + 2\text{H}_2\text{O} = 2\text{H}_3\text{O}^+ \ (a_{H^+} = ?) + 2e^-$$

Right (reduction):
$$\text{Hg}_2\text{Cl}_2 + 2e^- = 2\text{Cl}^- + 2\text{Hg} \qquad (9\text{–}32)$$

Overall reaction:
$$\text{H}_2 + \text{Hg}_2\text{Cl}_2 + 2\text{H}_2\text{O} = 2\text{H}_3\text{O}^+ + 2\text{Hg} + 2\text{Cl}^-$$

and the cell is represented as

$$\text{Pt, H}_2 \ (1 \text{ atm})|\text{H}_3\text{O}^+ \ (a_{H^+} = ?) \ \| \ \text{KCl (sat), Hg}_2\text{Cl}_2|\text{Hg}$$

in which $(a_{H^+} = ?)$ stands for the hydrogen ion activity of the test solution, the pH of which is being determined.

The emf of the cell is

$$E_{cell} = E_{H_2\rightarrow 2H_3O^+} + E_{Hg_2Cl_2\rightarrow 2Hg} \qquad (9\text{–}33)$$

The potential of the hydrogen electrode at 25° C and at a partial pressure of the hydrogen gas of 1 atm is written

$$E_{H_2} = E'^o_{H_2\rightarrow H_3O^+} - 0.0592 \log \frac{a_{H_3O^+}}{1 \text{ atm}}$$

Under these conditions, $E^o = 0$, from Table 9–1, and the equation becomes

$$E_{H_2} = -0.0592 \log a_{H_3O^+}$$

and since $\text{pH} = -\log a_{H_3O^+}$

$$E_{H_2} = 0.0592 \text{ pH}$$

The potential of the saturated KCl calomel electrode in the reduction reaction of equation (9–32) is $+0.242$ volt at 25° C. Hence, from equation (9–33),

$$E_{cell} = 0.0592 \text{ pH} + 0.242$$

TABLE 9–2. *National Bureau of Standards Reference Buffer Solutions at 25° C*

Composition	pH	Dilution Value (change in pH on dilution with an equal volume of water)	Buffer Capacity, β
Potassium tetraoxalate, 0.05 M	1.68	+0.19	0.070
Potassium hydrogen phthalate, 0.05 M	4.01	+0.05	0.016
Potassium dihydrogen phosphate and disodium hydrogen phosphate, anhydrous, each 0.025 M	6.86	+0.08	0.029
Borax (sodium tetraborate, decahydrate), 0.01 M	9.18	+0.01	0.020

and

$$pH = \frac{E_{cell} - 0.242}{0.0592} \qquad (9\text{-}34)$$

Example 9–11. A solution is placed between the hydrogen electrode and the calomel electrode in Figure 9–6. The emf of the cell is +0.963 volt at 25° C. What is the pH of the solution?

$$pH = \frac{0.963 - 0.242}{0.0592} = 12.2$$

The Glass Electrode. The glass membrane electrode is typical of the membrane-type electrodes described on p. 192. It is now the most widely used pH-indicating electrode. The conventional electrode includes an acidic electrolyte solution of 0.1 N HCl, and an internal silver–silver chloride reference electrode, as depicted in Figure 9–3. The complete cell, using a saturated calomel reference electrode (abbreviated SCE), can be represented as

Ag|AgCl, 0.1N HCl|glass membrane|

$$\underset{(a_{H_3O^+} = ?)}{\text{unknown solution}} \| \text{KCl (sat), Hg}_2\text{Cl}_2|\text{Hg}$$

The pH of the unknown solution is obtained from the cell emf if the pH of the internal solution, 0.1 N HCl, is constant. The emf of this cell at 25° C results from the sum of four separate potentials, arising at separate interfaces:

$$E_{cell} = E_{SCE} + E_{ASYM} - E_{AgCl,Ag}$$
$$+ \, 0.059 \, (pH_{unknown} - pH_{HCl \; solution}) \quad (9\text{-}35)$$

where E_{SCE} arises at the boundary, Hg$_2$Cl$_2$|Hg; E_{ASYM}, known as the asymmetry potential, comes from the two boundaries of the glass membrane and is equivalent to differences in resistance that arise owing to variations in manufacture; and $E_{AgCl,Ag}$ arises at the boundary Ag|AgCl. The pH$_{HCl \; solution}$ term comes from the 0.1-N HCl solution, while the pH$_{unknown}$ is the pH of the solution being determined. The asymmetry potential may be associated with the mechanical properties of the glass membrane, which can effect unequal mobility or absorption of ions on the two sides of the membrane. Although the E_{ASYM} potential varies from one glass membrane to another, it can be considered constant for a particular cell arrangement using one glass electrode, and equation (9–35) can be simplified at 25° C to

$$E_{cell} = E_{constant} + 0.0592 \, pH(unknown) \quad (9\text{-}36)$$

or

$$pH = \frac{E_{cell} - E_{constant}}{0.0592} \qquad (9\text{-}37)$$

$E_{constant}$ is the sum of all the boundary potentials in the cell plus the constant potential arising from the 0.1-N HCl solution.

The value of $E_{constant}$ cannot normally be determined accurately because of the variation in E_{ASYM} from one glass electrode to another; however, this is not neces-sary inasmuch as the pH meter can be standardized using a reference buffer solution, as listed in Table 9–2. The pH of a reference buffer, measured with the glass electrode and cell just described, is

$$pH_s = \frac{E_s - E_{constant}}{0.0592} \qquad (9\text{-}38)$$

in which pH$_s$ is the pH and E_s is the emf of the NBS reference buffer solution. Subtracting (9–38) from (9–37) to eliminate the undetermined $E_{constant}$ results in the expression

$$pH - pH_s = \frac{E_{cell} - E_s}{0.0592}$$

or

$$pH = pH_s + \frac{E_{cell} - E_s}{0.0592} \qquad (9\text{-}39)$$

Equation (9–39) is the *operational* or practical definition of pH now accepted by the NBS and the British Standards Institute.

In the actual measurement of pH, a *standardization dial* on the pH meter is adjusted manually until the needle on the scale reads the pH of a reference buffer solution. For accurate determinations, it is best to use two reference buffers, one with a pH below and the other with a pH above that for the unknown solution. The pH meter is similar in operation to the potentiometer discussed previously, except that it functions with a high input resistance, associated with the glass electrode. A diagram of a representative instrument is shown in Figure 9–7.

The chemical composition of the membrane of the glass electrode is critical for a correct potential response to the pH of a solution. At high pH values, a negative deviation from the theoretic potential is often found with glass membranes containing a high proportion of sodium ions, as shown in Figure 9–8. This "sodium error" is due to the fact that, at a high pH, the electrode potential can be partially determined by sodium ions in solution. In strongly acid solutions, a

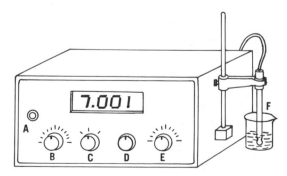

Fig. 9–7. Schematic diagram of a pH meter. A, On-off stand-by switch; B, temperature compensation; C, pH-millivolt switch; D, standardization dial; E, asymmetry or % slope dial; F, combination electrode.

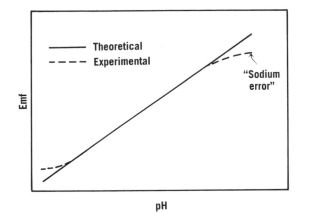

Fig. 9-8. The relationship between the cell emf and the pH for a glass electrode. (From W. C. Purdy. *Electroanalytical Methods in Biochemistry*, McGraw-Hill, New York, 1965, p. 44, used with the permission of McGraw-Hill Book Company.)

positive deviation from the theoretic emf also may be encountered. This error is believed to be due to a decrease in the activity of water, which may be associated with a decrease in the ability of the solution to hydrate the membrane surface and the ions in solution.

Electrodes currently available reduce the "sodium error" by incorporating a high proportion of lithium ions into the glass lattice. The glass electrode has an advantage over other electrodes in that it is not affected by oxidation–reduction systems since there is no exchange of electrons across the membrane, although it can be affected by cation exchange between the glass and the solution. The lithium ions incorporated in the glass do not exchange with other cations in the glass, unlike the sodium ion. This decrease in the ion-exchange property produces a more stable glass lattice with a decreased sodium ion exchange at high pH values and, therefore, a reduction in the alkaline error. A typical structure of a glass used in glass electrodes, as visualized by Perley,[4] is sketched in Figure 9-9. The composition of glass membranes for potentiometry is discussed by Purdy.[5]

A modern innovation in pH electrodes is the *combination electrode*. This incorporates a reference electrode junction next to a glass membrane so that both electrodes are within a single body. This provides a

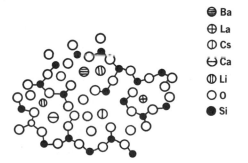

⊖	Ba
⊕	La
◑	Cs
⊖	Ca
⊕	Li
○	O
●	Si

Fig. 9-9. The structure of glass used in glass electrodes. (After G. E. Perley, Anal. Chem. **21**, 392, 1949).

compact electrochemical system that can be used with small or poorly accessible samples. A recent development involves the use of a fiber-optics sensor that allows the measurement of pH within a single living cell (Chem. Eng. News, Nov. 2, 1992).

Instructions for the determination of pH using the glass electrode are given in some detail by Bates.[6] Useful information on the determination of pH and the use of buffer solutions for the standardization of pH meters are given in the U.S. Pharmacopeia, XXII, pp. 1598, 1599.

A Summary of pH Definitions. The reader should be reminded that pH has been defined in three distinctly different ways in this book.

1. It was first introduced on pages 149, 150, according to Sörensen's definition of pH = $-\log [H_3O^+]$.

2. It was then shown on page 150 that the *activity*, rather than the concentration, of hydrogen ions should be used, and the definition became pH = $-\log a_{H_3O^+}$.

3. Unfortunately, however, it is not possible by experimental means to measure the activity of a single ion. For this reason, the pH scale in the United States and Great Britain is now defined in terms of a reference standard buffer that has been assigned an arbitrary pH value so as to conform as closely as possible to the thermodynamic definition pH = $-\log a_{H_3O^+}$.

This last definition, known as the *operational* or experimental pH, does not correspond exactly to the pH on the activity scale since the junction potentials of the cells used cannot be eliminated. Consequently, pH is not a true physical constant but rather a practical scale of acidity and alkalinity measured in an appropriate cell that is calibrated by use of a reference standard buffer.

Finally, it should be observed that the pH numbers obtained by measuring solutions containing colloids and nonaqueous solvents have little correspondence with pH on the activity scale, and they should be specified as *arbitrary pH numbers*. These arbitrary values may be useful for control purposes to ensure uniformity of acidity or alkalinity of marketed products as long as the conditions are specified and it is recognized that the pH values do not correspond to the operational definition.

Ion-Selective Electrodes.[2] Electrodes that exhibit a selective and sensitive response to certain ions in solution are known as ion-selective electrodes. In this sense, the glass electrode just discussed is an ion-selective electrode since it is particularly sensitive to H_3O^+ ions. By carefully controlling the glass composition, it was discovered that electrodes could be constructed that showed enhanced sensitivity to certain monovalent cations, for example, K^+ or Na^+, compared with hydrogen ions. The glass surface can act as an ion exchanger, and certain ions can be held strongly at surface-binding sites depending on the glass composition. In addition, ion mobility through the glass can be controlled by modifications in the glass lattice structure. Through glass composition and structure, a membrane can be made selective for certain ions. With these membrane electrodes, complete selectivity cannot be achieved, since the glass response cannot be made completely independent of hydrogen or other ions in solution. Nonetheless, the selectivity is usually adequate for many applications.

The sensing barrier of the ion-selective electrode operates through the selective exchange of ions between two solutions on either side of the barrier. Potentials arise owing to concentration differences between the solutions as well as from the resistance of the barrier. Salt crystals, liquids, and enzymes, as well as glass membranes, have been used either by themselves or incorporated into some structural matrix, such as a plastic, to form a sensing barrier.

An example of the salt-type of barrier is the fluoride-sensitive electrode, which uses a fluoride salt of one of the lanthanum elements (see periodic table, inside front cover) as an insoluble membrane. For example, a crystal containing LaF_3, praseodymium or europium fluoride (PrF_3 or EuF_3), can be sealed into the end of an electrode. An inner filling solution of a known activity, a, of NaF is used with an internal reference electrode, such as silver–silver chloride. The entire electrode can be represented as

Internal reference electrode	NaF(a)	LaF_3 crystal	External test solution (F^-, unknown concentration)

Figure 9–10 shows the construction of a typical fluoride

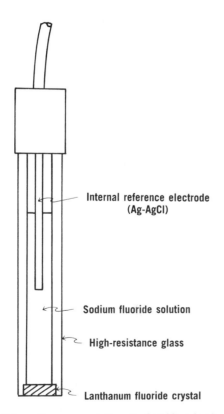

Fig. 9–10. Schematic representation of a fluoride-selective electrode.

electrode. The potential difference cross the LaF_3 crystal is due exclusively to the conductance of F^- ions, unless lanthanum ions are present in appreciable concentration in the test solution. The electrode is practically free of interferences and can be considered selective for fluoride ion. For biologic samples, fluoride concentrations as low as 10^{-6} M can be determined quickly, usually with only a dilution or solubilization step, after calibration. Accuracy of the method is usually within $\pm10\%$ for solution pH values between 4 and 8. Interferences are limited to hydroxide ions present at higher pH values, fluoride complexes, and hydrofluoric acid formation at lower pH values.

Membrane barriers can also be constructed from electrically neutral, and water-insoluble, sensors. The compound is incorporated into a plastic matrix such as a polyvinyl chloride (PVC) membrane. This is accomplished simply by mixing the sensor with a suitable solvent, adding the PVC, mixing, and then removing the solvent. The membrane produced can be incorporated directly as a barrier. One of the most selective sensors being used is the antibiotic valinomycin.

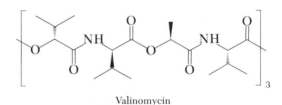

Valinomycin

This antibiotic has a 36-membered ring structure and acts as a selective complexing agent for potassium ions. The electrode mechanism involves cation exchange across the antibiotic membrane to produce a potential between solutions on either side. The valinomycin electrode shows a selectivity of 4000:1 for K^+ over Na^+ ions and selectivity of 20,000:1 for K^+ over H^+ ions. It has a linear potential response over the region from about 10^{-5} to 10^{-1} M for potassium ions. The electrode can be represented as:

Internal reference electrode	KCl (known concentration)	Valinomycin membrane	External test solution (K^+, unknown concentration)

Charged ion exchangers, such as phosphate diesters, may also be used as sensors. In this case, the compound can be dissolved in an appropriate solution that is in contact with a porous membrane that acts as a barrier and a junction to the test solution.

An enzyme may be incorporated into a polyacrylonitrile plastic film to act as part of a sensing barrier. For example, urease, which converts urea to ammonium ions by the reaction

$$Urea + H_2O \xrightarrow{\text{urease}} HCO_3^- + NH_4^+ \quad (9\text{–}40)$$

can be used. The immobilized enzyme in the plastic matrix is attached to a glass membrane electrode. The glass membrane in this case is sensitive to ammonium

TABLE 9–3. *Some Ions Detectable with Commercially Available Ion-Selective Electrodes**

	Minimum Detectable Concentration (*M*)	Possible Interfering Ions
Cations		
Cadmium	10^{-7}	Silver, mercuric, or cupric
Calcium	10^{-5}	Zinc, ferrous
Copper	10^{-7}	Silver, mercuric, cadmium, ferric or high levels of chloride or bromide
Lead	10^{-7}	Silver, mercuric, cupric, high levels of cadmium or ferric
Potassium	10^{-5}	Cesium, ammonium, hydrogen, silver
Silver	10^{-7}	Mercuric
Sodium	10^{-6}	Cesium, lithium, hydrogen, silver, rubidium, thallium
Anions		
Bromide	5×10^{-6}	Sulfide, iodide
Chloride	5×10^{-5}	Perchlorate, sulfide, bromide, iodide, cyanide
Cyanide	10^{-6}	Sulfide, chloride, iodide
Fluoride	10^{-6}	Hydroxide
Fluoroborate	10^{-5}	—
Iodide	2×10^{-7}	Sulfide
Nitrate	10^{-5}	Bromide, iodide, nitrite
Perchlorate	10^{-5}	—
Sulfide	10^{-7}	—
Thiocyanate	10^{-6}	Hydroxide, iodide, sulfide

*Adapted from the *Guide to Electrodes and Instrumentation,* Orion Research, Cambridge, Mass.

ions. The ammonium ions formed from the enzyme reaction migrate through the plastic membrane to the glass surface where they are detected through a change in potential. This electrode can detect urea in solution over a linear response range from approximately 10^{-4} to 10^{-2} *M*.

Typical ions detectable with ion-selective electrodes are listed in Table 9–3. Potential interferences from other ions in solution as well as minimum detectable concentrations are also listed.

All the ion-selective electrodes produce a response that is directly proportional to the logarithm of the activity of the ion. That is, from equation (9–36) at 25° C:

$$E_{\text{cell}} = E_{\text{constant}} + \frac{0.0592}{n} \log (a) \qquad (9\text{–}41)$$

in which a is the activity of the ion being monitored. In practice, the concentration of the ion is determined from a calibration curve, which relates E_{cell} on the y axis to standard ionic concentrations on the x axis. A typical calibration curve for fluoride ion is shown in Figure 9–11. In this case, the ionic strength of the standards has been adjusted to that of the test solutions by treating each with an appropriate buffer of high molarity. This eliminates errors that might be produced when analyzing solutions of widely varying ionic strengths. The emf of a cell incorporating an ion-selective electrode is usually determined with an expanded-scale pH meter. Such a pH meter can be used with a high-resistance input and allows any 100-mV portion of the voltmeter's scale to be expanded to the full scale, thus increasing the accuracy of the emf reading. Of course, like the ordinary pH meter, the voltmeter draws an infinitesimally small current from the electrochemical cell. This current is so small that it produces no distortion in cell emf, and the reading can

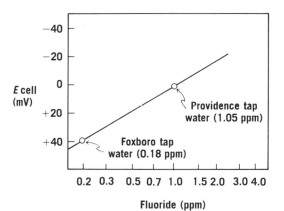

Fig. 9–11. Determination of fluoride in municipal water supplies using ionic-strength buffering. (Adapted from T. S. Light, in *Ion-Selective Electrodes,* R. A. Durst, Ed. N.B.S. Special Publication 314, Washington D.C., U.S. Government Printing Office, 1969.)

be considered essentially as a potentiometric determination.

Ion-selective electrodes have been used to determine the dissolution rate of tablets containing alkali metal ions,[7] and the release of sodium phenobarbital through a dialysis membrane has been studied by monitoring the dialyzed solution with a sodium-selective electrode.[8] Such applications can provide a rapid and continuous determination of the release rate of a drug from a formulation and may be particularly useful in monitoring slow-release preparations.[9]

Potentiometric Titration.[10] A glass electrode and a suitable reference electrode, such as the calomel electrode, can be used with a pH or millivoltmeter to measure cell emf for potentiometric acid–base titrations. The change in potential of the glass electrode is measured as the volume of titrant of a known concentration is added. The titration curves obtained by plotting E_{cell}, usually in millivolts, against the volume of titrant added are similar to those shown in Figure 8–1 (p. 175). When the endpoint is not marked by a sharp inflection in the curve, it is more desirable to plot the slope of the emf versus the volume of acid or base added, that is, $\Delta E/\Delta V$ against volume V. $\Delta E'$ can be obtained directly from the pH meter for a set change in volume, ΔV. A differential titration curve is obtained, Figure 9–12, the maximum point of which represents the endpoint of the titration.

An ion-selective electrode also may be used with a suitable reference electrode for potentiometric titrations. For example, ethylenediaminetetraacetic acid (EDTA) can be determined in solution by titrating with a standard calcium ion solution.

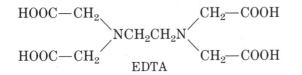

The calcium-EDTA complex is formed during the titration until the endpoint is reached, whereupon free calcium ion in solution can be detected with a calcium-selective indicating electrode. This endpoint is observed as a sudden increase in the electrode signal, analogous to the inflection observed in the previous acid–base titration.

Potentiometric Determination of Dissociation Constants.[10] The titration curve may be used to obtain a *rough* estimation of the dissociation constant of a weak acid by invoking the Henderson–Hasselbalch equation from Chapter 8:

$$pH = pK_a + \log \frac{[salt]}{[acid]} \qquad (9{-}42)$$

This equation is useful over a limited range for relatively dilute buffers. In practice, at the equivalence point of the titration where [salt] = [acid], the second term of the right-hand side of the equation becomes zero, and pH = pK_a. For a more exact determination of pK_a, the buffer equation should be used in its general form:

$$pH = pK_a + \log \frac{[salt]}{[acid]} + \log \gamma_A^- \qquad (9{-}43)$$

in which γ_A^- is the activity coefficient of the anion (p. 132). Introducing the Debye–Hückel expression (pp. 135, 170), the formula becomes

$$pH = pK_a + \log \frac{[salt]}{[acid]} - \frac{Az^2\sqrt{\mu}}{1 + a_iB\sqrt{\mu}} \qquad (9{-}44)$$

in which A, a_i, and B are constants and μ is the ionic strength. One experimental procedure involves "half-neutralizing" the acidic drug by titrating with sodium hydroxide until [salt] = [acid] and the [salt]/[acid] ratio becomes unity, whereby the second term on the right-hand side of equation (9–44) becomes zero, and

$$pH = pK_a - \frac{Az^2\sqrt{\mu}}{1 + a_iB\sqrt{\mu}} \qquad (9{-}45)$$

sodium chloride is added in varying amounts to produce solutions of different ionic strengths. The pH of each solution is determined, and the results are plotted against μ to yield a curve as shown in Figure 9–13. In this figure, phenobarbital is the weak acid, and sodium phenobarbital the salt. Extrapolating the line to the intercept of the vertical axis where $\mu = 0$ gives a close approximation to the thermodynamic dissociation con-

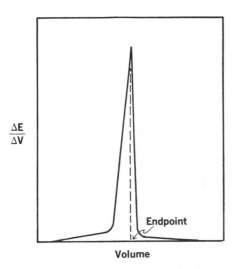

Fig. 9–12. Results of a potentiometric titration plotted as a differential curve of $\Delta E/\Delta V$ against the volume of titrant added.

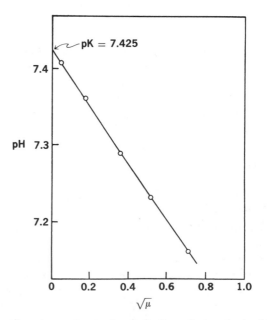

Fig. 9–13. Approximate determination of the thermodynamic dissociation constant of phenobarbital.

stant, pK_a, of the drug. An equation similar to (9–45) can be written for weak bases, and their pK_b values can be determined by an analogous procedure.

For the accurate pK_a or pK_b determination of an acid–base pair of unequal strength, correction should be made for the undissociated weak acid or base, as described by Benet and Goyan.[11]

Example 9–12. Calculate the dissociation constant and pK_a of valproic acid,

$$CH_3-CH_2-CH_2 \atop CH_3-CH_2-CH_2 \Big\rangle CH-COOH$$
Valproic acid

for a cell

$Pt|H_2$ (P = 1 atm)|valproic acid $(10^{-6}\ m)$,
sodium valproate $(10^{-8}\ m)$, H^+ $(?m)$ ‖ H^+ $(a = 1)|H_2$ (P = 1 atm)|Pt

which develops an emf of +0.175 volt.

As shown, the cell has a standard hydrogen electrode as the cathode (i.e., $E_{cathode} = 0.000$ volt). The reaction occurring at the hydrogen anode depends on the hydrogen ion activity according to the oxidation,

$$H_2 = 2H^+ + 2e^-$$

so

$$E_{anode} = E° - \frac{0.0592}{2} \log \frac{a_{H^+}{}^2}{P = 1\ atm} = 0.000 - 0.0296 \log \frac{a_{H^+}{}^2}{1}$$

Since

$$E_{cell} = E_{anode} + E_{cathode}$$
$$E_{cell} = 0.175 = 0.000 - 0.0296 \log a_{H^+}{}^2 - 0.000$$

Therefore, after rearrangement,

$$\log a_{H^+}{}^2 = -\frac{0.175}{0.0296}$$
$$a_{H^+}{}^2 = 1.22 \times 10^{-6}$$

and, if the activity coefficient is considered to be nearly unity under relatively dilute conditions, then $[H^+] = 1.11 \times 10^{-3}\ m$. Since the valproic acid is mostly undissociated under acidic conditions,

$$K_a = \frac{[H^+][valproate^-]}{[valproic\ acid]} = \frac{(1.11 \times 10^{-3})(10^{-8})}{(10^{-6})}$$
$$= 1.11 \times 10^{-5}\ approximately$$

and, therefore, the pK_a is about 4.96.

By using a method similar to the ionic strength method previously described in this section, Krahl[12] determined the dissociation constants of a number of substituted barbituric acids. Improved determinations have been introduced since 1940; a more recent listing of barbiturate pK_a values is provided by Prankerd and others in Table 7–6. Spectrophotometric methods are also used for determining pK_a values, as described on pages 81, 82 in Chapter 4. The pK_a of estrogens has been determined using a pH meter and a spectrophotometric assay procedure developed by Hurwitz and Liu.[13] A thorough description of potentiometric methods used for pK_a measurements is given by Albert and Serjeant,[14] and the determination of pK_a by various methods is reviewed by Cookson.[15]

The exact determination of the thermodynamic dissociation constant of a weak electrolyte involves the use of cells without liquid junctions. Such cells are described by Buck,[16] and methods using such cells are discussed by Harned and Owen.[17]

Hydrogen Ion Concentration in Oxidation—Reduction. Hydrogen ion concentrations must be considered in certain oxidation–reduction (redox) reactions, such as the oxidation

$$Mn^{2+} + 6H_2O = MnO_2 + 4H_3O^+ + 2e^- \quad (9-46)$$

The oxidation–reduction potential is given the symbol E_D. For the oxidation of Mn^{2+} at 25° C the oxidation–reduction potential is

$$E_D = -E° - \frac{0.0592}{2} \log \frac{a^4_{H_3O^+}}{a_{Mn^{2+}}} \quad (9-47)$$

which shows the influence of the hydrogen ion activity on E_D.

A number of reversible organic oxidation–reduction reactions of the quinone type involve acid–base equilibria and hence are influenced by hydrogen ions. As shown on page 192, the hydroquinone–quinone reaction is written as

$$\underset{\substack{\text{Hydro-}\\\text{quinone}\\\text{(reductant)}}}{H_2Q} + 2H_2O = \underset{\substack{\text{Quinone}\\\text{(oxidant)}}}{Q} + 2H_3O^+ + 2e^- \quad (9-48)$$

The potential for the *oxidation* is therefore

$$E_D = -E° - \frac{RT}{2F} \ln \frac{a_Q a^2_{H_3O^+}}{a_{H_2Q}} \quad (9-49)$$

or, in general,

$$E_D = -E° - \frac{RT}{2F} \ln \frac{a_{Ox}}{a_{Red}} - \frac{RT}{F} \ln a_{H_3O^+} \quad (9-50)$$

from which it is seen that increasing the hydrogen ion activity, or decreasing the pH, reduces E_D. If the pH of the system is held constant, the last term of equation (9–50) may be combined with $E°$ to yield a standard potential $E°'$, characteristic of the system at a fixed hydrogen ion activity or pH, which for an oxidation yields

$$E_D = -E°' - \frac{RT}{2F} \ln \frac{Ox}{Rd} \quad (9-51)$$

The standard potentials $E°'$ for some organic oxidation–reduction systems of importance to pharmacy and the biologic sciences are listed in Table 9–4, together with the pH at which they were determined.

The decomposition processes of many drugs in formulations can be described as oxidation–reduction reactions. For example, the decomposition of apomorphine in tablets can occur via the following reaction:

TABLE 9–4. *Standard Reduction Potentials at Specified pH Values for Some Oxidation–Reduction Systems**

Redox System	$E^{\circ\prime}$ (volt)	pH	Temperature (°C)
Homogentisic acid	+0.570	1.98	25
Epinephrine	+0.380	7.0	30
	+0.791	0.29	30
Vitamin K_1	+0.363	0.2 N HCl +95% alcohol	20
Cytochrome C	+0.256	6.77	30
Ascorbic acid	+0.115	5.2	30
	+0.136	4.58	30
Methylene blue	+0.011	7.0	30
Riboflavin	−0.208	7.0	30
	−0.117	5.0	30

*The algebraic sign of the $E^{\circ\prime}$ values in this table and throughout this chapter correspond to the reduction potentials as defined in the text.

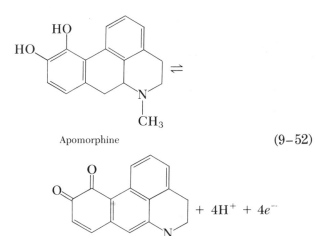

$$\text{Apomorphine} \qquad (9\text{–}52)$$

$$+ \, 4H^+ + 4e^-$$

Because of the participation of hydrogen ions in this reaction, the decomposition is pH dependent. It has been found that apomorphine is more stable in acidic formulations and rapidly decomposes in basic or neutral solutions. In general, the stability of many drugs in aqueous solutions often depends on the pH of the solution. Usually, pH must be controlled in liquid formulations to inhibit redox reactions, and for most drugs this requires a low pH. Stability and oxidation will be discussed in more detail later in this chapter. Chapter 12 treats the kinetics of drug stability.

McCreery[18] has shown that oxidation potentials of chlorpromazine metabolites at selected pH values can be associated with their pharmacologic features. Additionally, Marzullo and Hine[19] have associated redox mechanisms with opiate receptor function. Such conclusions, which associate redox potentials with drug actions at particular pH values, are important for drugs acting as neurotransmitters and help to explain mechanisms of drug–receptor interaction.

Titration Curves of Oxidation–Reduction Systems. An inorganic or organic oxidation–reduction system may be titrated by placing the solution in a cell containing a platinum and a suitable reference electrode, such as the calomel electrode. The potentiometric titration may be performed by adding measured quantities of either a powerful reducing agent, such as titanous chloride, to a buffered solution of the oxidized form of a compound, or an oxidizing agent, such as potassium dichromate, to the reduced form. If a 1N calomel electrode is used, the value 0.280 volt at 25° C is subtracted from E_{cell} to obtain E_D at any stage of the titration. Typical curves resulting from plotting the potential E_D of the inert electrode against the volume of reducing agent, or the percent reduction, are shown in Figure 9–14. When the system is 50% reduced, Ox/Red = 1 and $E_D = E^{\circ\prime}$ at a definite hydrogen ion activity. The slopes of the curves depend on n, the number of electrons transferred, and the vertical position of each curve on the graph depends on the value of $E^{\circ\prime}$. Oxidation–reduction systems are said to be *poised* to the maximum extent at half-reduction, just as acid–base systems show maximum buffer capacity at half-neutralization. A system that resists changes in E_D on the addition of oxidizing or reducing agents exhibits good *poising action*.

If an organic substance has two forms of different colors corresponding to its reversible oxidation–reduction couple, it may be useful as an indicator of the endpoint for an oxidation–reduction titration. Such indicators should show a color change that corresponds to a change in potential of the system rather than a change in concentration of one of the reactants. Most of these indicator redox systems depend on hydrogen ion concentration. For example, the redox indicator methylene blue undergoes the following reaction under neutral conditions (pH = 7) with $E^{\circ\prime} = +0.011$:

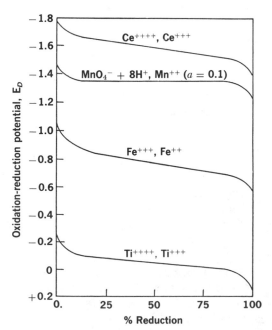

Fig. 9–14. Oxidation–reduction titration curves.

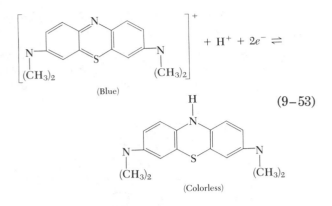

(Blue)

$$+ H^+ + 2e^- \rightleftharpoons \qquad (9\text{-}53)$$

(Colorless)

For changes in the hydrogen ion activity, the E_D range at which a color change of blue (oxidized form) to colorless (reduced form) occurs for this indicator at 25° C is given by

$$E_D = E° \pm \frac{0.0592}{n} + 0.0592 \log a_{H^+} \qquad (9\text{-}54)$$

This equation is derived from (9–50), in which a color change is defined as occuring for the ratio between

$$\frac{1}{10} \le \frac{a_{Ox}}{a_{Red}} \le 10 \qquad (9\text{-}55)$$

which is equivalent to a range of $\pm \dfrac{0.0592}{n}$ at 25° C for the second term on the right side of equation (9–50). From equation (9–54), the E_D range for methylene blue at pH 7 is calculated as approximately $+0.040$ to -0.019 volt. An oxidation–reduction indicator is useful within the narrow range of $E°' \pm 0.059$ when n is unity. Some commonly used indicators are listed in Table 9–5.

Oxidation–Reduction in Stages and the Use of Potential Mediators. Some oxidation–reduction reactions proceed in steps, particularly when n, the number of electrons between the oxidized and reduced states, is large. The oxidation–reduction reactions of many organic compounds involve a transfer of two electrons, which may be transported together or in consecutive steps. If two stages are involved, the oxidation titration curve shows two equivalence points, and the curve is similar to that

for a dibasic acid, such as H_2CO_3, titrated with the strong base, NaOH.

When n is large, the oxidation–reduction reaction may be slow, and the measured emf will be in doubt, since a truly reversible system is not attained. Under these circumstances, an easily oxidized or reduced substance may be added to act as a *potential mediator*. Ti^{3+} and I_3^- react together sluggishly except in the presence of certain indicators, acting as mediators, which accept electrons one by one from Ti^{3+} and donate them in pairs to the triiodide ion.[20]

Oxidation–Reduction in Pharmacy. Some pharmaceutical compounds are affected significantly by oxidation and reduction. These include ascorbic acid, riboflavin, vitamin K, epinephrine, vitamin E, morphine, and chlorpromazine. Additionally, fats and oils are susceptible to redox mechanisms. A limited number of examples are given here to show the kind of oxidation–reduction that can occur with medicinal compounds.

Ascorbic acid in aqueous solution oxidizes slowly in contact with air according to the following reversible reaction:

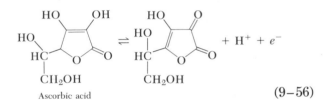

Ascorbic acid

$$+ H^+ + e^- \qquad (9\text{-}56)$$

This reaction is somewhat faster under acid conditions owing to hydrogen ion catalysis. The dehydration product can undergo further irreversible hydrolysis in alkaline solution to form diketogulonic acid and, eventually, oxalic acid, $(COOH)_2$, among other products. As the decomposition proceeds, the ascorbic acid solution turns from light yellow to a deep red color.

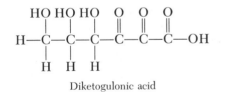

Diketogulonic acid

Ball[21] found that adding a small amount of a potential mediator, such as methylene blue, which has an $E°'$ value similar to that of the ascorbic acid system, creates a thermodynamically reversible system. By using a suitable oxidizing agent and mediator and buffering the system well in the acid range, one obtains $E°'$ from the E_D value at the point where 50% of the compound is oxidized according to equation (9–51). At a pH of 4.58 and a temperature of 30° C, the value of $E°'$ for the ascorbic acid system is $+0.1362$ volt.

Riboflavin, vitamin B_2, is also subject to a redox mechanism according to the reversible reaction.

TABLE 9–5. *Reduction Potentials of Some Oxidation-Reduction Indicators*

Substance	$E°'$ (reduction potential) (volt)	pH
p-Nitrodiphenylamine	+1.06	0
o-Toluidine	+0.87	0
Diphenylamine-4-sulfonate (Na salt)	+0.85	0
2,6-Dichloroindophenol (Na salt)	+0.217	7
Methylene blue	+0.011	7
Indigo trisulfonate (Na salt)	−0.081	7
Cresyl violet	−0.173	7

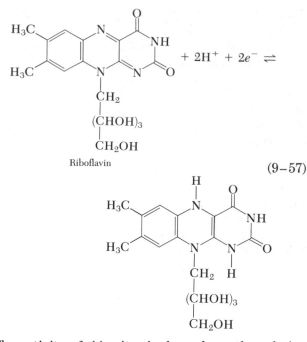

Riboflavin (9–57)

The activity of this vitamin depends on the relative amount of the dihydro product in a formulation. Dry preparations of riboflavin are quite stable; however, the redox reaction becomes significant when the vitamin is dissolved in aqueous solution, especially alkaline solutions that are exposed to sunlight. Both riboflavin and ascorbic acid have greatest stability, that is, the lowest rate of oxidation–reduction, when buffered on the acid side to pH 5 and 6, respectively.

In addition to pH control, oxidation or reduction can be controlled by the addition of compounds that are more easily oxidized or reduced, respectively, than the particular drug. In many instances, *antioxidants* are added to formulations to prevent the oxidation of a particular drug. Antioxidants must be oxidized more easily than the compound they are meant to protect. In a closed container, the antioxidant acts as a reducing agent to eventually consume the oxygen that is present. In many instances, combinations of antioxidants are used to increase their effectiveness. Typical water-soluble antioxidants include sodium bisulfate, ascorbic acid (used here *because* of its ability to oxidize), sodium sulfite, sodium metabisulfite, cysteine hydrochloride, thioglycolic acid, and sulfur dioxide. Oil-soluble antioxidants include ascorbyl palmitate, butylated hydroxyanisole (BHA), butylated hydroxytoluene (BHT), lecithin, propyl gallate, and α-tocopherol. The sulfite ion in aqueous solution undergoes oxidation according to the reaction

$$SO_3^{2-} + 2OH^- = SO_4^{2-} + 2e^- + H_2O \quad (9\text{–}58)$$

This reaction has a reduction potential, $E°$, of -0.93 volt, which is equivalent to a standard oxidation potential, in accord with the way the reaction is written, of $+0.93$ volt. Sulfite is a useful antioxidant for drugs that undergo redox reactions with smaller posi-

tive oxidation potentials, in other words, drugs that are less easily oxidized.

Example 9–13. Is a solution containing 10^{-2} M sulfite ion useful to prevent oxidation of 10^{-3} M ascorbic acid in a pH 7 aqueous solution at 25° C? K_1 for ascorbic acid at 25°C is 8.5×10^{-5}. K_2 is insignificant and may be neglected.

For the sulfite reaction:

$$K = \frac{[SO_4^{2-}]}{[SO_3^{2-}][OH^-]^2}$$

At pH 7, the OH^- and H_3O^+ concentrations must be equal so,

$$K_{(pH=7)} = \frac{[SO_4^{2-}]}{[SO_3^{2-}][H_3O^+]^2}$$

If we assume that the differences between activities and concentrations for the various species are small, the sulfite oxidation potential and concentration can be substituted in a slightly modified version of equation (9–50) to give, at 25° C,

$$E_D = -E° - \frac{0.0592}{2} \log \frac{[SO_4^{2-}]}{[SO_3^{2-}]} + 0.0592 \log [H_3O^+]$$

At pH 7, $[H_3O^+] = 10^{-7}$ M, and if we assume that the $[SO_4^{2-}]$ term should not exceed 10^{-7} M, that is, the sulfate level is being governed only by the availability of hydroxide ion to drive reaction (9–57), then

$$E_D = -E° - \frac{0.0592}{2} \log \frac{(10^{-7})}{(10^{-2})} + 0.0592 \log (10^{-7})$$

or

$$E_D = 0.93 + 0.15 - 0.41 = +0.67 \text{ volt}$$

It is of interest to note that if the $[SO_4^{2-}]$ term becomes somewhat larger, which would occur as oxidation proceeds, the second term on the right-hand side of the equation becomes smaller, which is consistent with a decrease in the oxidation potential.

For ascorbic acid, which is a dibasic acid, the $E°$ reduction potential value at 25° C is approximately -0.383 volt. Since the oxidation of ascorbic acid is similar to the hydroquinone redox reaction discussed on page 205 equation (9–50) becomes

$$E_D = -E° - \frac{0.0592}{2} \log \frac{[Ox]}{[\text{Ascorbic acid}]} - 0.0592 \log [H_3O^+]$$

For [Ox], one obtains

$$[Ox] = K_a[\text{Red}]/[H_3O^+]$$

Thus

$$[Ox] = 8.5 \times 10^{-5}[10^{-3}]/10^{-7} = 0.85$$

at equilibrium and

$$E_D = -E° - \frac{0.0592}{2} \log \frac{(0.85)}{10^{-3}} - 0.0592 \log(10^{-7})$$

$$= 0.383 - 0.087 + 0.414 = +0.710 \text{ volt}$$

At the beginning of the oxidation, [Ox] must be small compared with [Red]. If we assume that [Ox] is 10^{-7} M, comparable to $[H_3O^+]$, then before significant oxidation has occurred,

$$E_D = -E° - \frac{0.0592}{2} \log \frac{(10^{-7})}{(10^{-3})} - 0.0592 \log (10^{-7})$$

$$E_D = 0.383 + 0.118 + 0.414 = +0.915 \text{ volt}$$

Both the E_D value at the start of the oxidation and at equilibrium for ascorbic acid are greater than the E_D for sulfite. Therefore, the sulfite would not be effective as an antioxidant under the stated conditions. This implies that, at the concentrations specified at 25° C, ascorbic acid is a greater reducing agent than sulfite, and the oxidation of ascorbic acid would proceed *before* that of sulfite under the stated conditions. To prevent oxidation of ascorbic acid, some other compound should be chosen and the pH adjusted to a more acidic

TABLE 9-6. *Standard Potentials of Some Compounds that Readily Undergo Oxidation—Reduction**

	$E°$ (reduction potential) (volt)	$E°$ (Oxidation Potential) (volt)	Structure
Epinephrine	+0.808	−0.808	
Adrenalone	+0.909	−0.909	
Pyrogallol	+0.713	−0.713	
Catechol	+0.792	−0.792	

*From E. G. Ball and T. T. Chen, J. Biol. Chem. **102**, 691, 1933.

value. For example, dimercaptopropanol and various metal chelating agents have been found to reduce the rate of ascorbic acid oxidation under acidic conditions.[22] Such compounds are useful in pharmaceutical applications only if they are nontoxic.

Oxidation–reduction potentials are related to chemical structure, as shown in Table 9–6 for some hydroxyaromatic compounds. The more readily the reduced form loses electrons to yield the oxidized form, the better a reducing agent it is. Thus, pyrogallol, with its oxidation potential of −0.713 volt, is more easily oxidized, that is, it is a greater reducing agent, than catechol, with an oxidation potential of −0.792 volt. This greater ease of oxidation is related to the additional hydroxy group in the pyrogallol molecule.

Moore[23] has described a photooxidation system that can determine the relative efficiency of an antioxidant. The system measures the rate of a photochemically induced model oxidation reaction, the oxidation of benzaldehyde, after a known amount of an antioxidant is added. This method has been used to determine the efficiencies of a number of phenolic compounds with results that differ somewhat from the results in Table 9–6. For example, catechol is reported to be a more efficient antioxidant than pyrogallol. This implies that the relative efficiency of an antioxidant depends upon the specific mechanism of oxidation. Further work with other model systems may help to establish the relative dependency of antioxidation efficiency on oxidation conditions.

A number of new electrochemical methods and apparatus have been introduced into pharmaceutical analysis, and some of these are useful for the study of oxidation–reduction systems. Electron transfer in redox reactions may be measured today by *voltammetry* (current plotted against voltage), *chronoamperometry* (current plotted against time), *rotating electrode* techniques, and others. Studies[24-27] of antitumor activity, carcinogenesis, and antiviral and herbicidal activities provide examples of some applications of oxidation–reduction and voltammetry in analytic pharmaceutical chemistry. For a discussion of these rapidly advancing methods, refer to the literature[28,29] and the references given there to modern electroanalytic instrumentation.

References and Notes

1. C. D. Ferris, *Introduction to Bioelectrodes*, Plenum Press, New York, 1974, Chapter 4.
2. R. A. Durst, in *Ion-Selective Electrodes in Analytical Chemistry*, H. Freiser, Ed., Plenum Press, New York, 1978, Chapter 5; K. A. Connors, *A Textbook of Pharmaceutical Analysis*, 3rd Edition, Wiley, New York, 1982, pp. 134–139.
3. R. G. Bates, *Determination of pH: Theory and Practice*, Wiley, New York, 1973; C. C. Westcott, *pH Measurements*, Academic Press, New York, 1978; K. A. Connors, *A Textbook of Pharmaceutical Analysis*, 3rd Edition, Wiley, New York, 1982, p. 123.
4. G. A. Perley, Anal. Chem. **21**, 394, 1949.
5. W. C. Purdy, *Electroanalytical Methods in Biochemistry*, McGraw-Hill, New York, 1965, Chapter 3.
6. R. G. Bates, *Electrometric pH Determinations*, Wiley, New York, 1964, Chapter 9.
7. W. H. Thomas, J. Pharm. Pharmacol. **25**, 27, 1973.
8. W. H. Thomas and R. McCormack, J. Pharm. Pharmacol. **23**, 490, 1971.
9. G. J. Moody and J. D. R. Thomas, in *Ion-Selective Electrodes in Analytical Chemistry*, H. Freiser, Ed., Plenum Press, New York, 1978, Chapter 12, p. 409.
10. A. Albert and E. P. Serjeant, *The Determination of Ionization Constants*, 3rd Edition, Chapman and Hall, New York, 1984, Chapters 2 and 3; K. A. Connors, *A Textbook of Pharmaceutical Analysis*, 3rd Edition, Wiley, New York, 1982, p. 139.

11. L. Z. Benet and J. E. Goyan, J. Pharm. Sci. **56**, 665, 1967.
12. M. E. Krahl, J. Phys. Chem. **44**, 449, 1940.
13. A. R. Hurwitz and S. T. Liu, J. Pharm. Sci. **66**, 624, 1977.
14. A. Albert and E. P. Serjeant, *The Determination of Ionization Constants*, Chapman and Hall, London, 1971; ibid, 3rd Edition, 1984.
15. R. F. Cookson, Chem. Rev. **74**, 5, 1974.
16. R. P. Buck, in *Ion-Selective Electrodes in Analytical Chemistry*, H. Freiser, Ed., Plenum Press, New York, 1978, Chapter 1, p. 83.
17. H. S. Harned and B. B. Owen, Chem. Rev. **25**, 31, 1939.
18. R. L. McCreery, J. Pharm. Sci. **66**, 357, 1977.
19. G. Marzullo and B. Hine, Science, **208**, 1171, 1980.
20. P. A. Schaffer, J. Phys. Chem. **40**, 1021, 1936.
21. E. G. Ball, J. Biol. Chem. **118**, 219, 757, 1937.
22. K. A. Connors, G. L. Amidon and V. J. Stella, *Chemical Stability of Pharmaceuticals*, Wiley, New York, 1986, p. 217.
23. D. E. Moore, J. Pharm. Sci. **65**, 1447, 1976.
24. M. D. Ryan, R. G. Scamehorn and P. Kovacic, J. Pharm. Sci. **74**, 492, 1985.
25. R. Kenley, S. E. Jackson, J. C. Martin and G. C. Visor, J. Pharm. Sci. **74**, 1082, 1985.
26. M. M. Mossoba, M. Alizadeh and P. L. Gutierrez, J. Pharm. Sci. **74**, 1249, 1985.
27. P. W. Crawford, W. O. Foye, M. D. Ryan, and P. Kovacic, J. Pharm. Sci. **76**, 481, 1987.
28. R. N. Adams, J. Pharm. Sci. **58**, 1171, 1969.
29. R. V. Smith and J. T. Stewart, *Textbook of Biopharmaceutic Analysis*, Lea & Febiger, Philadelphia, 1981, Chapter 8.
30. E. G. Ball and T. T. Chen, J. Biol. Chem. **102**, 691, 1933.
31. R. Chang, *Physical Chemistry with Applications to Biological Systems*, Macmillan, New York, 1981, p. 308.
32. D. Eisenberg and D. Crothers, *Physical Chemistry with Applications to the Life Sciences*, Benjamin/Cummings, Menlo Park, Ca., 1979, p. 381.

Problems

9–1. Calculate the emf of the following cell at 25° C.

$$Zn|Zn^{2+} \ (a = 0.2) \ \| \ Cu^{2+} \ (a = 0.1)|Cu$$

Answer: 1.091 volt

9–2. For a cell consisting of one half-cell with a nickel electrode dipping into a solution of Ni^{2+} ions ($a = 0.1$) and the other half-cell a cadmium electrode dipping into a solution of Cd^{2+} ions ($a = 0.5$) at 25° C, which electrode must be the cathode and which the anode?

Answer: The cadmium electrode is the anode.

9–3. Calculate the oxidation potential of a finely divided iron electrode in an acidic solution of ferrous ion. The ferrous ion concentration is 0.50 M and the activity coefficient is 0.40. $E^\circ_{Fe \rightarrow Fe^{2+}} = 0.440$ (for oxidation) as seen in Table 9–1. The activity of the ferrous ion is obtained from the molar concentration and the activity coefficient. The electrons transported, n, is 2. The activity for solid iron, Fe, is unity.

Answer: $E_{electrode} = 0.461$ volt

9–4. Compute the emf of an iron-nickel cell:

$$Fe + Ni^{2+} \rightarrow Fe^{2+} + Ni$$

in which the activity of ferrous is 0.2 and that of ionic nickel is 0.4. The two half-cells may be combined as

$$Fe|Fe^{2+} \ (a = 0.2) \ \| \ Ni^{2+} \ (a = 0.4)|Ni$$

The electron transfer n is equal to 2.

Answer: $E^\circ_{cell} = 0.210$ volt; $E_{cell} = 0.219$ volt

9–5. Calculate E°_{cell} for an electrochemical cell consisting of a lithium electrode and a lead electrode each immersed in a solution of its ions at an activity of 1.00 at 25° C. (a) Represent the electrodes of the cell and write the cell reaction. (b) Calculate E°_{cell}. (c) Oxidation is to take place at the left electrode. Reverse the electrodes so that the oxidation cell now becomes reduction and vice versa. Calculate E°_{cell} under these conditions. It is possible for this reaction to occur? Is it easier for lead to be oxidized than lithium?

Answers: (a) $Li|Li^+ \ (a = 1) \ \| \ Pb^{2+} \ (a = 1)|Pb$; (b) $E^\circ_{cell} = 2.919$ volt; (c) this part is left for the student to answer.

9–6. Calculate the E°_{cell} for the reaction

$$Zn^{2+} \ (a = 1) + Cu \rightarrow Cu^{2+} \ (a = 1) + Zn$$

in which the half-cell reactions are

$$\frac{1}{2}Zn^{2+} \ (a = 1) + e^- \rightarrow Zn; \text{ and } \frac{1}{2}Cu^{2+} \ (a = 1) + e^- \rightarrow \frac{1}{2}Cu$$

Will copper reduce zinc in such a cell?

Answer: $E^\circ_{cell} = -1.100$ volts. The copper reduction potential in Table 9–1 is more positive than the zinc reduction potential. Therefore copper is more easily reduced than zinc, and a copper electrode cannot reduce a zinc electrode.

9–7. The standard emf E° of a cell consisting of a hydrogen gas electrode as the anode and a silver–silver chloride electrode as the cathode in an aqueous solution of HCl is 0.223 volt at 25° C. When the electrodes are immersed in a 0.50-M solution of HCl the mean ionic activity coefficient $\gamma_\pm$ is 0.77. (a) Write the overall cell reaction and the two half-cell representations. (b) Calculate the emf E of the cell at 25° C.

Answers: (a) see equations under Standard EMF of Cells, page 195; (b) $E = 0.272$ volt

9–8. Will mercurous mercury reduce ferric to ferrous iron at 25° C when both half-cells are at unit activity? This case is known as an oxidation–reduction system because it consists of mercurous, mercuric, ferrous, and ferric ions in solution. The two reduction reactions and their corresponding standard potentials at 25° C are found in Table 9–1:

$$Hg^{2+} + e^- = \frac{1}{2}Hg_2^{2+} \qquad E^\circ = +0.907$$

$$Fe^{3+} + e^- = Fe^{2+} \qquad E^\circ = +0.771$$

Answer: The half cell potential E° for the mercury electrode is more positive than that of the iron electrode. Mercury is reduced more easily than iron and therefore cannot reduce the iron.

9–9. Consider a concentration cell consisting of two lead electrodes immersed in lead sulfate solutions at 25° C with activities of 0.023 and 0.075:

$$Pb|Pb^{2+} \ (a_1 = 0.023) \ \| \ Pb^{2+} \ (a_2 = 0.075)|Pb$$

Calculate (a) the E°_{cell} and (b) the cell emf, E_{cell}.

Answers: (a) $E^\circ_{cell} = 0$, as for all concentration cells; (b) $E_{cell} = 0.015$ volt

9–10. As observed in Table 3–1, electrical energy consists of an intensity factor (electromotive force in volts) multiplied by a capacity factor (the quantity of electrical charge in coulombs). In terms of free energy change, the amount of work $-\Delta G$ done by an electrochemical cell operating reversibly is equal to the electromotive force E_{cell} multiplied by the charge transferred, i.e., n moles or gram equivalents, Eq, times the Faraday constant F in coulombs per mole:

$$-\Delta G = E_{cell} \text{ (volt)} \times (n \text{ Eq of charge transferred}) \times$$
$$F \text{ (96,500 coulombs/Eq)}$$

The resulting units on the free energy change are therefore volts × coulombs or joules.

(a) What is the free energy change ΔG for the cell reaction

$$I^- + AgCl = AgI + Cl^-$$

in which the standard emf is $E_{cell} = +0.361$ volt? This is not the standard potential, E°_{cell} (pp. 195, 196).

(b) The standard potential E° for the cell is $+0.379$ volt at 25° C. What is the value of the equilibrium constant, K (p. 194, equation (9–11)) and what is the value of ΔG°?

Answers: (a) $\Delta G = -34{,}837$ J/mole or -8326 cal/mole; (b) $K = 2.55 \times 10^6$, $\Delta G^\circ = -8740$ cal/mole or $-36{,}568$ J/mole

9–11. A concentration cell at 25° C is represented as

Ag, AgBr|Br⁻ ($a_1 = 0.02$) ∥ Br⁻ ($a_2 = 0.15$)|AgBr, Ag

What is the emf of this cell?

Answer: 0.052 volt

9–12. Calculate the electromotive force of the concentration cell

$$Zn|ZnSO_4 \,(0.01m) \parallel ZnSO_4 \,(0.1 \text{ m})|Zn$$

Hint: It will be necessary to change molalities to activities by reference to Table 6–1, p. 133.

Answer: $E_{cell} = 0.017$ volt

9–13. The pH of a solution containing benzylpenicillin and the potassium salt of this drug, both in a concentration of 0.02 mole/liter, was found to be 2.71 at 25° C. Compute the dissociation constant at this ionic strength, assuming that the average a_i value is 3×10^{-8}, B is 0.33×10^8, and A is 0.509 (equation 9–45, p. 204 and Table 6–4, p. 136).

Answer: $K_a = 1.69 \times 10^{-3}$

9–14. Instead of using the "half-neutralization" method for the determination of dissociation constants, equation (9–44) can be used directly if the concentration of acid and salt are known. The pH of a mixture containing 0.005 M of a new barbituric acid derivative and 0.01 M of its sodium salt was found to be 7.66 at 25° C. Compute the dissociation constant of the barbiturate at 25° C. The average a_i value is 2×10^{-8} and B is 0.33×10^8. A at 25° C is 0.509. (See Tables 6–3 and 6–4, p. 136).

Answer: $K_a = 3.92 \times 10^{-8}$

9–15. In *Example 9–4* we have a cell consisting of a hydrogen gas electrode as anode and a silver–silver bromide electrode as cathode in a solution of hydrobromic acid:

$$Pt|H_2 \,(1 \text{ atm})|HBr \,(0.0004 \text{ M})|AgBr|Ag$$

with an overall cell reaction of

$$AgBr + \frac{1}{2}H_2 = H^+ + Ag + Br^-$$

The cell emf, E, is found to be 0.4745 volt and the $E°$ value is 0.071 volt. Since the solid phases are assigned an activity of unity and the pressure of hydrogen gas is 1 atm, the emf of the cell can be written

$$E = E° - 0.0592 \log a_{H^+} a_{Br^-}$$

Calculate the mean ionic activity coefficient, $\gamma_\pm$, for the solution of HBr in this reaction.

Answer: $\gamma_\pm = 0.977$

9–16. Ball and Chen[30] oxidized a 0.002 M solution of epinephrine with a 0.002 normal ceric sulfate solution in the presence of 0.5 M sulfuric acid. The pH of the solution was 0.29 and the temperature 30° C.

(a) When 39.86% epinephrine was oxidized, i.e., [Ox] = 39.86%, and the remaining 60.14% was in the reduced form, i.e., [Rd] = 60.14%, the observed E_D was −0.7850 volt.

(b) When [Ox] = 71.5% and [Rd] = 28.5%, the observed E_D was −0.8030 at 30° C.

Compute $E°'$ for each case at 30° C.

Answers: **(a)** $E°' = -0.790$ volt; **(b)** $E°' = -0.791$ volt

9–17. A solution contains Fe^{3+} and Fe^{2+} in the ratio $a_{Fe^{2+}}:a_{Fe^{3+}}$ of 10:1. Compute E_D, the redox potential, at 25° C. *Hint:* See *Example 9–3.*

Answer: 0.712 volt

9–18. What is the useful E_D range at 25° C for the oxidation-reduction indicator diphenylamine-4-sulfonate (Na salt) in a solution at pH 8, assuming the hydrogen ion activity is the same as its concentration? *Note:* We find $E°'$ is equal to +0.85 at a pH of 0; we must calculate $E°'$ for pH 8. Then add and subtract the quantity 0.0592 to obtain the useful range. See equations (9–54) and (9–55).

Answer: +0.436 to +0.317 volt

9–19. (a) In the oxidation of ascorbic acid with potassium ferricyanide at 30° C, the E_D value observed when ascorbic acid was oxidized 35.43% was −0.1284 volt. What is the $E°'$ value?

(b) The E_D value observed when ascorbic acid was oxidized 90.79% was −0.1670 volt. Compute $E°'$ for this case.

(c) Using the average $E°'$ thus obtained, calculate $E°$ for a solution buffered at pH 4.58.

Answers: **(a)** $E°' = -0.1362$; **(b)** $E°' = -0.1371$; **(c)** $E_{av}^{o'} = -0.1367$; $E° = E_{av}^{o'} + 0.06016 \,pH = -0.1367 + (0.06016)(4.58) = 0.1388$ volt

9–20. In the assay of ascorbic acid in orange juice, Ball and Chen[30] titrated 10 mL of orange juice with 0.1 N potassium ferricyanide in 40 mL of an acetate buffer containing 0.001 M thionine as a potential mediator. The ferricyanide solution was standardized against a reference standard ascorbic acid, and each milliliter of the ferricyanide solution was found to be equivalent to 0.87 mg of ascorbic acid in orange juice. If 6.8 mL of ferricyanide was required to reach the endpoint, what is the concentration of ascorbic acid in a 100-mL sample of orange juice?

Answer: 59.2 mg

9–21. From *Problem 9–16* it is observed that the $E°'$ value of epinephrine at 30° C and pH 0.29 is −0.791. The oxidation potential of the system may be represented by the equation

$$E° = E°' + 0.06 \,pH$$

Compute $E°$ for epinephrine using this data, and compare your answer with the oxidation potential in Table 9–6.

Answer: $E° = -0.774$ volt

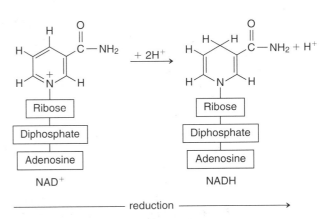

9–22.[31,32] In the oxidation of metabolites in the mitochondria of aerobic cells, nicotinamide adenine dinucleotide (NAD^+) serves as an oxidizing agent and is reduced to NADH, as shown in the above reaction. The $E°'$ value for the reaction at 25° C is −0.320 volt, with both NAD^+ and NADH at 1 M concentration ($a \cong 1$). A modification of the Nernst equation, viz. equation (9–51), is required to calculate E_D, the oxidation–reduction potential. Obtain the value of E_D when the reaction is conducted at a pH 1.0 (i.e., $[H^+] = 0.1$).

Answer: $E_D = -0.350$ volt

9–23. Calculate the equilibrium constant K and the standard free energy change $\Delta G°'$ for the biologic reduction of acetaldehyde to ethyl alcohol in which NADH serves as the electron donor or reducing agent for the reaction[31]

$$acetaldehyde + NADH + H^+ = ethyl \; alcohol + NAD^+$$

at 25° C. The standard potentials $E°'$ are

$$CH_3CHO + 2H^+ + 2e^- = C_2H_5OH \qquad E°' = -0.197$$

$$NAD^+ + 2H^+ + 2e^- = NADH + H^+ \qquad E°' = -0.320$$

Hint: Subtraction of these two half-cell $E°'$ values gives the overall cell $E°'$. $E°' = E°'_{left} - E°'_{right} = 0.123$ volt. Also $\ln K = \dfrac{nFE°'}{RT}$, $n = 2$.

Answer: $K = 1.44 \times 10^4$; at 298.15° K, $\Delta G°' = -23,739$ J/mole = −5674 cal/mole

10
Solubility and Distribution Phenomena

General Principles
Solvent—Solute Interactions
Solubility of Gases in Liquids
Solubility of Liquids in Liquids

Solubility of Nonionic Solids in Liquids
Distribution of Solutes Between Immiscible
Solvents

The topic of solutions was introduced in Chapter 5. We must now look at solutions in a more quantitative manner so as to understand the theory and applications of the phenomenon of solubility. Such knowledge is important to the pharmacist, for it permits him to choose the best solvent medium for a drug or combination of drugs, helps in overcoming certain difficulties that arise in the preparation of pharmaceutical solutions, and, furthermore, can serve as a standard or test of purity. A detailed study of solubility and related properties also yields information about the structure and intermolecular forces of drugs.

The solubility of a compound depends upon the physical and chemical properties of the solute and the solvent, as well as upon such factors as temperature, pressure, the pH of the solution, and, to a lesser extent, the state of subdivision of the solute.

Of the nine possible types of mixtures, based on the three states of matter (p. 102), only gases in liquids, liquids in liquids, and solids in liquids are of particular pharmaceutical importance and will be considered in this chapter.

GENERAL PRINCIPLES

Definitions. A *saturated solution* is one in which the solute is in equilibrium with the solid phase (solute). *Solubility* is defined in quantitative terms as the concentration of solute in a saturated solution at a certain temperature, and in a qualitative way, it may be defined as the spontaneous interaction of two or more substances to form a homogeneous molecular dispersion.

An *unsaturated* or *subsaturated* solution is one containing the dissolved solute in a concentration below that necessary for complete saturation at a definite temperature.

A *supersaturated solution* is one that contains more of the dissolved solute than it would normally contain at a definite temperature, were the undissolved solute present. Some salts such as sodium thiosulfate and sodium acetate can be dissolved in large amounts at an elevated temperature and, upon cooling, fail to crystallize from the solution. Such supersaturated solutions can be converted to stable saturated solutions by seeding the solution with a crystal of solute, by vigorous agitation, or by scratching the walls of the container. Supersaturation presumably occurs when the small nuclei of the solute required for the initiation of crystal formation are more soluble than larger crystals, making it difficult for the nuclei to form and grow with resultant failure of crystallization.

The Phase Rule. Solubility may be described in a concise manner by use of Gibbs' phase rule, which was described on page 37.

$$F = C - P + 2 \qquad (10-1)$$

in which F is the *number of degrees of freedom*, that is, the number of independent variables (usually temperature, pressure, and concentration) that must be fixed to completely determine the system, C is the smallest number of components that are adequate to describe the chemical composition of each phase, and P is the number of phases. The application of the phase rule to the miscibility of liquids is described on pages 40, 41 and the application to solutions of solids in liquids is given on p. 41.

Solubility Expressions. The solubility of a drug may be expressed in a number of ways. The U.S. Pharmacopeia and National Formulary list the solubility of drugs as the number of milliliters of solvent in which 1 gram of

TABLE 10–1. *Terms of Approximate Solubility*

Term	Parts of Solvent Required for 1 Part of Solute
Very soluble	Less than 1 part
Freely soluble	1 to 10 parts
Soluble	10 to 30 parts
Sparingly soluble	30 to 100 parts
Slightly soluble	100 to 1000 parts
Very slightly soluble	1000 to 10,000 parts
Practically insoluble, or insoluble	More than 10,000 parts

solute will dissolve. For example, the solubility of boric acid is given in the U.S. Pharmacopeia as follows: 1 g of boric acid dissolves in 18 mL of water, in 18 mL of alcohol, and in 4 mL of glycerin. Solubility is also quantitatively expressed in terms of molality, molarity, and percentage (p. 103).

For substances whose solubilities are not definitely known, the values are described in pharmaceutical compendia by the use of certain general terms, as given in Table 10–1. Solubilities of drugs are found expressed in various units in the *Merck Index*. For exact solubilities of many substances, the reader is referred to the works of Seidell, Landolt–Bornstein, *International Critical Tables*, Lange's *Handbook of Chemistry*, and the *CRC Handbook of Chemistry and Physics*. Techniques suitable for accurately determining the solubilities of solid compounds in liquids and the mutual solubilities of two liquids have been described by Mader and Grady.[1]

SOLVENT–SOLUTE INTERACTIONS

The reader should review pages 22 to 24 in Chapter 2 on intermolecular forces before continuing with this section. The pharmacist knows that water is a good solvent for salts, sugars, and similar compounds, whereas mineral oil and benzene are often solvents for substances that are normally only slightly soluble in water. These empiric findings are summarized in the statement: "like dissolves like." Such a maxim is satisfying to most of us, but the occasional inquisitive student may be troubled by this vague idea of "likeness." If he sets out to learn in what manner the solute and solvent are alike, he will find himself in a fascinating area of scientific investigation that is still in an unsettled state. The advanced student who is interested in this subject may wish to consult the books by Hildebrand and Scott,[2] Leussing,[3] and Dack.[4]

Polar Solvents. The solubility of a drug is due in large measure to the polarity of the solvent, that is, to its dipole moment. Polar solvents dissolve ionic solutes and other polar substances. Accordingly, water mixes in all proportions with alcohol and dissolves sugars and other polyhydroxy compounds.

Hildebrand has shown, however, that a consideration of dipole moments alone is not adequate to explain the solubility of polar substances in water. The ability of the solute to form hydrogen bonds is a far more influential factor than is the polarity as reflected in a high dipole moment. Although nitrobenzene has a dipole moment of 4.2×10^{-18} esu cm and phenol a value of only 1.7×10^{-18} esu cm, nitrobenzene is soluble only to the extent of 0.0155 mole/kg in water, while phenol is soluble to the extent of 0.95 mole/kg at 20° C.

Water dissolves phenols, alcohols, aldehydes, ketones, amines, and other oxygen- and nitrogen-containing compounds that can form hydrogen bonds with water.

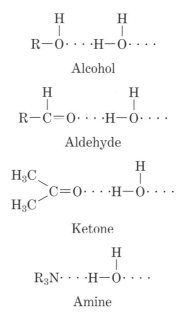

A difference in acidic and basic character of the constituents in the Lewis electron donor–acceptor sense also contributes to specific interactions in solutions.

The molecules of water in ice are joined together by hydrogen bonds to yield a tetrahedral structure. Although some of the hydrogen bonds are broken when ice melts, water still retains its ice-like structure in large measure at ordinary temperatures. This quasi-crystalline structure is broken down when water is mixed with another substance that is capable of hydrogen bonding. When ethyl alcohol and water are mixed, the hydrogen bonds between the water molecules are replaced partly by hydrogen bonds between water and alcohol molecules.

In addition to the factors already enumerated, the solubility of a substance also depends on structural features such as the ratio of the polar to nonpolar groups of the molecule. As the length of a nonpolar chain of an aliphatic alcohol increases, the solubility of the compound in water decreases. Straight-chain monohydroxy alcohols, aldehydes, ketones, and acids with more than four or five carbons cannot enter into the hydrogen-bonded structure of water and hence are only slightly soluble. When additional polar groups are present in the molecule, as found in propylene glycol, glycerin, and tartaric acid, water solubility increases greatly. Branching of the carbon chain reduces the nonpolar effect and leads to increased water solubility. Tertiary butyl alcohol is miscible in all proportions with water, whereas *n*-butyl alcohol dissolves to the extent of about 8 g/100 mL of water at 20° C.

In brief, polar solvents such as water act as solvents according to the following mechanisms.[5]

(a) Owing to their high dielectric constant, namely about 80 for water, polar solvents reduce the force of attraction between oppositely charged ions in crystals such as sodium chloride (p. 30). Chloroform has a dielectric constant of 5 and benzene one of about 2; hence, ionic compounds are practically insoluble in these solvents.

(b) Polar solvents break covalent bonds of potentially strong electrolytes by acid–base reactions since these solvents are amphiprotic (p. 143). For example, water brings about the ionization of HCl as follows:

$$HCl + H_2O \rightarrow H_3O^+ + Cl^-$$

Weak organic acids are not ionized appreciably by water; their partial solubility is attributed instead to the hydrogen bond formation with water. Phenols and carboxylic acids, however, are readily dissolved in solutions of strong bases.

$$R-\overset{\overset{\displaystyle O}{\|}}{C}-OH + H_2O \rightarrow \text{negligible}$$

$$R-\overset{\overset{\displaystyle O}{\|}}{C}-OH + NaOH \rightarrow R-\overset{\overset{\displaystyle O}{\|}}{C}-O^-Na^+$$

(c) Finally, polar solvents are capable of solvating molecules and ions through dipole interaction forces, particularly hydrogen-bond formation, which leads to the solubility of the compound. The solute must be polar in nature since it often must compete for the bonds of the already associated solvent molecules if it is to win a place in the associated structure. The ion–dipole interaction between the sodium salt of oleic acid and water may be depicted as

$$C_{17}H_{33}-\overset{\overset{\displaystyle O}{\|}}{C}-O^-Na^+ + n\,\boxed{H_2O} \rightleftharpoons$$

Nonpolar Solvents. The solvent action of nonpolar liquids, such as the hydrocarbons, differs from that of polar substances. Nonpolar solvents are unable to reduce the attraction between the ions of strong and weak electrolytes because of the solvents' low dielectric constants. Nor can the solvents break covalent bonds and ionize weak electrolytes since they belong to the group known as aprotic solvents (p. 143), and they cannot form hydrogen bridges with nonelectrolytes. Hence, ionic and polar solutes are not soluble or are only slightly soluble in nonpolar solvents.

Nonpolar compounds, however, can dissolve nonpolar solutes with similar internal pressures (p. 224) through induced dipole interactions. The solute molecules are kept in solution by the weak van der Waals–London type of forces (p. 22). Thus, oils and fats dissolve in carbon tetrachloride, benzene, and mineral oil. Alkaloidal bases and fatty acids also dissolve in nonpolar solvents.

Semipolar Solvents. Semipolar solvents, such as ketones and alcohols, can *induce* a certain degree of polarity in nonpolar solvent molecules, so that, for

TABLE 10–2. *Polarity of Some Solvents and the Solutes That Readily Dissolve in Each Class of Solvent*

Dielectric Constant of Solvent ϵ (approx.)	Solvent	Solute
80	Water	Inorganic salts, organic salts
50	Glycols	Sugars, tannins
30	Methyl and ethyl alcohols	Caster oil, waxes
20	Aldehydes, ketones and higher alcohols, ethers, esters, and oxides	Resins, volatile oils, weak electrolytes including barbiturates, alkaloids, and phenols
5	Hexane, benzene, carbon tetrachloride, ethyl ether, petroleum ether	Fixed oils, fats, petrolatum, paraffin, other hydrocarbons
0	Mineral oil and fixed vegetable oils	

(Left side: Decreasing Polarity ↓ — Right side: Decreasing Water Solubility ↓)

example, benzene, which is readily polarizable, becomes soluble in alcohol. In fact, semipolar compounds may act as *intermediate solvents* to bring about miscibility of polar and nonpolar liquids. Accordingly, acetone increases the solubility of ether in water. Loran and Guth[6] studied the intermediate solvent action of alcohol on water–castor oil mixtures. Propylene glycol has been shown to increase the mutual solubility of water and peppermint oil and water and benzyl benzoate.[7]

Summary. The simple maxim that *like dissolves like* can now be rephrased by stating that the solubility of a substance may be predicted only in a qualitative way in most cases and only after considerations of polarity, dielectric constant, association, solvation, internal pressures, acid–base reactions, and other factors. In short, solubility depends on chemical, electrical, and structural effects that lead to mutual interactions between the solute and solvent.

A number of common solvent types are listed in the order of decreasing "polarity" in Table 10–2, together with corresponding solute classes. The term *polarity* is loosely used here to represent not only dielectric constants of the solvents and solutes but also the other factors enumerated previously.

SOLUBILITY OF GASES IN LIQUIDS

Pharmaceutical solutions of gases include hydrochloric acid, ammonia water, and effervescent preparations containing carbon dioxide that are dissolved and maintained in solution under positive pressure. Aerosol products in which the propellant is either carbon dioxide or nitrogen, some of which is dissolved under pressure, can also be considered to fall under this classification.

The solubility of a gas in a liquid is the concentration of the dissolved gas when it is in equilibrium with some of the pure gas above the solution. The solubility depends primarily on the *pressure, temperature, presence of salts*, and *chemical reactions* that the gas sometimes undergoes with the solvent.

Effect of Pressure. The pressure of a gas above the solution is an important consideration in gaseous solutions since it changes the solubility of the dissolved gas in equilibrium with it. The effect of the pressure on the solubility of a gas is expressed by *Henry's law*, which states that in a very dilute solution at constant temperature, the concentration of dissolved gas is proportional to the partial pressure of the gas above the solution at equilibrium. The partial pressure of the gas is obtained by subtracting the vapor pressure of the solvent from the total pressure above the solution. If C_2 is the concentration of the dissolved gas in grams per liter of solvent and p is the partial pressure in millimeters of the undissolved gas above the solution, Henry's relationship may be written as

$$C_2 = \sigma p \qquad (10\text{--}2)$$

in which σ is the inverse of the Henry's law constant, k (p. 109). It is sometimes referred to as the *solubility coefficient*. Mole fraction is more properly used here, but in dilute solutions, molarity may be used.

The significance of Henry's law for the pharmacist rests upon the fact that the solubility of a gas increases directly as the pressure on the gas, and conversely, that the solubility of the gas decreases, so that sometimes the gas escapes with violence when the pressure above the solution is released. This phenomenon is commonly recognized in effervescent solutions when the stopper of the container is removed.

Effect of Temperature. Temperature also has a marked influence on the solubility of a gas in a liquid. As the temperature increases, the solubility of most gases decreases, owing to the greater tendency of the gas to expand. The property of expansion, coupled with the pressure phenomenon, requires that the pharmacist exercise caution in opening containers of gaseous solutions in warm climates and under other conditions of elevated temperatures. A vessel containing a gaseous solution or a liquid with a high vapor pressure, such as ethyl nitrite, should be immersed in ice or cold water for some time to reduce the temperature and pressure of the gas before opening the container.

Salting Out. Gases are often liberated from solutions in which they are dissolved by the introduction of an electrolyte such as sodium chloride and sometimes by a nonelectrolyte such as sucrose. This phenomenon is known as *salting out*. The salting-out effect may be demonstrated by adding a small amount of salt to a "carbonated" solution. The resultant escape of gas is due to the attraction of the salt ions or the highly polar nonelectrolyte for the water molecules, which reduces the density of the aqueous environment adjacent to the gas molecules. Salting out may also occur in solutions of liquids in liquids and solids in liquids.

Effect of Chemical Reaction. Henry's law applies strictly to *gases* that are only slightly soluble in solution and that do not react in any way in the solvent. Gases such as hydrogen chloride, ammonia, and carbon dioxide show deviations as a result of chemical reaction between the gas and solvent, usually with a resultant increase in solubility. Accordingly, hydrogen chloride is about 10,000 times more soluble in water than is oxygen.

Solubility Calculations. The solubility of a gas in a liquid may be expressed either by the inverse *Henry's law constant* σ or by the *Bunsen absorption coefficient* α. The Bunsen coefficient is defined as the volume of gas in liters (reduced to standard conditions of $0°$ C and 760 mm pressure) that dissolves in 1 liter of solvent under a partial pressure of 1 atmosphere of the gas at a definite temperature.

$$\frac{V_{\text{gas,STP}}}{V_{\text{soln}}} = \alpha p \qquad (10\text{--}3)$$

TABLE 10–3. *Bunsen Coefficients (α) for Gases in Water at 0° and 25° C*

Gas	α	
	0° C	25° C
H_2	0.0215	0.0175
N_2	0.0235	0.0143
O_2	0.0478	0.0284
CO_2	1.713	0.759

in which V_{gas} is the volume of gas at standard temperature and pressure, STP, dissolved in a volume V_{soln} of solution at a partial gas pressure p. The Bunsen coefficients α for some gases in water at 0° and 25° C are found in Table 10–3. The application of Henry's law and the calculation of σ and α are illustrated in the following example.

Example 10–1. If 0.0160 g of oxygen dissolves in 1 liter of water at a temperature of 25° C and at an oxygen pressure of 300 mm Hg, calculate (a) σ and (b) the Bunsen coefficient, α

(a)

$$\sigma = \frac{C_2 \text{ (g/liter)}}{p \text{(mm Hg)}}$$

$$= \frac{0.0160}{300} = 5.33 \times 10^{-5}$$

(b) To compute the Bunsen coefficient, one must first reduce the volume of gas to STP. According to the ideal gas equation, $V = nRT/p$.

$$V_{gas,STP} = \frac{\dfrac{0.0160}{32} \times 0.08205 \times 273.15}{1 \text{ atm}}$$

$$= 0.0112 \text{ at STP}$$

and from equation (10–3)

$$\alpha = \frac{V_{gas}}{V_{soln}\,p} = \frac{0.0112}{1 \times \dfrac{300}{760}} = 0.0284$$

(c) How many grams of oxygen can be dissolved in 250 mL of aqueous solution when the total pressure above the mixture is 760 mm Hg? The partial pressure of oxygen in the solution is 0.263 atm, and the temperature is 25° C.

$$\sigma = 5.33 \times 10^{-5} = \frac{C_2 \text{ (g/liter)}}{(0.263 \times 760) \text{ mm}}$$

$$C_2 = 0.0107 \text{ g/liter or } 0.0027 \text{ g/250 mL}$$

Oxygen is carried in the human body (a) as dissolved gas in the contents of the red blood cells and (b) as O_2 molecules bound to the iron atom of the heme part of hemoglobin. Shown here is part of the heme molecule of

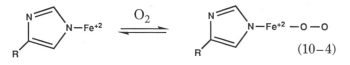

(10–4)

hemoglobin demonstrating the binding of two atoms of oxygen to the iron atom.[8] Hemoglobin is made up of four heme molecules and so has four iron atoms with which to bind four molecules of oxygen. The concentra-

tion of O_2 dissolved in the blood ([a] above) regulates the uptake and release of oxygen by the iron atoms in hemoglobin ([b] above).

Example 10–2. The partial vapor pressure[9], p, of oxygen in the blood is 75 mm Hg and the percent saturation of O_2 in the red blood cells has been determined to be 92.8%. What is the concentration of O_2 dissolved in the red blood cells (rbc's), exclusive of the binding of O_2 by the iron of hemoglobin?

The solubility coefficient, σ (inverse Henry's law constant), may be expressed in volume (cm³) at a definite temperature and pressure rather than mass (grams or moles) of gas dissolved in the solvent. The value of σ at 37° C for O_2 is 4.1×10^{-5} cm³ O_2/cm³ rbc content/mm Hg. Here, the solubility coefficient is actually more closely related to the Bunsen coefficient α than to the inverse Henry's law constant σ. From equation (10–2):

oxygen conc. $C_2 = (4.1 \times 10^{-5}$ cm³ solute/cm³ rbc/mm Hg)

$\times$ (75 mm Hg, O_2 pressure in blood)

$C_2 = 3.075 \times 10^{-3}$ cm³ O_2/cm³ rbc content

However, we learned above that O_2 in the rbc's is at only 92.8% of saturation. Therefore, $C_2 = 0.928 \times (3.075 \times 10^{-3}) = 2.85 \times 10^{-3}$ cm³ O_2/cm³ rbc content at a pressure of 75 mm Hg in the blood.

We now consider the second, and more significant, avenue for the transport of O_2 in the blood. The combining capacity has been determined to be 0.40 cm³ of O_2 per cm³ of rbc's; and at the partial pressure of oxygen of 75 mm Hg, the saturation of O_2 on the heme iron sites is not 100% but rather 18.7%. Thus,

(0.40 cm³ O_2/cm³ rbc content)(0.187) = 0.075 cm³

Although this may appear to be a small and inefficient binding of O_2 to hemoglobin, when compared with (a) above (the transport of O_2 by solution in the bulk content of the red blood cells), the hemoglobin binding as an O_2 transport system is 26 times more effective in carrying O_2 to the various tissues of the body:

$$\frac{0.075 \text{ cm}^3 \text{ O}_2/\text{cm}^3 \text{ rbc content}}{0.00285 \text{ cm}^3 \text{ O}_2/\text{cm}^3 \text{ rbc content}} = 26.3$$

Tables 10–4 and 10–5 give the k values for a number of gases in the solvents water and benzene. Several examples follow, showing the calculation of the Henry's law constant, k, and the solubilities of gases expressed in mole fraction, molality, or molarity and in grams of solute per liter of solution. The gaseous solutions that follow Henry's law are so dilute that essentially no difference exists between molarity and molality.

The Henry's law constant k as found in columns 3 and 4 of Table 10–4 may be represented as

$$k = \frac{p_2}{X_2}$$

$$= \frac{\text{pressure of gas (solute) in torrs or atmospheres}}{\text{mole fraction of the gas in solution}}$$

(10–5)

and the constant k in columns 5 and 6 as

$$k = \frac{p_2}{c \text{ or } m}$$

$$= \frac{\text{pressure of gas (solute) in torrs}}{\text{molarity, molality, or g/liter of gas in solution}}$$

(10–6)

TABLE 10–4. *Henry's Law Constants for Gases in Water at 25° C**

Gas	Molecular Weight	mm Hg (torrs) per Mole Fraction of Gas	Atm Pressure per Mole Fraction of Gas	mm Hg (torrs) per Molality or Molarity of Gas	mm Hg (torrs) per Gram of Gas per Kilogram H_2O or per Liter of Solution
H_2	2.02	5.34×10^7	7.03×10^4	9.62×10^5	4.76×10^5
He	4.00	1.10×10^8	1.45×10^5	1.99×10^6	4.98×10^5
N_2	28.01	6.51×10^7	8.57×10^4	1.17×10^6	4.18×10^4
O_2	32.00	3.30×10^7	4.34×10^4	5.94×10^5	1.86×10^4
CO	28.01	4.34×10^7	5.71×10^4	7.82×10^5	2.79×10^4
CO_2	44.01	1.25×10^6	1.64×10^3	2.24×10^4	5.09×10^2
CH_4	16.04	31.4×10^6	4.13×10^4	5.65×10^5	3.52×10^4
C_2H_6	30.07	23.0×10^6	3.03×10^4	4.15×10^5	1.38×10^4

*After F. Daniels and R. A. Alberty, *Physical Chemistry*, Wiley, New York, 1955, p. 200.

TABLE 10–5. *Henry's Law Constants for Gases in Benzene at 25° C**

Gas	mm Hg (torrs) per Mole Fraction of Gas
H_2	2.75×10^6
N_2	1.79×10^6
CO	1.22×10^6
CO_2	8.57×10^4
CH_4	4.27×10^5

*After F. Daniels and R. A. Alberty, *Physical Chemistry*, Wiley, New York, 1955, p. 200.

Although the k values for CO_2 are found in Table 10–4, this gas is too soluble to adhere well to Henry's law.

The inverse Henry's law constant σ is not listed for the gases in Table 10–4; it is obtained in each case simply by taking the reciprocal of k found in the table. The k values for gases dissolved in solvents other than water may be found in the literature. The k values for several gases in the solvent benzene, at 25° C, are listed in Table 10–5.

Example 10–3. *(a)* What is the solubility of oxygen in water at 1 atm pressure at a temperature of 25° C? Express the results in both molality and molarity.

Useful equations for converting from mole function X_2 to molality m and to molarity c are

$$m = \frac{1000\,X_2}{M_1(1 - X_2)} \quad \text{and} \quad c = \frac{1000\,\rho\,X_2}{M_1(1 - X_2) + M_2 X_2}$$

where M_1 is the molecular weight of the solvent, M_2 that of the solute, and ρ is the density of the solution. In a solution sufficiently dilute for Henry's law to apply, ρ is essentially 1.0 and $M_2 X_2$ may be ignored in the equation for c. Thus, molality and molarity are roughly equal in dilute solution.

Using k from Table 10–4, we find the solubility of O_2 in water at 1 atm and 25° C using the proportion

$$4.34 \times 10^4 \text{ atm/mole fraction} = \frac{1 \text{ atm}}{X_2}; \; X_2 = 2.30 \times 10^{-5}$$

molality, $m = \dfrac{1000(2.30 \times 10^{-5})}{18.015(1 - (2.30 \times 10^{-5}))} = 0.00128$ mole/kg H_2O

molality $\cong$ molarity, or $c \cong 0.00128$ mole/liter of solution.

(b) Calculate the Henry's law constant k for methane at 1 atm and 25° C, expressed in torr/(mole/kg H_2O).

From Table 10–4,

$$k_{(CH_4)} = 4.13 \times 10^4 \text{ atm/(mole fraction)} = \frac{1 \text{ atm}}{X_2}$$

$$X_2 = 1 \text{ atm}/(4.13 \times 10^4 \text{ atm/(mole fraction)})$$

$$= 2.42 \times 10^{-5} \text{ (mole fraction)}$$

Convert mole fraction of CH_4 to molality.

$$m = \frac{1000(2.42 \times 10^{-5})}{18.015(1 - (2.42 \times 10^{-5}))} = 1.344 \times 10^{-3} \text{ mole/kg } H_2O$$

k in torr/(mole/kg H_2O) is therefore

$$k = \frac{1 \text{ atm} \times 760 \text{ torr/atm}}{1.344 \times 10^{-3} \text{ mole/kg } H_2O} = \frac{760}{1.344 \times 10^{-3}}$$

$$= 5.65 \times 10^5 \text{ torr/(mole/kg } H_2O)$$

(c) Obtain the Henry's law constant for hydrogen, molecular weight $H_2 = 2.02$ g/mole, at a pressure in torrs at 25° C. Express k in torr/(g/liter), where g/liter is essentially equal to g/kg of water in a solution sufficiently dilute for Henry's law to apply. One obtains

$$k_{(H_2)} = \frac{760 \text{ torr}}{X_2 \text{ (mole fraction)}} = 5.34 \times 10^7 \text{ torr/(mole fraction)}$$

$$X_2 = 760 \text{ torr}/(5.34 \times 10^7 \text{ torr/(mole fraction)})$$

$$= 1.42 \times 10^{-5} \text{ (mole fraction)}$$

$$m = \frac{1000(1.87 \times 10^{-8})}{18.015(1 - (1.87 \times 10^{-8}))} = 7.88 \times 10^{-4} \text{ mole/kg } H_2O$$

$$\cong 7.88 \times 10^{-4} \text{ mole/liter}$$

To convert moles to grams, we write $g = $ mole $\times$ mol. wt.

$$7.88 \times 10^{-4} \text{ mole/liter} \times 2.02 \text{ g/mole} = 1.59 \times 10^{-3} \text{ g/liter}$$

$$k = \frac{760 \text{ torr}}{1.59 \times 10^{-3} \text{ g/L}} = 4.77 \times 10^5 \text{ torr/(g/liter)}$$

(d) Using the value of k you got in *(c)*, calculate the grams of hydrogen gas dissolved in a liter of aqueous solution at an external pressure of the gas of 1 atm (760 torr) at 25° C.

$$k = 4.77 \times 10^5 \text{ torr/(g/liter)} = \frac{760 \text{ torr}}{c \text{ (g/liter)}}$$

$$c = 760 \text{ torr}/(4.77 \times 10^5 \text{ torr/(g/liter)})$$

$$c = 0.00160 \text{ g/liter.}$$

(e) To obtain the Henry's law constant, k, for a gas at a temperature other than 25° C, we proceed as follows.

The solubility of O_2 in water at 1 atm pressure and 0° C is 0.070 g/liter. To express k in torr/(g/liter) we simply write

$$k = 760 \text{ torr}/(0.070 \text{ g/liter}) = 1.09 \times 10^4 \text{ torr/(g/l)}$$

In these examples involving the Henry's law constants, the term *mole fraction* is placed after the values of X_2 to indicate that the numbers are expressed as mole fractions—that is, as ratios of moles—and therefore are dimensionless, having no physical units associated with them.

SOLUBILITY OF LIQUIDS IN LIQUIDS

Frequently two or more liquids are mixed together in the preparation of pharmaceutical solutions. For example, alcohol is added to water to form hydroalcoholic solutions of various concentrations: volatile oils are mixed with water to form dilute solutions known as aromatic waters; volatile oils are added to alcohol to yield spirits and elixirs; ether and alcohol are combined in collodions; and various fixed oils are blended into lotions, sprays, and medicated oils.

Ideal and Real Solutions. According to Raoult's law, $p_i = p_i° X_i$, the partial pressure p_i of a component in a liquid mixture at a definite temperature is equal to the vapor pressure in the pure state multiplied by the mole fraction of the component in the solution. The mixture is said to be ideal when both components of a binary solution obey Raoult's law over the whole range of composition. If one of the components shows a negative deviation, it can be demonstrated by the use of thermodynamics that the other component must also show negative deviation (cf. Fig. 5–2, p. 108). The corresponding statement can also be made for positive deviations from Raoult's law.

Negative deviations lead to increased solubility and are frequently associated with hydrogen bonding between polar compounds (p. 23). The interaction of the solvent with the solute is known as *solvation*. Positive deviations, leading to decreased solubility, are interpreted as resulting from association of the molecules of one of the constituents to form double molecules (dimers) or polymers of higher order. Hildebrand, however, suggests that positive deviation is better accounted for in most cases by the difference in the cohesive forces of the molecules of each constituent. These attractive forces, which may occur in gases, liquids, or solids, are called *internal pressures*.

When the vapor is assumed to be nearly ideal, the internal pressure in cal/cm^3 is obtained by using the equation

$$P_i = \frac{\Delta H_v - RT}{V} \qquad (10\text{--}7)$$

in which ΔH_v is the heat of vaporization and V is the molar volume of the liquid at temperature T.

Example 10–4. The molar heat of vaporization of water at 25° C is 10,500 cal and V is approximately 18.01 cm^3. The gas constant R is 1.987 cal/mole deg. Compute the internal pressure of water.

$$P_i = \frac{10,500 - (1.987 \times 298.2)}{18.01}$$

$$= 550 \text{ cal/cm}^3 \text{ or } 22,700 \text{ atm}$$

A familiarity with calculations such as those appearing on pages 3 and 4 should allow the student to make this conversion from cal/cm^3 to atmospheres.

When the internal pressures or cohesive forces of the constituents of a mixture such as hexane and water are quite different, the molecules of one constituent cannot mingle with those of the other, and partial solubility results. Polar liquids have high cohesive forces, that is, large internal pressures, and they are solvents only for compounds of similar nature. Nonpolar substances with low internal pressures are "squeezed out" by the powerful attractive forces existing between the molecules of the polar liquid. This results in positive deviation from Raoult's law as shown in Figure 5–3 on page 108. It must be remarked that limited solubility of nonpolar solutes in highly polar solvents, and particularly in those solvents that associate through hydrogen bonds, cannot be attributed entirely to a difference of internal pressures. These factors will be considered in more detail on page 229.

Liquid–liquid systems may be divided into two categories according to the solubility of the substances in one another: (1) complete miscibility and (2) partial miscibility. The term *miscibility* refers to the mutual solubilities of the components in liquid–liquid systems.

Complete Miscibility. Polar and semipolar solvents, such as water and alcohol, glycerin and alcohol, and alcohol and acetone, are said to be completely miscible since they mix in all proportions. Nonpolar solvents such as benzene and carbon tetrachloride are also completely miscible. Completely miscible liquid mixtures in general create no solubility problems for the pharmacist and need not be considered further.

Partial Miscibility. When certain amounts of water and ether or water and phenol are mixed, two liquid layers are formed, each containing some of the other liquid in the dissolved state. The phenol–water system has been discussed in detail in Chapter 2, and the student at this point should review the section dealing with the phase rule. It is sufficient here to reiterate the following points. (1) The mutual solubilities of partially miscible liquids are influenced by temperature. In a system such as phenol and water, the mutual solubilities of the two conjugate phases increase with temperature until, at the critical solution temperature (or upper consolute temperature), the compositions become identical. At this temperature, a homogeneous or single-phase system is formed. (2) From a knowledge of the phase diagram, more especially the tie lines that cut the binodal curve, it is possible to calculate both the composition of each component in the two conjugate phases and the amount of one phase relative to the other. *Example 10–5* gives an illustration of such a calculation.

Example 10–5. A mixture of phenol and water at 20° C has a total composition of 50% phenol. The tie line at this temperature cuts the binodal at points equivalent to 8.4 and 72.2% *w/w* phenol (taken from Fig. 2–14, p. 40). What is the weight of the aqueous layer and of the phenol layer in 500 g of the mixture and how many grams of phenol are present in each of the two layers?

Let Z be the weight in grams of the aqueous layer. Therefore, $(500 - Z)$ is the weight in grams of the phenol layer, and the sum of the percentages of phenol in the two layers must equal the overall composition of 50% or 500 × 0.50 = 250 g.

$$Z(8.4/100) + (500 - Z)(72.2/100) = 250$$

weight of aqueous layer, $Z = 174$ g

weight of phenol layer $(500 - Z) = 326$ g

The weight of phenol in the aqueous layer is

$$174 \times 0.084 = 15 \text{ g}$$

and the weight of phenol in the phenolic layer is

$$326 \times 0.722 = 235 \text{ g}$$

In the case of some liquid pairs, the solubility may increase as the temperature is lowered, and the system will exhibit a *lower consolute temperature*, below which the two members are soluble in all proportions and above which two separate layers form (Fig. 2–15, p. 41). Another type, involving a few mixtures such as nicotine and water (see Fig. 2–16, p. 41), shows both an upper and a lower consolute temperature with an intermediate temperature region in which the two liquids are only partially miscible. A final type exhibits no critical solution temperature; the pair, ethyl ether and water, for example, has neither an upper nor a lower consolute temperature and shows partial miscibility over the entire temperature range at which the mixture exists.

Influence of Foreign Substances.[10] The addition of a substance to a binary liquid system produces a ternary system, that is, one having three components. If the added material is soluble in only one of the two components or if the solubilities in the two liquids are markedly different, the mutual solubility of the liquid pair is decreased. If the original binary mixture has an upper critical solution temperature, the temperature is raised; if it has a lower consolute temperature, it is lowered by the addition of the third component. For example, if 0.1 *M* naphthalene is added to a mixture of phenol and water, it dissolves only in the phenol and raises the consolute temperature about 20°; if 0.1 *M* potassium chloride is added to a phenol–water mixture, it dissolves only in water and raises the consolute temperature approximately 8°. This latter case illustrates the salting-out effect previously referred to under solutions of gases.

When the third substance is soluble in both of the liquids to roughly the same extent, the mutual solubility of the liquid pair is increased; an upper critical solution temperature is lowered and a lower critical solution temperature is raised. The addition of succinic acid or sodium oleate to a phenol–water system brings about such a result. The increase in mutual solubility of two partially miscible solvents by another agent is ordinarily referred to as *blending*. When the solubility in water of a nonpolar liquid is increased by a micelle-forming surface-active agent, the phenomenon is called *micellar solubilization* (p. 410).

Three-Component Systems. The principles underlying systems that may contain one, two, or three partially miscible pairs have been discussed in detail in Chapter

2. Further examples of three-component systems containing one pair of partially miscible liquids are water, CCl_4, and acetic acid; and water, phenol, and acetone. Loran and Guth[6] made a study of the three-component system, water, castor oil, and alcohol, to determine the proper proportions for use in certain lotions and hair preparations, and a triangular diagram is shown in their report. A similar titration with water of a mixture containing peppermint oil and polyethylene glycol is shown in Figure 10–1.[7] Ternary diagrams have also found use in cosmetic formulations involving three liquid phases.[11] Gorman and Hall[12] determined the ternary-phase diagram of the system, methyl salicylate, isopropanol, and water (Fig. 10–2.).

Dielectric Constant and Solubility. Paruta and associates[13] have studied the solubility of barbiturates, parabens, xanthines, and other classes of drugs in a range of solvents of various dielectric constants. The solubility of caffeine in a mixture of dioxane and water as determined in two laboratories is shown in Figure 10–3. The solubility is plotted against dielectric constant, and against solvent solubility parameter, δ, to be discussed later. Gorman and Hall[12] obtained a linear relationship when they plotted log mole fraction of the solute, methyl salicylate, versus the dielectric constant of isopropanol–water mixtures, as seen in Figure 10–4.

Molecular Connectivity. Kier and Hall[14] investigated the solubility of liquid hydrocarbons, alcohols, ethers, and esters in water. They used a topologic (structural) index χ, or chi, which takes on values that depend on the structural features and functional groups of a particular molecule. The technique used by Kier and Hall is referred to as *molecular connectivity*. A zero-order chi term, $^0\chi$, first-order chi term, $^1\chi$, and higher-order chi terms are used to describe a molecule. The $^1\chi$ term is obtained by summing the bonds weighted by the reciprocal square root number of each bond. In the case of propane,

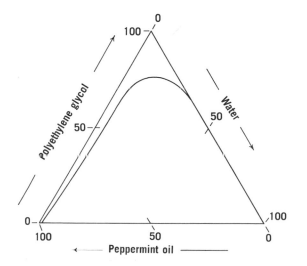

Fig. 10–1. A triangular diagram showing the solubility of peppermint oil in various proportions of water and polyethylene glycol.

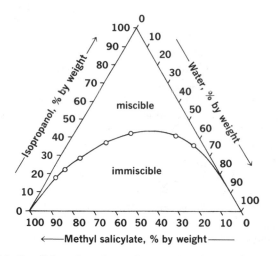

Fig. 10–2. Triangular phase diagram for the three component system, methyl salicylate–isopropanol–water. (From W. G. Gorman and G. D. Hall, J. Pharm. Sci. **53**, 1017, 1964, reproduced with permission of the copyright owner.)

$$\underset{H_3C}{\overset{①}{}}\overset{CH_2}{\underset{②}{}}\overset{③}{\underset{CH_3}{}}$$

disregarding attached hydrogens, carbon 1 is connected through one bond to the central carbon, which is joined to the other carbons by two bonds. The reciprocal square root "valence" is therefore $(1 \cdot 2)^{-1/2} = 0.707$ for the left bond. The right-hand bond has the same reciprocal square root valence, or 0.707. These are summed to yield

$$^1\chi = 0.707 + 0.707 = 1.414$$

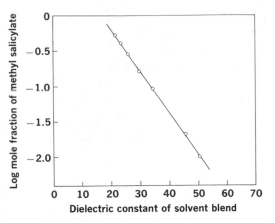

Fig. 10–3. Caffeine in dioxane–water mixtures at 25° C. Solubility profiles were obtained from two studies, A[13] and B.[34] Solubility in mg/mL is plotted against both dielectric constant (upper scale) and solvent solubility parameter (lower scale). (From A. Martin, A. N. Paruta, and A. Adjei, J. Pharm. Sci. **70**, 1115, 1981, reproduced with permission of the copyright owner.)

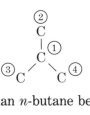

Fig. 10–4. Solubility of methyl salicylate in isopropanol–water blends of differing dielectric constants. (From W. G. Gorman and G. D. Hall, J. Pharm. Sci. **53**, 1017, 1964, reproduced with permission of the copyright owner.)

for *n*-butane, considering only the carbon atoms and their bonds,

$$\underset{C}{\overset{①}{}}\overset{C}{\underset{②}{}}\underset{C}{\overset{③}{}}\overset{C}{\underset{④}{}}$$

$$^1\chi = (1 \cdot 2)^{-1/2} + (2 \cdot 2)^{-1/2} + (1 \cdot 2)^{-1/2} = 1.914$$

Isobutane,

$$\overset{②}{C}$$
$$\underset{③}{\overset{①}{C}}\underset{C}{}\overset{④}{C}$$

has a different $^1\chi$ than *n*-butane because of its branching:

$$^1\chi = (1 \cdot 3)^{-1/2} + (1 \cdot 3)^{-1/2} + (1 \cdot 3)^{-1/2} = 1.732$$

For calculating second- and higher-order χ indexes and applications of molecular connectivity in pharmacy, refer to the book by Kier and Hall.[14]

$^1\chi$ may be used to correlate the molal solubilities of aliphatic hydrocarbons, alcohols, and esters in water, using regression analysis (see Chapter 1, p. 15, for regression analysis). The equation found[14] to fit the data for alkanes at 25° C is

$$\ln S = -1.505 - 2.533\, ^1\chi \qquad (10-8)$$

We learned that the $^1\chi$ value of isobutane was 1.732. Using this value in equation (10–8) yields

$$\ln S = -5.8922; \quad S = 2.76 \times 10^{-3}\ \text{molal}$$

The experimentally observed solubility of isobutane in water at 25° C is 2.83×10^{-3} molal.

Molecular Surface Area and Solubility. Amidon and associates[15] have published a number of papers dealing with the solubility of liquid nonelectrolytes in polar solvents. They investigated the aqueous solubility of hydrocarbons, alcohols, esters, ketones, ethers, and carboxylic acids. The method consisted of regression analysis, in which ln (solubility) of the solute is correlated with the total surface area (TSA) of the solute. Excluding olefins, the equation that gave the best correlation with 158 compounds was

$$\log \text{(solubility)} = 0.0168 \text{ (TSA)} + 4.44 \quad (10-9)$$

The TSA of a compound was calculated using a computer program prepared earlier by Hermann.[16,17] Elaborations on the Hermann approach involved dividing the TSA of the solute into *hydrocarbon* and *functional group* surface-area contributions (HYSA and FGSA, respectively).

The following equation was developed by Amidon et al.[15] for calculating molal solubility of hydrocarbons and alcohols in water at 25° C:

$$\ln \text{(solubility)} = -0.0430 \text{ (HYSA)}$$
$$- 0.0586 \text{ (FGSA)} + 8.003 \text{ } (I) + 4.420 \quad (10-10)$$

in which (FGSA) is the surface area for the hydroxyl group. It was found that an indicator variable, I, was needed in equation (10–10) to handle the alcohols. I was given a value of 1 if the compound was an alcohol and 0 if it was a hydrocarbon (no OH groups present).

Example 10–6. Calculate the molar solubility in water at 25° C for *n*-butanol and for cyclohexane using equation (10–10). Determine the percent difference from the observed values. The observed solubilities and the surface areas calculated with the modified computer program of Hermann are found in Table 10–6.

For *n*-butanol:

$$\ln \text{(solubility)} = -0.0430 \text{ (212.9)}$$
$$-0.0586 \text{ (59.2)} + (8.003) \text{ (l)} + 4.420$$
$$\ln \text{(solubility)} = -0.20082$$

Molal solubility = 0.818 (error = 18.7%

from the observed value, 1.006)

For cyclohexane:

$$\ln \text{(solubility)} = -0.0430 \text{ (279.1)} -0.586(0) + (8.003) \text{ (0)} + 4.420$$
$$= -7.5813$$

Molal solubility = 5.1×10^{-4} (error = 22.8%

from the observed value, 6.61×10^{-4})

The method of Amidon et al. may prove applicable for predicting solubilities of complex organic drug molecules that have limited solubility in water.

TABLE 10–6. *Molecular Surface Areas of Alcohols and Hydrocarbons*

	HYSA (angstroms)^2	FGSA (angstroms)^2	Observed Solubility (molal)
n-butanol	212.9	59.2	1.006
Cyclohexanol	240.9	49.6	3.8×10^{-1}
Cyclohexane	279.1	—	6.61×10^{-4}
n-Octane	383	—	5.80×10^{-6}

Key: HYSA = hydrocarbon surface area; FGSA = functional group surface area (OH group in the case of an alcohol).

SOLUBILITY OF SOLIDS IN LIQUIDS

Systems of solids in liquids include the most frequently encountered and probably the most important type of pharmaceutical solutions. The solubility of a solid in a liquid cannot be predicted in a wholly satisfactory manner as yet, except possibly for ideal solutions, because of the complicating factors that must be taken into account.

Pharmaceutical solutions consist of a wide variety of solutes and solvents, as listed in Table 10–2. We shall begin with the ideal solution, proceeding then to regular solutions of nonpolar or moderately polar character and finally to solutions of high polarity, in which solvation and association result in marked deviation from ideal behavior.

In this limited treatment, only the highlights of the derivations are sketched out, and the resulting equations are given without a detailed development of each step in the formulation. It is hoped, however, that the worked examples will show the usefulness of the various equations and that the selected references will lead the interested reader to the original literature where details can be found.

Ideal Solutions. The solubility of a solid in an ideal solution depends on temperature, melting point of the solid, and molar heat of fusion ΔH_f, that is, the heat absorbed when the solid melts. In an ideal solution, the heat of solution is equal to the heat of fusion, which is assumed to be a constant independent of the temperature. Ideal solubility is not affected by the nature of the solvent. The equation derived from thermodynamic considerations for an ideal solution of a solid in a liquid is

$$-\log X_2{}^i = \frac{\Delta H_f}{2.303R} \left(\frac{T_0 - T}{TT_0} \right) \quad (10-11)$$

in which $X_2{}^i$ is the ideal solubility of the solute expressed in mole fraction, T_0 is the melting point of the solid solute in absolute degrees, and T is the absolute temperature of the solution.* The superscript ^{i} in the symbol $X_2{}^i$ refers to an ideal solution, and the subscript $_2$ designates the mole fraction as that of the solute. At temperatures above the melting point, the solute is in the liquid state, and, in an ideal solution, the liquid solute is miscible in all proportions with the solvent. Therefore, equation (10–11) no longer applies when $T > T_0$. The equation is also inadequate at temperatures considerably below the melting point where ΔH_f can no longer be used.

Example 10–7. What is the solubility of naphthalene at 20° C in an ideal solution? The melting point of naphthalene is 80° C, and the molar heat of fusion is 4500 cal/mole.

---

*Hildebrand and Scott[2] show that calculated results compare better with experimental values if terms involving ΔC_p, the difference in heat capacities of the solid and liquid, are also included in the equation.

$$\log X_2{}^i = -\frac{4500}{2.303 \times 1.987} \frac{(353 - 293)}{293 \times 353}$$

$$X_2{}^i = 0.27$$

The mole fraction solubility can be converted to molality (provided the molecular weight M_1 of the solvent is known) by means of the relationship

$$m = \frac{1000 X_2}{M_1(1 - X_2)}$$

The value of X_2 in *Example 10–7* may be compared with the results of Scatchard.[18] He found that the mole fraction solubility of naphthalene was 0.24 in benzene, 0.23 in toluene, and 0.21 in carbon tetrachloride at 20° C.

Equation (10–11) can also be written as

$$\log X_2{}^i = -\frac{\Delta H_f}{2.303 R} \frac{1}{T} + \text{constant} \quad (10\text{–}12)$$

Therefore, a plot of the logarithm of the solubility, expressed in mole fraction, against the reciprocal of the absolute temperature results in a straight line with a slope of $-\Delta H_f/2.303R$ for an ideal solution. By this means, the molar heat of fusion of various drugs may be obtained from their solubility in ideal solutions.

The molar heat of fusion is determined most conveniently in a differential scanning calorimeter (see p. 47). The Drug Standards Laboratory of the United States Pharmacopeial Convention in Washington, D. C., has determined the ΔH_f values for a number of drugs, and these, together with values from other sources, are found in Table 10–7.

Phase Diagrams and the Ideal Solubility Equation.[19] The phase diagram for the system thymol–salol, shown in Figure 2–17 (p. 42), may be constructed with the help of the ideal solubility equation (equations (10–11) and (10–12)). Conversely, if the points along the two lines of Figure 2–17 are obtained experimentally, they may be used together with the ideal solubility equation (equation (10–11) or (10–12)) to calculate the heats of fusion ΔH_f of substances such as salol and thymol, which are completely miscible in the liquid state, immiscible as solids, and form eutectic mixtures. Phase diagrams, such as Figure 2–17, have been used to study matrix-type dosage forms, changes in the solubility of drug mixtures as a function of temperature and composition, and to locate the eutectic point for mixtures of various pharmaceutical excipients.[20–23]

Example 10–8.[24,25] To demonstrate the use of the ideal solubility equation (equation (10–11)), we begin by calculating several points on the phase diagram, Figure 2–17, first taking thymol as the solute and salol as the solvent. This puts us on the right-hand side of the graph. The heat of fusion ΔH_f of thymol is 4126 cal/mole, the melting point is 51.5° C (324.7° K), and the molecular weight is 150.2 g/mole. The melting point of salol is 42.0° C (315.2° K), and its molecular weight is 214.2 g/mole.

(a) Let us calculate the ideal solubilities of thymol, expressed as mole fraction, at 20°, 30°, and 40° C, using the ideal solubility equation (equation (10–11)). Once the mole fraction solubilities are obtained

TABLE 10–7. *Heats of Fusion for Drugs and Other Molecules** *

	ΔH_f (cal/mole)
Anthracene	6,897
Benzoic acid	4,302
Butyl *p*-hydroxybenzoate	6,410
Brompheniramine maleate	11,200
Caffeine	5,044
Cannabidiol	4,660
Cetyl alcohol	8,194
Chlorpromazine hydrochloride	6,730
Estradiol cypionate	7,030
Iodine	3,740
Meprobamate	9,340
Methoxyphenamine hydrochloride	6,960
Methyl *p*-aminobenzoate	5,850
Methyl *p*-hydroxybenzoate	5,400
Methyltestosterone	6,140
Myristic acid	10,846
Naphthalene	4,440
Phenanthrene	4,456
Phenylephrine hydrochloride	6,800
Phenytoin	11,300
p-Aminobenzoic acid	5,000
p-Hydroxybenzoic acid	7,510
Protriptyline hydrochloride	6,140
Stearic acid	13,524
Sulfadiazine	9,740
Sulfamethoxazole	7,396
Sulfapyridine	8,930
Sulfisomidine	10,780
Sulfur	4,020
Testolactone	6,760
Testosterone	6,190
Testosterone enanthate	5,260
Testosterone propionate	5,290
Theobromine	9,818
Theophylline	7,097
Thiopental	7,010
Tolbutamide	6,122

*Data from the Drug Standards Laboratory of the U.S. Pharmacopeial Convention (courtesy U.S. Pharmacopeial Drug Research and Testing Laboratories); *Handbook of Chemistry and Physics*, R. C. Weast, Ed., CRC, Cleveland, Ohio, 1975, pp. 717–719; S. H. Yalkowsky, G. L. Flynn and T. G. Slunick, J. Pharm. Sci. **61**, 852, 1972; K. C. James and M. Roberts, J. Pharm. Pharmacol. **20**, 1045, 1968; S. S. Yang and J. K. Guillory, J. Pharm. Sci. **61**, 26, 1972. (See S. S. Yang and J. K. Guillory, J. Pharm. Sci. **61**, 26, 1972, and H. O. Lin and J. K. Guillory, J. Pharm. Sci. **59**, 973, 1970, for the effect of polymorphism on the ΔH_f of sulfonamides.)

they may be converted to molalities, $m = 1000 X_2/M_1(1 - X_2)$, and from molalities to weight percent (%[w/w]). The three points may be plotted on the right-hand side of a graph, patterned after Figure 2–17, and a straight line drawn through the points.

The approach taken with thymol as solute and salol as solvent at 40° C (313.2° K) is as follows:

$$\ln X_2 = \frac{-4126}{1.9872}\left(\frac{324.7 - 313.2}{324.7 \cdot 313.2}\right) = -0.235$$

The anti-ln (that is, the exponential, e^x), of ln X_2, −0.235, at 40° C is

$$X_2{}^{40°} = 0.791 \text{ or } 72.63\% \text{ (w/w)}$$

At 30° and 20° C, the X_2 values are

$$X_2{}^{30°} = 0.635$$

$$X_2{}^{20°} = 0.503$$

We now assume that phenyl salicylate (salol), molecular weight 214.2 g/mole, is the solute and thymol is the solvent. It is difficult to find the heat of fusion ΔH_f for salol in the literature; let us work backwards to calculate it. Knowing the melting point of salol, 42° C, and calculating its mole fraction near the temperature (melting point) for the pure liquid at, say, 35° C, we obtain, with the help of equation (10–11), a good estimate for the heat of fusion of salol. One gets a more accurate value for ΔH_f where the solute, salol, is in high concentration; that is, near the left-hand side of Figure 2–17.

(b) With salol as the solute (left side of the phase diagram) at 35° C (308.2° K), the solution contains 9% (w/w) thymol and 91% (w/w) salol. One converts to mole fraction of salol, using the equation

$$X_2 = \frac{n_2}{n_2 + n_1}$$

The mole n_2 of salol at 35° C is 91 g/214.2 g/mole = 0.4248 mole and the mole n_1 of thymol is 9 g/150.2 g/mole = 0.0599 mole. The mole fraction is therefore

$$X_2 = \frac{0.4248}{0.4248 + 0.0599} = 0.8764$$

$$\ln X_2 = -0.1319 = -\frac{\Delta H_f}{1.9872}\left(\frac{315.2 - 308.2}{315.2 \cdot 308.2}\right)$$

$$\Delta H_f \text{ (salol)} = 3639 \text{ cal/mole}$$

At 35° C the solution should behave nearly ideal, for salol is in the concentration of 91% (w/w), and the ΔH_f obtained should be a reasonable estimate of the heat of fusion of salol.

Nonideal Solutions. The activity of a solute in a solution is expressed as the concentration multiplied by the activity coefficient. When the concentration is given in mole fraction, the activity is expressed as

$$a_2 = X_2\gamma_2 \qquad (10\text{–}13)$$

in which γ_2 on the mole fraction scale is known as the rational activity coefficient (p. 132). Converting to logarithms, we have

$$\log a_2 = \log X_2 + \log \gamma_2 \qquad (10\text{–}14)$$

In an ideal solution, $a_2 = X_2{}^i$ since $\gamma_2 = 1$, and accordingly the ideal solubility, equation (10–14), may be expressed in terms of activity as

$$-\log a_2 = -\log X_2{}^i = \frac{\Delta H_f}{2.303RT}\left(\frac{T_0 - T}{T_0}\right) \qquad (10\text{–}15)$$

By combining equations (10–14) and (10–15), the mole fraction solubility of a solute in a nonideal solution, expressed in log form, becomes

$$-\log X_2 = \frac{\Delta H_f}{2.303R}\left(\frac{T_0 - T}{T_0 \, T}\right) + \log \gamma_2 \qquad (10\text{–}16)$$

Therefore, the mole fraction solubility in various solvents can be expressed as the sum of two terms: the solubility in an ideal solution and the logarithm of the activity coefficient of the solute. As a real solution becomes more ideal, γ_2 approaches unity, and equation (10–16) reduces to equation (10–15). Only rarely, however, does the experimentally determined solubility in real solutions compare favorably with the value calculated by use of the ideal solubility equation. The activity coefficient γ_2, depending on the nature of both the solute and the solvent as well as on the temperature of the solution, must be accounted for before the calculated solubility will correspond well with experimental values.

The log γ_2 term of equation (10–16) is obtained by considering the intermolecular forces of attraction that must be overcome, or the work that must be done, in removing a molecule from the solute phase and depositing it in the solvent. This process may be considered as occurring in three steps.[26]

1. The first step involves the removal of a molecule from the solute phase at a definite temperature. The work done in removing a molecule from a solute so that it passes into the vapor state requires breaking the bonds between adjacent molecules. The work involved in breaking the bond between two adjacent molecules is $2w_{22}$, in which the subscript $_{22}$ refers to the interaction between solute molecules. When the molecule escapes from the solute phase, however, the hole it has created closes, and one half of the energy is regained. The gain in potential energy or net work for the process is thus w_{22}, schematically represented as

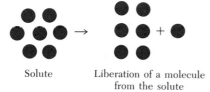

Solute   Liberation of a molecule
from the solute

2. The second step involves the creation of a hole in the solvent just large enough to accept the solute molecule. The work required for this step,

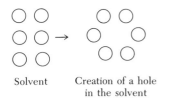

Solvent   Creation of a hole
in the solvent

is w_{11}, in which the subscript refers to the energy of interaction between solvent molecules.

3. The solute molecule is finally placed in the hole in the solvent,

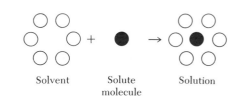

Solvent   Solute   Solution
molecule

and the gain in work or decrease of potential energy in this step is $-w_{12}$. The subscript $_{12}$ stands for the interaction energy of the solute with the solvent. The hole or cavity in the solvent, created in step 2, is now closed, and an additional decrease in energy, $-w_{12}$, occurs, involving net work in this final step of $-2w_{12}$.

The total work as given by this extremely simplified scheme is thus $(w_{22} + w_{11} - 2w_{12})$. The activity coefficient term of the solubility equation, however, has been shown by Scatchard and by Hildebrand and Wood[18] to be proportional also to the volume of the solute, considered as a supercooled liquid, and to the fraction of the total volume occupied by the solvent. The logarithm of the activity coefficient is given by the more elaborate expression

$$\ln \gamma_2 = (w_{22} + w_{11} - 2w_{12}) \frac{V_2 \Phi_1^2}{RT} \quad (10-17)$$

in which V_2 is the molar volume or volume per mole of (supercooled) liquid solute and Φ_1 is the volume fraction, or $X_1V_1/(X_1V_1 + X_2V_2)$ of the solvent. R is the gas constant, 1.987 cal/mole deg, and T is the absolute temperature of the solution.

The w terms in equation (10-17) are potential energies or terms representing attractive forces. Since van der Waals forces between molecules follow a geometric mean rule, the term w_{12} can be taken as approximately equal to the *geometric mean* of the solvent and solute terms. That is, the interaction between different molecules is equal to the square root of the product of the attractions among similar molecules, or

$$w_{12} = \sqrt{w_{11}w_{22}} \quad (10-18)$$

When this substitution is made in equation (10-17), it becomes

$$\ln \gamma_2 = [w_{11} - 2(w_{11}w_{22})^{1/2} + w_{22}] \frac{V_2 \Phi_1^2}{RT} \quad (10-19)$$

The terms within the brackets are seen to represent a perfect square, and equation (10-19) therefore becomes

$$\ln \gamma_2 = [(w_{11})^{1/2} - (w_{22})^{1/2}]^2 \frac{V_2 \Phi_1^2}{RT} \quad (10-20)$$

Equation (10-20) can be modified in the following manner. The w terms of equation (10-20) are approximately equal to the a/V^2 term in the van der Waals equation for nonideal gases and liquids (p. 27), and they serve as a measure of the *internal pressures* of the solvent and the solute in nonpolar or moderately polar nonideal solutions. The $(w)^{1/2}$ terms are known as *solubility parameters* and are designated by the symbols δ_1 and δ_2 for solvent and solute respectively. Equation (10-20) is thus written in terms of the common logarithm as

$$\log \gamma_2 = (\delta_1 - \delta_2)^2 \frac{V_2 \Phi_1^2}{2.303RT} \quad (10-21)$$

In dilute solutions, the volume fraction is nearly unity, and Φ_1^2 may be disregarded as a first approximation. When a rough calculation shows it to be significantly less than 1, a recalculation must be made taking into account the value of Φ_1. this correction will be described in the example to follow.

When the term for $\log \gamma_2$ is substituted in equation (10-16), the mole fraction solubility of a nonpolar or moderately polar solute is obtained as

$$-\log X_2 = \frac{\Delta H_f}{2.303RT} \left(\frac{T_0 - T}{T_0} \right)$$
$$+ \frac{V_2 \Phi_1^2}{2.303RT} (\delta_1 - \delta_2)^2 \quad (10-22)$$

If R is replaced by 1.987 cal/mole deg and T by 298° K at 25° C, the temperature most frequently employed, we obtain

$$-\log X_2 = \frac{\Delta H_f}{1364} \left(\frac{T_0 - 298}{T_0} \right)$$
$$+ \frac{V_2 \Phi_1^2}{1364} (\delta_1 - \delta_2)^2 \quad (10-23)$$

The solubility parameters, which express the cohesion between like molecules, may be calculated from heats of vaporization, internal pressures, surface tensions, and other properties, as described by Hildebrand and Scott.[27] The heat of vaporization in conjunction with the molar volume of the species, when available at the desired temperature, probably affords the best means for calculating the solubility parameter. It is roughly the square root of the internal pressure (p. 218) or

$$\delta = \left(\frac{\Delta H_v - RT}{V_l} \right)^{1/2} \quad (10-24)$$

in which ΔH_v is the heat of vaporization and V_l is the molar volume of the liquid compound at the desired temperature, R is the gas constant, and T is the absolute temperature. If the solute is a solid at this temperature, its molar volume must be obtained at elevated temperature where it is a liquid (i.e., at temperatures above the melting point) and extrapolated to the temperature under consideration. Where this method is not satisfactory for solids, other methods have been devised.[28,29]

Example 10-9. (a) Compute the solubility parameter of iodine and then (b) determine the mole fraction and molal solubility of iodine in carbon disulfide at 25° C.[30] (c) What is the activity coefficient of the solute in this solution? The heat of vaporization of liquid iodine extrapolated to 25° C is 11,493 cal/mole, the average heat of fusion ΔH_f is about 3600 cal at 25° C, the melting point of iodine is 113° C, and its molar volume V_2 is 59 cm³ at 25° C. The solubility parameter of carbon disulfide is 10.

(a)

$$\delta = \left(\frac{11,493 - 1.987 \times 298.2}{59} \right)^{1/2} = 13.6$$

(Notice that the delta value, δ, for iodine, viz .14, obtained from solubility data is somewhat different from the value, $\delta = 13.6$ (cal/cm³)$^{1/2}$, obtained here.)

(b) X_2 is first calculated assuming that Φ_1^2 is unity.

$$-\log X_2 = \frac{3,600}{1364} \left(\frac{386 - 298}{386} \right) + \frac{59}{1364} (10.0 - 13.6)^2$$

$$X_2 = 0.0689$$

Now the volume fraction Φ_1 is equal to $V_1(1 - X_2)/[V_1(1 - X_2) + V_2X_2]$ or, for iodine ($V_2 = 59$ cm^3) in carbon disulfide ($V_1 = 60$ cm^3),

$$\Phi_1 = 0.9322$$

Recalculating X_2 under (b) with $\Phi_1{}^2$ as $(0.9322)^2$ included in the second right-hand term of the solubility equation gives

$$X_2 = 0.0815$$

After six such replications (iterations) using a hand calculator, the result becomes $X_2 = 0.0845$. This procedure of repeated calculations is called *iteration*.[30] The experimental value for the solubility in carbon disulfide is recorded by Hildebrand and Scott[31] as 0.0546 at 25° C. The ideal mole fraction solubility $X_2{}^i$ of iodine is 0.250 at 25° C.

The calculated mole fraction solubility of iodine in carbon disulfide may be converted to molal concentration by use of the equation

$$m = \frac{1000\, X_2}{(1 - X_2)M_1} = \frac{1000 \times 0.085}{(1 - 0.085)(76.13)} = 1.22 \text{ mole/kg}$$

(c) By comparing equations (10–13) and (10–15), it becomes clear that the ideal solubility is related to the actual solubility at a definite temperature by the expression

$$a_2 = X_2{}^i = X_2\gamma_2$$

Therefore, the activity coefficient of the solute is

$$\gamma_2 = X_2{}^i/X_2 = 0.25/0.055 = 4.55$$

Hildebrand and Scott[31] include the solubility parameters for a number of compounds in their book. A table of solubility parameters has also been compiled by Hansen and Beerbower.[32] The approximate values for

some representative compounds of pharmaceutical interest are listed in Tables 10–8 and 10–9. $\delta_{(total)}$ is essentially the δ value for solvent and drug referred to in this section. δ_D, δ_P, and δ_H are partial solubility parameters introduced by Hansen and used for an extended theory of solubility, which is not treated here. The parameter δ_D accounts for nonpolar effects, δ_P for polar effects, and δ_H to express the hydrogen bonding nature of the solute or solvent molecules. The sum of the squares of the partial parameters gives the total cohesive energy density $\delta_{(total)}{}^2$,

$$\delta_{(total)}{}^2 = \delta_D{}^2 + \delta_P{}^2 + \delta_H{}^2 \qquad (10\text{--}25)$$

Kesselring et al.[33] have determined both total and partial solubility parameters using gas–liquid chromatography.

The more alike are the δ values of two components, the greater is the mutual solubility of the pair. For example, the δ value of phenanthrene is 9.8; for the solvent carbon disulfide, 10; and for normal hexane, 7.3. Therefore, phenanthrene would be expected to be more soluble in CS_2 than in $n\text{-}C_6H_{14}$. When the solubility parameter of the solute is identical to that of the solvent, the cohesive forces of the solute and the solvent are alike as long as hydrogen bonding and other

TABLE 10–8. *Molar Volume and Solubility Parameters for Some Liquid Compounds**,†

Liquid	V (cm^3/mole)	Solubility Parameter (cal/cm^3)$^{1/2}$			
		δ_D	δ_P	δ_H	$\delta_{(total)}$
n-Butane	101.4	6.9	0	0	6.9
n-Hexane	131.6	7.3	0	0	7.3
n-Octane	163.5	7.6	0	0	7.6
Diethyl ether	104.8	7.1	1.4	2.5	7.7
Cyclohexane	108.7	8.2	0	0.1	8.2
n-Butyl acetate	132.5	7.7	1.8	3.1	8.5
Carbon tetrachloride	97.1	8.7	0	0.3	8.7
Toluene	106.8	8.8	0.7	1.0	8.9
Ethyl acetate	98.5	7.7	2.6	3.5	8.9
Benzene	89.4	9.0	0	1.0	9.1
Chloroform	80.7	8.7	1.5	2.8	9.3
Acetone	74.0	7.6	5.1	3.4	9.8
Acetaldehyde	57.1	7.2	3.9	5.5	9.9
Carbon disulfide	60.0	10.0	0	0.3	10.0
Dioxane	85.7	9.3	0.9	3.6	10.0
1-Octanol	157.7	8.3	1.6	5.8	10.3
Nitrobenzene	102.7	9.8	4.2	2.0	10.9
1-Butanol	91.5	7.8	2.8	7.7	11.3
1-Propanol	75.2	7.8	3.3	8.5	12.0
Dimethylformamide	77.0	8.5	6.7	5.5	12.1
Ethanol	58.5	7.7	4.3	9.5	13.0
Dimethyl sulfoxide	71.3	9.0	8.0	5.0	13.0
Methanol	40.7	7.4	6.0	10.9	14.5
Propylene glycol	73.6	8.2	4.6	11.4	14.8
Ethylene glycol	55.8	8.3	5.4	12.7	16.1
Glycerin	73.3	8.5	5.9	14.3	17.7
Formamide	39.8	8.4	12.8	9.3	17.9
Water	18.0	7.6	7.8	20.7	23.4

*From C. Hansen and A. Beerbower, in *Encyclopedia of Chemical Technology*, Suppl. Vol., 2nd Edition, A. Standen, Ed., Wiley, New York, 1971, pp. 889–910.
δ_D, δ_P, and δ_H are partial solubility parameters defined briefly above. $\delta_{(total)}$ is essentially the solvent solubility parameter, δ_1, defined by Hildebrand and used throughout this section.

†It must be cautioned that a number of solvents in this table and throughout the book are not suitable as solvents in medicinal or nutritive products. Dioxane, for example, is both toxic and irritating to the skin.

TABLE 10–9. *Molar Volume and Solubility Parameters of Crystalline Compounds (Tentative Values)**

		Solubility Parameter (cal/cm³)^1/2			
Solid Compound	V (cm³/mole)	δ_D	δ_P	δ_H	$\delta_{(total)}$
Benzoic acid	104	8.9	3.4	4.8	10.7
Caffeine	144	10.1	3.5	9.1	14.1
Methyl paraben	145	9.3	4.4	6.0	11.8
Naphthalene	123	9.4	1.0	1.9	9.6
Phenobarbital	137	10.3	4.8	5.3	12.6
Sulfadiazine	182	9.5	4.8	6.6	12.5
Testosterone propionate	294	9.2	2.9	2.8	10.0
Tolbutamide	229	9.7	2.9	4.1	10.9

*Refer to the footnote in Table 10–8 for a definition of δ_D, δ_P, and δ_H. $\delta_{(total)}$ is essentially the solute δ_2 value referred to in this section.

complicating interactions are not involved. Then $\delta_1 - \delta_2 = 0$, and the last term of equation (10–23) becomes zero. The solubility of the solute then depends alone on the ideal solubility term of the equation, involving the heat of fusion, the melting point of the solute, and the temperature of the solution.

James et al.[29] investigated the solubility of testosterone esters in a number of aliphatic straight- and branched-chain alkanes, cyclic and aromatic hydrocarbons, and halogen derivatives. They determined the δ value of testosterone propionate and other esters and arrived at values of 9.5 to 10.0 (cal/cm³)^1/2 for testosterone propionate. The Hildebrand solubility theory was used with some success by James and his associates to predict the solubilities of steroidal esters in hydrocarbon solvents.

In the use of solubility parameters, a distinction should also be made between those compounds that form hydrogen bonds and those that do not. The δ values may be used to predict the miscibility of hydrogen-bonding solvents or of non–hydrogen-bonding solvents, but they are not always applicable when members of the two different classes are mixed.

The nonideal solutions to which the Scatchard–Hildebrand equation applies are called *regular solutions*. Regular solutions may be better understood by reference to several properties of ideal solutions. First, the molecules of an ideal solution exhibit complete freedom of motion and randomness of distribution in the solution. Secondly, an ideal solution forms with no change in heat content, that is to say, heat is not absorbed or evolved during the mixing process. Furthermore, there is no change in volume when the components of an ideal solution are mixed. The partial free energy change involved in the transfer of a mole of solute from the solute phase to a saturated solution is written, for an ideal solution, as

$$\overline{\Delta G_2} = RT \ln X_2 \qquad (10\text{–}26)$$

Since the change in heat content ΔH is zero

$$\overline{\Delta G_2} = \overline{\Delta H_2} - T\,\overline{\Delta S_2} = -T\,\overline{\Delta S_2} \qquad (10\text{–}27)$$

and the entropy for the solute in the ideal solution is

$$\overline{\Delta S_2} = -\overline{\Delta G_2}/T = -R \ln X_2 \qquad (10\text{–}28)$$

The molecules of regular solutions, like those of ideal solutions, possess sufficient kinetic energy to prevent ordering and a loss in entropy; and a regular solution, like an ideal solution, exhibits complete randomness. The entropy change in forming a regular solution is given by the same formula as that for an ideal solution,

$$\overline{\Delta S_2} = -R \ln X_2 \qquad (10\text{–}29)$$

On the other hand, owing to cohesion among the solute molecules and among the solvent molecules, regular solutions exhibit positive deviation from Raoult's law. Unlike ideal solutions, they absorb heat when the components are mixed. It can be shown from thermodynamic considerations that the heat change when 1 mole of solute is added to a large quantity of regular solution is equal to $RT \ln \gamma_2$, which may be set equal to the solubility parameter term in the solubility equation (cf. equation (10–21)):

$$\overline{\Delta H_2} = RT \ln \gamma_2 = V_2\Phi_1^2(\delta_1 - \delta_2)^2 \qquad (10\text{–}30)$$

These relationships can be used to derive the solubility expression, equation (10–22) as demonstrated in the following paragraph. For a nonideal solution, X_2 in equation (10–26) must be replaced by the activity a_2 or

$$\overline{\Delta G_2} = RT \ln a_2 \qquad (10\text{–}31)$$

From equations (10–15) and (10–31)

$$-\overline{\Delta G_2} = \frac{\Delta H_f(T_0 - T)}{T_0} \qquad (10\text{–}32)$$

Writing the familiar free energy equation

$$\overline{\Delta G_2} = \overline{\Delta H_2} - T\,\overline{\Delta S_2} \qquad (10\text{–}33)$$

or

$$T\,\overline{\Delta S_2} = -\overline{\Delta G_2} + \overline{\Delta H_2} \qquad (10\text{–}34)$$

gives

$$-RT \ln X_2 = \frac{\Delta H_f(T_0 - T)}{T_0} + V_2\Phi_1^2(\delta_1 - \delta_2)^2 \qquad (10\text{–}35)$$

by the application of equations (10–29), (10–30),

(10–32) and (10–34). Then equation (10–35) may be written as

$$-\log X_2 = \frac{\Delta H_f}{2.303RT}\left(\frac{T_0 - T}{T_0}\right) + \frac{V_2\Phi_1{}^2}{2.303RT}(\delta_1 - \delta_2)^2$$

which is identical with equation (10–22).

Extended Hildebrand Solubility Approach. A modification of the Scatchard–Hildebrand equation has been developed[34] and is referred to as the *extended Hildebrand solubility approach* (EHS). The extended method allows one to calculate the solubility of polar and nonpolar solutes in solvents ranging from nonpolar hydrocarbons to highly polar solvents such as alcohols, glycols, and water. Although formulated specifically for crystalline solids in liquid solution, the EHS approach should also apply to liquid–liquid and gas–liquid systems.

It is well recognized that the established regular solution theory, represented by equation (10–22), usually provides poor predictions of solubility for drugs and other crystalline solids in polar solvents. Polar systems are quite irregular, involving self-association of solute or solvent, solvation of the solute by the solvent molecules, or complexation of two or more solute species in the solution. The intermolecular attachments consist of hydrogen bonds, charge transfer complexes (Chapter 11), and other types of Lewis acid–base interactions.

The solubility equation used in the EHS approach is

$$-\log X_2 = -\log X_2{}^i + A(w_{11} + w_{22} - 2W) \quad (10\text{–}36)$$

in which the last term corresponds to the expression for $\log \gamma_2$, equation (10–17) of Hildebrand and Scatchard. In equation (10–36), A stands for $V_2\Phi_1{}^2/(2.303RT)$ and W is used for w_{12} from equation (10–17). The negative logarithm of the ideal solubility, $-\log X_2{}^i$, may be calculated from a knowledge of ΔH_f, T_0, and T as shown in equation (10–15).

Alternatively, it may be obtained from ΔS_f:

$$-\log X_2{}^i = \frac{\Delta S_f}{R}\log \frac{T_o}{T} \quad (10\text{–}37)$$

as suggested by Hildebrand et al.[35] ΔS_f, the entropy of fusion at the melting point, is determined using the expression

$$\Delta H_f = T_o\Delta S_f \quad (10\text{–}38)$$

According to the EHS approach, the term involving the logarithm of the activity coefficient γ_2 is partitioned into two terms, one representing mainly physical or van der Waals forces γ_v and an additional term γ_R representing residual, presumably stronger, forces:

$$\log \gamma_2 = \log \gamma_v + \log \gamma_R \quad (10\text{–}39)$$

in which

$$\log \gamma_v = A(\delta_1 - \delta_2)^2 = A(\delta_1{}^2 + \delta_2{}^2 - 2\delta_1\delta_2) \quad (10\text{–}40)$$

and

$$\log \gamma_R = A(2\delta_1\delta_2 - 2W) \quad (10\text{–}41)$$

Equation (10–39) is written, in terms of equations (10–40) and (10–41) as:

$$\log \frac{X_2{}^i}{X_2} = \log \gamma_2 = A(\delta_1 - \delta_2)^2 + 2A(\delta_1\delta_2 - W)$$

or

$$-\log X_2 = -\log X_2{}^i + A(\delta_1{}^2 + \delta_2{}^2 - 2W) \quad (10\text{–}42)$$

Investigators[34] have applied the EHS approach to polar and nonpolar solutes in individual solvents as well as mixed solvent systems.

Equation (10–42) differs from equation (10–22) in that the geometric mean is replaced by W. Equation (10–42) ordinarily provides an accurate prediction of the mole fraction solubility of a polar drug in binary solvent systems (i.e., two solvents mixed in various proportions) as demonstrated in *Examples 10–10* and *10–11*. W is obtained for a solute in a particular solvent system by rearranging equation (10–42):

$$\frac{\log (X_2{}^i/X_2)}{A} = \frac{\log \gamma_2}{A} = \delta_1{}^2 + \delta_2{}^2 - 2W$$

$$W = \frac{1}{2}(\delta_1{}^2 + \delta_2{}^2 - (\log \gamma_2)/A) \quad (10\text{–}43)$$

The solubility parameters, δ_1 and δ_2, are known quantities. Log γ_2 is obtained from a knowledge of the drug's ideal solubility, $X_2{}^i$, and its mole fraction solubility, X_2, in a particular solvent system. The observed solubilities of caffeine in mixtures of dioxane and water are shown in Figure 10–5 together with the back-calculated solubility curve obtained by use of the

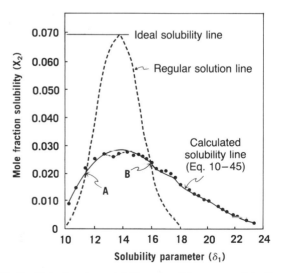

Fig. 10–5. Mole fraction solubility of caffeine at 25° C in dioxane–water mixtures. *A* and *B* are points at which real solubility equals regular solution solubility and $W = \delta_1\delta_2$. Filled circles are experimental solubility points. (From A. Adjei, J. Newburger and A. Martin, J. Pharm. Sci. **69**, 659, 1980, reproduced with permission of the copyright owner.)

TABLE 10–10. *Several Observed and Calculated Solubilities of Caffeine in Dioxane–Water Systems at 25° C**

Volume % water	δ_1	log X_2	A	W†	$W_{(calc)}$‡	$X_{2(obs)}$	$X_{2(calc)}$§
0	10.01	0.90646	0.10257	140.901	141.120	0.0085	0.0094
20	12.70	0.40443	0.09467	173.729	173.729	0.0270	0.0270
40	15.39	0.41584	0.09269	211.403	211.380	0.0263	0.0261
50	16.73	0.50555	0.09369	232.469	233.465	0.0214	0.0214
60	18.07	0.62665	0.09520	255.191	255.220	0.0162	0.0164
80	20.76	0.94347	0.09837	305.913	305.951	0.0078	0.0080
100	23.45	1.47643	0.10179	362.919	362.343	0.0023	0.0022

*$\delta_2 = 13.8$; $-\log X_2{}^i = 1.1646$.
†W is calculated from equation (10–43). Its units are cal/cm^3.
‡$W_{(calc)}$ is obtained using the quartic expression (10–45).
§$X_{2(calc)}$ is calculated using equation (10–42) with W replaced by $W_{(calc)}$.

extended Hildebrand approach. The calculations are illustrated in *Example 10–10*, part of the data for which are found in Tables 10–9 and 10–10.

Example 10–10. Compute the value of W for a solution of caffeine in the pure solvent, dioxane ($\delta = 10.01$), in pure water ($\delta = 23.45$), and in a 50:50 volume percent of dioxane and water ($\delta = 16.73$) at 25° C. ΔH_f is 5044 cal/mole, and $T_0 = 512°$ K. According to equation (10–38), $\Delta S_f = 9.85$ cal/mole deg. Using equation (10–37), the logarithm of the ideal mole fraction solubility, $-\log X_2{}^i$ is found to be 1.16460, or $X_2{}^i = 0.068376$. The molar volume, V_2, of caffeine is 144 cm^3/mole at 25° C. The volume fractions, ϕ_1, of dioxane, water, and a 50:50 mixture of dioxane and water are 0.985809, 0.982066, and 0.942190, respectively. Using the definition of A, following equation (10–36), one obtains A^* for caffeine in dioxane as 0.102570; in water, 0.101793; and in the 50:50 mixture, 0.093694.

The mole fraction solubilities of caffeine in the three solvents at 25° C are found experimentally to be 0.008491 in dioxane, 0.002285 in water, and 0.021372 in the 50:50 mixture of dioxane and water.

Using equation (10–43), one obtains for log γ_2/A for the three solutions

$$\frac{\log (0.068454/0.008491)}{0.102570} = 8.83728 \text{ in dioxane}$$

$$\frac{\log (0.068454/0.002285)}{0.101793} = 14.50505 \text{ in water}$$

and

$$\frac{\log (0.068454/0.021372)}{0.093694} = 5.39580 \text{ in the 50:50 mixture}$$

W values are then obtained again with the help of equation (10–43):

In dioxane:

$$8.83728 = (10.01)^2 + (13.8)^2 - 2W$$
$$W = 140.90141$$

In water:

$$14.50425 = (23.45)^2 + (13.8)^2 - 2W$$
$$W = 362.91913$$

In the 50:50 mixture:

$$5.39574 = (16.73)^2 + (13.8)^2 - 2W$$
$$W = 232.46858$$

The desirability of a theoretic approach is the ability to calculate solubilities of a drug in mixed and pure solvents, using only fundamental physical chemical properties of solute and solvent. Unfortunately, W at present cannot be obtained by a consideration of the molecular characteristics of the species in solution. It has been found, however, that when the experimentally derived W values (as calculated in *Example 10–10*) are regressed against a power series in δ_1, for the various solvents of the mixture, a polynomial equation is obtained that may be used for the accurate back-calculation of solubilities. A power series in the second degree (quadratic) may be used for this purpose. Using the complete set of 30 solubility values (see Table 10–10 for some of these), the quadratic equation is obtained:

$$W_{(calc)} = 79.411400 + 1.868572\delta_1 + 0.435648\delta_1{}^2 \tag{10–44}$$

The quartic equation is:

$$W_{(calc)} = 15.075279 + 17.627903\delta_1$$
$$- 0.966827\delta_1{}^2 + 0.053912\delta_1{}^3 - 0.000758\delta_1{}^4 \tag{10–45}$$

Using equation (10–44) or (10–45) and a hand calculator, one can readily calculate the solubility of caffeine in any combination of dioxane and water at 25° C.

Example 10–11†. Calculate the solubility of caffeine ($\delta_2 = 13.8$) at 25° C in a 40:60 volume percent mixture of dioxane and water. Use the quadratic expression, equation (10–44), to obtain $W_{(calc)}$.

One first obtains the δ_1 value of the 40:60 mixture of dioxane and water using the equation

$$\delta_1 = \phi_d \delta_d + \phi_w \delta_w$$

in which ϕ_d and ϕ_w are the volume fractions, 0.40 and 0.60, of the solvents dioxane and water and δ_d and δ_w are their solubility parameters.

$$\delta_1 = 0.40(10.01) + 0.60(23.45) = 18.07$$

Then $W_{(calc)}$ is obtained by back-calculation:

$$W_{(calc)} = 79.41140 + 1.86857(18.07) + 0.43565(18.07)^2$$
$$W_{(calc)} = 255.427 \qquad W_{(exp)} = 255.191$$

---

*A is obtained from a knowledge of $X_{2(obs)}$, and these values are used for convenience in this example. When the solubility is not known, it is necessary to obtain A by use of an iteration (replication) procedure as described on page 225.

†As mentioned in the footnote of Table 10–8, dioxane is externally irritating and internally toxic and cannot be used in drug or food products. It is chosen as a solvent in *Example 10–11* simply because it is miscible with water and has an appropriate solubility parameter. Such agents must be carefully tested for untoward effects before any use is made of them in man or animal.

This value for $W_{(calc)}$ is substituted in equation (10–42) in which $-\log X_2{}^i$ for caffeine is 1.1646 and A is 0.09520.

$$-\log X_2 = 1.1646 + 0.09520[(18.07)^2 + (13.8)^2 - 2(255.427)]$$

$$-\log X_2 = 1.74635$$

$$X_{2(calc)} = 0.0179 \qquad X_{2(exp)} = 0.0162$$

Some values, calculated as shown in *Examples 10–10* and *10–11*, are found in Table 10–10. The $X_{2(calc)}$ values in Table 10–10 were back-calculated using a quartic expression, equation (10–45), rather than the quadratic equation used in *Example 10–11*, which accounts for the small difference in results.

Solvation and Association in Solutions of Polar Compounds. We saw in equation (10–30) that heat must be absorbed when the solute is mixed with the solvent to form a regular solution. This happens because the squared term $(\delta_1 - \delta_2)^2$ can lead only to positive values (or zero). We can refer back to equation (10–17), however, where we find the term w_{12}, which expresses the interaction of the solute and solvent molecules. If we remove the restriction that this term must follow the rule of the geometric mean given in formula (10–18), we allow $2w_{12}$ to be $> w_{11} + w_{22}$ and ΔH may then become negative. This leads to a negative deviation from Raoult's law and applies when specific interactions, such as hydrogen bonding (p. 213), occur between the solute and the solvent. Such specific combinations of the solvent with the solute are known as *solvation*.

When the interaction occurs between like molecules of one of the components in a solution, the phenomenon is referred to as *association*. This type of interaction is exemplified by the dimerization of benzoic acid in some nonpolar solvents or the interlinking of water molecules by hydrogen bonding. It leads to positive heats of solution and to positive deviations from Raoult's law. The association of water molecules is reflected in a large w_{11} in equation (10–17). When water is mixed with a nonpolar solute, w_{11} is much larger than w_{22}, and w_{12} is small. Such a situation obviously leads to low solubility. The specific interaction effects, known as *solvation* and *association*, cannot be accounted for in a satisfactory way by the Scatchard–Hildebrand formula (equation (10–22)) but rather require a more refined treatment, which is outside the scope of this book.

Solubility and the Heat of Solution. Solubility as a function of temperature for nonelectrolytes, weak electrolytes, or strong electrolytes in highly nonideal solutions can be calculated using the *heat of solution*, ΔH_{soln}, instead of the heat of fusion in an expression analogous to the ideal solubility expression (equation (10–11), p. 221). For nonelectrolytes and weak electrolytes, the following equation is used[36,37]:

$$\ln (c''/c') = \frac{\Delta H_{soln}}{R} \frac{(T'' - T')}{(T'T'')} \qquad (10–46)$$

For strong electrolytes, R is replaced by νR, in which ν is the number of ions produced in the dissociation of the electrolyte. The terms c' and c'' are concentrations such as molar, molal, mole fraction, grams/liter, or percent. These concentration terms appear in equation (10–46) as ratios, c''/c', so as to cancel the concentration units, as long as the same units are used for both c' and c''. The concentration term c' corresponds to the Kelvin temperature T', and c'' corresponds to T''. ΔH_{soln} is the heat of solution in cal/mole and R is the universal gas constant expressed as 1.9872 cal mole^{-1} deg^{-1}.

Using equation (10–46), the solubility of a solute in a particular solvent can be determined at one temperature if the heat of solution ΔH_{soln} and the solubility at another temperature are known.

Example 10–12. The solubility of urea (molecular weight 60.06 g/mole) in water at 298° K is 1.20 g/g H_2O; the ΔH_{soln} for urea in water at 25° C is 2820 cal/mole. What is the molal solubility of urea at 5° C?

$$\ln (1.20) - \ln c' = \frac{2820}{1.9872} \left(\frac{298 - 278}{298 \cdot 278} \right)$$

$\ln c' = -0.16$ and $c' = 0.85$ g/g H_2O or 850 g/kg H_2O

850 g/kg $H_2O \div 60.06$ g/mole = 14.2 mole/kg H_2O

The experimental solubility of urea on the molal scale is 14.2 mole/kg H_2O.

Solubility of Strong Electrolytes. The effect of temperature on the solubility of some salts in water is shown in Figure 10–6. A rise in temperature increases the solubility of a solid that absorbs heat (*endothermic process*) when it dissolves. This effect conforms with the Le Chatelier principle, which states that a system tends to adjust itself in a manner so as to counteract a stress such as an increase of temperature. Conversely, if the solution process is *exothermic*, that is, if heat is evolved, the temperature of the solution rises and the container feels warm to the touch. The solubility in this case decreases with an elevation of the temperature, again following Le Chatelier's principle. Most solids belong to the class of compounds that absorb heat when they dissolve.

Sodium sulfate exists in the hydrated form, $Na_2SO_4 \cdot 10H_2O$, up to a temperature of about 32° C, the solution process (dissolution) is endothermic, and solu-

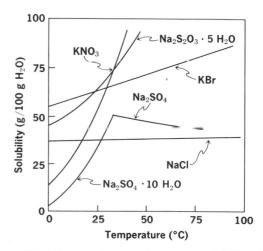

Fig. 10–6. The influence of temperature on the solubility of various salts.

bility increases with temperature. Above this point, the compound exists as the anydrous salt, Na_2SO_4, the dissolution is exothermic, and solubility decreases with an increase of temperature (Fig. 10–6). Sodium chloride does not absorb or evolve an appreciable amount of heat when it dissolves in water; thus, its solubility is not altered much by a change of temperature, and the heat of solution is approximately zero, as observed in Figure 10–6.

These phenomena can be explained in terms of the heat of solution, ΔH. The quantity ΔH is properly known as the *partial* or *differential heat of solution*. It is the heat absorbed per mole when a small quantity of solute is added to a large quantity of solution. It may also be defined as the rate of change of the heat of solution per mole of solute in a solution of any specified concentration. The *total* or *integral heat of solution* is the heat absorbed when 1 mole of solute is dissolved in enough solvent to produce a solution of specified concentration.

The heat of solution of a crystalline substance is the sum of the *heat of sublimation* of the solid, as given by the *crystal lattice energy*, and the *heat of hydration* (solvation) of the ions in solution (Table 10–11).

$$\Delta H \text{ (solution)} = \Delta H_{subl} + \Delta H_{hyd} \quad (10-47)$$

The lattice energy is the energy required to separate 1 mole of a crystal into its ions in the gaseous state or to vaporize the solid:

$$NaCl_{solid} \rightarrow Na^+_{gas} + Cl^-_{gas}$$

The heat of hydration is the heat liberated when the gaseous ions are hydrated; it is influenced by the radius of an ion, since for ions of the same valence, the smaller the ionic radius, the greater is the electrostatic field surrounding the ion and the larger is the heat of hydration. The hydration process can be represented as

$$Na^+_{gas} + Cl^-_{gas} \xrightarrow{H_2O} Na^+_{aq} + Cl^-_{aq}$$

If the heat of hydration, that is, the heat liberated when the ions are hydrated, is sufficient to provide the energy needed to overcome the lattice forces and thus "pull" the ions away from the crystal, the salt will be soluble. In an ideal solution, no hydration (solvation) occurs, and the heat absorbed is that alone that is required to transform the crystals to the liquid state. For this reason, only the heat of fusion ΔH_f is included in the ideal solubility expression, equation (10–11) on page 221.

The heats of solution and solubilities of some salts are shown in Table 10–11. A positive value of ΔH indicates an absorption of heat; a negative value signifies that heat is evolved. The heat of hydration and the lattice energy of sodium chloride are so similar that the process is only slightly endothermic and the temperature has little effect on the solubility. The large heat of solution of silver chloride (large endothermic value) accounts for the insolubility of the salt in water. This is due to the large lattice energy brought about by the great polarizability of the silver ion (p. 87).

Gibbs' phase rule, page 37, is applied to the solubility of a solid in a liquid in the following manner. Since the pressure is ordinarily fixed at 1 atm and hence need not be specified, the rule becomes

$$\mathbf{F} = C - P + 1$$

A subsaturated solution of sodium chloride in water, for example, consists of a single homogeneous phase and two components, salt and water. The number of degrees of freedom is thus $\mathbf{F} = 2 - 1 + 1 = 2$. This means that two variables, both temperature and composition, must be stated to define the system completely. When the solution is saturated with the solute, sodium chloride, and excess solute is present, two phases exist, and the number of degrees of freedom is $\mathbf{F} = 2 - 2 + 1 = 1$. Hence, the conclusion reached by applying the phase rule is that the solubility of sodium chloride in water has a fixed value at any specified temperature. This statement of course is true not only for this specific system but for solubility in general.

Solubility of Slightly Soluble Electrolytes. When slightly soluble electrolytes are dissolved to form saturated solutions, the solubility is described by a special constant, known as the *solubility product*, K_{sp}, of the compound. The solubility products of a number of substances used in pharmacy are listed in Table 10–12.

TABLE 10–11. *Heats of Solution and Solubility of Some Chlorides*

Compound	Crystal Energy (kcal/mole)	Heat of Hydration (kcal/mole)	ΔH_{soln}* (kcal/mole) (25° C)	Solubility (g/100 g H$_2$O) (20° C)
AgCl	207	−192	+15.0	1.5×10^{-4}
LiCl	199	−209	−10.0	78.5
NaCl	184	−183	+1.0	36.0
CsCl	152	−147	+5.0	186.5
KCl	167	−164	+3.0	23.8
KBr	161	−156	+5.0	65.0

*A negative value for ΔH, the heat of solution, indicates an evolution of heat (exothermic), and a positive value indicates an absorption of heat (endothermic) during solution.

TABLE 10–12. *Solubility Products of Some Slightly Soluble Electrolytes in Water*

Substance	Solubility Product K_{sp}	Temperature (°C)
Aluminum hydroxide	7.7×10^{-13}	25
Barium carbonate	8.1×10^{-9}	25
Barium sulfate	1×10^{-10}	25
Calcium carbonate	9×10^{-9}	25
Calcium sulfate	6.1×10^{-5}	20
Ferric hydroxide	1×10^{-36}	18
Ferrous hydroxide	1.6×10^{-14}	18
Lead carbonate	3.3×10^{-14}	18
Lead sulfate	1.1×10^{-8}	18
Magnesium carbonate	2.6×10^{-5}	12
Magnesium hydroxide	1.4×10^{-11}	18
Mercurous chloride	2×10^{-18}	25
Mercurous iodide	1.2×10^{-28}	25
Potassium acid tartrate	3.8×10^{-4}	18
Silver bromide	7.7×10^{-13}	25
Silver chloride	1.25×10^{-10}	25
Silver iodide	1.5×10^{-16}	25
Zinc hydroxide	1.8×10^{-14}	18
Zinc sulfide	1.2×10^{-23}	18

Silver chloride is an example of such a slightly soluble salt. The excess solid in equilibrium with the ions in saturated solution at a specific temperature is represented by the equation

$$AgCl_{solid} \rightleftharpoons Ag^+ + Cl^- \qquad (10\text{–}48)$$

and since the salt dissolves only with difficulty and the ionic strength is low, the equilibrium expression may be written in terms of concentrations instead of activities:

$$\frac{[Ag^+][Cl^-]}{[AgCl_{solid}]} = K \qquad (10\text{–}49)$$

Moreover, since the concentration of the solid phase is essentially constant,

$$[Ag^+][Cl^-] = K_{sp} \qquad (10\text{–}50)$$

The equation is only approximate for sparingly soluble salts, or in the presence of other salts, when activities rather than concentrations should be used. It does not hold for salts that are freely soluble in water such as sodium chloride.

As in the case of other equilibrium expressions, the concentration of each ion is raised to a power equal to the number of ions appearing in the formula. Thus, for aluminum hydroxide, $Al(OH)_3$,

$$Al(OH)_{3\ solid} \rightleftharpoons Al^{3+} + 3OH^-$$

$$[Al^{3+}][OH^-]^3 = K_{sp} \qquad (10\text{–}51)$$

Example 10–13. The measured solubility of silver chloride in water at 20° C is 1.12×10^{-5} mole/liter. This is also the concentration of the silver ion and the chloride ion, since silver chloride, being a strong electrolyte, is nearly completely dissociated. Calculate the solubility product of this salt.

$$K_{sp} = (1.12 \times 10^{-5}) \times (1.12 \times 10^{-5})$$
$$= 1.25 \times 10^{-10}$$

If an ion in common with AgCl, that is, Ag^+ or Cl^-, is added to a solution of silver chloride, the equilibrium is altered. The addition of sodium chloride, for example, increases the concentration of chloride ions so that momentarily

$$[Ag^+][Cl^-] > K_{sp}$$

and some of the AgCl precipitates from the solution until the equilibrium $[Ag^+][Cl^-] = K_{sp}$ is reestablished. Hence, the result of adding a *common ion* is to *reduce* the solubility of a slightly soluble electrolyte, unless, of course, the common ion forms a complex with the salt whereby the net solubility may be increased.

Example 10–14. What is the solubility x of silver chromate in moles/liter in an aqueous solution containing 0.04 M silver nitrate? The solubility of silver chromate in water is 8×10^{-5} and its solubility product is 2.0×10^{-12}. The dissociation of silver chromate may be represented as

$$Ag_2CrO_4 \rightleftharpoons 2Ag^+ + CrO_4^=$$
$$K_{sp} = 2.0 \times 10^{-12} = (2x + 0.04)^2 x = 4x^3 + 0.16x^2 + 0.0016x$$

Since the terms in x^3 and x^2 are so small that they may be neglected, the result is

$$x = [Ag_2CrO_4] = \frac{2.0 \times 10^{-12}}{1.6 \times 10^{-3}} = 1.25 \times 10^{-9}\ mole/liter$$

Salts having no ion in common with the slightly soluble electrolyte produce an effect opposite to that of a common ion: at moderate concentration, they *increase* rather than decrease the solubility because they lower the activity coefficient. As mentioned previously, the exact equilibrium expression involves activities. For silver chloride,

$$K_{sp} = a_{Ag^+} a_{Cl^-} \qquad (10\text{–}52)$$

Since activities may be replaced by the product of concentrations and activity coefficients,

$$K_{sp} = [Ag^+][Cl^-]\gamma_{Ag^+}\gamma_{Cl^-} = [Ag^+][Cl^-]\gamma^2_\pm$$

$$\frac{K_{sp}}{\gamma^2_\pm} = [Ag^+][Cl^-]$$

and

$$Solubility = [Ag^+] = [Cl^-] = \frac{\sqrt{K_{sp}}}{\gamma_\pm} \qquad (10\text{–}53)$$

Example 10–15. Calculate the solubility of silver chloride in a 0.1-M solution of ammonium sulfate. The ionic strength of 0.1 M $(NH_4)_2SO_4$ is 0.3, and the activity coefficient of a 1:1 electrolyte such as silver chloride at this ionic strength is about 0.70.

$$Solubility = \frac{\sqrt{1.2 \times 10^{-10}}}{0.70}$$
$$= 1.6 \times 10^{-5}\ mole/liter$$

Therefore, the addition of an electrolyte that does not have an ion in common with AgCl causes an increase in the solubility of silver chloride.

Other useful conclusions may be reached by use of the solubility product principle. If the pharmacist wishes to prevent precipitation of a slightly soluble salt in water, he may add some substance that will tie up and reduce the concentration of one of the ions. More of the salt will then pass from the undissolved to the dissolved state until the solubility product constant is reached and the equilibrium is reestablished. For example, if the ferric ion in a solution of the slightly soluble base, $Fe(OH)_3$, can be combined by complex formation with sodium citrate, more Fe^{3+} will pass into solution so as to keep K_{sp} constant. In this manner, the solubility of iron compounds is increased by citrates and similar compounds.

Solubility of Weak Electrolytes. Many important drugs belong to the class of weak acids and bases. They react with strong acids and bases and, within definite ranges of pH, exist as ions that are ordinarily soluble in water.

Although carboxylic acids containing more than five carbons are relatively insoluble in water, they react with dilute sodium hydroxide, carbonates, and bicarbonates to form soluble salts. The fatty acids containing more than 10 carbon atoms form soluble soaps with the alkali metals and insoluble soaps with other metal ions. They are soluble in solvents having low dielectric constants; for example, oleic acid ($C_{17}H_{33}COOH$) is insoluble in water but is soluble in alcohol and in ether.

Hydroxy acids, such as tartaric and citric acids, are quite soluble in water since they are solvated through their hydroxyl groups. The potassium and ammonium bitartrates are not very soluble in water, although most alkali metal salts of tartaric acid are soluble. Sodium citrate is used sometimes to dissolve water-insoluble acetylsalicylic acid since the soluble acetylsalicylate ion is formed in the reaction. The citric acid that is produced is also soluble in water, but the practice of dissolving aspirin by this means is questionable since the acetylsalicylate is also hydrolyzed rapidly.

Aromatic acids react with dilute alkalies to form water-soluble salts, but they may be precipitated as the free acids if stronger acidic substances are added to the solution. They may also be precipitated as heavy metal salts should heavy metal ions be added to the solution. Benzoic acid is soluble in sodium hydroxide solution, alcohol, and fixed oils. Salicylic acid is soluble in alkalies and in alcohol. The OH group of salicyclic acid cannot contribute to the solubility since it is involved in an intramolecular hydrogen bond (p. 24).

Phenol is weakly acidic and only slightly soluble in water but is quite soluble in dilute sodium hydroxide solution.

$$C_6H_5OH + NaOH \rightarrow C_6H_5O^- + Na^+ + H_2O$$

Phenol is a weaker acid than H_2CO_3 and is thus displaced and precipitated by CO_2 from its dilute alkali solution. For this reason, carbonates and bicarbonates cannot increase the solubility of phenols in water.

Many organic compounds containing a basic nitrogen atom in the molecule are important in pharmacy. These include the alkaloids, sympathomimetic amines, antihistamines, local anesthetics, and others. Most of these weak electrolytes are not very soluble in water but are soluble in dilute solutions of acids; such compounds as atropine sulfate and tetracaine hydrochloride are formed by reacting the basic compounds with acids. Addition of an alkali to a solution of the salt of these compounds precipitates the free base from solution if the solubility of the base in water is low.

The aliphatic nitrogen of the sulfonamides is sufficiently negative so that these drugs act as slightly soluble weak acids rather than as bases. They form water-soluble salts in alkaline solution by the following mechanism. The oxygens of the sulfonyl ($-SO_2-$) group withdraw electrons, and the resulting electron deficiency of the sulfur atom results in the electrons of the N:H bond being held more closely to the nitrogen atom. The hydrogen therefore is bound less firmly, and, in alkaline solution, the soluble sulfonamide anion is readily formed.

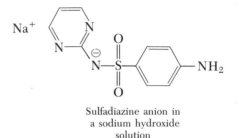

Sulfadiazine anion in
a sodium hydroxide
solution

The sodium salts of the sulfonamides are precipitated from solution by the addition of a strong acid, or by a salt of a strong acid and a weak base such as ephedrine hydrochloride.

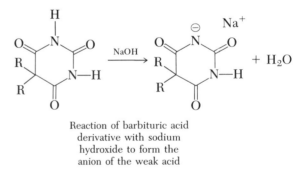

Reaction of barbituric acid
derivative with sodium
hydroxide to form the
anion of the weak acid

The barbiturates, like the sulfonamides, are weak acids because the electronegative oxygen of each acidic carbonyl group tends to withdraw electrons and to create a positive carbon atom. The carbon in turn attracts electrons from the nitrogen group and causes the hydrogen to be held less firmly. Thus, in sodium hydroxide solution, the hydrogen is readily lost, and the molecule exists as a soluble anion of the weak acid. Butler et al.[38] have demonstrated that, in highly alkaline solutions, the second hydrogen ionizes. The pK_1 for phenobarbital is 7.41 and the pK_2 is 11.77. Although the barbiturates are soluble in alkalies, they are precipitated as the free acids when a stronger acid is added and the pH of the solution is lowered.

Calculating the Solubility of Weak Electrolytes as Influenced by pH. From what has been said about the effects of acids and bases on solutions of weak electrolytes, it becomes evident that the solubility of weak electrolytes is strongly influenced by the pH of the solution. For example, a 1% solution of phenobarbital sodium is soluble at pH values high in the alkaline range. The soluble ionic form is converted into molecular phenobarbital as the pH is lowered, and below 8.3, the drug begins to precipitate from solution at room temperature. On the other hand, alkaloidal salts such as atropine sulfate begin to precipitate as the pH is elevated.

To ensure a clear homogeneous solution and maximum therapeutic effectiveness, the preparations should be adjusted to an optimum pH. The pH below which the salt of a weak acid, sodium phenobarbital, for example, begins to precipitate from aqueous solution is readily calculated in the following manner.

Representing the free acid form of phenobarbital as HP and the soluble ionized form as P^-, the equilibria in a saturated solution of this slightly soluble weak electrolyte are

$$HP_{solid} \rightleftharpoons HP_{sol} \qquad (10-54)$$

$$HP_{sol} + H_2O \rightleftharpoons H_3O^+ + P^- \qquad (10-55)$$

Since the concentration of the un-ionized form in solution HP_{sol} is essentially constant, the equilibrium constant for the solution equilibrium, equation (10-54) is

$$S_0 = [HP]_{sol} \qquad (10-56)$$

and the constant for the acid–base equilibrium, equation (10-55), is

$$K_a = \frac{[H_3O^+][P^-]}{[HP]} \qquad (10-57)$$

or

$$[P^-] = K_a \frac{[HP]}{[H_3O^+]} \qquad (10-58)$$

in which the subscript "sol" has been deleted from $[HP]_{sol}$, since no confusion should result from this omission.

The total solubility S of phenobarbital consists of the concentration of the undissociated acid [HP] and the conjugate base or ionized form $[P^-]$:

$$S = [HP] + [P^-] \qquad (10-59)$$

Substituting S_0 for [HP] from equation (10-56) and the expression from equation (10-58) for $[P^-]$ yields

$$S = S_0 + K_a \frac{S_0}{[H_3O^+]} \qquad (10-60)$$

$$S = S_0 \left(1 + \frac{K_a}{[H_3O^+]}\right) \qquad (10-61)$$

Equation (10-61) has been expressed in various forms by Krebs and Speakman[39] Albert,[40] Higuchi,[41] Kostenbauder et al.,[42] and others.

When the electrolyte is weak and does not dissociate appreciably, the solubility of the acid in water or acidic solutions is $S_0 = $ [HP], which, for phenobarbital is approximately 0.005 mole/liter, in other words, 0.12%.

The solubility equation may be written in logarithmic form, beginning with equation (10-60). By rearrangement, we obtain

$$(S - S_0) = K_a \frac{S_0}{[H_3O^+]}$$

$$\log (S - S_0) = \log K_a + \log S_0 - \log [H_3O^+]$$

and finally

$$pH_p = pK_a + \log \frac{S - S_0}{S_0} \qquad (10-62)$$

in which pH_p is the pH below which the drug separates from solution as the undissociated acid.

In pharmaceutical practice, a drug such as phenobarbital is usually added to an aqueous solution in the soluble salt form. Of the initial quantity of salt, sodium phenobarbital, that can be added to a solution of a certain pH, some of it is converted into the free acid HP and some remains in the ionized form P^- (equation (10-59). The amount of salt that can be added initially before the solubility [HP] is exceeded is therefore equal to S. As seen from equation (10-62), pH_p depends on the initial molar concentration S of salt added, the molar solubility of the undissociated acid S_0, and the pK_a. Equation (10-62) has been used to determine the pK_a of sulfonamides and other drugs (see references **49** to **52**). Solubility and pH data may also be used to obtain the pK_1 and pK_2 values of dibasic acids as suggested by Zimmerman[43] and by Blanchard et al.[44]

Example 10-16. Below what pH will free phenobarbital begin to separate from a solution having an initial concentration of 1 g of sodium phenobarbital per 100 mL at 25° C? The molar solubility S_0 of phenobarbital is 0.0050 and the $pK_a = 7.41$ at 25° C. The secondary dissociation of phenobarbital, referred to previously, may ordinarily be disregarded. The molecular weight of sodium phenobarbital is 254.

The molar concentration of salt initially added is

$$\frac{\text{g/liter}}{\text{mol. wt.}} = \frac{10}{254} = 0.039 \text{ mole/liter}$$

$$pH_p = 7.41 + \log \frac{(0.039 - 0.005)}{0.005} = 8.24$$

An analogous derivation may be carried out to obtain the equation for the solubility of a weak base as a function of the pH of a solution. The expression is

$$pH_p = pK_w - pK_b + \log \frac{S_0}{S - S_0} \qquad (10-63)$$

in which S is the concentration of the drug initially added as the salt and S_0 is the molar solubility of the free base in water. Here pH_p is the pH *above* which the drug begins to precipitate from solution as the free base.

The Influence of Solvents on the Solubility of Drugs.

Weak electrolytes may behave like strong electrolytes and like nonelectrolytes in solution. When the solution is of such a pH that the drug is entirely in the ionic form, it behaves as a solution of a strong electrolyte and solubility does not constitute a serious problem. However, when the pH is adjusted to a value at which un-ionized molecules are produced in sufficient concentration to exceed the solubility of this form, precipitation occurs. In this discussion, we are now interested in the solubility of nonelectrolytes and the undissociated molecules of weak electrolytes. The solubility of undissociated phenobarbital in various solvents is discussed here because it has been studied to some extent by pharmaceutical investigators.

Frequently a solute is more soluble in a mixture of solvents than in one solvent alone. This phenomenon is known as *cosolvency*, and the solvents that, in combination, increase the solubility of the solute are called *cosolvents*. Approximately 1 g of phenobarbital is soluble in 1000 mL of water, in 10 mL of alcohol, in 40 mL of chloroform, and in 15 mL of ether at 25° C. The solubility of phenobarbital in water–alcohol–glycerin mixtures is plotted on a semilogarithm grid in Figure 10–7 from the data of Krause and Cross.[45]

By drawing lines parallel to the abscissa in Figure 10–7 at a height equivalent to the required phenobarbital concentration, it is a simple matter to obtain the relative amounts of the various combinations of alcohol, glycerin and water needed to achieve solution. For example, at 22% alcohol, 40% glycerin, and the remainder water (38%), 1.5% *w/v* of phenobarbital is dissolved, as seen by following the vertical and horizontal lines drawn on Figure 10–7.

Combined Effect of pH and Solvents.

The solvent affects the solubility of a weak electrolyte in a buffered solution in two ways:

1. The addition of alcohol to a buffered aqueous solution of a weak electrolyte increases the solubility of the un-ionized species by adjusting the polarity of the solvent to a more favorable value.

2. Being less polar than water, alcohol decreases the dissociation of a weak electrolyte, and the solubility of the drug goes down as the dissociation constant is decreased (pK_a is increased).

Stockton and Johnson[46] and Higuchi et al.[47] studied the effect of an increase of alcohol concentration on the dissociation constant of sulfathiazole, and Edmonson and Goyan[48] investigated the effect of alcohol on the solubility of phenobarbital.

Agarwal and Blake[49] and Schwartz et al.[50] determined the solubility of phenytoin as a function of pH and alcohol concentration in various buffer systems and calculated the apparent dissociation constant. Kramer and Flynn[51] examined the solubility of hydrochloride salts of organic bases as a function of pH, temperature, and solvent composition. They described the determination of the pK_a of the salt from the solubility profile at various temperatures and in several solvent systems. Chowhan[52] measured and calculated the solubility of the organic carboxylic acid, naproxen, and its sodium, potassium, calcium, and magnesium salts. The observed solubilities were in excellent agreement with the pH-solubility profiles based on equation (10–62).

The results of Edmonson and Goyan[48] are shown in Figure 10–8, where one observes that the pK_a of phenobarbital, 7.41, is raised to 7.92 in a hydroalcoholic solution containing 30% by volume of alcohol. Furthermore, as can be seen in Figure 10–7 the solubility S_o of un-ionized phenobarbital is increased from 0.12 g/100 mL or 0.005 M in water to 0.64% or 0.0276 M in a 30%

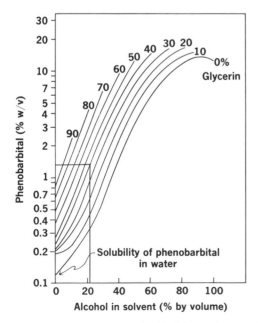

Fig. 10–7. The solubility of phenobarbital in a mixture of water, alcohol, and glycerin at 25° C. The vertical axis is a logarithmic scale representing the solubility of phenobarbital in g/100 mL. (After G. M. Krause and J. M. Cross, J. Am. Pharm. Assoc., Sci. Ed. **40**, 137, 1951, reproduced with permission of the copyright owner.)

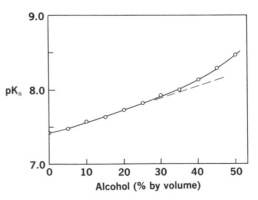

Fig. 10–8. The influence of alcohol concentration on the dissociation constant of phenobarbital. (After T. D. Edmonson and J. E. Goyan, J. Am. Pharm. Assoc., Sci. Ed. **47**, 810, 1958, reproduced with permission of the copyright owner.)

alcoholic solution. The calculation of solubility as a function of pH involving these results is illustrated in the following example.

Example 10–17. What is the minimum pH required for the complete solubility of the drug in a stock solution containing 6 g of phenobarbital sodium in 100 mL of a 30% by volume alcoholic solution? From equation (10–62):

$$pH_p = 7.92 + \log \frac{(0.236 - 0.028)}{0.028}$$

$$pH_p = 7.92 + 0.87 = 8.79$$

For comparison, the minimum pH for complete solubility of phenobarbital in an aqueous solution containing no alcohol is computed using equation (10–62).

$$pH_p = 7.41 + \log \frac{(0.236 - 0.005)}{0.005} = 9.07$$

From the calculations of *Example 10–17*, it is seen that although the addition of alcohol increases the pK_a, it also increases the solubility of the un-ionized form of the drug over that found in water sufficiently so that the pH may be reduced somewhat before precipitation occurs.

Equations (10–62) and (10–63) can be made more exact if activities are used instead of concentrations to account for interionic attraction effects. This refinement, however, is seldom required for practical work, in which the values calculated from the approximate equations just given serve as satisfactory estimates.

Influence of Surfactants. Weakly acidic and basic drugs may be brought into solution by the solubilizing action of surface-active agents. Solubilization of drugs in micelles is discussed as a colloidal phenomenon on pages 410 to 414, but it is appropriate here to describe the influence of surface-active agents on the solubility of drugs in quantitative terms along with the solubilizing effects of solvents, such as glycerin and ethanol.

Rippie et al.[53] investigated the micellar solubilization of weak electrolytic drugs by aqueous solutions of the nonionic surfactant polysorbate 80. The terminology of Rippie and associates is used in the following description of the theory.

The total solubility D_T of an acidic drug is expressed as the sum of the concentrations of species in solution:

$$D_T = (D) + (D^-) + [D] + [D^-] \quad (10{-}64)$$

in which (D) and (D^-) are nonionized acid and ionized acid, respectively, not in the micelles; $[D]$ and $[D^-]$ are nonionized and ionized acid, respectively, present in the micelles. The drug is considered to partition between the aqueous solution and the surfactant micelles according to the expression

$$K' = \frac{[D]_0}{(D)_0} \quad (10{-}65)$$

for the nonionized acid, and

$$K'' = \frac{[D^-]_0}{(D^-)_0} \quad (10{-}66)$$

for the ionized acid.

The subscript $_0$ represents concentrations expressed relative to individual phase volumes rather than the total volume of the system. In terms of total volume, equations (10–65) and (10–66) become

$$K' = \frac{[D][1 - (M)]}{(D)(M)} \quad (10{-}67)$$

$$K'' = \frac{[D^-][1 - (M)]}{(D^-)(M)} \quad (10{-}68)$$

The concentration term, (M), is the volume fraction of surfactant as micelles in solution; the amount in true solution would be small and can be neglected. Now, $1 - (M)$ can be set equal to unity in equations (10–67) and (10–68), yielding

$$[D] = K'(D)(M) \quad (10{-}69)$$

$$[D^-] = K''(D^-)(M) \quad (10{-}70)$$

The total drug solubility, $D_T{}^*$, in a solution at a definite pH and in the absence of the surfactant ($D_T{}^* \equiv S$ in equation (10–59)) is defined as

$$D_T{}^* = (D) + (D^-) \quad (10{-}71)$$

The fraction, $(D)/D_T{}^*$, of un-ionized drug in the aqueous phase is

$$\frac{(D)}{D_T{}^*} = \frac{(H^+)}{K_a + (H^+)} \quad (10{-}72)$$

or

$$D_T{}^* = (D) \frac{K_a + (H^+)}{(H^+)} \quad (10{-}73)$$

Using the relationships just given, Rippie et al.[53] obtained the expression

$$\frac{D_T}{D_T{}^*} = 1 + (M) \left[\frac{(H^+)K' + K_aK''}{K_a + (H^+)} \right] \quad (10{-}74)$$

in which D_T is total drug solubility in the presence of surfactant, according to equation (10–64). With equation (10–74), one may calculate total drug solubility in a solution of a definite pH and having a volume fraction (M) of surfactant present in the form of micelles.

Example 10–18. Calculate the solubility of sulfisoxazole at 25° C in (a) a pH 6.0 buffer and (b) a pH 6.0 buffer containing 4% by volume (i.e., 0.04 volume fraction) polysorbate 80 (Tween 80). The aqueous solubility of nonionized sulfisoxazole at 25° C is 0.15 g/liter, its $K_a = 7.60 \times 10^{-6}$, and the apparent partition coefficient of the molecular drug, K', and its anion, K'', between polysorbate 80 micelles and water are 79 and 15, respectively. (K' and K'' are dimensionless constants.)

(a) From equation (10–73), the total drug solubility at pH 6 in the absence of the surfactant is

$$D_T{}^* = 0.15 \text{ g/liter} \left[\frac{\begin{array}{c}(7.6 \times 10^{-6}) \text{ moles/liter} \\ + (1.0 \times 10^{-6}) \text{ moles/liter}\end{array}}{(1.0 \times 10^{-6}) \text{ moles/liter}} \right] = 1.29 \text{ g/liter}$$

(b) From equation (10–74), the total solubility of sulfisoxazole in a pH 6 buffer in the presence of 4% Tween 80 is

$$D_T = (1.29) \left\{ 1 + (0.04) \times \left[\frac{(1 \times 10^{-6})(79) + (7.6 \times 10^{-6})(15)}{(7.6 \times 10^{-6}) + (1 \times 10^{-6})} \right] \right\}$$

$$D_T = 2.45 \text{ g/liter}$$

The presence of the surfactant has almost doubled the concentration of the drug in solution.

The total solubility of a basic drug corresponding to that for an acidic drug, equation (10–64), in a solution containing a micellar surfactant, is

$$D_T = (D^+) + (D) + [D^+] + [D] \qquad (10\text{–}75)$$

in which D^+ is the cationic acid species and D is the nonionized base. The ionization of a molecular (nonionic) base, procaine, is represented as

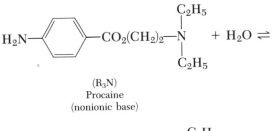

(R₃N)
Procaine
(nonionic base)

(R₃NH⁺)
Procaine cation
(ionic acid conjugate to
Procaine base)   (10–76)

The dissociation equilibrium for this reaction is written

$$K_b = \frac{[\text{R}_3\text{NH}^+][\text{OH}^-]}{[\text{R}_3\text{N}]} \qquad (10\text{–}77)$$

The dissociation also may be written in terms of the procaine cation to obtain the acid dissociation constant, K_a,

$$\text{R}_3\text{NH}^+ + \text{H}_2\text{O} \rightleftharpoons \text{R}_3\text{N} + \text{H}_3\text{O}^+ \qquad (10\text{–}78)$$

$$K_a = \frac{[\text{R}_3\text{N}][\text{H}_3\text{O}^+]}{[\text{R}_3\text{NH}^+]} \qquad (10\text{–}79)$$

As noted earlier in the text, the following relationship holds between a molecular base and its cationic acid (also between a molecular acid and its anionic base):

$$K_a K_b = K_w \qquad (10\text{–}80)$$

and

$$\text{p}K_a + \text{p}K_b = \text{p}K_w \qquad (10\text{–}81)$$

For a molecular base such as procaine,

$$(D) = D_T{}^* \left[\frac{K_a}{K_a + (\text{H}^+)} \right] \qquad (10\text{–}82)$$

$$(D^+) = D_T{}^* \left[\frac{\text{H}^+}{K_a + (\text{H}^+)} \right] \qquad (10\text{–}83)$$

and

$$\frac{D_T}{D_T{}^*} = 1 + (M) \left[\frac{K_a K' + (\text{H}^+)K''}{K_a + (\text{H}^+)} \right] \qquad (10\text{–}84)$$

in which (D) is the free acid not in the micelle, (D^+) is the cationic acid, conjugate to the molecular base, not in the micelle, and the other terms have the same meanings as defined earlier. The expressions permit the calculation of solubilization of a weakly basic drug, such as procaine, in aqueous solutions of a micellar solubilizing agent such as polysorbate 80.

Example 10–19. The aqueous solubility of procaine base at 25° C is 5 g/liter, its K_a is 1.4×10^{-9}, and the apparent partition coefficient for the molecular base is $K' = 30$; for its cationic acid, $K'' = 7.0$. Calculate the solubility of procaine in a pH 7.40 buffer containing 3% (w/v) polysorbate 80.

(a)

$$D_T{}^* = (D) \left[\frac{K_a + (\text{H}^+)}{K_a} \right] = (5.0) \left[\frac{(1.4 \times 10^{-9}) + (3.98 \times 10^{-8})}{(1.40 \times 10^{-9})} \right]$$

$$= 147.2 \text{ g/liter}$$

(b)

$$D_T = 147.2 \left\{ 1 + (0.03) \times \left[\frac{(1.4 \times 10^{-9})(30) + (3.98 \times 10^{-8})(7)}{(1.40 \times 10^{-9}) + (3.98 \times 10^{-8})} \right] \right\}$$

$$= 181.6 \text{ g/liter}$$

What is the fraction of the drug in the aqueous phase and the fraction in the micelles?

$$\frac{\text{Total drug in aqueous phase, } D_T{}^*}{\text{Total drug in aqueous phase and micelles, } D_T} = \frac{147.2 \text{ g/liter}}{181.6 \text{ g/liter}} = 0.81$$

Thus, the fraction 0.81 of procaine exists in the aqueous phase, and the remainder, 0.19, resides in the micelles. The solubility of procaine is increased by one quarter over that in aqueous buffer owing to the surfactant micelles.

Influence of Complexation in Multicomponent Systems. Many liquid pharmaceutical preparations consist of more than a single drug in solution. Fritz et al.[54] have shown that when several drugs together with pharmaceutical adjuncts interact in solution to form insoluble complexes, simple solubility profiles of individual drugs cannot be used to predict solubilities in mixtures of ingredients. Instead, the specific multicomponent systems must be studied to estimate the complicating effects of species interactions.

Influence of Other Factors on the Solubility of Solids. The size and shape of small particles (those in the micrometer range) also affect solubility. Solubility increases with decreasing particle size according to the approximate equation

$$\log \frac{s}{s_0} = \frac{2\gamma V}{2.303 RTr} \qquad (10\text{–}85)$$

in which s is the solubility of the fine particles; s_0 is the solubility of the solid consisting of relatively large particles; γ is the surface tension of the particles, which, for solids, unfortunately, is extremely difficult to obtain; V is the molar volume (volume in cm³ per mole of particles); r is the final radius of the particles in cm;

R is the gas constant (8.314×10^7 erg/deg mole); and T is the absolute temperature. The equation may be used for solid or liquid particles such as those in suspensions or emulsions. The following example is taken from the book by Hildebrand and Scott.[55]

Example 10–20. A solid is to be comminuted so as to increase its solubility by 10%, i.e., s/s_o is to become 1.10. What must be the final particle size, assuming that the surface tension of the solid is 100 dynes/cm and the volume per mole is 50 cm³? The temperature is 27° C.

$$r = \frac{2 \times 100 \times 50}{2.303 \times 8.314 \times 10^7 \times 300 \times 0.0414}$$

$$= 4.2 \times 10^{-6} \text{ cm} = 0.042 \ \mu\text{m}$$

The effects of particle size on the solubility of a solid have been reviewed in some detail by May and Kolthoff,[56] and the interested reader should refer to their report.

The configuration of a molecule and the kind of arrangement in the crystal also has some influence on solubility, and a symmetric particle may be less soluble than an unsymmetric one. This is because solubility depends in part on the work required to separate the particles of the crystalline solute. The molecules of the amino acid α-alanine form a compact crystal with high lattice energy and consequently low solubility. The molecules of α-amino-*n*-butyric acid pack less efficiently in the crystal, partly because of the projecting side chains, and the crystal energy is reduced. Consequently, α-amino-*n*-butyric acid has a solubility of 1.80 moles/liter and α-alanine only 1.66 moles/liter in water at 25° C, although the hydrocarbon chain of α-amino-*n*-butyric acid is the longer of the two compounds.

DISTRIBUTION OF SOLUTES BETWEEN IMMISCIBLE SOLVENTS

If an excess of liquid or solid is added to a mixture of two immiscible liquids, it will distribute itself between the two phases so that each becomes saturated. If the substance is added to the immiscible solvents in an amount insufficient to saturate the solutions, it will still become distributed between the two layers in a definite concentration ratio.

If C_1 and C_2 are the equilibrium concentrations of the substance in solvent$_1$ and solvent$_2$, the equilibrium expression becomes

$$\frac{C_1}{C_2} = K \qquad (10\text{–}86)$$

The equilibrium constant K is known as the *distribution ratio*, *distribution coefficient*, or *partition coefficient*. Equation (10–86), which is known as the *distribution law*, is strictly applicable only in dilute solutions in which activity coefficients may be neglected.

Example 10–21. When boric acid is distributed between water and amyl alcohol at 25° C, the concentration in water was found to be

0.0510 mole/liter and in amyl alcohol it was found to be 0.0155 mole/liter. What is the distribution coefficient?

$$K = \frac{C_{\text{H}_2\text{O}}}{C_{\text{alc}}} = \frac{0.0510}{0.0155} = 3.29$$

No convention has been established with regard to whether the concentration in the water phase or in the organic phase should be placed in the numerator. Therefore, the result may also be expressed as

$$K = \frac{C_{\text{alc}}}{C_{\text{H}_2\text{O}}} = \frac{0.0155}{0.0510} = 0.304$$

One should always specify in which of these two ways the distribution constant is being expressed.

A knowledge of partition is important to the pharmacist, for the principle is involved in several areas of current pharmaceutical interest. These include preservation of oil–water systems, drug action at nonspecific sites, and the absorption and distribution of drugs throughout the body. Certain aspects of these topics are discussed in the following sections.

Effect on Partition of Ionic Dissociation and Molecular Association. The solute may exist partly or wholly as associated molecules in one of the phases or it may dissociate into ions in either of the liquid phases. The distribution law applies only to the concentration of the species common to both phases, namely, the *monomer* or simple molecules of the solute.

Consider the distribution of benzoic acid between an oil phase and a water phase. When it is neither associated in the oil nor dissociated into ions in the water, equation (10–86) can be used to compute the distribution constant. When association and dissociation occur, however, the situation becomes more complicated. The general case in which benzoic acid associates in the oil phase and dissociates in the aqueous phase is shown schematically in Figure 10–9.

Two cases will be treated. *First,* according to Garrett and Woods,[57] benzoic acid is considered to be distributed between the two phases, peanut oil and water. Although benzoic acid undergoes dimerization (association to form two molecules) in many nonpolar solvents, it does not associate in peanut oil. It ionizes in water to

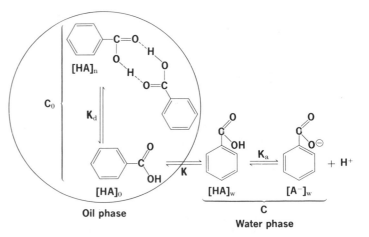

Fig. 10–9. Schematic representation of the distribution of benzoic acid between a water and an oil phase. (The oil phase is depicted as a magnified oil droplet in an oil-in-water emulsion.)

a degree, however, depending on the pH of the solution. Therefore, in Figure 10-9 for the case under consideration, C_o, the total concentration of benzoic acid in the oil phase, is equal to $[HA]_o$, the monomer concentration in the oil phase, since association does not occur in peanut oil.

The species common to both the oil and water phases are the unassociated and undissociated benzoic acid molecules. The distribution is expressed as

$$K = \frac{[HA]_o}{[HA]_w} = \frac{C_o}{[HA]_w} \quad (10\text{-}87)$$

in which K is the *true distribution coefficient* $[HA]_o = C_o$ is the molar concentration of the simple benzoic acid molecules in the oil phase, and $[HA]_w$ is the molar concentration of the undissociated acid in the water phase.

The total acid concentration obtained by analysis of the aqueous phase is

$$C_w = [HA]_w + [A^-]_w \quad (10\text{-}88)$$

and the experimentally observed or *apparent distribution coefficient* is

$$K' = \frac{[HA]_o}{[HA]_w + [A^-]_w} = \frac{C_o}{C_w} \quad (10\text{-}89)$$

As seen in Figure 10-9, the observed distribution coefficient depends on two equilibria: the distribution of the undissociated acid between the immiscible phases as expressed in equation (10-87), and the species distribution of the acid in the aqueous phase, which depends on the hydrogen ion concentration $[H_3O^+]$ and the dissociation constant K_a of the acid.

$$K_a = \frac{[H_3O^+][A^-]_w}{[HA]_w} \quad (10\text{-}90)$$

Association of benzoic acid in peanut oil does not occur, and K_d (the equilibrium constant for dissociation of associated benzoic acid into monomer in the oil phase) may be neglected in this case.

Given these equations and the fact that the concentration C of the acid in the aqueous phase before distribution, assuming equal volumes of the two phases, is*

---

*The meaning of C in equation (10-91) is understood readily by considering a simple illustration. Suppose one begins with 1 liter of oil and 1 liter of water, and after benzoic acid has been distributed between the two phases, the concentration C_o of benzoic acid in the oil is 0.01 mole/liter and the concentration C_w of benzoic acid in the aqueous phase is 0.01 mole/liter. Accordingly, there is 0.02 mole/2 liter or 0.01 mole of benzoic acid per liter of total mixture after distribution equilibrium has been attained. Equation (10-91) gives

$$C = C_o + C_w = 0.01 \text{ mole/liter} + 0.01 \text{ mole/liter}$$
$$= 0.02 \text{ mole/liter}$$

The concentration C obviously is not the total concentration of the acid in the mixture at equilibrium but, rather, twice this value. C is therefore seen to be the concentration of benzoic acid in the water phase (or the oil phase) *before* the distribution is carried out.

$$C = C_o + C_w \quad (10\text{-}91)$$

one arrives at the combined result,†

$$\frac{K_a + [H_3O^+]}{C_w} = \frac{K_a}{C} + \frac{K+1}{C}[H_3O^+] \quad (10\text{-}92)$$

Expression (10-92) is a linear equation of the form, $y = a + bx$, and therefore a plot of $(K_a + [H_3O^+])/C_w$ against $[H_3O^+]$ yields a straight line with a slope $b = (K + 1)/C$ and an intercept $a = K_a/C$. The true distribution coefficient K can thus be obtained over the range of hydrogen ion concentration considered. Alternatively, the true distribution constant could be obtained according to equation (10-87) by analysis of the oil phase and of the water phase at a sufficiently low pH ($\cong 2.0$) at which the acid would exist completely in the un-ionized form. One of the advantages of equation (10-92), however, is that the oil phase need not be analyzed; only the hydrogen ion concentration and C_w, the total concentration remaining in the aqueous phase at equilibrium, need be determined.

Example 10-22. According to Garrett and Woods,[57] the plot of $(K_a + [H_3O^+])/C_w$ against $[H_3O^+]$ for benzoic acid distributed between equal volumes of peanut oil and a buffered aqueous solution yielded a slope $b = 4.16$ and an intercept $a = 4.22 \times 10^{-5}$. The K_a of benzoic acid is 6.4×10^{-5}. Compute the true partition coefficient, K, and compare it with the value $K = 5.33$ obtained by the authors.

$$b = (K + 1)/C$$

or

$$K = bC - 1$$

---

†Equation (10-92) is obtained as follows. Substituting for $[A^-]_w$ from equation (10-90) into equation (10-89) gives

$$K' = \frac{[HA]_o}{[HA]_w + \frac{K_a[HA]_w}{[H_3O^+]}} = \frac{[HA]_o[H_3O^+]}{[HA]_w(K_a + [H_3O^+])} \quad (a)$$

Then $[HA]_w$ from equation (10-87) is substituted into (a) to eliminate $[HA]_o$ from the equation:

$$K' = \frac{[HA]_o[H_3O^+]}{[HA]_o/K(K_a + [H_3O^+])} = \frac{K[H_3O^+]}{K_a + [H_3O^+]} \quad (b)$$

The apparent distribution constant is eliminated by substituting equation (b) into equation (10-89) to give

$$\frac{K[H_3O^+]}{K_a + [H_3O^+]} = \frac{C_o}{C_w}$$

or

$$C_o = \frac{K[H_3O^+]C_w}{K_a + [H_3O^+]} \quad (c)$$

C_o is eliminated by substituting equation (c) into equation (10-91):

$$C = \frac{K[H_3O^+]C_w}{K_a + [H_3O^+]} + C_w$$
$$= \frac{K[H_3O^+]C_w + (K_a + [H_3O^+])C_w}{K_a + [H_3O^+]} \quad (d)$$

Rearranging equation (d) gives the final result:

$$\frac{K_a + [H_3O^+]}{C_w} = \frac{[H_3O^+](K + 1) + K_a}{C}$$

Since

$$a = K_a/C \quad \text{or} \quad C = \frac{K_a}{a}$$

the expression becomes

$$K = \frac{bK_a}{a} - 1 = \frac{bK_a - a}{a}$$

and

$$K = \frac{(4.16 \times 6.4 \times 10^{-5}) - 4.22 \times 10^{-5}}{4.22 \times 10^{-5}} = 5.31$$

Second, let us now consider the case in which the solute is associated in the organic phase and exists as simple molecules in the aqueous phase. If benzoic acid is distributed between benzene and acidified water, it exists mainly as associated molecules in the benzene layer and as undissociated molecules in the aqueous layer.

The equilibrium between simple molecules HA and associated molecules $(HA)_n$ in benzene is

$$(HA)_n \quad \rightleftharpoons \quad n(HA)$$

Associated molecules   Simple molecules

and the equilibrium constant expressing the dissociation of associated molecules into simple molecules in this solvent is

$$K_d = \frac{[HA]_o{}^n}{[(HA)_n]} \tag{10-93}$$

or

$$[HA]_o = \sqrt[n]{K_d}\sqrt[n]{[(HA)_n]} \tag{10-94}$$

Since benzoic acid exists predominantly in the form of double molecules in benzene, C_o may replace $[(HA)_2]$ where C_o is the total molar concentration of the solute in the organic layer. Then equation (10-94) may be written approximately as

$$[HA]_o \cong \text{constant} \times \sqrt{C_o} \tag{10-95}$$

In conformity with the distribution law as given in equation (10-87), the true distribution coefficient is always expressed in terms of simple species common to both phases, that is, in terms of $[HA]_w$ and $[HA]_o$. In the benzene–water system, $[HA]_o$ is given by equation (10-95), and the modified distribution constant becomes

$$K'' = \frac{[HA]_o}{[HA]_w} = \frac{\sqrt{C_o}}{[HA]_w} \tag{10-96}$$

The results for the distribution of benzoic acid between benzene and water, as given by Glasstone,[58] are found in Table 10-13.

A third case, involving both association in the organic phase and dissociation in the aqueous phase, might be treated at this point but will be deferred until a later section. It follows directly from the two cases already presented, as will be illustrated in *Example 10-25* dealing with preservative action. Various cases of

TABLE 10-13. *Distribution of Benzoic Acid between Benzene and Acidified Water at 6° C**

	The concentrations are expressed in moles per liter	
$[HA]_w$	C_o	$K'' = \sqrt{C_o}/[HA]_w$
0.00329	0.0156	38.0
0.00579	0.0495	38.2
0.00749	0.0835	38.6
0.0114	0.195	38.8

*From S. Glasstone, *Textbook of Physical Chemistry*, Van Nostrand, New York, 1946, p. 738.

distribution are treated most adequately by Davies and Hallam.[59]

Extraction. To determine the efficiency with which one solvent can extract a compound from a second solvent—an operation commonly employed in analytic chemistry and in organic chemistry—we follow Glasstone.[60] Suppose that w grams of a solute are extracted repeatedly from V_1 mL of one solvent with successive portions of V_2 mL of a second solvent, which is immiscible with the first. Let w_1 be the weight of the solute remaining in the original solvent after extracting with the first portion of the other solvent. Then the concentration of solute remaining in the first solvent is (w_1/V_1) g/mL and the concentration of the solute in the extracting solvent is $(w - w_1)/V_2$ g/mL. The distribution coefficient is thus

$$K = \frac{\text{concentration of solute}}{\text{in original solvent}}\Big/\frac{\text{concentration of solute}}{\text{in extracting solvent}}$$

$$K = \frac{w_1/V_1}{(w - w_1)V_2} \tag{10-97}$$

or

$$w_1 = w\frac{KV_1}{KV_1 + V_2} \tag{10-98}$$

The process can be repeated, and after n extractions[60]

$$w_n = w\left(\frac{KV_1}{KV_1 + V_2}\right)^n \tag{10-99}$$

By use of this equation, it can be shown that most efficient extraction results when n is large and V_2 is small, in other words, when a large number of extractions are carried out with small portions of extracting liquid. The development just described assumes complete immiscibility of the two liquids. When ether is used to extract organic compounds from water, this is not true; however, the equations provide approximate values that are satisfactory for practical purposes. The presence of other solutes, such as salts, may also affect the results by complexing with the solute or by salting out one of the phases.

Example 10–23. The distribution coefficient for iodine between water and carbon tetrachloride at 25° C is $K = C_{H_2O}/C_{CCl_4} = 0.012$. How many grams of iodine are extracted from a solution in water containing 0.1 g in 50 mL by one extraction with 10 mL of CCl_4? How many grams are extracted by two 5-mL portions of CCl_4?

$$w_1 = 0.10 \times \frac{0.012 \times 50}{(0.012 \times 50) + 10}$$

$$= 0.0057 \text{ g remain or } 0.0943 \text{ g are extracted}$$

$$w_2 = 0.10 \times \left(\frac{0.012 \times 50}{(0.012 \times 50) + 5}\right)^2$$

$$= 0.0011 \text{ g of iodine}$$

Thus, 0.0011 g of iodine remains in the water phase, and the two portions of CCl_4 have extracted 0.0989 g.

Solubility and Partition Coefficients. Hansch et al.[61] observed a relationship between aqueous solubilities of nonelectrolytes and partitioning. Yalkowsky and Valvani[62] obtained an equation to determine the aqueous solubility of liquid or crystalline organic compounds:

$$\log S = - \log K$$
$$-1.11 \frac{\Delta S_f \,(\text{mp} - 25)}{1364} + 0.54 \qquad (10\text{--}100)$$

in which S is aqueous solubility in moles/liter, K is the octanol–water partition coefficient, ΔS_f is the molar entropy of fusion, and mp is the melting point of a solid compound on the centigrade scale. For a liquid compound, mp is assigned a value of 25 so that the second right-hand term of equation (10–100) becomes zero.

The entropy of fusion and the partition coefficient may be estimated from the chemical structure of the compound. For rigid molecules, $\Delta S_f = 13.5$ entropy units (eu). For molecules with n greater than five nonhydrogen atoms in a flexible chain,

$$\Delta S_f = 13.5 + 2.5(n - 5) \text{ eu} \qquad (10\text{--}101)$$

Leo et al.[61] have provided partition coefficients for a large number of compounds. When experimental values are not available, group contribution methods (Leo et al.,[61] Rekker[63]) are available for estimating partition coefficients.

Example 10–24. Estimate the molar aqueous solubility of heptyl *p*-aminobenzoate, mp 75° C at 25° C.

$$H_2N - \langle \text{benzene ring} \rangle - \overset{\overset{\displaystyle O}{\|}}{C} - O - CH_2 - CH_2 - CH_2 - CH_2 - CH_2 - CH_2 - CH_3$$

It is first necessary to calculate ΔS_f and $\log K$.

There are nine nonhydrogens in the flexible chain (C, O, and seven carbons). Using equation (10–101), we obtain:

$$\Delta S_f = 13.5 + 2.5 \,(9 - 5) = 23.5 \text{ eu}$$

For the partition coefficient, Leo et al.[61] give $\log K$ of benzoic acid a value of 1.87, the contribution of NH_2 is -1.16, and $CH_2 = 0.50$ or $7 \times 0.50 = 3.50$ for the seven carbon atoms in the chain.

$$\log K \text{ (heptyl } p\text{-aminobenzoate)} = 1.87 - 1.16 + 3.50 = 4.21$$

These values are substituted into equation (10–100):

$$\log S = -4.21 - 1.11 \left(\frac{23.5 \,(75 - 25)}{1364}\right) + 0.54$$

$$\log S = -4.63$$
$$S_{(calc)} = 2.36 \times 10^{-5} \, M$$
$$S_{(obs)} = 2.51 \times 10^{-5} \, M$$

Preservative Action of Weak Acids in Oil–Water Systems. Solutions of foods, drugs, and cosmetics are subject to deterioration by the enzymes of microorganisms that act as catalysts in decomposition reactions. These enzymes are produced by yeasts, molds, and bacteria, and such microorganisms must be destroyed or inhibited to prevent deterioration. Sterilization and the addition of chemical preservatives are common methods used in pharmacy to preserve drug solutions against attack by various microorganisms. Benzoic acid in the form of its soluble salt, sodium benzoate, is often used for this purpose since it produces no injurious effects in humans when taken internally in small quantities.

Rahn and Conn[64] showed that the preservative or bacteriostatic action of benzoic acid and similar acids is due almost entirely to the undissociated acid and not to the ionic form. These investigators found that the yeast, *Saccharomyces ellipsoideus*, which grows normally at a pH of 2.5 to 7.0 in the presence of strong inorganic acids or salts, ceased to grow in the presence of undissociated benzoic acid when the concentration of the acid reached 25 mg/100 mL. The preservative action of undissociated benzoic acid as compared with the ineffectiveness of the benzoate ion is presumably due to the relative ease with which the un-ionized molecule penetrates living membranes, and conversely, the difficulty with which the ion does so. The undissociated molecule, consisting of a large nonpolar portion, is soluble in the lipoidal membrane of the microorganism and penetrates rapidly.

Bacteria in oil–water systems are generally located in the aqueous phase and at the oil–water interface. Therefore, the efficacy of a weak acid, such as benzoic acid, as a preservative for these systems is largely a result of the concentration of the undissociated acid in the aqueous phase.

To calculate the total concentration of benzoic acid that must be added to preserve an oil–water mixture, we proceed as follows. Let us take the peanut oil–water mixture considered by Garrett and Woods[57] and begin by writing the expression

$$C = qC_o + C_w = q[HA]_o + [HA]_w + [A^-]_w \qquad (10\text{--}102)$$

in which $q = V_o/V_w$, the volume ratio of the two phases, is needed when the volumes are not equal. C is the original concentration of the acid in the water phase before the aqueous solution is equilibrated with peanut oil. C_o is the molar concentration of the simple undissociated molecules in the oil, because the acid does not dimerize or dissociate in the organic phase. C_w, the molar concentration of benzoic acid in water, is equal to the sum of the two terms, $[HA]_w$ and $[A^-]_w$, in this ionizing solvent. It is furthermore assumed that concentrations are approximately equal to activities.

The distribution of total benzoic acid among the various species in this system depends upon the distribution coefficient K, the dissociation constant K_a of the acid in the aqueous phase, the phase volume ratio, and the hydrogen ion concentration of the aqueous phase. To account for the first effect, we introduce the term $K = [HA]_o/[HA]_w$ or $[HA]_o = K[HA]_w$ into equation (10–102). We write the dissociation constant, $K_a = [H_3O^+][A^-]_w/[HA]_w$, or the ionic species $[A^-]_w = K_a[HA]_w/[H_3O^+]$, to account for the influence of K_a and $[H_3O^+]$ and substitute it also into equation (10–102). The expression then becomes

$$C = Kq[HA]_w + [HA]_w + K_a[HA]_w/[H_3O^+] \quad (10–103)$$

Factoring out $[HA]_w$, we have

$$C = (Kq + 1 + K_a/[H_3O^+])[HA]_w \quad (10–104)$$

or

$$[HA]_w = \frac{C}{Kq + 1 + K_a/[H_3O^+]} \quad (10–105)$$

Equations (10–104) and (10–105) may be used to calculate the concentration C of total acid that must be added to the entire two-phase system to obtain a final specified concentration $[HA]_w$ of undissociated acid in the aqueous phase buffered at a definite pH or hydrogen ion concentration.[65]

Kazmi and Mitchell[66] and Bean et al.[67] have also proposed calculations for preserving solubilized and emulsified systems that are slightly different from that of Garrett and Woods.

Example 10–25. If benzoic acid is distributed between equal volumes of peanut oil and water, what must be the original concentration in the water phase in order that 0.25 mg/mL of undissociated acid remains in the aqueous phase buffered at a pH of 4.0? The partition coefficient $K = [HA]_o/[HA]_w$ is 5.33 and the dissociation constant of the acid in water is 6.4×10^{-5}. Since the two phases are present in equal amounts, $q = V_o/V_w = 1$. Equation (10–104) is employed.

$$C = \left(5.33 + 1 + \frac{6.4 \times 10^{-5}}{10^{-4}}\right) 0.25$$

$$= 1.74 \text{ mg/mL}$$

In the case in which benzoic acid exists as a dimer in the oil phase, the modified distribution coefficient is $K'' = (1/[HA]_w)\sqrt{C_o}$, therefore equation (10–102) becomes

$$C = K''^2 q[HA]_w^2 + [HA]_w$$
$$+ K_a[HA]_w/[H_3O^+] \quad (10–106)$$

and finally

$$C = K''^2 q[HA]_w + 1 + (K_a/[H_3O^+])[HA]_w \quad (10–107)$$

Example 10–26. How much undissociated benzoic acid (molecular weight 122 g/mole) remains in the aqueous phase of an emulsion consisting of 100 mL of benzene and 200 mL of water buffered at a pH of 4.2? Is this quantity sufficient to preserve the emulsion? The amount of benzoic acid initially added to the 200 mL of aqueous phase was 0.50 g. The dissociation constant of the acid is 6.4×10^{-5} ($pK_a =$

4.2), the hydrogen ion concentration of the solution is also 6.4×10^{-5}, and q is $V_o/V_w = 100/200 = 0.5$. The distribution coefficient $K'' = \sqrt{C_o}/[HA]_w \cong 38.5$ as seen in Table 10–13.

$$C = \left\{[(38.5)^2 \times 0.5 \times [HA]_w] + 1 + \frac{6.4 \times 10^{-5}}{6.4 \times 10^{-5}}\right\}[HA]_w$$

$$\frac{0.50 \text{ mole/liter}}{(122)(0.200)} = (741[HA]_w + 2)[HA]_w$$

$$741[HA]_w^2 + 2[HA]_w - 0.0205 = 0$$

$$[HA]_w = \frac{-2 + \sqrt{4 + 60.75}}{1482}$$

$$= 4.079 \times 10^{-3} \text{ mole/liter or } 0.0996 \text{ g/200 mL aqueous phase}$$

Drug Action and Partition Coefficients. At the turn of the century, Meyer and Overton proposed the hypothesis that narcotic action of a nonspecific drug is a function of the distribution coefficient of the compound between a lipoidal medium and water. Later it was concluded that narcosis was a function only of the concentration of the drug in the lipids of the cell. Thus, a wide variety of drugs of different chemical types should produce equal narcotic action at equal concentration in the lipoidal cell substance. Actually, as will be seen shortly, this is a restatement of the theory, first proposed by Ferguson and generally accepted today, that equal degrees of narcotic action should occur at equal thermodynamic activities of the drugs in solution.

The activity of a vapor is obtained approximately by use of the equation (p. 134)

$$\frac{p_{nar}}{p^\circ} = a_{nar} \quad (10–108)$$

If p_{nar} is the partial pressure of a narcotic in solution just necessary to bring about narcosis, and p° is the vapor pressure of the pure liquid, narcosis will occur at a thermodynamic activity of a_{nar}.

Example 10–27. The vapor pressure p° of pure propane is 13 atm and that of butane is 3 atm at 37° C. The partial vapor pressure of propane for narcosis in mice is 0.9 and that for butane is 0.2.[68] Compute the thermodynamic activities of these two compounds required for equinarcotic action.

(a) For propane:

$$a_{nar} = \frac{p_{nar}}{p^\circ} = \frac{0.9}{13} = 0.069$$

(b) For butane:

$$a_{nar} = \frac{p_{nar}}{p^\circ} = \frac{0.2}{3} = 0.067$$

A still more striking confirmation of the rule that equal degrees of narcosis occur at equal thermodynamic activities (rather than at equal partition coefficients as originally proposed by Meyer and Overton) is shown in Table 10–14. Here it is seen that ethanol, *n*-propanol, and *n*-butanol have distribution coefficients of the same order and all would be expected to show similar narcotic action. Thymol, on the other hand, has a partition coefficient roughly 10,000 times that of the straight-chain alcohols, although its narcotic action is equal to that of the normal alcohols.

TABLE 10–14. *Narcotic Action of Various Compounds*

Substance	Concentration of Compound in Water in Moles/Liter Required for Narcotic Action in Tadpoles	Partition Coefficient of Narcotic Compound $K = \dfrac{C_{\text{oleyl alcohol}}}{C_{\text{water}}}$	Approximate Activity of Narcotic in Water or Lipoidal Phase ($a_w \cong a_o$)
Ethanol	0.33	0.10	0.033
n-Propanol	0.11	0.35	0.039
n-Butanol	0.03	0.65	0.020
Thymol	0.000047	950	0.045

We can now show that although the distribution coefficients differ, the thermodynamic activities of the compounds are all approximately the same for equal narcotic action. The partition coefficient may be written

$$K = \frac{\text{concentration in organic phase}}{\text{concentration in water phase}} = \frac{a_o/\gamma_o}{a_w/\gamma_w} \quad (10\text{--}109)$$

The student will notice that partition coefficients may be written in terms of concentration rather than activities. Since the activities, a_o and a_w, are equal at equilibrium, K would always equal 1.0. It is the differences in *concentration* we are interested in, and K is therefore defined as expressed in equation (10–109).

When a system is in equilibrium with respect to a compound distributed between two phases, the activities of the solute in the two phases may be taken to be identical, or $a_o = a_w$. Therefore, from (10–109),

$$K = \frac{a/\gamma_o}{a/\gamma_w} = \frac{\gamma_w}{\gamma_o} \quad (10\text{--}110)$$

It can be assumed that the organic solution is approximately ideal so that γ_o is unity. Then, equation (10–110) reduces to

$$K \cong \gamma_w \quad (10\text{--}111)$$

or *the partition coefficient is equal to the activity coefficient* of the compound in the aqueous phase. Finally, when the narcotic concentration in water is multiplied by the activity coefficient, obtained from equation (10–111) in terms of the partition coefficient, the thermodynamic activity for narcosis is obtained:

$$\left(\begin{array}{c}\text{narcotic concentration}\\ \text{in the aqueous phase}\end{array}\right)$$

$$\times \text{ (partition coefficient)} = a_{\text{nar}} \quad (10\text{--}112)$$

This value for the narcotic in the external phase will also give the thermodynamic activity in the lipoidal or biophase since, as already noted, at equilibrium the activities in the two phases must be the same. The molar concentrations of the narcotics in the external aqueous phase are listed in Table 10–14 together with the oil–water partition coefficients. The thermodynamic activity, calculated according to equation (10–112), is shown in column 4 of Table 10–14. Since the

activity coefficients of the drugs in the lipoidal phase are considered to be approximately unity, the *concentrations* in the biophase should be roughly equal to the calculated activities. Therefore, the modified rule of Meyer that isonarcotic action occurs at equal concentrations of the drugs in the lipoidal phase is understandable.

The oil–water partition coefficient is an indication of the lipophilic or hydrophobic character of a drug molecule. Passage of drugs through lipid membranes and interaction with macromolecules at receptor sites sometimes correlate well with the octanol–water partition coefficient of the drug. In the last few sections, the student has been introduced to the distribution of drug molecules between immiscible solvents together with some important applications of partitioning and may wish to pursue the subject further; towards this end, references **69** through **72** provide information on the subject. Three excellent books[73,74,75] on solubility in the pharmaceutical sciences will be of interest to the serious student of the subject.

References and Notes

1. W. J. Mader and L. T. Grady, Determination of solubility, Chapter 5 in *Techniques of Chemistry, Physical Methods in Chemistry*, Vol. I, Part V, A. Weissberger and B. W. Rossiter, Eds., Wiley, New York, 1971; *Techniques of Chemistry*, Vol. II, *Organic Solvents*, 3rd Edition, J. A. Reddick and W. B. Bunger, Eds., Wiley-Interscience, New York, 1970.
2. J. H. Hildebrand and R. L. Scott, *Solubility of Nonelectrolytes*, Dover, New York, 1964.
3. D. L. Leussing, Solubility, Chapter 17 in *Treatise on Analytical Chemistry*, I. M. Kolthoff and P. J. Elving, Eds., Vol. I, Part I, Interscience Encyclopedia, New York, 1959.
4. M. R. J. Dack, Solution and solubilities, in *Techniques of Chemistry*, A. Weissberger, Ed., Vol. VIII, Parts I and II, Wiley, New York 1975, 1976.
5. S. M. McElvain, *Characterization of Organic Compounds*, Macmillan, New York, 1953, p. 49.
6. M. R. Loran and E. P. Guth, J. Am. Pharm. Assoc., Sci. Ed. **40**, 465, 1951.
7. W. J. O'Malley, L. Pennati and A. Martin, J. Am. Pharm. Assoc., Sci. Ed. **47**, 334, 1958.
8. *Harper's Review of Biochemistry*, D. W. Martin, Jr., *et al.*, Editors, Lange Medical, Los Altos, Calif., 1985, pp. 46, 47.
9. M. H. Jacobs, *Diffusion Processes*, Springer Verlag, New York, 1967, pp. 51, 52.
10. A. Findlay, *The Phase Rule*, 4th Edition, Dover, New York, 1951, p. 101.
11. R. J. James and R. L. Goldemberg, J. Soc. Cosm. Chem. **11**, 461, 1960.
12. W. G. Gorman and G. D. Hall, J. Pharm. Sci. **53**, 1017, 1964.

13. A. N. Paruta, B. J. Sciarrone and N. G. Lordi, J. Pharm. Sci. **54**, 838 (1965); A. N. Paruta, J. Pharm. Sci. **58**, 294, 1969; B. Laprade, J. W. Mauger, H. Peterson, Jr., et al., J. Pharm. Sci. **65**, 277, 1976; T. L. Breon, J. W. Mauger, G. E. Osborne, et al., Drug Develop. Commun. **2**, 521, 1976; K. S. Alexander, J. W. Mauger, H. Peterson, Jr. and A. N. Paruta J. Pharm. Sci. **66**, 42, 1977.

14. L. B. Kier and L. H. Hall, *Molecular Connectivity in Chemistry and Drug Research*, Academic Press, New York, 1976.; *Molecular Connectivity in Structure-Activity Analysis*, Wiley, New York, 1986.

15. G. L. Amidon, S. H. Yalkowsky and S. Leung, J. Pharm. Sci. **63**, 1858, 1974; G. L. Amidon, S. H. Yalkowsky, S. T. Anik and S. C. Valvani, J. Phys. Chem. **79**, 2239, 1975; S. C. Valvani, S. H. Yalkowsky and G. L. Amidon, J. Phys. Chem. **80**, 829, 1976.

16. R. B. Hermann, J. Phys. Chem. **76**, 2754, 1972. The computer program is available through the Quantum Chemical Program Exchange, Indiana University, Bloomington, Indiana. Also see Reference 17.

17. R. S. Pearlman, SAREA: Calculating Van der Waals Surface Areas, QCPE Bull. **1**, 15, 1981.

18. G. Scatchard, Chem. Rev. **8**, 321, 1931; J. H. Hildebrand and S. E. Wood, J. Chem. Phys. **1**, 817, 1933.

19. J. K. Guillory, University of Iowa, personal communication.

20. W. L. Chiou and S. Riegelman, J. Pharm. Sci: **60**, 1281, 1971.

21. W. L. Chiou and S. Niazi, J. Pharm. Sci. **62**, 498, 1973.

22. A. Brodin, A. Nyqvist–Mayer, T. Wadsten, et al. J. Pharm. Sci. **73**, 481, 1984.

23. A. A. Nyqvist-Mayer, A. F. Brodin and S. G. Frank, J. Pharm. Sci. **75**, 365, 1986.

24. R. E. Morris and W. A. Cook, J. Am. Chem. Soc. **57**, 2403, 1935.

25. H. R. Ellison, J. Chem. Ed. **55**, 406, 1978.

26. I. Langmuir, Colloid Symposium Monograph, **3**, 48, 1925; E. A. Moelwyn-Hughes, *Physical Chemistry*, 2nd Edition, Pergamon, New York, 1961, p. 775; T. Higuchi, Solubility, in *Pharmaceutical Compounding and Dispensing*. R. Lyman, Ed., Lippincott, Philadelphia, 1949, p. 176.

27. J. H. Hildebrand and R. L. Scott, *Solubility of Nonelectrolytes*, Dover, New York, 1964, Chapter 23.

28. M. J. Chertkoff and A. Martin, J. Pharm. Assoc., Sci. Ed. **49**, 444, 1960; S. Cohen, A. Goldschmidt, G. Shtacher, S. Srebrenik, and S. Gitter, Mol. Pharmacol. **11**, 379, 1975.

29. K. C. James, C. T. Ng and P. R. Noyce, J. Pharm. Sci. **65**, 656, 1976.

30. R. R. Wenner, *Thermochemical Calculations*, McGraw-Hill, New York, 1941, pp. 200, 201.

31. J. H. Hildebrand and R. L. Scott, ibid, p. 274; ibid, Appendix I.

32. C. M. Hansen and A. Beerbower, in *Encyclopedia of Chemical Technology*, Suppl. Vol., 2nd Edition, A. Standen, Ed., Wiley, New York, 1971, pp. 889–910.

33. N. Huu-Phuoc, H. Nam-Tran, M. Buchmann and U. W. Kesselring, Int. J. Pharm. **34**, 217, 1987; A. Munafo, M. Buchmann, H. Nam-Tran, and U. W. Kesselring, J. Pharm. Sci. **77**, 169, 1988.

34. A. Martin, J. Newburger and A. Adjei, J. Pharm. Sci. **68**, p. iv, Oct., 1979; J. Pharm. Sci. **69**, 487, 1980; A. Adjei, J. Newburger and A. Martin, J. Pharm. Sci. **69**, 659, 1980; A. Martin, A. N. Paruta and A. Adjei, J. Pharm. Sci. **70**, 1115, 1981.

35. J. H. Hildebrand, J. M. Prausnitz and R. Scott, *Regular and Related Solutions*, Van Nostrand Reinhold, New York, 1970, p. 22.

36. I. Schröder, Z. Phys. Chem. **11**, 449, 1893.

37. A. T. Williamson, Trans. Faraday Soc. **40**, 421, 1944.

38. T. C. Butler, J. M. Ruth and G. F. Tucker, J. Am. Chem. Soc. **77**, 1486, 1955.

39. H. A. Krebs and J. C. Speakman, J. Chem. Soc. 593, 1945.

40. A. Albert, *Selective Toxicity*, Wiley, New York, 1975.

41. T. Higuchi, Solubility, in *Pharmaceutical Compounding and Dispensing*, R. Lyman, Ed., Lippincott, Philadelphia, 1949, p. 179.

42. H. Kostenbauder, F. Gable and A. Martin, J. Am. Pharm. Assoc., Sci. Ed. **42**, 210, 1953.

43. I. Zimmerman, Int. J. Pharm. **31**, 69, 1986.

44. J. Blanchard, J. O. Boyle and S. Van Wagenen, J. Pharm. Sci. **77**, 548, 1988.

45. G. M. Krause and J. M. Cross, J. Am. Pharm. Assoc., Sci. Ed. **40**, 137, 1951.

46. J. R. Stockton and C. R. Johnson, J. Am. Chem. Soc. **33**, 383, 1944.

47. T. Higuchi, M. Gupta and L. W. Busse, J. Am. Pharm. Assoc., Sci. Ed. **42**, 157, 1953.

48. T. D. Edmonson and J. E. Goyan, J. Am. Pharm. Assoc., Sci. Ed. **47**, 810, 1958.

49. S. P. Agarwal and M. I. Blake, J. Pharm. Sci. **57**, 1434, 1968.

50. P. A. Schwartz, C. T. Rhodes and J. W. Cooper, Jr., J. Pharm. Sci. **66**, 994, 1977.

51. S. F. Kramer and G. L. Flynn, J. Pharm. Sci. **61**, 1896, 1972.

52. Z. T. Chowhan, J. Pharm. Sci. **67**, 1257, 1978.

53. E. G. Rippie, D. J. Lamb and P. W. Romig, J. Pharm. Sci. **53**, 1364, 1964; J. Y. Park and E. G. Rippie, J. Pharm. Sci. **66**, 858, **1977**.

54. B. Fritz, J. L. Lack and L. D. Bighley, J. Pharm. Sci. **60**, 1617, 1971.

55. J. H. Hildebrand and R. L. Scott, *Solubility of Nonelectrolytes*, Dover, New York, 1964, p. 417.

56. D. R. May, and I. M. Kolthoff, J. Phys. Colloid Chem. **52**, 836, 1948.

57. E. R. Garrett and O. R. Woods, J. Am. Pharm. Assoc., Sci. Ed. **42**, 736, 1953.

58. S. Glasstone, *Textbook of Physical Chemistry*, Van Nostrand, New York, 1946, p. 738.

59. M. Davies and H. E. Hallam, J. Chem. Educ. **33**, 322, 1956.

60. S. Glasstone, loc. cit., pp. 741–742.

61. C. Hansch, J. E. Quinlan and G. L. Lawrence, J. Org. Chem. **33**, 347, 1968; A. J. Leo, C. Hansch and D. Elkin, Chem. Revs., **71**, 525, 1971; C. Hansch and A. J. Leo, *Substituent Constants for Correlation Analysis in Chemistry and Biology*, Wiley, New York, 1979.

62. S. H. Yalkowsky and S. C. Valvani, J. Pharm. Sci. **69**, 912, 1980; G. Amidon, Int. J. Pharmaceut. **11**, 249, 1982.

63. R. F. Rekker, *The Hydrophobic Fragmental Constant*, Elsevier, New York, 1977; G. G. Nys and R. F. Rekker, Eur. J. Med. Chem. **9**, 361, 1974.

64. O. Rahn and J. E. Conn, Ind. Eng. Chem. **36**, 185, 1944.

65. J. Schimmel and M. N. Slotsky, Preservation of cosmetics, in *Cosmetics, Science and Technology*, M. S. Balsam and E. Sagarin, Eds., Vol. 3, 2nd Edition, Wiley, New York, 1974, pp. 405–407.

66. S. J. A. Kazmi and A. G. Mitchell, J. Pharm. Sci. **67**, 1260, 1978.

67. H. S. Bean, G. K. Konning and S. M. Malcolm, J. Pharm. Pharmacol. **21** Suppl., 173, 1969.

68. M. H. Seevers and R. M. Waters, Physical Revs. **18**, 447, 1938.

69. C. Hansch and W. J. Dunn, III, J. Pharm. Sci. **61**, 1, 1972; C. Hansch and J. M. Clayton, J. Pharm. Sci. **62**, 1, 1973; R. N. Smith, C. Hansch and M. M. Ames, J. Pharm. Sci. **64**, 599, 1975.

70. K. C. Yeh and W. I. Higuchi, J. Pharm. Soc. **65**, 80, 1976.

71. R. D. Schoenwald and R. L. Ward, J. Pharm. Sci. **67**, 787, 1978.

72. W. J. Dunn III, J. H. Block and R. S. Pearlman, Eds., *Partition Coefficient, Determination and Estimation*, Pergamon Press, New York, 1986.

73. K. C. James, *Solubility and Related Properties*, Marcel Dekker, New York, 1986.

74. D. J. W. Grant and T. Higuchi, *Solubility Behavior of Organic Compounds*, Wiley, New York, 1990. Volume 21 of the Techniques of Chemistry series, W. H. Saunders, Jr., series editor.

75. S. H. Yalkowsky and S. Banerjee, *Aqueous Solubility*, Marcel Dekker, New York, 1992.

76. P. Bustamante, Ph.D. thesis, *Solubility and Stability of Indomethacin*, University of Granada, Spain, 1980.

77. F. A. Shihab, F. W. Ezzedeen and S. J. Stohs, J. Pharm. Sci. **77**, 455, 1988.

78. Z. Liron, S. Srebrenik, A. Martin and S. Cohen, J. Pharm. Sci. **75**, 463, 1986.

79. F. Daniels and R. A. Alberty, *Physical Chemistry*, Wiley, New York, 1955, p. 282.

80. S.-Y. P. King, A. M. Basista and G. Torosian, J. Pharm. Sci. **78**, 95, 1989.

81. J. J. Sciarra, J. Autian and N. E. Foss, J. Am. Pharm. Assoc., Sci. Ed. **47**, 144, 1958.

82. R. Pinal and S. H. Yalkowsky, J. Pharm. Sci. **76**, 75, 1987.

83. S. H. Yalkowsky, S. C. Valvani and T. J. Roseman, J. Pharm. Sci. **72**, 866, 1983, and earlier papers referenced here.

84. A. K. Mitra and T. J. Mikkelson, J. Pharm. Sci. **77**, 771, 1988.

Problems*

10-1. The solubility of sulfamethoxypyridazine (SMP) in a 10% by volume mixture of dioxane and 90% by volume of water is 1.8 mg/mL at 25° C. Calculate **(a)** molarity, **(b)** molality, and **(c)** mole fraction of SMP. The density of the liquid, dioxane, is 1.0313 g/mL, of the solution 1.0086 g/mL, of water 0.9970 g/mL, and of the solvent mixture 1.0082 g/mL. The molecular weight of SMP is 280.32 g/mole, that of dioxane is 88.10, and that of water is 18.015.

Answers: **(a)** 6.421×10^{-3} M; **(b)** 6.378×10^{-3} m; **(c)** $X_2 = 1.251 \times 10^{-4}$

10-2. How many liters of carbon dioxide, reduced to standard conditions of temperature and pressure (25° C and 1 atm, respectively), will dissolve in 1 liter of water at 25° C when the partial pressure of the gas is 0.7 atm?

Answer: 0.53 liter

10-3. Henry's law $p_2 = kX_2$ was discussed in Chapter 5, page 109, and was used in *Problems 5-11, 5-12* and *5-13*. Rather than the Henry's law constant, k, its reciprocal, $\sigma = 1/k$ (pp. 215–216), is sometimes used in problems dealing with the solubility of gases in liquids. What is the solubility of oxygen in water at 25° C and a partial pressure of 610 mm Hg if the reciprocal Henry's law constant, $\sigma = 1/k$, is expressed as σ = concentration (g/liter H_2O)/pressure (mm Hg) = 5.38×10^{-5}?

Answer: 0.0328 g/liter

10-4. Divers ordinarily breathe from tanks of air containing 20% O_2 and 80% N_2. However, He (helium) is less soluble in the blood than N_2 and is now often used to replace N_2.

If the partial pressure of helium in the blood of a diver, using a tank of 20% O_2 and 80% He, is 187.5 mm Hg and the percent of saturation in the red blood cell content is found to be 85.5%, what is the amount of helium that dissolves in the blood? No helium is bound by the hemoglobin of the blood. Express the solubility in moles per kilogram of blood, assuming that the blood behaves as a solvent essentially the same as water. See Table 10–4 for the k value (the Henry's law constant) of helium. Assume that k at 25° C applies with little error at 37° C, the body temperature which is applicable here.

Answer: The concentration of He in the blood at 37° C and a pressure of 187.5 mm Hg is 8.06×10^{-5} moles/kg blood.

10-5. What is the mole fraction solubility of N_2 in water at 25° C and 1 atm pressure? What is the molal solubility? The molecular weight of water is 18.015 g/mole.

Answer: 9.37×10^{-6}, expressed as mole fraction; in molality, the result is 5.20×10^{-4} mole/kg H_2O

10-6. A diver, breathing a mixture of oxygen and helium, descends in a fresh-water lake at sea level to a depth of 30 meters. It is desired that the partial pressure of oxygen at this depth be 0.20 atm.

(a) What is the percent by volume of oxygen in the mixture at this depth? *Hint:* The pressure in atmospheres at a given depth may be computed from the expression: $g\rho h$, where ρ is the density of water, g is the gravity acceleration, and h is the depth (see *Problem 1–10*). Assume that $\rho = 1$ g/cm^3.

(b) At what depth will the diver be subjected to a pressure of 2.5 atmospheres, i.e., 1 atm in air above the lake plus 1.5 atm below the surface of the lake?

(c) At a depth of 50 meters below the surface of the lake what is the pressure in atmospheres? Remember to add on the 1 atm pressure in air above the lake. Incidentally, a diver can withstand a pressure for a short period of time of about 6 atm, corresponding to a depth of about 60 meters.

(d) As stated in Problem 10–4, divers often use a mixture of oxygen, 20% by volume, and helium, 80% by volume. Calculate the

mole fraction solubility of helium, He, in water (or in blood where the solubility is essentially the same as in water at 1 atm [in air]) and 25° C. The Henry's law constant for He in water at 25° C is 1.45×10^5 (atm/mole fraction).

(e) At a depth of 30 meters in the lake, the pressure is 3.9 atm and the partial pressure of He is 0.8×3.9 atm or 3.12 atm. The value, 0.8, corresponds to the percentage of He in the gas mixture, 80%. Compute the mole fraction solubility of He in the blood at a partial pressure of 3.12 atm, i.e., at a depth of 30 meters.

(f) Convert the solubility to molality, i.e., moles per kilogram of blood. The blood of an adult consists of approximately 6 kg. Calculate the total moles of He in the blood of the diver at a measured depth in the lake of 30 meters.

(g) Using the ideal gas law, $V_2 = nRT/P$, with R expressed as liter atmosphere per mole degree, and n as the number of moles of He in the blood at a partial pressure P of 3.12 atm, calculate the volume of He in the blood at a depth of 30 meters in the lake. The temperature T is that of the blood, 310° K.

(h) A diver must not surface too quickly, for the sudden decrease in pressure reduces the solubility and releases the gas from the blood as bubbles that may block the blood vessels and cause a painful and possibly life-threatening condition called "bends." What is the volume of He that is suddenly released as bubbles into the bloodstream if the diver surfaces rapidly so as to reduce the He pressure from $(2.3 + 1)$ atm to the surface (1 atm)? For this calculation, one may use the relation, $V_2/V_1 = P_2/P_1$ to obtain the volume of He in the blood at the surface of the lake.

Answers: **(a)** 5.1%; **(b)** 25.85 meter; **(c)** 5.8 atm; **(d)** 5.52×10^{-6}; **(e)** $X_2 = 2.15 \times 10^{-5}$; **(f)** 1.193×10^{-3} mole/kg blood—the total amount is 0.00716 mole He in the blood of an adult; **(g)** 58.4 mL of He in 6 kg of blood; **(h)** 106.5 mL of He released abruptly into the blood as bubbles.

10-7.† According to Chiou and Niazi,[21] succinic acid and griseofulvin form eutectic mixtures (see p. 42). The table here shows the melting temperatures of the mixtures, the compositions of which are given in percent, w/w. The molecular weights of succinic acid and griseofulvin are 118.09 g/mole and 352.8 g/mole, respectively.

Data for *Problem 10-7*

Succinic acid		Griseofulvin	
Temp. (°C)	% (w/w)	Temp. (°C)	% (w/w)
187.2	98	218	99
186.6	96	210	90
183.8	80	200	80
181	65	192	70
177.6	55	—	—
173.3	44	—	—

Plot the phase diagram using temperature in °C against mole fraction (see Fig 2–17, p. 42, for a similar diagram), and from it determine the melting points, T_o, in °C for the two pure components, their heats of fusion, °H_f, and the eutectic point of the mixture of succinic acid and griseofulvin.

The ideal solubility expression, equation (10–12), page 222, may be used as a linear regression equation to calculate ΔH_f for both compounds, using the two branches of the plot. The two melting points are obtained from the intercepts on the vertical axes of the

---

*Problems 10–4 and 10–6 are modified from J. W. Moncrief and W. H. Jones, *Elements of Physical Chemistry*, Addison-Wesley, Reading, Mass., 1977, p. 122 and R. Chang, *Physical Chemistry with Applications to Biological Systems*, 2nd ed., Macmillan, New York 1977, pp. 23, 24, 175.

---

†Dr. J. Kieth Guillory suggested this problem and kindly assisted in the preparation of problems from which this one was made.

graph or may be obtained from the two linear regression equations by setting $X_2^i = 1$. The eutectic point is found by extrapolating both lines to their common intersection. To begin the calculations, one should convert °C to °K and % (w/w) to mole fraction.

Answers:

Compound	ΔH_f (cal/mole)	T_o °K (°C)	T_o Literature value
Succinic acid	10,411	460.4 (187.3)	185–187° C
Griseofulvin	13,744	492.3 (219.3)	220° C

The eutectic point, obtained from the intersection of the two lines, corresponds to a mixture of 0.30 griseofulvin and 0.70 succinic acid on the mole fraction scale. The melting point of the eutectic mixture is 173° C.

10–8. At the critical solution temperature of 65.85° C for the phenol–water system, p. 40, the critical composition is 34% by weight of phenol. How many grams of water are dissolved in 1000 g of the solution at this temperature?

Answer: 660 g

10–9. A 200-g mixture of phenol and water at 55° C has a total composition of 20% by weight of phenol. The two liquids have the respective compositions of 13% and 60% phenol. What is the weight in grams of the aqueous layer and of the phenol layer and how many grams of phenol are present in each layer?

Answer: The aqueous layer weighs 170.2 g and contains 22.1 g of phenol; the phenol layer weighs 29.8 g and contains 17.9 g of phenol

10–10. Calculate the Kier–Hall[14] value $^1\chi$ for n-hexane. Using equation (10–8) for the solubility of aliphatic hydrocarbons in water, obtain the molar solubility of n-hexane.

Answer: $^1\chi = 2.914$; $\ln S = 8.886$; $S_{(calc)} = 1.38 \times 10^{-4}$ mole/liter; $S_{(obs)} = 1.11 \times 10^{-4}$ mole/liter

10–11. Using equation (10–10) from Amidon et al.,[15] calculate the molal solubility in water at 25° C of (a) cyclohexanol and (b) n-octane. Compute the percentage difference of the calculated from the observed solubilities. See Table 10–6 for the HYSA, the FGSA value for the hydroxyl group, and the observed solubilities for the two compounds, cyclohexanol and n-octane.

Answers: (a) 0.431 m (−13.4% error); (b) 5.85×10^{-6} m (−0.86% error)

10–12. The melting points and molar heat of fusion of three indomethacin polymorphs, I, II, and VII, are found in the table:[76]

Data for *Problem 10–12*

Indomethacin Polymorph	Melting point °C (°K)	ΔH_f cal/mole
I	158 (431)	9550
II	153 (426)	9700
VII	95 (368)	2340

Calculate the ideal mole fraction solubilities at 25° C of the three indomethacin polymorphs, and rank the solubilities in descending order. Is melting point or ΔH_f more useful in ordering the solubilities of the three polymorphs?

Answer: The ideal solubilities, ranked in decreasing order, are

Polymorph	VII	II	I
X_2^i	0.4716	0.0073	0.0069

10–13. Calculate the ideal mole fraction solubility, X_2^i of benzoic acid at 25° C. The melting point of benzoic acid is 122° C (395.15 °K) and the molar heat of fusion is 4139 cal/mole.

Answer: $X_2^i = 0.18$

10–14. The melting points (mp) and heat of fusion for the following three sulfonamides are

Data for *Problem 10–14*

Compound	mp °C (°K)	ΔH_f cal/mole
Sulfamethoxypyridazine	180.4 (453.55)	8110
Sulfameter	211.6 (484.75)	9792
Sulfisomidine	242.2 (515.35)	10781

Calculate the ideal solubilities of these three sulfonamide analogs at 25° C.

Answer:

Compound	Sulfamethoxypyridazine	Sulfameter	Sulfisomidine
X_2^i	0.0092	0.0017	0.00047

10–15. In 1893 Schröder[36] measured the solubility of naphthalene in chlorobenzene and obtained the following data for the mole fraction solubility X_2 of naphthalene at a number of temperatures, T, in degrees Kelvin (°K). The δ values (solubility parameter) of naphthalene and chlorobenzene are both 9.6 $(\text{cal/cm}^3)^{1/2}$.

Data for *Problem 10–15*

X_2^i	0.840	0.742	0.482	0.392	0.309	0.232
T (°K)	343.5	337.5	317.5	307.5	297.0	285.5

The melting point T_f of naphthalene is 80.2° C (353.4° K). It is assumed that the solubilities X_2 in the table are ideal solubilities, since the δ value of the solvent is equal to that of the solute. This assumption permits the use of equation (10–11) or (10–12) to obtain the heat of fusion and the entropy of fusion from the slope and intercept, respectively, of a plot of $1/T$ (x-axis) (°K^{-1}) versus $\ln X_2^i$ (y-axis). The intercept along the vertical $\ln X_2^i$ axis occurs where $1/T$ on the horizontal axis becomes zero, i.e., where T becomes infinite!

(a) Using linear regression, obtain the heat of fusion, ΔH_f, from the slope $\Delta H_f /R$, in which R is the gas constant, 1.9872 cal mole^{-1} deg^{-1}; $\Delta S_f/R$ allows calculation of the entropy of fusion from the integration constant of equation (10–12).

(b) Compare the ΔH_f value obtained from the slope of the regression line with the average ΔH_f obtained from use of equation (10–11), which yields six ΔH_f values.

Answers: (a) ΔH_f (from regression) = 4310 cal/mole; ΔS_f = 12.18 cal/(mole deg); (b) the average value of ΔH_f from the six values obtained by the use of equation (10–11) is 4382 cal/mole, about 2% larger than the value obtained using equation (10–12). The student's values may differ slightly depending on the rounding off of the decimals.

10–16. Benzoic acid forms an ideal solution in a mixture of 0.7 part of ethanol and 0.3 part of ethyl acetate. The mole fraction solubility at 25° C in this mixture is 0.179. The melting point of benzoic acid is 122.4° C. Calculate the heat of fusion of benzoic acid at 25° C.

Answer: ΔH_f = 4144 cal/mole. The CRC *Handbook of Chemistry and Physics*, 63rd ed., gives ΔH_f of benzoic acid as 4139 cal/mole.

10–17. Compute the mole fraction and the molal solubility of benzoic acid in ethyl acetate at 25° C assuming regular solution behavior. Refer to *Example 10–9* and Wenner[30] for the calculations involved. What is the activity and the activity coefficient of the solute in this solution? The solubility parameter of benzoic acid is 11.3 $(cal/cm^3)^{1/2}$ and the molar volume of the supercooled liquid at 25° C is 104.4 cm^3/mole. The solubility parameter of ethyl acetate may be obtained from its heat of vaporization ΔH_v at 25° C = 97.5 cal/g. The molar volume of ethyl acetate at 25° C is obtained from the molecular weight 88.1 divided by its density at 25° C, 0.90 g/cm^3. The heat of fusion of benzoic acid is 33.9 cal/g and the molecular weight is 122 g/mole. The melting point of benzoic acid is 122° C. For purposes of successive approximations, one may assume that $V_1 = V_2$ so that $\phi_1 \approx 1 - X_2$, although the full equation for ϕ, *Example 10–9*, is ordinarily used.

Answer: $X_2 = 0.082$; $a_2 = X_2^i = 0.18$; $\gamma = 2.21$

10–18. If the mole fraction solubility X_2 of naphthalene in chlorobenzene can be considered as the ideal solubility X_2^i for naphthalene, and if X_2^i is 0.444 for naphthalene in chlorobenzene at 40° C (313° K), a determination of the mole fraction solubility in other solvents at 40° C should allow calculation of the activity coefficient, γ_2, in each solvent. What is γ_2 for naphthalene at 40° C in each of the following solvents?

Data for *Problem 10–18*

Solvent	X_2 (40° C)
Acetone	0.378
Hexane	0.222
Methanol	0.0412
Acetic acid	0.117
Water	1.76×10^{-5}
Chlorobenzene	0.444

Relative to the γ_2 values, what might one conclude about the solubility of naphthalene in these various solvents?

Answers:

Solvent	γ_2 (40° C)
Acetone	1.2
Hexane	2.0
Methanol	10.8
Acetic acid	3.8
Water	2.5×10^4
Chlorobenzene	1.0

10–19. The units of solubility parameter (δ) in the cgs system are $(cal/cm^3)^{1/2}$. **(a)** Obtain a conversion factor to express δ in SI units, $(MPa)^{1/2}$. **(b)** Express the solubility parameter of chloroform, caffeine, tolbutamide, and hydrocortisone in SI units. The solubility parameters in cgs units are 9.3, 14.1, 10.9, and 12.4 $(cal/cm^3)^{1/2}$, respectively.

Answers: **(a)** the conversion factor is 1 $(cal/cm^3)^{1/2}$ = 2.0455 $(MPa)^{1/2}$; **(b)** the δ value for each drug above in SI units is, respectively, 19.0, 28.8, 22.3, and 25.4 $(MPa)^{1/2}$

10–20. The cgs system of units is ordinarily used in this chapter for the calculation of solubilities. However, it is sometimes useful to convert to SI units. For a solution of benzoic acid in water, necessary values are expressed in the cgs units as follows. The molar volume, V_2, for benzoic acid is 104.3 cm^3/mole and for water $V_1 = 18.015$ cm^3/mole. The heat of fusion of benzoic acid is 4302 cal/mole and the melting point is 395.6° K. The solubility parameters δ_1 and δ_2 for the solvent, water, and the solute, benzoic acid, are, respectively, 23.4 $(cal/cm^3)^{1/2}$ and 11.5 $(cal/cm^3)^{1/2}$. The gas constant R is given in the cgs system as 1.9872 cal deg^{-1} $mole^{-1}$. **(a)** Convert each of these quantities into the SI system of units. **(b)** Compute the mole fraction solubility of benzoic acid in water at 25° C from the Hildebrand equation using the SI units obtained. Assume that $\phi_1 = 1$. Convert the mole fraction to molality. *Hint:* Use the conversion factor obtained in *Problem 10–19* to express the solubility parameters in SI units.

Answers: **(a)** $V_2 = 104.3 \times 10^{-6}$ m^3/mole, $V_1 = 18.015 \times 10^{-6}$ m^3/mole, $\Delta H_f = 17999.6$ J/mole, $\delta_1 = 47.9$ $(MPa)^{1/2}$, $\delta_2 = 23.5$ $(MPa)^{1/2}$; **(b)** $X_2 = 3.04 \times 10^{-3}$, $m = 0.169$ mole/(kg H_2O).

10–21. The heat of vaporization of the solvent carbon disulfide is 6682 cal/mole and the molar volume is 60.4 cm^3/mole at 25° C. Compute the internal pressure and the solubility parameter of carbon disulfide.

Answer: $P_i \cong 101$ cal/cm^3; $\delta = 10$ $(cal/cm^3)^{1/2}$

10–22. It has been stated in the literature that the a/V^2 term in the van der Waals equation (equations (2–13) and (2–14), pp. 26, 27) is approximately equal to the cohesive energy density, i.e., to the square of the solubility parameter, δ, or $a = \delta^2 V^2$. The CRC *Handbook of Chemistry and Physics*, 63rd ed., page D-195, gives the value of a for n-hexane as 24.39 and a for benzene as 18.00 liter^2 atm mole^{-2}. Using these handbook values for the van der Waals a—the value for attractive forces between molecules—calculate the solubility parameter δ of n-hexane and of benzene.

The accepted δ values for these two liquids (see Table 10–8) are 7.3 and 9.1 $(cal\ cm^{-3})^{1/2}$, respectively. Do you agree that a/V^2 is a good estimate of δ^2? *Hint:* You will need the conversion factor, 1 liter atm = 24.2179 cal. Express the pressure in atmospheres, the volume in liters, and R as 0.08206 liter atm mole^{-1} deg^{-1}. The molar volume of benzene is 89.4 cm^3 mole^{-1} and the molar volume of n-hexane is 131.6 cm^3 mole^{-1}.

Answer: $(a/V^2)^{1/2} \stackrel{?}{=} \delta$(n-hexane) = 5.8 $(cal/cm^3)^{1/2}$; $(a/V^2)^{1/2} \stackrel{?}{=} \delta$(benzene) = 7.4 $(cal/cm^3)^{1/2}$

10–23. Calculate the solute–solvent interaction energy, W_{calc}, for a solution of caffeine in 20% water–80% dioxane (Table 10–10) at 25° C using equation (10–44). With this value for $W_{(calc)}$ and the solubility parameter of the mixed solvent (Table 10–10), calculate the solubility of caffeine in this mixture. The value for A is 0.09467 cm^3/cal, δ_2 (caffeine) = 13.8 $(cal/cm^3)^{1/2}$, and $-\log X_2^i = 1.1646$.

Answer: $W_{(calc)} = 173.4079$ cal/cm^3; $X_{2(calc)} = 0.024$. The results in Table 10–10, $W_{(calc)} = 173.729$ cal/cm^3 and $X_{2(calc)} = 0.027$, were obtained using the more accurate quartic expression, equation (10–45).

10–24. **(a)** What is the $W_{(calc)}$ value for caffeine in a mixture of dioxane and water having a δ_1 value of 17.07 $(cal/cm^3)^{1/2}$? This mixture contains 47.5% by volume of dioxane and 52.5% water. Calculate $W_{(calc)}$ using both the quadratic (equation 10–44) and the quartic (equation 10–45) expressions.

(b) The A value at 25° C is 0.093711 cm^3/cal. The δ_2 value of caffeine is 13.8 $(cal/cm^3)^{1/2}$. The negative log ideal solubility of caffeine at 25° C is $-\log X_2^i = 1.1646$. Calculate the solubility of caffeine in mole fraction and in moles/liter using both $W_{(calc)}$ results (quadratic and quartic) of part (a). The density ρ of the solution is 1.0493 g/cm^3. The molecular weight M_2 of caffeine is 194.19 g/mole, and that of dioxane 88.016 g/mole.

$$\text{Solubility in (moles/liter)} = \frac{1000\ \rho\ (X_2)}{M_1(1 - X_2) + X_2 M_2} \quad \text{(p. 104)}$$

M_1, the average molecular weight of the solvent at a volume percent of 47.5 dioxane, is given approximately by the use of molecular weights and volume fractions:

$M_1 = (88.10$ g/mole$)(0.475) + (18.015$ g/mole$)(0.525) \approx 51.3$ g/mole

Partial Answer: Using equation (10–45), $W_{(calc)}$ = 238.06175 cal/cm³; mole fraction solubility $X_{2(calc)}$ = 0.0200; molar solubility (calculated) = 0.39; molar solubility (experimental) = 0.40 mole/liter.

10–25. Calculate the values of W (equation 10–43), $\delta_1\delta_2$, and the ratio $W/\delta_1\delta_2$ for ketoprofen, an analgesic, in a 70:30 volume percent mixture (δ_1 = 10.32) and a 50:50 volume percent mixture (δ_1 = 11.00) of chloroform–ethanol at 25° C. The ideal solubility of ketoprofen is $X_2{}^i$ = 0.1516 and its molar volume V_2 = 196 cm³/mole. The solvent volume fraction ϕ_1 of the two mixtures is 0.6694 and 0.6820, respectively, and the mole fraction solubilities of ketoprofen in the mixtures are X_2 = 0.1848 and X_2 = 0.1622. The solubility parameter of ketoprofen, calculated from the peak solubility value in the chloroform–ethanol mixtures, is δ_2 = 9.8 (cal/cm³)$^{1/2}$.

Answer:

Mixture	A	W	$\delta_1\delta_2$	$W/\delta_1\delta_2$
70:30	0.0644	101.9389	101.136	1.0079
50:50	0.0668	108.7395	107.800	1.0087

Notice that the use of W instead of $\delta_1\delta_2$ in the Hildebrand equation gives the exact solubility of X_2 = 0.1848. The use of $-2\delta_1\delta_2$ instead of $-2W$ gives a result, X_2 = 0.0813, that is some 56% in error. $W/\delta_1\delta_2$ is nearly unity, viz. 1.0079, which means that W is only slightly different from $\delta_1\delta_2$. Yet, the very small difference causes the use of $-2W$ in the Hildebrand equation to give the exact solubility of ketoprofen in a 70:30 mixture of chloroform and ethanol, and the use of $-2\delta_1\delta_2$ to give a less exact solubility value.

10–26. Calculate the values of A, W, $\delta_1\delta_2$, and $W/\delta_1\delta_2$ for solutions of sulfamethoxypyridazine (SMP) in benzene, δ_1 = 9.07, and in benzyl alcohol, δ_1 = 11.64 (cal/cm³)$^{1/2}$, at 25° C. The ideal solubility $X_2{}^i$ of SMP is 9.1411 × 10^{-3}, and its molar volume, V_2, is 172.5 cm³/mole. The volume fractions ϕ_1 of the solvents benzene and benzyl alcohol are 0.9999 and 0.9757, respectively. The solubility parameter δ_2 of the solute, SMP, is 12.89. The mole fraction solubilities X_2 of SMP in benzene and in benzyl alcohol are 0.0636 × 10^{-3} and 14.744 × 10^{-3} respectively.

Answers:

Solvent	A cm³/cal	W cal/cm³	$\delta_1\delta_2$ cal/cm³	$W/\delta_1\delta_2$
Benzene	0.1264	115.6739	116.9123	0.9894
Benzyl alcohol	0.1204	151.6831	150.0396	1.0110

10–27. The presence of usual components such as sweetening agents in syrup formulas may affect the solubility of preservatives so that changes in temperature yield precipitation and leave the product unprotected. The molar solubility of sorbic acid used as a preservative was studied at 20° C and 37° C as a function of the concentration of glucose.[77]

Data for *Problem 10–27*: Molar Solubility of Sorbic Acid

% Glucose in water	20° C	37° C
0	0.013	0.022
15	0.011	0.019
30	0.009	0.016
45	0.007	0.014
60	0.005	0.011

(a) Plot on the same graph the molar solubility of sorbic acid at 20° C and 37° C (vertical axis) against the percent of glucose in water (horizontal axis) and find a quantitative relationship between these variables. Comment on your results.

(b) The change in the aqueous molar solubility, S, of sorbic acid with addition of glucose is determined by the standard free energy of transfer of sorbic acid from water (w) to the glucose solution (s). Show that these thermodynamic functions, $\Delta G°_{tr}$ and $\Delta H°_{tr}$, can be computed from the following expressions:

$$\Delta G°_{tr} = -RT \ln \frac{S_s}{S_w}$$

and

$$\ln \frac{(S_{s2}/S_{s1})}{(S_{w2}/S_{w1})} = \frac{\Delta H°_{tr}}{R} \left(\frac{T_2 - T_1}{T_1 T_2} \right)$$

(c) As an example, compute $\Delta G°_{tr}$ and $\Delta H°_{tr}$ for the transfer of sorbic acid from water to a 45% solution of glucose at both 20° C and 37° C. Compare your results to the *change in solubility* of sorbic acid from water to 45% glucose at both temperatures. *Hint:* Observe the sign and magnitude of these thermodynamic functions.

Partial Answer: **(c)** $\Delta G°_{tr}$ (20° C) = 360.6 cal/mole; $\Delta G°_{tr}$ (37° C) = 278.6 cal/mole; $\Delta H°_{tr}$ = 1775 cal/mole

10–28. Suppose you traveled to the hypothetical planet Ariston, where the temperature ranged from −100° to 0° C. You were asked to join the scientists at the Ariston National Laboratories to prepare a solution of solid carbon dioxide dissolved in ethanol at −80° C (193° K) to be used in a new rocket engine being developed. The melting point of CO_2 is −56° C and that of ethanol is −114.1° C. At −80° C, the normal room temperature on Ariston, CO_2 exists as a solid and ethanol as a liquid. The boiling point of ethanol is 78.5° C and it re-mains as a liquid from about −114° C to +78.5° C, where it becomes a gas.

(a) Calculate the ideal solubility of solid CO_2 at −80° C. The heat of fusion of CO_2 is 1900 cal/mole.

(b) The density of ethanol at several temperatures is given in the table:

Data for *Problem 10–28*

T (°K)	273.2	283.2	293.2	298.2	303.2
t (°C)	0	10	20	25	30
Density (g/cm³)	0.80625	0.79788	0.78945	0.78521	0.78097

Regress the density (y values) against t °C (x values) and compute the density and molar volume (cm³/mole) of ethanol at −80° C. The molecular weight of ethanol is 46.07 gram/mole.

(c) The solubility parameter at temperatures other than 25° C may be determined approximately for a liquid from the densities of the liquid at 25° C and at the new temperature.[78]

$$\delta_{T_1} = \delta_{25°} \left(\frac{\rho_{25°}}{\rho_{T_1}} \right)^{1.25}$$

Use the density of ethanol from the table above (at 25° C) and your result at −80° C, and compute δ for ethanol at −80° C; the δ value for ethanol at 25° C is 12.8 (cal/cm³)$^{1/2}$.

(d) Estimate the solubility of solid CO_2 in ethanol at −80° C under which conditions it is expected to form a regular solution. The heat of vaporization of CO_2 is 3460 cal/mole. Obtain the solubility parameter at −80° C from this value, knowing that the molar volume at −80° C is V_2 = 38 cm³/mole. The δ value for CO_2 may be calculated using the expression

$$\delta_{CO_2} = \left(\frac{\Delta H_2{}^v - RT}{V_2} \right)$$

where $\Delta H_2{}^v$ is the heat of vaporization, R is the gas constant 1.9872 cal/(mole deg), and T is the absolute temperature, 193° K. You will need the molar volume, V_1, of ethanol and its solubility parameter at $-80°$ C $(193°$ K) (see answers (b) and (c)). You can assume that the volume fraction ϕ_1 of ethanol is 1.00 for the first round of calculations. Then by six or more iteration steps, obtain the more correct solubility (see p. 224, 225).

(e) Once you have calculated the mole fraction solubility of CO_2 in ethanol at $-80°$ C, convert the solubility into units of molality. The molecular weight of CO_2 is 44.01 g/mole.

Answers: (a) X_2^i (CO_2, $-80°$ C) = 0.5782; (b) ρ (ethanol, $-80°$ C) = 0.87370, V_1 = 52.73 cm³/mole; (c) δ (ethanol, $-80°$ C) = 11.2 (cal/cm³)$^{1/2}$; δ (CO_2, $-80°$ C) = 9.0 (cal/cm³)$^{1/2}$; (d) X_2 (CO_2, $-80°$ C) = 0.4887 after eight iterations. If ϕ_1 is unity, we obtain the first result of iteration, viz. X_2 = 0.3579; (e) molality = 20.7 moles/kg

10–29. The solubility of sodium carbonate, decahydrate, $Na_2CO_3 \cdot 10H_2O$ (washing soda), is 21.52 g/100 g of water at 0° C, and the heat of solution ΔH_{soln} is 13,500 cal/mole. When a substance such as washing soda is added to ice at 0° C, the freezing point of water is lowered and a liquid solution of sodium carbonate is formed at 0° C. Calculate the solubility of sodium carbonate decahydrate at 25° C.

Answer: The solubility of $Na_2CO_3 \cdot 10H_2O$ is 43.13 g/(100 g H_2O) using equation (10–46). Note that Na_2CO_3 contributes three ions in solution, i.e., ν = 3. The experimental value is 50 g/(100 g H_2O) at 25° C, a 14% difference from the calculated value.

10–30. The solubility of $Ba(OH)_2 \cdot 8H_2O$ in water at three temperatures is reported by Daniels and Alberty[79] as follows:

Data for *Problem 10–30*

Temperature (°C)	0.0	10.0	20.0
Molal solubility	0.0974	0.1447	0.227

Use the modification of equation (10–46), that is,

$$\ln m_2 = -\frac{\Delta H_{soln}}{R}\frac{1}{T} + I$$

which provides the heat of solution, ΔH_{soln}, when a graph of the data is plotted with $\ln m_2$ (m_2 is the molality of the solute) on the vertical axis and $1/T$ (T is the absolute temperature) on the horizontal axis. The slope of the line, obtained by linear regression analysis and multiplied by R = 1.9872 cal mole^{-1} deg^{-1}, gives ΔH_{soln} in cal/mole. I in the equation is an integration constant and is the point of intersection on the vertical axis.

Use the equation above to obtain ΔH_{soln}, the heat of solution in the range of 0° C to 20° C and to predict the solubility of barium hydroxide octahydrate at 30° C in water.

Answer: ΔH_{soln} = 6719 cal/mole; calculated molal solubility at 30° C = 0.327 m; experimental solubility[79] = 0.326 m

10–31. If the solubility product of silver chromate is 2×10^{-12} at 25° C, what is the solubility in mole/liter of silver chromate?

Answer: 7.9×10^{-5} mole/liter

10–32. What is the solubility of the electrolyte, magnesium hydroxide, (a) in moles/liter and (b) in g/100 mL if the solubility product is 1.4×10^{-11}? The molecular weight of $Mg(OH)_2$ is 58.34.

Answers: (a) 1.5×10^{-4} mole/liter; (b) 8.8×10^{-4} g/dL. The symbol dL stands for deciliter = 100 mL.

10–33. Brequinar sodium dissociates as brequinar$^-$ and Na$^+$. Its apparent solubility product K'_{sp} = 0.0751. (a) Compute the solubility of this compound.[80] (b) Compute the solubility product K_{sp}, using the mean activity coefficient, $\gamma_\pm$. (c) Compute the solubility after addition of a 0.05-M solution of KCl.

Answers: (a) 0.274 mole/liter; (b) K_{sp} = 0.0335; (c) 0.280 mole/liter

10–34. the crystal lattice energy of AgCl is 207 kcal/mole and its heat of hydration is -192 kcal/mole. (a) What is the heat of solution of AgCl in kcal/mole and in kJ/mole (b) The solubility of AgCl in water at 10° C is 8.9×10^{-5} g/dL of solution. What is the solubility of AgCl at 25° C? AgCl dissociates into two ionic species in solution.

Answers: (a) ΔH_{soln} = 15 kcal/mole (Table 10–11); in kJ/mole; ΔH_{soln} = 62.8; (b) 1.74×10^{-4} g/dL of solution. The experimental value is 1.93×10^{-4} % (w/v).

Note: For the strong electrolytes such as NaCl and KBr, which are very soluble in water, the use of equation (10–46) does not give very reasonable results for solubility. As seen in this example, the solubility for a slightly soluble strong electrolyte such as silver chloride at various temperatures is reasonable in comparison with observed values (i.e., within 10%).

10–35. The crystal lattice energies of potassium bromide and potassium chloride are 673 and 699 kJ/mole; their heats of hydration are -651 kJ/mole and -686 kJ/mole, respectively. What is the heat of solution ΔH_{soln} of KBr and of KCl?. Express the results in kJ/mole, then convert to kcal/mole.

Answer: for KBr, ΔH_{soln} = 22 kJ/mole = 5.3 kcal/mole; for KCl, ΔH_{soln} = 13 kJ/mole = 3.1 kcal/mole

10–36. What is the solubility of barium sulfate in a solution having an ionic strength μ of 0.25 and $K_{sp} = 1 \times 10^{-10}$ at 25° C? The activity coefficient for a bi-bivalent salt at this ionic strength is 0.23.

Answer: 4.3×10^{-5} mole/liter

10–37. The solubility of boric acid in an aqueous solvent containing 25% by volume of sorbitol was found by Sciarra et al.[81] to be 2.08 molal at 35° C. The heat of solution of boric acid in this mixed solvent is 3470 cal/mole. Calculate the molal solubility of boric acid at 50° C in this solvent.

Answer: 2.71 molal

10–38. The molar solubility of sulfathiazole in water is 0.002, the pK_a is 7.12, and the molecular weight of sodium sulfathiazole is 304. What is the lowest pH allowable for complete solubility in a 5% solution of the salt?

Answer: pH_p = 9.03

10–39. What is the pH_p of a 2% w/v solution of sodium phenobarbital in a hydroalcoholic solution containing 15% by volume of alcohol? The solubility of phenobarbital in 15% alcohol is 0.22% w/v. The pK_a of phenobarbital in this solution is 7.6. The molecular weight of sodium phenobarbital is 254.22 g/mole and that of phenobarbital is 232.23 g/mole.

Answer: pH_p = 8.5

10–40. Calculate pH_p for a 0.5% solution of cocaine hydrochloride. The molecular weight of the salt is 339.8, and the molar solubility of the base is 5.60×10^{-3}. The pK_b of cocaine is 5.59.

Answer: pH_p = 8.20

10–41. Using data in Figures 10–7 and 10–8, calculate the minimum pH required for complete solubility of sodium phenobarbital in a solution containing 3 g of the drug in 100 mL of a mixed alcohol–water solvent. (a) Calculate pH_p, the minimum pH for the drug, in each aqueous solvent consisting of 10%, 20%, 30%, 40%, and 50% by volume of ethanol. (b) Plot pH_p versus percent by volume of alcohol in the solvent. The procedure may be checked by comparing the results with the calculations illustrated in *Example 10–17*, page 235. The molecular weight of phenobarbital is 232.23 g/mole and that of sodium phenobarbital is 254.22.

Answer:

% Alcohol	10	20	30	40	50
pH_p	8.73	8.63	8.55	8.02	*

*At about 50% alcohol and above, phenobarbital in a 3g/100 mL solution of the drug will not precipitate no matter how low the pH.

10–42. The molar solubility of codeine, S_0, in water at 25° C is approximately 0.0279 mole/liter; the pK_a of codeine (actually, the conjugate acid of the base, codeine) is 8.21 at 25° C; and the molecular weight of codeine phosphate $\cdot \frac{1}{2}H_2O$ (U.S.P.) is 406.37 dalton.* What

---

*Recall that the word *dalton* is another term for the units g/mole, i.e., for molecular weight units.

is the highest pH allowable for complete solubility in an aqueous solution of 60 mg of the salt per 5 mL of solution?

Answer: The pH above which the free base precipitates from solution is 9.45.

10–43. A prescription calls for 7 grains (1 gram = 15.432 grains) of phenobarbital in 60 mL of solution. The vehicle consists of 20% by volume of glycerin, 5% by volume of alcohol, and the balance water. From Figure 10–7 it is observed that about 25% by volume of alcohol is required in the solution to dissolve this quantity of phenobarbital. How much U.S.P. alcohol (95% by volume) must be added?

Answer: 13.3 mL

10–44. If a container of pure water is shaken in the air, the water will dissolve atmospheric carbon dioxide until the dissolved gas is in equilibrium with that in the air. At atmospheric pressure the solubility of CO_2 is found to be 1×10^{-5} mole/liter. The dissociation constant K_1 of carbonic acid is approximately equal to 4×10^{-7}. Compute the pH of water saturated with CO_2. *Hint:* $[H_3O^+] = \sqrt{K_1 c}$, in which c is the equilibrium concentration of the gas in water.

Answer: pH = 5.7

10–45. (a) Calculate the solubility at 25° C of sulfisoxazole in an aqueous buffer having a pH of 5.12. (b) Repeat the calculation for the pH 5.12 buffer solution when 3.0% Tween 80 is included in the solution. See *Example 10–18* for K_a, K', and K'', and for the aqueous solubility of nonionized sulfisoxazole at 25° C. (c) Calculate the fraction of sulfisoxazole solubilized in the Tween 80 micelles in this solution.

Answers: (a) 0.30 g/liter; (b) 0.723 g/liter; (c) 0.585

10–46. Calculate the molar solubility of butyl p-hydroxybenzoate (mp 68° C) in water at 25° C using equation (10–100), page 240. The log K for benzoic acid is 1.87; the contribution by an OH group is -1.16 and by a CH_2 group is 0.50, according to Leo et al.[61]

Answer: ΔS_f = 16.0 e.u. log $K_{(calc)}$ = 2.71, log S = -2.73, $S_{(calc)}$ = 1.86×10^{-3} M, $S_{(obs)}$ = 1.29×10^{-3} M

10–47. Pinal and Yalkowsky[82] extended their earlier equations[83] to estimate the aqueous solubility of weak electrolytes. The new equation is

$$\log S = -\frac{\Delta S_f(T_m - T)}{2.303RT} - \log K + \log \alpha + 0.8 \quad (10\text{–}113)$$

where T_m and T are respectively the absolute temperature at the melting point and the temperature at which the experiment is done. The other symbols have the same meaning as in equation (10–100), page 240; α is an ionization term defined as

$$\alpha = \left(1 + \frac{10^{-pK_a}}{10^{-pH}}\right)$$

for monoprotic acids.

(a) Compute the aqueous solubility of phenytoin (a derivative of hydantoin used as an antiepileptic drug) at pH 7.1 and 25° C. The pK_a of phenytoin is 8.30, the melting point is 296.9° C, and the partition coefficient K is 208.9. The entropy of fusion can be calculated according to equation (10–101), page 240, where n is the number of carbons in the longest hydrocarbon chain or flexible ring. Phenytoin has the formula

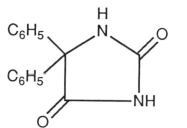

(b) Compute the partition coefficient in an octanol–water system for pentobarbital using the equation of Yalkowsky et al.[82] (equation (10–113)). The observed solubility of pentobarbital at 33° C and pH 8

is 0.01107 mole/liter. the pK_a is 8.07 and ΔS_f = 12.67 entropy units (e.u.) (i.e., 12.67 cal/mole deg). The melting point is 128.5° C.

Answers: (a) n, the number of carbons in the calculation of ΔS_f, is $n = 6$; ΔS_f = 16 e.u.; α = 1.063; log S = -4.6835; S, the aqueous solubility of phenytoin, = 2.07×10^{-5} mole/liter; (b) log K = 2.16; $K = 144.5$

10–48. If 0.15 g of succinic acid in 100 mL of ether is shaken with a 10-mL portion of water, how much succinic acid is left in the ether layer? The distribution coefficient K = (conc. in ether)/(conc. in water) = 0.125 at 25° C. How much succinic acid is left in the ether when the phase is extracted with an additional 10 mL of water?

Answer: 0.083 g after first extraction; 0.046 g after second extraction

10–49. How much benzoic acid, K_a = 6.3×10^{-5}, will remain undissociated in the aqueous phase of a 50% oil–water emulsion if the initial concentration of benzoic acid in the aqueous phase is 0.5%? The aqueous phase is buffered at pH 5 and the o/w partition coefficient = 5.33. Assume that benzoic acid remains as a monomer in the oil phase.

Answer: 0.396 mg/mL

10–50. Propionic acid is added to the aqueous phase of a 20% oil–water emulsion, and 0.65 mg/mL of free acid remains in the aqueous phase after equilibrium has been attained between the two phases. In a 20% emulsion, $q = V_o/V_w = 20/80 = 0.25$. The aqueous phase is buffered at pH 3.5. Propionic acid is found to dimerize in the oil phase and the distribution constant, $K'' = \sqrt{C}/[HA_w]$, is equal to 15.0. The K_a of propionic acid is 1.4×10^{-5}. Compute the initial concentration C of propionic acid to be introduced into the aqueous phase. The molecular weight of propionic acid is 74.08 g/mole.

Answer: C = 1.0 mg/mL

10–51. To determine the *intrinsic partition coefficient* K_{in} of pilocarpine base in a study of transcorneal permeation, the octanol–water aqueous buffer partition coefficient, K_{obs}, was obtained experimentally at various temperatures and pH values (Mitra and Mikkelson[84]). The results are presented in Table 10–15.

TABLE 10–15. *Observed Partition Coefficients K_{obs} at Various pH's and Temperatures. (Data for Problem 10–51)*

pH	6.25	6.50	6.70	6.85	7.00	7.25
$[H_3O^+]$ ($\times 10^7$)	5.62	3.16	2.00	1.41	1.00	0.56
T (°C)	Observed Partition Coefficients, K_{obs}					
27	0.24	0.38	0.52	0.63	0.72	0.89
30	0.31	0.46	0.62	0.78	0.84	1.06
40	—	0.65	0.88	1.06	1.23	1.49

(a) According to Mitra and Mikkelson,[84] the observed partition coefficient K_{obs} is related to the hydrogen ion concentration of the aqueous phase $[H_3O^+]$ by the expression

$$\frac{1}{K_{obs}} = \frac{1}{K_{in}K_a}[H_3O^+] + \frac{1}{K_{in}}$$

where the intrinsic partition coefficient K_{in} of the free base, pilocarpine is independent of pH. The term K_a is the ionization constant in water of the conjugate acid of pilocarpine, i.e., the pilocarpinium cation. Plot the reciprocal of the observed partition coefficient, $1/K_{obs}$, versus the hydrogen ion concentration, $[H_3O^+]$. Using linear regression analysis obtain the intrinsic partition coefficient, K_{in}, for pilocarpine base between octanol and an aqueous phosphate buffer, and the acidic ionization constant K_a for the pilocarpinium cation at temperatures 27°, 30°, and 40° C. The cation does not partition into octanol.

(b) The intrinsic partition coefficient of pilocarpine base in the logarithmic form $\ln K_{in}$ may be expressed in terms of the thermodynamic quantities $\Delta H°$, $\Delta S°$, and $\Delta G°$ using the van't Hoff equation:

$$\ln K_{in} = -\frac{\Delta H°}{R}\frac{1}{T} + \frac{\Delta S°}{R}$$

Regress $\ln K_{in}$ against $1/T$, at the three absolute temperatures 27° C = 300.15° K, 30° C = 303.15° K, and 40° C = 313.15° K. Solve for $\Delta H°$ and $\Delta S°$ and obtain $\Delta G°$ at the three temperatures. Interpret the magnitude and the sign of these three thermodynamic quantities as they relate to the partitioning process.

Answers: **(a)**

Temperature (°C)	K_{in}	K_a	pK_a
27	1.324	1.25×10^{-7}	6.90
30	1.433	1.54×10^{-7}	6.81
40	2.106	1.42×10^{-7}	6.85

(b) $\Delta H° = 6777$ cal/mole $= 6.8$ kcal/mole; $\Delta S° = 23$ cal/(mole deg); $\Delta G° = -159$ cal/mole at 27° C, -228 cal/mole at 30° C, and -460 cal/mole at 40° C

$\Delta H°$ is positive, which mitigates against the partitioning process, yet $\Delta S°$ is sufficiently positive to provide a spontaneous reaction. The negative $\Delta G°$ values corroborate the conclusion that the process is spontaneous (for the solute in its standard state). The large positive $\Delta S°$ value suggests that pilocarpine base is solvated in the aqueous phase in an orderly structure of water, which is broken down to a more random arrangement of drug and solvent in the octanol phase.

11
Complexation and Protein Binding

Metal Complexes
Organic Molecular Complexes
Inclusion Compounds
Methods of Analysis

Protein Binding
Thermodynamic Treatment of
Stability Constants

Complexes or coordination compounds, according to the classic definition, result from a donor-acceptor mechanism or Lewis acid–base reaction (p. 144) between two or more different chemical constituents. Any nonmetallic atom or ion, whether free or contained in a neutral molecule or in an ionic compound, that can donate an electron pair may serve as the donor. The acceptor, or constituent that accepts a share in the pair of electrons, is frequently a metallic ion, although it can be a neutral atom. Complexes may be divided broadly into two classes depending on whether the acceptor component is a metal ion or an organic molecule; these are classified according to one possible arrangement in Table 11–1. A third class, the inclusion/occlusion compounds, involving the entrapment of one compound in the molecular framework of another, is also included in the table.

Intermolecular forces involved in the formation of complexes are the van der Waals forces of dispersion, dipolar, and induced dipolar types. Hydrogen bonding provides a significant force in some molecular complexes, and coordinate covalence is important in metal complexes. Charge transfer and hydrophobic interaction are introduced later in the chapter.

METAL COMPLEXES

A satisfactory understanding of metal ion complexation is based upon a familiarity with atomic structure and molecular forces, and the reader would do well to go to texts on inorganic and organic chemistry to study those sections dealing with electronic structure and hybridization before proceeding.

Inorganic Complexes. This group constitutes the simple inorganic complexes first described by Werner in 1891. The ammonia molecules in hexamminecobalt III chloride, as the compound $[Co(NH_3)_6]^{3+}Cl_3^-$ is called, are known as the *ligands* and are said to be

TABLE 11–1. *Classification of Complexes*

I. Metal Ion Complexes
  A. Inorganic type
  B. Chelates
  C. Olefin type
  D. Aromatic type
    1. Pi (π) complexes
    2. Sigma (σ) complexes
    3. "Sandwich" compounds
II. Organic Molecular Complexes
  A. Quinhydrone type
  B. Picric acid type
  C. Caffeine and other drug complexes
  D. Polymer type
III. Inclusion/Occlusion Compounds
  A. Channel lattice type
  B. Layer type
  C. Clathrates
  D. Monomolecular type
  E. Macromolecular type

*This classification does not pretend to describe the mechanism or the type of chemical bonds involved in complexation. It is meant simply to separate out the various types of complexes that are discussed in the literature. A highly systematized classification of electron donor-acceptor interactions is given by R. S. Mulliken, J. Phys. Chem. **56**, 801, 1952.

coordinated to the cobalt ion. The *coordination number* of the cobalt ion, or number of ammonia groups coordinated to the metal ions is six. Other complex ions belonging to the inorganic group include $[Ag(NH_3)_2]^+$, $[Fe(CN)_6]^{4-}$, and $[Cr(H_2O)_6]^{3+}$.

Each ligand donates a pair of electrons to form a coordinate covalent link between itself and the central ion having an incomplete electron shell. For example,

$$Co^{3+} + 6:NH_3 = [Co(NH_3)_6]^{3+}$$

Hybridization plays an important part in coordination compounds in which sufficient bonding orbitals are not ordinarily available in the metal ion. The reader's understanding of hybridization will be refreshed by a brief review of the argument advanced for the quadrivalence of carbon. It will be recalled that the ground state configuration of carbon is

1s 2s 2p

This cannot be the bonding configuration of carbon, however, since it normally has four rather than two valence electrons. Pauling[1] suggested the possibility of *hybridization* to account for the quadrivalence. According to this mixing process, one of the 2s electrons is promoted to the available 2p orbital to yield four equivalent bonding orbitals:

1s 2s 2p

These are directed toward the corners of a tetrahedron, and the structure is known as an sp^3 hybrid because it involves one s and three p orbitals. In a double bond, the carbon atom is considered to be sp^2 hybridized, and the bonds are directed toward the corners of a triangle.

Orbitals other than the 2s and 2p orbitals can become involved in hybridization. The transition elements, such as iron, copper, nickel, cobalt, and zinc, seem to make use of their 3d, 4s, and 4p orbitals in forming hybrids. These hybrids account for the differing geometries often found for the complexes of the transition metal ions. Table 11–2 shows some compounds in which the

central atom or metal ion is hybridized differently and it shows the geometry that results.

Ligands such as $H_2O:$, $H_3N:$, $NC:^-$, or $Cl:^-$ donate a pair of electrons in forming a complex with a metal ion, and the electron pair enters one of the unfilled orbitals on the metal ion. A useful but not inviolate rule to follow in estimating the type of hybridization in a metal ion complex is to select that complex in which the metal ion has its 3d levels filled or that can use the lower-energy 3d and 4s orbitals primarily in the hybridization. For example, the ground-state electronic configuration of Ni^{2+} may be given by

3d   4s   4p

In combining with $4CN:^-$ ligands to form $[Ni(CN)_4]^{2-}$, the electronic configuration of the nickel ion may become either

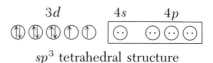

sp^3 tetrahedral structure

or

TABLE 11–2. *Bond Types of Representative Compounds*

Coordination Number	Orbital Configuration	Bond Type	Examples	
			Formula	Structure
2	sp	linear	O_2	O—O
3	sp^2	trigonal	BCl_3	
4	sp^3	tetrahedral	CH_4	
4	dsp^2	square planar	$Cu(NH_3)_4^{2+}$	
5	dsp^3	bipyramidal	PF_5	
6	d^2sp^3	octahedral	$Co(NH_3)_6^{3+}$	

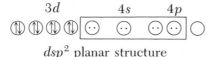

dsp^2 planar structure

in which the electrons donated by the ligand are shown as dots. The dsp^2 or square planar structure is predicted to be the complex formed since it uses the lower-energy 3d orbital. By the preparation and study of a number of complexes, Werner deduced many years ago that this is indeed the structure of the complex.

Similarly, the trivalent cobalt ion Co(III) has the ground state electronic configuration

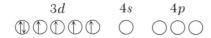

and one may inquire into the possible geometry of the complex $[Co(NH_3)_6]^{3+}$. The electronic configuration of the metal ion leading to filled 3d levels is

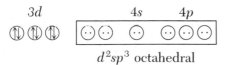

d^2sp^3 octahedral

and thus the d^2sp^3 or octahedral structure is predicted as the structure of this complex. Chelates (see following section) of octahedral structure can be resolved into optical isomers, and in an elegant study, Werner used this technique to prove that cobalt complexes are octahedral.

In the case of divalent copper Cu(II), which has the electronic configuration

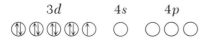

the formation of the complex $[Cu(NH_3)_4]^{2+}$ requires the promotion of one d electron of Cu^{2+} to a 4p level to obtain a filled 3d configuration in the complexed metal ion, and a dsp^2 or planar structure is obtained

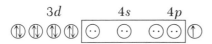

Although the energy required to elevate the d electron to the 4p level is considerable, the formation of a planar complex having the 3d levels filled entirely more than "pays" for the expended energy.

The metal ion Fe(III) has the ground-state configuration

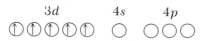

and in forming the complex $[Fe(CN)_6]^{3-}$, no electron promotion takes place

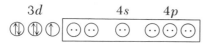

since no stabilization is gained over that which the d^2sp^3 configuration already possesses. Compounds of this type, in which the ligands lie "above" a partially filled orbital, are termed *outer-sphere complexes;* when the ligands lie "below" a partially filled orbital, as in the previous example, the compound is termed an *inner-sphere complex.* The presence of unpaired electrons in a metal ion complex can be detected by *electron spin resonance spectroscopy* (pp. 90, 91).

Chelates. A substance containing two or more donor groups may combine with a metal to form a special type of complex known as a *chelate* (Greek: kelos, claw). Some of the bonds in a chelate may be ionic or of the primary covalent type, while others are coordinate covalent links. When the ligand provides one group for attachment to the central ion, the chelate is called *monodentate.* Pilocarpine behaves as a monodentate ligand toward Co(II), Ni(II), and Zn(II) to form chelates of pseudotetrahedral geometry. The donor atom of the ligand is the pyridine-type nitrogen of the imidazole ring of pilocarpine (Fig. 3–4, p. 72, shows the pyridine-like nitrogen of pilocarpine). Molecules with two and three donor groups are called *bidentate* and *tridentate*, respectively.[2] Ethylenediaminetetraacetic acid (EDTA) has six points for attachment to the metal ion and is accordingly *hexadentate;* however, in some complexes, only four or five of the groups are coordinated.

Chelation places stringent steric requirements on both metal and ligands. Ions such as Cu(II) and Ni(II), which form square planar complexes, and Fe(III) and Co(III), which form octahedral complexes, can exist in either of two geometric forms. As a consequence of this isomerism only *cis-coordinated ligands*—ligands adjacent on a molecule—will be readily replaced by reaction with a chelating agent. Vitamin B₁₂ and the hemoproteins are incapable of reacting with chelating agents, because their metal is already coordinated in such a way that only the *trans*-coordination positions of the metal are available for complexation. In contrast, the metal ion in certain enzymes, such as alcohol dehydrogenase, which contains zinc, can undergo chelation, suggesting that the metal is bound in such a way as to leave two *cis* positions available for chelation.

Chlorophyll and hemoglobin, two extremely important compounds, are naturally occurring chelates involved in the life processes of plants and animals. Albumin is the main carrier of various metal ions and small molecules in the blood serum. The N-terminal portion of human serum albumin binds Cu(II) and Ni(II) with higher affinity than that of dog serum albumin. This fact partly explains why humans are less susceptible to copper poisoning than are dogs. The binding of copper to serum albumin is important since this metal is possibly involved in several pathologic conditions.[3] The synthetic chelating agent, ethylenediaminetetraacetic acid (Fig. 11–1), has been used to tie up or *sequester* iron and copper ions so that they cannot

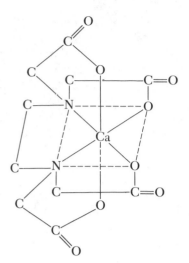

Fig. 11–1. Calcium ions sequestered by ethylenediaminetetraacetic acid (EDTA).

catalyze the oxidative degradation of ascorbic acid in fruit juices and in drug preparations. In the process of sequestration, the chelating agent and metal ion form a water-soluble compound. EDTA is widely used to sequester and remove calcium ions from hard water.

Chelation can be applied to the assay of drugs. A calorimetric method to assay procainamide in injectable solutions is based on the formation of a 1:1 complex of procainamide with cupric ion at pH 4 to 4.5. The complex absorbs visible radiation at a maximum wavelength of 380 nm.[4] The many uses to which metal complexes and chelating agents can be put are discussed by Martell and Calvin.[5]

ORGANIC MOLECULAR COMPLEXES

An organic coordination compound or molecular complex consists of constituents held together by weak forces of the donor–acceptor type or by hydrogen bonds.

The difference between complexation and the formation of organic compounds has been shown by Clapp.[6] The compounds, dimethylaniline and 2,4,6-trinitroanisole, react in the cold to give a molecular complex:

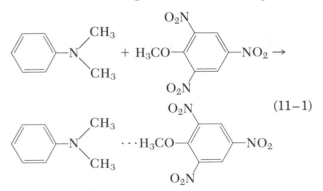

On the other hand, these two compounds react at an elevated temperature to yield a salt, the constituent

molecules of which are held together by primary valence bonds.

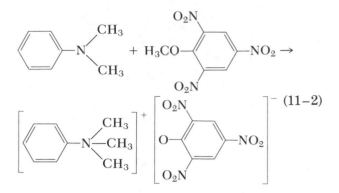

The dotted line in the complex of equation (11–1) indicates that the two molecules are held together by a weak secondary valence force. It is not to be considered as a clearly defined bond but rather as an overall attraction between the two aromatic molecules.

The type of bonding existing in molecular complexes in which hydrogen bonding plays no part is not fully understood, but it may be considered for the present as involving an electron donor–acceptor mechanism corresponding to that in metal complexes but ordinarily much weaker.

Many organic complexes are so weak that they cannot be separated from their solutions as definite compounds, and they are often difficult to detect by chemical and physical means. The energy of attraction between the constituents is probably less than 5 kcal/mole for most organic complexes. Since the bond distance between the components of the complex is usually greater than 3 Å, a covalent link is not involved. Instead, one molecule polarizes the other, resulting in a type of ionic interaction or charge transfer, and these molecular complexes are often referred to as *charge transfer complexes*. For example, the polar nitro groups of trinitrobenzene induce a dipole in the readily polarizable benzene molecule, and the electrostatic interaction that results leads to complex formation.

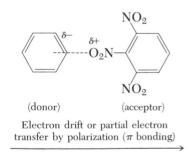

(donor)   (acceptor)

Electron drift or partial electron transfer by polarization (π bonding)

X-ray diffraction studies of complexes formed between trinitrobenzene and aniline derivatives have shown that one of the nitro groups of trinitrobenzene lies over the benzene ring of the aniline molecule, the intermolecular distance between the two molecules being about 3.3 Å. This result strongly suggests that the interaction involves π bonding between the π

electrons of the benzene ring and the electron-accepting nitro group.

A factor of some importance in the formation of molecular complexes is the steric requirement. If the approach and close association of the donor and acceptor molecules are hindered by steric factors, the complex is not likely to form. Hydrogen bonding and other effects must also be considered, and these are discussed in connection with the specific complexes considered on the following pages.

The difference between a *donor–acceptor* and a *charge-transfer* complex is that in the latter type resonance makes the main contribution to complexation, while in the former, London dispersion forces and dipole–dipole interactions contribute more to the stability of the complex. Resonance interaction is shown in Figure 11–2 as depicted by Bullock.[7] Trinitrobenzene is the acceptor, A, molecule and hexamethyl benzene is the donor, D. On the left side of the figure weak dispersion and dipolar forces contribute to the interaction of A and D; on the right side of the figure the interaction of A and D results from a significant transfer of charge, making the electron acceptor trinitrobenzene negatively charged (A$^-$) and leaving the donor hexamethylbenzene positively charged (D$^+$). The overall complex, Donor–Acceptor, is shown by the double-headed arrow to resonate between the uncharged D . . . A and the charged D$^+$ . . . A$^-$ moieties. If, as in the case of hexamethylbenzene–trinitrobenzene, the resonance is fairly weak, having an intermolecular binding energy ΔH of about -4700 calories, the complex is referred to as a *donor–acceptor complex*. If, on the other hand, resonance between the charge-transfer structure (D$^+$ . . . A$^-$) and the uncharged species (D . . . A) contributes greatly to the binding of the donor and acceptor molecule, the complex is called a *charge-transfer complex*. Finally, those complexes bound together by van der Waals forces, dipole–dipole interactions, and hydrogen bonding but lacking charge transfer are known simply as *molecular complexes*. In both charge-transfer and donor–acceptor complexes, new absorption bands occur in the spectra, as shown in Figure 11–13, p. 266. In this book we shall not attempt to separate the first two classes but rather refer to all interactions that produce absorption bands as charge-transfer or as electron donor–acceptor complexes without distinction. Those com-

plexes that do not show new bands are called molecular complexes.

Charge-transfer complexes are of importance in pharmacy. Iodine forms 1:1 charge-transfer complexes with the drugs disulfiram, chlomethiazole, and tolnaftate. These drugs have recognized pharmacologic actions of their own: disulfiram is used against alcohol addiction, clomethiazole is a sedative-hypnotic and anticonvulsant, and tolnaftate is an antifungal agent. Each of these drugs possesses a nitrogen–carbon–sulfur moiety (see the structure of tolnaftate below), and a complex may result from the transfer of charge from the pair of free electrons on the nitrogen and/or sulfur atoms of these drugs to the antibonding orbital of the iodine atom. Thus, by tying up iodine, molecules containing the N – C = S moiety inhibit thyroid action in the body.[8]

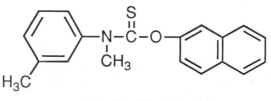

Tolnaftate (Tinactin)

Quinhydrone Complexes. The molecular complex that was referred to in Chapter 9 as quinhydrone is formed by mixing alcoholic solutions of equimolar quantities of benzoquinone and hydroquinone. The complex settles as green crystals. When an aqueous solution is saturated with quinhydrone, the complex dissociates into equivalent amounts of quinone and hydroquinone and is used as an electrode in pH determinations.

The 1:1 complex formed between benzoquinone and hydroquinone may be said to result from the overlap of the pi-framework of the electron-deficient quinone molecule with the pi-framework of the electron-rich hydroquinone molecule. Maximum overlap between the pi-frameworks is expected if the aromatic rings are parallel and are oriented in such a way as to have their centers directly over one another. Hydrogen bonding may contribute in stabilizing this complex, but it is not the sole means of association, since hydroquinone dimethyl ether also forms a colored adduct with quinone.

An interesting quinone is obtained from salicylic acid. This compound is readily oxidized, yielding blue-black quinhydrone compounds of the type

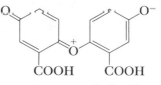

Quinhydrone of salicylic acid

Picric Acid Complexes. Picric acid, 2,4,6-trinitrophenol, $pK_a = 0.38$, reacts with strong bases to form salts

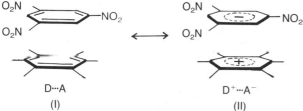

D···A
(I)

D$^+$···A$^-$
(II)

Fig. 11–2. Resonance in a donor–acceptor complex of trinitrobenzene and hexamethylbenzene. (From F. Y. Bullock, Charge transfer in biology, Chapter 3 in *Comprehensive Biochemistry*, M. Florkin and E. H. Stotz, Eds., Vol. 22 of *Bioenergetics*, Elsevier, N.Y., 1967, pp. 82–85, reproduced with permission of the copyright owner.)

and with weak bases to form molecular complexes. Butesin picrate (Abbott Laboratories), presumably a 2:1 complex, may be represented by the formula

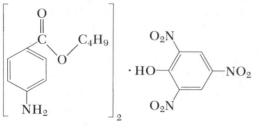

Butesin picrate

It is a yellow powder, insoluble in water but soluble in organic solvents. Butesin picrate is used as a 1% ointment for burns and painful skin abrasions. It combines the antiseptic property of picric acid and the anesthetic property of butesin.

It has been suggested that the stability of the complexes formed between carcinogenic agents and picric acid is related to carcinogenic activity, and any substitution on the carcinogen molecule that hinders picrate complexation also reduces carcinogenicity. Symmetric trinitrobenzene forms more complexes than does picric acid, and perhaps trinitrobenzene may also be used to provide a test for carcinogenicity.

Drug Complexes. Higuchi and his associates[9] have investigated the complexing of caffeine with a number of acidic drugs. They attribute the interaction between caffeine and a drug such as a sulfonamide or a barbiturate to a dipole–dipole force or hydrogen bonding between the polarized carbonyl groups of caffeine and the hydrogen atom of the acid. A secondary interaction probably occurs between the nonpolar parts of the molecules, and the resultant complex is "squeezed out" of the aqueous phase owing to the great internal pressure of water. These two effects lead to a high degree of interaction.

The complexation of esters is of particular concern to the pharmacist, since many important drugs belong to this class. The complexes formed between esters and amines, phenols, ethers and ketones, have been attributed to the hydrogen bonding between a nucleophilic carbonyl oxygen and an active hydrogen. This, however, does not explain the complexation of esters such as benzocaine, procaine, and tetracaine with caffeine, as reported by Higuchi et al.[10] There are no activated hydrogens on caffeine; the hydrogen in the number 8 position (formula I) is very weak ($K_a = 1 \times 10^{-14}$) and is not likely to enter into complexation. It might be suggested that, in the caffeine molecule, a relatively positive center exists that serves as a likely site of complexation. The caffeine molecule is numbered in I for convenience in the discussion. As observed in formula II, the nitrogen at the 2 position presumably can become strongly electrophilic or acidic just as it is in an imide, owing to the withdrawal of electrons by the

oxygens at position 1 and 3. An ester such as benzocaine also becomes polarized (formula III) in such a way that the carboxyl oxygen is nucleophilic or basic. The complexation can thus occur as a result of a dipole–dipole interaction between the nucleophilic carboxyl oxygen of benzocaine and the electrophilic nitrogen of caffeine.

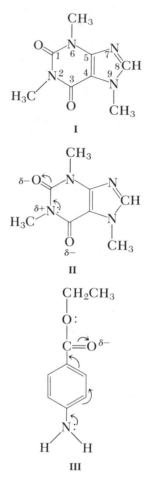

Caffeine forms complexes with organic acid *anions* that are more soluble than the pure xanthine, but the complexes formed with organic acids, such as gentisic acid, are less soluble than caffeine alone. Such insoluble complexes provide caffeine in a form that masks its normally bitter taste and should serve as a suitable state for chewable tablets. Higuchi and Pitman[11] synthesized 1:1 and 1:2 caffeine–gentisic acid complexes and measured their equilibrium solubility and rates of dissolution. Both the 1:1 and 1:2 complexes were less soluble in water than caffeine, and their dissolution rates were also less than that of caffeine. Chewable tablets formulated from these complexes should provide an extended-release form of the drug with improved taste.

York and Saleh[12] studied the effect of sodium salicylate on the release of benzocaine from topical vehicles, it being recognized that salicylates form molecular complexes with benzocaine. Complexation between drug and complexing agents can improve or impair drug absorption and bioavailability; the authors found that the presence of sodium salicylate significantly influenced the release of benzocaine, depending on the type of vehicle involved. The largest increase in absorption was observed for a water-miscible polyethylene glycol base.

Polymer Complexes. Polyethylene glycols, polystyrene, carboxymethylcellulose, and similar polymers containing nucleophilic oxygens can form complexes with various drugs. The incompatibilities of certain polyethers, such as the Carbowaxes®, Pluronics®, and Tweens® with tannic acid, salicylic acid, and phenol, can be attributed to these interactions. Marcus[13] has reviewed some of the interactions that may occur in suspensions, emulsions, ointments, and suppositories. The incompatibility may be manifested as a precipitate, flocculate, delayed biologic absorption, loss of preservative action, or other undesirable physical, chemical, and pharmacologic effects.

Plaizier-Vercammen et al.[14] have studied the interaction of povidone (PVP) with ionic and neutral aromatic compounds. Several factors affect the binding to PVP of substituted benzoic acid and nicotine derivatives. While ionic strength has no influence, the binding increases in phosphate buffer solutions and decreases as the temperature is raised.

Crosspovidone, a cross-linked insoluble PVP, is able to bind drugs owing to its dipolar character and porous structure. Frömming et al.[15] studied the interaction of crosspovidone with acetaminophen, benzocaine, benzoic acid, caffeine, tannic acid, and papaverine hydrochloride, among other drugs. The interaction is mainly due to any phenolic groups on the drug. Hexylresorcinol shows exceptionally strong binding, but the interaction is less than 5% for most drugs studied (32 drugs). Crosspovidone is a disintegrant in pharmaceutical granules and tablets. It does not interfere with gastrointestinal absorption because the binding to drugs is reversible.

Solutes in parenteral formulations may migrate from the solution and interact with the wall of a polymeric container. Hayward et al.[16] showed that the ability of a polyolefin container to interact with drugs depends linearly on the octanol–water partition coefficient of the drug. For parabens and drugs that exhibit fairly significant hydrogen bond donor properties, a correction term related to hydrogen-bonding formation is needed. Polymer–drug container interactions may result in loss of the active component in liquid dosage forms.

Polymer–drug complexes are used to modify biopharmaceutical parameters of drugs; the dissolution rate of ajmaline is enhanced by complexation with PVP. The interaction is due to the aromatic ring of ajmaline and the amide groups of PVP to yield a dipole–dipole induced complex.[17]

Some molecular organic complexes of interest to the pharmacist are found in Table 11–3. (Complexes involving caffeine are listed in Table 11–6.)

INCLUSION COMPOUNDS

The class of addition compounds known as *inclusion* or *occlusion* compounds results more from the architecture of molecules than from their chemical affinity. One of the constituents of the complex is trapped in the open lattice or cage-like crystal structure of the other to yield a stable arrangement.

Channel Lattice Type. The *choleic acids* (bile acids) can form a group of complexes principally involving deoxycholic acid in combination with paraffins, organic acids, esters, ketones, and aromatic compounds and with solvents such as ether, alcohol, and dioxane. The crystals of deoxycholic acid are arranged to form a channel into which the complexing molecule can fit (cf. Fig. 11–3). Such stereospecificity should permit the resolution of optical isomers. In fact, camphor has been partially resolved by complexation with deoxycholic

TABLE 11–3. *Some Molecular Organic Complexes of Pharmaceutical Interest**

Agent	Compounds That Form Complexes with the Agent Listed in the First Column
Polyethylene glycols	m-Hydroxybenzoic acid, p-hydroxybenzoic acid, salicylic acid, o-phthalic acid, acetylsalicylic acid, resorcinol, catechol, phenol, phenobarbital, iodine (in I_2 • KI solutions), bromine (in presence of HBr).
Povidone (polyvinyl-pyrrolidone, PVP)	Benzoic acid, m-hydroxybenzoic acid, p-hydroxybenzoic acid, salicylic acid, sodium salicylate, p-aminobenzoic acid, mandelic acid, sulfathiazole, chloramphenicol, phenobarbital.
Sodium carboxymethylcellulose	Quinine, benadryl, procaine, pyribenzamine.
Oxytetracycline and tetracycline	N-methylpyrrolidone, N,N-dimethylacetamide, γ-valerolactone, γ-butyrolactone, sodium p-aminobenzoate, sodium salicylate, sodium p-hydroxybenzoate, sodium saccharin, caffeine.

*Compiled from the results of T. Higuchi et al., J. Am. Pharm. Assoc., Sci. Ed. **43**, 393, 398, 456, 1954; ibid. **44**, 668, 1955, ibid. **45**, 157, 1956; ibid. **46**, 458, 587, 1957 and from J. L. Lach et al., Drug Standards **24**, 11, 1956. An extensive table of acceptor and donor molecules that form aromatic molecular complexes has been compiled by L. J. Andrews, Chem. Revs. **54**, 713, 1954. Also refer to T. Higuchi and K. A. Connors, Phase solubility techniques. *Advances in Analytical Chemistry and Instrumentation*, C. N. Reilley, Ed., New York, Wiley, 1965, pp. 117–212.

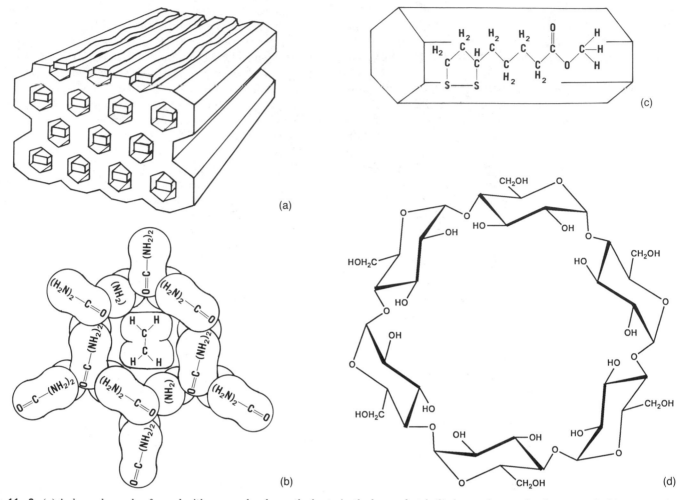

Fig. 11–3. (*a*) A channel complex formed with urea molecules as the host. As the lower sketch (*b*) shows, these molecules are packed in an orderly manner and held together by hydrogen bonds between nitrogen and oxygen atoms. The hexagonal channels, approximately 5 Å in diameter, provide room for guest molecules such as long chain hydrocarbons, as shown here. (From J. F. Brown, Jr., Sci. Am. **207**, 82, 1962. Copyright © 1962 by Scientific American, Inc. All rights reserved.) (*c*) A hexagonal channel complex (adduct) of methyl α-lipoate and 15 g of urea in methanol prepared with gentle heating. Needle crystals of the adduct separated overnight at room temperature. This inclusion compound or adduct begins to decompose at 63° C and melts at 163° C. Thiourea may also be used to form the channel complex. (From H. Mima and M. Nishikawa, J. Pharm. Sci. **53**, 931, 1964, reproduced with permission of the copyright owner.) (*d*) Cyclodextrin (cycloamylose, Schardinger dextrin). See *Merck Index*, Edition 11, Rahway, N.J., 1989, p. 425.

acid, and *dl*-terpineol has been resolved by the use of digitonin, which occludes certain molecules in a manner similar to that of deoxycholic acid.

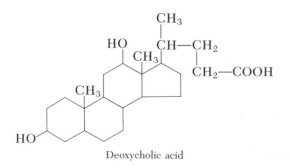

Deoxycholic acid

Urea and thiourea also crystallize in a channel-like structure permitting enclosure of unbranched paraffins, alcohols, ketones, organic acids, and other compounds, as shown in Figure 11–3*a* and *b*. The well-known starch-iodine solution is a channel-type complex consist-

ing of iodine molecules entrapped within spirals of the glucose residues.

Forman and Grady[18] found that monostearin, an interfering substance in the assay of dienestrol, could be extracted easily from dermatologic creams by channel-type inclusion in urea. They felt that urea inclusion might become a general approach for separation of long-chain compounds in assay methods. The authors reviewed the earlier literature on urea inclusion of straight-chain hydrocarbons and fatty acids.

Layer Type. Some compounds such as the clay montmorillonite, the principal constituent of bentonite, can trap hydrocarbons, alcohols, and glycols between the layers of their lattices.[19] Graphite can also intercalate compounds between its layers.

Clathrates.[20] The clathrates crystallize in the form of a cage-like lattice in which the coordinating compound is entrapped. Chemical bonds are not involved in these complexes, and only the molecular size of the encaged component is of importance. Ketelaar[21] observed that the stability of a clathrate may be related to the confinement of a prisoner. The stability of a clathrate is due to the strength of the structure, that is, to the high energy that must be expended to decompose the compound, just as a prisoner is confined by the bars that prevent his escape.

Powell and Palin[22] have made a detailed study of clathrate compounds and have shown that the highly toxic agent hydroquinone (quinol) crystallizes in a cage-like hydrogen-bonded structure, as seen in Figure 11–4. The holes have a diameter of 4.2 Å and permit the entrapment of one small molecule to about every two quinol molecules. Small molecules such as methyl alcohol, CO_2, and HCl may be trapped in these cages, but smaller molecules such as H_2 and larger molecules such as ethanol cannot be accommodated. It is possible that clathrates may be used to resolve optical isomers and to bring about other processes of molecular separation.

One official drug, warfarin sodium USP, is a clathrate of water, isopropyl alcohol, and sodium warfarin in the form of a white crystalline powder.

Monomolecular Inclusion Compounds. Cyclodextrins. Inclusion compounds are reviewed by Frank.[23] In addition to channel- and cage-type (clathrate) compounds, Frank adds classes of *mono-* and *macromolecular* inclusion compounds. Monomolecular inclusion compounds involve the entrapment of a single guest molecule in the cavity of one host molecule. Monomolecular host structures are represented by the cyclodextrins. These compounds are cyclic oligosaccharides

containing a minimum of six D-(+)-glucopyranose units attached by α-1,4 linkages produced by the action on starch of *Bacillus macerans* amylase. The natural α, β, and γ cyclodextrins (α-CD, β-CD, and γ-CD) consist of 6, 7, and 8 units of glucose, respectively.

Their ability to form inclusion compounds in aqueous solution is due to the typical arrangement of the glucose units (see Fig. 11–3*d*). As observed in cross-section in the figure, the cyclodextrin structure forms a torus or doughnut ring. The molecule actually exists as a truncated cone, which is seen in Figure 11–5*a*; it can accommodate molecules such as mitomycin C to form inclusion compounds (Fig. 11–5*b*). The interior of the cavity is relatively hydrophobic because of the CH_2 groups, whereas the cavity entrances are hydrophilic owing to the presence of the primary and secondary hydroxyl groups.[24,25] α-CD has the smallest cavity (internal diameter almost 5 Å). β-CD and γ-CD are the most useful for pharmaceutical technology owing to their larger cavity size (internal diameter almost 6 Å and 8 Å, respectively). Water inside the cavity tends to be squeezed out and to be replaced by more hydrophobic species. Thus, molecules of appropriate size and stereochemistry can be included in the cyclodextrin cavity by hydrophobic interactions. (See pp. 272–273). Complexation does not ordinarily involve the formation of covalent bonds. Some drugs may be too large to be accommodated totally in the cavity. As

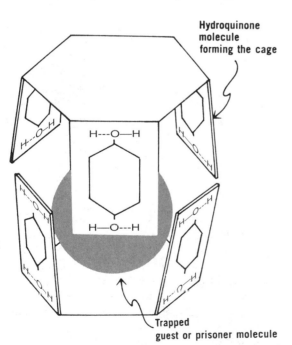

Fig. 11–4. Cage-like structure formed through hydrogen bonding of hydroquinone molecules. Small molecules such as methanol are trapped in the cages to form the clathrate. (Modified from J. F. Brown, Jr., Sci. Am. **207**, 82, 1962. Copyright © 1962 by Scientific American, Inc. All rights reserved.)

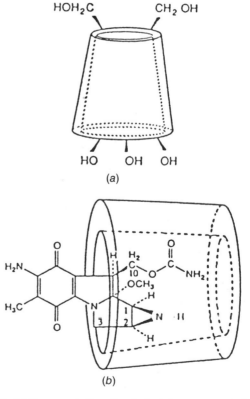

Fig. 11–5. (*a*) Representation of cyclodextrin as a truncated cone. (*b*) Mitomycin C partly enclosed in cyclodextrin to form an inclusion complex. (From O. Beckers, Int. J. Pharm. **52**, 240, 247, 1989, reproduced with permission of the copyright owner.)

shown in Figure 11–5*b*, mitomycin C interacts with γ-CD at one side of the torus. Thus, the aziridine ring

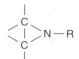

of mitomycin C is protected from degradation in acidic solution.[26] Bakensfield et al.[27] studied the inclusion of indomethacin with β-CD using an ^{1}(H-N)MR technique. The *p*-chlorobenzoyl part of indomethacin (shaded part of Fig. 11–6) enters the β-CD ring, whereas the substituted indol moiety (the remainder of the molecule) is too large for inclusion and rests against the entrance of the CD cavity.

Cyclodextrins are studied as solubilizing and stabilizing agents in pharmaceutical dosage forms. Lach and associates[28] used cyclodextrins to trap, stabilize, and solubilize sulfonamides, tetracyclines, morphine, aspirin, benzocaine, ephedrine, reserpine, and testosterone. The aqueous solubility of retinoic acid (0.5 mg/liter), a drug used topically in the treatment of acne,[29] is increased to 160 mg/liter by complexation with β-CD. Dissolution rate plays an important role in bioavailability of drugs, fast dissolution usually favoring absorption. Thus, the dissolution rate of famotidine,[30] a potent drug in the treatment of gastric and duodenal ulcers, and tolbutamide, an oral antidiabetic drug, are both increased by complexation with β-cyclodextrin.[31]

Cyclodextrins may increase or decrease the reactivity of the guest molecule depending on the nature of the reaction and the orientation of the molecule within the CD cavity. Thus, α-cyclodextrin tends to favor pH-dependent hydrolysis of indomethacin in aqueous solution, whereas β-cyclodextrin inhibits it.[27] Unfortunately, the water solubility of β-CD (1.8 g/100 mL at 25° C) is often insufficient to stabilize drugs at therapeutic doses, and is also associated with nephrotoxicity when CD is administered by parenteral routes.[32] The relatively low aqueous solubility of the cyclodextrins may be due to the formation of intramolecular hydrogen bonds between the hydroxyl groups (see Fig. 11–3*d*), which prevent their interaction with water molecules.[33]

Derivatives of the natural crystalline CD have been developed to improve aqueous solubility and to avoid

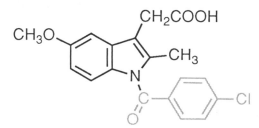

Fig. 11–6. Indomethacin (Indocin).

toxicity. Partial methylation (alkylation) of some of the OH groups in CD reduces the intermolecular hydrogen bonding, leaving some OH groups free to interact with water, thus increasing the aqueous solubility of CD.[33] According to Müller and Brauns,[34] a low degree of alkyl substitution is preferable. Derivatives with a high degree of substitution lower the surface tension of water, and this has been correlated with the hemolytic activity observed in some CD derivatives. Amorphous derivatives of β-CD and γ-CD are more effective as solubilizing agents for sex hormones than the parent cyclodextrins. Complexes of testosterone with amorphous hydroxypropyl β-CD allow an efficient transport of hormone into the circulation when given sublingually.[35] This route avoids both metabolism of the drug in the intestines and rapid *first-pass* decomposition in the liver (see Chapter 19), thus improving bioavailability.

In addition to hydrophilic derivatives, hydrophobic forms of β-CD have been found useful as sustained-release drug carriers. Thus, the release rate of the water-soluble calcium antagonist diltiazem was significantly decreased by complexation with ethylated β-CD. The release rate was controlled by mixing hydrophobic and hydrophilic derivatives of cyclodextrins at several ratios.[36] Ethylated β-CD has also been used to retard the delivery of isosorbide dinitrate, a vasodilator.[37]

Cyclodextrins may improve the organoleptic characteristics of oral liquid formulations. The bitter taste of suspensions of femoxetine, an antidepressant, is greatly suppressed by complexation of the drug with β-cyclodextrin.[38]

Molecular Sieves. Macromolecular inclusion compounds, or *molecular sieves* as they are commonly called, include zeolites, dextrins, silica gels, and related substances. The atoms are arranged in three dimensions to produce cages and channels. Synthetic zeolites may be made to a definite pore size so as to separate molecules of different dimensions, and they are also capable of ion exchange. See the review article by Frank[23] for a detailed discussion of inclusion compounds.

METHODS OF ANALYSIS[39]

A determination of the *stoichiometric ratio* of ligand-to-metal or donor-to-acceptor and a quantitative expression of the *stability constant* for complex formation are important in the study and application of coordination compounds. A limited number of the more important methods for obtaining these two quantities are presented here.

Method of Continuous Variation. Job[40] suggested the use of an additive property such as the spectrophotometric extinction coefficient (dielectric constant or the square of the refractive index may also be used) for the measurement of complexation. If the property for two species is sufficiently different and if no interaction occurs when the components are mixed, then the value of the property is the weighted mean of the values of the separate species in the mixture. This means that if the additive property, say dielectric constant, is plotted against the mole fraction from 0 to 1 for one of the components of a mixture where no complexation occurs, a linear relationship is observed, as shown by the dotted line in Figure 11–7. If solutions of two species A and B of equal molar concentration (and hence of a fixed total concentration of the species) are mixed and if a complex forms between the two species, the value of the additive property will pass through a maximum (or minimum), as shown by the upper curve in Figure 11–7. For a constant total concentration of A and B, the complex is at its greatest concentration at a point where the species A and B are combined in the ratio in which they occur in the complex. The line therefore shows a break or a change in slope at the mole fraction corresponding to the complex. The change in slope occurs at a mole fraction of 0.5 in Figure 11–7, indicating a complex of the 1:1 type.

When spectrophotometric absorbance is used as the physical property, the observed values, obtained at various mole fractions when complexation occurs, are usually subtracted from the corresponding values that would have been expected had no complex resulted. This difference D is then plotted against mole fraction, as shown in Figure 11–8. From such a curve, the molar ratio of the complex is readily obtained. By means of a calculation involving the concentration, and the property being measured, the stability constant of the formation may be determined by a method described by Martell and Calvin.[41] Another method, suggested by Bent and French,[42] is given here.

If the magnitude of the measured property, such as absorbance, is proportional only to the concentration of the complex MA_n, the molar ratio of ligand A to metal

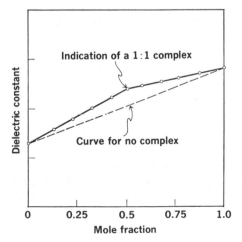

Fig. 11–7. A plot of an additive property against mole fraction of one of the species in which complexation between the species has occurred. The dotted line is that expected if no complex had formed. (C. H. Giles et al., J. Chem. Soc., 1952, 3799, should be referred to for similar figures.)

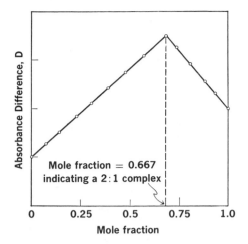

Fig. 11–8. A plot of absorbance difference against mole fraction showing the result of complexation.

M and the stability constant may be readily determined. The equation for complexation can be written as

$$M + nA = MA_n \qquad (11\text{–}3)$$

and the stability constant as

$$K = \frac{[MA_n]}{[M][A]^n} \qquad (11\text{–}4)$$

or in logarithmic form

$$\log [MA_n] = \log K + \log [M] + n \log [A] \qquad (11\text{–}5)$$

in which $[MA_n]$ is the concentration of the complex, $[M]$ the concentration of the uncomplexed metal, $[A]$ the concentration of the uncomplexed ligand, n the number of moles of ligand combined with one mole of metal ion, and K the equilibrium or *stability* constant for the complex. The concentration of a metal ion is held constant while the concentration of ligand is varied, and the corresponding concentration $[MA_n]$ of complex formed is obtained from the spectrophotometric analysis.[40] Now, according to equation (11–5), if $\log [MA_n]$ is plotted against $\log [A]$, the slope of the line yields the stoichiometric ratio or the number n of ligand molecules coordinated to the metal ion, and the intercept on the vertical axis allows one to obtain the stability constant, K, since $[M]$ is a known quantity.

Job restricted his method to the formation of a single complex; however, Vosburgh et al.[43] modified it so as to treat the formation of higher complexes in solution. Osman and Abu-Eittah[44] used spectrophotometric techniques to investigate 1:2 metal–ligand complexes of copper and barbiturates. A greenish-yellow complex is formed by mixing a blue solution of copper (II) with thiobarbiturates (colorless). By using the Job method, an apparent stability constant as well as the composition of the 1:2 complex was obtained.

pH Titration Method. This is one of the most reliable methods and can be used whenever the complexation is attended by a change in pH. The chelation of the cupric ion by glycine, for example, may be represented as

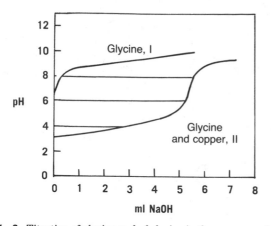

Fig. 11-9. Titration of glycine and of glycine in the presence of cupric ions. The difference in pH for a given quantity of base added indicates the occurrence of a complex.

$$Cu^{2+} + 2NH_3^+CH_2COO^-$$

$$= Cu(NH_2CH_2COO)_2 + 2H^+ \qquad (11-6)$$

Since two protons are formed in the reaction of equation (11-6), the addition of glycine to a solution containing cupric ions should result in a decrease in pH.

Titration curves can be obtained by adding a strong base to a solution of glycine, and to another solution containing glycine and a copper salt, and plotting the pH against the equivalents of base added. The results of such a potentiometric titration are shown in Figure 11-9. The curve for the metal–glycine mixture is well below that for the glycine alone, and the decrease in pH shows that complexation is occurring throughout most of the neutralization range. Similar results are obtained with other zwitterions and weak acids (or bases), such as *N,N'*-diacetylethylenediamine diacetic acid, which has been studied for its complexing action with copper and calcium ions.

The results can be treated quantitatively in the following manner to obtain stability constants for the complex. The two successive or stepwise equilibria between the copper ion or metal M and glycine or the ligand A may be written in general as

$$M + A = MA; \quad K_1 = \frac{[MA]}{[M][A]} \qquad (11-7)$$

$$MA + A = MA_2; \quad K_2 = \frac{[MA_2]}{[MA][A]} \qquad (11-8)$$

and the overall reaction (11-7 and 11-8) is

$$M + 2A = MA_2; \quad \beta = K_1K_2 = \frac{[MA_2]}{[M][A]^2} \qquad (11-9)$$

Bjerrum[45] called K_1 and K_2 the *formation constants*, while the equilibrium constant β for the overall reaction is known as the *stability constant*. A quantity n may now be defined. It is the number of ligand molecules bound to a metal ion. The *average* number of ligand groups bound per metal ion present is therefore designated $\overline{n}$ (n bar) and is written

$$\overline{n} = \frac{\text{(total concentration of ligand bound)}}{\text{(total concentration of metal ion)}} \qquad (11-10)$$

or

$$\overline{n} = \frac{[MA] + 2[MA_2]}{[M] + [MA] + [MA_2]} \qquad (11-11)$$

While n has a definite value for each species of complex (1 or 2 in this case), it may have any value between 0 and the largest number of ligand molecules bound, 2 in this case. The numerator of equation (11-11) gives the total concentration of ligand species bound. The second term in the numerator is multiplied by 2 since two molecules of ligand are contained in each molecule of the species, MA_2. The denominator gives the total concentration of metal present in all forms, both bound and free. For the special case in which $\overline{n} = 1$, equation (11-11) becomes

$$[MA] + 2[MA_2] = [M] + [MA] + [MA_2]$$

$$[MA_2] = [M] \qquad (11-12)$$

Employing the results in equations (11-9) and (11-12), we obtain the following relation:

$$\beta = K_1K_2 = \frac{1}{[A]^2} \quad \text{or} \quad \log \beta = -2 \log [A]$$

and finally

$$p[A] = \tfrac{1}{2} \log \beta \text{ at } \overline{n} = 1 \qquad (11-13)$$

in which p[A] is written for $-\log [A]$. Bjerrum has also shown that, to a first approximation,

$$p[A] = \log K_1 \text{ at } \overline{n} = \tfrac{1}{2} \qquad (11-14)$$

$$p[A] = \log K_2 \text{ at } \overline{n} = \tfrac{3}{2} \qquad (11-15)$$

It should now be possible to obtain the individual complex formation constants K_1 and K_2 and the overall stability constant β if one knows two values: $\overline{n}$ and p[A].

Equation (11-10) shows that the concentration of bound ligand must be determined before $\overline{n}$ can be evaluated. The horizontal distances represented by the lines in Figure 11-9 between the titration curve for glycine alone (curve I) and for glycine in the presence of Cu^{2+} (curve II) give the amount of alkali used up in the reactions (equations 11-16 and 11-17):

$$\text{(11-16)}$$

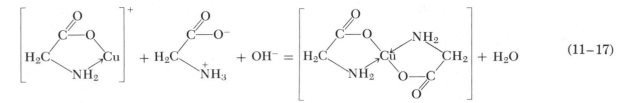

$$(11-17)$$

This quantity of alkali is exactly equal to the concentration of ligand bound at any pH, and, according to equation (11–10), when divided by the total concentration of metal ion, gives the value of $\bar{n}$.

The concentration of free glycine $[A]$ as the "base," $NH_2CH_2COO^-$, at any pH is obtained from the acid dissociation expression for glycine:

$$NH_3{}^+CH_2COO^- + H_2O = H_3O^+ + NH_2CH_2COO^-$$

$$K_a = \frac{[H_3O^+][NH_2CH_2COO^-]}{[NH_3{}^+CH_2COO^-]} \quad (11-18)$$

or

$$[NH_2CH_2COO^-] = [A] = \frac{K_a[HA]}{[H_3O^+]} \quad (11-19)$$

The concentration $[NH_3{}^+CH_2COO^-]$ or $[HA]$ of the acid species at any pH is taken as the difference between the initial concentration $[HA]_{init}$ of glycine and the concentration $[NaOH]$ of alkali added. Then

$$[A] = K_a \frac{([HA]_{init} - [NaOH])}{[H_3O^+]} \quad (11-20)$$

or

$$-\log [A] = p[A] = pK_a - pH$$
$$- \log ([HA]_{init} - [NaOH]) \quad (11-21)$$

in which $[A]$ is the concentration of the ligand, glycine.

Example 11–1. If 75-mL samples containing 3.34×10^{-2} mole/liter of glycine hydrochloride alone and in combination with 9.45×10^{-3} mole/liter of cupric ion are titrated with 0.259 N NaOH, the two curves I and II respectively, in Figure 11–9 are obtained. Compute $\bar{n}$ and p[A] at pH 3.50 and pH 8.00. The pK_a of glycine is 9.69 at 30° C.

(a) From Figure 11–9, the horizontal distance at pH 3.50 for the 75-mL sample is 1.60 mL NaOH, or 2.59×10^{-4} mole/mL $\times 1.60 = 4.15 \times 10^{-4}$ mole. For a 1-liter sample, the value would be 5.54×10^{-3} mole. The total concentration of copper ion per liter is 9.45×10^{-3} mole, and $\bar{n}$ from equation (11–10) is

$$\bar{n} = \frac{5.54 \times 10^{-3}}{9.45 \times 10^{-3}} = 0.59$$

From equation (11–21),

$$p[A] = 9.69 - 3.50 - \log [(3.34 \times 10^{-2}) - (5.54 \times 10^{-3})] = 7.75$$

(b) At pH 8.00, the horizontal distance between the two curves I and II in Figure 11–9 is equivalent to 5.50 mL of NaOH in the 75-mL sample or $2.59 \times 10^{-4} \times 5.50 \times 1000/75 = 19.0 \times 10^{-3}$ mole/liter.

$$\bar{n} = \frac{19.0 \times 10^{-3}}{9.45 \times 10^{-3}} = 2.01$$

$$p[A] = 9.69 - 8.00 - \log [(3.34 \times 10^{-2}) - (1.90 \times 10^{-2})] = 3.53$$

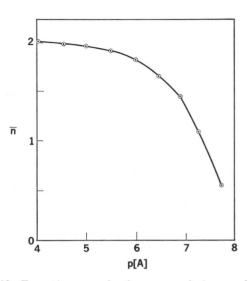

Fig. 11–10. Formation curve for the copper–glycine complex.

The values of $\bar{n}$ and p[A] at various pH values are then plotted as shown in Figure 11–10. The curve that is obtained is known as a *formation curve*. It is seen to reach a limit at $\bar{n} = 2$, signifying that the maximum number of glycine molecules that can combine with one atom of copper is two. From this curve at $\bar{n} = 0.5$, at $\bar{n} = \frac{3}{2}$, and at $\bar{n} = 1.0$, the approximate values for log K_1, log K_2, and log β respectively are obtained. A typical set of data for the complexation of glycine by copper is shown in Table 11–4. Log K_1, log K_2, and log β values for some metal complexes of pharmaceutical interest are given in Table 11–5.

TABLE 11–4. *Potentiometric Titration of Glycine Hydrochloride (3.34×10^{-2} mole/liter, pK$_a$ 9.69) and Cupric Chloride (9.45×10^{-3} mole/liter) in 75 mL Samples Using 0.259 N NaOH at 30° C*

pH	Δ mL NaOH (per 75-mL sample)	Moles OH$^-$, MA Complexed (mole/liter)	$\bar{n}$	p[A]
3.50	1.60	5.54×10^{-3}	0.59	7.66
4.00	2.90	10.1×10^{-3}	1.07	7.32
4.50	3.80	13.1×10^{-3}	1.39	6.85
5.00	4.50	15.5×10^{-3}	1.64	6.44
5.50	5.00	17.3×10^{-3}	1.83	5.98
6.00	5.20	18.0×10^{-3}	1.91	5.50
6.50	5.35	18.5×10^{-3}	1.96	5.02
7.00	5.45	18.8×10^{-3}	1.99	4.53
7.50	5.50	19.0×10^{-3}	2.03	4.03
8.00	5.50	19.0×10^{-3}	2.01	3.15

From the data in the last two columns of Table 11–4, the formation curve, Figure 11–10, is plotted, and the following results are obtained from the curve: log $K_1 = 7.9$, log $K_2 = 6.9$, and log $\beta = 14.8$ (average log β from the literature at 25° C is about 15.3).

TABLE 11–5. *Selected Constants for Complexes between Metal Ions and Organic Ligands**

Organic Ligand	Metal Ion	$\log K_1$	$\log K_2$	$\log \beta = \log K_1 K_2$
Ascorbic acid	Ca^{2+}	0.19	—	—
Nicotinamide	Ag^+	—	—	3.2
Glycine (aminoacetic acid)	Cu^{2+}	8.3	7.0	15.3
Salicylaldehyde	Fe^{2+}	4.2	3.4	7.6
Salicylic acid	Cu^{2+}	10.6	6.3	16.9
p-Hydroxybenzoic acid	Fe^{3+}	15.2	—	—
Methyl salicylate	Fe^{3+}	9.7	—	—
Diethylbarbituric acid (barbital)	Ca^{2+}	0.66	—	—
8-Hydroxyquinoline	Cu^{2+}	15	14	29
Pteroylglutamic acid (folic acid)	Cu^{2+}	—	—	7.8
Oxytetracycline	Ni^{2+}	5.8	4.8	10.6
Chlortetracycline	Fe^{3+}	8.8	7.2	16.0

*From J. Bjerrum, G. Schwarzenback, and L. G. Sillen, *Stability Constants,* Part I, Organic Ligands, The Chemical Society, London, 1957.

Pecar et al.[46] described the tendency of pyrrolidone 5-hydroxamic acid to bind the ferric ion to form mono, bis, and tris chelates. These workers later studied the thermodynamics of these chelates using a potentiometric method to determine stability constants. The method employed by Pecar et al. is known as the *Schwarzenbach method* and may be used, instead of the potentiometric method described here, when complexes are unusually stable. Sandmann and Luk[47] measured the stability constants for lithium catecholamine complexes by potentiometric titration of the free lithium ion. The results demonstrated that lithium forms complexes with the zwitterionic species of catecholamines at pH 9 to 10 and with deprotonated forms at pH values above 10. The interaction with lithium depends on the dissociation of the phenolic oxygen of catecholamines. At physiologic pH, the protonated species show no significant complexation. Some lithium salts such as lithium carbonate, lithium chloride, and lithium citrate are used in psychiatry.

Agrawal et al.[48] applied a pH titration method to estimate the average number of ligand groups per metal ion, $\bar{n}$, for several metal–sulfonamide chelates in dioxane–water. The maximum $\bar{n}$ values obtained indicate 1:1 and 1:2 complexes. The linear relationship between the pK_a of the drugs and the log of the stability constants of their corresponding metal ion complexes shows that the more basic ligands (drugs) give the more stable chelates with cerium IV, palladium II, and copper II. A potentiometric method was described in detail by Connors et al.[49] for the inclusion-type complexes formed between α-cyclodextrin and substituted benzoic acids.

Distribution Method. The method of distributing a solute between two immiscible solvents (p. 237) can be used to determine the stability constant for certain complexes. The complexation of iodine by potassium iodide may be used as an example to illustrate the method. The equilibrium reaction in its simplest form is

$$I_2 + I^- = I_3^- \qquad (11-22)$$

Addition steps also occur in polyiodide formation; for example, $2I^- + 2I_2 = I_6^{2-}$ may occur at higher concentrations, but it need not be considered here.

Example 11–2. When iodine is distributed between water (*w*) at 25°C and carbon disulfide as the organic phase (*o*), as depicted in Figure 11–11, the distribution constant $K(o/w) = C_o/C_w$ is found to be 625. When it is distributed between a 0.1250-*M* solution of potassium iodide and carbon disulfide, the concentration of iodine in the organic solvent is found to be 0.1896 mole/liter. The aqueous KI solution is analyzed, and the concentration of iodine is found to be 0.02832 mole/liter.

In summary, the results are:

Total concentration of I_2 in the aqueous layer (free + complexed iodine): 0.02832 mole/liter

Total concentration of KI in the aqueous layer (free + complexed KI): 0.1250 mole/liter

Concentration of I_2 in the CS_2 layer (free): 0.1896 mole/liter

Distribution coefficient, $K(o/w) = [I_2]_o / [I_2]_w = 625$

The species common to both phases is the free or uncomplexed iodine; the distribution law expresses only the concentration of *free* iodine, whereas a chemical analysis yields the *total* concentration of iodine in the aqueous phase. The concentration of free iodine in the aqueous phase is obtained as follows:

$$[I_2]_w = \frac{[I_2]_o}{K(o/w)} = \frac{0.1896}{625} = 3.034 \times 10^{-4} \text{ mole/liter}$$

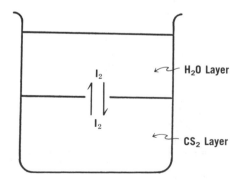

Fig. 11–11. The distribution of iodine between water and carbon disulfide.

To obtain the concentration of iodine in the complex and hence the concentration of the complex $[I_3^-]$, one subtracts the free iodine from the total iodine of the aqueous phase:

$$[I_2]_{complexed} = [I_2]_{w,\,total} - [I_2]_{w,\,free}$$
$$= 0.02832 - 0.000303$$
$$= 0.02802 \text{ mole/liter}$$

According to equation (11–22), I_2 and KI combine in equimolar concentrations to form the complex. Therefore,

$$[KI]_{complexed} = [I_2]_{complexed} = 0.02802 \text{ mole/liter}$$

KI is insoluble in carbon disulfide and remains entirely in the aqueous phase. The concentration of *free* KI is thus

$$[KI]_{free} = [KI]_{total} - [KI]_{complexed}$$
$$= 0.1250 - 0.02802$$
$$= 0.09698 \text{ mole/liter}$$

and finally

$$K = \frac{[\text{complex}]}{[I_2]_{free}\,[KI]_{free}}$$
$$= \frac{0.02802}{0.000303 \times 0.09698} = 954$$

Higuchi and his associates investigated the complexing action of caffeine, polyvinylpyrrolidone, and polyethylene glycols on a number of acidic drugs using the partition or distribution method. According to Higuchi and Zuck,[50] the reaction between caffeine and benzoic acid to form the benzoic acid–caffeine complex is

$$\text{Benzoic acid} + \text{caffeine} = (\text{benzoic acid} - \text{caffeine})$$

$$(11\text{–}23)$$

and the stability constant for the reactions at 0° C is

$$K = \frac{[\text{benzoic acid} - \text{caffeine}]}{[\text{benzoic acid}][\text{caffeine}]} = 37.5 \quad (11\text{–}24)$$

The results varied somewhat, the value 37.5 being an average stability constant. Guttman and Higuchi[51] later showed that caffeine exists in aqueous solution primarily as a monomer, dimer, and tetramer, which would account in part for the variation in K as observed by Higuchi and Zuck.

Solubility Method. According to the solubility method, excess quantities of the drug are placed in well-stoppered containers, together with a solution of the complexing agent in various concentrations, and the bottles are agitated in a constant-temperature bath until equilibrium is attained. Aliquot portions of the supernatant liquid are removed and analyzed.

Higuchi and Lach[52] used the solubility method to investigate the complexation of p-aminobenzoic acid (PABA) by caffeine. The results are plotted as shown in Figure 11–12, and the graph is explained as follows. The point A at which the line crosses the vertical axis is the solubility of the drug in water. With the addition of caffeine, the solubility of p-aminobenzoic acid rises linearly owing to complexation. At point B, the solution is saturated with respect to the complex and to the drug itself. The complex continues to form and to precipitate

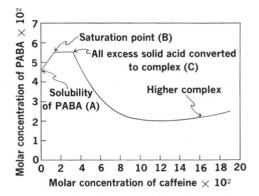

Fig. 11–12. The solubility of *para*-aminobenzoic acid in the presence of caffeine. (After T. Higuchi and J. L. Lach, J. Am. Pharm. Assoc., Sci. Ed. **43**, 525, 1954).

from the saturated system as more caffeine is added. At point C, all the excess solid PABA has passed into solution and has been converted to the complex. Although the solid drug is exhausted and the solution is no longer saturated, some of the PABA remains uncomplexed in solution, and it combines further with caffeine to form higher complexes such as (PABA–2 caffeine) as shown by the curve at the right of the diagram.

Example 11–3. The following calculations are made to obtain the stoichiometric ratio of the complex. The concentration of caffeine, corresponding to the plateau BC, equals the concentration of caffeine entering the complex over this range, and the quantity of p-aminobenzoic acid entering the complex is obtained from the undissolved solid remaining at point B. It is computed by subtracting the acid in solution at the saturation point B from the total acid initially added to the mixture, since this is the amount yet undissolved that can form the complex.

The concentration of caffeine in the plateau region is found from Figure 11–12 to be 1.8×10^{-2} mole/liter. The free undissolved solid PABA is equal to the total acid minus the acid in solution at point B, namely, $7.3 \times 10^{-2} - 5.5 \times 10^{-2}$ or 1.8×10^{-2} mole/liter, and the stoichiometric ratio is

$$\frac{\text{Caffeine in complex}}{\text{PABA in complex}} = \frac{1.8 \times 10^{-2}}{1.8 \times 10^{-2}} = 1$$

The complex formation is therefore written

$$\text{PABA} + \text{caffeine} \rightleftharpoons \text{PABA–caffeine} \quad (11\text{–}25)$$

and the stability constant for this 1:1 complex is

$$K = \frac{[\text{PABA–caffeine}]}{[\text{PABA}][\text{caffeine}]} \quad (11\text{–}26)$$

K may be computed as follows. The concentration of the complex [PABA–caffeine] is equal to the total acid concentration at saturation less the solubility [PABA] of the acid in water. The concentration [caffeine] in the solution at equilibrium is equal to the caffeine added to the system less the concentration that has been converted to the complex. The total acid concentration of saturation is 4.58×10^{-2} mole/liter when no caffeine is added (solubility of PABA), and is 5.312×10^{-2} mole/liter when 1.00×10^{-2} mole/liter of caffeine is added.

$$[\text{PABA–caffeine}] = (5.31 \times 10^{-2}) - (4.58 \times 10^{-2}) = 0.73 \times 10^{-2}$$
$$[\text{PABA}] = 4.58 \times 10^{-2}$$
$$[\text{caffeine}] = (1.00 \times 10^{-2}) - (0.73 \times 10^{-2}) = 0.27 \times 10^{-2}$$

therefore

$$K = \frac{[\text{PABA–caffeine}]}{[\text{PABA}][\text{caffeine}]} = \frac{0.73 \times 10^{-2}}{(4.58 \times 10^{-2})(0.27 \times 10^{-2})} = 59$$

The stability constants for a number of caffeine complexes obtained principally by the distribution and the solubility methods are found in Table 11–6. Stability constants for a number of other drug complexes have been compiled by Higuchi and Connors.[53] Kenley et al.[54] studied water-soluble complexes of various ligands with the antiviral drug acyclovir using the solubility method.

Spectroscopy and Change Transfer Complexation. Absorption spectroscopy in the visible and ultraviolet regions of the spectrum is commonly used to investigate electron donor–acceptor or charge-transfer complexation.[55,56] When iodine is analyzed in a noncomplexing solvent such as CCl_4, a curve is obtained with a single peak at about 520 nm. The solution is violet in color. A solution of iodine in benzene exhibits a maximum shift to 475 nm, and a new peak of considerably higher intensity for the charge-shifted band appears at 300 nm. A solution of iodine in diethyl ether shows a still greater shift to lower wavelength and the appearance of a new maximum. These solutions are red to brown in color. Their curves are observed in Figure 11–13. In benzene and ether, iodine is the electron acceptor and the organic solvent is the donor; in CCl_4, no complex is formed. The shift towards the ultraviolet region becomes greater as the electron donor solvent becomes a stronger electron-releasing agent. These spectra arise from the transfer of an electron from the donor to the acceptor in close contact in the excited state of the complex. The more easily a donor such as benzene or diethyl ether releases its electron, as measured by its ionization potential, the stronger it is as a donor. Ionization potentials of a series of donors produce a straight line when plotted against the frequency maxi-

TABLE 11–6. *Approximate Stability Constants of Some Caffeine Complexes in Water at 30° C*

Compound Complexed with Caffeine	Approximate Stability Constant
Suberic acid	3
Sulfadiazine	7
Picric acid	8
Sulfathiazole	11
o-Phthalic acid	14
Acetylsalicylic acid	15
Benzoic acid (monomer)	18
Salicylic acid	40
p-Aminobenzoic acid	48
Butylparaben	50
Benzocaine	59
p-Hydroxybenzoic acid	>100

*Compiled from T. Higuchi et al., J. Am. Pharm. Assoc., Sci. Ed., **42**, 138, 1953; ibid. **43**, 349, 524, 527, 1954; ibid. **45**, 290, 1956; ibid. **46**, 32, 1957. Over 500 such complexes with other drugs are recorded by Higuchi and Connors, Phase solubility techniques, in *Advances in Analytical Chemistry and Instrumentation*, C. N. Reilley, Ed., Wiley, Vol. 4, 1965, pp. 117–212.

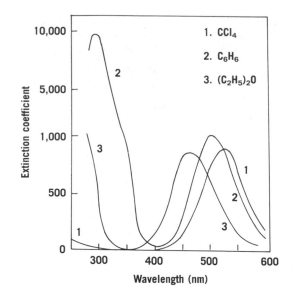

Fig. 11–13. Absorption curve of iodine in the noncomplexing solvent, (1) CCl_4, and the complexing solvents, (2) benzene, and (3) diethyl ether. (From H. A. Benesi and J. A. Hildebrand, J. Am. Chem. Soc. **70**, 2832, 1948.)

mum or charge-transfer energies (1 nm = 18.63 cal/mole) for solutions of iodine in the donor solvents.[55,56]

The complexation constant, K, may be obtained by use of visible and ultraviolet spectroscopy. The association between the donor D and acceptor A is represented as

$$D + A \underset{k_{-1}}{\overset{k_1}{\rightleftharpoons}} DA \qquad (11\text{–}27)$$

in which $K = \dfrac{k_1}{k_{-1}}$ is the equilibrium constant for complexation (stability constant), and k_1 and k_{-1} are the interaction rate constants. When two molecules associate according to this scheme and the absorbance A of the charge transfer band is measured at a definite wavelength, K is readily obtained from the *Benesi–Hildebrand equation*[57]:

$$\frac{A_0}{A} = \frac{1}{\epsilon} + \frac{1}{K\epsilon}\frac{1}{D_0} \qquad (11\text{–}28)$$

A_0 and D_0 are initial concentrations of the acceptor and donor species, respectively, in mole/liter, ϵ is the molar absorptivity of the charge-transfer complex at its particular wavelength, and K, the stability constant, is given in liter/mole or M^{-1}. A plot of A_0/A versus $1/D_0$ results in a straight line with a slope of $1/(K\epsilon)$ and an intercept of $1/\epsilon$, as observed in Figure 11–14.

Borazan et al.[58] investigated the interaction of nucleic acid bases (electron acceptors) with catechol, epinephrine, and isoproterenol (electron donors). Catechols have low ionization potentials and hence a tendency to donate electrons. Charge-transfer complexation was evident as demonstrated by ultraviolet absorption measurements. Assuming 1:1 complexes, the equilibrium constants K for charge-transfer inter-

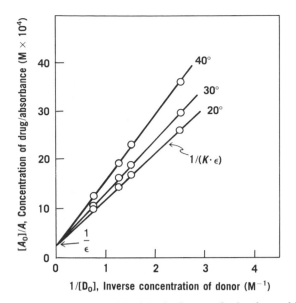

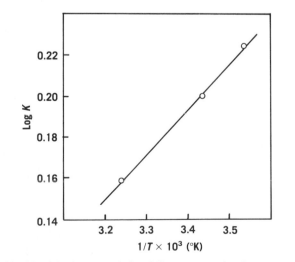

Fig. 11–14. A Benesi–Hildebrand plot to obtain the stability constant, K, from equation (11–28) for charge transfer complexation. (From M. A. Slifkin, Biochim. Biophys. Acta **109**, 617, 1965.)

action were obtained from Benesi–Hildebrand plots, Figure 11–14, at three or four temperatures, and $\Delta H°$ was obtained at these same temperatures from the slope of the line as plotted in Figure 11–15. The values of K and the thermodynamic parameters $\Delta H°$, $\Delta G°$, and $\Delta S°$ are found in Table 11–7. The thermodynamic values are calculated according to methods described on pages 274 to 277.

Example 11–4. When A_0/A is plotted against $1/D_0$ for catechol (electron-donor) solutions containing uracil (electron acceptor) in 0.1 N HCl at 6°, 18°, 25°, and 37° C, the four lines were observed to intersect the vertical axis at 0.01041. Total concentration, A_0, for uracil was $2 \times 10^{-2}\ M$, and D_0 for catechol ranged from 0.3 to 0.8 M. The slopes of the lines determined by the least-squares method, were

6° C	18° C	25° C	37° C
0.02125	0.02738	0.03252	0.04002

Fig. 11–15. Adenine–catechol stability constant for charge-transfer complexation measured at various temperatures at a wavelength of 340 nm. (From F. A. Al-Obeidi and H. N. Borazan, J. Pharm. Sci. **65**, 892, 1976, reproduced with permission of the copyright owner.)

TABLE 11–7. *Stability Constant, K, and Thermodynamic Parameters for Charge-Transfer Interaction of Nucleic Acid Bases with Catechol in Aqueous Solution.**

Temperature (°C)	K (M^{-1})	$\Delta G°$ (cal/mole)	$\Delta H°$ (cal/mole)	$\Delta S°$ (cal/(deg mole))
		Adenine–Catechol		
9	1.69	−294		
18	1.59	−264	−1015	−2.6
37	1.44	−226		
		Uracil–Catechol		
6	0.49	396		
18	0.38	560	−3564	−14
25	0.32	675		
37	0.26	830		

*From F. A. Al-Obeidi and H. N. Borazan, J. Pharm. Sci. **65**, 892, 1976, reproduced by permission of the copyright owner.

Calculate the molar absorptivity and the stability constants, K. Knowing K at these four temperatures, how does one proceed to obtain $\Delta H°$, $\Delta G°$, and $\Delta S°$?

The intercept, from the Benesi–Hildebrand equation, is the reciprocal of the molar absorptivity, or $1/(0.01041) = 96.1$. The molar absorptivity, ϵ, is a constant for a compound or a complex, independent of temperature or concentration. K is obtained from the slope of the four curves:

$$(1)\ 0.02125 = 1/(K \times 96.1);\ K = 0.49\ M^{-1}$$
$$(2)\ 0.02738 = 1/(K \times 96.1);\ K = 0.38\ M^{-1}$$
$$(3)\ 0.03252 = 1/(K \times 96.1);\ K = 0.32\ M^{-1}$$
$$(4)\ 0.04002 = 1/(K \times 96.1);\ K = 0.26\ M^{-1}$$

These K values are then plotted as their logarithms on the vertical axis of a graph against the reciprocal of the four temperatures, converted to degrees Kelvin. This is a plot of equation (11–49), and yields $\Delta H°$ from the slope of the line. $\Delta G°$ is calculated from log K at each of the four temperatures using equation (11–48), in which the temperature, T, is expressed in degrees Kelvin. $\Delta S°$ is finally obtained using equation (11–51), $\Delta G° = \Delta H° - T\,\Delta S°$. The answers to this sample problem are found in Table 11–7. The details of the calculation are explained in *Example 11–8*.

Webb and Thompson[59] studied the possible role of electron donor–acceptor complexes in drug receptor binding using quinoline and naphthalene derivatives as model electron donors and a trinitrofluorene derivative as the electron acceptor. The most favorable arrangement for the donor 8-aminoquinoline (heavy lines) and the acceptor 9-dicyanomethylene trinitrofluorene (light lines), as calculated by a quantum chemical method, is the arrangement:

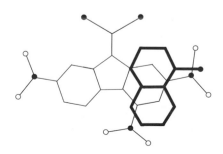

Filled circles are nitrogen and open circles oxygen atoms. The donor lies above the acceptor molecule at an intermolecular distance of about 3.35 Å and is attached by a binding energy of −5.7 kcal/mole. The negative sign signifies a positive binding force.

Other Methods. A number of other methods are available for studying the complexation of metal and organic molecular complexes. They include NMR and infrared spectroscopy, polarography, circular dichroism, kinetics, x-ray diffraction, and electron diffraction. Several of these will be discussed briefly in this section.

Complexation of caffeine with L-tryptophan in aqueous solution was investigated by Nishijo et al.[60] using ^{1}H−NMR spectroscopy. Caffeine interacts with L-tryptophan at a molar ratio of 1:1 by parallel stacking. Complexation is a result of polarization and π–π interactions of the aromatic rings. A possible mode of parallel stacking is shown in Figure 11–16. This study demonstrates that tryptophan, which is presumed to be the binding site in serum albumin for certain drugs, can interact with caffeine even as free amino acid. However, caffeine does not interact with other aromatic amino acids such as L-valine or L-leucine.

Borazan and Koumriqian[61] studied the coil–helix transition of polyadenylic acid induced by the binding of the catecholamines norepinephrine and isoproterenol using circular dichroism (see p. 98). Most mRNA molecules contain regions of polyadenylic acid, which are thought to increase the stability of mRNA and to favor genetic code translation. The change of the circular dichroism spectrum (see Chapter 4, p. 98) of polyadenylic acid was interpreted as being due to intercalative binding of catecholamines between the stacked adenine bases. These researchers suggested that catecholamines may exert a control mechanism through induction of the coil to helix transition of

polyadenylic acid which influences genetic code translation.

De Taeye and Zeegers-Huyskens[62] used infrared spectroscopy to investigate the hydrogen bonded complexes involving polyfunctional bases such as proton donors. This is a very precise technique to determine the thermodynamic parameters involved in the hydrogen bond formation and to characterize the interaction sites when the molecule has several groups available to form hydrogen bonds. Caffeine forms hydrogen bonded complexes with various proton donors: phenol, phenol derivatives, aliphatic alcohols, and water. From the infrared technique, the preferred hydrogen bonding sites are the carbonyl functions of caffeine. Seventy percent of the complexes is formed at the C=O(6) group and thirty percent of the complexes at the C=O(2) function of caffeine (see structure I, p. 256, for numbering of the atoms of caffeine). El Said et al.[63] used conductometric and infrared methods to characterize 1:1 complexes between uranyl acetate and tetracycline. The structure suggested for the uranyl-tetracycline complex is

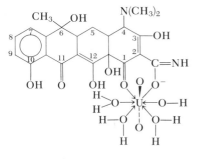

PROTEIN BINDING

The binding of drugs to proteins contained in the body can influence their action in a number of ways. Proteins may (a) facilitate the distribution of drugs throughout the body, (b) inactivate the drug by not enabling a sufficient concentration of free drug to develop at the receptor site, or (c) retard the excretion of a drug. The interaction of a drug with proteins may cause (a) the displacement of body hormones or a coadministered agent, (b) a configurational change in the protein, the structurally altered form of which is capable of binding a coadministered agent, or (c) the formation of a drug–protein complex that itself is biologically active. These topics are discussed in a number of reviews.[64,65] Among the plasma proteins, albumin is the most important owing to its high concentration relative to the other proteins and owing also to its ability to bind both acidic and basic drugs. Another plasma protein, α_1-acid glycoprotein, has been shown to bind numerous drugs; this protein appears to have greater affinity for basic than for acidic drug molecules.

A complete analysis of protein binding, including the multiple equilibria that are involved, would go beyond

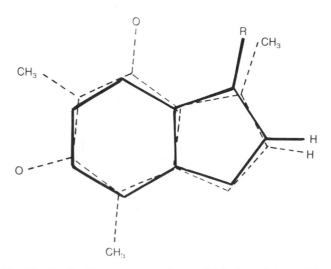

Fig. 11–16. Stacking of L-tryptophan (solid line) overlying caffeine (dashed line). The benzene ring of tryptophan is located above the pyrimidine ring of caffeine, and the pyrrole ring of L-tryptophan above the imidazole ring of caffeine. (From J. Nishijo, I. Yonetami, E. Iwamoto, et al., J. Pharm. Sci. **79**, 18, 1990, reproduced with permission of the copyright owner.)

our immediate needs. Therefore, only an abbreviated treatment is given here.

Binding Equilibria. The interaction between a group or free receptor P in a protein and a drug molecule D is written

$$P + D \rightleftharpoons PD \qquad (11-29)$$

The equilibrium constant, disregarding the difference between activities and concentrations, is

$$K = \frac{[PD]}{[P][D_f]} \qquad (11-30a)$$

or

$$K[P][D_f] = [PD] \qquad (11-30b)$$

in which K is the association constant, $[P]$ is the concentration of the protein in terms of free binding sites, $[D_f]$ is the concentration, usually given in moles, of free drug, sometimes called the ligand, and $[PD]$ is the concentration of the protein–drug complex. K varies with temperature and would be better represented as $K(T)$, $[PD]$, the symbol for bound drug is sometimes written as $[D_b]$ and $[D]$, the free drug, as $[D_f]$.

If the total protein concentration is designated as $[P_t]$, we can write

$$[P_t] = [P] + [PD]$$

or

$$[P] = [P_t] - [PD] \qquad (11-31)$$

Substituting the expression for $[P]$ from (11–31) into (11–30b) gives

$$[PD] = K[D_f]([P_t] - [PD]) \qquad (11-32)$$

$$[PD] + K[D_f][PD] = K[D_f][P_t] \qquad (11-33)$$

$$\frac{[PD]}{[P_t]} = \frac{K[D_f]}{1 + K[D_f]} \qquad (11-34)$$

Let r be the number of moles of drug bound $[PD]$ per mole of total protein $[P_t]$; then $r = [PD]/[P_t]$ or

$$r = \frac{K[D_f]}{1 + K[D_f]} \qquad (11-35)$$

The ratio r may also be expressed in other dimensions, such as milligrams of drug bound x per gram of protein m. Equation (11–35) is one form of the Langmuir adsorption isotherm to be found on page 381. Although it is quite useful for expressing protein binding data, it must not be concluded that obedience to this formula necessarily requires that protein binding be an adsorption phenomenon. Expression (11–35) can be converted to a linear form, convenient for plotting, by inverting it:

$$\frac{1}{r} = \frac{1}{K[D_f]} + 1 \qquad (11-36)$$

If v independent binding sites are available, the expression for r, equation (11–35), is simply v times that for a single site, or

$$r = v\frac{K[D_f]}{1 + K[D_f]} \qquad (11-37)$$

and equation (11–36) becomes

$$\frac{1}{r} = \frac{1}{vK}\frac{1}{[D_f]} + \frac{1}{v} \qquad (11-38)$$

Equation (11–38) produces what is called a *Klotz reciprocal plot*.[66]

An alternative manner of writing equation (11–37) is to rearrange it first to

$$r + rK[D_f] = vK[D_f] \qquad (11-39)$$

and subsequently to

$$\frac{r}{[D_f]} = vK - rK \qquad (11-40)$$

Data presented according to equation (11–40) are known as a *Scatchard plot*.[66,67] The binding of bis-hydroxycoumarin to human serum albumin is shown as a Scatchard plot in Figure 11–17.

Graphical treatment of data using equation (11–38) heavily weights those experimental points obtained at low concentrations of free drug D and may therefore lead to misinterpretations regarding the protein binding behavior at high concentrations of free drug. Equation (11–40) does not have this disadvantage and is the method of choice for plotting data. Curvature in these plots usually indicates the existence of more than one type of binding site.

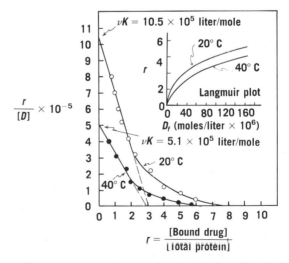

Fig. 11–17. A Scatchard plot showing the binding of bis-hydroxy-coumarin to human serum albumin at 20° and 40° C plotted according to equation (11–40). Extrapolation of the two lines to the horizontal axis, assuming a single class of sites with no electrostatic interaction, gives an approximate value of 3 for v. (From M. J. Cho, A. G. Mitchell and M. Pernarowski, J. Pharm. Sci. **60,** 196, 1971; **60,** 720, 1971, reproduced with permission of the copyright owner.) The insert is a Langmuir adsorption isotherm of the binding data plotted according to equation (11–35).

Equations (11–38) and (11–40) cannot be used for the analysis of data if the nature and the amount of protein in the experimental system is unknown. In these situations, Sandberg et al.[68] recommend the use of a slightly modified form of equation (11–40):

$$\frac{[D_b]}{[D_f]} = -K[D_b] + \nu K[P_t] \qquad (11-41)$$

in which $[D_b]$ is the concentration of bound drug. Equation (11–41) is plotted as the ratio $[D_b]/[D_f]$ versus $[D_b]$, and in this way K is determined from the slope while $\nu K[P_t]$ is determined from the intercept.

The Scatchard plot yields a straight line when only one class of binding sites is present. Frequently in drug binding studies, n classes of sites exist, each class i having ν_i sites with a unique association constant K_i. In such a case, the plot of $r/[D_f]$ vs. r is not linear but exhibits a curvature that suggests the presence of more than one class of binding sites. The data in Figure 11–17 were analyzed in terms of one class of sites for simplification. The plots at 20° and 40° C clearly show that multiple sites are involved. Blanchard et al.[69] reviewed the case of multiple classes of sites. Equation (11–37) is then written

$$r = \frac{\nu_1 K_1 [D_f]}{1 + K_1 [D_f]}$$

$$+ \frac{\nu_2 K_2 [D_f]}{1 + K_2 [D_f]} + \cdots \frac{\nu_n K_n [D_f]}{1 + K_n [D_f]} \qquad (11-42a)$$

or

$$r = \sum_{i=1}^{n} \frac{\nu_i K_i [D_f]}{1 + K_i [D_f]} \qquad (11-42b)$$

As previously noted, only ν and K need be evaluated when the site are all of one class. When n classes of sites exist, equation (11–42) may be written as

$$r = \sum_{i=1}^{n-1} \frac{\nu_i K_i [D_f]}{1 + K_i [D_f]} + \nu_n K_n [D_f] \qquad (11-43)$$

The binding constant K_n in the term on the right is small, indicating extremely weak affinity of the drug for the sites, but this class may have a large number of sites so as to be considered unsaturable.

Equilibrium Dialysis and Ultrafiltration. A number of methods are used to determine the amount of drug bound to a protein. Equilibrium dialysis, ultrafiltration, and electrophoresis are the classic techniques used, and in recent years other methods, such as gel filtration and nuclear magnetic resonance, have been used with satisfactory results. We shall discuss the equilibrium dialysis, ultrafiltration, and kinetic methods.

The equilibrium dialysis procedure was refined by Klotz et al.[70] for studying the complexation between metal ions or small molecules and macromolecules that cannot pass through a semipermeable membrane.

According to the equilibrium dialysis method, the serum albumin (or other protein under investigation) is placed in a Visking cellulose tubing (Visking Corporation, Chicago) or similar dialyzing membrane. The tubes are tied securely and suspended in vessels containing the drug in various concentrations. Ionic strength and sometimes hydrogen ion concentration are adjusted to definite values, and controls and blanks are run to account for the adsorption of the drug and the protein on the membrane.

If binding occurs, the drug concentration in the sac containing the protein is greater at equilibrium than the concentration of drug in the vessel outside the sac. Samples are removed and analyzed to obtain the concentrations of free and complexed drug.

Equilibrium dialysis is the classic technique for protein binding and remains the most popular method. Some potential errors associated with this technique are the possible binding of drug to the membrane, transfer of substantial amounts of drug from the plasma to the buffer side of the membrane, and osmotic volume shifts of fluid to the plasma side. Tozer et al.[71] developed mathematical equations to calculate and correct for the magnitude of fluid shifts. Briggs et al.[72] proposed a modified equilibrium dialysis technique to minimize experimental errors for the determination of low levels of ligand or small molecules.

Ultrafiltration methods are perhaps more convenient for the routine determination because they are less time-consuming. The ultrafiltration method is similar to equilibrium dialysis in that macromolecules such as serum albumin are separated from small drug molecules. Hydraulic pressure or centrifugation is used in ultrafiltration to force the solvent and the small molecules, unbound drug, through the membrane while preventing the passage of the drug bound to the protein. This ultrafiltrate is then analyzed by spectrophotometry or other suitable technique.

The concentration of the drug D_f that is free and unbound is obtained by use of the Beer's law equation (equation 4–9) and *Example 4–4*.

$$A = \epsilon bc \qquad (11-44)$$

in which A is the spectrophotometric absorbance (dimensionless), ϵ is the molar absorptivity, determined independently for each drug (see Table 4–4, p. 82), c (D_f in binding studies) is the concentration of the free drug in the ultrafiltrate in moles per liter, and b is the optical path length of the spectrophotometer cell, ordinarily 1 cm. The following example outlines the steps involved in calculating the Scatchard r value and the percent drug bound.

Example 11–5. The binding of sulfamethoxypyridazine to human serum albumin was studied at 25° C, pH 7.4, using the ultrafiltration technique. The concentration of the drug under study $[D_t]$ is 3.24×10^{-5} mole/liter and the human serum albumin concentration $[P_t]$ is 1.0×10^{-4} mole/liter. After equilibration the ultrafiltrate has an absorbance (A) of 0.559 at 540 nm in a 1-cm cell (b). The molar absorptivity (ϵ) of the drug is 5.6×10^4 liter mole^{-1} cm^{-1}. Calculate the Scatchard r value and the percent drug bound.

The concentration of free (unbound drug), $[D_f]$ is

$$[D_f] = \frac{A}{b\epsilon} = \frac{0.559}{(5.6 \times 10^4)1} = 0.99 \times 10^{-5} \text{ mole/liter}$$

The concentration of bound drug $[D_b]$ is

$$[D_b] = [D_t] - [D_f] = (3.24 \times 10^{-5}) - (0.99 \times 10^{-5}) = 2.25 \times 10^{-5} \text{ mole/liter}$$

The r value is

$$r = \frac{[D_b]}{[P_t]} = \frac{2.25 \times 10^{-5}}{1.0 \times 10^{-4}} = 0.225$$

The percent of bound drug is $[D_b]/[D_t] \times 100 = 69\%$

A potential error in ultrafiltration techniques may result from the drug binding to the membrane. The choice between ultrafiltration and equilibrium dialysis methods depends on the characteristics of the drug. The two techniques have been compared in several protein binding studies.[73-75]

Dynamic Dialysis. Meyer and Guttman[76] developed a kinetic method for determining the concentrations of bound drug in a protein solution. The method has found favor in recent years because it is relatively rapid, economical in terms of the amount of protein required, and readily applied to the study of competitive inhibition of protein binding. It is discussed here in some detail. The method, known as *dynamic dialysis*, is based on the rate of disappearance of drug from a dialysis cell that is proportional to the concentration of unbound drug. The apparatus consists of a 400-mL jacketed (temperature-controlled) beaker into which 200 mL of buffer solution are placed. A cellophane dialysis bag containing 7 mL of drug or drug–protein solution is suspended in the buffer solution. Both solutions are stirred continuously. Samples of solution external to the dialysis sac are removed periodically and analyzed spectrophotometrically, and an equivalent amount of buffer solution is returned to the external solution. The dialysis process follows the rate law:

$$\frac{-d[D_t]}{dt} = k[D_f] \qquad (11\text{--}45)$$

in which $[D_t]$ is the total drug concentration, $[D_f]$ the concentration of free or unbound drug in the dialysis sac, $-d[D_t]/dt$ the rate of loss of drug from the sac, and k the first-order rate constant (see Chapter 12) representative of the diffusion process. The factor k may also be referred to as the apparent permeability rate constant for the escape of drug from the sac. The concentration of unbound drug, $[D_f]$, in the sac (protein compartment) at a total drug concentration, $[D_t]$, is calculated using equation (11–45), knowing k and the rate $-d[D_t]/dt$ at a particular drug concentration, $[D_t]$. The rate constant k is obtained from the slope of a semilogarithmic plot of $[D_t]$ versus time when the experiment is conducted in the absence of the protein.

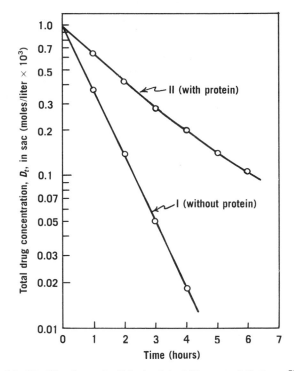

Fig. 11–18. The dynamic dialysis plot of Meyer and Guttman[76] for determining the concentration of bound drug in a protein solution.

Figure 11–18 illustrates the type of kinetic plot that can be obtained with this system. Note that in the presence of protein, Curve II, the rate of loss of drug from the dialysis sac, is slowed compared with the rate in the absence of protein, Curve I. In order to solve equation (11–45) for free drug concentration $[D_f]$, it is necessary to determine the slope of Curve II at various points in time. This is not done graphically but, rather, it is accurately accomplished by first fitting the time-course data to a suitable empiric equation, such as that given as equation (11–46), using a computer.

$$[D_t] = C_1 e^{-C_2 t} + C_3 e^{-C_4 t} + C_5 e^{-C_6 t} \qquad (11\text{--}46)$$

The computer fitting provides estimates of C_1 through C_6. The values for $d[D_t]/dt$ may then be computed from equation (11–47), which represents the first derivative of equation (11–46):

$$-\frac{d[D_t]}{dt} = C_1 C_2 e^{-C_2 t} + C_3 C_4 e^{-C_4 t} + C_5 C_6 e^{-C_6 t} \qquad (11\text{--}47)$$

Finally, once we have a series of $[D_f]$ values, computed from equations (11–47) and (11–45), corresponding to experimentally determined values of $[D_t]$ at each time t, we can proceed to calculate the various terms for the Scatchard plot.

Example 11–6.* Assume that the kinetic data illustrated in Figure 11–18 were obtained under the following conditions: Initial drug

---

Example 11–6 was prepared by Professor M. Meyer of the University of Tennessee.

concentration $[D_{t_0}] = 1 \times 10^{-3}$ mole/liter; protein concentration $= 1 \times 10^{-3}$ mole/liter. Assume also that the first-order rate constant (k) for the control (Curve I) was determined to be 1.0 hr^{-1} and that fitting of Curve II to equation (11–46) resulted in the following empiric constants: $C_1 = 5 \times 10^{-4}$ mole/liter, $C_2 = 0.6$ hr^{-1}, $C_3 = 3 \times 10^{-4}$ mole/liter, $C_4 = 0.4$ hr^{-1}, $C_5 = 2 \times 10^{-4}$ mole/liter, and $C_6 = 0.2$ hr^{-1}.

Calculate the Scatchard values (the Scatchard plot was discussed in the previous section) for r and $r/[D_f]$ if, during the dialysis in the presence of protein, the experimentally determined value for $[D_t]$ was 4.2×10^{-4} mole/liter at 2 hours. $r = [D_b]/P_t$, in which $[D_b]$ is drug bound and P_t is total protein concentration.

Using equation (11–47),

$$-\frac{d[D_t]}{dt} = k[D_f] = (5 \times 10^{-4})(0.6)e^{-0.6(2)}$$

$+ (3 \times 10^{-4})(0.4)e^{-0.4(2)} + (2 \times 10^{-4})(0.2)e^{-0.2(2)}$, where the (2) in the exponent stands for 2 hr.

Thus,

$$[D_f]_{2 \text{ hr}} = \frac{1.7 \times 10^{-4} \text{ mole/liter hr}^{-1}}{1.0 \text{ hr}^{-1}} = 1.7 \times 10^{-4} \text{ mole/liter}$$

It follows that at 2 hours,

$$[D_b] = [D_t] - [D_f] = 4.2 \times 10^{-4} \text{ mole/liter}$$
$$-1.7 \times 10^{-4} \text{ mole/liter} = 2.5 \times 10^{-4} \text{ mole/liter}$$

$$r = [D_b]/[P_t] = (2.5 \times 10^{-4})/(1 \times 10^{-3}) = 0.25$$

$$(r)/[D_f] = (0.25)/(1.7 \times 10^{-4}) = 1.47 \times 10^{3} \text{ liter/mole}$$

Additional points for the Scatchard plot would be obtained in a similar fashion, using the data obtained at various points throughout the dialysis. Accordingly, this series of calculations permits one to prepare a Scatchard plot (see Fig. 11–17).

Judis[77] investigated the binding of phenol and phenol derivatives by whole human serum using the dynamic dialysis technique and presented the results in the form of Scatchard plots.

Hydrophobic Interaction. Hydrophobic "bonding," first proposed by Kauzmann,[78] is actually not bond forma-tion at all, but rather the tendency of hydrophobic molecules or hydrophobic parts of molecules to avoid water because they are not readily accommodated in the hydrogen-bonding structure of water. Large hydrophobic species such as proteins avoid the water molecules in an aqueous solution insofar as possible by associating into micelle-like structures (Chapter 14) with the nonpolar portions in contact in the inner regions of the "micelles," the polar ends facing the water molecules. This attraction of hydrophobic species, resulting from their unwelcome reception in water, is known as hydrophobic bonding, or better, *hydrophobic interaction*. It involves van der Waals forces, hydrogen bonding of water molecules in a three-dimensional structure, and other interactions. Hydrophobic interaction is favored thermodynamically because of an increased disorder or entropy of the water molecules that accompanies the association of the nonpolar molecules, which squeeze out the water. Globular proteins are thought to maintain their ball-like structure in water because of the hydrophobic effect. Hydrophobic interaction is depicted in Figure 11–19.

Nagwekar and Kostenbauder[79] studied hydrophobic effects in drug binding using as a model of the protein a copolymer of vinylpyridine and vinylpyrrolidone. Kristiansen et al.[80] studied the effects of organic solvents in decreasing complex formation between small organic molecules in aqueous solution. They attributed the interactions of the organic species to a significant contribution by both hydrophobic bonding and the unique effects of the water structure. They suggested

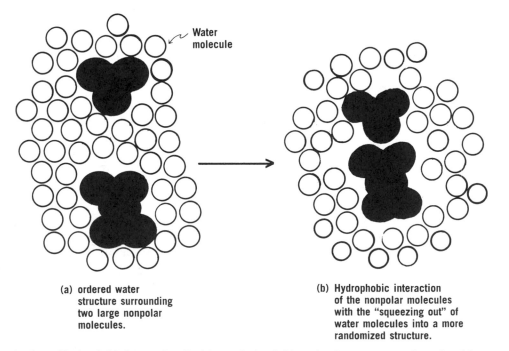

(a) ordered water
structure surrounding
two large nonpolar
molecules.

(b) Hydrophobic interaction
of the nonpolar molecules
with the "squeezing out" of
water molecules into a more
randomized structure.

Fig. 11–19. Schematic view of hydrophobic interaction. In (a), two hydrophobic molecules are separately enclosed in cages, surrounded in an orderly fashion by hydrogen-bonded molecules of water, $\bigcirc$. The state at (b) is somewhat favored by breaking of the water cages of (a) to yield a less ordered arrangement and an overall entropy increase of the system. Van der Waals attraction of the two hydrophobic species also contributes to the hydrophobic interaction.

that some nonclassic "donor–acceptor" mechanism may be operating to lend stability to the complexes formed.

Feldman and Gibaldi[81] studied the effects of urea, methylurea, and 1,3-dimethylurea on the solubility of benzoic and salicylic acids in aqueous solution. They concluded that the enhancement of solubility by urea and its derivatives was a result of hydrophobic bonding rather than complexation. Urea broke up the hydrogen-bonded water clusters surrounding the nonpolar solute molecules, increasing the entropy of the system and producing a driving force for solubilization of benzoic and salicylic acids. It may be possible that the ureas formed channel complexes with these aromatic acids as shown in Figure 11–3a, b, and c.

The interaction of drugs with proteins in the body may involve hydrophobic bonding at least in part, and this force in turn may affect the metabolism, excretion, and biologic activity of a drug.

Self-Association. Some drug molecules may self-associate to form dimers, trimers, or aggregates of larger sizes. A high degree of association may lead to formation of micelles, depending on the nature of the molecule (see Chapter 15). Doxorubicin forms dimers, the process being influenced by buffer composition and ionic strength. The formation of tetramers is favored by hydrophobic stacking aggregation.[82] Self-association may affect solubility, diffusion, transport through membranes, and therapeutic action. Insulin shows concentration-dependent self-association, which leads to complications in the treatment of diabetes. Aggregation is of particular importance in long-term insulin devices, where insulin crystals have been observed. The initial step of insulin self-association is a hydrophobic interaction of the monomers to form dimers, which further associate into larger aggregates. The process is favored at higher concentrations of insulin.[83] Addition of urea at nontoxic concentrations (1.0–3 mg/mL) has been shown to inhibit the self-association of insulin. Urea breaks up the "icebergs" in liquid water and associates with structured water by hydrogen bonding, taking an active part in the formation of a more open "lattice" structure.[84]

Sodium salicylate improves the rectal absorption of a number of drugs, all of them exhibiting self-association. Touitou and Fisher[85] chose methylene blue as a model for studying the effect of sodium salicylate on molecules that self-associate by a process of stacking. Methylene blue is a planar aromatic dye that forms dimers, trimers, and higher aggregates in aqueous solution. The workers found that sodium salicylate prevents the self-association of methylene blue. The inhibition of aggregation of porcine insulin by sodium salicylate results in a 7875-fold increase in solubility.[86] Commercial heparin samples tend to aggregate in storage depending on factors such as temperature and time in storage.[87]

Factors Affecting Complexation and Protein Binding. Kenley et al.[54] investigated the role of hydrophobicity in the formation of water-soluble complexes. The logarithm of the ligand partition coefficient between octanol and water was chosen as a measure of hydrophobicity of the ligand. The authors found a significant correlation between the stability constant of the complexes and the hydrophobicity of the ligands. Electrostatic forces were not considered as an important factor since all compounds studied were uncharged under the conditions investigated. Donor–acceptor properties expressed in terms of orbital energies (from quantum chemical calculations) and relative donor–acceptor strengths correlated poorly with the formation constants of the complex. It was suggested that ligand hydrophobicity is the main contribution to the formation of water-soluble complexes. Coulson and Smith[88] found that the more hydrophobic chlorobiocin analogs showed the highest percent of drug bound to human serum albumin. These workers suggested that chlorobiocin analogs bind to human albumin at the same site as warfarin. This site consists of two non-coplanar hydrophobic areas and a cationic group. Warfarin, an anticoagulant, serves as a model drug in protein binding studies because it is extensively but weakly bound. Thus, many drugs are able to compete with and displace warfarin from its binding sites. The displacement may result in a sudden increase of the free (unbound) fraction in plasma, leading to toxicity, since only the free fraction of a drug is pharmacologically active. Diana et al.[89] investigated the displacement of warfarin by nonsteroidal antiinflammatory drugs. Table 11–8 shows the variation of the stability constant K and the number of binding sites n of the complex albumin–warfarin after addition of competing drugs. Azapropazone decreases markedly the K value, suggesting that both drugs, warfarin and azapropazone, compete for the same binding site on albumin. Phenylbutazone also competes strongly for the binding site on albumin. Conversely, tolmetin may increase K, as suggested by the authors, by a conformational change in the albumin molecule which favors warfarin binding. The other drugs (see Table 11–8) decrease the K value of warfarin to a lesser extent, indicating that they do not share exclusively the same binding site as that of warfarin.

TABLE 11–8. *Binding Parameters (± S.D.) for Warfarin in the Presence of Displacing Drugs**

| Competing Drug | Racemic Warfarin | |
	n	$K \times 10^{-5} M^{-1}$
None	1.1 ± 0.0	6.1 ± 0.2
Azapropazone	1.4 ± 0.1	0.19 ± 0.02
Phenylbutazone	1.3 ± 0.2	0.33 ± 0.06
Naproxen	0.7 ± 0.0	2.4 ± 0.2
Ibuprofen	1.2 ± 0.2	3.1 ± 0.4
Mefenamic acid	0.9 ± 0.0	3.4 ± 0.2
Tolmetin	0.8 ± 0.0	12.6 ± 0.6

*F. J. Diana, K. Veronich and A. L. Kapoor, J. Pharm. Sci. **78**, 195, 1989.

Plaizier-Vercammen[90] studied the effect of polar organic solvents on the binding of salicylic acid to povidone. He found that in water–ethanol and water–propylene glycol mixtures, the stability constant of the complex decreased as the dielectric constant of the medium was lowered. Such a dependence was attributed to hydrophobic interaction and may be explained as follows. Lowering the dielectric constant decreases polarity of the aqueous medium. Since most drugs are less polar than water, their *affinity to the medium increases* when the dielectric constant decreases. As a result, the binding to the macromolecule is reduced.

Protein binding has been related to the solubility parameter δ of drugs (solubility parameter is defined on p. 224). Bustamante and Selles[91] found that the percent of drug bound to albumin in a series of sulfonamides showed a maximum at $\delta = 12.33$ cal$^{1/2}$ cm$^{-3/2}$. This value closely corresponds to the δ-value of the postulated binding site on albumin for sulfonamides and suggests that the closer the solubility parameter of a drug to the δ-value of its binding site, the greater the binding.

THERMODYNAMIC TREATMENT OF STABILITY CONSTANTS

The standard free energy change of complexation is related to the overall stability constant K (or any of the formation constants) by the relationship (pp. 70, 161).

$$\Delta G^\circ = -2.303 RT \log K \qquad (11\text{--}48)$$

The standard enthalpy change ΔH° may be obtained from the slope of a plot of $\log K$ versus $1/T$, following the expression

$$\log K = -\frac{\Delta H^\circ}{2.303\,R}\frac{1}{T} + \text{constant} \qquad (11\text{--}49)$$

When the values of K at two temperatures are known, the following equation may be used:

$$\log(K_2/K_1) = \frac{\Delta H^\circ}{2.303 R}\left(\frac{T_2 - T_1}{T_1 T_2}\right) \qquad (11\text{--}50)$$

The standard entropy change ΔS° is obtained from the expression

$$\Delta G^\circ = \Delta H^\circ - T\Delta S^\circ \qquad (11\text{--}51)$$

Andrews and Keefer[92] demonstrated that ΔH° and ΔS° generally become more negative as the stability constant for molecular complexation increases. As the binding between donor and acceptor becomes stronger, ΔH° would be expected to have a larger negative value. Apparently, the specificity of interacting sites or structural restraint also becomes greater, leading to a larger negative ΔS° value. Although the negative ΔS° value disfavors complexation, the negative ΔH° is large enough to overcome the unfavorable entropy contribution, leading to a negative ΔG°. See Table 11–11, row 4.

The results of Borazan et al.[58] in the charge-transfer complexation of nucleic acid bases with catechol are given in Table 11–7. These results run counter to the generalization just given. It is observed that the uracil–catechol complex exhibited both larger negative ΔH° and ΔS° than the adenine–catechol interaction, yet complexation constants for the uracil–catechol complex were much smaller than for the adenine interaction with catechol.

Nagwekar and Kostenbauder[79] used alkyl vinylpyridine–vinylpyrrolidone copolymers to test the strength of binding to a model drug, *p*-toluene sulfonic acid sodium (PTSAS), and to calculate thermodynamic parameters. The binding constants, K(liter/mole) and the thermodynamic values for interaction of PTSAS with various alkyl copolymers at 15° to 37° C are found in Table 11–9. In ascending the homologous series of alkyl copolymers, the binding constants increased in a sawtooth or zigzag manner, the K for a copolymer of an odd-numbered alkyl carbon chain being higher than for the next member of even carbon number. The K values and the thermodynamic functions (negative ΔG° and positive ΔH° and ΔS°), however, increased with increasing alkyl chain length for a series of odd or even alkyl copolymers. The binding process is endothermic (positive ΔH°), but the large increase in entropy on complexation resulted in a free energy that was negative.

The binding in these molecular complexes may be considered as a kind of hydrophobic interaction, the *p*-toluene sulfonic acid anion interacting with the positively charged vinylpyridine units to form a hydrophobic compound that squeezes out the water molecules that originally surrounded both the copolymer and PTSAS in an orderly iceberg-like structure (Fig. 11–20). When binding occurs between the copolymer molecules and PTSAS, the iceberg structure of water is partly destroyed and becomes less ordered. Presumably, this is the reason for the increase in entropy on complexation (positive ΔS°) as observed in Table 11–9.

Example 11–7. Basolo[93] obtained the following results for the complexation between ethylenediamine and the cupric ion: $\log K = 21.3$ at 0° C and $\log K = 20.1$ at 25° C. Compute ΔG°, ΔH°, and ΔS° at 25° C.

$$\Delta G^\circ = -2.303 RT \log K = -2.303 \times 1.987 \times 298 \times 20.1 =$$

$$-27.4 \text{ kcal/mole} \quad \log K_2 - \log K_1 = \frac{\Delta H^\circ}{2.303\,R}\left(\frac{298 - 273}{298 \times 273}\right)$$

$$\Delta H^\circ = \frac{(20.1 - 21.3)2.303 \times 1.987 \times 298 \times 273}{25} = -17.9 \text{ kcal/mole}$$

$$\Delta S^\circ = \frac{\Delta H^\circ - \Delta G^\circ}{T} = \frac{-17.9 + 27.4}{298} = +32 \text{ cal/(deg mole)}$$

The positive entropy change in *Example* 11–7 is characteristic of chelation. It occurs because the water molecules that are normally arranged in an orderly fashion around the ligand* and metal ion have acquired a more random configuration as a result of chelation, as in hydrophobic binding. This is referred to as a gain of

TABLE 11–9. *Binding Constants and Thermodynamic Functions for the Interaction of PTSAS with Various Alkyl Copolymers Over a Temperature Range of 15° to 37° C**

Temperature (°C)	K (liter/mole)	$\Delta G°$ (cal/mole)	$\Delta H°$ (cal/mole)	$\Delta S°$ (cal/(mole deg))
Ethyl Copolymer–PTSAS				
15	46.00	−2193		
30	46.66	−2316	458	9.21
37	50.00	−2414		
Propyl Copolymer–PTSAS				
15	61.00	−2354		
30	85.70	−2683	4068	22.32
37	102.14	−2853		
Butyl Copolymer–PTSAS				
15	52.84	−2272		
30	55.00	−2430	1373	12.64
37	63.28	−2558		
Pentyl Copolymer–PTSAS				
15	62.80	−2372		
30	111.00	−2837	5611	27.77
37	127.20	−2987		
Hexyl Copolymer–PTSAS				
15	63.36	−2377		
30	94.80	−2743	4728	24.41
37	108.08	−2888		

From J. B. Nagwekar and H. B. Kostenbauder, J. Pharm. Sci. **59, 751, 1970, reproduced by permission of the copyright owner.*

configurational entropy. The effect is shown clearly by Calvin and Melchior,[94] who complexed the salicylaldehyde-5-sulfonate ion (A) with the cupric ion. The ions are normally hydrated with a certain number of water molecules in aqueous solution, and these molecules are "squeezed out" when the complex is formed. Thus, the ordered arrangement of the solvent around the ions is lost and the entropy of the system increases. The process is represented as

$$Cu^{2+} \cdot (H_2O)_x + 2A \cdot (H_2O)_y = CuA_2 + z(H_2O);$$
$$\Delta S \cong + 100 \text{ cal/deg}$$

in which x and y are the number of water molecules bound and z is the number free in solution.

The decrease in ionic charge that usually accompanies complexation of polydentate ligands* (chelation) also decreases the possibility of hydration and leads to an additional increase in entropy. The entropy change involved in complexation of monodentate ligands and in electron donor–acceptor interactions (molecular complexation), on the other hand, usually is attended by a negative $\Delta S°$. This effect is due to an increased ordering of the species by complexation. These complexes are not ordinarily as stable as the chelates, and their formation is not attended by the same loss of solvent around the ions. Anthralin, an antipsoriatic drug, rapidly decomposes in aqueous solution near neutral pH to give principally dantron (Fig. 11–21). The thermodynamic parameters of the binding of dantron to bovine serum albumin at 25° C are $\Delta G° = -8.03$ kcal/mole, $\Delta H° = -11.8$ kcal/mole, and $\Delta S° = -12.6$ u.e.[95] The negative $\Delta S°$ value indicates that electrostatic forces are not important. (Electrostatic forces lead to positive entropies, which favor the binding process.) The large negative $\Delta H°$ as well as the negative $\Delta S°$ suggest

**The term *ligand* is from "ligate"—to bind—and is a general term meaning the agent that binds. The ligand referred to here is the large molecule attached to the central metal. Conversely, in molecular complexes the ligand is the drug (the small molecule) and the protein, polypeptide, and so on, constitutes the large molecule.*

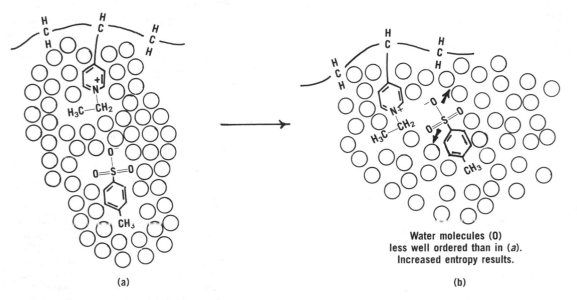

Water molecules (O) less well ordered than in (a). Increased entropy results.

(a) (b)

Fig. 11–20. Interaction of a *p*-toluene sulfonic acid anion with a positively charged vinylpyridine unit of a copolymer chain, with a squeezing out of water molecules. The ice-like cages of water molecules around the two ionic species (*a*) are disrupted on complexation of the anion and cation and in (*b*) the entropy of the system is increased, which favors the process. The open circles, O, represent partly hydrogen-bonded water molecules (see Fig. 11–19).

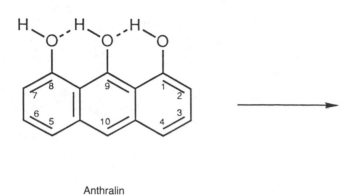

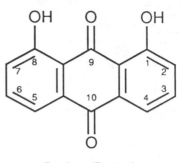

Anthralin

Danthron (Dantron)

Fig. 11–21. Decomposition of anthralin to yield dantron.

hydrogen bonding between dantron and its binding site in albumin. The carbonyl group in the 10-position of dantron (see Fig. 11–21) is able to hydrogen-bond to the tryptophan residue in bovine serum albumin, which

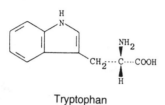

Tryptophan

could serve as a proton donor. The negative entropy does not favor complexation but, owing to hydrogen bonding, the large negative enthalpy is the driving force that leads to a negative free energy change (see Table 11–11, row 4).

Plaizier-Vercammen and De Nève[96] studied the interaction forces for the binding of several ligands to povidone and interpreted the thermodynamics of the binding. The influence of dissociation of the ligand on $\Delta G°$, $\Delta H°$, and $\Delta S°$ and on the equilibrium constant K is shown in Table 11–10. $\Delta H°$ becomes more negative and $\Delta S°$ decreases as the degree of dissociation increases. If the binding were exclusively due to hydrogen bonding, both $\Delta H°$ and $\Delta S°$ would be negative (see Table 11–11). However, $\Delta S°$ is positive, which can be due to either electrostatic or hydrophobic interactions (see Table 11–11). The fact that the dielectric constant of the medium has a positive influence on the binding (see

TABLE 11–10. *Binding Constants, K, and Thermodynamic Functions for the Interaction of Salicylamide (pK$_a$ = 8.2) with Povidone at 25° C**

pH	Degree of Dissociation	$K(M^{-1})$	$\Delta G°$ (kcal/mole)	$\Delta H°$ (kcal/mole)	$\Delta S°$ (kcal/mole)
5.0	0.00063	9.3	−5.4	−0.5	16.5
7.2	0.091	8.6	−5.4	−2.1	10.9
9.2	0.909	2.1	−4.5	−3.2	4.6

*From J. A. Plaizier-Vercammen and R. E. De Nève, J. Pharm. Sci. **71**, 552, 1982. The degree of dissociation is calculated using equation (13–77), page 342.

TABLE 11–11. *Positive and Negative Thermodynamic Functions Resulting from Several Kinds of Interactions*

Type of Interaction	Sign on		−$\Delta G°$ is Favored By
	$\Delta H°$	$\Delta S°$	
1. Electrostatic	~0	+	+$\Delta S°$
2. Hydrophobic	+	+	large +$\Delta S°$
3. Chelation (polydentate ligand)	−	+	+$\Delta S°$ and/or −$\Delta H°$
4. Donor–acceptor (hydrogen bonding and chelation [monodentate ligand])	−	−	−$\Delta H°$
5. Unfolding of proteins	+	+	+$\Delta S°$

problem 11–14) and that povidone has no ionizable groups suggest that hydrophobic rather than electrostatic interactions influence the binding. The positive $\Delta S°$ value is due to the disordering of the iceberg structure of water surrounding both the polymer and the drug. The negative $\Delta H°$ values can be due to van der Waals or hydrogen bonding interactions that together with the hydrophobic interaction lead to complex formation.

The value of $\Delta H°$ may be obtained from equation (11–49) by plotting log K versus $1/T$. The slope is $-\Delta H°/(2.303R)$ and is ordinarily calculated in analytic geometry by use of the two-point formula: slope = $\dfrac{Y_2 - Y_1}{X_2 - X_1}$. It is more correct, however, to linearly regress log K versus $1/T$ using the method of least squares. A number of inexpensive hand calculators available today do the linear least-squares method automatically, providing the slope and intercept of the line and statistical quantities such as the linear correlation coefficient, r.

Example 11–8. The association constants K at the temperatures, 6°, 18°, 25°, and 37° C for the interaction between uracil and catechol are found in Table 11–7. Calculate $\Delta H°$, $\Delta G°$, and $\Delta S°$ for this complexation reaction over the temperature range 6° to 37° C.

When the four log K values and the corresponding $1/T$ (in which T is in Kelvin degrees) are run on a hand calculator using equation (11–49) and a linear regression program, the slope obtained is −776.65, and $\Delta H°$ = −776.65 × 1.987 × 2.303 = −3554 cal/mole.

$\Delta H°$ is a constant over the temperature range 6° to 37° C for this complexation reaction. $\Delta G°$, on the other hand, (in which $\Delta G°$ =

$-2.303RT \log K$) has a different value for each temperature. Now $\Delta S° = - (\Delta G° - \Delta H°)/T$; therefore, $\Delta S°$ also might be expected to have different values at each temperature. Using these equations, $\Delta G°$ and $\Delta S°$ are calculated, and the results are

Thermodynamic Function	Temperature (°C)			
	6	18	25	37
$\Delta G°$ cal/mole	396	560	675	830
$\Delta S°$ cal/(mole deg)	−14	−14	−14	−14

From the values obtained, we learn that although $\Delta G°$ varies considerably for the four temperatures, $\Delta S°$, like $\Delta H°$, is reasonably constant. In fact, the constant in equation (11–49),

$$log K = -\frac{\Delta H°}{2.303R}\frac{1}{T} + \text{constant}$$

may actually be written as $\Delta S°/2.303R$. In other words,

$$\log K = -\frac{\Delta H°}{2.303R}\frac{1}{T} + \frac{\Delta S°}{2.303R} \qquad (11–52)$$

By comparing this equation with (11–48) and (11–51), we can verify that the constant of equation (11–49) is in fact $\Delta S°/2.303R$. Therefore, $\Delta S°$ remains essentially constant at about -14 cal/mole deg over this temperature range. From equation (11–52), it should be possible to calculate $\Delta S°$ from the intercept on the vertical axis on a plot of $\log K$ versus $(1/T)$. This is a long extrapolation from ambient temperatures to the vertical axis where $1/T = 0$ or $T = \infty$ and can be done only by least-squares analysis and a computer or hand calculator. A line estimated by eye and drawn with a ruler through the experimental points would create a large error in the extrapolated intercept. The least-square value obtained from equation (11–52) gives $\Delta S° = -14.4$ cal/mole deg, which agrees with the average value of -14 obtained in *Example 11–8*.

Table 11–11 summarizes, in a qualitative way, the values of $\Delta H°$ and $\Delta S°$ that would be expected depending on the kind of interaction occurring in the complex. Column 4 shows the main contribution, either $\Delta H°$ and/or $\Delta S°$, that is needed to get a negative (favorable) $\Delta G°$ value. For example, for donor–acceptor and hydrogen bonding interactions, a large negative $\Delta H°$ value overcomes the unfavorable (negative) entropy change, leading to a favorable negative $\Delta G°$ value. On the other hand, the positive entropy change is the main factor in the unfolding of proteins that yields a negative $\Delta G°$ in spite of the positive (unfavorable) $\Delta H°$ value.

References and Notes

1. L. Pauling, *The Nature of the Chemical Bond*, Cornell University Press, Ithaca, N.Y., 1940, p. 81.
2. G. Canti, A. Scozzafava, G. Ciciani and G. Renzi, J. Pharm. Sci. **69**, 1220, 1980.
3. P. Mohanakrishnan, C. F. Chignell and R. H. Cox, J. Pharm. Sci. **74**, 61, 1985.
4. J. E. Whitaker and A. M. Hoyt, Jr., J. Pharm. Sci. **73**, 1184, 1984.
5. A. E. Martell and M. Calvin, *Chemistry of the Metal Chelate Compounds*, Prentice Hall, N.Y., 1952.
6. L. B. Clapp, Organic molecular complexes, Chapter 17 in J. R. Bailar, Jr., Ed., *The Chemistry of the Coordination Compounds*, Reinhold, N.Y., 1956.
7. F. J. Bullock, Charge transfer in biology, Chapter 3 in *Comprehensive Biochemistry*, M. Florkin and E. H. Stotz, Eds., Vol. 22 of *Bioenergetics*, Elsevier, N.Y., 1967, pp. 82–85.
8. J. Buxeraud, A. C. Absil and C. Raby, J. Pharm. Sci. **73**, 1687, 1984.
9. T. Higuchi and J. L. Lach, J. Am. Pharm. Assoc., Sci. Ed. **43**, 349, 525, 527, 1954; T. Higuchi and D. A. Zuck, ibid. **42**, 132, 1953.
10. T. Higuchi and L. Lachman, J. Am. Pharm. Assoc., Sci. Ed. **44**, 521, 1955; L. Lachman, L. J. Ravin and T. Higuchi, ibid. **45**, 290, 1956; L. Lachman and T. Higuchi, ibid. **46**, 32, 1957.
11. T. Higuchi and I. H. Pitman, J. Pharm. Sci. **62**, 55, 1973.
12. P. York and A. Saleh, J. Pharm. Sci. **65**, 493, 1976.
13. A. Marcus, Drug Cosmet. Ind. **79**, 456, 1956.
14. J. A. Plaizier-Vercammen and R. E. De Nève, J. Pharm. Sci. **70**, 1252, 1981; J. A. Plaizier-Vercammen, ibid. **76**, 817, 1987.
15. K. H. Frömming, W. Ditter and D. Horn, J. Pharm. Sci. **70**, 738, 1981.
16. D. S. Hayward, R. A. Kenley and D. R. Jenke, Int. J. Pharm. **59**, 245, 1990.
17. T. Hosono, S. Tsuchiya and H. Matsumaru, J. Pharm. Sci. **69**, 824, 1980.
18. B. J. Forman and L. T. Grady, J. Pharm. Sci. **58**, 1262, 1969.
19. H. van Olphen, *Introduction to Clay Calloid Chemistry*, 2nd Edition, Wiley, N.Y., 1977, pp. 66–68.
20. *Merck Index*, 11th edition, Merck, Rahway, N.J., 1989, p. 365.
21. J. A. A. Ketelaar, *Chemical Constitution*, Elsevier, N.Y., 1958, p. 365.
22. H. M. Powell and D. E. Palin, J. Chem. Soc. **208**, 1947; ibid. **61**, 571, 815, 1948; ibid. 298, 300, 468, 1950; ibid. 2658, 1954.
23. S. G. Frank, J. Pharm. Sci. **64**, 1585, 1975.
24. K. Cabrera and G. Schwinn, American Laboratory, June, 1990, p. 22.
25. D. Duchêne and D. Wouessidjewe, Pharm. Tech. June, 1990, p. 26.
26. O. Beckers, J. H. Beijnen, E. H. G. Bramel, M. Otagiri, A. Bult and W. J. M. Underberg, Int. J. Pharm. **52**, 239, 1989.
27. T. Bakensfield, B. W. Müller, M. Wiese and J. Seydel, Pharm. Res. **7**, 484, 1990.
28. J. L. Lach and J. Cohen, J. Pharm. Sci. **52**, 137, 1963; W. A. Pauli and J. Lach, ibid. **54**, 1945, 1965; J. Lach and W. A. Pauli, ibid. **55**, 32, 1966.
29. D. Amdidouche, H. Darrouzet, D. Duchêne and M.-C. Poelman, Int. J. Pharm. **54**, 175, 1989.
30. M. A. Hassan, M. S. Suleiman and N. M. Najib, Int. J. Pharm. **58**, 19, 1990.
31. F. Kedzierewicz, M. Hoffman and P. Maincent, Int. J. Pharm. **58**, 22, 1990.
32. M. E. Brewster, K. S. Estes and N. Bodor, Int. J. Pharm. **59**, 231, 1990; M. E. Brewster, et al., J. Pharm. Sci. **77**, 981, 1988.
33. A. R. Green and J. K. Guillory, J. Pharm. Sci. **78**, 427, 1989.
34. B. W. Müller and U. Brauns, J. Pharm. Sci. **75**, 571, 1986.
35. J. Pitha, E. J. Anaissie and K. Uekama, J. Pharm. Sci. **76**, 788, 1987.
36. Y. Horiuchi, F. Hiriyama and K. Uekama, J. Pharm. Sci. **79**, 128, 1990.
37. F. Hirayama, N. Hirashima, K. Abe, K. Uekama, T. Ijitsu, and M. Ueno, J. Pharm. Sci. **77**, 233, 1988.
38. F. M. Andersen, H. Bungaard and H. B. Mengel, Int. J. Pharm. **21**, 51, 1984.
39. K. A. Connors, Complexometric titrations, Chapter 4 in *A Textbook of Pharmaceutical Analysis*, Wiley, N.Y., 1982; K. A. Connors, *Binding Constants*, Wiley, N.Y., 1987.
40. P. Job, Ann. Chim. **9**, 113, 1928.
41. A. E. Martell and M. Calvin, *Chemistry of the Metal Chelate Compounds*, Prentice-Hall, N.Y., 1952, p. 98.
42. M. E. Bent and C. L. French, J. Am. Chem. Soc. **63**, 568, 1941; R. E. Moore and R. C. Anderson, ibid. **67**, 168, 1945.
43. W. C. Vosburgh, et al., J. Am. Chem. Soc. **63**, 437, 1941; ibid. **64**, 1630, 1942.
44. A. Osman and R. Abu-Eittah, J. Pharm. Sci. **69**, 1164, 1980.

45. J. Bjerrum, *Metal Amine Formation in Aqueous Solution*, P. Haase and Son, Copenhagen, 1941.
46. M. Pecar, N. Kujundzic and J. Pazman, J. Pharm. Sci. **66**, 330, 1977; M. Pecar, et al., ibid. **64**, 970, 1975.
47. B. J. Sandmann and H. T. Luk, J. Pharm. Sci. **75**, 73, 1986.
48. Y. K. Agrawal, R. Giridhar and S. K. Menon, J. Pharm. Sci. **76**, 903, 1987.
49. K. A. Connors, S-F. Lin and A. B. Wong, J. Pharm. Sci. **71**, 217, 1982.
50. T. Higuchi and A. A. Zuck, J. Am. Pharm. Assoc., Sci. Ed. **42**, 132, 1953.
51. D. Guttman and T. Higuchi, J. Am. Pharm. Assoc., Sci. Ed. **46**, 4, 1957.
52. T. Higuchi and J. L. Lach, J. Am. Pharm. Assoc., Sci. Ed. **43**, 525, 1954.
53. T. Higuchi and K. A. Connors, Phase solubility techniques, in *Advances in Analytical Chemistry and Instrumentation*, C. N. Reilley, Ed., Vol. 4, Wiley, N.Y., 1965.
54. R. A. Kenley, S. E. Jackson, J. S. Winterle, Y. Shunko and G. C. Visor, J. Pharm. Sci. **75**, 648, 1986.
55. *Molecular Complexes*, Vol. 1, R. Foster, Ed., Elek, London, 1973.
56. M. A. Slifkin, *Charge Transfer Interactions of Biomolecules*, Academic Press, N.Y., 1971, Chapters 1,2.
57. H. A. Benesi and J. H. Hildebrand, J. Am. Chem. Soc. **70**, 2832, 1948.
58. F. A. Al-Obeidi and H. N. Borazan, J. Pharm. Sci. **65**, 892, 1976; ibid. **65**, 982, 1976; H. M. Taka, F. A. Al-Obeidi and H. N. Borazan, J. Pharm. Sci. **68**, 631, 1979; N. I. Al-Ani and H. N. Borazan, J. Pharm. Sci. **67**, 1381, 1978; H. N. Borazan and Y. H. Ajeena, J. Pharm. Sci. **69**, 990, 1980; ibid. **77**, 544, 1988.
59. N. E. Webb and C. C. Thompson, J. Pharm. Sci. **67**, 165, 1978.
60. J. Nishijo, I. Yonetami, E. Iwamoto, S. Tokura and K. Tagahara, J. Pharm. Sci. **79**, 14, 1990.
61. H. N. Borazan and S. N. Koumriqian, J. Pharm. Sci. **72**, 1450, 1983.
62. J. De Taeye and Th. Zeegers-Huyskens, J. Pharm. Sci. **74**, 660, 1985.
63. A. El-Said, E. M. Khairy and A. Kasem, J. Pharm. Sci. **63**, 1453, 1974.
64. A Goldstein, Pharmacol. Revs. **1**, 102, 1949.
65. J. J. Vallner, J. Pharm. Sci. **66**, 447, 1977.
66. C. K. Svensson, M. N. Woodruff and D. Lalka, in *Applied Pharmacokinetics*, 2nd Edition, W. E. Evans, J. J. Schentag and W. J. Jusko, Eds. Applied Therapeutics Inc., Spokane, Wash. 1986, Chapter 7.
67. G. Scatchard, Ann. N. Y. Acad. Sci. **51**, 660, 1949.
68. A. A. Sandberg, H. Rosenthal, S. L. Schneider and W. R. Slaunwhite, in *Steroid Dynamics*, T. Nakao, G. Pincus and J. F. Tait, Eds., Academic Press, N. Y., 1966, p. 33.
69. J. Blanchard, W. T. Fink and J. P. Duffy, J. Pharm. Sci. **66**, 1470, 1977.
70. I. M. Klotz, F. M. Walker and R. B. Puvan, J. Am. Chem. Soc. **68**, 1486, 1946.
71. T. N. Tozer, J. G. Gambertoglio, D. E. Furst, D. S. Avery and N. H. G. Holford, J. Pharm. Sci. **72**, 1442, 1983.
72. C. J. Briggs, J. W. Hubbard, C. Savage and D. Smith, J. Pharm. Sci. **72**, 918, 1983.
73. A. Zini, J. Barre, G. Defer, J. P. Jeanniot, G. Houin and J. P. Tillement, J. Pharm. Sci. **74**, 530, 1984.
74. E. Okezaki, T. Teresaki, M. Nakamura, O. Nagata, H. Kato and A. Tsuji, J. Pharm. Sci. **78**, 504, 1989.
75. J. W. Melten, A. J. Wittebrood, H. J. J. Williams, G. H. Faber, J. Wemer and D. B. Faber, J. Pharm. Sci. **74**, 692, 1985.
76. M. C. Meyer and D. E. Guttman, J. Pharm. Sci. **57**, 1627, 1968.
77. J. Judis, J. Pharm. Sci. **71**, 1145, 1982.
78. W. Kauzmann, Adv. Prot. Chem. **14**, 1, 1959.
79. J. B. Nagwekar and H. B. Kostenbauder, J. Pharm. Sci. **59**, 751, 1970.
80. H. Kristiansen, M. Nakano, N. I. Nakano and T. Higuchi, J. Pharm. Sci. **59**, 1103, 1970.
81. S. Feldman and M. Gibaldi, J. Pharm. Sci. **56**, 370, 1967.
82. M. Menozzi, L. Valentini, E. Vannini and F. Arcamone, J. Pharm. Sci. **73**, 6, 1984.
83. S. Sato, C. D. Ebert and S. W. Kim, J. Pharm. Sci. **72**, 228, 1983.
84. A. M. Saleh, A. R. Ebian and M. A. Etman, J. Pharm. Sci. **75**, 644, 1986.
85. E. Touitou and P. Fisher, J. Pharm. Sci. **75**, 384, 1986.
86. E. Touitou, F. Alhaique, P. Fisher, A. Memoli, F. M. Riccieri and E. Santucci, J. Pharm. Sci. **76**, 791, 1987.
87. T. J. Racey, P. Rochon, D. V. C. Awang and G. A. Neville, J. Pharm. Sci. **76**, 314, 1987.
88. J. Coulson and V. J. Smith, J. Pharm. Sci. **69**, 799, 1980.
89. F. J. Diana, K. Veronich and A. Kapoor, J. Pharm. Sci. **78**, 195, 1989.
90. J. A. Plaizier-Vercammen, J. Pharm. Sci. **72**, 1042, 1983.
91. P. Bustamante and E. Selles, J. Pharm. Sci. **75**, 639, 1986.
92. L. J. Andrews and R. M. Keefer, *Molecular Complexes in Organic Chemistry*, Holden Day, San Francisco, 1964.
93. F. Basolo, J. Am. Chem. Soc., **74**, 5243, 1952.
94. M. Calvin and M. C. Melchior, J. Am. Chem. Soc. **70**, 3270, 1948.
95. D. E. Wurster and S. M. Upadrashta, Int. J. Pharm. **55**, 221, 1989.
96. J. A. Plaizier-Vercammen and R. E. De Nève, J. Pharm. Sci. **71**, 552, 1982.
97. A. Albert, Biochem. J. **47**, 531, 1950.
98. T. Higuchi and A. A. Zuck, J. Am. Pharm. Assoc., Sci. Ed. **41**, 10, 1952.
99. T. Higuchi and J. L. Lach, J. Am. Pharm. Assoc., Sci. Ed. **43**, 465, 1954.
100. T. Higuchi and J. L. Lach, J. Am. Pharm. Assoc., Sci. Ed., **42**, 138, 1953.
101. T. Higuchi and A. A. Zuck, J. Am. Pharm. Assoc., Sci. Ed. **42**, 138, 1953.
102. G. Smulevich, A. Feis, G. Mazzi and F. F. Vincieri, J. Pharm. Sci. **77**, 523, 1988.
103. M. Mehdizadeh and D. J. W. Grant, J. Pharm. Sci. **73**, 1195, 1984.
104. F. A. Al-Obeidi and H. N. Borazan, J. Pharm. Sci. **65**, 982, 1976.
105. H. N. Borazan and Y. H. Ajeena, J. Pharm. Sci. **77**, 544, 1988.
106. M. W. Hanna and A. L. Askbaugh, J. Phys. Chem. **68**, 811, 1964.
107. J. Nishijo, et al., Chem. Pharm. Bull. **36**, 2735, 1988.
108. J. A. Plaizier-Vercammen and R. E. De Nève, J. Pharm. Sci. **71**, 552, 1982.
109. R. A. O'Reilly, J. Clin. Invest. **48**, 193, 1969.
110. M. C. Meyer and D. E. Guttman, J. Pharm. Sci. **57**, 895, 1968.
111. K. K. H. Chan, K. H. Vyas and K. D. Brandt, J. Pharm. Sci. **76**, 105, 1987.
112. T. Higuchi and A. A. Zuck, J. Am. Pharm. Assoc. **42**, 132, 1953.
113. M. J. Cho, A. G. Mitchell and M. Pernarowski, J. Pharm. Sci. **60**, 196, 1971.

Problems

11–1. Albert[97] studied the chelation of cadmium ion by asparagine. Potentiometric titration of 0.01 M asparagine, $pK_a = 8.85$, and 0.005 M cadmium sulfate was conducted in 50-mL samples by adding successive quantities of 0.1 N KOH. Plot the data of $\bar{n}$ versus p[A] and compute log K_1, log K_2, and log β. The data table is on p. 279. ($\bar{n}$, p[A], and β are defined on pp. 262–263).
Answer: log K_1 = 3.9, log K_2 = 2.97, log β = 6.87

11–2. Calvin and Melchior[94] investigated the chelation between the 5-salicylaldehydesulfonate ion and the cupric ion and obtained the following results; log K = 9.79 at 40° C and log K = 9.27 at 25° C. Calculate $\Delta H°$, $\Delta G°$, and $\Delta S°$ for the chelation process at 40° C. Give possible reasons for the entropy change $\Delta S°$ obtained by these investigators.
Answer: $\Delta H°$ = 14.8 kcal/mole, $\Delta G°$ = −14 kcal/mole, $\Delta S°$ = +92 cal/mole deg

11–3. The following results were obtained by Higuchi and Zuck[98] for the complex formed between caffeine and benzoic acid. In the analytic procedure, benzoic acid was distributed between water and a hydrocarbon solvent, Skellysolve-C.

Molar concentration of *free* benzoic acid in aqueous solution of caffeine obtained by partition study   11.94 × 10^{-3} mole/liter

Data for *Problem 11–1*

mL of 0.1 N NaOH	pH	$\bar{n}$	p[A]
0	4.81	—	—
0.25	6.12	0.10	4.75
0.50	6.50	0.20	4.40
1.0	6.85	0.40	4.10
1.5	7.20	0.57	3.80
2.0	7.45	0.74	3.62
2.5	7.70	0.93	3.45
3.0	7.95	1.11	3.30
3.5	8.21	1.26	3.16
4.0	8.50	1.42	3.05
4.5	8.93	1.56	2.92

Experimentally determined molar concentration of *total* undissociated benzoic acid in the aqueous phase, corrected for partial dissociation (free + complexed benzoic acid)	20.4×10^{-3} mole/liter
Original concentration of caffeine added (free + complexed caffeine)	2.69×10^{-2} mole/liter

Assuming that the stoichiometric ratio of the two species in the complex is 1:1, compute the association constant, K.
Answer: $K = 38.5$

11–4. Using the solubility method, Higuchi and Lach[99] studied the complexation between a polyethylene glycol and phenobarbital. The findings obtained at 30° C are given as follows:

Polyethylene glycol content of the complex formed in the plateau region of the solubility diagram	30×10^{-3} mole/liter
Total phenobarbital added	21.5×10^{-3} mole/liter
Phenobarbital dissolved at point B in the solubility diagram, Fig. 11–12	6.5×10^{-3} mole/liter

Compute the stoichiometric ratio [PGE]/[phenobarbital].
Answer: 2:1 complex

11–5. According to Higuchi and Lach,[100] the following results are obtained for the interaction of caffeine and sulfathiazole at 30° C.

Total sulfathiazole concentration at saturation when no caffeine is present (cf. Point A in Fig. 11–12, p. 265)	2.27×10^{-3} mole/liter
Total sulfathiazole concentration at saturation when 3.944×10^{-2} mole/liter of caffeine is added to the system	3.27×10^{-3} mole/liter

Compute the stability constant, assuming a 1:1 complex.
Answer: 11.5.

11–6. Higuchi and Zuck[101] investigated the complex formation betwene caffeine and butyl paraben by the solubility method. The results at 15° C are

Solubility of butyl paraben when no caffeine is present	0.58×10^{-3} M
Concentration of added caffeine	6.25×10^{-2} M
Solubility of butyl paraben when above amount of caffeine is present	3.72×10^{-3} M

Assuming that the complex has a stoichiometric ratio of 1:1, compute the stability constant.
Answer: $K = 91$

11–7. The formation of an inclusion complex of 1,8 dihydroxyanthraquinone with γ-cyclodextrin in aqueous solution was studied using the solubility technique[102] (see p. 265). The concentrations of anthraquinone derivative found after addition of several increments of γ-cyclodextrin to 10 mL of buffer containing an excess of the anthraquinone (1×10^{-3} M) are

Data for *Problem 11–7*

Cyclodextrin added ($\times 10^{3}$ M)	Anthraquinone found ($\times 10^{6}$ M)
2.37	2.56
7.89	8.72
11.58	12.56
15.79	15.60
18.95	15.81
22.63	16.41
30.0	16.41
38.0	13.84

(a) Obtain the phase diagram by plotting the concentration of the anthraquinone found (vertical axis) against the concentration of γ-cyclodextrin added (see Fig. 11–12 for a similar diagram).

(b) Compute the solubility of 1,8 dihydroxyanthraquinone.

(c) Compute the apparent stability constant K of the complex from the slope of the initial linear portion of the plot obtained in part (a). (Use the first five points.) K is obtained from the expression,[53] $K = $ slope/[intercept $(1 - $ slope$)$].

Answers: **(a)** The phase diagram should look similar to Figure 11–12 on p. 265; **(b)** $S_0 = 1.7 \times 10^{-6}$ M (the solubility in water reported by the authors is about 1×10^{-6} M); **(c)** $K = 479$ M^{-1}

11–8. Griseofulvin contains two keto groups, four ether oxygen atoms, and an aromatic ring, all capable of accepting protons to form hydrogen bonds. Griseofulvin has no proton donating groups so it acts only as a proton acceptor, A. The molar solubility of griseofulvin in isooctane, $[A_o] = 0.9358 \times 10^{-5}$ mole/liter, increases rapidly with increasing molar concentrations of hexanoic acid, $[D_t]$, an acidic donor, owing to the formation of a donor–acceptor complex, AD_m:

$$A + m D \rightleftharpoons AD_m$$

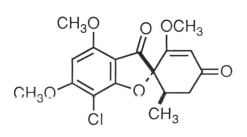

Griseofulvin

where m is the stoichiometric number of D molecules interacting with one A molecule. Mehdizadeh and Grant[103] determined the experimental solubilities of griseofulvin in isooctane with increasing concentrations of hexanoic acid, $[D_t]$; the data are shown in the following table:

Data for *Problem 11–8**

$[D_t]$, molar concentration of hexanoic acid (donor)	$[A_t]$ ($M \times 10^5$), concentration of griseofulvin (acceptor)
0.1632	2.317
0.465	4.178
0.784	7.762
1.560	20.902
3.118	77.581
4.693	207.16
6.316	435.18
7.855	858.98

*The concentrations given here are selected from among the 15 concentrations each of hexanoic acid and griseofulvin given in the original article.

The authors show that if only one complex species, AD_m, is considered, say $m = 2$, the increase in solubility $[A_t] - [A_o]$ of the acceptor (griseofulvin) in isooctane is proportional to the $m/2$ power of the total concentration of the donor (hexanoic acid), $[D_t]^{m/2}$, according to the following expression:

$$[A_t] - [A_o] = [AD_m] = K [D_t]^{m/2} \qquad (11\text{–}53)$$

where K includes K_m, the stability constant of the complex, K_d, the dimerization constant of hexanoic acid raised to the power $(-m/2)$, and an additional term, $2^{-m/2}$:

$$K = K_m K_d^{-m/2} 2^{-m/2} \qquad (11\text{–}54)$$

(a) Take the log of both sides of equation (11–53) and regress log $([A_t] - [A_o])$, the dependent variable, against log $[D_t]$, the independent variable. Compute the stoichiometric number m of the complex from the slope.

(b) Obtain the stability constant of the complex, K_m, using the intercept you got in part (a) and equation (11–54). The dimerization constant of hexanoic acid from a separate experiment is $K_d = 6000$ M^{-1}

Answers: **(a)** $m = 3.39$ (number of hexanoic acid molecules per griseofulvin molecule in the complex); **(b)** $K_m = 1248$ M^{-1}, the stability constant of the complex of the formula, AD_3. The number 3.39 is obtained by regression analysis and is therefore an average. It is assumed to be an integer value, $m = 3$, for the complex.

11–9. Al-Obeidi and Borazan[104] investigated the charge transfer complex formation between epinephrine and the nucleic acid bases adenine, thymine, and uracil by ultraviolet absorption spectrometry. Epinephrine is an electron donor, and the nucleic acid bases are assumed to act as electron acceptors.

Obtain the molar absorptivity ϵ and the equilibrium constant K (1/molarity) of the Benesi–Hildebrand equation (equation (11–28),

Data for *Problem 11–9*

$1/D_o$ (liter/mole)	1.0	2.0	3.0
A_o/A at 2° C	0.022	0.034	0.047
A_o/A at 18° C	0.029	0.047	0.066
A_o/A at 25° C	0.031	0.053	0.075
A_o/A at 37° C	0.037	0.065	0.093

p. 266) by plotting A_o/A versus $1/D_o$. A_o and D_o are the total concentrations of adenine and epinephrine, respectively. A is the absorbance of the complex at a definite wavelength. It is assumed that epinephrine forms 1:1 charge transfer complexes with these nucleic acid bases in acidified aqueous solution.

The accompanying table shows the values for A_o/A and $1/D_o$ for the adenine–epinephrine complex at four temperatures, as back-calculated from the K and ϵ values, Table 1, of the paper.[104]

Answer: See Table 1 in the paper, J. Pharm. Sci. **65**, 982, 1976.

11–10. Assuming 1:1 complexes and using the Benesi–Hildebrand equation, Al-Obeidi and Borazan[104] obtained the following stability constants, K (1/molarity) for thymine–epinephrine at three temperatures, at a wavelength of 314 nm:

Data for *Problem 11–10*

Temperature (°C)	2	18	37
K (M^{-1})	0.97	0.73	0.57

Calculate the standard free energy ($\Delta G°$), standard enthalpy ($\Delta H°$), and standard entropy ($\Delta S°$) changes for the complexation. Give an explanation for the magnitude and the arithmetic sign of these thermodynamic quantities.

Answer: Check your results against those in Table 1 of the paper in J. Pharm. Sci. **65**, 982, 1976. The discussion section of the paper will assist you in explaining the meaning of the $\Delta G°$, $\Delta H°$, and $\Delta S°$ values.

11–11. Al-Obeidi and Borazan[104] investigated the charge transfer complex formation between epinephrine and the nucleic acid bases adenine, thymine, and uracil by ultraviolet absorption spectrometry. Epinephrine is an electron donor, and the nucleic acid bases are assumed to act as electron acceptors.

Assuming 1:1 complexes and using the Benesi–Hildebrand equation, these workers obtained the following stability constants, K (M^{-1}), for adenine–epinephrine at four temperatures at a wavelength of 326 nm:

Data for *Problem 11–11*

T (°C)	2	18	25	37
K (M^{-1})	0.79	0.52	0.45	0.35

Calculate the standard free energy ($\Delta G°$), standard enthalpy ($\Delta H°$), and standard entropy ($\Delta S°$) changes for the complexation.

Answer: Compare your results with those in Table 1 of Al-Obeidi and Borazan, J. Pharm. Sci., **65**, 982, 1976.

11–12. The charge transfer complex between tryptamine and isoproterenol was studied in aqueous solution containing 0.1 M HCl at several temperatures.[105] The equilibrium constants K were obtained using the Benesi–Hildebrand equation

Data for *Problem 11–12*

T (°C)	5.0	15.0	25.0
K (M^{-1})	3.50	2.30	1.42

(a) Compute $\Delta G°$, $\Delta H°$, and $\Delta S°$. **(b)** Compute the absorbance of the complex A at 5° C from the Benesi–Hildebrand equation. The molar absorptivity ϵ of the complex is 66.0, the initial concentration of the acceptor (tryptamine) is 0.02 M, and the concentration of the donor (isoproterenol) is 0.5 M.

Answers: **(a)** $\Delta H° = -7.4$ kcal/mole, $\Delta S° = -24.2$ cal/(mole deg), $\Delta G°$ at 5° C $= -0.69$ kcal/mole; **(b)** the absorbance A of the charge-transfer band was calculated from the Benesi–Hildebrand equation and is 0.833 at 5° C

11–13. Hanna and Askbaugh[106] derived an expression to compute the apparent equilibrium constant of 1:1 π-molecular complexes from nuclear magnetic resonance data:

$$\frac{1}{\Delta^A_{obs}} = \frac{1}{K(\delta^A_c - \delta^A_m)} \frac{1}{C_D} + \frac{1}{\delta^A_c - \delta^A_m} \quad (11\text{--}55)$$

where C_D is the concentration of the donor on the molality scale, δ^A_c is the chemical shift (see Chapter 4, p. 92) of the acceptor in the pure complex form, and δ^A_m is the chemical shift of the acceptor in the uncomplexed form. Therefore, $\delta^A_c - \delta^A_m$ is the shift due to complexation. Δ^A_{obs} is the difference between the observed chemical shift and δ^A_m.

The equation requires that the concentration of the donor be much larger than that of the acceptor, and is analogous to the Benesi–Hildebrand equation (p. 266) except that the shift of acceptor protons on the pure complex replaces the molar absorptivity of the complex, and the concentration of acceptor does not appear.

Nishijo et al.[107] studied the complexation of theophylline with an aromatic aminoacid, L-tryptophan, in aqueous solution using proton nuclear magnetic resonance. L-Tryptophan is a constituent of serum albumin and was suggested to be the binding site on serum albumin for certain drugs. The authors added L-tryptophan to a fixed concentration of theophylline at 25° C.

Data for *Problem 11–13*

(Tryp), $1/C_D$ (M^{-1})	25	50	75	100
$1/\Delta^A_{obs}$	5.9	9.8	13.7	17.6

Compute the apparent equilibrium constant K and the complexation shift, $(\delta^A_c - \delta^A_m)$ using equation (11–55).

Answer: $K = 12.8$, $(\delta^A_c - \delta^A_m) = 0.50$

11–14. The binding or association constant K for the complex povidone-5-hydroxysalicylic acid was determined by equilibrium dialysis at 25° C and 35° C in solvent mixtures of ethanol and water. Using the *Klotz reciprocal plot* (equation (11–38), p. 269),

$$\frac{1}{r} = \frac{1}{\nu K'} \frac{1}{[D_f]} + \frac{1}{\nu}$$

Plaizier-Vercammen and De Nève[108] obtained $\nu K'$ as the slope of the line, plotting $1/r$ against $1/[D_f]$. K' is the binding constant in liters/mole and ν is the binding capacity, i.e, the number of binding sites per mole of the macromolecule, povidone. $[D_f]$ is the molar concentration of free ligand or drug and r is the moles of ligand bound per mole of povidone. The ν and K' are combined in this work to give $\nu K' = K$ as an association constant that measures the strength of binding of 5-hydroxysalicylic acid to povidone. The K values at various percent concentrations of ethanol in water and corresponding dielectric constants, D, at 25° C and 35° C, are given in the following table:

Data for *Problem 11–14*

% Ethanol in water	Dielectric Constant, D		$K \times 10^{-3}$ liter/mole	
	25° C	35° C	25° C	35° C
2.5	75.2	72.1	20.5	18.0
5.0	73.9	70.9	19.4	17.1
10.0	71.5	68.6	18.0	16.0
20.0	66.6	63.8	15.9	14.1

(a) Compute $\Delta H°$ and $\Delta S°$ over this temperature range, and $\Delta G°$ at both 25° C and 35° C for each mixture.

(b) On the same graph, plot $\Delta G°$ and $\Delta H°$ obtained in (a) as a function of dielectric constant. Two lines will be obtained for $\Delta G°$ versus dielectric constant, D; one for 25° C and a second for 35° C. The values of $\Delta H°$ at various D values are the same at 25° C and 35° C and yield a single line on this plot, as will become evident from the results of the calculations made.

(c) Give a plausible explanation in terms of intermolecular interaction for the binding of 5-hydroxysalicylic acid to povidone, using the magnitude and the signs of the thermodynamic quantities. Compare your answers with the information given on pp. 272–273 and 275–277, Table 11–11, and in J. Pharm. Sci. **71,** 552, 1982.

Partial Answer: **(a)** The thermodynamic values at 2.5% ethanol are:

Partial Answer for *Problem 11–14*

% Ethanol in water	$\Delta H°$ kcal/mole	$\Delta S°$ cal/(mole deg)	$\Delta G°$ kcal/mole	
			25° C	35° C
2.5	−2.38	+11.8	−5.88	−6.00

11–15. The binding of warfarin to human serum albumin was studied at pH 6, ionic strength 0.170. The following values were found by O'Reilly.[109] For a definition of symbols, see page 269 of this book.

Data for *Problem 11–15*

[PD] μmole/L	[D_f] μmole/L	$r/[D_f]$ L/μmole	r
9.1	3.0	0.13	0.40
17.8	6.4	0.11	0.72
30.2	17.2	0.08	1.35
46.1	50.8	0.04	2.00

(a) Obtain the Scatchard plot, equation (11–40), using this data and compute K and ν using linear regression; it is the number of independent binding sites. Express K in L/mole, were L stands for liters.

(b) Assume that the concentration of protein is unknown, and compute K from [PD] and [D_f] equation (11–41). Compare the constant K obtained in (a) and (b). Compute [P_t] (total concentration of protein) using the number of binding sites obtained in (a). See equation (11–41) on page 270.

Answers: **(a)** $K = 0.0552$ L/μmole = 55,200 L/mole; $\nu = 2.75$; **(b)** $K = 0.0602$ L/μmole = 60,200 L/mole; using $\nu = 2.75$ from (a), [P_t] = 22.2 μmole/L

11–16. In a study by Meyer and Guttman[110] of the binding of caffeine to bovine serum albumin by the equilibrium dialysis method, 2.8×10^{-4} M of albumin was allowed to equilibrate with 1×10^{-4} M of caffeine. After equilibrium was established, 0.7×10^{-4} M of caffeine was contained in the dialysis bag, while 0.3×10^{-4} M of caffeine was found in the external solution. Calculate r, the ratio of bound to total protein. What is the fraction bound, β, of caffeine?

Answer: $r = 0.14$; $\beta = 0.571$

11.17. Chan and his associates[111] investigated the in vitro protein binding of diclofenac sodium, a nonsteroidal antiinflammatory drug, by equilibrium dialysis and plotted the results according to the Scatchard equation (equation (11–42b)) used to describe two classes of sites:

$$r = \frac{\nu_1 K_1 [D_f]}{1 + K_2 [D_f]} + \frac{\nu_2 K_2 [D_f]}{1 + K_2 [D_f]}$$

These workers used a statistical method known as *nonlinear regression* on the data given below to calculate the parameters ν_1, ν_2, K_1, and K_2. The number of binding sites ν_1 and ν_2 found for the two classes of sites are 2.26 and 10.20, respectively. The corresponding association constants are $K_1 = 1.32 \times 10^5$ M^{-1} and $K_2 = 3.71 \times 10^3$ M^{-1}

Using the equation given above, calculate the values of r (dimensionless) for the following free drug concentrations: $[D_f]$ in millimole/liter ($\times 10^3$) = 1.43, 4.7, 16, 63, 132.4, 303.4, and 533.2.

Plot $r/[D_f]$ (liter/millimole) versus r to obtain what is called a *Scatchard plot*. Compare your results with those of Chan et al. To obtain an answer to this problem, the student may compare his or her calculated $r/[D_f]$ values with the $r/[D_f]$ abscissa values read from the graph of Chan et al.

Hint: Use the same units on K_1, K_2, and $[D_f]$ to calculate r.

Partial Answer: for $[D_f] = 1.43 \times 10^{-3}$ millimole/liter (1.43×10^{-6} mole/liter), $r = 0.41$; $r/[D_f] = 289$ (liter/millimole)

11-18. The number of binding sites and the association constant for the binding of sulfamethoxypyridazine to albumin at pH 8 can be obtained from the data given as follows:

Data for Problem 11-18

$r = [D_b/P_t]$	0.23	0.46	0.66	0.78
$[D_f] \times 10^4$ (mole/liter)	0.10	0.29	0.56	1.00

where $[D_b]$ is the concentration of drug bound, also referred to as $[PD]$, and $[P_t]$ is the total protein concentration. What values are obtained for the number of binding sites ν and for the association constant K?

Answer: $\nu = 1$; $K = 26{,}821$

11-19. The effect of phenylbutazone in displacing acetaminophen from its binding sites on human serum albumin (HSA) was studied by the ultrafiltration method (p. 270) at 37° C and pH 7.4, with a constant concentration of acetaminophen, $[D_t] = 3.97 \times 10^{-4}$ mole/liter, and with increasing concentrations of phenylbutazone $[D'_t]$. After ultrafiltration the absorbance A of the free fraction of acetaminophen, corresponding to several concentrations of phenylbutazone, is

Data for Problem 11-19

Case	I	II	III	IV
$D'_t \times 10^4$ mole/liter	0	0.65	3.89	6.48
A	0.683	0.782	0.809	0.814

The table also shows the absorbance of acetaminophen in the absence of phenylbutazone, $D'_t = 0$. The molar absorptivity, ϵ, of acetaminophen at 420-nm wavelength in a cell of path length $b = 1$ cm is 2.3×10^3 liter mole^{-1} cm^{-1}. The HSA concentration $[P_t]$ is 5.8×10^{-4} mole/liter.

Calculate the percent decrease in the Scatchard r values for acetaminophen and the percent bound at different concentrations of phenylbutazone, D'_t, shown in the table.

Partial Answer: In case I (see the table above), the concentration, $[D_f] = A/\epsilon b$, of unbound acetaminophen in the absence of phenylbutazone, $[D'_t] = 0$, is 2.97×10^{-4} mole/liter. The concentration $[D_b]$ of bound acetaminophen is 1.00×10^{-4} mole/liter. The r value, $[D_b]/[P_t] = 0.17$, and the percent bound ($[D_b]/[D_t]) \times 100 = 25\%$.

In case II (in the presence of phenylbutazone, $[D_t] = 0.65 \times 10^{-4}$ mole/liter), the concentration of unbound acetaminophen is $[D_f] = A/(\epsilon b) = 0.782/(2.03 \times 10^3)(1) = 3.4 \times 10^{-4}$ mole/liter. $[D_b]$ is (3.97×10^{-4}) − (3.4×10^{-4}) = 0.57×10^{-4} mole/liter and $r = (0.57 \times 10^{-4})/(5.8 \times 10^{-4}) = 0.10$.

11-20.* In a study of protein binding, using the dynamic dialysis method of Meyer and Guttman,[76] 2×10^{-3} mole/liter of drug was placed in a dialysis sac. In the absence of protein, the following values for $[D_t]$ were determined:

Data (a) for Problem 11-20

Time (hr)	2.0	4.0
$[D_t]$ mole/liter $\times 10^3$	0.74	0.27

Equation (11-45) may be written as

$$\ln [D_t] = \ln [D_f] - kt$$

Compute k, the slope, from the two-point formula using the data given in the table above.

When the dialysis study was repeated in the presence of 5×10^{-4} mole/liter of protein, the rate of loss of drug from the dialysis sac was again determined. The resulting data were fit by computer to equation (11-46) and the following empiric constants were obtained:

$$C_1 = 1 \times 10^{-3} \text{ mole/liter}, \quad C_2 = 0.2 \text{ hr}^{-1},$$
$$C_3 = 6 \times 10^{-4} \text{ mole/liter}, \quad C_4 = 0.1 \text{ hr}^{-1},$$
$$C_5 = 4 \times 10^{-4} \text{ mole/liter}, \quad C_6 = 0.05 \text{ hr}^{-1}$$

The experimentally determined values for $[D_t]$ in the presence of protein were as follows at 1, 3, and 5 hours:

Data (b) for Problem 11-20

Time (hr)	1	3	5
$[D_t]$ mole/liter $\times 10^3$	1.74	1.34	1.04

Calculate the three values of the Scatchard terms r and $r/[D_f]$, which can be determined from these data. Although many more points than three are required to prepare a satisfactory Scatchard plot, sketch these three points on a plot of $r/[D_f]$ versus r to obtain a rough idea of the curve that would result. See Figure 11-17, page 269, for the general shape of a Scatchard plot.

Answer: At 1 hr, $r = 2.53$, $r/[D_f] = 5.35 \times 10^3$ liter/mole; at 3 hr, $r = 1.99$, $r/[D_f] = 5.80 \times 10^3$ liter/mole; at 5 hr, $r = 1.58$, $r/[D_f] = 6.31 \times 10^3$ liter/mole

11-21. Higuchi and Zuck[112] investigated the complex formed between caffeine and benzoic acid and obtained the following results: $K = 29$ at 0° C and $K = 18$ at 30° C. Compute $\Delta H°$, $\Delta G°$, and $\Delta S°$ at 30° C. What significance can be attributed to each of these values? See Table 11-11.

Answer: $\Delta H° = -2.62$ kcal/mole, $\Delta G° = -1.74$ kcal/mole, $\Delta S° = -2.9$ cal/mole deg.

11-22. The data in Table 11-12 are similar to those obtained by Cho et al.[113] using equilibrium dialysis for the binding of bishydroxycoumarin to human serum albumin (HSA). The concentration of HSA was 0.20% (2.90×10^{-5} mole/liter). The pH was held at 7.4 by the use of a tris (hydroxymethyl) aminomethane–hydrochloric acid buffer, and ionic strength was maintained at 0.15. Using the data of Table 11-12 at 20° C and 40° C,

(a) plot $r = $ [Drug bound]/[Total HSA] against free drug concentration, $[D_f]$, to obtain what is known as a *Langmuir isotherm*. The HSA concentration is 2.9×10^{-5} mole/liter.

(b) Plot $r/[D_f]$ on the vertical axis of a graph and r on the horizontal axis to obtain a Scatchard plot as represented by equation (11-40). You will obtain a curve rather than a straight line.

Problem 11-20 was prepared by Professor M. Meyer of the University of Tennessee.

TABLE 11-12. *Bishydroxycoumarin Interaction with Human Serum Albumin* at 20° C and 40° C (Data for Problem 11-22)*

$[D_b]$	$[D_f]$		20° C		40° C	
			$\dfrac{r}{[D_f]} \times 10^{-5}$			$\dfrac{r}{[D_f]} \times 10^{-5}$
moles/liter $\times 10^6$	moles/liter $\times 10^6$	r †		r		
23.20	1.000	0.8	8.0	0.6	4.0	
29.00	1.430	1.0	7.0	1.1	3.1	
34.80	2.000	1.2	6.0	1.7	2.3	
40.60	2.690	1.4	5.2	1.9	1.5	
52.20	4.290	1.8	4.2	2.5	1.1	
63.80	6.880	2.2	3.2	3.1	0.7	
92.80	14.55	3.2	2.2	3.9	0.5	
116.0	33.33	4.0	1.2	4.9	0.3	
145.0	62.50	5.0	0.8	5.7	0.1	
174.0	150.00	6.0	0.4			

*Serum albumin concentration, 2.9×10^{-5} mole/liter.
†$r = D_b$/albumin concentration.

(c) Determine ν, the average number of the first type of binding sites at 20° C and 40° C, and round off the values of ν to obtain integer numbers. Use the roughly linear part of the Scatchard plot, i.e., the first five points given in Table 11-12. The intercept on the ordinate is νK, from which K may be obtained at the two temperatures.

(d) Using the first five values of Table 11-12, compute the association constant, K, for the first type of binding sites of bishydroxycoumarin on human serum albumin, at both 20° C and 40° C. You may use either the two-point formula or regression analysis.

(e) The authors obtained $K = 3.5 \times 10^5$ liter/mole and 1.7×10^5 for the binding constants at 20° C and 40° C, respectively. Using these values, estimate the standard free energy changes, $\Delta G°$, for the interactions at 20° C and 40° C from the expression, $\Delta G° = -RT \ln K$.

(f) Calculate the standard enthalpy change, $\Delta H°$, using the association constants at the two temperatures, and the equation

$$\ln \frac{K_{20°}}{K_{40°}} = -\frac{\Delta H°}{R} \left(\frac{1}{293.15} - \frac{1}{313.15} \right)$$

(g) Obtain the standard entropy change $\Delta S°$ for the complexation using $\Delta G° = \Delta H° - T \Delta S°$.

(h) Give a plausible explanation for the magnitude and sign of the thermodynamic quantities obtained.

Answers: Compare your results with those obtained by Cho et al.[113] Table I. For example, the authors obtain $\Delta G° = -7.43$ kcal/mole at 20°C. See Table 11-11, p. 276, to help you explain the results obtained.

12
Kinetics

Rates and Orders of Reactions
Influence of Temperature and Other Factors on
    Reaction Rates

Decomposition and Stabilization of Medicinal
    Agents
Kinetics in the Solid State
Accelerated Stability Analysis

In this chapter a study is made of the rates and mechanisms of reactions with particular emphasis on decomposition and stabilization of drug products. The experimental investigation of the possible breakdown of new drugs is not a simple matter. However, a small expenditure of time and energy in this direction can yield results that may save the pharmaceutical industry both money and reputation. Applications of kinetics in pharmacy result in the production of more stable drug preparations, the dosage and rationale of which may be established on sound scientific principles.

Although the manufacturer is primarily responsible for assuring the stability of marketed products, the community pharmacist also must have some understanding of stability characteristics to handle and store products under the proper conditions. He or she must also recognize that alterations may occur when a drug is combined with other ingredients. For example, if thiamine hydrochloride, which is most stable at a pH of 2 to 3 and is unstable above pH 6, is combined with a buffered vehicle of say pH 8 or 9, the vitamin is rapidly inactivated.[1] Knowing the rate at which a drug deteriorates at various hydrogen ion concentrations allows one to choose a vehicle that will retard or prevent the degradation.

Thus, as a result of current research involving the kinetics of drug systems, the pharmacist is able to assist the physician and patient regarding the proper storage and use of medicinal agents. This chapter brings out a number of factors that bear upon the formulation, stabilization, and administration of drugs. Concentration, temperature, light, and catalysts are important in relation to the speed and the mechanism of reactions and will be discussed in turn.

RATES AND ORDERS OF REACTIONS

The rate, velocity, or speed of a reaction is given by the expression, dc/dt, where dc is the increase or decrease of concentration over an infinitesimal time interval, dt. According to the law of mass action, the rate of a chemical reaction is proportional to the product of the molar concentration of the reactants each raised to a power usually equal to the number of molecules, a and b, of the substances A and B undergoing reaction. In the reaction

$$aA + bB + \ldots = \text{Products} \qquad (12\text{--}1)$$

the rate of the reaction is

$$\text{Rate} = -\frac{1}{a}\frac{d(A)}{dt}$$

$$= -\frac{1}{b}\frac{d(B)}{dt} = \ldots k(A)^a(B)^b \ldots \qquad (12\text{--}2)$$

in which k is the *rate constant*.

The overall *order* of a reaction is the sum of the exponents ($a + b$, for example, in equation (12–2) of the concentration terms, A and B. The order with respect to one of the reactants, A or B, is the exponent a or b of that particular concentration term. In the reaction of ethyl acetate with sodium hydroxide in aqueous solution, for example,

$$CH_3COOC_2H_5 + NaOH_{soln} \rightarrow CH_3COONa + C_2H_5OH$$

the rate expression is

$$\text{Rate} = -\frac{d[CH_3COOC_2H_5]}{dt}$$

$$= -\frac{d[NaOH]}{dt} = k[CH_3COOC_2H_5]^1[NaOH]^1$$

$$(12-3)$$

The reaction is first-order ($a = 1$) with respect to ethyl acetate and first-order ($b = 1$) with respect to sodium hydroxide solution; overall the reaction is second-order ($a + b = 2$).

Suppose that in this reaction, sodium hydroxide as well as water was in great excess and ethyl acetate was in a relatively low concentration. As the reaction proceeded, ethyl acetate would change appreciably from its original concentration, whereas the concentrations of NaOH and water would remain essentially unchanged since they are present in great excess. In this case the contribution of sodium hydroxide to the rate expression is considered constant and the reaction rate can be written as

$$-\frac{d(CH_3COOC_2H_5)}{dt} = k'(CH_3COOC_2H_5) \qquad (12-4)$$

in which $k' = k(NaOH)$. The reaction is then said to be *pseudo–first-order*, for it depends only on the first power ($a = 1$) of the concentration of ethyl acetate. In general, when one of the reactants is present in such great excess that its concentration may be considered constant or nearly so, the reaction is said to be of *pseudo-order*.

Example 12–1. In the reaction of acetic anhydride with ethyl alcohol to form ethyl acetate and water,

$$(CH_3CO)_2O + 2C_2H_5OH = 2CH_3CO_2C_2H_5 + H_2O$$

the rate of reaction is

$$\text{Rate} = -\frac{d([CH_3CO]_2O)}{dt}$$

$$= k([CH_3CO]_2O)(C_2H_5OH)^2 \qquad (12-5)$$

What is the order of the reaction with respect to acetic anhydride? With respect to ethyl alcohol? What is the overall order of the reaction?

If the alcohol, which serves here as the solvent for acetic anhydride, is in large excess such that a small amount of ethyl alcohol is used up in the reaction, write the rate equation for the process and state the order.

Answer: The reaction appears to be first-order with respect to acetic anhydride, second-order with respect to ethyl alcohol, and overall third-order. However, since alcohol is the solvent its concentration remains essentially constant and the rate expression may be written

$$-\frac{d([CH_3CO]_2O)}{dt} = k'([CH_3CO]_2O) \qquad (12-6)$$

Kinetically the reaction is therefore pseudo–first-order as noted by S. Glasstone, *Textbook of Physical Chemistry*, Van Nostrand, 1946, pp. 1051, 1052.

Molecularity.
A reaction whose overall order is measured may be considered to occur through several steps or elementary reactions. Each of the elementary reactions has a stoichiometry giving the number of molecules taking part in that step. Since the order of an elementary reaction gives the number of molecules coming together to react in the step, it is common to refer to this order as the *molecularity* of the elementary reaction. If, on the other hand, a reaction proceeds through several stages, the term molecularity is not used in reference to the observed rate law: one step may involve two molecules, a second step only one molecule, and a subsequent step one or two molecules. Hence order and molecularity are ordinarily identical only for elementary reactions. Bimolecular reactions may or may not be second-order.

In simple terms molecularity is the number of molecules, atoms, or ions reacting in an elementary process. In the reaction

$$Br_2 \rightarrow 2Br$$

the process is *unimolecular*, since the single molecule, Br_2, decomposes to form two bromine atoms. In the single-step reaction

$$H_2 + I_2 \rightarrow 2HI$$

the process is *bimolecular*, since two molecules, one of H_2 and one of I_2, must come together to form the product HI. *Termolecular* reactions—that is, processes in which three molecules must come together simultaneously—are rare.

Chemical reactions that proceed through more than one step are known as *complex reactions*. The overall order determined kinetically may not be identical with the molecularity, for the reaction consists of several steps, each with its own molecularity. For the overall reaction

$$2NO + O_2 \rightarrow 2NO_2$$

the order has been found experimentally to be 2. The reaction is not termolecular, in which two molecules of NO would collide simultaneously with one molecule of O_2. Instead, the mechanism is postulated to consist of two elementary steps, each being bimolecular:

$$2NO \rightarrow N_2O_2$$

$$N_2O_2 + O_2 \rightarrow 2NO_2$$

Specific Rate Constant. The constant k appearing in the rate law associated with a single-step (elementary) reaction is called the *specific rate constant* for that reaction. Any change in the conditions of the reaction, for example, temperature, solvent, or a slight change in one of the reacting species, will lead to a rate law having a different value for the specific rate constant. Experimentally, a change of specific rate constant corresponds simply to a change in the slope of the line given by the rate equation. Variations in the specific rate constant are of great physical significance, for a change in this constant necessarily represents a change at the molecular level as a result of a variation in the reaction conditions. This is further discussed on pages 295–301.

Rate constants derived from reactions consisting of a number of steps of different molecularity are functions of the specific rate constants for the various steps. Any change in the nature of a step due to a modification in the reaction conditions or in the properties of the molecules taking part in this step could lead to a change in the value of the overall rate constant. At times, variations in an overall rate constant can be used to provide useful information about a reaction, but quite commonly, anything that affects one specific rate constant will affect another; hence, it is quite difficult to attach significance to variations in the overall rate constant for these reactions.

Units of the Basic Rate Constants. To arrive at units for the rate constants appearing in zero-, first-, and second-order rate laws, the equation expressing the law is rearranged to have the constant expressed in terms of the variables of the equation. Thus, for a zero-order reaction,

$$k = -\frac{dA}{dt} = \frac{\text{moles/liter}}{\text{second}}$$

$$= \frac{\text{moles}}{\text{liter second}} = \text{moles liter}^{-1}\text{ second}^{-1}$$

for a first-order reaction,

$$k = -\frac{dA}{dt}\frac{1}{A} = \frac{\text{moles/liter}}{\text{second-moles/liter}}$$

$$= \frac{1}{\text{second}} = \text{second}^{-1}$$

and for a second-order reaction,

$$k = -\frac{dA}{dt}\frac{1}{A^2} = \frac{\text{moles/liter}}{\text{second (moles/liter)}^2}$$

$$= \frac{\text{liter}}{\text{mole-second}} = \text{liter second}^{-1}\text{ mole}^{-1}$$

where A is the molar concentration of the reactant. It is an easy matter to replace the units, moles/liter, by any other units (e.g., pressure in atmospheres), to obtain the proper units for the rate constants if quantities other than concentration are being measured.

Zero-Order Reactions. Garrett and Carper[2] found that the loss in color of a multisulfa product (as measured by the decrease of spectrophotometric absorbance at a wavelength of 500 nm) followed a zero-order rate. The rate expression for the change of absorbance A with time is therefore

$$-\frac{dA}{dt} = k_0 \qquad (12-7)$$

in which the minus sign signifies that the absorbance is decreasing (i.e., the color is fading). The velocity of

fading is seen to be constant and independent of the concentration of the colorant used. The rate equation may be integrated between the initial absorbance A_0 corresponding to the original color of the preparation at $t = 0$, and A_t, the absorbance after t hours:

$$\int_{A_0}^{A_t} dA = -k_0 \int_0^t dt$$

$$A_t - A_0 = -k_0 t$$

or

$$A_t = A_0 - k_0 t \qquad (12-8)$$

The initial concentration corresponding to A_0 is ordinarily written as a and the concentration remaining at time t as c.

When this linear equation is plotted with c on the vertical axis against t on the horizontal axis, the slope of the line is equal to $-k_0$. Garrett and Carper obtained a value for k of 0.00082 absorbance decrease per hour at 60° C, signifying that the color was fading at this constant rate independent of concentration.

The half-period, or *half-life* as it is usually called, is the time required for one half of the material to disappear; it is the time at which A has decreased to $\frac{1}{2}A$. In the present illustration, $A_0 = 0.470$ and $\frac{1}{2}A_0 = 0.235$.

$$t_{1/2} = \frac{\frac{1}{2}A_0}{k_0} = \frac{0.235}{8.2 \times 10^{-4}} = 2.9 \times 10^2 \text{ hr.}$$

Suspensions. Apparent Zero-Order Kinetics.[3] Suspensions are another case of zero-order kinetics, in which the concentration in solution depends on the drug's solubility. As the drug decomposes in solution, more drug is released from the suspended particles so that the concentration remains constant. This concentration is, of course, the drug's equilibrium solubility in a particular solvent at a particular temperature. The important point is that the amount of drug in solution remains constant despite its decomposition with time. The reservoir of solid drug in suspension is responsible for this constancy.

The equation for an ordinary solution, with no reservoir of drug to replace that depleted, is the first-order expression, equation (12–11) (see p. 287):

$$\frac{-d[A]}{dt} = k[A]$$

in which A is the concentration of drug remaining undecomposed at time t, and k is known as a first-order rate constant. When the concentration $[A]$ is rendered constant, as in the case of a suspension, we may write

$$k[A] = k_0 \qquad (12-9)$$

so that the first-order rate law (12–11) becomes

$$-\frac{d[A]}{dt} = k_0 \qquad (12-10)$$

Equation (12–10) obviously is a zero-order equation. It is referred to as an *apparent zero-order equation*, being zero-order only because of the suspended drug reservoir that ensures constant concentration. Once all the suspended particles have been converted into drug in solution, the system changes to a first-order reaction.

Example 12–2. A prescription for a liquid aspirin preparation is called for. It is to contain 325 mg/5 mL or 6.5 g/100 mL. The solubility of aspirin at 25° C is 0.33 g/100 mL; therefore, the preparation will definitely be a suspension. The other ingredients in the prescription cause the product to have a pH of 6.0. The first-order rate constant for aspirin degradation in this solution is 4.5×10^{-6} sec^{-1}. Calculate the zero-order rate constant. Determine the shelf life for the liquid prescription, assuming that the product is satisfactory until the time at which it has decomposed to 90% of its original concentration (i.e., 10% decomposition) at 25° C.

Answer: $k_0 = k \times$ [aspirin in solution], from equation (12–9)

$$k_0 = (4.5 \times 10^{-6}\ \text{sec}^{-1}) \times (0.33\ \text{g/100 mL})$$

$$k_0 = 1.5 \times 10^{-6}\ \text{g/100 mL sec}^{-1}$$

$$*t_{90} = \frac{0.10[A]_0}{k_0} = \frac{(0.10)(6.5\ \text{g/100 mL})}{(1.5 \times 10^{-6}\ \text{g/100 mL sec}^{-1})}$$

$$= 4.3 \times 10^5\ \text{sec} = 5.0\ \text{days}$$

First-Order Reactions. In 1918, Harned showed that the decomposition rate of hydrogen peroxide, catalyzed by 0.02 *M* KI, was proportional to the concentration of hydrogen peroxide remaining in the reaction mixture at any time. The data for the reaction

$$2H_2O_2 = 2H_2O + O_2$$

are given in Table 12–1. Although two molecules of hydrogen peroxide appear in the stoichiometric equation as just written, the reaction was found to be first-order. The rate equation is written

$$-\frac{dc}{dt} = kc \tag{12–11}$$

in which c is the concentration of hydrogen peroxide remaining undecomposed at time t, and k is the first-order velocity constant. Integrating equation (12–11) between concentration c_0 at time $t = 0$ and concentration c at some later time t, we have

$$\int_{c_0}^{c} \frac{dc}{c} = -k \int_{0}^{t} dt$$

$$\ln c - \ln c_0 = -k(t - 0)$$

$$\ln c = \ln c_0 - kt \tag{12–12}$$

Converting to common logarithms yields

$$\log c = \log c_0 - kt/2.303 \tag{12–13}$$

$$k = \frac{2.303}{t} \log \frac{c_0}{c} \tag{12–14}$$

TABLE 12–1. *Decomposition of Hydrogen Peroxide at 25° C in Aqueous Solution Containing 0.02 M KI.*

t (minutes)	$a - x$	k (min^{-1})
0	57.90	—
5	50.40	0.0278
10	43.90	0.0277
25	29.10	0.0275
45	16.70	0.0276
65	9.60	0.0276
∞	0	—

H. S. Harned, J. Am. Chem. Soc. 40, 1462, 1918.

In exponential form, equation (12–12) becomes

$$c = c_0 e^{-kt} \tag{12–15}$$

and equation (12–13) becomes

$$c = c_0 10^{-kt/2.303} \tag{12–16}$$

Equations (12–15) and (12–16) express the fact that, in a first-order reaction, the concentration decreases exponentially with time. As shown in Figure 12–1, the concentration begins at c_0 and decreases as the reaction becomes progressively slower. The concentration asymptotically approaches a final value c_∞ as time proceeds toward infinity.

Equation (12–14) is often written as

$$k = \frac{2.303}{t} \log \frac{a}{(a - x)} \tag{12–17}$$

in which the symbol a is customarily used to replace c_0, x is the decrease of concentration in time t, and $(a - x) = c$.

The specific reaction rates listed in Table 12–1 were calculated by using equation (12–17). Probably the best way to obtain an average k for the reaction is to plot the logarithm of the concentration against the time, as shown in Figure 12–2. The linear expression in equation (12–13) shows that the slope of the line is $-k/2.303$ from which the rate constant is obtained. If a straight line is obtained, it indicates that the reaction is

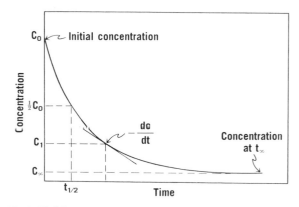

Fig. 12–1. Fall in concentration of a decomposing drug with time. In addition to C_0 and C_∞, $\frac{1}{2}C_0$ and the corresponding time, $t_{1/2}$, are shown. The rate of decrease of concentration with time $-dC/dt$ at an arbitrary concentration C_1 is also shown.

*The equation for t_{90} is obtained by substituting $0.9[A]_0$ for $[A]$ into the zero-order equation $[A] = [A]_0 - k_0 t$.

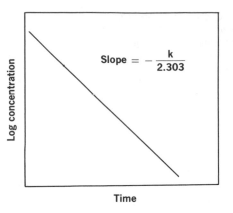

Fig. 12-2. A linear plot of log *C* versus time for a first-order reaction.

first-order. The tests for the order of a reaction are discussed in more detail on page 289.

Once the rate constant is known, the concentration of reactant remaining at a definite time may be computed as demonstrated in the following examples.

Example 12-3. The catalytic decomposition of hydrogen peroxide may be followed by measuring the volume of oxygen liberated in a gas burette. From such an experiment, it was found that the concentration of hydrogen peroxide remaining after 65 minutes, expressed as the volume in milliliters of gas evolved, was 9.60 from an initial concentration of 57.90.

(*a*) Calculate *k* using equation (12-14).

(*b*) How much hydrogen peroxide remained undecomposed after 25 minutes?

(*a*)

$$k = \frac{2.303}{65} \log \frac{57.90}{9.60} = 0.0277 \text{ min}^{-1}$$

(*b*)

$$0.0277 = \frac{2.303}{25} \log \frac{57.90}{c}; \quad c = 29.01$$

Example 12-4. A solution of a drug contained 500 units per milliliter when prepared. It was analyzed after a period of 40 days and was found to contain 300 units per milliliter. Assuming the decomposition is first-order, at what time will the drug have decomposed to one half its original concentration?

(*a*)

$$k = \frac{2.303}{40} \log \frac{500}{300} = 0.0128 \text{ day}^{-1}$$

(*b*)

$$t = \frac{2.303}{0.0128} \log \frac{500}{250} = 54.3 \text{ days}$$

Half-Life. The period of time required for a drug to decompose to one half the original concentration as calculated in *Example 12-3* is the half-life, $t_{1/2}$, for a first-order reaction:

$$t_{1/2} = \frac{2.303}{k} \log \frac{500}{250} = \frac{2.303}{k} \log 2$$

$$t_{1/2} = \frac{0.693}{k} \qquad (12-18)$$

In *Example 12-4*, the drug has decomposed 250 units/milliliter in the first 54.3 days. Since the half-life is a constant, independent of the concentration, it remains

at 54.3 days regardless of the amount of drug yet to be decomposed. In the second half-life of 54.3 days, half of the remaining 250 units or an additional 125 units/milliliter are lost; in the third half-life, 62.5 units/milliliter are decomposed, and so on.

The student should now appreciate the reason for stating the half-life rather than the time required for a substance to decompose completely. Except in a zero-order reaction, theoretically it takes an infinite period of time for a process to subside completely, as illustrated graphically in Figure 12-1. Hence, a statement of the time required for complete disintegration would have no meaning. Actually the rate ordinarily subsides in a finite period of time to a point at which the reaction may be considered to be complete, but this time is not accurately known, and the half-life, or some other fractional-life period, is quite satisfactory for expressing reaction rates.

The same drug may exhibit different orders of decomposition under various conditions. Although the deterioration of hydrogen peroxide catalyzed with iodine ions is first-order, it has been found that decomposition of concentrated solutions stabilized with various agents may become zero-order. In this case, in which the reaction is independent of drug concentration, decomposition is probably brought about by contact with the walls of the container or some other environmental factor.

Second-Order Reactions. The rates of bimolecular reactions, which occur when two molecules come together

$$A + B \rightarrow \text{products}$$

are frequently described by the second-order equation. When the speed of the reaction depends on the concentrations of *A* and *B* with each term raised to the first power, the rate of decomposition of *A* is equal to the rate of decomposition of *B*, and both are proportional to the product of the concentrations of the reactants:

$$-\frac{d[A]}{dt} = -\frac{d[B]}{dt} = k[A][B] \qquad (12-19)$$

If *a* and *b* are the initial concentrations of *A* and *B* and *x* is the concentration of each species reacting in time *t*, the rate law may be written

$$\frac{dx}{dt} = k(a - x)(b - x) \qquad (12-20)$$

in which *dx/dt* is the rate of reaction, and (*a − x*) and (*b − x*) are the concentrations of *A* and *B* remaining at time *t*. When, in the simplest case, both *A* and *B* are present in the same concentration so that *a = b*,

$$\frac{dx}{dt} = k(a - x)^2 \qquad (12-21)$$

Equation (12-21) is integrated, using the conditions that *x* = 0 at *t* = 0 and *x* = *x* at *t* = *t*.

$$\int_0^x \frac{dx}{(a-x)^2} = k \int_0^t dt$$

$$\left(\frac{1}{a-x}\right) - \left(\frac{1}{a-0}\right) = kt$$

$$\frac{x}{a(a-x)} = kt \qquad (12\text{-}22)$$

or

$$k = \frac{1}{at}\left(\frac{x}{a-x}\right) \qquad (12\text{-}23)$$

When, in the general case, A and B are not present in equal concentrations, integration of equation (12-20) yields

$$\frac{2.303}{a-b} \log \frac{b(a-x)}{a(b-x)} = kt \qquad (12\text{-}24)$$

or

$$k = \frac{2.303}{t(a-b)} \log \frac{b(a-x)}{a(b-x)} \qquad (12\text{-}25)$$

It can be seen by reference to equation (12-22) that when $x/a(a-x)$ is plotted against t, a straight line results if the reaction is second-order. The slope of the line is k. When the initial concentrations, a and b, are not equal, a plot of $\log b(a-x)/a(b-x)$ against t should yield a straight line with a slope of $(a-b)k/2.303$. The value of k can thus be obtained. It is readily seen from equation (12-23) or (12-25) that the units in which k must be expressed for a second-order reaction are $1/(\text{mole/liter}) \times 1/\text{sec}$ where the concentrations are given in mole/liter and the time in seconds. The rate constant k in a second-order reaction therefore has the dimensions, liter/(mole sec) or liter mole^{-1} sec^{-1}.

Example 12-5. Walker[4] investigated the saponification of ethyl acetate at 25° C:

$$CH_3COOC_2H_5 + NaOH \rightarrow CH_3COONa + C_2H_5OH$$

The initial concentrations of both ethyl acetate and sodium hydroxide in the mixture were 0.01000 M. The change in concentration x of alkali during 20 minutes was 0.000566 mole/liter; therefore $(a-x) = 0.01000 - 0.00566 = 0.00434$.

Compute (a) the rate constant and (b) the half-life of the reaction.
(a) Using equation (12-23)

$$k = \frac{1}{0.01 \times 20} \frac{(0.00566)}{(0.00434)} = 6.52 \text{ liter mole}^{-1} \text{ min}^{-1}$$

(b) The half-life of a second-order reaction is

$$t_{1/2} = \frac{1}{ak} \qquad (12\text{-}26)$$

It can be computed for the reaction only when the initial concentrations of the reactants are identical. In the present example,

$$t_{1/2} = \frac{1}{0.01 \times 6.52} = 15.3 \text{ min}$$

Determination of Order. The order of a reaction may be determined by several methods.

Substitution Method. The data accumulated in a kinetic study may be substituted in the integrated form of the equations that describe the various orders. When the equation is found in which the calculated k values remain constant within the limits of experimental variation, the reaction is considered to be of that order.

Graphic Method. A plot of the data in the form of a graph as shown in Figure 12-2 may also be used to ascertain the order. If a straight line results when concentration is plotted against t, the reaction is zero-order. The reaction is first-order if $\log(a-x)$ versus t yields a straight line; and it is second-order if $1/(a-x)$ versus t gives a straight line (in the case in which the initial concentrations are equal). When a plot of $1/(a-x)^2$ against t produces a straight line, with all reactants at the same initial concentration, the reaction is third-order.

Half-life Method. In a zero-order reaction, the half-life is proportional to the initial concentration, a, as observed in Table 12-2. The half-life of a first-order reaction is independent of a; $t_{1/2}$ for a second-order reaction, in which $a = b$, is proportional to $1/a$; and in a third-order reaction, in which $a = b = c$, it is proportional to $1/a^2$. The relationship between these results shows that, in general, the half-life of a reaction in which the concentrations of all reactants are identical is

$$t_{1/2} \propto \frac{1}{a^{n-1}} \qquad (12\text{-}27)$$

in which n is the order of the reaction. Thus if two reactions are run at different initial concentrations, a_1 and a_2, the half-lives $t_{1/2(1)}$ and $t_{1/2(2)}$ are related as follows:

$$\frac{t_{1/2(1)}}{t_{1/2(2)}} = \frac{(a_2)^{n-1}}{(a_1)^{n-1}} = \left(\frac{a_2}{a_1}\right)^{n-1} \qquad (12\text{-}28)$$

or in logarithmic form

$$\log \frac{t_{1/2(1)}}{t_{1/2(2)}} = (n-1) \log \frac{a_2}{a_1} \qquad (12\text{-}29)$$

and finally

$$n = \frac{\log(t_{1/2(1)}/t_{1/2(2)})}{\log(a_2/a_1)} + 1 \qquad (12\text{-}30)$$

The half-lives are obtained graphically by plotting a versus t at two different initial concentrations and reading the time at $\frac{1}{2}a_1$ and $\frac{1}{2}a_2$. The values for the half-lives and the initial concentrations are then substi-

TABLE 12-2. *Rate and Half-Life Equations*

Order	Integrated Rate Equation	Half-Life Equation
0	$x = kt$	$t_{1/2} = \dfrac{a}{2k}$
1	$\log \dfrac{a}{(a-x)} = \dfrac{k}{2.303} t$	$t_{1/2} = \dfrac{0.693}{k}$
2	$\dfrac{x}{a(a-x)} = kt$	$t_{1/2} = \dfrac{1}{ak}$
3	$\dfrac{2ax - x^2}{a^2(a-x)^2} = 2kt$	$t_{1/2} = \dfrac{3}{2}\dfrac{1}{a^2 k}$

tuted into equation (12–30), from which the order n is obtained directly. Rather than using different initial concentrations, two concentrations during a single run may also be taken as a_1 and a_2 and the half-lives $t_{1/2(1)}$ and $t_{1/2(2)}$ determined in terms of these. If the reaction is first-order, $t_{1/2(1)} = t_{1/2(2)}$ since the half-life is independent of concentration in a first-order reaction. Then $\log (t_{1/2(1)}/t_{1/2(2)}) = \log 1 = 0$, and one can see from equation (12–30) that

$$n = 0 + 1 = 1$$

Complex Reactions. Many reactions cannot be expressed by simple zero-, first-, and second-, or third-order equations. They involve more than one step or elementary reaction and accordingly are known as *complex reactions*. These processes include reversible, parallel, and consecutive reactions:

(1) Reversible reaction:

$$A + B \underset{k_{-1}}{\overset{k_1}{\rightleftharpoons}} C + D$$

(2) Parallel or side reactions:

$$A \overset{k_1}{\underset{k_2}{\swarrow}} \begin{array}{c} B \\ C \end{array}$$

(3) Series or consecutive reactions:

$$A \overset{k_1}{\longrightarrow} B \overset{k_2}{\longrightarrow} C$$

Reversible Reactions. The simplest reversible reaction is one in which both the forward and the reverse steps are first-order processes:

$$A \underset{k_r}{\overset{k_f}{\rightleftharpoons}} B$$

Although at first this equation appears to be that for an equilibrium between A and B, it must be pointed out that an equilibrium situation requires that the concentrations of A and B do not change with time. Since this expression is intended to explain a kinetic process, it must follow that the equation describes the approach to equilibrium. That is, the situation represented is one in which A decreases to form B and some of the product B reverts back to A. According to this description, the *net* rate at which A decreases will be given by the rate at which A decreases in the forward step less the rate at which A increases in the reverse step:

$$-\frac{dA}{dt} = k_f A - k_r B \qquad (12-31)$$

this rate law may be integrated by noting that

$$A_0 - A = B \qquad (12-32)$$

Substitution of equation (12–32) into equation (12–31) affords, upon integration,

$$\ln \frac{k_f A_0}{(k_f + k_r)A - k_r A_0} = (k_f + k_r)t \qquad (12-33)$$

Equation (12–33) may be simplified by introducing the equilibrium condition:

$$k_f A_{eq} = k_r B_{eq} \qquad (12-34)$$

in which

$$A_0 - A_{eq} = B_{eq} \qquad (12-35)$$

Equations (12–34) and (12–35) may be used to solve for the equilibrium concentration in terms of the starting concentration:

$$A_{eq} = \frac{k_r}{k_f + k_r} A_0 \qquad (12-36)$$

Use of equation (12–36) in equation (12–33) enables a simple form of the rate law to be given:

$$\ln \frac{A_0 - A_{eq}}{A - A_{eq}} = (k_f + k_r)t \qquad (12-37)$$

or

$$\log \frac{A_0 - A_{eq}}{A - A_{eq}} = \frac{(k_f + k_r)}{2.303} t \qquad (12-38)$$

Equation (12–38) has the advantage that the approach of A to equilibrium can be followed over a much wider range of concentrations than if an attempt is made to obtain the first-order rate constant k_f in the early stages of the reaction when $B \approx 0$. The equation corresponds to a straight line intersecting at zero and having a slope given by $\dfrac{k_f + k_r}{2.303}$. Since the equilibrium constant of the reaction is given by

$$K = \frac{k_f}{k_r} - \frac{B_{eq}}{A_{eq}} \qquad (12-39)$$

both the forward and reverse rate constants can be evaluated once the slope of the line and the equilibrium constant have been determined.

The tetracyclines and certain of their derivatives undergo a reversible isomerization at a pH in the range of 2 to 6. This isomerization has been shown to be an epimerization, resulting in *epitetracyclines*, which show much less therapeutic activity than the natural form. Considering only that part of the tetracycline molecule undergoing change, the transformation can be represented by the equation

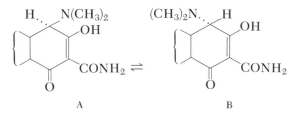

The natural configuration of tetracycline has the $N(CH_3)_2$ group above the plane and the H group below

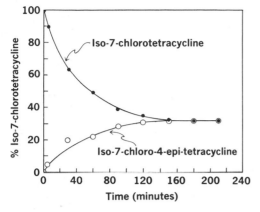

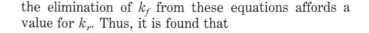

Fig. 12-3. Approach to equilibrium in the reversible epimerizations of iso-7-chloro-*epi*-tetracycline (○—○—○) and iso-7-chlorotetracycline (●—●—●). (After J. D. McCormick, S. M. Fox, L. L. Smith, *et al.* J. Am. Chem. Soc. **79**, 2849, 1957.)

the plane of the page. Under acidic conditions, the natural compound *A* is converted reversibly to the *epi*-isomer *B*.

McCormick et al.[5] followed the epimerization of iso-7-chlorotetracycline and its *epi*-isomer and noted that each isomer led to the same equilibrium distribution of isomers (Fig. 12–3). In the solvent dimethylformamide containing 1 *M* aqueous NaH_2PO_4 at 25° C, the equilibrium distribution consisted of 32% iso-7-chlorotetracycline and 68% iso-7-chloro-4-*epi*-tetracycline, which gives an equilibrium constant

$$K = \frac{B_{eq}}{A_{eq}} = \frac{68}{32} = 2.1$$

The data used to arrive at Figure 12–3, when plotted according to equation (12–38), give the line shown in Figure 12–4. The slope of this line is 0.010 min⁻¹. Since from equation (12–38) the slope *S* is

$$S = \frac{k_f + k_r}{2.30} = 0.010 \text{ min}^{-1}$$

and from equation (12–39)

$$K = \frac{B_{eq}}{A_{eq}} = \frac{k_f}{k_r} = 2.1$$

Fig. 12-4. Reversible epimerization of iso-7-chlorotetracycline in dimethylformamide containing 1 *M* NaH_2PO_4 at 25° C.

the elimination of k_f from these equations affords a value for k_r. Thus, it is found that

$$\frac{2.1k_r + k_r}{2.30} = 0.010 \text{ min}^{-1}$$

or

$$k_r = \frac{(0.010)(2.30)}{2.1 + 1} = 0.007 \text{ min}^{-1}$$

From this value, k_f is found to be

$$k_f = 2.30S - k_r = (2.30)(0.010) - 0.007$$
$$= 0.016 \text{ min}^{-1}$$

Parallel or Side Reactions. Parallel reactions are common in drug systems, particularly when organic compounds are involved. General acid–base catalysis, to be considered later (p. 303), belongs to this class of reactions.

The base-catalyzed degradation of prednisolone will be used here to illustrate the parallel-type process. Guttman and Meister[6] investigated the degradation of the steroid prednisolone in aqueous solutions containing sodium hydroxide as a catalyst. The runs were carried out at 35° C, and the rate of disappearance of the dihydroxyacetone side chain was followed by appropriate analytic techniques. The decomposition of prednisolone was found to involve parallel pseudo–first-order reactions with the appearance of acidic and neutral steroidal products.

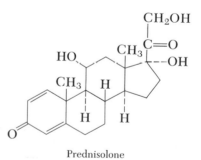

Prednisolone

The mechanism of the reaction may be represented as

$$\begin{array}{c}
\qquad \xrightarrow{k_1} A \qquad\qquad (12\text{–}40) \\
P \\
\qquad \xrightarrow{k_2} N \qquad\qquad (12\text{–}41)
\end{array}$$

in which *P*, *A*, and *N* are the concentrations of prednisolone, an acid product, and a neutral product, respectively.

The corresponding rate equation is

$$-\frac{dP}{dt} = k_1P + k_2P = kP \qquad (12\text{–}42)$$

in which $k = k_1 + k_2$. This first-order equation is integrated to give

$$\ln(P_0/P) = kt \qquad (12\text{–}43)$$

or

$$P = P_0 e^{-kt} \qquad (12-44)$$

The rate of formation of the acidic product can be expressed as

$$\frac{dA}{dt} = k_1 P = k_1 P_0 e^{-kt} \qquad (12-45)$$

Integration of equation (12-45) yields

$$A = A_0 + \frac{k_1}{k} P_0 (1 - e^{-kt}) \qquad (12-46)$$

in which A is the concentration of the acid product at time t, and A_0 and P_0 are the initial concentrations of the acid and prednisolone, respectively. Actually, A_0 is equal to zero since no acid is formed before the prednisolone begins to decompose. Therefore,

$$A = \frac{k_1}{k} P_0 (1 - e^{-kt}) \qquad (12-47)$$

Likewise for the neutral product,

$$N = \frac{k_2}{k} P_0 (1 - e^{-kt}) \qquad (12-48)$$

Equations (12-47) and (12-48) suggest that for the base-catalyzed breakdown of prednisolone, a plot of the concentration A or N against $(1 - e^{-kt})$ should yield a straight line. At $t = 0$, the curve should pass through the origin, and at $t = \infty$, the function should have a value of unity. the value for k, the overall first-order rate constant, was obtained by a plot of log [prednisolone] against the time at various concentrations of sodium hydroxide. It was possible to check the validity of expression (12-47) using the k values that were now known for each level of hydroxide ion concentration. A plot of the acidic material formed against $(1 - e^{-kt})$ yielded a straight line passing through the origin as predicted by equation (12-47). The value of k_1, the rate constant for the formation of the acidic product, was then calculated from the slope of the line.

$$k_1 = \text{slope} \times k/P_0 \qquad (12-49)$$

and the value of k_2, the rate constant for the formation of the neutral degradation product, was obtained by subtracting k_1 from k. The data, as tabulated by Guttman and Meister,[6] are found in Table 12-3.

The stability of hydrocortisone was explored by Allen and Gupta[7] in aqueous and oil vehicles, water-washable

ointment bases, and emulsified vehicles in the presence of other ingredients, at elevated temperatures and at

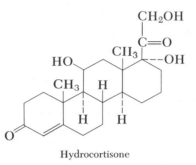

Hydrocortisone

various degrees of acidity and basicity. Hydrocortisone was unstable at room temperature in aqueous vehicles on the basic side of neutrality; alcohol and glycerin appeared to improve the stability. The decomposition in water and propylene glycol was pseudo–first-order. In highly acidic and basic media and at elevated temperatures, the decomposition of hydrocortisone was of a complex nature, following a parallel scheme.

Series or Consecutive Reactions. Consecutive reactions are common in radioactive series in which a parent isotope decays by a first-order process into a daughter isotope, and so on through a chain of disintegrations. We shall take a simplified version of the degradation scheme of glucose as illustrative of consecutive-type reactions. The depletion of glucose in acid solution may be represented by the scheme[8]

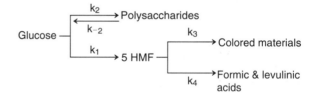

which is seen to involve all of the complex-type reactions–reversible, parallel, and consecutive processes. At low concentrations of glucose and acid catalyst, the formation of polysaccharides may be neglected. Furthermore, owing to the indefinite nature

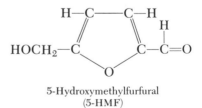

5-Hydroxymethylfurfural
(5-HMF)

TABLE 12-3. *Rate Constants for the Base-Catalyzed Degradation of Prednisolone in Air at 35° C*

NaOH (Normality)	k (hr^{-1})	k_1 (hr^{-1})	k_2 (hr^{-1})
0.01	0.108	0.090	0.018
0.02	0.171	0.137	0.034
0.03	0.233	0.181	0.052
0.04	0.258	0.200	0.058
0.05	0.293	0.230	0.063

of the breakdown products of 5-HMF, these may be combined together and referred to simply as constituent C. The simplified mechanism is therefore written as the series of reactions:

$$A \xrightarrow{k_1} B \xrightarrow{k_2} C$$

in which A is glucose, B is 5-HMF and C is the final breakdown products. The rate of decomposition of glucose is given by the equation

$$-dA/dt = k_1 A \qquad (12\text{--}50)$$

The rate of change in concentration of 5-HMF is

$$dB/dt = k_1 A - k_2 B \qquad (12\text{--}51)$$

and that of the breakdown products is

$$dC/dt = k_2 B \qquad (12\text{--}52)$$

When these equations are integrated and proper substitutions made, we obtain

$$A = A_0 e^{-k_1 t} \qquad (12\text{--}53)$$

$$B = \frac{A_0 k_1}{k_2 - k_1}(e^{-k_1 t} - e^{-k_2 t}) \qquad (12\text{--}54)$$

and

$$C = A_0\left[1 + \frac{1}{k_1 - k_2}(k_2 e^{-k_1 t} - k_1 e^{-k_2 t})\right] \qquad (12\text{--}55)$$

By the application of equations (12–53), (12–54), and (12–55), the rate constants k_1 and k_2 and the concentration of breakdown products C can be determined. Glucose is found to decompose by a first-order reaction. As glucose is depleted, the concentration of 5-HMF increases rapidly at the beginning of the reaction and then increases at a slower rate as time progresses. The decomposition products of 5-HMF increase slowly at first, indicating an induction or lag period, and then increase at a greater rate. These later products are responsible for the discoloration of glucose solutions that occurs when the solutions are sterilized at elevated temperatures.

Kinetic studies such as these have considerable practical application in pharmacy. When the mechanism of the breakdown of parenteral solutions is better understood, the manufacturing pharmacist should be able to prepare a stable product having a long shelf-life. Large supplies of glucose injection and similar products can then possibly be stockpiled for use in times of emergency.

Mauger et al.[9] studied the degradation of hydrocortisone hemisuccinate at 70° C over a narrow pH range and found the reaction to be another example of the consecutive first-order type. At pH 6.9, the rate constant k_1 was 0.023 hr^{-1} and k_2 was 0.50 hr^{-1}.

The Steady-State Approximation. Michaelis–Menten Equation. A number of kinetic processes cannot have their rate laws integrated exactly. In situations such as these, it is useful to postulate a reasonable reaction sequence and then to derive a rate law that applies to the postulated sequence of steps. If the postulate is reasonably accurate and reflects the actual steps involved in the reaction, the observed kinetics for the reaction should match the curve given by the derived rate law.

The *steady-state approximation* is commonly used to reduce the labor in deducing the form of a rate law. We will illustrate this approximation by deriving the Michaelis–Menten equation.

Michaelis and Menten[10] assumed that the interaction of a substrate S with an enzyme E to yield product P followed a reaction sequence given by

$$E + S \underset{k_2}{\overset{k_1}{\rightleftharpoons}} (E \cdot S) \xrightarrow{k_2} P$$

According to this scheme, the rate of product formation is

$$\frac{dP}{dt} = k_3(E \cdot S) \qquad (12\text{--}56)$$

We have no easy means of obtaining the concentration of enzyme–substrate complex, so it is necessary that this concentration be expressed in terms of easily measurable quantities. In an enzyme study, we can usually measure S, P, and E_0, the total concentration of enzyme.

The rate of formation of $(E \cdot S)$ is

$$\frac{d(E \cdot S)}{dt} = k_1(E)(S) - k_2(E \cdot S) - k_3(E \cdot S) \qquad (12\text{--}57)$$

or

$$\frac{d(E \cdot S)}{dt} = k_1(E)(S) - (k_2 + k_3)(E \cdot S) \qquad (12\text{--}58)$$

If the concentration of $E \cdot S$ is constant throughout most of the reaction and is always much less than the concentrations of S and P, we can write

$$\frac{d(E \cdot S)}{dt} = 0 \qquad (12\text{--}59)$$

It follows from equations (12–58) and (12–59) that

$$(E \cdot S)_{ss} = \frac{k_1(E)(S)}{k_2 + k_3} \qquad (12\text{--}60)$$

in which the subscript ss is used to designate the concentration referred to as the *steady-state* value.

The total concentration of enzyme E_0 is the sum of the concentrations of enzyme, both free E and bound $E \cdot S$,

$$E_0 = E + (E \cdot S)_{ss} \qquad (12\text{--}61)$$

Eliminating E from equations (12–60) and (12–61), we obtain

$$(E \cdot S)_{ss} = \frac{k_1 S E_0}{(k_2 + k_3) + k_1 S} \qquad (12\text{--}62)$$

or

$$(E \cdot S)_{ss} = \frac{SE_0}{K_m + S} \quad (12\text{--}63)$$

in which

$$K_m = \frac{k_2 + k_3}{k_1} \quad (12\text{--}64)$$

Thus, under steady-state conditions, the rate of product formation is given by

$$\frac{dP}{dt} = \frac{k_3 S E_0}{K_m + S} \quad (12\text{--}65)$$

which may be recognized as the Michaelis–Menten equation. The Michaelis–Menten constant K_m indicates the tendency of the enzyme-substrate complex to decompose to starting substrate or to proceed to product, relative to the tendency of the complex to be formed.

It is useful to introduce a maximum velocity for the Michaelis–Menten scheme, namely $(dP/dt)_{maximum}$, which is usually written as V_m. When S is very large, all enzyme E_o is present as $E \cdot S$; that is, all enzyme is combined with the substrate and the reaction proceeds at maximum velocity. From equation (12–56), dP/dt becomes V_m, and $V_m = k_3 E_o$, since $E \cdot S$ is equivalent to E_o. Accordingly, from equation (12–65)

$$V = V_m \frac{S}{k_m + S} \quad (12\text{--}66)$$

Equation (12–66) may be inverted to obtain a linear expression, known as the *Lineweaver–Burk equation:*

$$\frac{1}{V} = \frac{K_m + S}{V_m \cdot S} \quad (12\text{--}67)$$

$$\frac{1}{V} = \frac{1}{V_m} + \frac{K_m}{V_m} \frac{1}{S} \quad (12\text{--}68)$$

From equation (12–68) we see that a plot of $1/V$ versus $1/S$ yields a straight line with an intercept on the vertical axis of $1/V_m$ and a slope of K_m/V_m (Fig. 12–5). Knowing V_m from the intercept and obtaining K_m/V_m as the slope, it is possible to calculate K_m, the *Michaelis constant.*

Example 12–6. The velocity V of an enzymatic reaction at increasing substrate concentration [S] was experimentally determined and is recorded here:

V [μg/(ℓ min)]	0.0350	0.0415	0.0450	0.0490	0.0505
[S] (molarity, M)	0.0025	0.0050	0.0100	0.0167	0.0333

(a) Following the Lineweaver–Menten equation, plot $1/V$ versus $1/[S]$ using the data given below, and calculate V_m and K_m using linear regression analysis. The data for the Lineweaver–Burk plot and the regression analysis are:

1/V [min/(μg/ℓ)]	28.57	24.10	22.22	20.41	19.80
1/[S] (ℓ/mole)	400	200	100	59.88	30.0

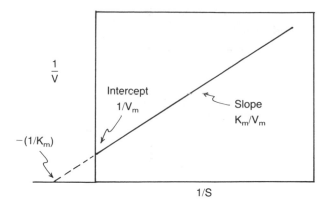

Fig. 12–5. A Lineweaver-Burk plot of Michaelis–Menten kinetics showing the calculation of K_m by two means.

(b) Extrapolate the line to the horizontal axis (x-axis) where the intercept is $-1/K_m$. Read $-1/K_m$ as accurately as possible by eye and obtain K_m as its reciprocal. Compare this value with that obtained by linear regression in (a) above.

Answer: (a) Linear regression analysis yields the expression

$$1/V = 19.316 + 0.0234 \; 1/[S]; \; r^2 = 0.990$$

Intercept, $1/V_m = 19.316$; $V_m = 0.0518$ μg/(ℓ-min)

Slope $= K_m/V_m = 0.0234$ (ℓ-min/μg) M

$K_m = 0.0234$ (ℓ-min/μg) M $\times$ 0.0518 μg/ℓ-min

$\quad = 0.0012$ M

(b) $-1/K_m$ by extrapolation $= -823$ M^{-1}

$\quad$ K$_m = 0.0012$ M

Michaelis–Menten kinetics is used not only for enzyme reactions but also for biochemical processes in the body involving carriers that transport substances across membranes such as blood capillaries and the renal tubule. It is assumed, for example, that L-tyrosine is absorbed from the nasal cavity into systemic circulation by a carrier-facilitated process, and Michaelis–Menten kinetics is applied to this case in Chapter 19, *Problem 19–8.*

Rate-Determining Step. In a reaction sequence in which one step is much slower than all the subsequent steps leading to product, the rate at which the product is formed may depend on the rates of all the steps preceding the slow step but does not depend on any of the steps following. The slowest step in a reaction sequence is called, somewhat misleadingly, the *rate-determining step* of the reaction.

Consider the following mechanistic pathway,

$$A \underset{k_2}{\overset{k_1}{\rightleftharpoons}} B \text{ (step 1 and step 2)}$$

$$B + C \xrightarrow{k_3} D \text{ (step 3)}$$

$$D \xrightarrow{k_4} P \text{ (step 4)}$$

which may be postulated for the observed overall reaction

$$A + C \rightarrow P$$

If the concentrations of the intermediates B and D are small, we may apply the steady-state approximation to evaluate their steady-state concentrations. These are given by

$$B_{ss} = \frac{k_1 A}{k_2 + k_3 C}$$

and

$$D_{ss} = \frac{k_1 k_3 AC}{k_4(k_2 + k_3 C)}$$

For the rate of formation of product, we can write

$$\frac{dP}{dt} = k_4 D_{ss}$$

or

$$\frac{dP}{dt} = \frac{k_1 k_3 AC}{(k_2 + k_3 C)} \qquad (12\text{--}69)$$

If, in the mechanistic sequence, step 3 is the slow step (the rate-determining step), we may say that $k_2 \gg k_3 C$, *and equation (12–69) is simplified to a second-order expression,*

$$\frac{dP}{dt} = \frac{k_1 k_3 AC}{k_2} = k_0 AC \qquad (12\text{--}70)$$

On the other hand, if step 2, the reverse reaction, is the slow step, then $k_3 C \gg k_2$, and equation (12–69) reduces to a first-order expression,

$$\frac{dP}{dt} - \frac{k_1 k_3 AC}{k_3 C} = k_1 A \qquad (12\text{--}71)$$

Thus we see that reactions may exhibit a simple first- or second-order behavior, yet the detailed mechanism for these reactions may be quite complex.

INFLUENCE OF TEMPERATURE AND OTHER FACTORS ON REACTION RATES

Temperature. A number of factors other than concentration may affect the reaction velocity. Among these are temperature, solvents, catalysts, and light. The speed of many reactions increases about two to three times with each 10° rise in temperature. The effect of temperature on reaction rate is given by the equation, first suggested by Arrhenius,

$$k = Ae^{-E_a/RT} \qquad (12\text{--}72)$$

or

$$\log k = \log A - \frac{E_a}{2.303} \frac{1}{RT} \qquad (12\text{--}73)$$

in which k is the specific reaction rate, A is a constant known as the *Arrhenius factor* or the *frequency factor*, E_a is the *energy of activation*, R is the gas constant, 1.987 calories/deg mole, and T is the absolute temperature. The constants, A and E_a, will be considered further in later sections of the chapter. They may be evaluated by determining k at several temperatures and plotting $1/T$ against $\log k$. As seen in equation

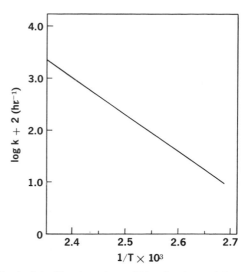

Fig. 12–6. A plot of $\log k$ against $1/T$ for the thermal decomposition of glucose.

(12–73), the slope of the line so obtained is $-E_a/2.303R$, and the intercept on the vertical axis is $\log A$, from which E_a and A may be obtained.

The data, obtained from a study of the decomposition of glucose solutions between 100° and 140° C in the presence of 0.35 N hydrochloric acid, are plotted in this manner, as shown in Figure 12–6.* It should be observed that since the *reciprocal* of the absolute temperature is plotted along the horizontal axis, the temperature is actually *decreasing* from left to right across the graph. It is sometimes advantageous to plot $\log t_{1/2}$ instead of $\log k$ on the vertical axis. The half-life for a first-order reaction is related to k by equation (12–18), $t_{1/2} = 0.693/k$, and in logarithmic form

$$\log k = \log 0.693 - \log t_{1/2} \qquad (12\text{--}74)$$

Substituting equation (12–74) into equation (12–73) gives

$$\log t_{1/2} = \log 0.693 - \log A + \frac{E_a}{2.303R} \frac{1}{T}$$

or

$$\log t_{1/2} = \frac{E_a}{2.303R} \frac{1}{T} + \text{constant}$$

and $E_a/2.303R$ is obtained as the slope of the line resulting from plotting $\log t_{1/2}$ against $1/T$. Higuchi et al.[11] plotted the results of the alkaline hydrolysis of procaine in this manner, as shown in Figure 12–7.

E_a may also be obtained by writing equation (12–73) for a temperature T_2 as

---

*Notice that $\log k + 2$ is plotted on the vertical axis of Figure 12–6. This is a convenient way of eliminating negative values along the axis. For example, if $k = 1.0 \times 10^{-2}$, 2.0×10^{-2}, etc., the logarithmic expressions are $\log 1.0 + \log 10^{-2}$, $\log 2.0 + \log 10^{-2}$, ... or $0.0 - 2 = -2$, $0.3 - 2 = -1.7$, etc. The negative signs may be eliminated along the vertical axis if 2 is added to each value; hence the label, $\log k + 2$.

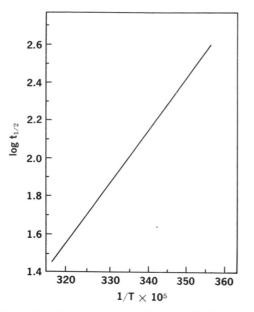

Fig. 12–7. A plot of log $t_{1/2}$ against $1/T$ for the alkaline hydrolysis of procaine. (After T. Higuchi et al[11].)

$$\log k_2 = \log A - \frac{E_a}{2.303R}\frac{1}{T_2}$$

and for another temperature T_1 as

$$\log k_1 = \log A - \frac{E_a}{2.303R}\frac{1}{T_1}$$

Subtracting these two expressions yields

$$\log \frac{k_2}{k_1} = \frac{E_a}{2.303R}\left(\frac{T_2 - T_1}{T_2 T_1}\right)$$

Example 12–7. The rate constant k_1 for the decomposition of 5-hydroxymethylfurfural at 120° C (393° K) is 1.173 hr^{-1} or 3.258×10^{-4} sec^{-1} and k_2 at 140° C (413° K) is 4.860 hr^{-1}. What is the activation energy E_a in kcal/mole and the frequency factor A in sec^{-1} for the breakdown of 5-HMF within this temperature range?

$$\log \frac{4.860}{1.173} = \frac{E_a}{2.303 \times 1.987}\left(\frac{413 - 393}{413 \times 393}\right)$$

$$E_a = 23 \text{ kcal/mole}$$

At 120° C, using equation (12–73), one obtains

$$\log (3.258 \times 10^{-4} \text{ sec}^{-1}) = \log A - \frac{23,000 \text{ cal}}{2.303 \times 1.987}\frac{1}{393}$$

$$A = 2 \times 10^9 \text{ sec}^{-1}$$

Classic Collision Theory of Reaction Rates. The Arrhenius equation is largely an empiric relation giving the effect of temperature on an observed rate constant. Relations of this type are observed for unimolecular and bimolecular reactions and often are also observed for complex reactions involving a number of bimolecular and unimolecular steps. Although it is extremely difficult, in most cases, to attach significance to the temperature dependence of complex reactions, the temperature dependence of uni- and bimolecular reactions appears to reflect a fundamental physical requirement that must be met for a reaction to occur.

The manner by which temperature affects molecular motion may be understood by considering a hypothetic situation in which all the molecules of a substance are moving in the same direction at the same velocity. If a molecule deviates from its course, it will collide with another molecule, causing both molecules to move off in different directions with different velocities. A chain of collisions between molecules can then occur, which finally results in random motion of all the molecules. In this case, only a certain fraction of the molecules have a velocity equivalent to the initial velocity of the ordered system. The net result is that for a fixed number of molecules at a given temperature, and therefore at a definite total energy, a distribution of molecular velocities varying from zero upward is attained. Since kinetic energy is proportional to the square of velocity, the distribution of molecular velocities corresponds to the distribution of molecular energies, and the fraction of the molecules having a given kinetic energy can be expressed by the *Boltzmann distribution law*

$$f_i = \frac{N_i}{N_T} = e^{-E_i/RT} \qquad (12\text{–}75)$$

From the Boltzmann distribution law we note that of the total number of moles N_T of a reactant, N_i moles have a kinetic energy given by E_i. The collision theory of reaction rates postulates that a collision must occur between molecules for a reaction to occur and, further, that a reaction between molecules does not take place unless the molecules are of a certain energy. By this postulate, the rate of a reaction can be considered proportional to the number of moles of reactant having sufficient energy to react, that is

$$\text{Rate} = PZN_i \qquad (12\text{–}76)$$

The proportionality constant in this relation is divided into two terms: the collision number Z which for a reaction between two molecules is the number of collisions per second per cubic centimeter, and the steric or probability factor P, which is included to take into account the fact that not every collision between molecules leads to reaction. That is, P gives the probability that a collision between molecules will lead to product.

Substituting for N_i in equation (12–76) yields

$$\text{Rate} = (PZe^{-E_i/RT})N_T \qquad (12\text{–}77)$$

which, when compared with the general rate law

$$\text{Rate} = k(\text{concentration of reactants}) \qquad (12\text{–}78)$$

leads to the conclusion that

$$k = (PZ)e^{-E_i/RT} \qquad (12\text{–}79)$$

Thus, collision state theory interprets the Arrhenius A factor in terms of the frequency of collision between molecules

$$A = PZ \qquad (12\text{–}80)$$

and the Arrhenius activation energy E_a as the minimum kinetic energy a molecule must possess in order to undergo reaction,

$$E_a = E_i \qquad (12-81)$$

Yang[12] has shown the error possible in determining the activation energy E_a and the predicted shelf-life when the kinetic order in an accelerated stability test (pp. 313–315) is incorrectly assigned; for example, when an actual zero-order reaction can equally well be described by a first-order degradation.

Transition State Theory. An alternative to the collision theory is the *transition state theory* or absolute rate theory, according to which an equilibrium is considered to exist between the normal reactant molecules and an activated complex of these molecules. Decomposition of the activated complex leads to product. For an elementary bimolecular process, the reaction may be written as

$$\underset{\substack{\text{Normal reactant}\\\text{molecules}}}{A + B} \quad \rightleftharpoons \quad \underset{\substack{\text{Activated reactant}\\\text{molecules in the}\\\text{transition state}\\\text{(activated complex)}}}{[A \cdots B]^{\ddagger}} \quad \rightarrow \quad \underset{\substack{\text{Product}\\\text{molecules}}}{P} \qquad (12-82)$$

A double dagger is used to designate the activated state, namely $[A \cdots B]^{\ddagger}$

The rate of product formation in this theory is given by

$$\text{Rate} = v[A \cdots B]^{\ddagger} \qquad (12-83)$$

in which v is the frequency with which an activated complex goes to product. Since an equilibrium exists between the reactants and the activated complex,

$$K^{\ddagger} = \frac{[A \cdots B]^{\ddagger}}{[A][B]} \qquad (12-84)$$

and this expression can be rearranged to

$$[A \cdots B]^{\ddagger} = K^{\ddagger}[A][B] \qquad (12-85)$$

Hence,

$$\text{Rate} = [vK^{\ddagger}][A][B] \qquad (12-86)$$

The general rate law for a bimolecular reaction is

$$\text{Rate} = k[A][B] \qquad (12-87)$$

so it follows that

$$k = vK^{\ddagger} \qquad (12-88)$$

It will be recalled from previous thermodynamic considerations (p. 70) that

$$\Delta G^{\circ} = -RT \ln K \qquad (12-89)$$

or

$$K = e^{-\Delta G^{\circ}/RT} \qquad (12-90)$$

and (p. 65)

$$\Delta G^{\circ} = \Delta H^{\circ} - T \, \Delta S^{\circ} \qquad (12-91)$$

Replacing the ordinary K for present purposes with $K^{\ddagger}$, and by making similar substitutions for the thermodynamic quantities, it follows that

$$k = ve^{-\Delta G^{\ddagger}/RT} \qquad (12-92)$$

and

$$k = (ve^{\Delta S^{\ddagger}/R})e^{-\Delta H^{\ddagger}/RT} \qquad (12-93)$$

where $\Delta G^{\ddagger}$, $\Delta S^{\ddagger}$, and $\Delta H^{\ddagger}$ are the respective differences between the standard free energy, entropy, and enthalpy in the transition state and in the normal reactant state.

In this theory, the Arrhenius A factor is related to the entropy of activation of the transition state:

$$A = ve^{\Delta S^{\ddagger}/R} \qquad (12-94)$$

and the Arrhenius activation energy E_a is related to the enthalpy of activation of the transition state:

$$E_a = \Delta H^{\ddagger} = \Delta E^{\ddagger} + P \, \Delta V^{\ddagger} \qquad (12-95)$$

For most practical purposes, $\Delta V^{\ddagger} = 0$; hence

$$E_a = \Delta E^{\ddagger} \qquad (12-96)$$

In principle, the transition state theory gives the influence of temperature on reaction rates by the general equation

$$k = (ve^{\Delta S^{\ddagger}/R})e^{-\Delta E^{\ddagger}/RT} \qquad (12-97)$$

in which the frequency of decomposition of the transition state complex v may vary depending on the nature of the reactants. Eyring[13] has shown that the quantity v may be considered, to a good approximation, as a universal factor for reactions, depending only on temperature, and that it may be written,

$$v = \left(\frac{RT}{Nh}\right) \qquad (12-98)$$

in which R is the molar gas constant, T is the absolute temperature, N is Avogadro's number, and h is Planck's constant. The factor (RT/Nh) has a value of about 10^{12} to $10^{13} \sec^{-1}$ at ordinary temperatures ($\cong 2 \times 10^{10}T$). In many unimolecular gas reactions in which $\Delta S^{\ddagger}$ is zero so that $e^{\Delta S^{\ddagger}/R} = 1$, the rate constant ordinarily has a value of about $10^{13}e^{-E_a/RT}$ or

$$k \cong \frac{RT}{Nh} e^{-\Delta H^{\ddagger}/RT} \cong 10^{13}e^{-E_a/RT} \qquad (12-99)$$

When the rate deviates from this value, it can be considered as resulting from the $e^{\Delta S^{\ddagger}/R}$ factor. When the activated complex represents a more probable arrangement of molecules than found in the normal reactants $\Delta S^{\ddagger}$ is positive and the reaction rate will be greater than normal. Conversely, when the activated complex results only after considerable rearrangement of the structure of the reactant molecules, making the complex a less probable structure, $\Delta S^{\ddagger}$ is negative, and the reaction will be slower than predicted from equation (12–99). The collision theory and the transition state theory are seen to be related by comparing equations (12–80), (12–94), and (12–98). One concludes that

$$PZ = \frac{RT}{Nh} e^{\Delta S^{\ddagger}/R} \qquad (12\text{–}100)$$

The collision number Z is identified with RT/Nh and the probability factor P with the entropy term $e^{\Delta S^{\ddagger}/R}$.

Example 12–8. In the study of the acid-catalyzed hydrolysis of procaine, Marcus and Baron[14] obtained the first-order reaction rate k from a plot of log c versus t, and the activation energy E_a from an Arrhenius plot of log k versus $1/T$. The values were $k = 38.5 \times 10^{-6}$ sec^{-1} at 97.30° C and $E_a = 16.8$ kcal/mole.

Compute $\Delta S^{\ddagger}$ and the frequency factor A using equations (12–93) and (12–94), and the probability factor P. It is first necessary to obtain RT/Nh at 97.30° C or about 371° K:

$$v = \frac{RT}{Nh} = \frac{8.31 \times 10^7 \text{ erg/mole deg} \times 371 \text{ deg}}{6.62 \times 10^{-27} \text{ erg sec/molecule}}$$
$$\times 6.02 \times 10^{23} \text{ molecule/mole}$$
$$= 7.74 \times 10^{12} \text{ sec}^{-1}$$

Then, from equation (12–93), in which

$$\Delta H^{\ddagger} \cong E_a,$$

$$38.5 \times 10^{-6} = 7.74 \times 10^{12} e^{\Delta S^{\ddagger}/1.987} \times e^{-16,800/(1.987 \times 371)}$$

$$\Delta S^{\ddagger} = -24.73 \text{ cal/mole deg}$$

and from equation (12–94)

$$A = 7.74 \times 10^{12} e^{-33.9/1.987} = 3.05 \times 10^7 \text{ sec}^{-1}$$

Finally, from the discussion accompanying equation (12–100)

$$P = e^{-33.9/1.987} = 3.9 \times 10^{-6}$$

Tables of e^{-x} values, available in handbooks of chemistry and physics, are convenient for handling calculations such as these, but hand calculators give the results directly.

Marcus and Baron[14] compared the kinetics of the acid-catalyzed hydrolyses of procainamide, procaine, and benzocaine. They found that the frequency factors for procainamide and procaine were considerably lower than the values expected for compounds of this type. Procainamide and procaine are diprotonated species in acid solution, that is, they have taken on two protons, and hydrolysis in the presence of an acid involves the interaction of positively charged ions, namely the diprotonated procaine molecule and the hydronium ion:

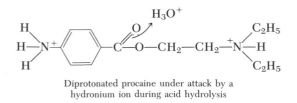

Diprotonated procaine under attack by a
hydronium ion during acid hydrolysis

According to the authors, the two positively charged protonated centers on the procaine molecule exert a considerable repulsive effect on the attacking hydronium ions. This repulsion results in a low frequency factor. The $\Delta S^{\ddagger}$ is unusually negative (cf. *Example 12–8*) perhaps for the following reason. When the third

proton finally attaches itself, the activated complex that results is a highly charged ion. The activated molecule is markedly solvated, reducing the freedom of the solvent and decreasing the entropy of activation. This effect, too, tends to lower the frequency factor.

Effect of the Solvent. The influence of the solvent on the rate of decomposition of drugs is a topic of great importance to the pharmacist. Although the effects are complicated and generalizations cannot usually be made, it appears that the reaction of nonelectrolytes is related to the relative internal pressures or solubility parameters of the solvent and solute (p. 224). The influence of the ionic strength and the dielectric constant of the medium on the rate of ionic reactions also are significant and will be discussed in subsequent sections.

Solutions are ordinarily nonideal, and equation (12–84) should be corrected by including activity coefficients. For the bimolecular reaction,

$$A + B \rightleftharpoons [A \cdots B]^{\ddagger} \rightarrow \text{Products}$$

the thermodynamic equilibrium constant should be written in terms of activities as

$$K^{\ddagger} = \frac{a^{\ddagger}}{a_A a_B} = \frac{C^{\ddagger}}{C_A C_B} \frac{\gamma^{\ddagger}}{\gamma_A \gamma_B} \qquad (12\text{–}101)$$

in which $a^{\ddagger}$ is the activity of the species in the transition state and a_A and a_B are the activities of the reactants in their normal state. Then the following expressions, analogous to equations (12–83) and (12–86), are obtained:

$$\text{Rate} = \frac{RT}{Nh} C^{\ddagger} = \frac{RT}{Nh} K^{\ddagger} C_A C_B \frac{\gamma_A \gamma_B}{\gamma^{\ddagger}} \qquad (12\text{–}102)$$

and

$$k = \frac{\text{Rate}}{C_A C_B} = \frac{RT}{Nh} K^{\ddagger} \frac{\gamma_A \gamma_B}{\gamma^{\ddagger}}$$

or

$$k = k_o \frac{\gamma_A \gamma_B}{\gamma^{\ddagger}} \qquad (12\text{–}103)$$

in which $k_0 = RTK^{\ddagger}/Nh$ is the rate constant in an infinitely dilute solution, that is, one that behaves ideally. It will be recalled from knowledge gained in previous chapters that the activity coefficients may relate the behavior of the solute in the solution under consideration to that of the solute in an infinitely dilute solution. When the solution is ideal the activity coefficients become unity and $k_0 = k$ in equation (12–103). This condition was tacitly assumed in equation (12–86).

Now, the activity coefficient γ_2 of a not too highly polar nonelectrolytic solute in a dilute solution is given by the expression (p. 224)

$$\log \gamma_2 = \frac{V_2}{2.303RT} (\delta_1 - \delta_2)^2 \qquad (12\text{–}104)$$

in which V_2 is the molar volume of the solute and δ_1 and δ_2 are the solubility parameters for the solvent and solute, respectively. The volume fraction term, Φ^2 on page 224 is assumed here to have a value of unity.

Writing equation (12–103) in logarithmic form

$$\log k = \log k_0 + \log \gamma_A + \log \gamma_B - \log \gamma^{\ddagger} \qquad (12\text{–}105)$$

and substituting for the activity coefficients from (12–104) gives

$$\log k = \log k_0 + \frac{V_A}{2.303RT}(\delta_1 - \delta_A)^2$$
$$+ \frac{V_B}{2.303RT}(\delta_1 - \delta_B)^2$$
$$- \frac{V^{\ddagger}}{2.303RT}(\delta_1 - \delta^{\ddagger})^2 \qquad (12\text{–}106)$$

in which V_A, V_B, $V^{\ddagger}$, and the corresponding δ_A, δ_B, and $\delta^{\ddagger}$ are the molar volumes and solubility parameters of reactant A, reactant B, and the activated complex $(A \cdots B)^{\ddagger}$ respectively. The quantity δ_1 is the solubility parameter of the solvent.

Thus it is seen that the rate constant depends on the molar volumes and the solubility parameter terms. Since these three squared terms $(\delta_1 - \delta_A)^2$, $(\delta_1 - \delta_B)^2$, and $(\delta_1 - \delta^{\ddagger})^2$ represent the differences between solubility parameters or internal pressures of the solvent and the reactants, and the solvent and the activated complex, they may be symbolized respectively as $\Delta\delta_A$, $\Delta\delta_B$, and $\Delta\delta^{\ddagger}$. The molar volumes do not vary significantly, and the rate constant therefore depends primarily on the difference between $(\Delta\delta_A + \Delta\delta_B)$ and $\Delta\delta^{\ddagger}$. This is readily seen by writing equation (12–106) as

$$\log k = \log k_0 + \frac{V}{2.303RT}(\Delta\delta_A + \Delta\delta_B - \Delta\delta^{\ddagger})$$

It is assumed that the properties of the activated complex are quite similar to those of the products, so that $\Delta\delta^{\ddagger}$ may be taken as a squared term expressing the internal pressure difference between the solvent and the products. This equation indicates that if the internal pressure or "polarity" of the products is similar to that of the solvent, so that $\Delta\delta^{\ddagger} \cong 0$, and the internal pressures of the reactants are unlike that of the solvent, so that $\Delta\delta_A$ and $\Delta\delta_B > 0$, then the rate will be large in this solvent relative to the rate in an ideal solution. If, conversely, the reactants are similar in "polarity" to the solvent so that $\Delta\delta_A$ and $\Delta\delta_B \cong 0$, whereas the products are not similar to the solvent, that is, $\Delta\delta^{\ddagger} > 0$, then $(\Delta\delta_A + \Delta\delta_B) - \Delta\delta^{\ddagger}$ will have a sizable negative value and the rate will be small in this solvent.

As a result of this analysis, it can be said that polar solvents—those with high internal pressures—tend to accelerate reactions that form products having higher internal pressures than the reactants. If, on the other hand, the products are less polar than the reactants, they are accelerated by solvents of low polarity or internal pressure and retarded by solvents of high internal pressure. To illustrate this principle, the reaction between ethyl alcohol and acetic anhydride may be used:

$$C_2H_5OH + (CH_3CO)_2O$$
$$= CH_3COOC_2H_5 + CH_3COOH$$

The activated complex, resembling ethyl acetate, is less polar than the reactants, and accordingly, the reaction should be favored in a solvent having a relatively low solubility parameter. The rate constants for the reaction in various solvents are given in Table 12–4 together with the solubility parameters of the solvents.[15] The reaction slows down in the more polar solvents as predicted.

Influence of Ionic Strength. In a reaction between ions, the reactants A and B have charges z_A and z_B, and the activated complex $(A \cdots B)^{\ddagger}$ has a charge of $(z_A + z_B)$. A reaction involving ions may be represented as

$$A^{z_A} + B^{z_B} \rightleftharpoons [A \cdots B]^{\ddagger(z_A + z_B)} \rightarrow \text{Products}$$

The activity coefficient γ_i of an ion in a dilute aqueous solution ($< 0.01 M$) at $25°$ C is given by the Debye–Hückel equation (p. 135) as

$$\log \gamma_i = -0.51 z_i^2 \sqrt{\mu} \qquad (12\text{–}107)$$

in which μ is the ionic strength. Therefore, we can write

$$\log \gamma_A + \log \gamma_B - \log \gamma^{\ddagger}$$
$$= -0.51 z_A^2 \sqrt{\mu} - 0.51 z_B^2 \sqrt{\mu} + 0.51(z_A + z_B)^2 \sqrt{\mu}$$
$$= -0.51\sqrt{\mu}[z_A^2 + z_B^2 - (z_A^2 + 2z_A z_B + z_B^2)]$$
$$= 0.51 \times 2z_A z_B \sqrt{\mu} = 1.02 z_A z_B \sqrt{\mu} \qquad (12\text{–}108)$$

Substituting into equation (12–105) results in the expression, at $25°$ C,

$$\log k = \log k_0 + 1.02 z_A z_B \sqrt{\mu} \qquad (12\text{–}109)$$

in which k_0 is the rate constant in an infinitely dilute solution in which $\mu = 0$. It follows from equation (12–109) that a plot of $\log k$ against $\sqrt{\mu}$ should give a straight line with a slope of $1.02 z_A z_B$. If one of the reactants is a neutral molecule, $z_A z_B = 0$ and the rate constant as seen from equation (12–109) should then be independent of the ionic strength in dilute solutions.

TABLE 12–4. *Influence of Solvents on Rate Constants*

Solvent	Solubility Parameter δ	k at $50°$ C
Hexane	7.3	0.0119
Carbon tetrachloride	8.6	0.0113
Chlorobenzene	9.5	0.0053
Benzene	9.2	0.0046
Chloroform	9.3	0.0040
Nitrobenzene	10.0	0.0024

Good agreement has been obtained between experiment and theory as expressed by equation (12–109).

If the reacting molecules are uncharged in a solution having a reasonable ionic strength, the rate expression is

$$\log k = \log k_0 + b\mu \qquad (12\text{–}110)$$

in which b is a constant obtained from experimental data. Carstensen[16] has considered the various ionic strength effects in pharmaceutical solutions.

Influence of Dielectric Constant. The effect of the dielectric constant on the rate constant of an ionic reaction, extrapolated to infinite dilution where the ionic strength effect is zero, is often a necessary piece of information in the development of new drug preparations. One of the equations by which this effect may be determined is

$$\ln k = \ln k_{\epsilon=\infty} - \frac{N z_A z_B e^2}{R T r^{\ddagger}} \frac{1}{\epsilon} \qquad (12\text{–}111)$$

in which $k_{\epsilon=\infty}$ is the rate constant in a medium of infinite dielectric constant, N is Avogadro's number, z_A and z_B are the charges on the two ions, e is the unit of electric charge, $r^{\ddagger}$ is the distance between ions in the activated complex, and ϵ is the dielectric constant of the solution, equal approximately to the dielectric constant of the solvent in dilute solutions. The term $\ln k_{\epsilon=\infty}$ is obtained by plotting $\ln k$ against $1/\epsilon$ and extrapolating to $1/\epsilon = 0$, that is, to $\epsilon = \infty$. Such a plot, according to equation (12–111), should yield a straight line with a positive slope for reactant ions of opposite sign and a negative slope for reactants of like sign. For a reaction between ions of opposite sign, an increase in dielectric constant of the solvent results in a decrease in the rate constant. For ions of like charge, on the other hand, an increase in dielectric constant results in an increase in the rate of the reaction.

When a reaction occurs between a dipole molecule and an ion A, the equation is

$$\ln k = \ln k_{\epsilon=\infty} + \frac{N z_A^2 e^2}{2RT} \left(\frac{1}{r_A} - \frac{1}{r^{\ddagger}} \right) \frac{1}{\epsilon} \qquad (12\text{–}112)$$

in which z_A is the charge on the ion A, r_A is the radius of the ion, and $r^{\ddagger}$ is the radius of the activated complex. Equation (12–112) predicts that a straight line should be obtained when $\ln k$ is plotted against $1/\epsilon$, the reciprocal of the dielectric constant. Since $r^{\ddagger}$, being the radius of the combined ion and neutral molecule in the transition state, will be larger than r_A, the radius of the ion, the second term on the right side of the equation will always be positive, and the slope of the line will consequently be positive. Therefore, $\ln k$ will increase with increasing values of $1/\epsilon$, that is, the rate of reaction between an ion and a neutral molecule will increase with *decreasing* dielectric constant of the medium. This relationship, however, does not hold if different solvents are used or if the solutions are not dilute, in which ionic strength effects become significant.

The orientation of the solvent molecules around the solute molecules in solution will result in an effect that has not been accounted for in the equations given previously. When a solvent-mixture is composed of water and a liquid of low dielectric constant, water molecules will be oriented about the ions in solution, and the dielectric constant near the ion will be considerably greater than that in the bulk of the solution. Thus, when $\ln k$ is plotted against the reciprocal of the dielectric constant of the solvent mixture, deviations from the straight line predicted by equations (12–111) and (12–112) will frequently result.

A number of studies relating the dielectric constant of the solvent medium to the rate of reactions have been undertaken. Several investigations involving compounds of pharmaceutical interest are briefly reviewed here.

Amis and Holmes[17] studied the effect of the dielectric constant on the acid inversion of sucrose. When the dielectric constant was reduced by adding dioxane* to the aqueous solvent, the rate of the reaction was found to increase in accord with the theory of ion–dipole reactions as expressed by (12–112).

To determine the effect of dielectric constant on the rate of glucose decomposition in acidic solution, Heimlich and Martin[8] carried out tests in dioxane*–water mixtures. The results shown in Table 12–5 are those expected for a reaction between a positive ion and a dipole molecule. As observed in the table, the dielectric constant of the medium should be an important consideration in the stabilization of glucose solutions, since replacing water with a solvent of lower dielectric constant markedly increases the rate of breakdown of glucose. Marcus and Taraszka[18] studied the kinetics of the hydrogen-ion–catalyzed degradation of the antibiotic chloramphenicol in water–propylene glycol systems. The decrease in dielectric constant resulted in an increase in the rate of the reaction, a finding that agrees with the requirements for an ion–dipole reaction.

These findings have considerable pharmaceutical significance. The replacement of water with other solvents is often used in pharmacy as a means of stabilizing drugs against possible hydrolysis. The results of the investigations reviewed here suggest, however, that the use of a solvent mixture of lowered dielectric constant actually may increase rather than decrease the rate of decomposition. On the other hand, as pointed out by Marcus and Taraszka, a small increase in decomposition rate due to the use of nonaqueous solvents may be outweighed by enhancement of solubility of the drug in the solvent of lower dielectric constant. Thus, there is a need for thorough kinetic studies and cautious interpretations of the results before one can predict the optimum conditions for stabilizing drug products.

---

*Dioxane is toxic and cannot be used in pharmaceutical preparations. See Merck Index, 11th ed., p. 3297, 1989.

TABLE 12–5. *Decomposition of 0.278-M Solutions of Glucose at pH 1.27 and 100° C in Dioxane–Water Mixtures**

Dioxane % by Weight	Dielectric Constant of the Solvent at 100° C	Rate Constant $k \times 10^5$ hr^{-1}
0	55	4.58
9.98	48	4.95
29.74	35	6.34
49.32	22	10.30

*See footnote on page 300.

Catalysis. As already noted, the rate of a reaction is frequently influenced by the presence of a catalyst. Although the hydrolysis of sucrose in the presence of water at room temperature proceeds with a decrease in free energy, the reaction is so slow as to be negligible. When the hydrogen ion concentration is increased by adding a small amount of acid, however, inversion proceeds at a measurable rate.

A *catalyst* is therefore defined as a substance that influences the speed of a reaction without itself being altered chemically. When a catalyst decreases the velocity of a reaction, it is called a *negative catalyst*. Actually, negative catalysts often may be changed permanently during a reaction, and should be called *inhibitors* rather than catalysts.

Since a catalyst remains unaltered at the end of a reaction, it does not change the overall $\Delta G°$ of the reaction and hence, according to the relationship

$$\Delta G° = -RT \ln K$$

it cannot change the position of the equilibrium of a reversible reaction. The catalyst increases the velocity of the reverse reaction to the same extent as the forward reaction, so that although the equilibrium is reached more quickly in the presence of the catalyst, the equilibrium constant

$$K = k_{\text{forward}}/k_{\text{reverse}}$$

remains the same and the product yield is not changed.

Catalysis is considered to operate in the following way. The catalyst combines with the reactant known as the *substrate* and forms an intermediate known as a *complex*, which then decomposes to regenerate the catalyst and yield the products. In this way, the catalyst decreases the energy of activation by changing the mechanism of the process, and the rate is accordingly increased. Alternatively, a catalyst may act by producing free radicals such as $CH_3 \cdot$, which bring about fast *chain reactions*. Chain reactions are reactions consisting of a series of steps involving free atoms or radicals that act as intermediates. The chain reaction is begun by an initiating step and stopped by a chain-breaking or terminating step. Negative catalysts, or inhibitors, frequently serve as chain breakers in such reactions. Antiknock agents act as inhibitors in the explosive reactions attending the combustion of motor fuels.

Catalytic action may be homogeneous or heterogeneous and may occur in either the gaseous or liquid state. *Homogeneous catalysis* occurs when the catalyst and the reactants are in the same phase. Acid–base catalysis, the most important type of homogeneous catalysis in the liquid phase, will be discussed in some detail in the next section.

Heterogeneous catalysis occurs when the catalyst and the reactants form separate phases in the mixture. The catalyst may be a finely divided solid such as platinum, or it may be the walls of the container. The catalysis occurs at the surface of the solid and is therefore sometimes known as *contact catalysis*. The reactant molecules are adsorbed at various points or *active centers* on the rough surface of the catalyst. Presumably, the adsorption weakens the bonds of the reactant molecules and lowers the activation energy. The activated molecules then can react, and the products diffuse away from the surface.

Catalysts may be *poisoned* by extraneous substances that are strongly adsorbed at the active centers of the catalytic surface where the reactants would normally be held during reaction. Carbon monoxide is known to poison the catalytic action of copper in the hydrogenation of ethylene. Other substances, known as *promoters*, are found to increase the activity of a catalyst. For example, cupric ions promote the catalytic action of ferric ions in the decomposition of hydrogen peroxide. The exact mechanism of promoter action is not understood, although the promoter is thought to change the properties of the surface so as to enhance the adsorption of the reactants and thus increase the catalytic activity.

Specific Acid–Base Catalysis. Solutions of a number of drugs undergo accelerated decomposition upon the addition of acids or bases. If the drug solution is buffered, the decomposition may not be accompanied by an appreciable change in the concentration of acid or base, so that the reaction may be considered to be catalyzed by hydrogen or hydroxyl ions. When the rate law for such an accelerated decomposition is found to contain a term involving the concentration of hydrogen ion or the concentration of hydroxyl ion, the reaction is said to be subject to *specific acid–base catalysis*.

As an example of specific acid–base catalysis, we may consider the pH dependence for the hydrolysis of esters. In acidic solution, we can consider the hydrolysis to involve an initial equilibrium between the esters and a hydrogen ion followed by a rate-determining reaction with water, *R:*

$$S + H^+ \rightleftharpoons SH^+$$

$$SH^+ + R \rightarrow P$$

This general reaction scheme assumes that the products, *P*, of the hydrolysis reaction do not recombine to form ester.

For the generalized reaction, the rate of product formation is given by

$$\frac{dP}{dt} = k[SH^+][R] \qquad (12\text{–}113)$$

The concentration of the conjugate acid SH^+ can be expressed in terms of measurable quantities, because the pre-equilibrium requires that

$$K = \frac{[SH^+]}{[S][H^+]} \quad (12\text{--}114)$$

Thus,

$$[SH^+] = K[S][H^+] \quad (12\text{--}115)$$

and it follows that

$$\frac{dP}{dt} = kK[S][H^+][R] \quad (12\text{--}116)$$

Since water, R, is present in great excess, equation (12–116) reduces to the apparent rate law

$$\frac{dP}{dt} = k_1[S][H^+] \quad (12\text{--}117)$$

in which

$$k_1 = kK[R] \quad (12\text{--}118)$$

The hydrogen ion concentration term in equation (12–117) indicates that the process is a specific hydrogen-ion–catalyzed reaction.

By studying the acid-catalyzed hydrolysis of an ester at various concentrations of hydrogen ion—that is, by hydrolyzing the ester in buffer solutions of differing pH—we can obtain a rate–pH profile for the reaction. At a given pH, an apparent first-order reaction is observed:

$$\frac{dP}{dt} = k_{obs}[S] \quad (12\text{--}119)$$

in which

$$k_{obs} = k_1[H^+] \quad (12\text{--}120)$$

Taking logarithms of equation (12–120)

$$\log k_{obs} = \log [H^+] + \log k_1 \quad (12\text{--}121)$$

or, equivalently,

$$\log k_{obs} = -(-\log [H^+]) + \log k_1 \quad (12\text{--}122)$$

We finally arrive at the expression

$$\log k_{obs} = -pH + \log k_1 \quad (12\text{--}123)$$

Thus, a plot of $\log k_{obs}$ against the pH of the solution in which the reaction is run gives a line of slope equal to -1.

Consider, now, the specific hydroxide-ion–catalyzed decomposition of an ester, S. We may write the general reaction as

$$S + OH^- \rightarrow P$$

and the rate of product (P) formation is therefore given by

$$\frac{dP}{dt} = k_2[S][OH^-] \quad (12\text{--}124)$$

Under buffer conditions, an apparent first-order reaction is again observed:

$$\frac{dP}{dt} = k_{obs}[S] \quad (12\text{--}125)$$

in which now

$$k_{obs} = k_2[OH^-] \quad (12\text{--}126)$$

or, since

$$K_w = [H^+][OH^-] \quad (12\text{--}127)$$

$$k_{obs} = \frac{k_2 K_w}{[H^+]} \quad (12\text{--}128)$$

Taking the logarithm of equation (12–128)

$$\log k_{obs} = -\log [H^+] + \log k_2 K_w \quad (12\text{--}129)$$

we find that

$$\log k_{obs} = pH + \log k_2 K_w \quad (12\text{--}130)$$

In this case, a plot of $\log k_{obs}$ against pH should be linear with a slope equal to $+1$.

Figure 12–8 shows the rate–pH profile for the specific acid–base–catalyzed hydrolysis of methyl-*dl-o*-phenyl-2-piperidylacetate.[19] It is noted that an increase in pH from 1 to 3 results in a linear decrease in rate, as expected from equation (12–123), for specific hydrogen ion catalysis, while a further increase in pH from about 3 to 7 results in a linear increase in rate, as expected from equation (12–130), for specific hydroxide ion catalysis. Near pH 3, a minimum is observed that cannot be attributed to either hydrogen ion or hydroxyl ion participation in the reaction. This minimum is indicative of a solvent catalytic effect; that is, un-ionized water may be considered as the reacting species. Because of the pH independence of this reaction, the rate law is given by

$$\frac{dP}{dt} = k_0[S] \quad (12\text{--}131)$$

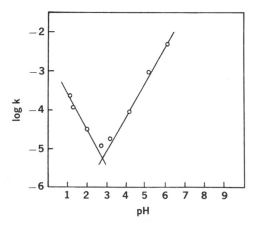

Fig. 12–8. Rate–pH profile for the specific acid–base catalyzed hydrolysis of methyl-dl-o-phenyl-2-piperidylacetate. (After S. Siegel, L. Lachmann, and L. Malspeis, J. Pharm. Sci. 48, 431, 1959, reproduced with permission of the copyright owner.)

so that

$$k_{\text{obs}} = k_0 \qquad (12\text{--}132)$$

Sometimes a minimum plateau extends over a limited pH region, indicating that solvent catalysis is the primary mode of reaction in this region.

Solvent catalysis may occur simultaneously with specific hydrogen ion or specific hydroxide ion catalysis, especially at pH values that are between the pH regions in which definitive specific ion and solvent catalytic effects are observed. Since each catalytic pathway leads to an increase in the same product, the rate law for this intermediate pH region may be written

$$\frac{dP}{dt} = (k_0{}' + k_1[\text{H}^+])[\text{S}] \qquad (12\text{--}133)$$

or

$$\frac{dP}{dt} = (k_0 + k_2[\text{OH}^-])[\text{S}] \qquad (12\text{--}134)$$

depending, respectively, on whether the pH is slightly lower or slightly higher than that for the solvent catalyzed case.

We may now summarize the pH dependency of specific acid–base–catalyzed reactions in terms of the general rate law

$$\frac{dP}{dt} = (k_0 + k_1[\text{H}^+] + k_2[\text{OH}^-])[\text{S}] \qquad (12\text{--}135)$$

for which

$$k_{\text{obs}} = k_0 + k_1[\text{H}^+] + k_2[\text{OH}^-] \qquad (12\text{--}136)$$

At low pH, the term $k_1[\text{H}^+]$ is greater than k_0 or $k_2[\text{OH}^-]$ because of the greater concentration of hydrogen ions, and specific hydrogen ion catalysis is observed. Similarly, at high pH at which the concentration of $[\text{OH}^-]$ is greater, the term $k_2[\text{OH}^-]$ outweighs the k_0 and $k_1[\text{H}^+]$ terms, and specific hydroxyl ion catalysis is observed. When the concentrations of H^+ and OH^- are low, or if the products $k_1[\text{H}^+]$ and $k_2[\text{OH}^-]$ are small in value, only k_0 is important, and the reaction is said to be *solvent catalyzed*. If the pH of the reaction medium is slightly acidic, so that k_0 and $k_1[\text{H}^+]$ are important and $k_2[\text{OH}^-]$ is negligible, both solvent and specific hydrogen ion catalysis operate simultaneously. A similar result is obtained when the pH of the medium is slightly alkaline, a condition that could allow concurrent solvent and specific hydroxide ion catalysis.

General Acid–Base Catalysis. In most systems of pharmaceutical interest, buffers are used to maintain the solution at a particular pH. Often, in addition to the effect of pH on the reaction rate, there may be catalysis by one or more species of the buffer components. The reaction is then said to be subject to *general acid* or *general base catalysis* depending, respectively, on whether the catalytic components are acidic or basic.

The rate–pH profile of a reaction that is susceptible to general acid–base catalysis exhibits deviations from the behavior expected on the basis of equations (12–123) and (12–130). For example, in the hydrolysis of the antibiotic streptozotocin, rates in phosphate buffer exceed the rate expected for specific base catalysis. This effect is due to a general base catalysis by phosphate anions. Thus, the alkaline branch of the rate–pH profile for this reaction is a line whose slope is different from 1 (Fig. 12–9).[20]

Other factors, such as ionic strength or changes in the pK_a of a substrate may also lead to apparent deviations in the rate–pH profile. Verification of a general acid or general base catalysis may be made by determining the rates of degradation of a drug in a series of buffers that are all at the same pH (i.e., the ratio of salt to acid is constant) but that are prepared with an increasing concentration of buffer species. Windheuser and Higuchi,[21] using acetate buffer, found that the degradation of thiamine is unaffected at pH 3.90, where the buffer is principally acetic acid. At higher pH values, however, the rate increases in direct proportion to the concentration of acetate. In this case, acetate ion is the general base catalyst.

Webb et al.[22] demonstrated the general catalytic action of acetic acid, sodium acetate, formic acid, and sodium formate in the decomposition of glucose. The equation for the overall rate of decomposition of glucose in water in the presence of acetic acid HAc and its conjugate base Ac⁻ can be written

$$-\frac{dG}{dt} = k_0[G] + k_{\text{H}}[\text{H}^+][G] + k_A[\text{HAc}][G]$$
$$+ k_{\text{OH}}[\text{OH}^-][G] + k_B[\text{Ac}^-][G] \qquad (12\text{--}137)$$

in which $[G]$ is the concentration of glucose, k_0 is the specific reaction rate in water alone, and the other k values, known as *catalytic coefficients*, represent the specific rates associated with the various catalytic

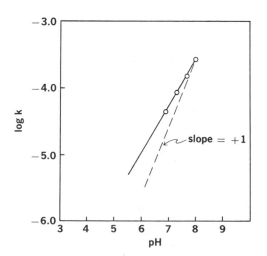

Fig. 12–9. Rate–pH profile of a reaction susceptible to general base catalysis. (After E. R. Garrett, J. Pharm. Sci. **49**, 767, 1960, reproduced with permission of the copyright owner.)

species. The overall first-order rate constant k, which involves all effects, is written as follows:

$$k = -\frac{dG/dt}{[G]} = k_0 + k_H[H^+] + k_A[HAc]$$
$$+ k_{OH}[OH^-] + k_B[Ac^-] \quad (12-138)$$

or, in general,

$$k = k_0 + \Sigma k_i c_i \quad (12-139)$$

in which c_i is the concentration of the catalytic species i and k_i is the corresponding catalytic coefficient. In reactions in which only specific acid–base effects occur, that is, in which only $[H^+]$ and $[OH^-]$ act as catalysts, the equation is

$$k = k_0 + k_H[H^+] + k_{OH}[OH^-] \quad (12-140)$$

Example 12–9. A sample of glucose was decomposed at 140° C in a solution containing 0.030 M HCl. The velocity constant k was found to be 0.0080 hr^{-1}. If the spontaneous rate constant k_0 is 0.0010 hr^{-1}, compute the catalytic coefficient k_H. The catalysis due to hydroxyl ions in this acidic solution may be considered as negligible.

The data are substituted in equation (12–140):

$$0.0080 \text{ hr}^{-1} = 0.0010 \text{ hr}^{-1} + k_H \text{ M}^{-1}\text{hr}^{-1} (0.030) \text{ M}$$

$$k_H = \frac{0.0080 \text{ hr}^{-1} - 0.0010 \text{ hr}^{-1}}{0.030 \text{ M}} = 0.233 \text{ M}^{-1} \text{ hr}^{-1}$$

In 1928, Brönsted[23] showed that a relationship exists between the catalytic power as measured by the catalytic coefficients and the strength of general acids and bases as measured by their dissociation constants. The catalytic coefficient for a weak acid is related to the dissociation constant of the acid by the expression

$$k_A = aK_a^\alpha \quad (12-141)$$

and the corresponding equation for catalysis by a weak base is

$$k_B = bK_a^{-\beta} \quad (12-142)$$

K_a is the dissociation constant of the weak acid, and a, b, α, and β are constants for a definite reaction, solvent, and temperature. From this relationship, the catalytic effect of a Brönsted–Lowry acid or base on the specific reaction rate can ·be predicted if the dissociation constant of the weak electrolyte is known. The relationships in equations (12–141) and (12–142) hold because both the catalytic power and the dissociation constant of a weak electrolyte depend on the ability of a weak acid to donate a proton or a weak base to accept a proton.

Noncatalytic salts can affect the rate constant directly through their influence on ionic strength as expressed by equation (12–109). Secondly, salts also affect the catalytic action of some weak electrolytes because, through their ionic strength effect, they change the classic dissociation constant K_a of equations (12–141) and (12–142). These two influences, known respectively as the *primary* and *secondary salt effects*, are handled in a kinetic study by carrying out the reaction under conditions of constant ionic strength, or

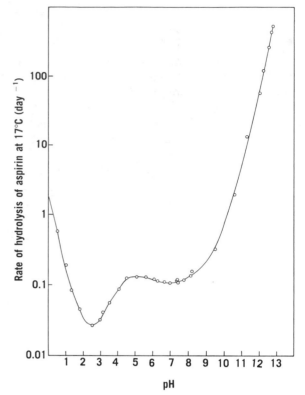

Fig. 12–10. Rate–pH profile for the hydrolysis of acetylsalicylic acid at 17° C. (After I. J. Edwards, Trans. Faraday Soc. **46**, 723, 1950.)

by obtaining a series of k values at decreasing ionic strengths and extrapolating the results to $\mu = 0$.

An interesting rate–pH profile, shown in Figure 12–10, is obtained for the hydrolysis of acetylsalicylic acid. In the range of pH 0 to about 4, there is clearly specific acid–base catalysis and a pH-independent solvolysis, as first reported by Edwards.[24] Above pH 4, there is a second pH-independent region, the plateau extending over at least 3 pH units. Fersht and Kirby[25] and others have provided suggestions for the presence of this plateau.

The hydrolysis of hydrochlorothiazide was investi-

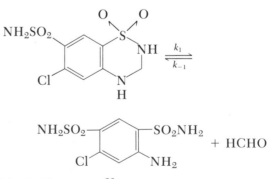

gated by Mollica et al.[26] over a pH range from 1 to 13. The reaction was found to be reversible (p. 290), the fraction that had reacted at equilibrium X_e being about 0.4. The pH profile provides a complex curve (Fig. 12–11) indicating multiple steps and an intermediate involved in the reaction.

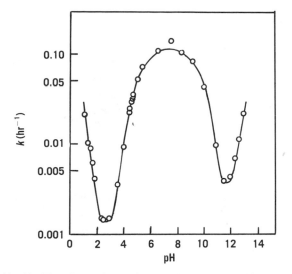

Fig. 12–11. The pH profile for the hydrolysis of hydrochlorothiazide. (From J. A. Mollica, C. R. Rohn and J. B. Smith, *J. Pharm. Sci.* **58**, 636, 1969, reproduced with permission of copyright owner.)

DECOMPOSITION AND STABILIZATION OF MEDICINAL AGENTS

In recent years, various institutions and manufacturing companies have initiated programs to study systematically the decomposition of drugs. Some of the findings, not already referred to in this chapter, are briefly reviewed here. The interested reader should consult the original papers for the details of the methods and results.

Pharmaceutical decomposition can be classified as hydrolysis, oxidation, isomerization, epimerization, and photolysis, and these processes may affect the stability of drugs in liquid, solid, and semisolid products. Mollica et al.[27] have reviewed the many effects that the ingredients of dosage forms and environmental factors may have on the chemical and physical stability of pharmaceutical preparations.

Hou and Poole[28] investigated the kinetics and mechanism of hydrolytic degradation of ampicillin in solution at 35° C and 0.5 ionic strength. The decomposition observed over a pH range of 0.8 to 10.0 followed first-order kinetics and was influenced by both specific and general acid–base catalysis. The pH–rate profile exhibited maximum stability in buffer solutions at pH 4.85 and in nonbuffered solutions at pH 5.85. The degradation rate is increased by the addition of various carbohydrates such as sucrose to the aqueous solution of ampicillin.[29] The Arrhenius plot shows the activation energy E_a to be 18 kcal/mole at pH 5 for the hydrolysis of ampicillin.

Alcohol is found to slow hydrolysis because of the decrease in the dielectric constant of the solvent. The half-life for the degradation of ampicillin in an acidified aqueous solution at 35° C is 8 hours; in a 50% alcohol solution the half-life is 13 hours.

Higuchi et al.[30] reported that chloramphenicol decomposed through hydrolytic cleavage of the amide linkage according to the reaction shown here.

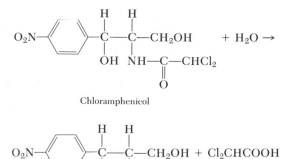

Chloramphenicol

The rate of degradation was low and independent of pH between 2 and 7 but was catalyzed by general acids and bases, including HPO_4^{2-} ions, undissociated acetic acid, and a citrate buffer. Its maximum stability occurs at pH 6 at room temperature, its half-life under these conditions being approximately 3 years. Below pH 2 the hydrolysis of chloramphenicol is catalyzed by hydrogen ions. In alkaline solution the breakdown is affected by both specific and general acid–base catalysis.[31]

The activation energy for the hydrolysis at pH 6 is 24 kcal/mole, and the half-life of the drug at pH 6 and 25° C is 2.9 years.

Beijnen et al.[32] investigated the stability of doxorubicin in aqueous solution using a stability-indicating

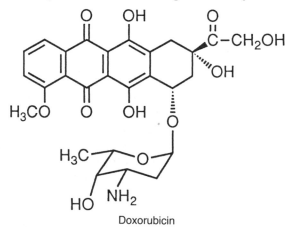

Doxorubicin

high-performance liquid chromatographic (HPLC) assay procedure. Doxorubicin has been used with success against various human neoplasms for the past 20 years. The decomposition of the drug has not been studied in depth, for it presents difficulties in analysis. It chelates with metal ions, self-associates in concentrated solutions, adsorbs to surfaces such as glass, and undergoes oxidative and photolytic decomposition.

Beijnen and associates studied the degradation kinetics of doxorubicin as a function of pH, buffer effects, ionic strength, temperature, and drug concentration. The decomposition followed pseudo–first-order kinetics at constant temperature and ionic strength at various pH values. The pH–rate profile showed maximum stability of the drug at about pH 4.5. Some study was made of the degradation in alkaline solution, other systematic work having been done only with degradation of doxorubicin in acid solution below pH 3.5. Work has also been reported on the stability of doxorubicin infusions used in clinical practice.

Steffansen and Bundgaard[33] studied the hydrolysis of erythromycin and erythromycin esters in aqueous

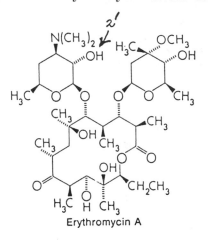

Erythromycin A

solution. Erythromycin is an antibiotic that acts against gram-positive and some gram-negative bacteria. It has the disadvantage of degradation in an acidic environment, as found in the stomach; and various methods have been suggested to protect the drug as it passes through the gastrointestinal tract. Most recent among these protective actions is the conversion of erythromycin into esters at the 2′ position. These are known as *prodrugs* (p. 513), since they are inactive until erythromycin is released from the esters by enzymatic hydrolysis in the body.

Vinckier et al.[34] studied the decomposition kinetics of erythromycin as a function of buffer type and concentration, ionic strength, pH, and temperature. Erythromycin was found to be most stable in a phosphate buffer and least stable in a sodium acetate buffer. Changes in ionic strength showed only a negligible effect on the kinetics of erythromycin. Log k–pH profiles were obtained over the pH range of about 2 to 5 and showed linearity with a slope of approximately 1, indicating specific acid catalysis in the decomposition of erythromycin at 22° C. Specific base catalysis occurs at higher pH values. Erythromycin base is most stable at pH 7 to 7.5.[35]

Atkins et al.[36] have also made a study of the kinetics of erythromycin decomposition in aqueous acidic and neutral buffers. They conclude that pH is the most important factor in controlling the stability of erythromycin A in acidic aqueous solutions.

The degradation of mitomycin C in acid solution was studied by Beijnen and Underberg.[37] Mitomycin C shows both strong antibacterial and antitumor activity. Degradation in alkaline solution involves the removal of an amino group and replacement by a hydroxyl group,

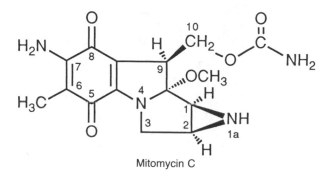

Mitomycin C

but the breakdown of mitomycin C is more complicated in acid solution, involving ring opening and the formation of two isomers, namely *trans* and *cis* mitosene (structures I and II).

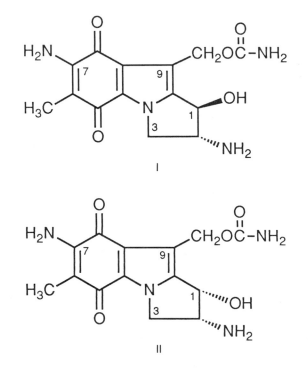

To study the mechanism of degradation the authors designed an HPLC assay that allows quantitative separation of the parent drug and its decomposition products.

The kinetics of mitomycin C in acid solution was studied at 20° C. To obtain pH values below 3 the solutions were acidified with aqueous perchloric acid, and for the pH range of 3 to 6 they were buffered with an acetic acid–acetate buffer. The degradation of mitomycin C shows first-order kinetics over a period of more than 3 half-lives.

The influence of pH and buffer species on the decomposition of mitomycin C is expressed as

$$k = k_o + k_H[\text{H}^+] + k_A[\text{HAc}] + k_B[\text{Ac}^-] \qquad (12\text{--}143)$$

in which k_o is the first-order constant for decomposition in water alone and k_H is a second-order rate constant (catalytic coefficient) associated with catalysis due to the [H$^+$]. The second-order rate constants k_A and k_B

are catalytic coefficients for catalysis by the buffer components, [HAc] and [Ac⁻], respectively (equation [12–138], p. 304). The term $k_{OH}[OH^-]$ is neglected because this study is conducted only in the acid region of the pH scale.

The log (rate-constant)–pH profile for the decomposition of mitomycin C at 20° C is seen in Figure 12–12. In other work, Beijnen and associates have shown that the inflection point in the curve is associated with the $pK_a = 2.6$ for mitomycin C. The straight-line portions of the curve—that is, below pH = 0 and above pH = 3—both exhibit slopes of approximately −1. Slopes of −1 in this region of the profile are an indication of specific acid catalysis for decomposition of the neutral form of mitomycin C (MMC) and for the protonated form (MMCH⁺).

Procaine decomposes mainly by hydrolysis, the degradation being due primarily to the breakdown of the uncharged and singly charged forms.[38] The reaction of procaine is catalyzed by hydrogen and hydroxyl ions. Both the free base and the protonated form are subject to specific base catalysis. Marcus and Baron[39] obtained an activation energy $E_a = 16.8$ kcal/mole for procaine at 97.30°. Garrett[40] has reviewed the degradation and stability of procaine.

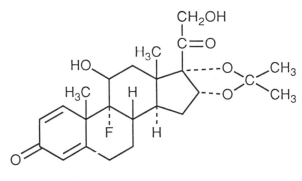

Triamcinolone Acetonide

Triamcinolone acetonide, a glucocorticoid (adrenal cortex) hormone, is a potent antiinflammatory agent when applied topically as a cream or suspension. Das Gupta[41] studied the stability of water–ethanol solutions at various pH values, buffer concentrations, and ionic strengths. The decomposition of triamcinolone acetonide followed first-order kinetics, the rate constant k_{obs} varying with the pH of phosphate, sodium hydroxide, and hydrochloric acid buffer solutions. The optimum pH for stability was found from a pH–rate profile to be about 3.4 and to be related to the concentration of the phosphate buffer. In the hydrochloric acid buffer solution, triamcinolone acetonide underwent hydrolysis to form triamcinolone and acetone. A study of the reaction in solvents of varying ionic strength showed that log k_{obs} decreased linearly with increasing values of $\sqrt{\mu}$, suggesting that reaction occurs between the protonated [H⁺] form of the drug and the phosphate buffer species, $H_2PO_4^-/HPO_4^{2-}$.

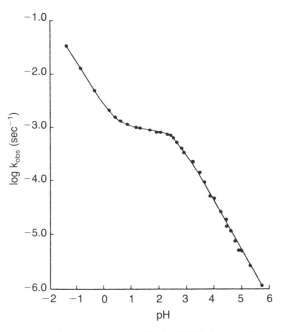

pH rate constant profile for MMC degradation at 20°C.

Fig. 12–12. pH–rate constant profile for mitomycin C decomposition. (From J. H. Beijnen and W. J. M. Underberg, Int. J. Pharm. **24**, 219, 1985, reproduced with permission of the copyright owner.)

Vincristine and vinblastine are natural alkaloids used as cytotoxic agents in cancer chemotherapy (Fig. 12–13). Vendrig et al.[42] investigated the degradation kinetics of vincristine sulfate in aqueous solution within the pH range of −2.0 to 11 at 80° C. The drug exhibited first-order kinetics under these conditions; the rate constant k_{obs} was calculated using the first-order equation (equation [12–14], p. 287) at various pH values in order to plot the pH profile as seen in Figure 12–14. The degradation rates were found to be independent of buffer concentration and ionic strength within the pH range investigated. Vincristine appears to be most stable in aqueous solution between pH 3.5 and 5.5 at 80° C.

The effect of temperature on the degradation of vincristine at various pH values from 1.2 to 8.2 and within the temperature range of 60° to 80° C was assessed using the Arrhenius equation [equation (12–72) or (12–73), p. 295]. The activation energy Ea and the Arrhenius factor A are given in Table 12–6.

Example 12–10. Vendrig et al.[42] listed the activation energies in kJ mole⁻¹ for vincristine from pH 1.2 to 8.2. Convert the values for E_a given below to quantities expressed in cal/mole, as found in Table 12–6:

pH	1.2	3.5	5.2	7.0	8.2
E_a (kJ · mole⁻¹)	62	84	73	106	116

The conversion of units is obtained by writing a sequence of ratios so as to change SI to cgs units. For the first value above, that of E_a at pH 1.2:

$$62 \, \frac{kJ}{mole} \times \frac{1000 \, J}{kJ} \times \frac{10^7 \, erg}{J} \times \frac{1 \, cal}{4.184 \times 10^7 \, erg}$$

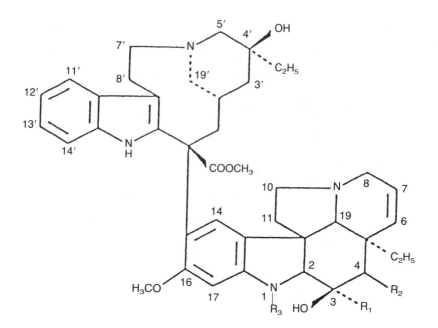

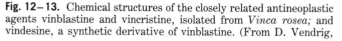

	R₁	R₂	R3
VINBLASTINE	$COOCH_3$	$OCOCH_3$	CH_3
VINCRISTINE	$COOCH_3$	$OCOCH_3$	CHO
VINDESINE	$CONH_2$	OH	CH_3

Fig. 12–13. Chemical structures of the closely related antineoplastic agents vinblastine and vincristine, isolated from *Vinca rosea;* and vindesine, a synthetic derivative of vinblastine. (From D. Vendrig, J. H. Beijnen, O. van der Houwen and J. Holthuis, Int. J. Pharm. **50**, 190, 1989, reproduced with permission of the copyright owner.)

or

$$62 \text{ mole}^{-1} \times 1000 \times 10^7 \times (1 \text{ cal}/4.184 \times 10^7) = 14818 \text{ cal/mole}$$

or

$$E_a = 1.4818 \times 10^4 \text{ cal/mole} \simeq 15 \text{ kcal/mole}$$

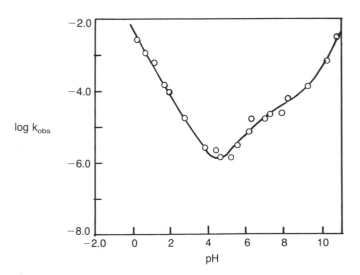

Fig. 12–14. Log k–pH profile for the decomposition of vincristine. (From D. Vendrig, J. H. Beijnen, O. van der Houwen and J. Holthuis, Int. J. Pharm. **50**, 194, 1989, reproduced with permission of the copyright owner.)

In the *CRC Handbook of Chemistry and Physics*, we find the conversion factor, 1 J = 0.239045 cal; therefore, we can make the direct conversion:

$$62000 \text{ J/mole} \times 0.239045 \text{ cal/J} = 14821 \text{ cal/mole}$$

or

$$E_a = 1.4821 \times 10^4 \text{ cal/mole}.$$

The kinetic study of the autoxidation of ascorbic acid is an interesting research story that began about 50 years ago. Some of the reports are reviewed here as an illustration of the difficulties encountered in the study of free radical reactions. Although the decomposition kinetics of ascorbic acid probably has been studied more thoroughly than that of any other drug, we are only now beginning to understand the mechanism of the autoxidation. The overall reaction may be represented as

TABLE 12–6. *Activation Energies and Arrhenius Factors for Vincristine at Various pH Values at 80° C*[42]

pH	E_a cal/mole $\times 10^{-4}$	A (sec^{-1})
1.2	1.482	1×10^6
3.5	2.008	9×10^6
5.2	1.745	4×10^5
7.0	2.534	9×10^{10}
8.2	2.773	9×10^{12}

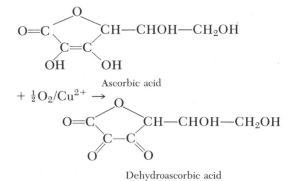

Ascorbic acid

Dehydroascorbic acid

One of the first kinetic studies of the autoxidation of ascorbic acid to dehydroascorbic acid was undertaken in 1936 by Barron et al.[43] These investigators measured the oxygen consumed in the reaction, using a Warburg type of vessel and a manometer to obtain the rate of decomposition of ascorbic acid. They found that when great care was taken to free the solution of traces of copper, ascorbic acid was not oxidized by atmospheric oxygen at a measurable rate except in alkaline solutions. Cupric ion was observed to oxidize ascorbic acid rapidly to dehydroascorbic acid, and KCN and CO were found to break the reaction chain by forming stable complexes with copper.

Dekker and Dickinson[44] suggested a scheme for oxidation of ascorbic acid by the cupric ion and obtained the following equations for the decomposition:

$$-\frac{d[H_2A]}{dt} = k\,\frac{[Cu^{2+}][H_2A]}{[H^+]^2} \qquad (12\text{–}144)$$

and in the integrated form,

$$k = \frac{2.303[H^+]^2}{[Cu^{2+}]t}\log\frac{[H_2A]_0}{[H_2A]} \qquad (12\text{–}145)$$

in which $[H_2A]_0$ is the initial concentration, and $[H_2A]$ is the concentration of ascorbic acid at time t. The experimental results compared favorably with those calculated from equation (12–145), and it was assumed that the initial reaction involved a slow oxidation of the ascorbate ion by cupric ion to a semiquinone, which was immediately oxidized by oxygen to dehydroascorbic acid. As the reaction proceeded, however, the specific reaction rate k was found to increase gradually.

Dekker and Dickinson observed that the reaction was retarded by increasing the initial concentration of ascorbic acid, presumably because ascorbic acid depleted the free oxygen. When oxygen was continually bubbled through the mixture, the specific rate of decomposition did not decrease with increasing ascorbic acid concentration.

Weissberger et al.[45] showed that the autoxidation of ascorbic acid involved both a singly and a doubly charged anion of L-ascorbic acid. Oxygen was found to react with the divalent ion at atmospheric pressure about 10^5 times as fast as with the monovalent ion of the acid at ordinary temperatures when metal catalysis was repressed. When copper ions were added to the reaction mixture, however, it was found that only the singly charged ion reaction was catalyzed. Copper was observed to be an extremely effective catalyst, since 2×10^{-4} mole/liter increased the rate of the monovalent ion reaction by a factor of 10,000.

Nord[46] showed that the rate of the copper-catalyzed autoxidation of ascorbic acid was a function of the concentrations of the monovalent ascorbate anion, the cuprous ion, the cupric ion, and the hydrogen ion in the solution. The kinetic scheme proposed by Nord appears to compare well with experimental findings.

Blaug and Hajratwala[47] observed that ascorbic acid degraded by aerobic oxidation according to the log rate constant–pH profile of Figure 12–15. The effects of buffer species were eliminated, so that only the catalysis due to hydrogen and hydroxyl ions was considered. Dehydroascorbic acid, the recognized breakdown product of ascorbic acid, was found to decompose further into ketogulonic acid, which then formed threonic and oxalic acids.

According to Rogers and Yacomeni,[48] ascorbic acid exhibits maximum degradation at pH 4 and minimum degradation at pH 5.6 in citric acid–phosphate buffers in the presence of excess oxygen at 25° C. The pH–rate profile can be fit closely to the experimental points using first- and second-order rate constants; $k_1 = 5.7 \times 10^{-6}\,M^{-1}s^{-1}$, $k_2 = 1.7\,s^{-1}$, and $k_3 = 7.4 \times 10^{-5}\,M^{-1}s^{-1}$ in the rate expression

$$k = k_1\,[H^+] + k_2 + k_3\,[OH^-] \qquad (12\text{–}146)$$

in which k_2 is the first-order solvent catalysis term, ordinarily written k_o, and k_1 and k_3 are the catalytic coefficients.

Takamura and Ito[49] studied the effect of metal ions and flavonoids on the oxidation of ascorbic acid, using polarography at pH 5.4. Transition metal ions increased the rate of first-order oxidation; the rate was increased by 50% in the presence of Cu^{2+}. Flavonoids are yellow

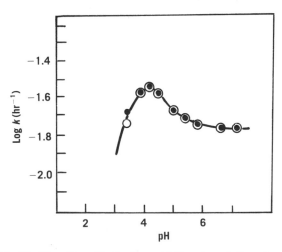

Fig. 12–15. The pH profile for the oxidative degradation of ascorbic acid. (From S. M. Blaug and B. Hajratwala, J. Pharm. Sci. **61**, 556, 1972; **63**, 1240, 1974, reproduced with permission of the copyright owner.) Key: ●, calculated rate constant; ○, rate constant extrapolated to zero buffer concentration where only the effect of hydrogen and/or hydroxyl ions is accounted for.

pigments found in higher plants. The flavonoid constituents, rutin and hesperidan, were used in the past to reduce capillary fragility and bleeding.[50] Takamura and Ito found that flavonoids inhibited the Cu^{2+}-catalyzed oxidation in the order of effectiveness: 3-hydroxyflavone < rutin < quercitin. This order of inhibition corresponded to the order of complexation of Cu^{2+} by the flavonoids, suggesting that the flavonoids inhibit Cu^{2+}-catalyzed oxidation by tying up the copper ion in solution.

Oxidation rates under conditions similar to those in pharmaceutical systems were examined by Fyhr and Brodin.[51] They investigated the iron-catalyzed oxidation of ascorbic acid at 35° C, at pH values of 4 to 6, at partial pressures of oxygen of 21 kPa (21 kilopascal), and at iron concentrations between 0.16 and 1.25 ppm. These workers found the oxidation of ascorbic acid to be first-order with respect to the total ascorbic acid concentration. Trace-element analysis was used to follow changes in iron concentration.

Akers[52] studied the *standard oxidation potentials* (pp. 207–209) of antioxidants in relation to stabilization of epinephrine in aqueous solution. He found that ascorbic acid or a combination of 0.5% thiourea with 0.5% acetylcysteine was the most effective in stabilizing parenteral solutions of epinephrine.

Thoma and Struve[53] attempted to protect epinephrine solutions from oxidative degradation by the addition of redox stabilizers (antioxidants) such as ascorbic acid. Sodium metabisulfite, $Na_2S_2O_5$, prevented discoloration of epinephrine solutions but improved the stability only slightly. The best stabilization of epinephrine in solution was provided by the use of nitrogen.

The decomposition of a new antiasthmatic agent (abbreviated here as HPAMB), which acts therapeutically by contraction of vascular and pulmonary smooth muscles, was investigated in the presence and absence of the antioxidant ascorbic acid, in phosphate buffer (pH 7.9), and in aqueous solution (pH 7.1).[54] As observed in Figure 12–16, the drug broke down rapidly

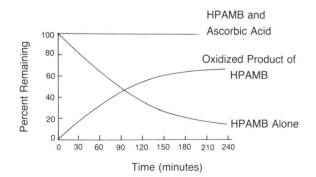

Fig. 12–16. Decomposition of HPAMB alone and in the presence of ascorbic acid. The curve for the oxidized product resulting from HPAMB breakdown is also shown. (From A. B. C. Yu and G. A. Portman, J. Pharm. Sci. **79**, 915, 1990, reproduced with permission of the copyright owner.)

at 25° C in water in the absence of ascorbic acid, whereas no loss in drug concentration occurred in the presence of 0.1% ascorbic acid. In two nonaqueous solvents, ethanol and dimethyl sulfoxide, the oxidative decomposition rate of HPAMB was much slower than in aqueous solution.

Influence of Light. Photodegradation. Light is not classified as a catalyst, and its effect on chemical reactions is treated as a separate topic. Light energy, like heat, may provide the activation necessary for a reaction to occur. Radiation of the proper frequency and of sufficient energy must be absorbed to activate the molecules. The energy unit of radiation is known as the *photon* and is equivalent to 1 *quantum* of energy. Photochemical reactions do not depend on temperature for activation of the molecules; therefore, the rate of activation in such reactions is independent of temperature. After a molecule has absorbed a quantum of radiant energy, however, it may collide with other molecules, raising their kinetic energy, and the temperature of the system will therefore increase. The initial photochemical reaction may often be followed by thermal reactions.

The study of photochemical reactions requires strict attention to control of the wavelength and intensity of light and the number of photons actually absorbed by the material. Reactions that occur by photochemical activation are usually complex and proceed by a series of steps. The rates and mechanisms of the stages can be elucidated through a detailed investigation of all factors involved, but in this elementary discussion of the effect of light on pharmaceuticals, we will not go into such considerations.

Examples of photochemical reactions of interest in pharmacy and biology are the irradiation of ergosterol and the process of photosynthesis. When ergosterol is irradiated with light in the ultraviolet region, vitamin D is produced. In photosynthesis, carbon dioxide and water are combined in the presence of a photosensitizer, chlorophyll. Chlorophyll absorbs visible light, and the light then brings about the photochemical reaction in which carbohydrates and oxygen are formed.

Some studies involving the influence of light on medicinal agents are reviewed here.

Moore[55] described the kinetics of photooxidation of benzaldehyde as determined by measuring the oxygen consumption with a polarographic oxygen electrode. Photooxidation of drugs is initiated by ultraviolet radiation according to one of two classes of reactions. The first is a free radical chain process in which a sensitizer, for example, benzophenone, abstracts a hydrogen atom from the drug. The free radical drug adds a molecule of oxygen and the chain is propagated by removing a hydrogen atom from another molecule of oxidant, a hydroperoxide, which may react further by a nonradical mechanism. The scheme for initiation, propagation, and termination of the chain reaction is shown in Figure 12–17.

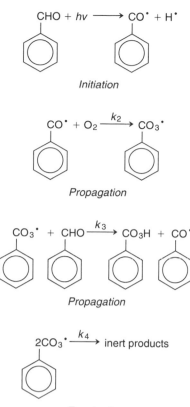

Fig. 12–17. Steps in the photooxidation of benzaldehyde. (From D. E. Moore, J. Pharm. Sci. **65**, 1449, 1976. Reproduced with permission of the copyright owner.)

The second class of photooxidation is initiated by a dye such as methylene blue.

A manometer is usually used to measure the rate of absorption of oxygen from the gas phase into a stirred solution of the oxidizing drug. In some cases, as in the oxidation of ascorbic acid, spectrophotometry may be used if the absorption spectra of the reactant and product are sufficiently different. An oxygen electrode or galvanic cell oxygen analyzer has also been used to measure the oxygen consumption.

Earlier studies of the photooxidation of benzaldehyde in *n*-decane solution showed that the reaction involved a free radical mechanism. Moore proposed to show whether a free radical process also occurred in a dilute aqueous solution and to study the antioxidant efficiency of some polyhydric phenols. The photooxidation of benzaldehyde was found to follow a free radical mechanism, and efficiency of the polyhydric phenolic antioxidants ranked as follows: catechol > pyrogallol > hydroquinone > resorcinol > *n*-propyl gallate. These antioxidants could be classified as retarders rather than inhibitors for they slowed the rate of oxidation but did not inhibit the reaction.

Asker et al.[56] investigated the photostabilizing effect of DL-methionine on ascorbic acid solution. A 10-mg% concentration of DL-methionine was found to enhance the stability of a 40-mg% solution of ascorbic acid buffered by phosphate but not by citrate at pH 4.5.

Uric acid was found[57] to produce a photoprotective effect in buffered and unbuffered solutions of sulfathiazole sodium. The addition of 0.1% sodium sulfite assisted in preventing the discoloration of the sulfathiazole solution prepared in either a borate or a phosphate buffer.

Furosemide (Lasix) is a potent diuretic, available as tablets and as a sterile solution for injection. It is fairly stable in alkaline solution but degrades rapidly in acid solution.

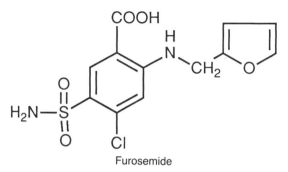

Furosemide

Irradiation of furosemide with 365 nm of ultraviolet light in alkaline solutions and in methanol results in photooxidation and reduction, respectively, to yield a number of products. The drug is relatively stable in ordinary daylight or under fluorescent (room) lighting, but has a half-life of only about 4 hours in direct sunlight. Bundgaard et al.[58] discovered that it is the un-ionized acid form of furosemide that is most sensitive to photodegradation. In addition to investigating the photoliability of furosemide, these workers also studied the degradation of the ethyl, dimethylglycolamide, and diethylglycolamide esters of furosemide and found them to be very unstable in solutions of pH 2 to 9.5 in both daylight and artificial room lighting. The half-lives of photodegradation for the esters were 0.5 to 1.5 hours.

Andersin and Tammilehto[59] noted that apparent first-order photokinetics had been shown by other workers for adriamycin, furosemide, menadione, nifedipine, sulfacetamide, and theophylline. Photodegradation of the tromethamine* salt of ketorolac, an analgesic and antiinflammatory agent, appeared in ethanol to be an exception;[59] it showed apparent first-order kinetics at low concentrations, ≤2.0 μg/mL, of the drug (Fig. 12–18a). When the concentration of ketorolac tromethamine became ≥10 μg/mL, however, the kinetics exhibited non–first-order rates. That is to say, the plots of drug concentration versus irradiation time were no longer linear but rather were bowed at these higher concentrations (Fig. 12–18b).[60]

Nifedipine is a calcium antagonist used in coronary artery disease and in hypertension; unfortunately, it is sensitive to light both in solution and in the solid state.

*Tromethamine is "tris buffer," or TRIS, aminohydroxymethylpropanediol.

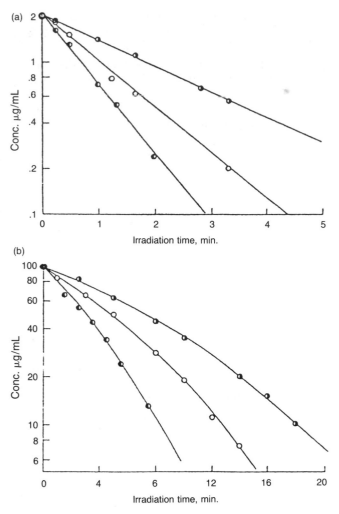

Fig. 12-18. A semilogarithmic plot of the photolysis of ketorolac tromethamine in ethyl alcohol. Key: ◑ under argon; ○ under air; ◐ under oxygen. *(a)* At low drug concentrations; *(b)* at high drug concentrations. (From L. Gu, H. Chiang and D. Johnson, Int. J. Pharm. **41**, 109, 1988. Reproduced with permission of the copyright owner.)

Matsuda et al.[61] studied the photodegradation of nifedipine in the solid state when exposed to the radiation of mercury vapor and fluorescent light sources. The drug decomposed into four compounds, the main photoproduct being a nitrosopyridine. It readily degraded in ultraviolet and visible light with maximum decomposition occurring at a wavelength of about 380 nm $(3.80 \times 10^{-7}$ meter). The rate of degradation of nifedipine was much faster when exposed to a mercury vapor lamp than when subjected to the rays of a fluorescent lamp; however, the degradation in the presence of both light sources exhibited first-order kinetics. The drug is more sensitive to light when in solution. The photodecomposition of nifedipine in the crystalline solid state was found to be directly related to the *total irradiation intensity*. The total intensity was used as a convenient parameter to measure accelerated photodecomposition of nifedipine in the solid state and thus to estimate its photostability under ordinary conditions of light irradiation.

The photosensitivity of the dye FD&C Blue No. 2 causes its solution to fade and gradually to become colorless. Asker and Collier[62] studied the influence of an ultraviolet absorber, uric acid, on the photostability of FD&C Blue No. 2 in glycerin and triethanolamine. They found that the greater the concentration of uric acid in triethanolamine the more photoprotection was afforded the dye. Glycerin was not a suitable solvent for the photoprotector since glycerin accelerates the rate of color fading, possibly owing to its dielectric constant effect.

As would be expected for a reaction that is a function of light radiation and color change rather than concentration, these reactions follow zero-order kinetics. Photodegradation reactions of chlorpromazine, menadione, reserpine, and colchicine are also kinetically zero-order.

Asker and Colbert[63] assessed the influence of various additives on the photostabilizing effect that uric acid has on solutions of FD&C Blue No. 2. The agents tested for their synergistic effects belong to the classes: antioxidants, chelating agents, surfactants, sugars, and preservatives. It was found that the antioxidants DL-methionine and DL-leucine accelerated the photodegradation of the FD&C Blue No. 2 solutions. The addition of the surfactant Tween 80 (polysorbate 80) increased the photodegradation of the dye, as earlier reported by Kowarski[64] and other workers. Lactose has been shown by these authors and others to accelerate the color loss of FD&C Blue No. 2, and the addition of uric acid retards the photodegradation caused by the sugar. Likewise, methylparaben accelerates the fading of the blue color and the addition of uric acid counteracts this color loss. Chelating agents, such as disodium edetate (EDTA disodium) significantly increased the rate of color loss of the dye. EDTA disodium has also been reported to increase the rate of degradation of epinephrine, physostigmine, and isoproterenol, and it accelerates the photodegradation of methylene blue and riboflavin. Acids, such as tartaric and citric, tend to increase the fading of dye solutions.

Asker and Jackson[65] found a photoprotective effect by dimethyl sulfoxide on FD&C Red No. 3 solutions exposed to long- and short-wave ultraviolet light. Fluorescent light was more detrimental to photostability of the dye solution than were the ultraviolet light sources.

KINETICS IN THE SOLID STATE

The breakdown of drugs in the solid state is an important topic, but it has not been studied extensively in pharmacy. The subject has been reviewed by Garrett,[66] Lachman,[67] and Carstensen,[68] and is discussed here briefly.

Pure Solids. The decomposition of pure solids, as contrasted with the more complex mixture of ingredients in a dosage form, has been studied, and a number of theories have been proposed to explain the shapes of the curves obtained when decomposition of the compound is plotted against time. Carstensen and Musa[69] described the decomposition of solid benzoic acid derivatives, such as aminobenzoic acid, which broke down into the liquid, aniline, and the gas, carbon dioxide. The plot of concentration of decomposed drug vs. time yielded a sigmoidal curve (Fig. 12–19). After liquid begins to form, the decomposition becomes a first-order reaction in the solution. Such single-component pharmaceutical systems can degrade by either zero-order or first-order reaction, as observed in Figure 12–19. It is often diffficult to determine which pattern is being followed when the reaction cannot be carried through a sufficient number of half-lives to differentiate between zero- and first-order.

Solid Dosage Forms. The decomposition of drugs in solid dosage forms is understandably more complex than decay occurring in the pure state of the individual compound. The reactions may be zero- or first-order, but in some cases, as with pure compounds, it is difficult to distinguish between the two. Tardif[70] observed that ascorbic acid decomposed in tablets followed a pseudo-first-order reaction.

In tablets and other solid dosage forms, the possibility exists for solid–solid interaction. Carstensen et al.[71] have devised a program to test for possible incompatibilities of the drug with excipients present in the solid mixture. The drug is blended with various excipients in the presence and absence of 5% moisture, sealed in vials, and stored for 2 weeks at 55° C. Visual observation is done and the samples are tested for chemical interaction using thin-layer chromatography. The method is qualitative but, in industrial preformulation, provides a useful screening technique to uncover possible incompatibilities between active ingredient and

pharmaceutical additives before deciding upon a suitable dosage form.

Lach and associates[72] used diffuse reflectance spectroscopy to measure interactions of additives and drugs in solid dosage forms. Blaug and Huang[73] used this spectroscopic technique to study the interaction of spray-dried lactose with dextroamphetamine sulfate.

Goodhart and associates[74] studied the fading of colored tablets by light (photolysis reaction) and plotted the results as color difference at various light energy values expressed in foot-candle hours.

Lachman, Cooper, and their associates[75] conducted a series of studies on the decomposition of FD&C colors in tablets and established a pattern of three separate stages of breakdown. The photolysis was found to be a surface phenomenon, causing fading of the tablet color to a depth of about 0.03 cm. Interestingly, fading did not occur further into the coating with continued light exposure, and the protected contents of the color-coated tablets were not adversely affected by exposure to light.

As noted by Monkhouse and Van Campen[76] solid-state reactions exhibit characteristics quite different than reactions in the liquid or gaseous state since the molecules of the solid are in the crystalline state. The quantitative and theoretical approaches to the study of solid-state kinetics is at its frontier, which, when opened, will probably reveal a new and fruitful area of chemistry and drug science. The authors[76] classify solid-state reactions as *addition* when two solids, A and B, interact to form the new solid AB. For example, picric acid reacts with naphthols to form what is referred to as *picrates*. A second kind of solid-state reaction is an *exchange* process in which solid A reacts with solid BC to form solid AB and release solid C. Solid–gas reactions constitute another class in which the oxidation of solid ascorbic acid and solid fumagillin are notable examples. Other types of solid-state processes include polymorphic transitions, sublimation, dehydration, and thermal decomposition.

Monkhouse and Van Campen[76] review the experimental methods used in solid-state kinetics, including reflectance spectroscopy, x-ray diffraction, thermal analysis, microscopy, dilatometry, and gas pressure–volume analysis. The review closes with sections on handling solid-state reaction data, temperature effects, application of the Arrhenius plot, equilibria expressions involved in solid-state degradation, and use of the van't Hoff equation for, say, a solid drug hydrate in equilibrium with its dehydrated form.

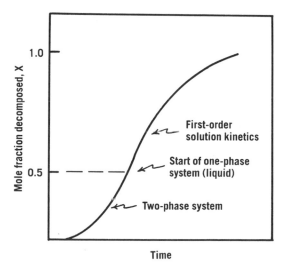

Fig. 12–19. Decomposition of a pure crystalline solid such as potassium permanganate, which involves gaseous reaction products. (From J. T. Carstensen, *J. Pharm. Sci.* **63**, 4, 1974, reproduced with permission of the copyright owner.)

ACCELERATED STABILITY ANALYSIS

In the past it was the practice in many pharmaceutical manufacturing companies to evaluate the stability of pharmaceutical preparations by observing them for a year or more, corresponding to the normal time that

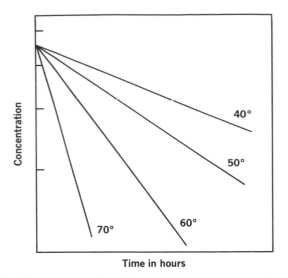

Fig. 12–20. Accelerated breakdown of a drug in aqueous solution at elevated temperature.

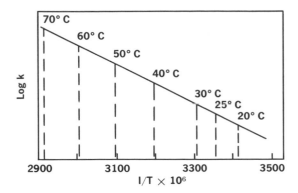

Fig. 12–21. Arrhenius plot for predicting drug stability at room temperatures.

$$t = \frac{2.303}{2.09 \times 10^{-5}} \log \frac{94}{45} = 3.5 \times 10^4 \text{ hr} \cong 4 \text{ years}$$

they would remain in stock and in use. Such a method was time-consuming and uneconomical. Accelerated studies at higher temperatures were also used by most companies, but the criteria were often arbitrary and were not based on fundamental kinetic principles. For example, some companies used the rule that the storage of liquids at 37° C accelerated the decomposition at twice the normal-temperature rate, while other manufacturers assumed that it accelerated the breakdown by 20 times normal. Levy[77] has pointed out that such arbitrary temperature coefficients of stability cannot be assigned to all liquid preparations and other classes of pharmaceuticals. The prediction of shelf-life must come instead from carefully designed analysis of the various ingredients in each product if the results are to be meaningful.

The method of accelerated testing of pharmaceutical products based on the principles of chemical kinetics was demonstrated by Garrett and Carper.[2] According to this technique, the k values for the decomposition of a drug in solution at various elevated temperatures are obtained by plotting some function of concentration against time, as seen in Figure 12–20 and already discussed in the early sections of this chapter. The logarithms of the specific rates of decomposition are then plotted against the reciprocals of the absolute temperatures as shown in Figure 12–21, and the resulting line is extrapolated to room temperature. The $k_{25°}$ is used to obtain a measure of the stability of the drug under ordinary shelf conditions.

Example 12–11. The initial concentration of a drug decomposing according to first-order kinetics is 94 units/mL. The specific decomposition rate k obtained from an Arrhenius plot is 2.09×10^{-5} hr^{-1} at room temperature, 25° C. Previous experimentation has shown that when the concentration of the drug falls below 45 units/mL it is not sufficiently potent for use and should be removed from the market. What expiration date should be assigned to this product?

$$t = \frac{2.303}{k} \log \frac{c_0}{c}$$

Free and Blythe and, more recently, Amirjahed[78] and his associates have suggested a similar method in which the fractional life-period (cf. *Example 12–2*) is plotted against reciprocal temperatures, and the time in days required for the drug to decompose to some fraction of its original potency at room temperature is obtained. The approach is illustrated in Figures 12–22 and 12–23. As observed in Figure 12–22, the log percent of drug remaining is plotted against time in days, and the time for the potency to fall to 90% of the original value, (i.e., t_{90}), is read from the graph. In Figure 12–23, the log time to 90% is then plotted against $1/T$, and the time at 25° C gives the shelf-life of the product in days. The decomposition data illustrated in Figure 12–22 result in a t_{90} value of 199 days. Shelf-life and expiration dates are estimated in this way; Baker and Niazi[79] have pointed out limitations of the method.

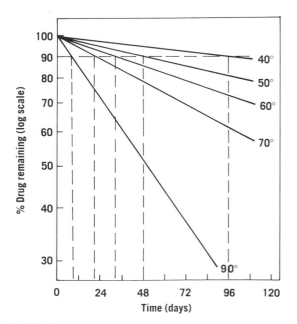

Fig. 12–22. Time in days required for drug potency to fall to 90% of original value. These times, designated t_{90}, are then plotted on a log scale in Figure 12–23.

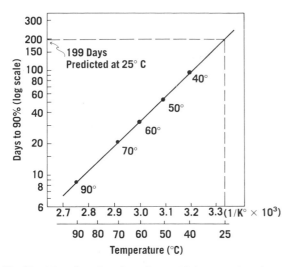

Fig. 12–23. A log plot of t_{90} (i.e., time to 90% potency) on the vertical axis against reciprocal temperature (both Kelvin and centigrade scales are shown) on the horizontal axis.

By either of these methods, the *overage*, that is, the excess quantity of drug that must be added to the preparation to maintain at least 100% of the labeled amount during the expected shelf-life of the drug, can be easily calculated and added to the preparation at the time of manufacture.

An improved approach to stability evaluation is that of nonisothermal kinetics, introduced by Rogers[80] in 1963. The activation energy, reaction rates, and stability predictions are obtained in a single experiment by programming the temperature to change at a predetermined rate. Temperature and time are related through an appropriate function, such as

$$1/T = 1/T_0 + at \qquad (12\text{–}147)$$

where T_0 is the initial temperature and a is a reciprocal heating rate constant. At any time during the run, the Arrhenius equation for time zero and time t may be written

$$\ln k_t = \ln k_0 - \frac{E_a}{R}\left(\frac{1}{T_t} - \frac{1}{T_0}\right) \qquad (12\text{–}148)$$

and substituting (12–147) into (12–148) yields

$$\ln k_t = \ln k_0 - \frac{E_a}{R}(at) \qquad (12\text{–}149)$$

Since temperature is a function of the time, t, a measure of stability, k_t, is directly obtained over a range of temperatures. A number of variations have been made on the method,[81–84] and it is now possible to change the heating rate during a run or combine programmed heating rate with isothermal studies and receive printouts of activation energy, order of reaction, and stability estimates for projected times and at various temperatures.

Although kinetic methods need not involve detailed studies of mechanism of degradation in the prediction of stability, they do demand the application of sound scientific principles if they are to be an improvement over extended room-temperature studies. Furthermore, before an older method, although somewhat less than wholly satisfactory, is discarded, the new technique should be put through a preliminary trial period and studied critically. Some general precautions regarding the use of accelerated testing methods are appropriate at this point.

In the first place, it should be re-emphasized that the results obtained from a study of the degradation of a particular component in a vehicle cannot be applied arbitrarily to other liquid preparations in general. As Garrett[85] has pointed out, however, once the energy of activation is known for a component, it probably is valid to continue to use this value although small changes of concentration (e.g., addition of overage) or slight formula changes are made. The known activation energy and a single-rate study at an elevated temperature may then be used to predict the stability of that component at ordinary temperatures.

Testing methods based on the Arrhenius law are valid only when the breakdown is a thermal phenomenon with an activation energy of about 10 to 30 kcal/mole. If the reaction rate is determined by diffusion or photochemical reactions, or if the decomposition is due to freezing, contamination by microorganisms, excessive agitation during transport, and so on, an elevated temperature study is obviously of little use in predicting the life of the product. Nor can elevated temperatures be used for products containing suspending agents such as methylcellulose that coagulate on heating, proteins that may be denatured, and ointments and suppositories that melt under exaggerated temperature conditions. Emulsion breaking involves aggregation and coalescence of globules, and some emulsions are actually more stable at elevated temperatures at which Brownian movement is increased. Lachman et al.[86] reviewed the stability testing of emulsions and suspensions and the effects of packaging on the stability of dosage forms.

Statistical methods should be used to estimate the errors in rate constants, particularly when assays are based on biologic methods; this is accomplished by the method of least squares as discussed by Garrett[85] and by Westlake.[87]

The investigator should be aware that the order of a reaction may change during the period of the study. Thus, a zero-order degradation may subsequently become first-order, second-order, or fractional-order, and the activation energy may also change if the decomposition proceeds by several mechanisms. At certain temperatures, autocatalysis (i.e., acceleration of decomposition by products formed in the reaction), may occur so as to make room temperature stability predictions from an elevated temperature study impractical.

In conclusion, the investigator in the product development laboratory must recognize the limitations of accelerated studies, both the classic and the more recent kinetic type, and must distinguish between those cases in which reliable prognosis can be made and those in which, at best, only a rough indication of product stability can be obtained. Where accelerated methods are not applicable, extended aging tests must be employed under various conditions to obtain the desired information.

References and Notes

1. K. A. Connors, G. L. Amidon and V. J. Stella, *Chemical Stability of Pharmaceuticals*, 2nd Edition, Wiley, N.Y., 1986, pp. 764–773.
2. E. R. Garrett and R. F. Carper, J. Am. Pharm. Assoc., Sci. Ed. **44**, 515, 1955.
3. K. A. Connors, G. L. Amidon and V. J. Stella, ibid., p. 15.
4. J. Walker, Proc. Roy. Soc. A. **78**, 157, 1906.
5. J. R. D. McCormick, S. M. Fox, L. L. Smith, et al., J. Am. Chem. Soc. **79**, 2849, 1957.
6. D. E. Guttman and P. D. Meister, J. Am. Pharm. Assoc., Sci. Ed. **47**, 773, 1958.
7. A. E. Allen and V. D. Gupta, J. Pharm. Sci. **63**, 107, 1974; V. D. Gupta, ibid. **67**, 299, 1978.
8. K. R. Heimlich and A. Martin, J. Am. Pharm. Assoc., Sci. Ed. **49**, 592, 1960.
9. J. W. Mauger, A. N. Paruta and R. J. Gerraughty, J. Pharm. Sci. **58**, 574, 1969.
10. L. Michaelis and M. L. Menten, Biochem. Z. **49**, 333, 1913.
11. T. Higuchi, A. Havinga and L. W. Busse, J. Am. Pharm. Assoc., Sci. Ed. **39**, 405, 1950.
12. W. Yang, Drug Dev. Ind. Pharm. **7**, 717, 1981.
13. H. Eyring, Chem. Rev. **10**, 103, 1932; ibid. **17**, 65, 1935.
14. A. D. Marcus and S. Baron, J. Am. Pharm. Assoc., Sci. Ed. **48**, 85, 1959.
15. M. Richardson and F. G. Soper, J. Chem. Soc. **1873**, 1929; F. G. Soper and E. Williams, ibid. **2297**, 1935.
16. J. T. Carstensen, J. Pharm. Sci. **59**, 1141, 1970.
17. E. S. Amis and C. Holmes, J. Am. Chem. Soc. **63**, 2231, 1941.
18. A. D. Marcus and A. J. Taraszka, J. Am. Pharm. Assoc., Sci. Ed. **48**, 77, 1959.
19. S. Siegel, L. Lachman and L. Malspeis, J. Pharm. Sci. **48**, 431, 1959.
20. E. R. Garrett, J. Pharm. Sci. **49**, 767, 1960; J. Am. Chem. Soc. **79**, 3401, 1957.
21. J. J. Windheuser and T. Higuchi, J. Pharm. Sci. **51**, 354, 1962.
22. N. E. Webb, Jr., G. J. Sperandio and A. Martin, J. Am. Pharm. Assoc. Sci. Ed. **47**, 101, 1958.
23. J. N. Brönsted and K. J. Pedersen, Z. Physik. Chem. **A108**, 185, 1923; J. N. Brönsted, Chem. Rev. **5**, 231, 1928; R. P. Bell, *Acid-Base Catalysis*, Oxford University, Oxford, 1941, Chapter 5.
24. L. J. Edwards, Trans. Faraday Soc. **46**, 723, 1950; ibid. **48**, 696, 1952.
25. A. R. Fersht and A. J. Kirby, J. Am. Chem. Soc., **89**, 4857, 1967.
26. J. A. Mollica, C. R. Rehm and J. B. Smith, J. Pharm. Sci. **58**, 636, 1969.
27. J. A. Mollica, S. Ahuja and J. Cohen, J. Pharm. Sci., **67**, 443, 1978.
28. J. P. Hou and J. W. Poole, J. Pharm. Sci. **58**, 447, 1969; ibid., **58**, 1510, 1969.
29. K. A. Connors and J. A. Mollica, J. Pharm. Sci. **55**, 772, 1966; S. L. Hem, E. J. Russo, S. M. Bahal and R. S. Levi, J. Pharm. Sci. **62**, 267, 1973.
30. T. Higuchi and C. D. Bias, J. Am. Pharm. Assoc., Sci. Ed. **42**, 707, 1953; T. Higuchi, A. D. Marcus and C. D. Bias, ibid. **43**, 129, 530, 1954.
31. K. C. James and R. H. Leach, J. Pharm. Pharmacol. **22**, 607, 1970.
32. J. H. Beijnen, O. A. G. J. van der Houwen and W. J. M. Underberg, Int. J. Pharm. **32**, 123, 1986.
33. B. Steffansen and H. Bundgaard, Int. J. Pharm. **56**, 159, 1989.
34. C. Vinckier, R. Hauchecorne, Th. Cachet, G. Van den Mooter and J. Hoogmartens, Int. J. Pharm. **55**, 67, 1989; Th. Cachet, G.

Van den Mooter, R. Hauchecorne, et al., Int. J. Pharm. **55**, 59, 1989.
35. K. A. Connors, G. L. Amidon and V. J. Stella, *Chemical Stability of Pharmaceuticals*, 2nd Edition, Wiley, New York, pp. 457–462.
36. P. Atkins, T. Herbert and N. Jones, Int. J. Pharm. **30**, 199, 1986.
37. J. H. Beijnen and W. J. M. Undenberg, Int. J. Pharm. **24**, 219, 1985.
38. T. Higuchi, A. Havinga and L. W. Busse, J. Am. Pharm. Assoc., Sci. Ed. **39**, 405, 1950.
39. A. D. Marcus and S. Baron, J. Am. Pharm. Assoc., Sci. Ed. **48**, 85, 1959.
40. E. R. Garrett, J. Pharm. Sci. **51**, 811, 1962.
41. V. Das Gupta, J. Pharm. Sci. **72**, 1453, 1983.
42. D. E. M. M. Vendrig, J. H. Beijnen, O. A. G. J. van der Houwen and J. J. M. Holthuis, Int. J. Pharm. **50**, 189, 1989.
43. E. S. Barron, R. H. De Meio and F. Klemperer, J. Biol. Chem. **112**, 624, 1936.
44. A. O. Dekker and R. G. Dickinson, J. Am. Chem. Soc. **62**, 2165, 1940.
45. A. Weissberger, J. E. Lu Valle and D. S. Thomas, Jr., J. Am. Chem. Soc. **65**, 1934, 1943; A. Weissberger and J. E. Lu Valle, ibid. **66**, 700, 1944.
46. H. Nord, Acta Chem. Scand. **9**, 442, 1955.
47. S. M. Blaug and B. Hajratwala, J. Pharm. Sci. **61**, 556, 1972; ibid. **63**, 1240, 1974.
48. A. R. Rogers and J. A. Yacomeni, J. Pharm. Pharmacol. **23S**, 218S, 1971.
49. K. Takamura and M. Ito, Chem. Pharm. Bull. **25**, 3218, 1977.
50. V. E. Tyler, L. R. Brady and J. E. Robbers, *Pharmacognosy*, 7th Edition, Lea & Febiger, Philadelphia, p. 97.
51. P. Fyhr and A. Brodin, Acta Pharm. Suec. **24**, 26, 1987; Chem. Abs. **107**, 46, 202y, 1987.
52. M. J. Akers, J. Parenteral Drug Assoc. **33**, 346, 1979.
53. K. Thoma and M. Struve, Pharm. Acta Helv. **61**, 34, 1986; Chem. Abs. **104**, 174, 544m, 1986.
54. A. B. C. Yu and G. A. Portmann, J. Pharm. Sci. **79**, 913, 1990.
55. D. E. Moore, J. Pharm. Sci. **65**, 1447, 1976.
56. A. F. Asker, D. Canady and C. Cobb, Drug Dev. Ind. Pharm. **11**, 2109, 1985.
57. A. F. Asker and M. Larose, Drug Dev. Ind. Pharm. **13**, 2239, 1987.
58. H. Bundgaard, T. Norgaard and N. M. Neilsen, Int. J. Pharm. **42**, 217–224, 1988.
59. R. Andersin and S. Tammilehto, Int. J. Pharm. **56**, 175, 1989.
60. L. Gu, H.–S. Chiang and D. Johnson, Int. J. Pharm. **41**, 105, 1988.
61. Y. Matsuda, R. Teraoka and I. Sugimoto, Int. J. Pharm. **54**, 211, 1989.
62. A. F. Asker and A. Collier, Drug Dev. Ind. Pharm. **7**, 563, 1981.
63. A. F. Asker and D. Y. Colbert, Drug Dev. Ind. Pharm. **8**, 759, 1982.
64. C. R. Kowarski, J. Pharm. Sci. **58**, 360, 1969.
65. A. F. Asker and D. Jackson, Drug Dev. Ind. Pharm. **12**, 385, 1986.
66. E. R. Garrett, J. Pharm. Sci. **51**, 811, 1962; Kinetics and mechanisms in stability of drugs, in *Advances in Pharmaceutical Sciences*, H. S. Bean, A. H. Beckett and J. E. Carless, Eds., Vol. 2, Academic Press, New York, 1967, pp. 77–84.
67. L. Lachman, J. Pharm. Sci. **54**, 1519, 1965.
68. J. T. Carstensen, *Theory of Pharmaceutical Systems*, Vol. 2, Academic Press, New York, 1973, Chapter 5; J. Pharm. Sci. **63**, 1, 1974.
69. J. Carstensen and M. Musa, J. Pharm. Sci. **61**, 1112, 1972.
70. R. Tardif, J. Pharm. Sci. **54**, 281, 1965.
71. J. Carstensen, J. Johnson, W. Valentine and J. Vance, J. Pharm. Sci. **53**, 1050, 1964.
72. J. L. Lach and M. Bornstein, J. Pharm. Sci. **54**, 1731, 1965; M. Bornstein and J. L. Lach, ibid. **55**, 1033, 1966; J. L. Lach and M. Bornstein, ibid. **55**, 1040, 1966; M. Bornstein, J. P. Walsh, B. J. Munden and J. L. Lach, ibid. **56**, 1419, 1967; M. Bornstein, J. L. Lach and B. J. Munden, ibid. **57**, 1653, 1968; W. Wu, T. Chin and J. L. Lach, ibid. **59**, 1122, 1234, 1970; J. J. Lach and L. D. Bigley, J. Pharm. Sci. **59**, 1261, 1970; J. D. McCallister, T. Chin and J. L. Lach, ibid. **59**, 1286, 1970.

73. S. M. Blaug and W-T. Huang, J. Pharm. Sci. **61,** 1770, 1972.
74. M. Everhard and F. Goodhard, J. Pharm. Sci. **52,** 281, 1963; F. Goodhard, M. Everhard and D. Dickcius, ibid. **53,** 388, 1964; F. Goodhard, H. Lieberman, D. Mody and F. Ninger, ibid. **56,** 63, 1967.
75. R. Kuramoto, L. Lachman and J. Cooper, J. Am. Pharm. Assoc., Sci. Ed. **47,** 175, 1958; T. Urbanyi, C. Swartz and L. Lachman, J. Pharm. Sci. **49,** 163, 1960; L. Lachman et al., ibid. **50,** 141, 1961; C. Swartz, L. Lachman, T. Urbanyi and J. Cooper, ibid. **50,** 145, 1961; C. Swartz and J. Cooper, ibid. **51,** 89, 1962; J. Cooper and C. Swartz, ibid. **51,** 321, 1962; C. Swartz et al. ibid. **51,** 326, 1962.
76. D. C. Monkhouse and L. Van Campen, Drug Dev. Ind. Pharm. **10,** 1175, 1984.
77. G. Levy, Drug Cosmet. Ind. **76,** 472, 1955.
78. S. M. Free, Considerations in sampling for stability, presented at Am. Drug Manuf. Assoc., Nov. 1955; R. H. Blythe, Product Formulation and Stability Prediction. Presented at the Production Section of the Canadian Pharmaceutical Manufacturers Association, April 1957. A. K. Amirjahed, J. Pharm. Sci. **66,** 785, 1977.
79. S. Baker and S. Niazi, J. Pharm. Sci. **67,** 141, 1978.
80. A. R. Rogers, J. Pharm. Pharmacol. **15,** 101T, 1963.
81. S. P. Eriksen and H. Stalmach, J. Pharm. Sci. **54,** 1029, 1965.
82. H. V. Maulding and M. A. Zoglio, J. Pharm. Sci. **59,** 333, 1970; M. A. Zoglio, H. V. Maulding, W. H. Streng and W. C. Vincek, ibid. **64,** 1381, 1975.
83. B. W. Madsen, R. A. Anderson, D. Herbison-Evans and W. Sneddon, J. Pharm. Sci. **63,** 777, 1974.
84. B. Edel and M. O. Baltzer, J. Pharm. Sci. **69,** 287, 1980.
85. E. R. Garrett, J. Am. Pharm. Assoc., Sci. Ed. **45,** 171, 470, 1956.
86. L. Lachman, P. DeLuca and M. J. Akers, Kinetic principles and stability testing, Chapter 26 in *The Theory and Practice of Industrial Pharmacy*, 3rd Edition, L. Lachman, H. A. Lieberman and J. L. Kanig, Eds., Lea & Febiger, Philadelphia, 1986, pp. 789–795.
87. W. J. Westlake, in *Current Concepts in the Pharmaceutical Sciences: Dosage Form Design and Bioavailability*, J. Swarbrick, Ed., Lea & Febiger, Philadelphia, 1973, Chapter 5.
88. K. A. Connors, G. L. Amidon and L. Kennon, *Chemical Stability of Pharmaceuticals*, 2nd Ed., Wiley, New York, 1986, p. 201.
89. C. R. Kowarski and H. I. Ghandi, J. Pharm. Sci. **64,** 696, 1975.
90. C.-H. Chiang, C.-Y. Wu and H.-S. Huang, J. Pharm. Sci. **76,** 914, 1987.
91. P. Zvirblis, I. Socholitsky and A. A. Kondritzer, J. Am. Pharm. Assoc., Sci. Ed. **45,** 450, 1956; ibid. **46,** 531, 1957.
92. J. V. Swintosky et al., J. Am. Pharm. Assoc., Sci. Ed. **45,** 34, 37, 1956.
93. A. J. Ross, M.-V. C. Go, D. L. Casey and D. J. Palling, J. Pharm. Sci. **76,** 306, 1987.
94. J. G. Strom, Jr. and H. W. Jun, J. Pharm. Sci. **69,** 1261, 1980.
95. J. Zheng and J.-f Zhang, Acta Pharm. Sin. **22,** 278, 1987.
96. Kissinger, Anal. Chem. **29,** 1702, 1957.
97. M. N. Khan, J. Pharm. Sci. **73,** 1767, 1984.
98. A. Martin, J. Newburger and A. Adjei, J. Pharm. Sci. **69,** 487, 1980.
99. H. Bundgaard and J. Møss, J. Pharm. Sci. **78,** 122, 1989.
100. M. F. Powell, J. Pharm. Sci. **75,** 901, 1986.
101. A. Albert and E. P. Serjeant, *The Determination of Ionization Constants*, 3rd Edition, Chapman and Hall, New York, 1984, p. 75.
102. S. M. Berge, N. L. Henderson and M. J. Frank, J. Pharm. Sci. **72,** 59, 1983.
103. G. B. Smith and F. F. Schoenewaldt, J. Pharm. Sci. **70,** 272, 1981.
104. R. E. Notari, J. Pharm. Sci. **56,** 804, 1967.
105. D.-P. Wang, Y.-H. Tu and L. V. Allen, Jr., J. Pharm. Sci. **77,** 972, 1988.
106. V. D. Gupta, Drug Dev. Ind. Pharm. **8,** 869, 1982.
107. V. D. Gupta, J. Pharm. Sci. **73,** 565, 1984.
108. V. D. Gupta, Int. J. Pharm. **10,** 249, 1982.
109. D. Brooke, J. A. Scoptt and R. J. Bequette, Am. J. Hosp. Pharm. **32,** 44, 1975.

Problems*

12-1. The time and amount of decomposition of 0.056 M glucose at 140° C in an aqueous solution containing 0.35 N HCl was found to be

Data for *Problem 12–1*

Time (hr.)	Glucose, remaining (mole/liter $\times 10^2$)
0.5	5.52
2	5.31
3	5.18
4	5.02
6	4.78
8	4.52
10	4.31
12	4.11

What is the order, the half-life, and the specific reaction rate of this decomposition? Can one unquestionably determine the order from the data given?

Answer: If first order, $k = 0.026$ hr^{-1}, $t_{1/2} = 26.8$ hr

12-2. According to Connors et al.,[88] the first-order rate constant, k_1, for the decomposition of ampicillin at pH 5.8 and 35° C is $k_1 = 2 \times 10^{-7}$ sec^{-1}. The solubility of ampicillin is 1.1 g/100 mL. If it is desired to prepare a suspension of the drug containing 2.5 g/100 mL, calculate (a) the zero-order rate constant, k_o, and (b) the shelf-life, i.e., the time in days required for the drug to decompose to 90% of its original concentration (at 35° C) in solution. (c) If the drug is formulated in solution rather than a suspension at this pH and temperature, what is its shelf-life? *Note:* 100 mL = 1 deciliter = 1 dL.

Answers: (a) $k_o = (2.2 \times 10^{-7}$ g dL^{-1} sec^{-1}; (b) $t_{90} = 13.2$ days at 35° C (zero-order breakdown); (c) $t_{90} = 6.1$ days at 35° C (first-order breakdown).

12-3. (a) Menadione (vitamin K_3) is degraded by exposure to light, which is called *photodegradation* or *photolysis*. The rate constant of decomposition is $k = 4.863 \times 10^{-3}$ min^{-1}. Compute the half-life.

(b) The formation of a complex of menadione with the quaternary ammonium compound cetylethylmorpholinium ethosulfate (I) in aqueous solution slows the rate of photodegradation by ultraviolet light. The rate of decomposition of 5.19×10^{-5} M of menadione containing a 5% (w/v) of the complexing agent (I) is as follows (the data are based on the paper by Kowarski and Ghandi[89]):

Time (min)	10	20	30	40
Menadione remaining (mole/liter $\times 10^5$)	5.15	5.11	5.07	5.03

Compute the k value, $t_{1/2}$, and the percent decrease of k and increase of $t_{1/2}$ in the presence of the complexing agent.

Problem 12–14 was provided by Professor Z. Zheng, Shanghai Medical University, Shanghai, China. Problems 12–33, 12–34, and 12–35 were prepared by Professor V. D. Gupta, University of Houston. Problem 12–36 was suggested by J. K. Guillory, University of Iowa.

(c) What is the concentration after 5 hours with and without complexing agent? Use ln rather than log throughout the problem.

Answer: **(a)** $t_{1/2}$ = 142.5 min or 2 hr 22 min; **(b)** k = 7.87 10^{-4} min^{-1}, $t_{1/2}$ = 880.56 min or 14 hr 41 min; k decreases by 84% and $t_{1/2}$ increases by 518%; **(c)** without (I) 1.2×10^{-5} M; with addition of (I), 4.10×10^{-5} M

12–4. Garrett and Carper[2] determined the zero-order rate constant for the degradation of the colorants in a multisulfa preparation. The results obtained at various temperatures are:

°C	40	50	60	70
k	0.00011	0.00028	0.00082	0.00196

(a) Plot these results according to the Arrhenius relationship and compute the activation energy E_a.

(b) Extrapolate the results to 25° C to obtain k at room temperature. You can also use regression analysis to answer (a) and (b).

(c) The rate of decrease of absorbance of the colored preparation at a wavelength of 500 nm was found to be zero-order and the initial absorbance A_o was 0.470. This preparation should be rejected when the spectrophotometric absorbance A falls to a value of 0.225. Therefore, to predict the absorbance of the preparation at any time t hr after preparation, the zero-order equation $A = A_o - kt$ is used. Calculate the predicted life of the preparation at 25° C.

Answers: **(a)** E_a = 20.8 kcal/mole; **(b)** k at 25° C = 1.99×10^{-5} absorbance units per hour (using regression analysis); **(c)** predicted life = 513 days (ca. 1.4 years)

12–5. In the saponification of methyl acetate at 25° C, the molar concentration of sodium hydroxide remaining after 75 min was 0.00552 M. The initial concentration of ester and of base was each 0.01 M. Calculate the second-order rate constant and the half-life of the reaction.

Answer: k = 1.082 (liter/mole) min^{-1}; $t_{1/2}$ = 92.4 min

12–6. Assume that under acidic conditions a compound undergoes reaction according to the following mechanism:

$$(1) \ A + H^+ \underset{2}{\overset{1}{\rightleftarrows}} AH^+$$

$$(2) \ AH^+ \overset{3}{\rightarrow} B$$

$$(3) \ B \overset{4}{\rightarrow} \text{Products}$$

(a) What is the expression giving the steady-state concentration of B?

(b) What is the expression giving the steady-state concentration of AH^+ if the total concentration of acid added to the reaction mixture $[H^+_T]$ is related to the acid present during the reaction, both free $[H^+]$ and bound $[AH^+]$, by the equation

$$[H^+_T] = [H^+] + [AH^+]$$

(c) Give the rate law expressing the rate of formation of products if, instead of measuring the total concentration of acid added to the reaction mixture, a pH meter is used to measure the concentration of "free" acid $[H^+]$. Use the results of parts (a) and (b). See under Rate Determining Step, page 294 for help in solving this problem.

Answers: **(a)**

$$B_{ss} = \frac{k_3}{k_4}[AH^+];$$

(b)

$$[AH^+]_{ss} = \frac{k_1[A][H^+_T]}{k_1[A] + (k_2 + k_3)}.$$

(c)

$$\text{rate} = \frac{d[P]}{dt} = \left(\frac{k_1 k_3}{k_2 + k_3}\right)[A][H^+]$$

12–7. Diacetyl nadolol, used in ophthalmic preparations for glaucoma therapy, hydrolyzes in a series or consecutive reactions represented as $A \overset{k_1}{\rightarrow} B \overset{k_2}{\rightarrow} C$ where B and C are the intermediate and final

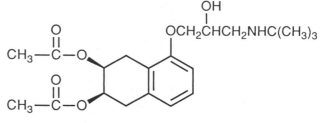

Diacetyl Nadolol

products, acetyl nadolol and nadolol, respectively. The apparent rate constants, k_1 and k_2, are first-order constants. The rate of decomposition $A \rightarrow B$ is given at pH 7.55 and 55° C by Chiang et al.[90]

Data for *Problem 12–7*

A (mM)	0.23	0.19	0.16	0.13	0.09	0.06
t (hr)	5	10	15	20	30	40

where mM in the table above stands for millimolar.

(a) Compute k_1 using least squares.

(b) The rate constant in the second step, k_2, was found by nonlinear regression analysis to be 0.0243 hr^{-1}. On the same graph plot the concentration of A remaining and the concentrations of B and C appearing as A hydrolyzes, versus the time in hours as given in the table. Prepare a table of concentrations of A, B, and C at various times, t, using the appropriate equations in the section on the complex reactions in this chapter, pages 290 to 293.

(c) Compute $t_{1/2}$ for A. What are the concentrations of B and C at this time?

Partial Answers: **(a)** k_1 = 0.0383 hr^{-1}; **(b)** at t = 5 hr, B = 0.046 mM and C = 0.004 mM; at t = 10 hr, B = 0.079 mM and C = 0.011 mM; **(c)** $t_{1/2}$ for A = 18.1 hr; the concentrations of B and C at 18.1 hr are 0.110 mM and 0.03 mM, respectively.

12–8. The initial stage of decomposition for a new drug according to a consecutive reaction was found to be first order. The initial concentration C_0 of the solution was 0.050 mole/liter and after 10 hours at 40° C, the drug concentration C was 0.015 mole/liter. Compute the specific rate at 40° C. What is the drug concentration after 2 hours? If the k value for this reaction at 20° C is 0.0020 hr^{-1}, what is the activation energy and the Arrhenius factor A for the reaction?

Answer: k = 0.120 hr^{-1}; concentration after 2 hours = 0.039 mole/liter, E_a = 37.4 kcal/mole, A = 1.5×10^{25} sec^{-1}

12–9. The hydrolysis of atropine base was found by Zvirblis et al.[91] to be first-order with respect to the base. The degradation constant k at 40° C was 0.016 sec^{-1}. If the energy of activation E_a is 7.7 kcal/mole, what is the Arrhenius factor A? What does the value of E_a suggest about the stability of atropine base at 40° C?

Answer: A = 3.8×10^3 sec^{-1}

12–10. The following data for the first-order decomposition of penicillin are obtained from Swintosky et al.[92]

Data for *Problem 12–10*

First-order rate constant, k, hr^{-1}	0.0216	0.0403	0.119
Temperature (°C)	37	43	54

Plot the results and compute the activation energy. What is the Arrhenius factor A?

Answer: $E_a = 20.3$ kcal/mole, $A = 1.2 \times 10^9$ sec^{-1} (using regression analysis)

12–11. The rate constant, k_{OH^-}, for the base catalysis of cibenzoline, a new antiarrhythmic agent, varies with temperature as follows:[93]

Data for *Problem 12–11*

Temp. (°C)	25	35	50	80
k_{OH^-} (M^{-1} hr^{-1})	15.5	78.0	275	2100

Compute the Arrhenius factor, A, and the energy of activation, E_a

Answer: $E_a = 18.$ kcal/mole, $A = 3.54 \times 10^{14}$ sec^{-1}

12–12. The first-order degradation of glucose in acid solution results in the formation of 5-hydroxymethylfurfural (5-HMF), and 5-HMF yields additional breakdown products that give the straw color to glucose solutions stored for long periods of time at high temperatures. These conditions exist, for example, in military warehouses and medical units.

The values of the rate constant for the breakdown of glucose in 0.35 N HCl solution at 110 to 150° C are given in the table.

Data for *Problem 12–12**

°C	°K	1/T (°K^{-1})	k (hr^{-1})	ln k
110	383	0.00261	0.0040	−5.521
130	403	0.00248	0.0267	−3.623
150	423	0.00236	0.1693	−1.776

*From K. R. Heimlich and A. Martin, J. Am. Pharm. Assoc., Sci. Ed. **49**, 592, 1960.

Calculate the activation energy and the Arrhenius factor A for glucose in acid solution tested experimentally for accelerated breakdown over the temperature range of 110° to 150° C.

Answer: $E_a = 29.8$ kcal/mole, $A = 3.71 \times 10^{14}$ hr^{-1}

12–13. Methenamine is used to treat urinary tract infections, its antibacterial activity being derived from formaldehyde, which is produced upon hydrolysis in acidic media. About 0.75 mg/mL is the physiologic concentration of methenamine following a normal dose in humans. Methenamine circulates in the blood (pH 7.4) as the intact drug without degradation but is rapidly converted to formaldehyde when it reaches the acidic urine.

The Arrhenius activation energy, $E_a = \Delta E^{\ddagger}$ at pH 5.1, obtained in vitro at several temperatures, is 12 kcal/mole and the Arrhenius factor A at 37.5° C is 2×10^7 hr^{-1} (Strom and Jun[94]).

(a) Compute the entropy of activation, $\Delta S^{\ddagger}$, and the first-order rate of the reaction, k. Compute the free energy of activation, $\Delta G^{\ddagger}$ from equation (12–91). Assume that $E_a = \Delta H^{\ddagger} = \Delta E^{\ddagger}$.

(b) The drug remains in the bladder for about 6 hours and the effective concentration of formaldehyde is about 20 μg/mL. Compute the concentration of formaldehyde in the bladder after 6 hr assuming that the concentration of methenamine in the urine is that of the drug in plasma (0.75 mg/mL).

(c) When does formaldehyde reach the effective concentration, 20 μg/mL, in urine?

(d) Note that $\Delta H^{\ddagger}$ is a large positive value, $\Delta S^{\ddagger}$ is a relatively large negative value, $\Delta G^{\ddagger}$ is therefore positive, and the Arrhenius factor is small relative to A values normally found. Rationalize these factors in terms of the conversion of methenamine in the body to formaldehyde. See *Example 12–8* and the paragraph following it to assist you in your reasoning.

Answers: **(a)** $\Delta S^{\ddagger} = -41.5$ cal/mole, $k = 0.072$ hr^{-1}; $\Delta G^{\ddagger} = 24.9$ kcal/mole; **(b)** 0.26 mg/mL; **(c)** 22.5 min

12–14. In a differential scanning calorimetric experiment of thermal degradation of cefamandole naftate, Zheng et al.[95] obtained the following data:

Data for *Problem 12–14*

Heating rate, β (°C/min)	5	2	1	0.5
Degradation peak temp., T_m (°K)	472	466	460	475

Let $x' = 1/T_m$ and $y' = \ln \dfrac{\beta}{T_m^2}$. One then casts the data in the transposed form:

Data for *Problem 12–14*

$x = x' \times 10^3$	2.119	2.146	2.174	2.188
$y = y' + 13$	2.2955	1.4048	0.7375	0.0575

Now one carries out regression analysis of y against x where the slope is $-E_a/R$, and solve for E_a. The degradation peak temperature T_m of a drug molecule depends on the rate of heating β in a differential scanning calorimeter; thus the slope is

$$-\frac{E_a}{R} = \frac{dy}{dx} = \frac{d\ln(\beta/T_m^2)}{d(1/T_m)}.$$

In this way one can obtain E_a values and rapidly scan a series of drug analogs for their stability or breakdown. This method is known as the Kissinger approach.[96]

Answer: $E_a = 61.6$ kcal/mole

12–15. The specific rate constant for the hydrolysis of procaine at 40° C is 0.011 sec^{-1} and the energy of activation is $E_a = 13,800$ cal/mole. Using the equation

$$k = \frac{RT}{Nh} e^{\Delta S^{\ddagger}/R} \, e^{-\Delta H^{\ddagger}/RT}$$

in which $\Delta H^{\ddagger} \approx E_a$, compute the entropy of activation $\Delta S^{\ddagger}$. Using the equation $\Delta G^{\ddagger} = \Delta H^{\ddagger} - T\Delta S^{\ddagger}$, compute the free energy of activation for the hydrolysis of procaine at 40° C. *Note:* The units in the above equation must cancel R in the terms $exp(\Delta S^{\ddagger}/R)$, and R in $exp(-\Delta H^{\ddagger}/RT)$ should be expressed as 1.9872 cal mole^{-1} deg^{-1} and in RT/Nh as 8.314×10^7 erg deg^{-1} mole^{-1}.

Answer: $\Delta S^{\ddagger} = -23.5$ e.u.; $\Delta G^{\ddagger} = 21.2$ kcal/mole

12–16. The first-order rate constant k for the acid-catalyzed hydrolysis of benzocaine is 140×10^{-6} sec^{-1}, and the energy of activation E_a is 18.6 kcal/mole at 97.3° C. Compute the entropy of activation $\Delta S^{\ddagger}$, the Arrhenius factor A, and the probability factor P.

Answer: $\Delta S^{\ddagger} = -26.4$ cal/(mole deg); $A = 1.31 \times 10^7$ sec^{-1}; $P = 1.7 \times 10^{-6}$

12–17.[†] The observed alkaline hydrolysis rate constants k_{obs} of maleimide[97] in dioxane–water mixtures (v/v %) at 30° C, containing 0.03 M NaOH, are given, on page 320, together with the solubility parameters[98] of the solvent mixtures, δ_1 (dioxane–water).

Plot k_{obs} (vertical axis) against the delta value, δ_1. Then plot the *log* of k_{obs} versus δ_1 on the same graph and find a simple linear relationship between the two variables. Does the addition of dioxane protect maleimide against hydrolysis? Explain. (The solubility parameter is related to polarity, as explained on pages 298–299; the larger is δ_1 the greater is the polarity of the dioxane–water mixture).

---

†Maleimide reacts with the sulfhydryl group of proteins and may one day become a useful drug. This problem deals with the chemical kinetics of the alkaline hydrolysis of an imide in an aqueous solvent, the dielectric constant of which is altered by the addition of dioxane.

Data for *Problem 12-17*

% (v/v) Dioxane	δ_1 (cal/cm^3)$^{1/2}$	$k_{obs} \times 10^3$ s^{-1}	log k_{obs}
5	22.78	10.68	−1.971
10	22.11	9.219	−2.035
15	21.43	7.612	−2.1185
20	20.76	6.572	−2.182
25	20.09	5.476	−2.262
30	19.42	4.580	−2.339
40	18.07	3.217	−2.493
50	16.73	2.223	−2.653
60	15.39	1.573	−2.803
70	14.04	1.199	−2.921

Would the toxicity of dioxane prevent its use in pharmaceutical products? See *Merck Index*, 11th ed., 1989, p. 521.

Partial Answer: log k_{obs} = 0.111 δ_1 − 4.504. A log k_{obs} against δ_1 plot results in a straight line.

12-18. The effect of ionic strength (μ) on the observed degradation rates of cefotaxime sodium, a potent third-generation cephalosporin, was studied in aqueous solution at several pH values, with the following results:[102]

Data for *Problem 12-18**

Ionic strength μ	$k_{obs} \times 10^3$ hr^{-1} (25° C)		
	pH 2.23	pH 5.52	pH 8.94
0.2	7.99	3.28	22.6
0.4	7.82	3.30	25.6
0.5	7.82	3.24	25.5
0.7	8.07	3.25	27.1
0.9	7.79	3.17	28.3

*Data from S. M. Berge, N. L. Henderson and M. J. Frank, J. Pharm. Sci. **72**, 59, 1983.

(a) Does a primary salt effect exist at any of the pH values under study? If so, compute the rate constant k_o by plotting log k_{obs} versus $\sqrt{\mu}$ and extrapolating to $\mu = 0$.

(b) When you regress log k_{obs} versus ($\sqrt{\mu}/(1 + \sqrt{\mu})$) instead of $\sqrt{\mu}$ at pH 8.94, the slope agrees better with the theoretical value, $Az_A z_B$, where $A_{(theor.)}$ = 0.51 at 29° C. Why? See Carstensen.[16]

Answers: **(a)** k_o = 0.019 hr^{-1}; **(b)** check your answer with page 299, equation (12-109) and page 136, *Example 6-14.* The rate constant k_o changes to 0.0156 hr^{-1} when $\sqrt{\mu}/(1 - \sqrt{\mu})$ replaces $\sqrt{\mu}$ on the x-axis and the slope A becomes 0.5295, similar to the theoretical A value.

12-19. The following data were obtained for the decomposition of 0.056 M glucose at 140° C at various concentrations of the catalysts, HCl:

Data for *Problem 12-19*

k_{obs} (hr^{-1})	normality, [H$_3$O$^+$]
0.00366	0.0108
0.00580	0.0197
0.00818	0.0295
0.01076	0.0394
0.01217	0.0492

Plot the results and, from the graph, obtain k_o and the catalytic constant k_H. It may be assumed that hydroxyl ion catalysis is negligible in this acidic solution.

Answer: k_H = 0.229 M^{-1} hr^{-1} or liter mole^{-1} hr^{-1}; k_o = 0.00135 hr^{-1} by linear regression analysis. Extrapolation by eye yields 0.0013 hr^{-1}.

12-20. The moieties, —CH$_2$NHCH$_3$, —CH$_2$N, and —CH$_2$NO, were attached to a model peptide to form a prodrug known as a Mannich base (compounds 7, 8, and 9, respectively, of Bundgaard and Møss[99]). The pH–rate profile for the hydrolysis of the Mannich bases (Figure 12-24) exhibits sigmoidal shapes. The points of the three curves can be calculated using the equation

$$k = \frac{k_1 K_a}{[H^+] + K_a} + \frac{k_2 [H^+]}{[H^+] + K_a}$$

in which k_1 and k_2 are the first-order rate constants for degradation of the Mannich base, B, and the conjugate acid, BH^+, respectively. K_a is the ionization constant of the protonated Mannich base. The values at 37° C given by the authors for compound 9 are k_1 (min^{-1}) = 2.5 × 10^{-3}, k_2 (min^{-1}) = 1.0 × 10^{-2}, and pK_a = 5.1; Ka = 7.94 × 10^{-6}.

Calculate k, the first-order rate constant for the degradation of the Mannich base, compound 9, at pH 4. Check your answer at pH 4 by reading the log k value from Figure 12-24, and converting it to the rate constant k (min^{-1}) for hydrolysis. The student may care to calculate the k values for compounds 7 and 8. The rate data for the breakdown of compound 7 are: k$_1$ = 0.024 (min^{-1}), k$_2$ = 1.8 × 10^{-4} (min^{-1}) and pK_a = 7.2. The values for compound 8 are k$_1$ = 0.42 (min^{-1}), k$_2$ = 1.7 × 10^{-3} (min^{-1}) and pK_a = 7.2.

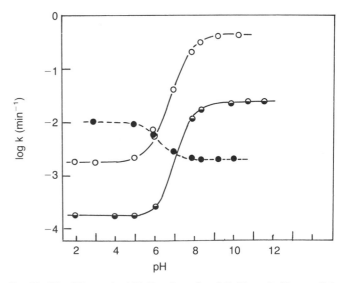

Fig. 12-24. (Figure 3 of H. Bundgaard and J. Møss, J. Pharm. Sci. **78**, 122, 1989. pH profile for the Mannich base derivatives 7(◐), 8(○) and 9(●) in aqueous solution at 37° C. (Reproduced with permission of the copyright owner and altered according to the authors.)

Answer: From Figure 12–24, log $k = -3.75$; $k = 1.78 \times 10^{-4}$ min^{-1}. From the calculation using the above equation, $k = 1.95 \times 10^{-4}$ min^{-1} for compound 7 at pH 4.

12–21. The degradation constant k_{obs} (sec^{-1}) for codeine sulfate may be calculated at 25° C using the expression

$$k_{obs} \text{ (sec}^{-1}) = k_{H^+}[H^+] + k_{OH^-}[OH^-] + k_o =$$
$$2.46 \times 10^{-11}[H^+] + 3.22 \times 10^{-9}[OH^-] + 7.60 \times 10^{-11}$$

The constants k_{H^+} and k_{OH^-} associated with the concentrations of $[H^+]$ and $[OH^-]$ are expressed in M^{-1} sec^{-1}, where M^{-1} stands for reciprocal moles per liter, and k_o is in sec^{-1}. Calculate the observed rate constant k_{obs} (sec^{-1}) for the decomposition of codeine at 25° C in codeine sulfate solutions, at pH 0.0, 2.0, 8.0, 10. Powell[100] shows that codeine sulfate solutions are subjected to general acid–base catalysis due to a buffer consisting of the phosphate ions, Na$_2$HPO$_4$ and NaH$_2$PO$_4$. Plot the log k_{obs} versus pH and compare with Figure 1, page 902 in the report by Powell. *Note:* At pH = 0.0, $[H^+] = 1$ M. Above this concentration (> 1 M), pH values become negative. However, below pH 0 we do not use minus pH values but rather an acidity function known as H_o (see Albert and Serjeant[101]).

Partial Answer: At pH = 2.0, $[H^+] = 0.01$ M, $[OH^-] = 1.0 \times 10^{-12}$ M, $k_{obs} = 7.62 \times 10^{-11}$ sec^{-1}, log $k_{obs} = -10.12$. At pH = 8.0, $[H^+] = 10^{-8}$ M, $[OH^-] = 10^{-6}$ M, $k_{obs} = 7.60 \times 10^{-11}$ sec^{-1}, log $k_{obs} = -10.12$

12–22. The hydrolysis of the prostaglandin, fenprostalene, in aqueous solution was studied at 80° C varying the buffer system. The total buffer concentration as well as the ionic strength was kept constant. Metal ions (Cu^{2+} or Fe^{3+}) were added to some solutions. The dependence of k_{obs} on the pH is given below (See **Data for Problem 12–22**).

(a) Do the buffer systems, Cu^{2+} or Fe^{3+}, influence hydrolysis?

(b) Plot log k_{obs} versus pH and compute the catalytic constants k_1 and k_2 corresponding to the left and the right branches of the "V"-shaped plot. *Hint:* You will need two equations; one for the left branch of the line, another for the right branch. Using regression analysis, compute the intercept of each branch. Combine these intercepts with equations (12–123) and (12–130) to obtain the second-order rate constants for acid, $k_1 = k_{H^+}$ and base, $k_2 = k_{OH^-}$. K_w at 80° C is 12.63×10^{-14}.

Partial Answers: **(a)** The hydrolysis is due to specific acid-base catalysis. The regression equations of part **(b)** will substantiate this. **(b)** $k_1 = 5.62 \times 10^{-3}$ M^{-1} sec^{-1}; $k_2 = 6.10$ M^{-1} sec^{-1}.

12–23. The pH–rate profile of cefotaxime sodium (log k_{obs} versus pH) at ionic strength $\mu = 0.5$ shows roughly slopes of -1, zero, and $+1$ within the pH ranges 0–4, 4–7, and 7–10, respectively.[102] **(a)** What kind of catalysis presumably occurs at each of the three pH ranges? **(b)** What is the value of the pH-independent rate constant

if k_{obs} at pH 6 is 3.064×10^{-3} M^{-1} hr^{-1}? **(c)** Compute k_{obs} at pH 8. The specific acid and base constants are $k_{H^+} = 0.4137$ M^{-1} hr^{-1} and $k_{OH^-} = 1616.5$ M^{-1} hr^{-1}, where M stands for molarity (see equation (12–136)). The OH^- concentration at pH 8 and $\mu = 0.5$ is 1.38×10^{-6} M.

Answers: **(a)** Check your results with pages 302–303; **(b)** $k_o = 3.064 \times 10^{-3}$ M^{-1} hr^{-1}; **(c)** $k_{obs} = 5.29 \times 10^{-3}$ hr^{-1}

12–24. Equation (12–128) may be written in logarithmic form to produce equation (12–130).

$$log \, k_{obs} = pH + log(K_w \, k_{OH^-})$$

This equation allows one to compute k_{OH^-} from the intercept of a regression of log k_{obs} against pH. Use the data of Khan[97] for the effect of pH on the alkaline hydrolysis rate constant of a new drug, maleimide, given in the table at the bottom of this page.

(a) Plot log k_{obs} (vertical axis) against pH. **(b)** Using least squares, compute the specific catalytic constant k_{OH^-} from the intercept.

Partial Answer: **(b)** The regression equation is log $k_{obs} = 0.8689$ pH $- 11.150$. The value of k_{OH^-} is 7.08×10^2 sec^{-1}.

12–25. Strom and Jun[94] studied the kinetics of the hydrolysis of methenamine to produce formaldehyde in citrate–phosphate buffers from pH 2.0 to 7.4 at 37.5° C. The reaction half-life for the conversion of methenamine to formaldehyde was found to be pH dependent, decreasing from 13.8 hr at pH 5.8 to 1.6 hr at pH 2.0. **(a)** Using the data of the following table, plot the pH–rate profile from pH 2.0 to pH 5.8 and compute $t_{1/2}$ at these pH values.

Data (a) for *Problem 12–25*

k (hr$^{-1} \times 10^2$)	43.3	22.4	18.6	8.36	5.01
pH	2.0	3.4	4.6	5.1	5.8

(b) Prepare an Arrhenius plot of ln k against $1/T$ for the degradation of methenamine at various temperatures. Calculate the activation energy, E_a and the Arrhenius A factor at pH 5.1 over a range of temperatures from 37.5° to 67° C. The required data is as follows:

Data (b) for *Problem 12–25*

Temp. (°C)	37.5	47	57	67
k (hr^{-1})	0.0836	0.111	0.233	0.427

Partial Answer: **(a)** At pH 2, $t_{1/2} = 1.60$ hr; **(b)** $E_a = 11.9$ kcal/mole; $A = 1.87 \times 10^7$ hr^{-1} at pH 5

Data for *Problem 12–22**

Buffer	HCl	Formate			Phosphate			Carbonate
Metal ion	—	Fe^{3+}	—	Cu^{2+}	Fe^{3+}	Cu^{2+}	—	—
$k_{obs} \times 10^7$ sec^{-1}	3360	35	22.1	21.6	18.6	21.4	84.5	8350
pH	1.15	2.99	3.21	3.22	6.51	6.57	7.21	9.22

*Selected data from D. M. Johnson, W. F. Taylor, G. Thompson and R. A. Pritchard, J. Pharm. Sci. 72, 946, 1983.

Data for *Problem 12–24*

pH	8.39	8.51	8.84	8.88	9.13	9.36	9.68	9.89	10.08
$k_{obs} \times 10^3$	0.1514	0.1750	0.330	0.3124	0.6510	0.9310	2.059	2.633	4.057

12–26. Thienamycin is an antibiotic with a structure somewhat related to the penicillins. Its decomposition accelerates as the concentration is increased; and a derivative, N-formimidoylthienamycin (imipemide, imipenen) has been introduced to improve the

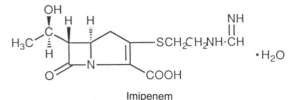

Imipenem

stability and broad spectrum of activity. Smith and Schoenewaldt[103] studied the stability of imipenen in aqueous solution at 25° C and 40° C. A first-order reaction of ring opening occurred in dilute solution (1 or 2 mg/mL) and a second-order reaction became evident at higher concentrations. The pseudo–first-order rate constants k, hr^{-1}, at 25° C and 40° C are given in the following table at buffer pH from 5.0 to 8.0. The reaction rates were independent of general acid–base buffer effects, and the effect of ionic strength on rate was insignificant.

Data for *Problem 12–26*

Buffer pH	5.0	6.0	7.0	8.0
k (hr^{-1}), 25° C	0.0315	0.0069	0.0040	0.0083
k (hr^{-1}), 40° C	0.111	0.0257	0.0169	0.0462

The equation describing the rate–pH profiles of the drug at 25° and 40° C is

$$k_{obs} = k_1 [H^+] + k_2 K_w/[H^+] + k_o \quad (12\text{–}150)$$

in which k_{obs} is the experimentally determined first-order rate constant k at a definite pH, k_1 and k_2 are the second-order rate constants for hydrogen ion and hydroxyl ion catalysis, k_o is the first-order rate constant for water or "spontaneous" decomposition. $K_w/[H^+]$ is written in place of $[OH^-]$, where K_w is the ionization constant of water. Knowing the pH, one has by experiment both $[H^+]$ and $[OH^-] = K_w/[H^+]$. At 25° C, $K_w \cong 10^{-14.00}$ and at 40° C, $K_w = 10^{-13.54}$ (see p. 148).

(a) Plot the experimentally obtained points on the pH-profiles for the pseudo–first-order rate constants at 25° C and 40° C using the data of the table above. Draw the line obtained by use of equation (12–150) to determine how well the theory fits the experimental results. Using multiple least-squares regression, compute the values of k_o, k_1, and k_2 at both 25° C and 40° C. The researchers obtained the following results using a statistical method known as nonlinear regression.

Data for *Problem 12–26*

Temperature	k_o (hr^{-1})	k_1 (M^{-1} hr^{-1})	k_2 (M^{-1} hr^{-1})
40° C	0.01565	9730	10300
25° C	0.00403	2780	4150

Use the coefficients k_o, k_1, and k_2 to back-calculate $k_{25°}$ and $k_{40°}$.

Partial Answer: $k_{25°} = 0.0315$ hr^{-1} at pH 5, $k_{25°} = 0.0083$ at pH 8, $k_{40°} = 0.111$ at pH 5.

12–27. Notari[104] has studied the hydrolytic deamination of cytosine arabinoside in buffer solutions of varying composition prepared so as to maintain the pH and the ionic strength constant. He has reported the following data for the hydrolysis at 70° C:

Data for *Problem 12–27*

	Buffer composition			
pH	NaH$_2$PO$_4$·H$_2$O	Na$_2$HPO$_4$	NaCl	k, hr^{-1}
6.15	0.120	0.012	0.000	0.00311
	0.048	0.0048	0.094	0.00171
	0.024	0.0024	0.125	0.00118
6.90	0.040	0.040	0.000	0.00113
	0.029	0.029	0.043	0.000872
	0.016	0.016	0.092	0.000619

Using these data, determine which species in the buffer solution is functioning as a catalytic agent. Give your reasoning for choosing this agent. *Hint:* Plot k versus [NaH$_2$PO$_4$] and versus [Na$_2$HPO$_4$] on the same graph. If one or other of these catalytic species produces parallel lines at the two pH values, catalysis by this species is occurring.*

Answer: The H$_2$PO$_4^-$ ion is acting as a catalyst.

12–28. The degradation of phentolamine hydrochloride in phosphate buffer at pH 5.9 to 7.2 and 90° C is attributed to both the buffer species H$_2$PO$_4^-$/HPO$_4^{2-}$ and specific base catalysis. The value of the specific base catalysis constant k_{OH^-} was found to be 4.28×10^6 liter mole^{-1} hr^{-1}. The catalytic coefficients of the species H$_2$PO$_4^-$ and HPO$_4^{2-}$ are $k_1 = 0.036$ and $k_2 = 1.470$ liter mole^{-1} hr^{-1}, respectively, and the total buffer concentration is 0.1 mole/liter. The equation for the overall rate constant is

$$k_{obs} = k_{OH^-}[OH^-] + k_1[H_2PO_4^-] + k_2[HPO_4^{2-}] \quad (12\text{–}151)$$

The solvent effect is negligible and $k_o = 0$ (based in part on Wang et al.[105]).

(a) Compute the overall hydrolysis rate constant k at the pH values of 6, 6.5, 7, and 7.2 using the appropriate expression. At the pH range of 5.9 to 7 you can use the second dissociation constant of phosphoric acid, p$K_{a2} = 7.21$, to obtain the concentration of H$_2$PO$_4^-$ and HPO$_4^{2-}$ at each pH value. Disregard the effect of the solvent alone. Then calculate the k_{obs} values at pH 6.5, 7.0 and 7.2. Finally convert the k values into log k and plot them versus pH.

(b) Plot the logarithm of the calculated k values against pH.

Partial Answer: **(a)** At pH 6, $k_{obs} = 0.0547$ hr^{-1}; at pH 6.5, $k_{obs} = 0.162$ hr^{-1}.

Hint: See page 303 and equations (12–138) and (12–139). To compute [H$_2$PO$_4^-$] and [HPO$_4^{2-}$] at each pH one uses the buffer equation

$$pH = pK_a + \log ([HPO_4^{2-}] / [H_2PO_4^-]) \quad (12\text{–}152)$$

in which pK_a is the second dissociation constant of H$_3$PO$_4$ (p. 147). At pH 6, one obtains [HPO$_4^{2-}$]/[H$_2$PO$_4^-$] = 0.062/1. Thus for 1 mole of buffer mixture, one has 0.062/(1 + 0.062) = 0.058 mole HPO$_4^{2-}$ and (1 − 0.058) = 0.942 mole H$_2$PO$_4^-$. Calculate the [H$_2$PO$_4^-$] and [HPO$_4^{2-}$] values at pH 6.0, 6.5, 7.0, and 7.2 for 0.1 mole/liter of buffer. The total rate constant at pH, say, 6 where $[OH^-] = 10^{-8}$ is $k_{(pH\ 6)} = (4.28 \times 10^6 \times 10^{-8}) + (0.036 \times 0.0942) + (1.470 \times 0.0058) = 0.0547$ hr^{-1}. Then, calculate the k_{obs} values at pH 6.5, 7.0, and 7.2.

(b) Finally, plot the log k_{obs} values versus pH.

12–29. The hydrolysis of mitomycin (see structure on p. 306 and Fig. 11–5*b*), an antitumor antibiotic, at pH 3.5 is due to the catalytic effect of water, the specific contribution of H$^+$ ions, and the effect of the phosphate buffer. At this pH value, phosphate buffers consist almost exclusively of H$_2$PO$_4^-$ ions so that the expression for k_{obs} is

---

*Dr. Keith Guillory, University of Iowa, suggested the test in *Problem 12–27* to determine what species is acting as the catalyst.

$$k_{obs} = k_o + k_{H^+}[H^+] + k_{H_2PO_4^-}[H_2PO_4^-]$$

The dependence of k_{obs} on the concentration of $H_2PO_4^-$ at a constant pH 3.5 is given in the table below.

Data for *Problem 12–29* **

$[H_2PO_4^-]$ (M)	0.01	0.05	0.1	0.2	0.3	0.4
$k_{obs} \times 10^3$ sec^{-1}	1.295	1.317	1.344	1.398	1.452	1.56

*From W. J. M. Underberg and H. Lingeman, J. Pharm. Sci. **72**, 549, 1983.

Note: k_o and k_{H^+} are constants and since the pH is held at 3.5 $[H^+]$ is also constant.

(a) Plot k_{obs} versus $[H_2PO_4^-]$ and compute the equation of the line and the catalytic coefficient $k_{H_2PO_4^-}$ of $H_2PO_4^-$ from the slope.

(b) Compute k_{H^+} at pH 3.5, knowing that $k_o = 1 \times 10^{-6}$ sec^{-1}

Answers: (a) $k_{H_2PO_4^-} = 5.4 \times 10^{-4}$ M^{-1} sec^{-1}; (b) $k_{H^+} = 4.08$ M^{-1} sec^{-1}

12–30. The degradation in methanol of chlorthalidone, an oral diuretic sulfonamide, is catalyzed by ferric ions. The observed rate constants in methanol as solvent vary with the $FeCl_3$ concentration as follows:

Data (a) for *Problem 12–30* †

$[FeCl_3] \times 10^4$ M	0.64	1.93	3.78	4.96	6.22
k_{obs}, hr^{-1}	0.019	0.081	0.21	0.26	0.36

†From N. K. Pandit and J. S. Hinderliter, J. Pharm. Sci. **74**, 857, 1985.

The addition of acetic acid to a chlorthalidone–methanol solution containing 6.15×10^{-4} mole/liter of $FeCl_3$ also influences hydrolysis. The variation of the observed rate constants with increasing concentrations of acetic acid, expressed as $[H^+]$, are as follows:

Data (b) for *Problem 12–30*

$[H^+] \times 10^7$	0.52	1.60	1.98	2.30
k_{obs}, hr^{-1}	0.436	0.672	0.764	0.772

The total k_{obs}, when both $[H^+]$ and $[FeCl_3]$ vary can therefore be represented as

$$k_{total} = k_o + k_M[M] + k'_M[M][H^+] \quad (12\text{–}153)$$

where k_o is the first-order rate constant due to the catalytic effect of the solvent alone (methanol), k_M (M^{-1} sec^{-1}) is the pseudo–second-order constant for the metal ion catalyzed reaction, [M] is the concentration in mole/liter of $FeCl_3$, and k'_M (M^{-2} sec^{-1}) is the pseudo–third-order constant for the metal ion and acid-catalyzed reaction.

(a) Plot k_{obs} (vertical axis) against $[FeCl_3]$ from the first table of this problem and compute the equation of the line from which k_M is obtained. (b) Plot k_{obs} versus $[H^+]$ from the second table, and compute k'_M. *Hint:* Apply the general equation (12–153) given above to each part of the problem. That is, include the appropriate terms in the slope and intercept you get in (a) and (b).

Answer: (a) $k_M = 0.169$ M^{-1} sec^{-1}; (b) $k'_M = 9.03 \times 10^5$ M^{-2} sec^{-1}

12–31. A new drug product is found to be ineffective after it has decomposed 30%. The original concentration of one sample was 5.0 mg/mL; when assayed 20 months later, the concentration was found to be 4.2 mg/mL. Assuming that the decomposition is first order, what would be the expiration time on the label? What is the half-life of this product?

Answer: Expiration, 41 mo.; half-life = 79.5 mo.

12–32. Using the temperature lines of Figure 12–21, obtain the time necessary for a drug to decompose from 100% to 80% at the temperatures 50°, 60°, 70° and 90° C. Plot log (t_{80}) vs. the reciprocal of the absolute temperature (Figure 12–22) and determine the time in days required for the drug to degrade to 80% of its 100% value at 25° C

Answer: ca. 400 days.

12–33. The decomposition of ethacrinic acid in the presence of ammonium ion was determined to be reversible.[106] From the following k_f (forward) and k_r (reverse) values at 25° C determine the k_{obs}, k_o, and $k_{NH_4^+}$ values. *Hint:* You may solve the two equations simultaneously. You will need two equations: $k_{obs} = k_f/k_r$ and $k_{obs} = k_o + k_{NH_4^+}[NH_4^+]$.

Data for *Problem 12–33*

Value (hr^{-1})	Remarks
$k_r = 0.101$ $k_f = 0.026$	$[NH_4^+]$ concentration 0.04 M
$k_r = 0.108$ $k_f = 0.052$	$[NH_4^+]$ concentration 0.08 M

Answer: $k_{obs} = 0.257$ hr^{-1} at 0.04 M $[NH_4^+]$ and 0.482 hr^{-1} at 0.08 M $[NH_4^+]$; $k_{NH_4^+} = 5.625$ liter mole^{-1} hr^{-1}; $k_o = 0.032$ hr^{-1}

12–34. The hydrolysis of cefotaxime sodium at 25° C is first order[107]; and $k_{obs} = k_o + k_{H^+}[H^+] + k_{OH^-}[OH^-]$. The pH has very little effect in the range of 4.3 to 6.2 and k_{obs} in this pH range has the value 0.056 day^{-1}. The ionic strength and the phosphate buffer used have no effect on the decomposition constant. The k_{obs} values at pH 1.5 and 8.5 are 0.625 day^{-1} and 0.16 day^{-1}, respectively. Compute k_o, k_{H^+} and k_{OH^-} values.

Answer: $k_o = 0.056$ day^{-1}; $k_{H^+} = 18.0$ M^{-1} day^{-1}; and $k_{OH^-} = 3.3 \times 10^4$ M^{-1} day^{-1}

12–35. The hydrolysis of cocaine is catalyzed by the phosphate buffer.[108] The hydrolysis may be expressed using the following equation:

$$k_{obs} = k[OH^-] + k_2[H_2PO_4^-] + k_3[HPO_4^{2-}]$$

The equation may be rearranged to

$$k_{obs} = k + [H_2PO_4^-](k_2 + k_3/q)$$

where $k = k_1[OH^-]$ and is a constant at constant pH and

$$q = \frac{[H_2PO_4^-]}{[HPO_4^{2-}]}$$

On plotting k_{obs} (day^{-1}) versus $[H_2PO_4^{2-}]$ expressed in molar concentration, straight lines were obtained at the two pH values of 6.35 and 5.90. The q values at these pH values can be determined. The slope of the plots at pH values of 6.35 and 5.90 were 0.155 and 0.0556, respectively. (a) Compute the k_2 and k_3 values. (b) Which buffer ion is catalyzing the reaction?

Answers: (a) $k_3 = 1.09$ M^{-1} day^{-1}, $k_2 = 0.001$ M^{-1} day^{-1}; (b) HPO_4^{2-} catalyzes the reaction

12–36. Cyclophosphamide monohydrate is available as a sterile blend of dry drug and sodium chloride packaged in vials. A suitable aqueous vehicle is added and the sterile powder dissolved with agitation before the product is used parenterally. However, cyclophosphamide monohydrate is only slowly soluble in water, and a hospital pharmacist inquired concerning the advisability of briefly (for 15 min) warming the solution to 70° C to facilitate dissolution. Brooke et al. addressed this problem.[109] Assuming that degradation to 95% of the labeled amount is permitted for this compound, and given k at 25° C = 0.028 day^{-1}, $E_a = 25.00$ kcal/mole, what answer would you give?

Answer: $t_{95\%} = 10.4$ min. Degradation has occurred to the extent of 5% in 10.4 min, so heating at 70° C for a full 15 min would not be advisable. Brooke et al.[109] found by actual assay that heating at 50° C or 60° C produced less than 5% decomposition.

13
Diffusion and Dissolution

Free diffusion or passive transport of substances through liquids, solids, and membranes is a process of considerable importance in the pharmaceutical sciences. Topics of mass transport phenomena applying to pharmacy are dissolution of drugs from tablets, powders, and granules; lyophilization, ultrafiltration, and other mechanical processes; release from ointments and suppository bases; passage of water vapor, gases, drugs, and dosage form additives through coatings, packaging, films, plastic container walls, seals, and caps; and permeation and distribution of drug molecules in living tissues.

Diffusion. *Diffusion* is defined as a process of mass transfer of individual molecules of a substance, brought about by random molecular motion and associated with a concentration gradient. Flow of molecules through a barrier such as a polymeric membrane is a particularly convenient way to study diffusion processes. The passage of matter through a barrier (Fig. 13–1) may occur by simple molecular permeation or by movement through pores and channels. Molecular diffusion or permeation through nonporous media depends on dissolution of the permeating molecules in the bulk membrane (Fig. 13–1a), whereas a second process may involve passage of a substance through solvent-filled pores of a membrane (Fig. 13–1b) and is influenced by the relative sizes of the penetrating molecules and the diameter of the pores. The transport of a drug through a polymeric membrane involves dissolution of the drug in the matrix of the membrane and is an example of simple molecular diffusion. Passage of steroidal molecules, substituted with hydrophilic groups, through human skin may predominantly involve transport through hair follicles, sebum ducts, and sweat pores in the epidermis (see Fig. 13–22). Perhaps a better representation of a membrane on the molecular scale is a matted arrangement of polymer strands with branch-

ing and intersecting channels as shown in Figure 13–1c. Depending on the size and shape of the diffusing molecules, they may pass through the tortuous pores formed by the overlapping strands of polymer. If too large for such channel transport, the diffusant may dissolve in the polymer matrix and pass through the film by simple diffusion.

Dialysis. Hwang and Kammermeyer[1] define *dialysis* as a separation process based on unequal rates of passage of solutes and solvent through microporous membranes, carried out in batch or continuous mode. *Hemodialysis* is used in kidney malfunction to rid the blood of metabolic waste products (small molecules) while preserving the high-molecular-weight components of the blood.

Osmosis. A process related to dialysis, *osmosis* was originally defined as the passage of both solute and solvent across a membrane, but now refers to an action in which only the solvent is transferred. The solvent passes through the semipermeable membrane to dilute the solution containing solute and solvent (see p. 116). The passage of solute together with solvent now is called *diffusion* or *dialysis*.

Ultrafiltration. Ultrafiltration is used to separate colloidal particles and macromolecules by the use of a membrane. Hydraulic pressure is employed to force the solvent through the membrane while the microporous membrane prevents the passage of large solute molecules. Ultrafiltration is similar to a process called *reverse osmosis*, but a much higher osmotic pressure is developed in reverse osmosis, which is used in desalination of brackish water. Ultrafiltration is used in the pulp and paper industry and in research to purify albumin and enzymes. *Microfiltration*, a process that employs membranes of slightly larger pore size, 100 nanometers to several micrometers, removes bacteria from intravenous injections, foods, and drinking wa-

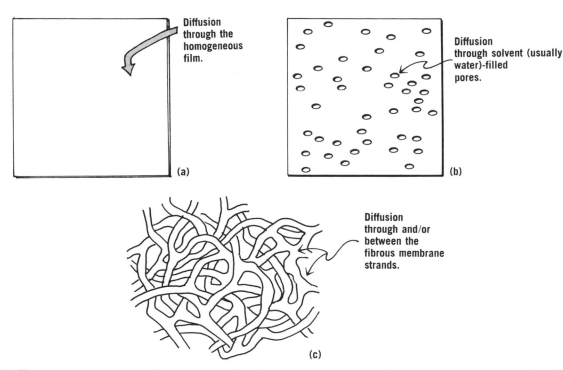

Fig. 13–1. *(a)* Homogeneous membrane without pores. *(b)* Membrane of dense material with straight-through pores, as found in certain filter barriers such as Nucleopore. *(c)* Cellulose membrane used in filtration processes, showing intertwining nature of fibers and tortuous channels.

ter.[2] In ordinary osmosis as well as in dialysis, separation is spontaneous and does not involve the high applied pressures of ultrafiltration and reverse osmosis.

Flynn et al.[3] differentiate between a membrane and a barrier. A *membrane* is a film separating the phases, and material passes by passive, active, or facilitated transport across this film. The term *barrier* applies in a more general sense to the region or regions that offer resistance to passage of a diffusing material, the total barrier being the sum of individual resistances of membranes or the component films of laminae interposed between a donor and a receptor chamber.

STEADY-STATE DIFFUSION

Fick's First Law. The amount M of material flowing through a unit cross-section, S, of a barrier in unit time, t, is known as the flux, J.

$$J = \frac{dM}{S \cdot dt} \qquad (13\text{--}1)$$

The flux in turn is proportional to the concentration gradient, dC/dx:

$$J = -D\frac{dC}{dx} \qquad (13\text{--}2)$$

in which D is the *diffusion coefficient* of a penetrant (also called the *diffusant*) in cm²/sec, C its concentration in g/cm³, and x the distance in cm of movement perpendicular to the surface of the barrier. In equation (13–1), the mass, M, is usually given in grams or moles, the barrier surface, S, in cm², and the time, t, in seconds. The units on J are g cm^{-2} sec^{-1}. The SI units of kilogram and meter are sometimes used, and the time may be given in minutes, hours, or days. The negative sign of equation (13–2) signifies that diffusion occurs in a direction (the positive x direction) opposite to that of increasing concentration. That is to say, diffusion occurs in the direction of decreasing concentration of diffusant; thus, the flux is always a positive quantity.

The diffusion constant, D, or *diffusivity* as it is often called, does not ordinarily remain constant, for it may change in value at higher concentrations. D is also affected by temperature, pressure, solvent properties, and the chemical nature of the diffusant. Therefore, D is referred to more correctly as a *diffusion coefficient* rather than as a constant. Equation (13–2) is known as *Fick's first law*.

Fick's Second Law. One often wants to examine the rate of change of diffusant concentration at a point in the system. An equation for mass transport that emphasizes the change in *concentration* with time at a definite location rather than the *mass* diffusing across a unit area of barrier in unit time, is known as *Fick's second law*. This diffusion equation is derived as follows. The concentration C in a particular volume element, (see Figs. 13–2 and 13–3) changes only as a result of net flow of diffusing molecules into or out of the region. A difference in concentration results from a difference in input and output. The concentration of diffusant in the volume element changes with time, that

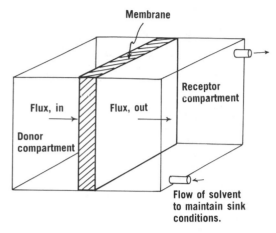

Fig. 13–2. Diffusion cell. Donor compartment contains diffusant at concentration C.

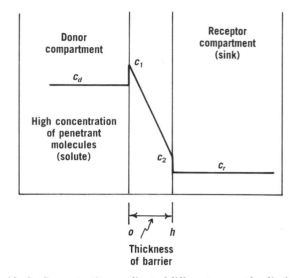

Fig. 13–3. Concentration gradient of diffusant across the diaphragm of a diffusion cell. It is normal for the concentration curve to increase or decrease sharply at the boundaries of the barrier since, in general, c_1 is different from c_d and c_2 is different from c_r. c_1 would be equal to c_d, for example, only if $K = c_1/c_d$ had a value of unity.

is, $\Delta C/\Delta t$, as the flux or amount diffusing changes with distance, $\Delta J/\Delta x$, in the x direction, or*

$$\frac{\partial C}{\partial t} = -\frac{\partial J}{\partial x} \qquad (13\text{–}3)$$

Differentiating the first-law expression, equation (13–2), with respect to x, one obtains

$$-\frac{\partial J}{\partial x} = D\,\frac{\partial^2 c}{\partial x^2} \qquad (13\text{–}4)$$

Substituting $\partial C/\partial t$ from equation (13–3) into equation (13–4) results in Fick's second law, namely

$$\frac{\partial C}{\partial t} = D\,\frac{\partial^2 c}{\partial x^2} \qquad (13\text{–}5)$$

Equation (13–5) represents diffusion only in the x direction. If one wishes to express concentration changes of diffusant in three dimensions, Fick's second law is written in the general form

$$\frac{\partial C}{\partial t} = D\left(\frac{\partial^2 C}{\partial x^2} + \frac{\partial^2 C}{\partial y^2} + \frac{\partial^2 C}{\partial z^2}\right) \qquad (13\text{–}6)$$

This expression is not usually needed in pharmaceutical problems of diffusion, however, since movement in one direction is sufficient to describe most cases. Fick's second law states that the change in concentration with time in a particular region is proportional to the change in the concentration gradient at that point in the system.

Steady State. An important condition in diffusion is that of the *steady state*. Fick's first law, equation (13–2), gives the flux (or rate of diffusion through unit area) in the steady state of flow. The second law refers in general to a change in concentration of diffusant with time, at any distance, x (i.e., a nonsteady state of flow). Steady state may be described, however, in terms of the second law, equation (13–5). Consider the diffusant

originally dissolved in a solvent in the left-hand compartment of the cell shown in Figure 13–2. Solvent alone is placed on the right-hand side of the barrier, and the solute or penetrant diffuses through the central barrier from solution to solvent side (donor to receptor compartment). In diffusion experiments, the solution in the receptor compartment is constantly removed and replaced with fresh solvent to keep the concentration at a low level. This is referred to as "sink conditions," the left compartment being the source and the right compartment the sink.

Originally, the diffusant concentration will fall in the left compartment and rise in the right compartment until the system comes to an equilibrium, based on the rate of removal of diffusant from the sink and the nature of the barrier. When the system has been in existence a sufficient time, the concentration of diffusant in the solutions at the left and right of the barrier become constant with respect to time, but obviously not the same in the two compartments. Then within each diffusional slice perpendicular to the direction of flow, the rate of change of concentration, dC/dt, will be zero, and by the second law,

$$\frac{dC}{dt} = D\,\frac{d^2C}{dx^2} = 0 \qquad (13\text{–}7)$$

C is the concentration of the permeant in the barrier expressed in mass/cm³. Equation (13–7) demonstrates that since D is not equal to zero, $d^2C/dx^2 = 0$. When a second derivative such as this equals zero, one concludes that there is no change in dC/dx. In other words, the concentration gradient across the membrane dC/dx is constant, signifying a linear relationship between concentration, C, and distance, x. This is shown in Figure 13–3 (in which the distance x is equal to h) for drug diffusing from left to right in the cell of Figure

*Concentration and flux are often written as $C(x,t)$ and $J(x,t)$, respectively, to emphasize that these parameters are functions of both distance x and time t.

13–2. Concentration will not be rigidly constant but rather is likely to vary slightly with time, and then dC/dt is not exactly zero. The conditions are referred to as a "quasi-stationary" state, and little error is introduced by assuming steady state under these conditions.

Fick adapted the two diffusion equations, (13–2) and (13–5), to the transport of matter from the laws of heat conduction. Equations of heat conduction are found in the book by Carslaw.[4] General solutions to these differential equations yield complex expressions; simple equations are used here for the most part, and worked examples are provided so that the careful reader will have no difficulty in following the arguments of dissolution and diffusion.

If a diaphragm separates the two compartments of a diffusion cell of cross-sectional area S and thickness h, and if the concentrations in the membrane on the left (donor) and on the right (receptor) sides are C_1 and C_2, respectively (Fig. 13–3), the first law of Fick may be written

$$J = \frac{dM}{S\,dt} = D\left(\frac{C_1 - C_2}{h}\right) \qquad (13-8)$$

in which $(C_1 - C_2)/h$ approximates dC/dx. The gradient $(C_1 - C_2)/h$ within the diaphragm must be assumed to be constant for a quasi-stationary state to exist. Equation (13–8) presumes that the aqueous boundary layers (so-called static or unstirred aqueous layers) on both sides of the membrane do not significantly affect the total transport process.

The concentrations C_1 and C_2 within the membrane ordinarily are not known but can be replaced by the partition coefficient multiplied by the concentration C_d on the donor side or C_r on the receiver side, as follows. The distribution or partition coefficient, K, is given by

$$K = \frac{C_1}{C_d} = \frac{C_2}{C_r} \qquad (13-9)$$

Hence,

$$\frac{dM}{dt} = \frac{DSK(C_d - C_r)}{h} \qquad (13-10a)$$

and, if sink conditions hold in the receptor compartment, $C_r \cong 0$,

$$\frac{dM}{dt} = \frac{DSKC_d}{h} = PSC_d \qquad (13-10b)$$

in which

$$P = \frac{DK}{h} \quad \text{(cm/sec)} \qquad (13-11)$$

It is noteworthy that the permeability coefficient, also called the *permeability*, P, has units of linear velocity.[*]

In some cases, it is not possible to determine D, K, or h independently and thereby to calculate P. It is a relatively simple matter, however, to measure the rate of barrier permeation and to obtain the surface area S and concentration C_d in the donor phase and the amount of permeant M in the receiving sink. One can then obtain P from the slope of a linear plot of M versus t:

$$M = PSC_d t \qquad (13-12a)$$

providing that C_d remains relatively constant throughout time. If C_d changes appreciably with time, one recognizes that $C_d = M_d/V_d$, the amount of drug in the donor phase divided by the donor phase volume, and then one obtains P from the slope of $\log C_d$ versus t:

$$\log C_d = \log C_d(0) - \frac{PSt}{2.303V_d} \qquad (13-12b)$$

The flux J of equation (13–8) is actually proportional to a gradient of thermodynamic activity rather than concentration. The activity will change in different solvents, and the diffusion rate of a solvent at a definite concentration may vary widely depending on the solvent employed. The thermodynamic activity of a drug may be held constant ($a = 1$) in a delivery form by using a saturated solution in the presence of excess solid drug. Unit activity ensures constant release of the drug at a rate that depends on the membrane permeability and the geometry of the dosage form. Figure 13–4 shows the rate of delivery of two steroids from a device, providing constant drug activity and what is known as "zero-order release." The reader is familiar with zero-order process from a study of kinetics (Chapter 12). If excess solid is not present in the delivery form, the activity decreases as the drug diffuses out of the device, the release rate falls exponentially, and the process is referred to as first-order release, analogous to the well-known reaction in chemical kinetics. First-order release from dosage forms is discussed by Baker and Lonsdale.[5]

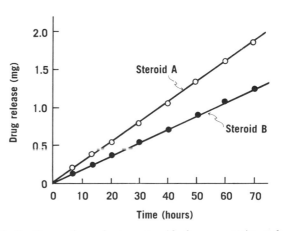

Fig. 13–4. Drug release for two steroids from a matrix or device providing zero-order release. (After R. W. Baker and H. K. Lonsdale, in *Controlled Release of Biologically Active Agents*, A. C. Tanquary and R. E. Lacey, Eds., Plenum Press, New York, 1974, p. 30.)

---

*Confusion arises when the permeability coefficient is defined by $P = DK$(cm²/sec) as used when D and K are not independently known. Equation (13–11), including h in the denominator, is the conventional definition of permeability.

A constant-activity dosage form may not exhibit a steady-state process from the initial time of release. Figure 13–5 is a plot of the amount of butylparaben penetrating through guinea pig skin from a dilute aqueous solution of the penetrant. It is observed that the curve of Figure 13–5 is convex to the time axis in the early stage and then becomes linear. The early stage is the nonsteady-state condition. At later times, the rate of diffusion is constant, the curve is essentially linear, and the system is at steady state. When the steady-state portion of the line is extrapolated to the time axis, as shown in Figure 13–5, the point of intersection is known as the *lag time*, t_L. This is the time required for a penetrant to establish a uniform concentration gradient within the membrane separating the donor from the receptor compartments.

In the case of a time lag, the straight line of Figure 13–5 may be represented by a modification of equation (13–10):

$$M = \frac{SDKC_d}{h}(t - t_L) \qquad (13-13)$$

The lag time, t_L, is given by

$$t_L = \frac{h^2}{6D} \qquad (13-14a)$$

and its measurement provides a means of calculating the diffusivity D, presuming a knowledge of the membrane thickness h. Also, knowing P, the thickness h can be calculated from

$$t_L = \frac{h}{6P} \qquad (13-14b)$$

Example 13–1. A newly synthesized steroid is allowed to pass through a siloxane membrane, having a cross-sectional area S of 10.36 cm^2 and a thickness h of 0.085 cm, in a diffusion cell at 25° C. From the horizontal intercept of a plot of $Q = M/S$ vs. t, the lag time t_L is found

to be 47.5 minutes. The original concentration C_0 is 0.003 mmole/cm.^{3} The amount of steroid passing through the membrane in 4.0 hours is 3.65×10^{-3} mmole.

(a) Calculate the parameter, DK, and the permeability, P.

$$Q = \frac{3.65 \times 10^{-3}\ \text{mmole}}{10.36\ \text{cm}^2} = 0.35 \times 10^{-3}\ \text{mmole/cm}^2$$

$$= DK\left(\frac{0.003\ \text{mmole/cm}^3}{0.085\ \text{cm}}\right)\left[4.0\ \text{hr} - \left(\frac{47.5}{60}\right)\text{hr}\right]$$

$DK = 0.0031\ \text{cm}^2/\text{hr} = 8.6 \times 10^{-7}\ \text{cm}^2/\text{sec}$

$P = DK/h = (8.6 \times 10^{-7}\ \text{cm}^2/\text{sec})/0.085\ \text{cm} = 1.01 \times 10^{-5}\ \text{cm/sec}$

(b) Using the lag time, $t_L = h^2/6D$, calculate the diffusion coefficient.

$$D = \frac{h^2}{6t_L} = \frac{(0.085)^2\ \text{cm}^2}{6 \times 47.5\ \text{min}}$$

$$= 25.4 \times 10^{-6}\ \text{cm}^2/\text{min}$$

or

$$= 4.23 \times 10^{-7}\ \text{cm}^2/\text{sec}$$

(c) Combining the permeability, Equation (13–11), with the value of D from (b), calculate the partition coefficient, K.

$$K = \frac{Ph}{D} = \frac{(1.01 \times 10^{-5}\ \text{cm/sec})(0.085\ \text{cm})}{4.23 \times 10^{-7}\text{cm}^2/\text{sec}} = 2.03$$

Partition coefficients have already been discussed in the chapter on solubility.

Diffusivity depends on the resistance to passage of a diffusing molecule. Gas molecules diffuse rapidly through air and other gases. Diffusivities in liquids are smaller, and in solids still smaller. Gas molecules pass slowly and with great difficulty through metal sheets and crystalline barriers. Diffusivities are a function of the molecular structure of the diffusant as well as the barrier material. Diffusion coefficients for gases and liquids passing through water, chloroform, and polymeric materials are found in Table 13–1. Approximate diffusion coefficients and permeabilities for drugs passing from a solvent in which they are dissolved (water, unless otherwise specified) through natural and synthetic membranes are found in Table 13–2.

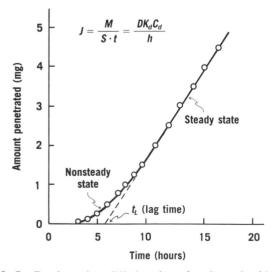

Fig. 13–5. Butyl paraben diffusing through guinea pig skin from aqueous solution. Steady-state and nonsteady-state regions are shown. (From H. Komatsu and M. Suzuki, J. Pharm. Sci. **68**, 596, 1979, reproduced with permission of the copyright owner.)

TABLE 13–1. *Diffusion Coefficients of Compounds in Various Media**

Diffusant	Partial Molar Volume (cm^3/mole)	$D \times 10^6$ (cm^2/sec)	Medium or Barrier (temperature, °C)
Ethanol	40.9	12.4	Water (25°)
n-Pentanol	89.5	8.8	Water (25°)
Formamide	26	17.2	Water (25°)
Glycine	42.9	10.6	Water (25°)
Sodium lauryl sulfate	235	6.2	Water (25°)
Glucose	116	6.8	Water (25°)
Hexane	103	15.0	Chloroform (25°)
Hexadecane	265	7.8	Chloroform (25°)
Methanol	25	26.1	Chloroform (25°)
Acetic acid dimer	64	14.2	Chloroform (25°)
Methane	22.4	1.45	Natural rubber (40°)
n-Pentane	—	6.9	Silicone rubber (50°)
Neopentane	—	0.002	Ethycellulose (50°)

*From G. L. Flynn, S. H. Yalkowsky, and T. J. Roseman, J. Pharm. Sci. **63**, 507, 1974, reproduced with permission of the copyright owner.

TABLE 13–2. *Drug Diffusion and Permeability Coefficients*

Drug	Membrane Diffusion Coefficient (cm²/sec)	Membrane Permeability Coefficient (cm/sec)	Pathway	Temperature (°C)	Reference
Benzoic acid	—	36.6×10^{-4}	Absorption from rat jejunum	37	a
Butyl p-aminobenzoate	2.7×10^{-6}	—	From aqueous solution through silastic membrane	37	b
Chloramphenicol	—	$\dagger 1.87 \times 10^{-6}$	Through mouse skin	25	c
	—	5.02×10^{-6}	Through mouse skin	37	c
Ethynodiol diacetate	3.94×10^{-7} (3.4×10^{-2} cm²/day)	—	Release from silastic matrix	25	d
Estrone	—	20.7×10^{-4}	Absorption from rat jejunum	37	a
Fluocinolone acetonide	1.11×10^{-8} (4×10^{-5} cm²/hr)	—	From 30% propylene glycol— 70% water solvent through a polyethylene membrane	25	e
Hydrocortisone	—	0.56×10^{-4}	Absorption from rat jejunum	37	a
	—	5.8×10^{-5}	Absorption from rabbit vaginal tract	37	f
Medroxyprogesterone acetate	3.7×10^{-7}	—	Release from silastic matrix	25	g
Nicotinamide	—	1.54×10^{-4}	Absorption from rat jejunum	37	a
Octanol	—	12×10^{-4}	Absorption from rat jejunum	37	a
Octanoic acid	—	39×10^{-4}	Absorption from rat jejunum	37	a
Progesterone	—	7×10^{-4}	Absorption from rabbit vaginal tract	37	a
Prostaglandin, 15(S)-methyl- PGF$_{2d}$	—	0.58×10^{-4}	In situ absorption from rat jejunum	37	a
Salicylates	1.69×10^{-6}	—	Diffusion across cellulose membrane	37	h
Salicylic acid	—	10.4×10^{-4}	Absorption from rat jejunum	37	a
Testosterone	—	20×10^{-4}	Absorption from rat jejunum	37	a
Water	2.8×10^{-10}	2.78×10^{-7}	Diffusion into human skin layers	37	i

a. N. F. H. Ho, J. Y. Park, W. Morozowich and W. I. Higuchi, Physical model approach to design of drugs with improved intestinal absorption, in *Design of Biopharmaceutical Properties Through Pro-drugs and Analogs,* E. B. Roche, Ed., American Pharmaceutical Association, Academy of Pharmaceutical Sciences, Washington, D.C., 1977, Chapter 8, pp. 154–155.
b. G. L. Flynn and S. H. Yalkowsky, J. Pharm. Sci. **61**, 838, 1972.
c. A. J. Aguiar and M. A. Weiner, J. Pharm. Sci. **58**, 210, 1969.
d. Y. W. Chien, in *Sustained and Controlled Release Drug Delivery Systems,* J. R. Robinson, Ed., Marcel Dekker, New York, 1978, Chapter 4.
e. J. S. Turi, D. Danielson and W. Wolterson, J. Pharm. Sci. **68**, 275, 1979.
f. N. F. H. Ho, L. Suhardja, S. Hwang, E. Owada, A. Molokhia, G. L. Flynn, W. I. Higuchi and J. Y. Park, J. Pharm. Sci. **65**, 1578, 1976.
g. T. J. Roseman, J. Pharm. Sci. **61**, 46, 1972; Y. W. Chien, H. J. Lambert and D. E. Grant, J. Pharm. Sci. **63**, 365, 1974.
h. K. F. Farng and K. G. Nelson, J. Pharm. Sci. **66**, 1611, 1977.
i. R. J. Scheuplein, J. Invest. Dermatol. **45**, 334, 1965.

In the chapter on colloids, p. 401, we will see that the molecular weight and the radius of a spherical protein can be obtained from a knowledge of its diffusivity.

PROCEDURES AND APPARATUS

A number of experimental methods and diffusion cells have been reported in the literature. Examples of those used mainly in pharmaceutical and biologic transport studies are introduced here.

Cells of simple construction, such as the one reported by Karth et al.[6] (Fig. 13–6), are probably best for diffusion work. They are made of glass or clear plastic, are easy to assemble and clean, and allow visibility of the liquids and rotating stirrer. They may be thermostated and lend themselves to automatic sample collection and assay. The donor chamber is filled with drug solution. Samples are collected from the receptor compartment in an automatic fraction collector and subsequently assayed spectrophotometrically. Experi-

ments may be run for hours under these controlled conditions.

Biber and Rhodes[7] constructed a Plexiglas three-compartment diffusion cell for use with either synthetic or isolated biologic membranes. The drug was allowed to diffuse from the two outer donor compartments in a central receptor chamber. Results were reproducible and compared favorably with those from other workers. The three-compartment design created greater membrane surface exposure and improved analytic sensitivity.

The permeation through plastic film of water vapor and of aromatic organic compounds from aqueous solution may be investigated in two-chamber glass cells similar in design to those used for studying drug solutions in general. Nasim et al.[8] reported on the permeation of 19 aromatic compounds from aqueous solution through polyethylene films. Higuchi and Aguiar[9] studied the permeability of water vapor through enteric coating materials using a glass diffusion cell and a McLeod gauge to measure changes in pressure across the film.

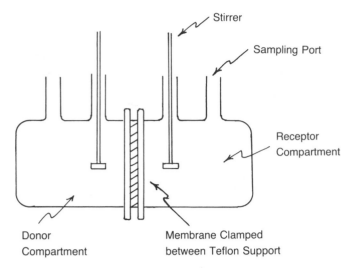

Fig. 13-6. Simple diffusion cell. (After M. G. Karth, W. I. Higuchi and J. L. Fox, J. Pharm. Sci. **74**, 612, 1985, reproduced with permission of the copyright owner.)

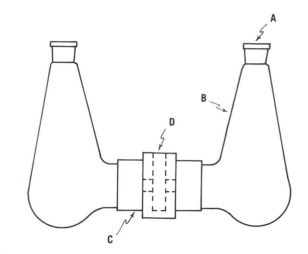

Fig. 13-7. Diffusion cell for permeation through stripped skin layers. The permeant may be in the form of a gas, liquid, or gel. Key: *A*, glass stopper; *B*, glass chamber; *C*, aluminum collar; *D*, membrane and sample holder. (From D. E. Wurster, J. A. Ostrenga and L. E. Matheson, Jr., J. Pharm. Sci. **68**, 1406, 1410, 1979, reproduced with permission of the copyright owner.)

The sorption of gases and vapors may be determined by use of a microbalance enclosed in a temperature-controlled and evacuated vessel that is capable of weighing within a sensitivity of $\pm 2 \times 10^{-6}$ g. The gas or vapor is introduced at controlled pressures into the glass chamber containing the polymer or biologic film of known dimensions, suspended on one arm of the balance. The mass of diffusant sorbed at various pressures by the film is recorded directly.[10] The rate of approach to equilibrium sorption permits easy calculation of the diffusion coefficients for gases and vapors.

In studying percutaneous absorption, animal or human skin, ordinarily obtained by autopsy, is employed. Scheuplein[11] described a cell for skin penetration experiments made of Pyrex and consisting of two halves, a donor and a receptor chamber, separated by a sample of skin supported on a perforated plate and securely clamped in place. The liquid in the receptor was stirred by a Teflon-coated bar magnet. The apparatus was submerged in a constant-temperature bath, and samples were removed periodically and assayed by appropriate means. For compounds such as steroids, penetration was slow, and radioactive methods were found necessary to determine the low concentrations.

Wurster et al.[12] developed a permeability cell to study the diffusion through stratum corneum (stripped from the human forearm) of various permeants, including gases, liquids, and gels. The permeability cell is shown in Figure 13-7. During diffusion experiments it was kept at constant temperature and gently shaken in the plane of the membrane. Samples were withdrawn from the receptor chamber at definite times and analyzed for the permeant.

The kinetics and equilibria of liquid and solute absorption into plastics, skin, and chemical and other biologic materials may be determined simply by placing sections of the film in a constant-temperature bath of the pure liquid or solution. The sections are retrieved at various times, excess liquid is removed with absorbant tissue, and the film samples are accurately weighed in tared weighing bottles. A radioactive-counting technique also may be used with this method to analyze for drug remaining in solution and, by difference, the amount sorbed into the film.

Partition coefficients are determined simply by equilibrating the drug between two immiscible solvents in a suitable vessel at a constant temperature and removing samples from both phases, if possible, for analysis.[13] Addicks et al.[14] described a new flow-through cell, Grass and Sweetana[15] proposed a diffusion cell for the study of gastrointestinal permeation, and Addicks et al.[16] designed a cell that yields results more comparable to the diffusion of drugs under clinical conditions. Equilibrium solubilities of drug solutes are also required in diffusion studies, and these are obtained as described earlier (Chapter 10).

DISSOLUTION

Biopharmaceutics and the modern design of dosage forms, as dealt with later in Chapter 19, are based partly on principles of dissolution and diffusion theory. The present chapter lays a foundation for the study of these topics by way of presenting concepts, illustrations, and worked examples. Dissolution is introduced first, followed by examples of diffusion from the literature, with applications of both subjects to pharmaceutical problems.

Dissolution Rate. When a tablet or other solid drug form is introduced into a beaker of water or into the gastrointestinal tract, the drug begins to pass into solution from the intact solid. Unless the tablet is a contiguous polymeric device, the solid matrix also disintegrates into granules, and these granules deaggregate in turn into fine particles. Disintegration, deaggregation, and dissolution may occur simultaneously with the release of a drug from its delivery form. These steps are separated for clarification as depicted in Figure 13–8.

The effectiveness of a tablet in releasing its drug for systemic absorption depends somewhat on the rate of disintegration of the dosage forms and deaggregation of the granules. Ordinarily of more importance, however, is the dissolution rate of the solid drug. Frequently, dissolution is the limiting or rate-controlling step in bioabsorption for drugs of low solubility, because it is often the slowest of the various stages involved in release of the drug from its dosage form and passage into systemic circulation. Dissolution has been reviewed by Wurster and Taylor,[17] Wagner,[18] and Leeson and Carstensen.[19] Release rate processes in general are discussed by W. Higuchi.[20]

The rate at which a solid dissolves in a solvent was proposed in quantitative terms by Noyes and Whitney in 1897 and elaborated subsequently by other workers. The equation may be written as

$$\frac{dM}{dt} = \frac{DS}{h}(C_s - C) \qquad (13\text{–}15)$$

or

$$\frac{dC}{dt} = \frac{DS}{Vh}(C_s - C) \qquad (13\text{–}16)$$

in which M is the mass of solute dissolved in time t, dM/dt the mass rate of dissolution (mass/time), D the diffusion coefficient of the solute in solution, S the surface area of the exposed solid, h the thickness of the diffusion layer, C_s the solubility of the solid (i.e., concentration of a saturated solution of the compound at the surface of the solid and at the temperature of the experiment), and C the concentration of solute in the bulk solution and at time t. The quantity dC/dt is the dissolution rate and V the volume of solution.

In dissolution or mass transfer theory, it is assumed that an *aqueous diffusion layer* or *stagnant liquid film* of thickness h exists at the surface of a solid undergoing dissolution, as observed in Figure 13–9. This thickness h represents a stationary layer of solvent in which the solute molecules exist in concentrations from C_s to C. Beyond the static diffusion layer, at x greater than h, mixing occurs in the solution, and the drug is found at a uniform concentration, C, throughout the bulk phase.

At the solid surface–diffusion layer interface, $x = 0$, the drug in the solid is in equilibrium with drug in the diffusion layer. The gradient, or change in concentration with distance across the diffusion layer, is constant, as shown by the straight downward-sloping line. This is the gradient represented in equations (13–15) and (13–16) by the term $(C_s - C)/h$. The similarity of the Noyes–Whitney equation to Fick's first law is evident in equation (13–15).

When C is considerably less than the drug's solubility, C_s, the system is represented by *sink conditions*, and concentration C may be eliminated from equations (13–15) and (13–16). Equation (13–15) then becomes

$$dM/dt = DSC_s/h \qquad (13\text{–}17)$$

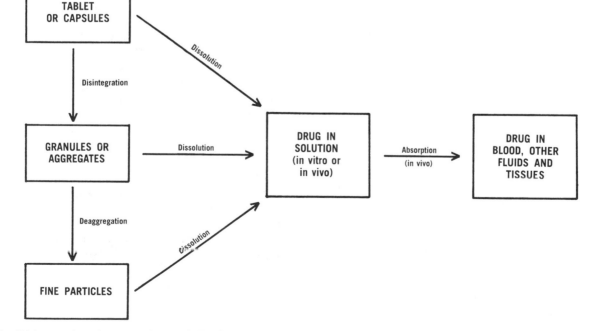

Fig. 13–8. Disintegration, deaggregation, and dissolution stages as a drug leaves a tablet or granular matrix. (From John G. Wagner, *Biopharmaceutics and Relevant Pharmacokinetics*, published by Drug Intelligence Publications, Inc., 1241 Broadway, Hamilton, IL 62341, p. 99, with permission of the copyright owner.)

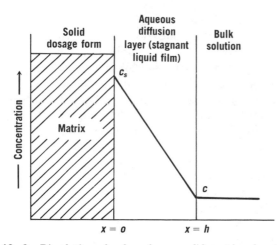

Fig. 13-9. Dissolution of a drug from a solid matrix, showing the stagnant diffusion layer between the dosage form surface and bulk solution.

In the derivation of equations (13-15) and (13-16), it was assumed that h and S were constant, but this is not the case. The static diffusion layer thickness is altered by the force of agitation at the surface of the dissolving tablet and will be referred to later. The surface area S obviously does not remain constant as a powder, granule, or tablet dissolves, and it is difficult to obtain an accurate measure of S as the process continues. In experimental studies of dissolution, the surface may be controlled by placing a compressed pellet in a holder that exposes a surface of constant area. Although this ensures better adherence to the requirements of equations (13-15), (13-16), and (13-17) and provides valuable information on the drug, it does not simulate the actual dissolution of the material in practice.

Dissolution of Tablets, Capsules, and Granules. A number of methods for the in vitro and in vivo testing of dosage forms have been suggested.[21,22] The purpose of an in vitro dissolution study is to provide a fast and inexpensive method that correlates with the performance of a dosage form in human subjects, and a number of studies towards this end have been reported in the literature.[23] Various dissolution apparatus and methods are described in some detail in the latter work.[22] The Hansen paddle equipment and a research apparatus provide two convenient systems, as shown in Figure 13-10a and b. As observed, the apparatus are similar except that the surface area of the tablet or compacted material in Figure 13-10b remains constant as the drug dissolves. This design has advantages in research and product formulation. Furthermore, exact hydrodynamic conditions are maintained by the fixed position of stirrer and sample holder. Much attention has been paid to the rotating disk, a modification of the apparatus in Figure 13-10b, in which the tablet in its holder is attached to a rotating shaft of a precision variable-speed motor.[24] The paddle of Figure 13-10b is not required in the rotating-disk apparatus. The paddle equipment of Figure 13-10a is currently known as the

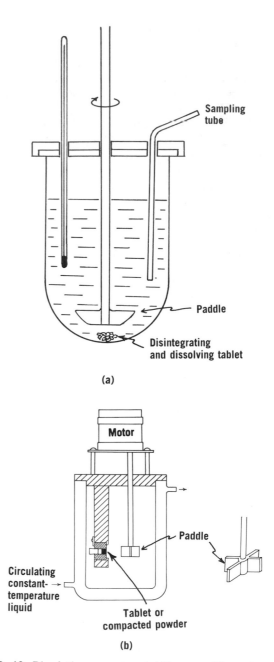

Fig. 13-10. Dissolution apparatus. *(a)* Hansen paddle equipment for granules and tablets. *(b)* Research design to ensure a constant surface area of tablet or compacted powder as the drug dissolves and diffuses out of the dosage form. (From A. P. Simonelli, S. C. Mehta and W. I. Higuchi, J. Pharm. Sci. **58**, 538, 1969, reproduced with permission of the copyright owner.)

USP Dissolution Apparatus 2, and a rotating basket apparatus (not shown) is referred to as USP Dissolution Apparatus 1.

In calculating the diffusion coefficient and dissolution rate constant, the application of equations (13-15) to (13-17) is demonstrated by way of the following two examples.

Example 13-2. A preparation of drug granules weighing 0.55 g and having a total surface area of 0.28 m² (0.28 × 10⁴ cm²) is allowed to dissolve in 500 mL of water at 25° C. After the first minute, 0.76 g have passed into solution. The quantity D/h may be referred to as a dissolution rate constant, k.

If the solubility C_s of the drug is 15 mg/mL at 25° C, what is k? From equation (13–17), M changes linearly with t initially, and

$$\frac{dM}{dt} = \frac{760 \text{ mg}}{60 \text{ sec}} = 12.67 \text{ mg/sec}$$

$$12.67 \text{ mg/sec} = k \times 0.28 \times 10^4 \text{ cm}^2 \times 15 \text{ mg/cm}^3$$

$$k = 3.02 \times 10^{-4} \text{ cm/sec}$$

In this example, 0.760 g dissolved in 500 mL after a time of 1 minute or 760 mg/500 mL = 1.5 mg/cm³. This value is one tenth of the drug's solubility and may be omitted from equation (13–15) without introducing significant error, shown by employing the full equation (13–15):

$$k = \frac{12.67 \text{ mg/sec}}{(0.28 \times 10^4 \text{ cm}^2)(15 \text{ mg/cm}^3 - 1.5 \text{ mg/cm}^3)}$$

$$k = 3.35 \times 10^{-4} \text{ cm/sec}$$

When this result is compared with 3.02×10^{-4} cm/sec, obtained using the less exact expression, it signifies that "sink conditions" are in effect, and the concentration term C may be omitted from the rate equation.

Example 13–3. The diffusion layer thickness in *Example 13–2* is estimated to be 5×10^{-3} cm. Calculate D, the diffusion coefficient, using the relation $k = D/h$.

$$D = (3.35 \times 10^{-4} \text{ cm/sec}) \times (5 \times 10^{-3} \text{ cm})$$

$$= 1.68 \times 10^{-6} \text{ cm}^2/\text{sec}$$

The reader will find additional examples in the book by Carstensen.[25]

Powder Dissolution: The Hixson–Crowell Cube Root Law. For a drug powder consisting of uniformly sized particles, it is possible to derive an equation that expresses the rate of dissolution based on the cube root of the weight of the particles. The radius of the particle is not assumed to be constant.

The particle (sphere) shown in Figure 13–11 has a radius r and a surface area $4\pi r^2$. Through dissolution, the radius is reduced by dr, and the infinitesimal volume of this section lost is

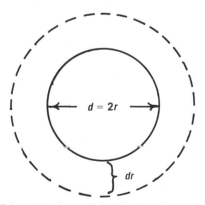

Fig. 13–11. Schematic of a particle, showing change in surface area and volume as the particle dissolves. The volume dV dissolved in dt seconds is given by: thickness × surface area = $dr \times 4\pi r^2$. (After J. T. Carstensen, *Pharmaceutics of Solids and Solid Dosage Forms*, Wiley, New York, 1977, p. 75.)

$$dV = 4\pi r^2 \, dr \qquad (13–18)$$

For N such particles, the volume loss is

$$dV = 4N\pi r^2 \, dr \qquad (13–19)$$

The surface area of N particles is

$$S = 4N\pi r^2 \qquad (13–20)$$

Now, the infinitesimal mass change as represented by the Noyes–Whitney law, equation (13–15), is

$$-dM = kSC_s \, dt \qquad (13–21)$$

in which k is used for D/h as in *Example 13–2*. The drug's density multiplied by the infinitesimal volume change, $\rho \, dV$, may be set equal to dM, or

$$-\rho \, dV = kSC_s \, dt \qquad (13–22)$$

Equations (13–19) and (13–20) are substituted into equation (13–22) to yield

$$-4\rho N\pi r^2 \, dr = 4N\pi r^2 \, kC_s \, dt \qquad (13–23)$$

Equation (13–23) is divided through by $4N\pi r^2$ to give

$$-\rho \, dr = kC_s \, dt \qquad (13–24)$$

Integration with $r = r_0$ at $t = 0$ produces the expression

$$r = r_0 - \frac{kC_s t}{\rho} \qquad (13–25)$$

The radius of spherical particles may be replaced by the mass of N particles by using the relationship (see inside front cover for volume of a sphere).

$$M = N\rho(\pi/6)d^3 \qquad (13–26)$$

in which $d = 2r$, the diameter of the particle. Taking the cube root of equation (13–26) yields

$$M^{1/3} = [N\rho(\pi/6)]^{1/3}d \qquad (13–27)$$

The diameter d of equation (13–27) is substituted for $2r$ into (13–25), giving

$$M_0^{1/3} - M^{1/3} = \kappa t \qquad (13–28)$$

in which

$$\kappa = [N\rho(\pi/6)]^{1/3}\frac{2kC_s}{\rho} = \frac{M_0^{1/3}}{d}\frac{2kC_s}{\rho} \qquad (13–29)$$

M_0 is the original mass of the drug particles. Equation (13–28) is known as the Hixson–Crowell cube root law,[26] and κ is the cube root dissolution rate constant.

Example 13–4. A specially prepared tolbutamide powder of fairly uniformly sized particles, with a diameter of 150 μm*, weighted 75 mg. Dissolution of the drug was determined in 1000 mL of water at 25° C as a function of time. Determine the value of κ, the cube root dissolution rate constant, at each time interval and calculate the average value of κ. The data and results are set forward in Table 13–3.

---

*The symbol, μm, stands for micrometer and is equal to 10^{-6} meters.

TABLE 13–3.   *Dissolution of Tolbutamide Powder*[27]

Time (min)	Concentration Dissolved (mg/mL)	Weight Undissolved (grams) M	$M_0^{1/3} - M^{1/3}$	κ (g$^{1/3}$/min)
0	0	$M_0 = 0.0750$	0	—
10	0.01970	0.0553	0.0406	0.0041
20	0.0374	0.0376	0.0866	0.0043
30	0.0510	0.0240	0.1332	0.0044
40	0.0595	0.0155	0.1724	0.0043
50	0.0650	0.0100	0.2063	0.0041

$$\kappa_{av} = \frac{\Sigma\kappa}{5} = \frac{0.0212}{5} = 0.00424 \text{ g}^{1/3}/\text{min}$$

In the situation in which the aqueous diffusion layer thickness about a spherical particle is comparable to or larger than the size of the sphere, for example, micronized particles less than 50 μm in diameter, the change in particle radius with time becomes

$$r^2 = r_0^2 - \frac{2DC_s t}{\rho} \qquad (13-30)$$

and the estimated time for complete dissolution, τ, (i.e., when $r^2 = 0$) is

$$\tau = \frac{\rho r_0^2}{2DC_s} \qquad (13-31)$$

Example 13–5. In clinical practice, diazepam injection (a sterile solution of diazepam in a propylene glycol–ethanol–water cosolvent system) is often diluted manyfold with normal saline injection. An incipient precipitation of diazepam occurs invariably upon addition of saline followed by complete dissolution within a minute upon shaking. With C_s in water = 3 mg/mL, $\rho \cong 1.0$ g/mL, and $D = 5 \times 10^{-6}$ cm^2/sec, calculate the time for complete dissolution when $r_0 = 10$ μm (10×10^{-4} cm).

$$\tau = \frac{(1 \text{ g/mL})(10 \times 10^{-4} \text{ cm})^2}{2(5 \times 10^{-6} \text{ cm}^2/\text{sec})(3 \times 10^{-3} \text{ g/mL})}$$

$$= 33 \text{ sec}$$

If $r_0 = 25$ μm, $\tau = 208$ sec.

Convective Diffusion. Convection, the transfer of heat (energy) and the presence of agitation accompanying the movement of a fluid, may be combined with diffusion to provide a *convective diffusion model* for the study of dissolution.[28] The convective diffusion model, unlike the simpler Noyes–Whitney and Nernst–Brünner approaches, takes into consideration such factors as flow rate, mixing (agitation), and the dimensions of the dosage form. Nelson and Shah[29] have investigated the convective diffusion model for the dissolution of alkyl *p*-aminobenzoates as test compounds. De Smidt et al.[30] also used a convective diffusion model in the study of the dissolution kinetics of griseofulvin in solutions of the solubilizing agent sodium dodecylsulfate.

Example 13–6. The above workers[29] introduced a drug dissolution rate approach to model the rates of dissolution of alkyl *p*-aminobenzoates in a specially designed diffusion cell. The model is based on convective diffusion, the equations of which may be used to calculate R, the rate of diffusion or permeation rate:

$$R = 0.808 \, D^{2/3} C_s \alpha^{1/3} b L^{2/3} \qquad (13-32)$$

for a *rectangular tablet surface* of width b and length L in the direction of flow, and

$$R = 2.157 \, D^{2/3} C_s \alpha^{1/3} r^{5/3} \qquad (13-33)$$

for a *circular tablet surface* of radius r. In these equations D is the diffusivity or diffusion coefficient, C_s is the solubility, and α is the rate of shear as the solvent is pumped over the dissolving surface. The rate of shear is calculated from $\alpha = 6Q/H^2W$, where Q is the flow rate and H and W are the height and width, respectively, of a channel in the diffusion cell to allow the flow of solvent (water) over the dissolving tablet.

Experiments on dissolution rate, R, were carried out at 37° C with rectangular tablet surfaces containing the drug model ethyl *p*-aminobenzoate. The long axis of the rectangular surface was 25.4 mm and the short axis 3.175 mm.

(*a* and *b*) Compute the rate of dissolution R with the long axis L placed perpendicular to the direction of flow, and then with the long axis placed parallel to the direction of flow. The flow rate Q is 14.9 mL/min; the diffusivity and solubility of the drug are $D = 9.86 \times 10^{-6}$ cm^2/sec and $C_s = 7.27 \times 10^{-6}$ mole/cm^3; and $H^2W = 0.3506$ cm^3.

(*c*) The experiment is repeated but using a disk with a circular surface of area equal to the surface area of the rectangle referred to above. Compute R expressing the results in mole/min.

(*d*) What differences do you find between this model and the classic stagnant or unstirred diffusion layer model? You may care to refer to the articles[29] to check the answers given here.

(*a*) The rate of shear is

$$\alpha = 6Q/H^2W = 6 \times 14.9 \text{ cm}^3\text{min}^{-1}/0.3506 \text{ cm}^3 = 255.0 \text{ min}^{-1}$$

For the long axis perpendicular to flow, $b = 2.54$ cm and $L = 0.3175$ cm. Then,

$$R = 0.808(9.86 \times 10^{-6} \text{ cm}^2/\text{sec} \times 60 \text{ sec/min})^{2/3} \times$$
$$(7.27 \times 10^{-6} \text{ mole/cm}^3) \times (255. \text{ min}^{-1})^{1/3} \times$$
$$(2.54 \text{ cm}) \times (0.3175 \text{ cm})^{2/3}$$
$$= 3.10 \times 10^{-7} \text{ mole/min}$$

(*b*) For the long axis parallel to the flow, $b = 0.3175$ cm and $L = 2.54$ cm.

$$R = 0.808(9.86 \times 10^{-6} \text{ cm}^2/\text{sec} \times 60 \text{ sec/min})^{2/3} \times$$
$$(7.27 \times 10^{-6} \text{ mole/cm}^3) \times (255. \text{ min}^{-1})^{1/3} \times$$
$$(0.3175 \text{ cm}) \times (2.54 \text{ cm})^{2/3}$$
$$= 1.55 \times 10^{-7} \text{ mole/min}$$

For the long axis perpendicular to the flow, R is twice the value when the long axis is parallel to the flow, as observed in (*a*) and (*b*) above:

$$R = 3.10 \times 10^{-7}/(1.55 \times 10^{-7}) = 2.0$$

(*c*) The surface area of the rectangular tablet is 2.54 cm × 0.3175 cm = 0.806 cm^2, which is also the surface area of the circular tablet or disk. Therefore, the radius, r, of the circular surface is $\pi r^2 = 0.806$ or $r = 0.507$ cm., and the rate R of diffusion or permeation for a tablet of circular surface (equation 13–33) is

$$R = 2.157(9.86 \times 10^{-6} \times 60 \text{ cm}^2/\text{min})^{2/3} \times$$
$$(7.27 \times 10^{-6} \text{ mole/cm}^3) \times (255. \text{ min}^{-1})^{1/3} \times$$
$$(0.507 \text{ cm})^{5/3}$$
$$= 2.26 \times 10^{-7} \text{ mole/min}$$

(*d*) The convective diffusion model, the *CD* model, which takes into account fluid flow as well as diffusion, has several parameters in common with the classic diffusion model. These include the solubility, C_s, diffusion coefficient or diffusivity, D, and the dimensions of a rectangular or circular surface, b, L, and r. In the classic model, R is proportional to D, while in the *CD* model R is proportional to $D^{2/3}$. In the classic model, R is proportional to the surface area, S, of a rectangle or disk; in the *CD* model R is proportional to a reduced function of surface area; that is, $bL^{2/3}$ or $r^{5/3}$. A new parameter, α, the rate of shear over the dissolving surface, is introduced in the *CD* model; it is calculated from the flow rate and the dimension of the diffusion cell.

DRUG RELEASE

Release from dosage forms and subsequent bioabsorption are controlled by the physical chemical properties of drug and delivery form, and the physiologic and physical chemical properties of the biologic system. Drug concentration, aqueous solubility, molecular size, crystal form, protein binding, and pK_a are among the physical chemical factors that must be understood to design a delivery system that exhibits controlled or sustained-release characteristics.[31]

The release of a drug from a delivery system involves factors of both dissolution and diffusion. As the reader has already observed in this chapter, the foundations of diffusion and dissolution theories bear many resemblances. Dissolution rate has been discussed as it influences drug release; the remainder of the chapter emphasizes principles of diffusion as related to the transport of drugs from dosage matrices, through the walls of containers and packages, and into the body by pathways through the gastrointestinal mucosa, skin, vagina, buccal cavity, and other sites of entry into the body.

Drugs in Polymer Matrices. A powdered drug is homogeneously dispersed throughout the matrix of an erodible tablet. The drug is assumed to dissolve in the polymer matrix and to diffuse out from the surface of the device. As the drug is released, the distance for diffusion becomes increasingly greater. The boundary that forms between drug and empty matrix therefore recedes into the tablet as drug is eluted. A schematic illustration of such a device is shown in Figure 13–12a. Figure 13–12b shows a granular matrix with interconnecting pores or capillaries. The drug is leached out of this device by entrance of the surrounding medium. Figure 13–12c depicts the concentration profile and shows the receding depletion zone that moves to the center of the tablet as the drug is released.

Higuchi[32] developed an equation for the release of a drug from an ointment base and later[33] applied it to diffusion of solid drugs dispersed in homogeneous and granular matrix dosage systems (Fig. 13–12).

Fick's first law,

$$\frac{dM}{S\,dt} = \frac{dQ}{dt} = \frac{DC_s}{h} \qquad (13\text{–}34)$$

may be applied to the case of a drug embedded in a polymer matrix, in which dQ/dt* is the rate of drug released per unit area of exposed surface of the matrix. Since the boundary between the drug matrix and the

---

*dM is amount of drug diffusing; dQ is introduced here to represent dM/S, in which S is surface area of the boundary.

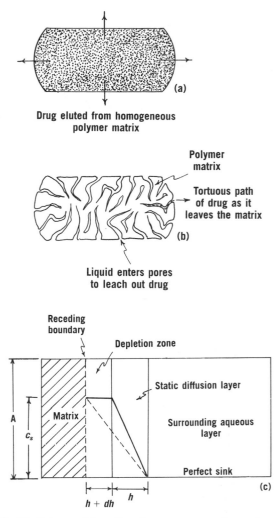

Fig. 13–12. Release of drug from homogeneous and granular matrix dosage forms. *(a)* Drug eluted from a homogeneous polymer matrix. *(b)* Drug leached from a heterogeneous or granular matrix. *(c)* Schematic of the solid matrix and its receding boundary as drug diffuses from the dosage form. (From T. Higuchi, J. Pharm. Sci. **50**, 874, 1961, reproduced with permission of the copyright owner.)

drug-depleted matrix recedes with time, the thickness of the empty matrix, dh, through which the drug diffuses also increases with time.

Whereas C_s is the solubility or saturation concentration of drug in the matrix, A is the total concentration (amount per unit volume), dissolved and undissolved, of drug in the matrix.

As drug passes out of a homogeneous matrix, a in Figure 13–12, the boundary of drug (represented by the dotted vertical line in Figure 13–12c) moves to the left by an infinitesimal distance, dh. The infinitesimal amount, dQ, of drug released because of this shift of the front is given by the approximate linear expression:

$$dQ = A\,dh - \tfrac{1}{2}C_s\,dh \qquad (13\text{–}35)$$

Now dQ of equation (13–35) is substituted into equation (13–34), integration is carried out, and the resulting equation is solved for h. The steps of the derivation as given by Higuchi[32] are

$$(A - \tfrac{1}{2}C_s)\, dh = \frac{DC_s}{h}\, dt \qquad (13\text{–}36)$$

$$\frac{2A - C_s}{2DC_s} \int h\, dh = \int dt \qquad (13\text{–}37)$$

$$t = \frac{(2A - C_s)}{4DC_s}\, h^2 + C \qquad (13\text{–}38)$$

The integration constant, C, may be evaluated at $t = 0$ at which $h = 0$, giving

$$t = \frac{(2A - C_s)h^2}{4DC_s} \qquad (13\text{–}39)$$

$$h = \left(\frac{4DC_s t}{2A - C_s}\right)^{1/2} \qquad (13\text{–}40)$$

The amount of drug depleted per unit area of matrix, Q, at time t, is obtained by integrating equation (13–35) to yield

$$Q = hA - \tfrac{1}{2}hC_s \qquad (13\text{–}41)$$

Substituting equation (13–40) into (13–41) produces the result

$$Q = \left(\frac{DC_s t}{2A - C_s}\right)^{1/2} (2A - C_s) \qquad (13\text{–}42)$$

which is known as the *Higuchi equation:*

$$Q = [D(2A - C_s)C_s t]^{1/2} \qquad (13\text{–}43)$$

The instantaneous rate of release of a drug at time t is obtained by differentiating equation (13–43) to yield

$$\frac{dQ}{dt} = \frac{1}{2}\left[\frac{D(2A - C_s)C_s}{t}\right]^{1/2} \qquad (13\text{–}44)$$

Ordinarily, $A \gg C_s$, and equation (13–43) reduces to

$$Q = (2ADC_s t)^{1/2} \qquad (13\text{–}45)$$

and equation (13–44) becomes

$$\frac{dQ}{dt} = \left(\frac{ADC_s}{2t}\right)^{1/2} \qquad (13\text{–}46)$$

for the release of a drug from a homogeneous polymer matrix-type delivery system. Equation (13–45) indicates that the amount of drug released is proportional to the square root of A, the total amount of drug in unit volume of matrix; D, the diffusion coefficient of the drug in the matrix; C_s, the solubility of drug in polymeric matrix; and t, the time.

The rate of release, dQ/dt, can be altered by increasing or decreasing the drug's solubility C_s in the polymer by complexation. The total concentration A of drug that the physician prescribes is also seen to affect the rate of drug release.

Example 13–7. (*a*) What is the amount of drug per unit area, Q, released from a tablet matrix at time $t = 120$ minutes? The total concentration of drug in the homogeneous matrix, A, is 0.02 g/cm³.

The drug's solubility C_s is 1.0×10^{-3} g/cm³ in the polymer. The diffusion coefficient D of the drug in the polymer matrix at 25° C is 6.0×10^{-6} cm²/sec or 360×10^{-6} cm²/min.

Equation (13–45) is used:

$$Q = [2(0.02 \text{ g/cm}^3)(360 \times 10^{-6} \text{ cm}^2/\text{min})$$
$$\times (1.0 \times 10^{-3} \text{ g/cm}^3)(120 \text{ min})]^{1/2}$$
$$= 1.3 \times 10^{-3} \text{ g/cm}^2$$

(*b*) What is the instantaneous rate of drug release occurring at 120 minutes?

$$dQ/dt = \left[\frac{(0.02)(360 \times 10^{-6})(1.0 \times 10^{-3})}{2 \times 120}\right]^{1/2}$$
$$= 5.5 \times 10^{-6} \text{ g cm}^{-2} \text{ min}^{-1}$$

Release from Granular Matrices: Porosity and Tortuosity. The release of a solid drug from a granular matrix (Fig. 13–12b) involves the simultaneous penetration of the surrounding liquid, dissolution of drug, and leaching out of the drug through interstitial channels or pores. A granule is, in fact, defined as a porous rather than a homogeneous matrix. The volume and length of the opening in the matrix must be accounted for in the diffusional equation, leading to a second form of the Higuchi equation:

$$Q = \left[\frac{D\epsilon}{\tau}(2A - \epsilon C_s)C_s t\right]^{1/2} \qquad (13\text{–}47)$$

in which ϵ is the porosity of the matrix and τ is the tortuosity of the capillary system, both parameters being dimensionless quantities.

Porosity, ϵ, is the fraction of matrix that exists as pores or channels into which the surrounding liquid can penetrate. The porosity term, ϵ, found in equation (13–47) is the total porosity of the matrix after the drug has been extracted. This is equal to the initial porosity, ϵ_0, due to pores and channels in the matrix before the leaching process begins, and the porosity created by extracting the drug. If A g/cm³ of drug is extracted from the matrix and the drug's specific volume or reciprocal density is $1/\rho$ cm³/g, then the drug's concentration, A, is converted to volume fraction of drug that will create an additional void space or porosity in the matrix once it is extracted. The total porosity of the matrix, ϵ, becomes

$$\epsilon = \epsilon_0 + A(1/\rho) \qquad (13\text{–}48)$$

The initial porosity ϵ_0 of a compressed tablet may be considered to be small (a few percent) relative to the porosity A/ρ created by the dissolution and removal of the drug from the device. Therefore, the porosity frequently is calculated conveniently by disregarding ϵ_0 and writing

$$\epsilon \cong A/\rho \qquad (13\text{–}49)$$

Tablet porosity and its measurement and applications in pharmacy are discussed in more detail on pages 442 to 446.

Equation (13–47) differs from equation (13–43) only in the addition of ϵ and τ. Equation (13–43) is applicable to release from a homogeneous tablet that gradually erodes and releases the drug into the bathing medium. Equation (13–47) applies instead to a drug-release mechanism based upon entrance of the surrounding medium into a polymer matrix, where it dissolves and leaches out the soluble drug, leaving a shell of polymer and empty pores. In equation (13–47), diffusivity is multiplied by porosity, a fractional quantity, to account for the decrease in D brought about by empty pores in the matrix. The apparent solubility of the drug C_s is also reduced by the volume fraction term, which represents porosity.

Tortuosity, τ, is introduced into equation (13–47) to account for an increase in the path length of diffusion due to branching and bending of the pores, as compared to the shortest "straight-through" pores. Tortuosity tends to reduce the amount of drug released in a given interval of time, and so it appears in the denominator under the square root sign. A straight channel has a tortuosity of unity, and a channel through spherical beads of uniform size has a tortuosity of 2 or 3. At times, an unreasonable value of, say, 1000 is obtained for τ, as Desai et al.[34a] have noted. When this occurs, the pathway for diffusion evidently is not adequately described by the concept of tortuosity, and the system must be studied in more detail to determine the factors controlling matrix permeability. Methods for obtaining diffusivity, porosity, tortuosity, and other quantities required in an analysis of drug diffusion are given by Desai et al.[34b]

Equation (13–47) has been adapted to describe the kinetics of lyophilization,[35] commonly called *freeze-drying*, of a frozen aqueous solution containing drug and an inert matrix-building substance (e.g., mannitol or lactose). The process involves the simultaneous change in the receding boundary with time, phase transition at the ice–vapor interface governed by the Clausius–Clapeyron pressure–temperature relationship, and water vapor diffusion across the pore path length of the dry matrix under low temperature and vacuum conditions.

Multilayer Diffusion. Diffusion across biologic barriers may involve a number of layers consisting of separate membranes, cell contents, and fluids of distribution. The passage of gaseous or liquid solutes through the walls of containers and plastic packaging materials is also frequently treated as a case of multilayer diffusion.

Higuchi[32] considered the passage of a topically applied drug from its vehicle through the lipoidal and lower hydrous layers of the skin. Two barriers, in series, the lipoidal and the hydrous skin layers of thickness h_1 and h_2, are shown in Figure 13–13. The resistance R to diffusion in each layer is equal to the reciprocal of the permeability coefficient P_i of that particular layer. Permeability P was defined earlier

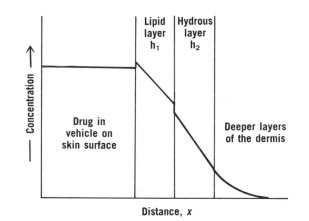

Fig. 13–13. Passage of a drug on the skin's surface through a lipid layer, h_1, and a hydrous layer, h_2, and into the deeper layers of the dermis. The curve of concentration against distance changes sharply at the two boundaries because the two partition coefficients have values other than unity.

(equation [13–11]) as the diffusion coefficient D multiplied by the partition coefficient K, and divided by the membrane thickness, h. For a particular lamina, i,

$$P_i = D_i K_i / h_i$$

and

$$R_i = 1/P_i = h_i/(D_i K_i) \qquad (13\text{–}50)$$

in which R_i is the resistance to diffusion. The total resistance R is the reciprocal of the total permeability, P, and is additive for a series of layers. It is written in general as

$$R = R_1 + R_2 + \cdots R_n \qquad (13\text{–}51a)$$

$$1/P = 1/P_i + 1/P_2 \cdots + 1/P_n \qquad (13\text{–}51b)$$

$$R = 1/P = h_1/D_1 K_1 \\ + h_2/D_2 K_2 + \cdots + h_n/D_n K_n \qquad (13\text{–}51c)$$

in which K_i is the distribution coefficient for layer i relative to the next corresponding layer, $i + 1$, of the system.[36] The total permeability for the two-ply model of the skin is obtained by taking the reciprocal of equation (13–51c), expressed in terms of two layers, to yield

$$P = \frac{D_1 K_1 D_2 K_2}{h_1 D_2 K_2 + h_2 D_1 K_1} \qquad (13\text{–}52)$$

The lag time to steady state for a two-layer system is

$$t_L = \frac{\dfrac{h_1^2}{D_1}\left(\dfrac{h_1}{6D_1 K_1} + \dfrac{h_2}{2D_2 K_2}\right) + \dfrac{h_2^2}{D_2}\left(\dfrac{h_1}{2D_1 K_1} + \dfrac{h_2}{6D_2 K_2}\right)}{(h_1/D_1 K_1 + h_2/D_2 K_2)} \qquad (13\text{–}53)$$

When the partition coefficients K_i of the two layers are essentially the same and one of the h/D terms, say 1, is much larger than the other, however, the time lag equation for the bilayer skin system reduces to the simple time lag expression

$$t_L = h_1^2/6D_1 \qquad (13\text{--}54)$$

Membrane Control and Diffusion Layer Control. A multilayer case of special importance is that of a membrane between two aqueous phases with stationary or stagnant solvent layers in contact with the donor and receptor sides of the membrane (Fig. 13–14).

The permeability of the total barrier, consisting of the membrane and two static aqueous diffusion layers, is

$$P = \frac{1}{R} = \frac{D_m K D_a}{h_m D_a + 2h_a D_m K}$$

$$= \frac{1}{h_m/D_m K + 2h_a/D_a} \qquad (13\text{--}55)$$

This expression is analogous to equation (13–52). In equation (13–55), however, only one partition coefficient K appears, that giving the ratio of concentrations of the drug in the membrane and in the aqueous solvent, $K = C_3/C_4 = C_3/C_2$. The flux J through this three-ply barrier is simply equal to the permeability P multiplied by the concentration gradient $(C_1 - C_5)$, that is, $J = P(C_1 - C_5)$. The receptor serves as a sink (i.e., $C_5 = 0$), and the donor concentration C_1 is assumed to be constant, providing a steady-state flux.[37]

$$J = \frac{1}{S}\frac{dM}{dt} = \frac{D_m K D_a C_1}{h_m D_a + 2h_a D_m K} \qquad (13\text{--}56)$$

In equations (13–55) and (13–56), D_m and D_a are membrane and aqueous solvent diffusivities, h_m is the membrane thickness, and h_a the thickness of the aqueous diffusion layer, as observed in Figure 13–14. M is the amount of permeant reaching the receptor, and

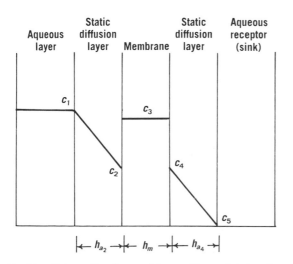

Fig. 13–14. Schematic of a multilayer (three-ply) barrier. The membrane is found between two static aqueous diffusion layers. (From G. L. Flynn, O. S. Carpenter and S. H. Yalkowsky, J. Pharm. Sci. **61**, 313, 1972, reproduced with permission of the copyright owner.)

S is the cross-sectional area of the barrier. It is important to release that h_a is physically influenced by the hydrodynamics in the bulk aqueous phases. The higher the degree of stirring, the thinner is the stagnant aqueous diffusion layer; the slower the stirring, the thicker is this aqueous layer.

Equation (13–56) is the starting point for considering two important cases of multilayer diffusion, namely, diffusion under *membrane control* and diffusion under *aqueous diffusion layer control*.

Membrane Control. When the membrane resistance to diffusion is much greater than the resistances of the aqueous diffusion layers, that is, $R_m > R_a$ by a factor of at least 10, or correspondingly, $P_m \ll P_a$, the rate-determining step (slowest step) is diffusion across the membrane. This is reflected in equation (13–56) when $h_m D_a \gg 2h_a D_m$. Thus, equation (13–56) reduces to

$$J = \left(\frac{K D_m}{h_m}\right) C_1 \qquad (13\text{--}57)$$

Equation (13–57) represents the simplest case of membrane control of flux.

Aqueous Diffusion Layer Control. When $2h_a K D_m \gg h_m D_a$, equation (13–56) becomes

$$J = \left(\frac{D_a}{2h_a}\right) C_1 \qquad (13\text{--}58)$$

and it is now said that the rate-determining barriers to diffusional transport are the stagnant aqueous diffusion layers. This statement means that the concentration gradient that controls the flux now resides in the aqueous diffusion layers rather than in the membrane. From the relationship, $2h_a K D_m \gg h_m D_a$, it is observed that membrane control shifts to diffusion layer control when the partition coefficient K becomes sufficiently large.

Flynn and Yalkowsky[37] demonstrated a transfer from membrane to diffusion-layer control in a homologous series of *n*-alkyl *p*-aminobenzoates (PABA esters). The concentration gradient is almost entirely within the silicone rubber membrane for the short-chain PABA

$$H_2N-\!\!\!\left\langle\!\!\!\bigcirc\!\!\!\right\rangle\!\!\!-\overset{\displaystyle O}{\overset{\displaystyle \|}{C}}-O-CH_2-CH_2-CH_2-CH_3$$

n-Butyl p–aminobenzoate

esters. As the alkyl chain of the ester is lengthened proceeding from butyl to pentyl to hexyl, the concentration no longer drops across the membrane. Rather, the gradient is now found in the aqueous diffusion layers, and diffusion-layer control takes over as the dominant factor in the permeation process.

Example 13–8. The steady-state flux J for hexyl *p*-aminobenzoate was found to be 1.60×10^{-7} mmole cm^{-2} sec^{-1}. D_a is 6.0×10^{-6} cm^2 sec^{-1} and the concentration of the PABA ester, C, is 1.0 mmole liter^{-1}. The system is in diffusion-layer control, so equation (13–58) applies. Calculate the thickness of the static diffusion layer, h_a.

$$J = \left(\frac{D_a}{2h_a}\right) C \quad \text{or} \quad h_a = \left(\frac{D_a}{2J}\right) C$$

$$h_a = \frac{6.0 \times 10^{-6} \text{ cm}^2 \text{ sec}^{-1}}{2(1.60 \times 10^{-7} \text{ mmole cm}^{-2} \text{ sec}^{-1})} \times$$

$$(1.0 \times 10^{-3} \text{ mmole cm}^{-3}) = 0.019 \text{ cm}$$

One observes from equations (13–57) and (13–58) that, under sink conditions, steady-state flux is proportional to concentration, C, in the donor phase whether the flux-determining mechanism is under membrane or diffusion-layer control. Equation (13–58) shows that the flux is independent of membrane thickness h_m and other properties of the membrane when under static diffusion layer control.

The maximum flux obtained in a membrane preparation depends on the solubility, or limiting concentration, of the PABA homolog. The maximum flux may therefore be obtained using equation (13–56), in which C is replaced by C_s, the solubility of the permeating compound:

$$J_{\max} = \left[\frac{D_m K D_a}{h_m D_a + 2h_a K D_m}\right] C_s \quad (13–59)$$

The maximum steady-state flux, $J_{\max}$, for saturated solutions of the PABA esters is plotted against the ester chain length in Figure 13–15.[37] The plot exhibits peak flux between $n = 3$ and $n = 4$ carbons, that is, between propyl and butyl p-aminobenzoates. The peak in Figure 13–15 suggests in part the solubility characteristics of the PABA esters, but primarily reflects the change from membrane to static diffusion layer control of flux. For the methyl, ethyl, and propyl esters, the concentration gradient in the membrane gradually

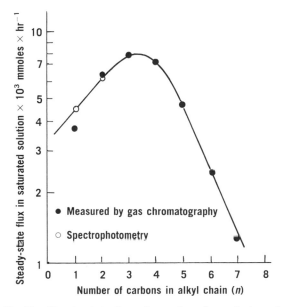

Fig. 13–15. Steady-state flux of a series of p-aminobenzoic acid esters. Maximum flux occurs between the esters having three and four carbons and is due to a change from membrane to diffusion-layer control, as explained in the text. (From G. L. Flynn and S. H. Yalkowsky, J. Pharm. Sci. **61**, 838, 1972, reproduced with permission of the copyright owner.)

decreases and shifts, in the case of the longer-chain esters, to a concentration gradient in the diffusion layers.

By using a well-characterized membrane such as siloxane of known thickness and a homologous series of PABA esters, these workers[37] were able to study the various factors: solubility, partition coefficient, diffusivity, diffusion lag time, and the effects of membrane and diffusion-layer control. From such carefully designed and conducted studies, it is possible to predict the roles played by various physicochemical factors as they relate to diffusion of drugs through plastic containers, as they influence release rates from sustained delivery forms, and as they influence absorption and excretion processes for drugs distributed in the body.

Lag Time under Diffusion-Layer Control. Flynn et al.[36] showed that the lag time for ultrathin membranes under conditions of diffusion-layer control may be represented as

$$t_L = \frac{(\Sigma h_a)^2}{6D_a} \quad (13–60)$$

in which Σh_a is the sum of the thicknesses of the aqueous diffusion layers on the donor and receptor sides of the membrane. The correspondence of t_L, equation (13–60), for systems under membrane control (equation [13–57]) is evident. The lag time for *thick* membranes operating under diffusion layer control is

$$t_L = \frac{h_m h_{a1} h_{a2} K}{(h_{a1} + h_{a2}) D_a} \quad (13–61)$$

When the diffusion layers, h_{a1} and h_{a2}, are of the same thickness, the lag time reduces to

$$t_L = \frac{h_m h_a K}{2D_a} \quad (13–62)$$

The partition coefficient, which was shown earlier to be instrumental in converting the flux from membrane to diffusion-layer control, now appears in the numerator of the lag-time equation. A large K signifies lipophilicity of the penetrating drug species. As one ascends a homologous series of PABA esters, for example, the larger lipophilicity increases the onset time for steady-state behavior; in other words, lengthening of the ester molecule increases the lag time, once the system is in diffusion-layer control. The sharp increase in lag time for PABA esters with alkyl chain length beyond C_4 is shown in Figure 13–16.

Soluble Drugs in Topical Vehicles and Matrices. The original Higuchi model[32,33] does not provide a fit to experimental data when the drug has a significant solubility in the tablet or ointment base. The model can be extended to drug release from homogeneous solid or semisolid vehicles, however, using a quadratic expression introduced by Bottari et al.[38]

$$Q^2 + 2DRA^*Q - 2DA^*C_s t = 0 \quad (13–63)$$

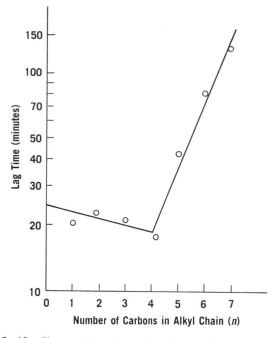

Fig. 13–16. Change in lag time of *p*-aminobenzoic acid esters with alkyl chain length. (From G. L. Flynn and S. H. Yalkowsky, J. Pharm. Sci. **61**, 838, 1972, reproduced with permission of the copyright owner.)

in which

$$A^* = A - \tfrac{1}{2}(C_s + C_v) \qquad (13\text{–}64)$$

Q is the amount of drug released per unit area of the dosage form, D an effective diffusivity of the drug in the vehicle, A the total concentration of drug, C_s the solubility of drug in the vehicle, C_v the concentration of drug at the vehicle–barrier interface, and R the diffusional resistance afforded by the barrier between the donor vehicle and the receptor phase. A^* is an effective A as defined in equation (13–64) and is used when A is only about three or four times greater than C_s.

When

$$Q^2 \geqslant 2DRA^*Q \qquad (13\text{–}65)$$

equation (13–63) reduces to one form of the Higuchi equation (equation [13–45]):

$$Q = (2A^*DC_st)^{1/2} \qquad (13\text{–}65a)$$

Under these conditions, resistance to diffusion R is no longer significant at the interface between vehicle and receptor phase. When C_s is not negligible in relation to A, the vehicle-controlled model of Higuchi becomes

$$Q = [D(2A - C_s)C_st]^{1/2} \qquad (13\text{–}65b)$$

as derived earlier (p. 336).

The quadratic expression of Bottari (equation [13–63]) should allow one to determine diffusion of drugs in ointment vehicles or homogeneous polymer matrices when C_s becomes significant in relation to A. The approach of Bottari et al.[38] follows.

Being a second-degree power series in Q, equation (13–63) may be solved using the well-known quadratic approach. One writes

$$aQ^2 + bQ + c = 0 \qquad (13\text{–}66)$$

in which, with reference to equation (13–63), a is unity, $b = 2DRA^*$, and $c = -2DA^*C_st$. Equation (13–66) has the well-known solution

$$Q = \frac{-b \pm \sqrt{b^2 - 4ac}}{2a} \qquad (13\text{–}67)$$

or

$$Q = \frac{-2DRA^* + \sqrt{(2DRA^*)^2 + (2DA^*C_st)}}{2} \qquad (13\text{–}68)$$

in which the positive root is taken for physical significance. If a lag time occurs, t in equation (13–68) is replaced by $(t - t_L)$ for the steady-state period. Bottari et al.[38] obtained satisfactory values for b and c by use of a least-square fit of equation (13–63) involving the release of benzocaine from suspension-type aqueous gels. R, the diffusional resistance, is determined from steady-state permeation, and C_v is then obtained from the expression

$$C_v = R(dQ/dt) \qquad (13\text{–}69)$$

The application of equation (13–63) is demonstrated in the following example.

Example 13–9. (a) Calculate Q, the amount in milligrams of micronized benzocaine released per cm^2 of surface area from an aqueous gel after 9000 seconds (2.5 hours) in a diffusion cell. Assuming that the total concentration A is 10.9 mg/mL, the solubility C_s is 1.31 mg/mL, $C_v = 1.05$ mg/mL, the diffusional resistance R of a silicone rubber barrier, separating the gel from the donor compartment, is 8.10×10^3 sec/cm, and the diffusivity D of the drug in the gel is 9.14×10^{-6} cm^2/sec. From equation (13–64),

$$A^* = 10.9 \text{ mg/mL} - \tfrac{1}{2}(1.31 + 1.05) \text{ mg/mL} = 9.72 \text{ mg/mL}$$

Then

$$DRA^* = (9.14 \times 10^{-6} \text{ cm}^2/\text{sec}) \times (8.10 \times 10^3 \text{ sec/cm})(9.72 \text{ mg/mL})$$
$$= 0.7196 \text{ mg cm}^{-2}$$
$$DA^*C_st = (9.14 \times 10^{-6})(9.72)(1.31)(9000) = 1.047 \text{ mg}^2/\text{cm}^4$$
$$Q = -0.7196 + [(0.7196)^2 + 2(1.047)]^{1/2} \text{ mg/cm}^2$$
$$= -0.7196 + [1.616] = 0.90 \text{ mg/cm}^2$$

The $Q_{(calc)}$ of 0.90 mg/cm^2 compares well with $Q_{(obs)} = 0.88$ mg/cm^2.

A slight increase in accuracy may be obtained by replacing $t = 9000$ sec with $t = (9000 - 405)$ sec, in which the lag time $t = 405$ sec is obtained from a plot of experimental Q values versus $t^{1/2}$. This correction yields a $Q_{(calc)} = 0.87$ mg/cm^2.

(b) Calculate Q using equation (13–65b) and compare the result with that obtained in (a).

$$Q = \{(9.14 \times 10^{-6})[(2 \times 10.9) - 1.31](1.31)(9000)\}^{1/2}$$
$$= 1.49 \text{ mg/cm}^2$$

Paul and coworkers[39] have studied cases in which A, the matrix loading of drug per unit volume in a polymeric dosage form, may be greater than, equal to, or less than the equilibrium solubility C_s of the drug in a matrix. The model is a refinement of the original

Higuchi approach,[32,33] providing an accurate set of equations that describe release rates of drugs, fertilizers, pesticides, antioxidants, and preservatives in commercial and industrial applications, over the entire range of ratios of A to C_s.

A Capsule-Type Device. A silastic capsule, as depicted in Figure 13–17a, has become a popular sustained and controlled delivery form in pharmacy and medicine.[40-42] The release of a drug from a silastic capsule is shown schematically in Figure 13–17b. The molecules of the crystalline drug lying against the inside wall of the capsule leave their crystals, pass into the polymer wall by a dissolution process, diffuse through the wall, and pass into the liquid diffusion layer and the medium surrounding the capsule. The concentration differences across the polymer wall of thickness h_m and the stagnant diffusion layer of thickness h_a are represented by the lines, $C_p - C_m$ and $C_s - C_b$, respectively. C_p is the solubility of the drug in the polymer and C_m the concentration at the polymer-solution interface, that is, the concentration of drug in the polymer in contact with the solution. C_s, on the other hand, is the concentration of the drug in the solution at the polymer–solution interface, and it is seen in Figure 13–17b to be somewhat below the solubility of drug in polymer at the interface. There is a real difference between the solubility of the drug in the polymer and in the solution, although both exist at the interface. Finally, C_b is the concentration of the drug in the bulk solution surrounding the capsule.

To express the rate of drug release under sink conditions, Chien[40] used the following expression:

$$Q = \left[\frac{K_r D_a D_m}{K_r D_a h_m + D_m h_a}\right] C_p t \qquad (13-70)$$

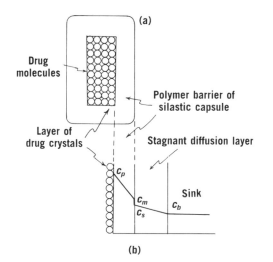

(a)

Drug molecules

Polymer barrier of silastic capsule

Layer of drug crystals

Stagnant diffusion layer

C_p

Sink

C_m C_b
C_s

(b)

Fig. 13–17. Diffusion of drug from silastic capsule. *(a)* Drug in capsule surrounded by polymer barrier; *(b)* diffusion of drug through polymer wall and stagnant aqueous diffusion layer and into the receptor compartment at sink-conditions. (After Y. W. Chien, in *Sustained and Controlled Release Drug Delivery Systems,* J. R. Robinson, Ed., Marcel Dekker, New York, 1978, p. 229; Chem. Pharm. Bull. 24, 147, 1976.)

which is an integrated form analogous to equation (13–56). In equation (13–70), Q is the amount of drug released per unit surface area of the capsule, and K_r is the partition coefficient, defined as

$$K_r = C_s/C_p \qquad (13-71)^*$$

When diffusion through the capsule membrane or film is the limiting factor in drug release, that is, when $K_r D_a h_m \gg D_m h_a$, equation (13–70) reduces to

$$Q = \left(\frac{D_m}{h_m}\right) C_p t \qquad (13-72)$$

and when the limiting factor is passage through the diffusion layer ($D_m h_a \gg K_r D_a h_m$):

$$Q = \left(\frac{D_a}{h_a}\right) C_s t = \left(\frac{K_r D_a}{h_a}\right) C_p t \qquad (13-73)$$

The right-hand expression may be written because $C_s = K_r C_p$ as defined earlier, in equation (13–71).

The rate of drug release, Q/t, for a polymer-controlled process may be calculated from the slope of a linear Q-versus-t plot, and from equation (13–72) is seen to equal $C_p D_m/h_m$. Likewise, Q/t, for the diffusion-layer–controlled process, resulting from plotting Q versus t, is found to be $C_s D_a/h_a$. Furthermore, a plot of the release rate, Q/t versus C_s, the solubility of the drug in the surrounding medium, should be linear with a slope of D_a/h_a.

Example 13–10. The partition coefficient, $K_r = C_s/C_p$, of progesterone is 0.022; the solution diffusivity $D_a = 4.994 \times 10^{-2}$ cm²/day; the silastic membrane diffusivity $D_m = 14.26 \times 10^{-2}$ cm²/day; the solubility of progesterone in the silastic membrane, C_p, is 513 μg/cm³; the thickness of the capsule membrane, h_m, is 0.080 cm, and that of the diffusion layer, h_a, as estimated by Chien, is 0.008 cm.

Calculate the rate of release of progesterone from the capsule and express it in μg/cm² per day. Compare the calculated result with the observed value, $Q/t = 64.50$ μg/cm² per day. Using equation (13–70),

$$Q/t = \frac{C_p K_r D_a D_m}{K_r D_a h_m + D_m h_a},$$

$$Q/t = \frac{\begin{matrix}(513 \text{ μg/cm}^3)(0.022)(4.994 \times 10^{-2} \text{ cm}^2/\text{day}) \\ \times (14.26 \times 10^{-2} \text{ cm}^2/\text{day})\end{matrix}}{\begin{matrix}(0.022)(4.994 \times 10^{-2} \text{ cm}^2/\text{day})(0.080 \text{ cm}) \\ + (14.26 \times 10^{-2} \text{ cm}^2/\text{day})(0.008 \text{ cm})\end{matrix}}$$

$$Q/t = \frac{0.08037}{0.00123} = 65.34 \text{ μg/cm}^2 \text{ per day}$$

In the example just given, (*a*) is $K_r D_a h_m \gg D_m h_a$ or (*b*) is $D_m h_a \gg K D_a h_m$? (*c*) What conclusion can be drawn regarding matrix or diffusion-layer control?

---

*Contrary to convention, the partition coefficient K_r in equation (13–71) is defined as the water/lipid distribution coefficient. Thus, K_r decreases here as the compound becomes more hydrophobic. The K as used previously, for example, in equations (13–50), (13–55), and (13–61), is the lipid/water distribution coefficient such that K increases with increasing hydrophobicity of the compound. C_m varies with time and eventually equals C_p. Therefore, the equilibrium partition coefficient does not involve C_m, but rather, the equilibrium values C_p and C_s.

$$K_r D_a h_m = 8.79 \times 10^{-5}; \quad D_m h_a = 1.14 \times 10^{-3}$$

$$D_m h_a / (K_r D_a h_m + D_m h_a)$$

$$= (1.14 \times 10^{-3})/[(8.79 \times 10^{-5})$$

$$+ (1.14 \times 10^{-3})] = 0.93$$

Therefore, $D_m h_a \gg K_r D_a h_m$, and the system is 93% under aqueous diffusion-layer control. It should thus be possible to use the simplified equation (13–73):

$$Q/t = \frac{K_r D_a C_p}{h_a} = \frac{(0.022)(4.994 \times 10^{-2})(513)}{0.008}$$

$$= 70.45 \ \mu g/cm^2 \text{ per day}$$

Although $D_m h_a$ is larger than $K_r D_a h_m$ by about one order of magnitude (i.e., $D_m h_a / K D_a h_m = 13$), it is evident that a considerably better result is obtained by using the full expression, equation (13–70).

Example 13–11. Two new contraceptive steroid esters, *A* and *B*, were synthesized, and the parameters determined for release from polymeric capsules are[40]

K_r	D_a (cm²/day)	D_m (cm²/day)	C_p (µg/cm³)	h_a(cm)	$Q/t_{(obs)}$ µg/cm² per day
A	0.15	25×10^{-2}	2.6×10^{-2}	100	0.008	24.50
B	0.04	4.0×10^{-2}	3.0×10^{-2}	85	0.008	10.32

Using equation (13–70) and the quantities in the table given, calculate values of h_m in cm for these capsule membranes.

$$Q/t = \frac{C_p K_r D_a D_m}{K_r D_a h_m + D_m h_a}$$

$$(Q/t)(K_r D_a h_m + D_m h_a) = C_p K_r D_a D_m$$

$$(Q/t)(K_r D_a h_m) = C_p K_r D_a D_m - D_m h_a (Q/t)$$

$$h_m = \frac{C_p K_r D_a D_m - D_m h_a (Q/t)}{(Q/t) K_r D_a}$$

For capsule *A*:

$$h_m = \frac{(100)(0.15)(25 \times 10^{-2})(2.6 \times 10^{-2})}{- (2.6 \times 10^{-2})(0.008)(24.50)}{(24.50)(0.15)[(25 \times 10^{-2})}$$

$$h_m = \frac{0.0924}{0.9188} \text{ cm} = 0.101 \text{ cm}$$

Note that all units cancel except cm in the equation for h_m. The reader should carry out the calculations for compound *B*. (*Answer:* 0.097 cm.)

DIFFUSION PRINCIPLES IN BIOLOGIC SYSTEMS

Gastrointestinal Absorption of Drugs. Drugs pass through living membranes according to two main classes of transport, passive and active. Passive transfer involves a simple diffusion driven by differences in drug concentration on the two sides of the membrane. In intestinal absorption, for example, the drug travels in most cases by passive transport from a region of high concentration in the gastrointestinal tract to a region of low concentration in the systemic circulation.

Active transport requires an energy source such as an enzyme or biochemical carrier to ferry the drug across the membrane; transport can proceed from regions of *low* concentration to regions of *high* concentration through the "pumping action" of these biologic transport systems. Other special mechanisms include convective and ion-pair transport. We will make limited use of specialized carrier systems, and will concentrate attention mainly on passive diffusion.

Many drugs are weakly acidic or basic, and the ionic character of the drug and the biologic compartments and membranes have an important influence on the transfer process. From the Henderson–Hasselbalch relationship (p. 170) for a weak acid,

$$pH = pK_a + \log \frac{[A^-]}{[HA]}$$

in which [HA] is the concentration of the nonionized weak acid and [A⁻] is the concentration of its conjugate base. For a weak base, the equation is (p. 170)

$$pH = pK_a + \log \frac{[B]}{[BH^+]}$$

in which [B] is the concentration of the base and [BH⁺] that of its conjugate acid. pK_a is the dissociation exponent for the weak acid in each case. For the weak base, $pK_a = pK_w - pK_b$.

The percent ionization of a weak acid is the ratio of concentration of drug in the ionic form (I) to total concentration of drug in ionic (I) and undissociated (U) form, multiplied by 100:

$$\% \text{ Ionized} = \frac{I}{I + U} \times 100 \qquad (13–74)$$

The Henderson–Hasselbalch equation for weak acid therefore may be written as

$$\frac{U}{I} = 10^{(pK_a - pH)} = \text{antilog } (pK_a - pH) \qquad (13–75)$$

or

$$U = I \text{ antilog } (pK_a - pH) \qquad (13–76)$$

Substituting U into the equation for percent ionization yields:

$$\% \text{ Ionized} = \frac{100}{1 + \text{antilog } (pK_a - pH)} \qquad (13–77)$$

Similarly, for a weak molecular base,

$$\% \text{ Ionized} = \frac{100}{1 + \text{antilog } (pH - pK_a)} \qquad (13–78)$$

In equation (13–77), pK_a refers to the weak acid, while in (13–78), pK_a signifies the acid that is conjugate to the weak base.

The percentage ionization at various pH values of a weak acid, sulfisoxazole, $pK_a \cong 5.0$, is found in Table 13–4. At a point at which the pH is equal to the drug's pK_a, equal amounts are present in the ionic and molecular forms.

TABLE 13–4. *Percent Sulfisoxazole, pK$_a$ ~ 5.0, Dissociated and Undissociated at Various pH Values*

pH	% Dissociated	% Undissociated
2.0	0.100	99.900
4.0	9.091	90.909
5.0	50.000	50.000
6.0	90.909	9.091
8.0	99.900	0.100
10.0	99.999	0.001

pH-Partition Hypothesis. Biologic membranes are predominantly lipophilic, and drugs penetrate these barriers mainly in their molecular, undissociated form. Brodie and his associates[43] were the first workers to apply the principle, known as the *pH-partition hypothesis*, that drugs are absorbed from the gastrointestinal tract by passive diffusion depending on the fraction of undissociated drug at the pH of the intestines. It is reasoned that the partition coefficient between membranes and gastrointestinal fluids is large for the undissociated drug species and favors transport of the molecular form from the intestine through the mucosal wall and into the systemic circulation.

The pH-partition principle has been tested in a large number of in vitro and in vivo studies, and it has been found to be only partly applicable in real biologic systems.[43,44] In many cases, the ionized as well as the un-ionized form partitions into, and is appreciably transported across, lipophilic membranes. It is found for some drugs, such as sulfathiazole, that the in vitro permeability coefficient for the ionized form may actually exceed that for the molecular form of the drug.

Transport of a drug by diffusion across a membrane such as the gastrointestinal mucosa is represented by Fick's law:

$$-\frac{dM}{dt} = \frac{D_m SK}{h}(C_g - C_p) \qquad (13-79)$$

in which M is the amount of drug in the gut compartment at time t, D_m is diffusivity in the intestinal membrane, S the area of the membrane, K the partition coefficient between membrane and aqueous medium in the intestine, h the membrane thickness, C_g the concentration of drug in the intestinal compartment, and C_p the drug concentration in the plasma compartment at time t. The gut compartment is kept at a high concentration and has a large volume relative to the plasma compartment so as to make C_g a constant. C_p, being relatively small, may be omitted. Equation (13–79) then becomes

$$-\frac{dM}{dt} = D_m SK\, C_g/h \qquad (13-80)$$

The left-hand side of (13–80) is converted into concentration units, C (mass/unit volume) $\times$ V (volume). On the right-hand side of (13–80), the diffusion constant,

membrane area, partition coefficient, and membrane thickness are combined to yield a *permeability coefficient*. These changes lead to a pair of equations:

$$-V\frac{dC_g}{dt} = P_g C_g \qquad (13-81a)$$

$$-V\frac{dC_p}{dt} = P_p C_g \qquad (13-81b)$$

in which C_g and P_g of equation (13–81a) are the concentration and permeability coefficient, respectively, for drug passage from intestine to plasma. In equation (13–81b), C_p and P_p are corresponding terms for the reverse passage of drug from plasma to intestine. Since the gut volume V and gut concentration C_g are constant, dividing (13–81a) by (13–81b) yields

$$\frac{dC_g/dt}{dC_p/dt} = \frac{P_g}{P_p} \qquad (13-82)$$

Equation (13–82) demonstrates that the ratio of absorption rates in the intestine-to-plasma and the plasma-to-intestine directions equals the ratio of permeability coefficients.

In a study by Turner et al.,[44] results show that undissociated drugs pass freely through the intestinal membrane in either direction by simple diffusion, in agreement with the pH-partition principle. Drugs that are partly ionized show an increased permeability ratio indicating favored penetration from intestine to plasma. Completely ionized drugs, either negatively or positively charged, show permeability ratios P_g/P_p of about 1.3, that is, a greater passage from gut to plasma than from plasma to gut. This suggests that penetration of ions is associated with sodium ion flux. Their forward passage P_g is apparently due to a coupling of the ions with sodium transport, which mechanism then ferries the drug ions across the membrane, in conflict with the simple pH-partition hypothesis.

Colaizzi and Klink[45] have investigated the pH-partition behavior of the tetracyclines, a class of drugs having three separate pK$_a$ values, which complicates the principles of pH-partition. The lipid solubility and relative amounts of the ionic forms of a tetracycline at physiologic pH may have a bearing on the biologic activity of the various tetracycline analogs used in clinical practice.

Modification of the pH-Partition Principle. Ho, Higuchi and coworkers[46] also have shown that the pH-partition principle is only approximate, assuming as it does that drugs are absorbed through the intestinal mucosa in the nondissociated form alone. Absorption of relatively small ionic and nonionic species through the aqueous pores and the aqueous diffusion layer in front of the membrane must be considered.[47] Other complicating factors, such as metabolism of the drug in the gastrointestinal membrane, absorption in micellar form, and enterohepatic circulatory effects, must also be accounted for in any model that is proposed to reflect in vivo processes.

Ho, Higuchi, and their associates[47] have investigated the gastrointestinal absorption of drugs using diffusional principles and a knowledge of the physiologic factors involved. They employed an in situ preparation, as shown in Figure 13–18, known as the modified Doluisio method for in situ rat intestinal absorption. (The original rat intestinal preparation[48] employed two syringes without the mechanical pumping modification.)

The model used for the absorption of a drug through the mucosal membrane of the small intestine is shown in Figure 13–19. The aqueous boundary layer is in series with the biomembrane, which is composed of lipid regions and aqueous pores in parallel. The final reservoir is a sink consisting of the blood. The flux of a drug permeating the mucosal membrane is

$$J = P_{app} (C_b - C_{blood}) \quad (13-83)$$

or, since the blood reservoir is a sink, $C_{blood} \cong 0$;

$$J = P_{app} C_b \quad (13-84)$$

in which P_{app} is the apparent permeability coefficient (cm/sec) and C_b is the total drug concentration in bulk solution in the lumen of the intestine.

The apparent permeability coefficient is given by

$$P_{app} = \frac{1}{\dfrac{1}{P_{aq}} + \dfrac{1}{P_m}} \quad (13-85)$$

in which P_{aq} is the permeability coefficient of the drug in the aqueous boundary layer (cm/sec), and P_m is the effective permeability coefficient for the drug in the lipoidal and polar aqueous regions of the membrane (cm/sec).

The flux may be written in terms of drug concentration C_b in the intestinal lumen by combining with it a term for the volume, or

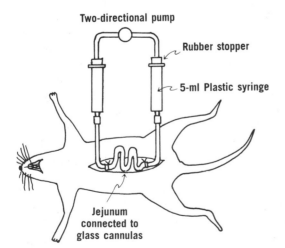

Fig. 13–18. Modified Doluisio technique for in situ rat intestinal absorption. (From N. F. H. Ho et al., in *Gastrointestinal Absorption of Drugs*, A. J. Aguiar, Ed., American Pharmaceutical Association, Academy of Pharmaceutical Sciences, Washington, D.C., 1981, reproduced with permission of the copyright owner.)

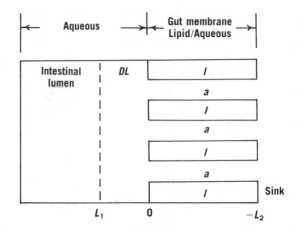

Fig. 13–19. Model for the absorption of a drug through the mucosa of the small intestine. The intestinal lumen is on the left, followed by a static aqueous diffusion layer, *DL*. The gut membrane consists of aqueous pores *a* and lipoidal regions *l*. The distance from the membrane wall to the systemic circulation (sink) is marked off from 0 to $-L_2$; the distance through the diffusion layer is 0 to L_1. (From N. F. H. Ho, W. I. Higuchi and J. Turi, J. Pharm. Sci. **61**, 193, 1972, reproduced with permission of the copyright owner.)

$$J = - \frac{V}{S} \cdot \frac{dC_b}{dt} \quad (13-86)$$

in which S is the surface area and V is the volume of the intestinal segment. The first-order disappearance rate K_u (sec^{-1}) of the drug in the intestine is found in the expression

$$\frac{dC_b}{dt} = -K_u C_b \quad (13-87)$$

Substituting equation (13–87) into (13–86) gives

$$J = \frac{V}{S} \cdot K_u C_b \quad (13-88)$$

and from equations (13–84) and (13–85), together with (13–88), yields

$$P_{app} = \frac{1}{\dfrac{1}{P_{aq}} + \dfrac{1}{P_m}} = \frac{V}{S} K_u \quad (13-89)$$

or

$$K_u = \frac{S}{V} \cdot \frac{P_{aq}}{1 + \dfrac{P_{aq}}{P_m}} \quad (13-90)$$

Consideration of two cases, (1) aqueous boundary layer control and (2) membrane control, results in simplification of equation (13–90).

(1) When the permeability coefficient of the intestinal membrane (i.e., the velocity of drug passage through the membrane in cm/sec) is much greater than that of the aqueous layer, the aqueous layer will cause a slower passage of the drug and become a rate-limiting barrier. (The slower passage is always the rate-determining process.) Therefore, P_{aq}/P_m will be much less than unity, and equation (13–90) reduces to

$$K_{u,max} = (S/V)P_{aq} \quad (13-91)$$

K_u is now written as $K_{u,max}$ because the maximum possible diffusional rate constant is determined by passage across the aqueous boundary layer.

(2) If, on the other hand, the permeability of the aqueous boundary layer is much greater than that of the membrane, P_{aq}/P_m will become much larger than unity, and equation (13–90) reduces to

$$K_u = (S/V)P_m \qquad (13-92)$$

The rate-determining step for transport of drug across the membrane is now under membrane control. When neither P_{aq} nor P_m is much larger than the other, the process is controlled by the rate of drug passage through both the stationary aqueous layer and the membrane. Figures 13–20 and 13–21 show the absorption studies of n-alkanol and n-alkanoic acid homologs that concisely illustrate the biophysical interplay of pH, pK_a, solute lipophilicity via carbon chain length, membrane permeability of the lipid and aqueous pore pathways, and permeability of the aqueous diffusion layer as influenced by the hydrodynamics of the stirred solution.

Example 13–12. Calculate the first-order rate constant, K_u, for transport of an aliphatic alcohol across the mucosal membrane of the rat small intestine if $S/V = 11.2$ cm^{-1}, $P_{aq} = 1.5 \times 10^{-4}$ cm/sec, and $P_m = 1.1 \times 10^{-4}$ cm/sec,

$$K_u = (11.2) \frac{1.5 \times 10^{-4} \text{ cm/sec}}{1 + \dfrac{1.5 \times 10^{-4} \text{ cm/sec}}{1.1 \times 10^{-4} \text{ cm/sec}}} = 11.2 \left(\frac{1.5 \times 10^{-4}}{2.3636} \right)$$

$$K_u = 7.1 \times 10^{-4} \text{ sec}^{-1}$$

For a weak electrolytic drug, the absorption rate constant K_u is[47]

$$K_u = \frac{S}{V} \cdot \frac{P_{aq}}{1 + \dfrac{P_{aq}}{P_0 X_s + P_p}} \qquad (13-93)$$

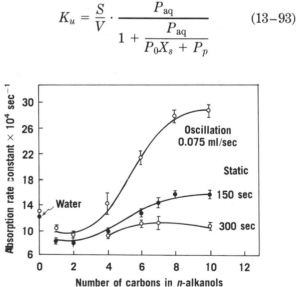

Fig. 13–20. First-order absorption rate constant for a series of n-alkanols under various hydrodynamic conditions (static or low stirring rates and oscillation or high stirring of fluid at 0.075 mL/sec) in the jejunum, using the modified Doluisio technique. (From N. F. H. Ho, J. Y. Park, W. Morozowich and W. I. Higuchi, in *Design of Biopharmaceutical Properties Through Prodrugs and Analogs*, E. B. Roche, Ed., American Pharmaceutical Association, Academy of Pharmaceutical Sciences, Washington, D.C., 1977, p. 148, reproduced with permission of the copyright owner.)

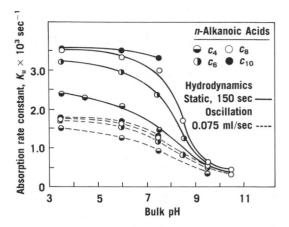

Fig. 13–21. First-order absorption rate constants of alkanoic acids versus buffered pH of the bulk solution in the rat gut lumen, using the modified Doluisio technique. Hydrodynamic conditions are shown in the figure. (From N. F. H. Ho, J. Y. Park, W. Morozowich and W. I. Higuchi, in *Design of Biopharmaceutical Properties Through Prodrugs and Analogs*, E. B. Roche, Ed., American Pharmaceutical Association, Academy of Pharmaceutical Sciences, Washington, D.C., 1977, p. 150, reproduced with permission of the copyright owner.)

in which P_m of the membrane is now separated into a term P_0, the permeability coefficient of the lipoidal pathway for nondissociated drug, and P_p, the permeability coefficient of the polar or aqueous pathway for both ionic and nonionic species.

$$P_m = P_0 X_s + P_p \qquad (13-94)$$

The fraction of nondissociated drug species, X_s, at the pH of the membrane surface in the aqueous boundary is

$$X_s = \frac{[H^+]_s}{[H^+]_s + K_a} = \frac{1}{1 + \text{antilog}(pH_s - pK_a)} \qquad (13-95)$$

for weak acids, and

$$X_s = \frac{K_a}{[H^+]_s + K_a} = \frac{1}{1 + \text{antilog}(pK_a - pH_s)} \qquad (13-96)$$

for weak bases. The student should note the relationship between equations (13–95) and (13–77) and between (13–96) and (13–78). K_a is the dissociation constant of a weak acid or of the acid conjugate to a weak base, and $[H^+]_s$ is the hydrogen ion concentration at the membrane surface, where s stands for surface. The surface pH_s is not necessarily equal to the pH of the buffered drug solution[47] since the membrane of the small intestine actively secretes buffer species (principally CO_2^{2-} and HCO_3^-). It is only at a pH of about 6.5 to 7.0 that the surface pH is equal to the buffered solution pH. One readily recognizes that for nonelectrolytes, X_s becomes unity, and also that for large molecules such as steroids, P_p is insignificant.

Example 13–13. A weakly acidic drug having a $K_a = 1.48 \times 10^{-5}$ is placed in the duodenum in a buffered solution of pH 5.0. Assume $[H^+]_s = 1 \times 10^{-5}$ in the duodenum, $P_{aq} = 5.0 \times 10^{-4}$ cm/sec, $P_0 = 1.14 \times 10^{-3}$ cm/sec, $P_p = 2.4 \times 10^{-5}$ cm/sec, and $S/V = 11.20$ cm^{-1}. Calculate the absorption rate constant, K_u, using equation (13–93). First, from equation (13–94),

Calculate the absorption rate constant, K_u, using equation (13–93). First, from equation (13–94),

$$X_s = \frac{[1 \times 10^{-5}]}{[1 \times 10^{-5}] + 1.48 \times 10^{-5}} = 0.403$$

Then

$$K_u = (11.2)\frac{5.0 \times 10^{-4}}{1 + \dfrac{5.0 \times 10^{-4}}{(1.14 \times 10^{-3})0.403 + 2.4 \times 10^{-5}}}$$

$$K_u = 2.75 \times 10^{-3} \text{ sec}^{-1}$$

Transcorneal Permeation. In gastrointestinal absorption *(Example 13–12)* the permeability coefficient is divided into P_0 as the lipoidal pathway for undissociated drug and P_p for the polar pathway for both ionic and nonionic species. In an analogous way, P can be divided for corneal penetration of a weak base into two permeation coefficients: P_B for the un-ionized species and P_{BH^+} for its ionized conjugated acid. The following example demonstrates the use of these two permeability coefficients.

Mitra and Mikkelson[49] studied the transcorneal permeation of pilocarpine using an in vitro rabbit corneal preparation clamped into a special diffusion cell. The permeability (permeability coefficient) P as determined experimentally is given at various pH values in Table 13–5.

Example 13–14. (a) Compute the un-ionized fraction, f_B, of pilocarpine at the pH values found in Table 13–5, using equation (13–96). The pK_a of pilocarpine (actually the pK_a of the conjugate acid of the weak base, pilocarpine, and known as the pilocarpinium ion) is 6.67 at 34° C.

(b) The relationship between the permeability P and the un-ionized fraction f_B of pilocarpine base over this range of pH values is given by the equation

$$P = P_B f_B + P_{BH^+} f_{BH^+} \qquad (13–97)$$

where B stands for base and BH^+ for its ionized or conjugate acid form. Noting that $f_{BH^+} = 1 - f_B$, equation (13–97) can be written

$$P = P_{BH^+} + (P_B - P_{BH^+})f_B \qquad (13–98)$$

Obtain the permeability for the protonated species P_{BH^+} and the uncharged base P_B using least-squares linear regression on equation (13–98) in which P, the total permeability, is the dependent variable and f_B the independent variable.

(c) Obtain the ratio of the two permeability coefficients, P_{BH^+}/P_B. *Answers:*

(a) The calculated f_B values are given at the various pH values:

pH, donor solution	4.67	5.67	6.24	6.40	6.67	6.91	7.04	7.40
f_B	0.01	0.09	0.27	0.35	0.50	0.64	0.70	0.84

(b) Upon linear regression, equation (13–98) becomes

$$P = 4.836 \times 10^{-6} + 4.897 \times 10^{-6} f_B$$

$$\text{Intercept} = 4.836 \times 10^{-6} = P_{BH^+}$$

TABLE 13–5. *Permeability Coefficients at Various pH Values*

pH, donor solution	4.67	5.67	6.24	6.40	6.67	6.91	7.04	7.40
$P \times 10^6$ cm/sec	4.72	5.44	6.11	6.81	7.06	7.56	8.79	8.85

$$\text{Slope} = 4.897 \times 10^{-6} = (P_B - 4.836 \times 10^{-6})$$
$$P_B = 9.733 \times 10^{-6} \text{ cm/sec}$$

(c) The ratio $P_B/P_{BH^+} \cong 2$. The permeability of the un-ionized form is seen to be about twice that of the ionized form. The reader should now be in a position to explain the result under (c) above based on the pH-partition hypothesis.

Percutaneous Absorption. Percutaneous penetration, that is, passage through the skin, involves (a) dissolution of a drug in its vehicle, (b) diffusion of solubilized drug (solute) from the vehicle to the surface of the skin, and (c) penetration of the drug through the layers of the skin, principally the stratum corneum. Figure 13–22 shows the various structures of the skin involved in percutaneous absorption. The slowest step in the process usually involves passage through the stratum corneum; therefore, this is the rate that limits or controls the permeation.*

Scheuplein[50] found that the average permeability constant, P_s, for water into skin was 1.0×10^{-3} cm/hr and the average diffusion constant, D_s, was 2.8×10^{-10} cm²/sec. (The subscript, s, on D stands for "skin.") Water penetration into the stratum corneum appears to alter the barrier only slightly, primarily by its effect on the pores of the skin. The stratum corneum is considered to be a dense homogeneous film. Small polar nonelectrolytes penetrate into the bulk of the stratum corneum and bind strongly to its components; diffusion of most substances through this barrier is quite slow. Diffusion, for the most part, is transcellular rather than occurring through channels between cells or through sebaceous pores and sweat ducts (Fig. 13–22, *A* rather than *B*, *C*, and *E*). Stratum corneum, normal and even hydrated, is a most impermeable biologic membrane; this is one of its important features in living systems.

It is an oversimplification to assume that one route prevails under all conditions.[50] Yet after steady-state conditions have been established, transdermal diffusion through the stratum corneum most likely predominates. In the early stages of penetration, diffusion through the appendages (hair follicles, sebaceous and sweat ducts) may be significant. These *shunt* pathways are even important in steady-state diffusion in the case of large polar molecules, as noted in the following.

Scheuplein et al.[51] investigated the percutaneous absorption of a number of steroids. They found that the skin's main barrier to penetration by steroid molecules was the stratum corneum. The diffusion coefficient, D_s, for these compounds was approximately 10^{-11} cm²/sec, several orders of magnitude smaller than for most nonelectrolytes. This small value of D_s resulted in low permeability of the steroids. The addition of polar groups to the steroid molecule reduced the diffusion constant still more. For the polar steroids, sweat and sebaceous ducts appeared to play a more important part

---

*Appreciable amounts of some drugs, such as steroids, may also penetrate the skin through sebaceous ducts ordinarily associated with hairs on the skin surface (transfollicular absorption).

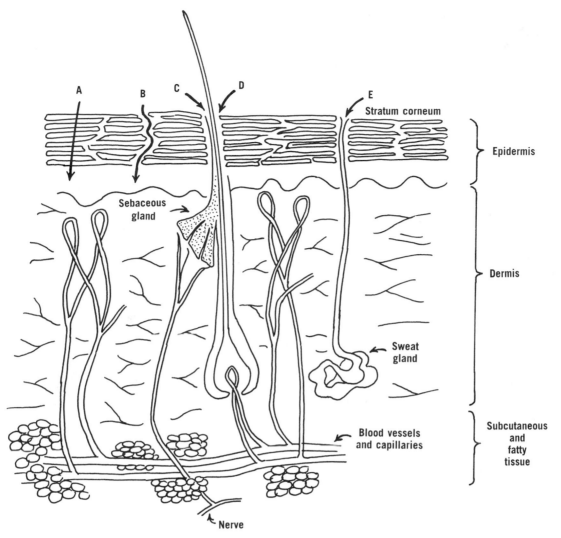

Fig. 13–22. Skin structures involved in percutaneous absorption. Thickness of layers is not drawn to scale. Key to sites of percutaneous penetration: *A*, transcellular; *B*, diffusion through channels between cells; *C*, through sebaceous ducts; *D*, transfollicular; *E*, through sweat ducts.

in percutaneous absorption than diffusion through the bulk stratum corneum.

The studies of Flynn, Higuchi, Ho, and coworkers[52] demonstrate the methods used to characterize the permeability of different sections of the skin. Distinct protein and lipid domains appear to have a role in the penetration of drugs into the stratum corneum. The uptake of a solute may depend on the characteristics of the protein region, the lipid pathway, or a combination of these two domains in the stratum corneum, and depends on the lipophilicity of the solute. The lipid content of the stratum corneum is important in the uptake of lipophilic solutes but is not involved in the attraction of hydrophilic drugs.[53]

The proper choice of vehicle is important in ensuring bioavailability of topically applied drugs. Turi et al.[54] studied the effect of solvents—propylene glycol in water and polyoxypropylene 15 stearyl ether in mineral oil—on the penetration of diflorasone diacetate (a steroid ester) into the skin. The percutaneous flux of the drug was observed to be reduced by the presence of excess solvent in the base. Optimum solvent concentra-

tions were determined for products containing both 0.05% and 0.1% diflorasone diacetate.

The important factors influencing the penetration of a drug into the skin are (1) concentration of dissolved drug C_s, since penetration rate is proportional to concentration; (2) partition coefficient K between the skin and vehicle, which is a measure of the relative affinity of the drug for skin and vehicle; and (3) diffusion coefficients, which represent the resistance of drug molecule movement through vehicle D_v and skin D_s barriers. The relative magnitude of the two diffusion coefficients, D_v and D_s, determines whether release from vehicle or passage through the skin is the rate-limiting step.[54,55]

For diflorasone diacetate in propylene glycol–water (a highly polar base) and in polyoxypropylene 15 stearyl ether in mineral oil (a nonpolar base), the skin was found to be the rate-limiting barrier. The diffusional equation for this system is

$$-\frac{dC_v}{dt} = \frac{SK_{vs}D_sC_v}{Vh} \qquad (13-99)$$

in which C_v is the concentration of dissolved drug in the vehicle (g/cm^3); S is surface area of application (cm^2); K_{sv} the skin-vehicle partition coefficient of diflorasone diacetate; D_s the diffusion coefficient of the drug in the skin (cm^2/sec); V the volume of the drug product applied (cm^3); and h the thickness of the skin barrier (cm).

The diffusion coefficient and skin barrier thickness may be replaced by a resistance R_s to diffusion in the skin:

$$R_s = h/D_s \qquad (13\text{--}100)$$

and equation (13-99) becomes

$$-\frac{dC_v}{dt} = \frac{SK_{vs}C_v}{VR_s} \qquad (13\text{--}101)$$

In a percutaneous experimental procedure, Turi et al.[54] measured the drug in the receptor rather than in the donor compartment of an in vitro diffusion apparatus, the barrier of which consisted of hairless mouse skin. At steady-state penetration,

$$-V\frac{dC_v}{dt} = V_R \cdot \frac{dC_R}{dt} \qquad (13\text{--}102)$$

The rate of loss of drug from the vehicle in the donor compartment is equal to the rate of gain of drug in the receptor compartment. With this change, equation (13-101) is integrated to yield

$$M_R = \left(\frac{SK_{vs}C_v}{R_s}\right)t \qquad (13\text{--}103)$$

in which M_R is the amount of diflorasone diacetate in the receptor solution at time t. The flux, J, is

$$J = \frac{M_R}{S \cdot t} = \frac{K_{vs}C_v}{R_s} \qquad (13\text{--}104)$$

The steady-state flux for a 0.05% diflorasone diacetate formulation containing various proportions (weight fractions) of polyoxypropylene 15 stearyl ether in mineral oil is shown in Figure 13-23. The skin–vehicle partition coefficient was measured for each vehicle formulation. The points represent the experimental values obtained with the diffusion apparatus; the line was calculated using equation (13-104). The point at 0 weight fraction of the ether cosolvent is due to low solubility and slow dissolution rate of the drug in mineral oil and may be disregarded. Beyond a critical concentration, about 0.2 weight fraction of polyoxypropylene 15 stearyl ether, penetration rate decreases. The results[54] indicated that one application of the topical steroidal preparation per day was adequate and that the 0.05% concentration was as effective as the 0.1% preparation.

Example 13-15. A penetration study of 5.0×10^{-3} g/cm^3 diflorasone diacetate solution was conducted at 27° C in the diffusion cell of Turi et al.[54] using a solvent of 0.4 weight fraction of polyoxypropylene 15 stearyl ether in mineral oil. The partition coefficient K_{vs} for the drug distributed between hairless mouse skin

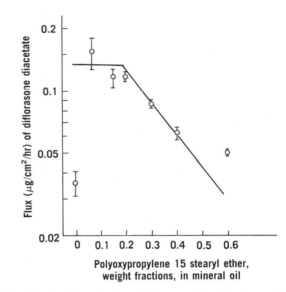

Fig. 13–23. Steady-state flux of diflorasone diacetate in a mixture of polyoxypropylene 15 stearate ether in mineral oil. (From J. S. Turi, D. Danielson and W. Wolterson, J. Pharm. Sci. **68**, 275, 1979, reproduced with permission of the copyright owner.)

and vehicle was found to be 0.625. The resistance R_s of the drug in the mouse skin was determined to be 6666 hr/cm. The diameter of a circular section of mouse skin used as the barrier in the diffusion cell was 1.35 cm.* Calculate (a) the flux, $J = M_R/(S \cdot t)$, in g/cm^2/hr, and (b) the amount M_R in μg of diflorasone diacetate that diffused through the hairless mouse skin in 8 hours.

Using equation (13-104)

(a)

$$J = \frac{K_{vs}C_v}{R_s} = \frac{(0.625)(5.0 \times 10^{-3} \text{ g/cm}^3)}{6666 \text{ hr/cm}}$$

$$J = 4.69 \times 10^{-7} \text{ g/cm}^2/\text{hr}$$

(b)

$$M_R = J \times S \times t$$
$$M_R = (4.69 \times 10^{-7} \text{ g/cm}^2/\text{hr}) \times \tfrac{\pi}{4}(1.35\text{cm})^2 (8 \text{ hr})$$
$$M_R = 5.37 \times 10^{-6} \text{ g} = 5.37 \text{ μg}$$

Ostrenga and his associates[56] studied the nature and composition of topical vehicles as they relate to the transport of a drug through the skin. They varied D_s, K_{vs}, and C_v in order to improve skin penetration of two topical steroids, fluocinonide and fluocinolone acetonide, incorporated into various propylene glycol–water gels. In vivo penetration and in vitro diffusion using abdominal skin removed at autopsy were studied. It was concluded that clinical efficacy of topical steroids can be estimated satisfactorily from in vitro data regarding release, diffusion, and the physical chemical properties of drug and vehicle.

The diffusion, D_s, of the drug in the skin barrier can be influenced by components of the vehicle (mainly solvents and surfactants), and an optimum partition coefficient may be obtained by altering the affinity of the vehicle for the drug.

---

*The area S of a circle, expressed in diameter, is $S = (\tfrac{1}{4})\pi d^2$. (See inside front cover.)

The in vitro rate of skin penetration of the drug, dQ/dt, at 25° C is obtained experimentally at definite times, and the cumulative amount penetrating (measured in radioactive disintegrations per minute) is plotted against time in minutes or hours. After steady state has been attained, the slope of the straight line yields the rate, dM/dt. The lag time is obtained by extrapolating the steady-state line to the time axis.

In vitro penetration of human cadaver skin and in vivo penetration of fluocinolone acetonide from propylene glycol gels into living skin are compared in Figure 13–24. It is observed that the shapes and peaks of the two curves are approximately similar. Thus, in vitro studies using human skin sections should serve as a rough guide to the formulation of acceptable bases for these steroidal compounds.

Ostrenga et al.[56] were able to show a relationship between release of the steroid from its vehicle, in vitro penetration through human skin obtained at autopsy, and in vivo vasoconstrictor activity of the drug depending on compositions of the vehicle. The correlations obtained suggest that information obtained from diffusion studies can assist in the design of effective topical dosage forms. Some useful guidelines are (a) all the drug should be in solution in the vehicle, (b) the solvent mixtures must maintain a favorable partition coefficient so that the drug is soluble in the vehicle and yet has a great affinity for the skin barrier into which it penetrates, and (c) the components of the vehicle should

favorably influence the permeability of the stratum corneum.

Sloan and coworkers[57] studied the effect of vehicles having a range of solubility parameters, δ (see pp. 224–228), on the diffusion of salicylic acid and theophylline through hairless mouse skin. They were able to correlate the partition coefficient K for the drugs between the vehicle and skin calculated from solubility parameters (see *Problem 13–16*, p. 359) and the permeability coefficient P, obtained experimentally from the diffusion data. The results obtained with salicylic acid, a soluble molecule, and with theophylline, a poorly soluble molecule with quite different physical chemical properties, were practically the same.

In the studies of skin permeation described thus far, efforts have been made to increase percutaneous absorption processes. It is important, however, that some compounds not be absorbed. Pharmaceutical adjuvants such as antimicrobial agents, antioxidants, coloring agents, and drug solubilizers, although ideally they should remain in the vehicle on the skin's surface, can penetrate the stratum corneum.

Parabens, typical preservatives incorporated into cosmetics and topical dosage forms, may cause allergic reactions if absorbed into the dermis. Komatsu and Suzuki[58] studied the in vitro percutaneous absorption of butylparaben (butyl *p*-hydroxybenzoate) through guinea pig skin. Disks of dorsal skin were placed in a diffusion cell between a donor and receptor chamber, and the penetration of ^{14}C-butylparaben was determined by the fractional collection of samples from the cell's receptor side and measurement of radioactivity in a liquid scintillation counter.

When butylparaben was incorporated into various vehicles containing polysorbate 80, propylene glycol, and polyethylene glycol 400, a constant diffusivity was obtained averaging $3.63(\pm 0.47$ S.D.$) \times 10^{-4}$ cm^2/hr.

The partition coefficient, K_{vs}, for the paraben between vehicle and skin changed markedly depending upon the vehicle. For a 0.015% (w/v) aqueous solution of butyl paraben, K_{vs} was found to be 2.77. For a 0.1% (w/v) solution of the preservative containing 2% (w/v) of polysorbate 80 and 10% (w/v) propylene glycol in water, the partition coefficient dropped to 0.18. There was no apparent complexation between these solubilizers and butylparaben, according to the authors.

The addition of either propylene glycol or polyethylene glycol 400 to water was found to increase the solubility of paraben in the vehicle and to reduce its partition coefficient between vehicle and skin. By this means, skin penetration of butylparaben could be retarded, maintaining the preservative in the topical vehicle where it was desired.

In the case of polysorbate 80, Komatsu and Suzuki[58] found that this surfactant, too, reduced preservative absorption, maintaining the antibacterial action of the paraben in the vehicle. These workers concluded that the action of polysorbate 80 was a balance of complex

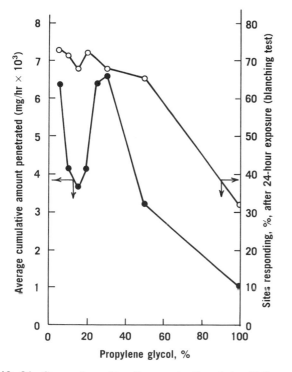

Fig. 13–24. Comparison of in vitro penetration of steroid through a skin section and in vivo skin blanching test. Key: ●, in vitro method: ○, in vivo method. (From J. Ostrenga, C. Steinmetz and B. Poulsen, J. Pharm. Sci. **60**, 1177, 1971, reproduced with permission of the copyright owner.)

factors, which is difficult for the product formulator to predict and manage.

Buccal Absorption. Using a wide range of organic acids and bases as drug models, Beckett and Moffat[59] studied the penetration of drugs into the lipid membrane of the mouths of humans. In harmony with the pH-partition hypothesis, absorption was related to the pK_a of the compound and its lipid–water partition coefficient.

Ho and Higuchi[60] applied one of the earlier mass transfer models[61] to the analysis of the buccal absorption of *n*-alkanoic acids.[62] They utilized the aqueous–lipid phase model in which the weak acid species are transported across the aqueous diffusion layer and, subsequently, only the nonionized species pass across the lipid membrane. Unlike the intestinal membrane, the buccal membrane does not appear to possess significant aqueous pore pathways, and the surface pH is essentially the same as the buffered drug solution pH. Buccal absorption is assumed to be a first-order process owing to the nonaccumulation of drug on the blood side.

$$\ln \frac{C}{C_0} = -K_u t \qquad (13–105)$$

in which C is the aqueous concentration of the *n*-alkanoic acid in the donor or mucosal compartment. The absorption rate constant, K_u, is

$$K_u = \frac{S}{V} \cdot \frac{P_{aq}}{1 + \dfrac{P_{aq}}{P_0 X_s}} \qquad (13–106)$$

the terms of which have been previously defined. Recall that $X_s = 1/(1 + 10^{pH_s - pK_a})$ or by equation (13–95) is $X_s = 1/(1 + \text{antilog }(pH_s - pK_a))$ and is the fraction of un-ionized weak acid at pH_s.

With $S = 100$ cm^2, $V = 25$ cm^3, $P_{aq} = 1.73 \times 10^{-3}$ cm/sec, $P_0 = 2.27 \times 10^{-3}$ cm/sec, $pK_a = 4.84$, and $pH_s = 4.0$, equations (13–95) and (13–106) yield for caproic acid an absorption rate constant:

$$K_u = \frac{100}{25} \left(\frac{1.73 \times 10^{-3}}{1 + \dfrac{1.73 \times 10^{-3}}{2.27 \times 10^{-3} \times 0.874}} \right)$$

$$= 3.7 \times 10^{-3} \text{ sec}^{-1}$$

Buccal absorption rate constants constructed according to the model of Ho and Higuchi agreed well with experimental values. The study shows an excellent correspondence between diffusional theory and in vivo absorption and suggests a fruitful approach for structure–activity studies, not only for buccal membrane permeation but for bioabsorption in general.

Uterine Diffusion. Drugs such as progesterone and other therapeutic and contraceptive compounds may be delivered in microgram amounts into the uterus by means of diffusion-controlled forms (intrauterine device, IUD). In this way the patient is automatically and continuously provided medication or protected from pregnancy for days, weeks, or months.[63]

Ho, Flynn, Higuchi and their associates[64a] performed in situ vaginal drug absorption studies using the rabbit doe as an animal model to develop more effective uterine drug delivery systems. A solution of a model drug was perfused through a specially constructed cell and implanted in the vagina of the doe (Fig. 13–25), and the drug disappearance was monitored. The drug release followed first-order kinetics, and the results permitted the calculation of apparent permeability coefficient and diffusion layer thickness.

The drug may also be implanted in the vagina in a silicone matrix (Fig. 13–26) and drug release at any time can be calculated using a quadratic expression,[64a]

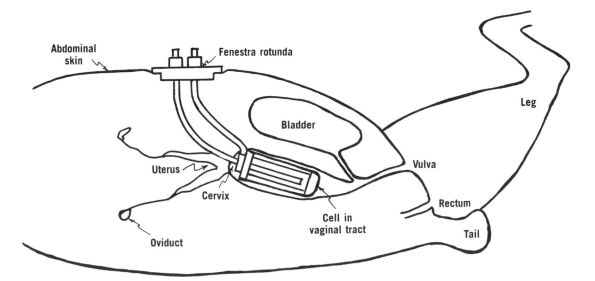

Fig. 13–25. Implanted rib-cage cell in vaginal tract of rabbit. (From T. Yotsuyanagi et al., J. Pharm. Sci. **64**, 71, 1975, reproduced with permission of the copyright owner.)

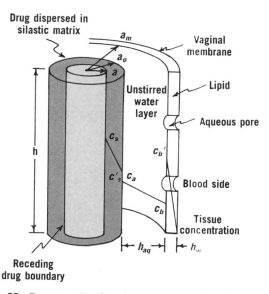

Fig. 13–26. Contraceptive drug in a water-insoluble silicone polymer matrix. Dimensions and sections of the matrix are shown together with concentration gradients across the drug release pathway. (From S. Hwang et al., J. Pharm. Sci. 65, 1578, 1976, reproduced with permission of the copyright owner.)

$$\left(\frac{1}{2\pi h a_0{}^2 A}\right) M^2 + \frac{D_e K_s}{a_0}\left(\frac{1}{P_{aq}} + \frac{1}{P_m}\right) M$$
$$- (2\pi h D_e C_s t) = 0 \qquad (13\text{--}107)$$

The method of calculation may be shown, using the data of Hwang et al.,[64b] which are found in Table 13–6. When the aqueous diffusion layer, h_{aq}, is 100 μm, the aqueous permeability coefficient P_{aq} is 7×10^{-4} cm/sec; this value is used in the following example. The length h of the silastic cyclinder (see Fig. 13–26) is 6 cm, its radius, a_0, is 1.1 cm, and the initial amount of drug per unit volume of plastic cylinder, or loading concentration, A, is 50 mg/cm^3.

Equation (13–107) is of the quadratic form, $aM^2 + bM + c = 0$, in which, for progesterone,

$$a = \frac{1}{2\pi h a_0{}^2 A}$$

$$= \frac{1}{(2)(3.1416)(6 \text{ cm})(1.1 \text{ cm})^2(50 \text{ mg/cm}^3)}$$

$$= 0.000438 \text{ mg}^{-1}$$

$$b = \frac{D_e K_s}{a_0}\left(\frac{1}{P_{aq}} + \frac{1}{P_m}\right) = \frac{(4.5 \times 10^{-7} \text{ cm}^2/\text{sec})(50.2)}{1.1 \text{ cm}}$$

$$\cdot \left(\frac{1}{7 \times 10^{-4} \text{ cm/sec}} + \frac{1}{7 \times 10^{-4} \text{ cm/sec}}\right)$$
$$= 0.0587 \text{ (dimensionless)}$$

$$c = -2\pi h D_e C_s t = -2(3.1416)(6 \text{ cm})$$
$$\times (4.5 \times 10^{-7} \text{ cm}^2/\text{sec})(0.572 \text{ mg/cm}^3)$$
$$\times \left(\frac{86,400 \text{ sec}}{\text{day}}\right) (t \text{ days}) = -0.8384 \times t \text{ (days)}$$

How much progesterone is released in 5 days? In 20 days? The quadratic formula to be used here is

$$M = \frac{-b + \sqrt{b^2 - 4ac}}{2a}$$

After 5 days,

$$c = -0.8384 \text{ mg/day} \times 5 \text{ days} = -4.1920 \text{ mg},$$

and

$$M = \frac{-0.0587 + \sqrt{(0.0587)^2 - (4)(0.000438)(-4.1920)}}{2(0.000438)}$$

$$= 51.6 \text{ mg}$$

After 20 days, $c = -0.8384$ mg/day $\times$ 20 days $= -16.77$ mg.

$$M = \frac{-0.0587 + \sqrt{(0.0587)^2 - (4)(0.000438)(-16.77)}}{2(0.000438)}$$

$$= 139.8 \text{ mg}$$

Okada et al.[65] have carried out detailed studies on the vaginal absorption of hormones, as reported in four papers.

THERMODYNAMICS OF DIFFUSION

Permeation of gases, liquids, and solutes through membranes requires an energy of activation (p. 295) for the small molecules to move through the matrix of the barrier material. This fact is expressed in the Arrhenius equation:[66]

$$P = P_0 e^{-E_p/RT} \qquad (13\text{--}108)$$

$$\ln P = \ln P_0 - E_p/RT \qquad (13\text{--}109)$$

in which P_0 is a factor independent of temperature and proportional to the number of molecules entering the

TABLE 13–6. *Physical Parameters for the Release of Progesterone and Hydrocortisone from a Silicone Matrix for Vaginal Absorption in the Rabbit* [64b]

	Progesterone	Hydrocortisone
Solubility in matrix, C_s (mg/cm^3)	0.572	0.014
Diffusion coefficient in matrix, D_e (cm^2/sec)	4.5×10^{-7}	4.5×10^{-7}
Silicone–water partition coefficient, K_s	50.2	0.05
Permeability coefficient of rabbit vaginal membrane, P_m (cm/sec)	7×10^{-4}	5.8×10^{-5}
P_{aq} (when $h_{aq} = 100$ μm)	7×10^{-4}	7×10^{-4}
P_{aq} (when $h_{aq} = 1000$ μm)	0.7×10^{-4}	0.7×10^{-4}

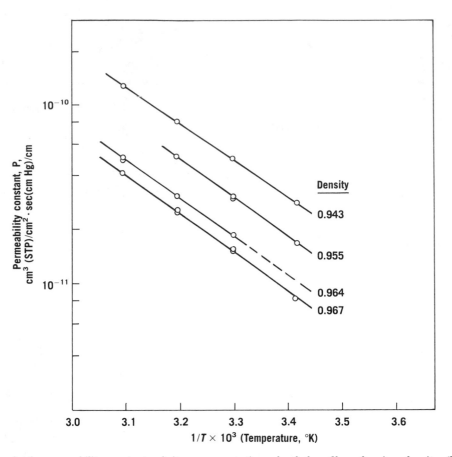

Fig. 13–27. Arrhenius-like plot for permeability constants of nitrogen permeating polyethylene films of various density. (From A. S. Michaels and R. B. Parker, J. Polym. Sci. **41**, 53, 1959.)

film and to the probability that these molecules have sufficient energy to engage in the diffusion process. E_p is the energy of activation for permeation in calories/mole, and R and T have their usual meaning.

Michaels and Parker[67] determined the permeability of oxygen, nitrogen, and other gases in polyethylene films of different densities. The Arrhenius plot (Fig. 13–27) demonstrates the constant energy of activation and corresponding decrease in permeability of nitrogen as density of the polyethylene film is increased by greater short-chain branching of the polymer structure.

E_p values vary from 5 to 20 kcal/mole for permeation through liquids and polymeric barriers, respectively. Higuchi and Aguiar[68] obtained a value of 8 kcal/mole for the permeation of water vapor into wax-like enteric tablet coatings.

Activation energies have also been obtained in the study of the diffusion of liquids across biologic membranes. Blank et al.[69] showed that the apparent activation energies E_p for permeation through human skin (autopsy specimens) by lower alcohols (ethanol to pentanol) and higher or less polar alcohols (hexanol to octanol) are 16.5 kcal/mole and 10 kcal/mole, respectively. The less polar alcohols penetrate the skin more rapidly and exhibit permeability similar to ethers and ketones. The polar compounds with higher activation

energies have lower permeability constants, as might be expected. The slopes of the lines in Figure 13–28 may be used to calculate the activation energies with the aid of equation (13–109). The uppermost line has a break at 14.2° C, the penetration of octanol appearing to show a higher activation energy at lower temperatures,

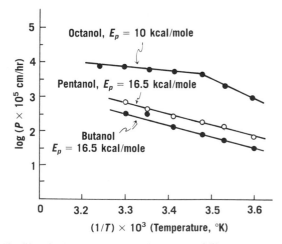

Fig. 13–28. Arrhenius-like plot (log permeability constant versus reciprocal absolute temperature) for diffusion of normal alkanols through autopsy specimens of human skin. (From I. H. Blank, R. J. Scheuplein and D. J. McFarlane, J. Invest. Dermatol. **49**, 582, 1967. © 1967, The Williams & Wilkins Co., Baltimore.)

that is, between 4.6° C ($1/T = 3.60 \times 10^{-3}$) and 14.2° C ($1/T = 3.48 \times 10^{-3}$°K). Temperature dependency of permeation can provide valuable information about the nature of the barrier and the mechanism of transport.

Autian[70] reviewed the importance of plastics in pharmacy and clinical practice and treated the theory of diffusion and sorption of drugs and environmental vapors in polymeric packaging materials. See the chapter by Autian in *Dispensing of Medication*[70] for reference to diffusion in plastic materials as it applies to clinical pharmacy.

FICK'S SECOND LAW

Fick's first law (equation (13–2), p. 325) has been used throughout this chapter as a starting point in the development of equations to describe the diffusion of drugs through natural and polymeric membranes. However, there are many diffusion problems in which the first law of Fick is not applicable, and the second law (equation (13–5), pp. 325, 326),

$$\frac{\partial u}{\partial t} = D \frac{\partial^2 u}{\partial x^2}$$

must be used. Here we use u instead of C to express concentration. The symbol ∂ signals that *partial derivatives* are being used since u is a function of both t and x. The second law is used to express diffusion in cylinders and spheres, as well as through flat plates. The simplest form of the second law diffusion equation is

$$\frac{\partial u}{\partial t} = D\left(\frac{\partial^2 u}{\partial r^2} + \frac{1}{r}\frac{\partial u}{\partial r}\right) \qquad (13–110)$$

for symmetrical diffusion outward from the axis of a cylinder, in which r is the radius of the cylinder.

For diffusion proceeding symmetrically about the center of a sphere of radius r, the partial differential equation, representing Fick's second law in its simplest form, is

$$r\frac{\partial u}{\partial t} = D\left(r\frac{\partial^2 u}{\partial r^2} + 2\frac{\partial u}{\partial r}\right) \qquad (13–111)$$

The equations for diffusion in cylinders and spheres are discussed by Crank[71] and by Jacobs.[72]

Although the derivation of equations based on Fick's second law is in most cases beyond the mathematical scope of this book, it is of value to present some equations and obtain their solutions. Such exercises give the student practice in calculations for diffusion problems that are more complicated than those derived from Fick's first law.

Diffusion in a Closed System. Determination of D. A simple apparatus (Fig. 13–29) was used by Graham (1861), one of the pioneers in diffusion studies, to obtain diffusion coefficients D for solutes in various solvents.

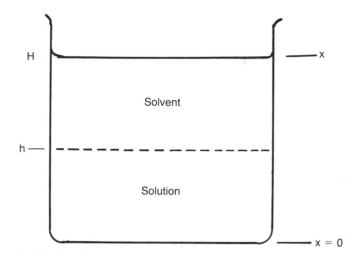

Fig. 13–29. Simple apparatus of Graham for early diffusion studies. (From M. H. Jacobs, *Diffusion Processes*, Springer-Verlag, New York, 1976, p. 24.)

The coefficients for some solutes diffusing through various media are listed in Table 13–1. In the apparatus depicted in Figure 13–29, the height of the solution is h, the combined height of solution and solvent is H, and the distance traversed by the solute is x. The concentration of solute at a position x and time t in the solution is u and its initial concentration is u_o. From the experimental values of u, x, and t, it is possible to determine the diffusion coefficient D for the solute in the solvent.

Initially—that is, at time $t = 0$ sec—the concentration u is equal to u_o (moles or grams per cm^3) in the cell from position $x = 0$ to $x = h$ (cm), and $u = 0$ from $x = h$ to $x = H$. These statements are known as *initial conditions*. In a case in which h is taken equal to $H/2$, that is, both solution and solvent are of equal volume, the equation for u is[72]

$$u = \frac{u_o}{2} + \frac{2u_o}{\pi}\left[\cos\left(\frac{\pi x}{H}\right)e^{-\frac{\pi^2 Dt}{H^2}}\right.$$
$$\left. - \frac{1}{3}\cos\frac{3\pi x}{H}e^{-\frac{9\pi^2 Dt}{H^2}} + \cdots\right] \qquad (13–112)$$

Equation (13–112) is simplified if we choose x, the position of sampling in the cell, to be $H/6$; the second cosine term in the parenthesis of equation (13–112) becomes $\cos(\pi/2) = \cos 90° = $ zero. This leaves only the first cosine term, $\cos(\pi/6) = \cos 30° = 0.866$. Thus, taking $x = H/6$, we have

$$u = \frac{u_o}{2} + \frac{2\,u_o}{\pi}\left(0.866\,e^{-\frac{\pi^2 Dt}{H^2}}\right) \qquad (13–113)$$

The reader is reminded that with trigonometric functions such as $\cos(\pi/6)$, pi is given in degrees; that is, $\pi = 180°$ and $\pi/6 = 30°$, whereas in a term such as $2\,u_o/\pi$ or $e^{-(\pi^2 Dt)/H^2}$ the value of π is 3.14159 . . .

Example 13–16. A new water-soluble drug, corazole, is placed in a Graham diffusion cell (see Fig. 13–29) at an initial concentration, $u_o = 0.030$ mmole/cm^3, to determine its diffusion coefficient in water at 25° C. The height of the solution h in the cell is 2.82 cm and the total height of aqueous solution and overlying water is $H = 5.64$ cm. A sample is taken at a depth of $x = H/6$ cm at time $t = 4.3$ hours (15480 sec) and is found by spectrophotometric analysis to have a concentration $u = 0.0225$ mmole/cm^3. D is obtained by rearranging equation (13–113):

$$D = -\left[\ln\left(\frac{u - u_o/2}{0.866(2\,u_o/\pi)}\right)\right] \cdot \frac{H^2}{\pi^2 t}$$

$$= (-0.79113)\frac{(-31.8096)}{(9.8696)(15480)}$$

$$= 16.47 \times 10^{-5} \text{ cm}^2/\text{sec}$$

Diffusion in Systems with One Open Boundary. The Graham cell for the determination of diffusion coefficients is an example of a closed system. In pharmaceutics, physiology, and biochemistry, systems with one or two open boundaries are of more interest than the closed-boundary system. In 1850 Graham introduced a system with one open and one closed boundary, as shown in Figure 13–30. Insignificant mixing occurs between the solution and the water because of differences in density. The condition at the interface between the solution and the water layer, known as a *boundary condition*, is expressed as "$u = o$ when $x = h$." A second boundary condition states that the change in concentration u with the change in position x is zero, or in mathematical notation, $(\partial u/\partial x) = 0$. This occurs at the bottom of the cell, for the solute cannot pass out through the bottom. In addition to the two boundary conditions, it is useful to specify an *initial condition*, as was done for the closed cell treated earlier. The initial condition is often taken as uniformity of concentration within the solution in the inner vessel of the cell; that is, $u = u_o$ at $t = 0$.

For a system with one open and one closed surface and in which the amount, $M_{o,t}$, of solute escaping

between time 0 and time t is expressed by the equation[72]

$$M_{o,t} = u_o A h \left[1 - \frac{8}{\pi^2}\left(e^{-\frac{\pi^2 Dt}{4h^2}} + \frac{1}{9}e^{-\frac{9\pi^2 Dt}{4h^2}} + \cdots\right)\right]$$

$$(13–114)$$

in which A is the cross-sectional area of the inner cell of height h (see Fig. 13–30), and the other terms have been defined in connection with equations (13–112) and (13–113).

Example 13–17. Calculate the total amount $M_{o,t}$ of the new drug corazole that escapes between times $t = 0$ and $t = 2.70$ hours (9720 sec) from the cell with one open boundary (see Fig. 13–30). The area A of the cell is 8.27 cm^2, and its height is $h = 2.65$ cm. The original concentration of the drug in the cell is $u_o = 0.0437$ g/cm^3. The total amount of drug M in the cell is the concentration in g/cm^3 multiplied by $A \times h$, the volume of the cell: 0.0437 g/cm^3 $\times$ 8.27 cm^2 $\times$ 2.65 cm = 0.9577 g. The diffusion coefficient D of the drug corazole in water at 25° C is 16.5×10^{-5} cm^2/sec, as found in Example 13–16.

Inserting these values into equation (13–114) yields

$$M_{o,t} = (0.0437 \text{ g/cm}^3 \times 8.27 \text{ cm}^2 \times 2.65 \text{ cm}) \times$$
$$\left[1 - \frac{8}{\pi^2}\left(e^{-\frac{\pi^2(16.5 \times 10^{-5}\text{cm}^2/\text{sec})(9720 \text{ sec})}{4 \times 7.0225 \text{ cm}^2}} + \right.\right.$$
$$\left.\left. \frac{1}{9}e^{-\frac{9\pi^2(16.5 \times 10^{-5}\text{ cm}^2/\text{sec})(9720 \text{ sec})}{4 \times 7.0225 \text{ cm}^2}} + \cdots\right)\right].$$
$$M_{o,t} = 0.9577 \text{ gram} \times 0.53805 = 0.51529 \text{ gram}.$$

Thus we arrive at the result that in a cell containing 0.0437 g/cm^3 or 0.9577 g of total drug, 0.5153 g diffuses out in 2.7 hours.

The diffusion of macromolecules, such as proteins, is discussed in the chapter on colloids.

DIFFUSION AND ECOLOGY

Diffusional processes have wide application not only in physical and chemical sciences but also in biology, in which living systems, such as animal colonies, are subject to diffusion as well as aggregation or consolidation. Diffusion is a random process by which atoms and molecules, colloidal and coarse particles, and even *living members of populations* diffuse or spread out with time. In the book *Diffusion and Ecological Problems*, Okubo[73] considers such diverse subjects as diffusion and dispersal of spores by the winds, distribution of fish eggs in the sea, migration of turtles, diffusion factors in the homing of birds, insect swarming and fish schooling, and animal movements on their home ranges. An important means of communication between animals is through the release of olfactory or gustatory signals and their transmission through the environment. These processes may be treated in terms of passive diffusion models.

In Figure 13–31, Okubo applies the principles of diffusion to the ventilation of animal burrows. The main opening of the tunnel of the prairie dog is on a mound, and the emergency exit at a lower level. This design apparently provides the most efficient diffusion of air

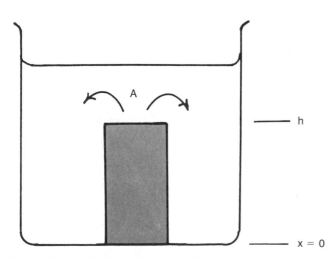

Fig. 13–30. Diffusion apparatus with one open and one closed boundary. (M. H. Jacobs, *Diffusion Processes*, Springer-Verlag, New York, 1976, p. 47.)

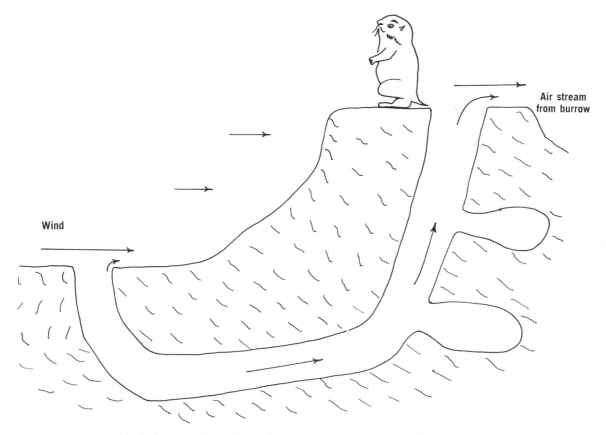

Fig. 13–31. Ventilation of a prairie dog's burrow by action of the wind. (From A. Okubo, *Diffusion and Ecological Problems: Mathematical Models*, Springer-Verlag, Berlin, 1980, p. 43.)

and ventilation for the burrow of the prairie dog. The difference in the height of the two openings produces a "viscous sucking" by the wind on the stagnant air in the burrow, according to Bernoulli's law. This is the principle of the Venturi tube, used to expel liquid medication from a spray atomizer. Diffusion theory has been used by Wilson and Kilgore[74] to calculate the concentration gradient of respiratory gases in small animal burrows. The interested student should see Okubo[73] for other examples of diffusion in biologic systems.

References and Notes

1. S. T. Hwang and K. Kammermeyer, *Membranes in Separations (Techniques of Chemistry)*, A. Weissberger, Ed., Wiley-Interscience, New York, 1975, pp. 23–28.
2. V. T. Stannett et al. Recent advances in membrane science and technology, in *Advances in Polymer Science*, Vol. 32, Springer-Verlag, Berlin, 1979, pp. 71–122; D. R. Paul and G. Morel, Membrane technology, in *Encyclopedia of Chemical Technology*, 3rd Ed., Kirk & Othmer, Eds., Vol. 15, Wiley, New York, 1981, pp. 92–131.
3. G. L. Flynn, S. H. Yalkowsky and T. J. Roseman, J. Pharm. Sci. **63**, 479, 1974.
4. H. Carslaw, *Mathematical Theory of the Conduction of Heat*, Macmillan, New York, 1921.
5. R. W. Baker and H. K. Lonsdale, in *Controlled Release of Biologically Active Agents*, A. C. Tanquary and R. E. Lacey, Eds., Plenum Press, New York, 1974, pp. 30–33.
6. M. G. Karth, W. I. Higuchi and J. L. Fox, J. Pharm. Sci. **74**, 612, 1985.
7. M. Z. Biber and C. T. Rhodes, J. Pharm. Sci. **65**, 564, 1976.

8. K. Nasim, N. C. Meyer and J. Autian, J. Pharm. Sci. **61**, 1775, 1972.
9. T. Higuchi and A. Aguiar, J. Am. Pharm. Assoc., Sci. Ed. **48**, 574, 1959.
10. J. Crank and G. S. Park, *Diffusion in Polymers*, Academic Press, New York, 1968, pp. 20–23.
11. R. Scheuplein, J. Invest. Dermatol. **45**, 334, 1965.
12. D. E. Wurster, J. A., Ostrenga and L. E. Matheson, Jr., J. Pharm. Sci. **68**, 1406, 1410, 1979.
13. Y. C. Martin, *Quantitative Drug Design*, Marcel Dekker, New York, 1978, pp. 76–81.
14. W. J. Addicks, G. L. Flynn and N. Weiner, Pharm. Res. **4**, 337, 1987.
15. G. M. Grass and S. A. Sweetana, Pharm. Res. **5**, 372, 1988.
16. W. J. Addicks, G. L. Flynn, N. Weiner and C-M. Chiang, Pharm. Res. **5**, 377, 1988.
17. D. E. Wurster and P. W. Taylor, J. Pharm. Sci. **54**, 169, 1965.
18. J. G. Wagner, *Biopharmaceutics and Relevant Pharmacokinetics*, Drug Intelligence, Hamilton, Ill., 1971, pp. 98–147.
19. L. J. Leeson and J. T. Carstensen, *Dissolution Technology*, Academy of Pharmaceutical Sciences, Washington, D.C., 1974.
20. W. I. Higuchi, J. Pharm. Sci. **56**, 315, 1967.
21. J. P. Skelley, G. L. Amidon, W. H. Barr, et al., J. Pharm. Sci. **79**, 849, 1991.
22. J. McGinity, S. Stavchansky and A. Martin, Bioavailability in tablet technology, in *Pharmaceutical Dosage Forms: Tablets*, H. A. Lieberman and L. Lachman, Eds. Vol. II, Marcel Dekker, New York, 1981.
23. M. K. T. Yau and M. C. Meyer, J. Pharm. Sci. **70**, 1017, 1981; V. P. Shah, V. K. Prasad, T. Alston, B. E. Cabana, R. P. Gural, and M. C. Meyer, J. Pharm. Sci. **72**, 306, 1983; P. J. McNamara, T. S. Foster, G. A. Digenis, R. B. Patel, W. A. Craig, P. G. Welling, R. S. Rapaka, V. K. Prasad, and V. P. Shah, Pharm. Res. **4**, 150, 1987.
24. G. Levy and B. A. Sahli, J. Pharm. Sci. **51**, 58, 1962; J. H. Wood, J. E. Syarto and H. Letterman, J. Pharm. Sci. **54**, 1068, 1965; J. H. de Smidt, et al. J. Pharm. Sci. **75**, 497, 1986.

25. J. T. Carstensen, *Pharmaceutics of Solids and Solid Dosage Forms*, Wiley, New York, 1977, Chapter III.
26. A. Hixson and J. Crowell, Ind. Eng. Chem. **23**, 923, 1931.
27. M. J. Miralles, Dissolution rates of tolbutamide coprecipitates, M. S. Thesis, University of Texas, August, 1980.
28. V. Levich, *Physicochemical Hydrodynamics*, Prentice-Hall, Englewood Cliffs, N.J., 1982.
29. K. G. Nelson and A. C. Shah, J. Pharm. Sci. **64**, 610, 1518, 1975.
30. J. H. de Smidt, J. C. A. Offringa and D. J. A. Crommelin, J. Pharm. Sci. **76**, 711, 1987.
31. J. R. Robinson, *Sustained and Controlled Release Drug Delivery Systems*, Marcel Dekker, New York, 1978,
32. T. Higuchi, J. Soc. Cosm. Chem. **11**, 85, 1960.
33. T. Higuchi, J. Pharm. Sci. **50**, 874, 1961.
34. (a) S. J. Desai, A. P. Simonelli and W. I. Higuchi, J. Pharm. Sci. **54**, 1459, 1965; (b) S. J. Desai, P. Singh, A. P. Simonelli and W. I. Higuchi, J. Pharm. Sci. **55**, 1224, 1230, 1235, 1966.
35. N. F. H. Ho and T. J. Roseman, J. Pharm. Sci. **68**, 1170, 1979.
36. G. L. Flynn, S. H. Yalkowsky and T. J. Roseman, J. Pharm. Sci. **63**, 479, 1974.
37. G. L. Flynn and S. H. Yalkowsky, J. Pharm. Sci. **61**, 838, 1972.
38. F. Bottari, G. DiColo, E. Nannipieri, et al., J. Pharm. Sci. **63**, 1779, 1974; ibid. **66**, 927, 1977.
39. D. R. Paul and S. K. McSpadden, J. Memb. Sci. **1**, 33, 1976; S. K. Chandrasekaran and D. R. Paul, J. Pharm. Sci. **71**, 1399, 1982.
40. Y. W. Chien, in *Sustained and Controlled Release Drug Delivery Systems*, J. R. Robinson, Ed., Marcel Dekker, New York, 1978, Chapter 4; Y. W. Chien, Chem. Pharm. Bull. **24**, 147, 1976.
41. C. K. Erickson, K. I. Koch, C. S. Metha and J. W. McGinity, Science, **199**, 1457, 1978; J. W. McGinity, L. A. Hunke and A. Combs, J. Pharm. Sci. **68**, 662, 1979.
42. Y. W. Chien, *Novel Drug Delivery Systems: Biomedical Applications and Theoretical Basis*, Marcel Dekker, New York, 1982, Chapter 9.
43. B. B. Brodie and C. A. M. Hogben, J. Pharm. Pharmacol. **9**, 345, 1957; P. A. Shore, B. B. Brodie and C. A. M. Hogben, J. Pharmacol. Exp. Ther. **119**, 361, 1957; L. S. Shanker, D. J. Tocco, B. B. Brodie and C. A. M. Hogben, ibid. **123**, 81, 1958; C. A. M. Hogben, D. J. Tocco, B. B. Brodie and L. S. Shanker, ibid. **125**, 275, 1959; L. S. Shanker, J. Med. Chem. **2**, 343, 1960; L. S. Shanker, Ann. Rev. Pharmacol. **1**, 29, 1961.
44. R. H. Turner, C. S. Mehta and L. Z. Benet, J. Pharm. Sci. **59**, 590, 1970.
45. J. L. Colaizzi and P. R. Klink, J. Pharm. Sci. **58**, 1184, 1969.
46. A. Suzuki, W. I. Higuchi and N. F. H. Ho, J. Pharm. Sci. **59**, 644, 651, 1970; N. F. H. Ho, W. I. Higuchi and J. Turi, J. Pharm. Sci. **61**, 192, 1972; N. F. H. Ho and W. I. Higuchi, J. Pharm. Sci. **63**, 686, 1974.
47. (a) N. F. H. Ho, J. Y. Park, G. E. Amidon, et al., in *Gastrointestinal Absorption of Drugs*, A. J. Aguiar, Ed., American Pharmaceutical Association, Academy of Pharmaceutical Sciences, Washington, D.C., 1981; (b) W. I. Higuchi, N. F. H. Ho, J. Y. Park, and I. Komiya, in *Drug Absorption*, L. F. Prescott and W. S. Nimmo, Eds., Adis Press, Balgowlah, NSW 2093, Australia, 1981, pp. 35–60; (c) N. F. H. Ho, J. Y. Park, W. Morozowich and W. I. Higuchi, in *Design of Biopharmaceutical Properties Through Prodrugs and Analogs*, E. B. Roche, Ed., American Pharmaceutical Association, Academy of Pharmaceutical Sciences, Washington, D.C., 1977, Chapter 8.
48. J. T. Doluisio, F. N. Billups, L. W. Dittert, E. T. Sugita and V. J. Swintosky, J. Pharm. Sci. **58**, 1196, 1969.
49. A. K. Mitra and T. J. Mikkelson, J. Pharm. Sci. **77**, 771, 1988.
50. R. J. Scheuplein, J. Invest. Dermatol. **45**, 334, 1965; R. J. Scheuplein, J. Invest. Dermatol. **48**, 79, 1967; R. J. Scheuplein and I. H. Blank, Physiol. Rev. **51**, 702, 1971.
51. R. J. Scheuplein, I. H. Blank, G. J. Brauner and D. J. MacFarlane, J. Invest. Dermatol. **52**, 63, 1969.
52. C. D. Yu, J. L. Fox, N. F. H. Ho and W. I. Higuchi, J. Pharm. Sci. **68**, 1341, 1347, 1979; ibid. **69**, 772, 1980; H. Durrheim, G. L. Flynn, W. I. Higuchi and C. R. Behl, J. Pharm. Sci. **69**, 781, 1980; G. L. Flynn, H. Durrheim and W. I. Higuchi, J. Pharm. Sci. **70**, 52, 1981; C. R. Behl, G. L. Flynn, T. Kurihara, N. Harper, W. Smith, W. I. Higuchi, N. F. H. Ho and C. L. Pierson, J. Invest. Dermatol. **75**, 346, 1980.
53. P. V. Raykar, M-C. Fung, and B. D. Anderson, Pharm. Res., **5**, 140, 1988.
54. J. S. Turi, D. Danielson, and W. Wolterson, J. Pharm. Sci. **68**, 275, 1979.
55. S. H. Yalkowsky and G. L. Flynn, J. Pharm. Sci. **63**, 1276, 1974.
56. J. Ostrenga, C. Steinmetz and B. Poulsen, J. Pharm. Sci. **60**, 1175, 1180, 1971.
57. K. B. Sloan, K. G. Siver, and S. A. M. Koch, J. Pharm. Sci. **75**, 744, 1986.
58. H. Komatsu and M. Suzuki, J. Pharm. Sci. **68**, 596, 1979.
59. A. H. Beckett and A. C. Moffat, J. Pharm. Pharmacol. **20**, 239S, 1968.
60. N. F. H. Ho and W. I. Higuchi, J. Pharm. Sci. **60**, 537, 1971.
61. A. Suzuki, W. I. Higuchi and N. F. H. Ho, J. Pharm. Sci. **59**, 644, 651, 1970.
62. G. L. Flynn, N. F. H. Ho, S. Hwang, E. Owada, A. Motokhia, C. R. Behl, W. I. Higuchi, T. Yotsuyanagi, Y. Shah and J. Park, in *Controlled Release Polymeric Formulations*, D. R. Paul and F. W. Harris, Eds., American Chemical Society, Washington, DC, 1976, pp. 87–122.
63. S. K. Chandrasekaran, H. Benson and J. Urquhart, in *Sustained and Controlled Release Drug Delivery Systems*, J. R. Robinson, Ed., Marcel Dekker, New York, 1978, pp. 572–574.
64. (a) T. Yotsuyanagi, A. Molakhia, S. Hwang, N. F. H. Ho, C. L. Flynn and W. I. Higuchi, J. Pharm. Sci. **64**, 71, 1975; (b) S. Hwang, E. Owada, T. Yotsuyanagi, L. Suhardja, Jr., N. F. H. Ho, G. L. Flynn, W. I. Higuchi and J. V. Park, J. Pharm. Sci. **65**, 1574, 1578, 1976.
65. H. Okada, I. Yamazaki, Y. Ogawa, S. Hirai, T. Yashiki and H. Mima, J. Pharm. Sci. **71**, 1367, 1982; H. Okada, I. Yamazaki, T. Yashiki and H. Mima, ibid. **72**, 75, 1983; H. Okada, T. Yashiki and H. Mima, ibid. **72**, 173, 1983; H. Okada, I. Yamazaki, T. Yashiki, T. Shimamoto and H. Mima, ibid. **73**, 298, 1984.
66. D. F. Othmer and G. J. Frohlich, Ind. Eng. Chem. **47**, 1034, 1955.
67. A. S. Michaels and R. B. Parker, J. Polym. Sci. **41**, 53, 1959.
68. T. Higuchi and A. Aguiar, J. Am. Pharm. Assoc., Sci. Ed. **48**, 574, 1959.
69. I. H. Blank, R. J. Scheuplein and D. J. McFarlane, J. Invest. Dermatol. **49**, 582, 1967.
70. J. Autian, Plastics medication, Chapter 15 in *Dispensing of Medication*, E. W. Martin, Ed., Mack, Easton, Penn., 1971.
71. J. Crank, *The Mathematics of Diffusion*, 2nd Edition, Oxford, Oxford University Press, 1975, Chapters 5 and 6.
72. M. H. Jacobs, *Diffusion Processes*, Springer-Verlag, New York, 1967, p. 43, and p. 49, equation 39 where we use the symbol M to replace Jacobs' term, Q.
73. A. Okubo, *Diffusion and Ecological Problems: Mathematical Models*, Springer-Verlag, Berlin, 1980.
74. K. J. Wilson and D. L. Kilgore, J. Theor. Biol. **71**, 73, 1978.
75. S. Esezobo, S. Zubair and N. Pilpel, J. Pharm. Pharmacol. **41**, 7, 1989.
76. K. G. Nelson and A. C. Shah, J. Pharm. Sci. **66**, 137, 1977.
77. A. C. Shah and K. G. Nelson, J. Pharm. Sci. **64**, 1518, 1975; ibid. **76**, 799, 1987.
78. Y. W. Chien et al., J. Pharm. Sci. **63**, 365, 1974.
79. A. C. Shah and K. G. Nelson, J. Pharm. Sci. **69**, 210, 1980.
80. S. Borodkin and F. E. Tucker, J. Pharm. Sci. **64**, 1289, 1975.
81. K. F. Farng and K. G. Nelson, J. Pharm. Sci. **66**, 1611, 1977.
82. S. S. Davis, Experientia, **26**, 671, 1970.
83. A. Adjei, J. Newburger, S. Stavchansky and A. Martin, J. Pharm. Sci. **73**, 742, 1984.
84. K. Tojo, C. C. Chiang and Y. W. Chien, J. Pharm. Sci. **76**, 123, 1987.
85. A. J. Aguiar and M. A. Weiner, J. Pharm. Sci. **58**, 210, 1969.
86. Z. Liron and S. Cohen, J. Pharm. Sci. **73**, 534, 1984; ibid. **73**, 538, 1984.
87. N. F. H. Ho et al., J. Pharm. Sci. **65**, 1578, 1976.
88. C. D. Yu, W. I. Higuchi, N. F. H. Ho, J. L. Fox and G. L. Flynn, J. Pharm. Sci. **69**, 770, 1980.

Problems

13–1. The diffusion coefficient of tetracycline in a hydroxyethyl methacrylate–methyl methacrylate copolymer film in a mole ratio of 2:98 is $D = 8.0(\pm 4.7)^* \times 10^{-9}$ cm²/sec and the partition coefficient

---

*The quantities in parentheses ± are standard deviations. That is, for example, the diffusion coefficient ranges from $(8.0 - 4.7) \times 10^{-9}$ to $(8.0 + 4.7) \times 10^{-9}$ based on a variability of ± 1 standard deviation (4.7) from the mean D value of 8.

K for tetracycline between the membrane and the reservoir is $6.8(\pm5.9) \times 10^{-3}$. The membrane thickness h of the trilaminar device is 1.40×10^{-2} cm, and the concentration of tetracycline in the core, C_o, is 0.02 g/cm^3 of the core material. Using equation (13–73), p. 341, calculate the release rate Q/t in units of μg cm^{-2} of tetracycline per day.

Answer: $Q/t = 6.71$ μg cm^{-2} day^{-1}

13–2. Diffusion of fluocinolone acetonide occurred from a 30% propylene glycol–water solution through a circular section of a polyethylene membrane in a two-compartment glass cell. The thickness h of the membrane was 0.076 cm and its diameter was 2.21 cm. The partition coefficient of the drug between the membrane and the solution was 1.28 at 25° C and C_v was 0.025 g/100 cm^3. A plot of drug amount (in grams) permeating versus time in hours produced a straight line (after steady state was established) with a lag time t_L of 25.0 hours. Calculate (a) the diffusion coefficient, knowing h and t_L, and (b) dQ/dt in μg/(cm^2 hr), using the expression $dQ/dt = DKC_v/h$.

Answers: (a) 3.85×10^{-5} cm^2/hr; (b) $dQ/dt = 1.62 \times 10^{-7}$ g/(cm^2 hr), or 0.162 μg/(cm^2 hr)

13–3. Esezobo et al.[75] studied the effect of concentration of binder on the dissolution rates of acetaminophen tablets using the integrated form of the Noyes–Whitney equation

$$\ln\left(\frac{C_s}{C_s - C}\right) = -kt$$

where C_s is the concentration of the solute at saturation (solubility), C is the concentration at time t, and k is the dissolution rate constant. The data are found in the following table.

Data for *Problem 13–3*

t (min)	$\ln\left(\dfrac{C_s}{C_s - C}\right)$		
	no binder	2.5% PVP	5% PVP
5	0.125	0.145	0.10
10	0.43	0.29	0.20
15	0.645	0.453	0.30
20	0.86	0.58	0.40
30	1.25	0.87	0.60
40	—	1.16	0.80

Plot $\ln\left(\dfrac{C_s}{C_s - C}\right)$ (vertical axis) against t and compute the dissolution rate constant k from the slope for the acetaminophen tablets with no binder and in the presence of 2.5% and 5% PVP.

Answer: With no binder, $k = 0.041$ min^{-1}; with 2.5% PVP, $k = 0.029$ min^{-1}; with 5% PVP, $k = 0.020$ min^{-1}.

13–4. A new fast-dissolving tolbutamide tablet was prepared and tested for rate of dissolution. The milligram amounts (m) of drug dissolved at various times are given here:

Data for *Problem 13–4*

time (min)	2	4	6	8	10	15
m (mg)	14.4	18.8	21.3	25.9	28.2	32.9

(a) Plot the results on rectangular graph paper (m versus t) and on semilog paper (log m versus t) and finally plot m versus $t^{1/2}$. Which method yields a straight line?

(b) Using regression analysis and the data that give a linear relationship, calculate the correlation coefficient, the intercept, and the slope, k, the dissolution rate constant.

(c) An intercept gives the value of the ordinate of a graph at the point at which the quantity on the horizontal axis is zero. How is it possible that the milligrams of tolbutamide dissolved at 0 min$^{1/2}$ is 3.3872 mg? Give several possible explanations.

Partial Answer: (b) $r^2 = 0.9922$, slope = $k = 7.706$ mg/(min)$^{1/2}$, intercept = 3.387 mg

13–5. A 0.625-g sample of acetohexamide powder was dissolved in 1000 cm^3 of water in a paddle-type dissolution apparatus at 30° C. The dissolution rate data are found in the table below. They are presumed to follow the Hixson–Crowell law.

Data for *Problem 13–5*

Time (min)	Concentration (mg/mL)	Weight Undissolved in gram (g)	$M_o^{1/3} - M^{1/3}$	κ in $g^{1/3}$/min
0	0	$M_o = 0.625$	0	—
2	0.159	0.466	0.080	0.040
4	0.288	0.337	0.159	
6	0.390	0.235	0.238	
8	0.468	0.157	0.315	
10	0.528	0.097	0.396	

(a) Calculate κ for each time period to fill in the last column of the table. Then add these separate κ values and divide by the number to obtain an average κ.

(b) Regress ($M_o^{1/3} - M^{1/3}$) versus time in minutes and obtain κ as the slope of the least-squares line. Which of these methods is the better for obtaining κ? Give reasons for your preference.

Answers: (a) $\kappa_{(av)} = 0.0397$ g$^{1/3}$/min; (b) $\kappa = 0.0394$ $g^{1/3}$/min

13–6. Nelson and Shah[76] applied their convective diffusion model (see *Example 13–6*) to the permeation rate (rate of diffusion), R, of butamben through a dimethicone membrane under conditions of aqueous diffusion layer control (p. 338). For a circular membrane, the permeation rate is given by the convective diffusion (CD) equation:

$$R = 2.157\, D_a^{2/3} C_s \alpha^{1/3} r^{5/3} \qquad (13\text{–}115)$$

where D_a is the diffusivity (diffusion coefficient) of the solute in the aqueous layer, C_s is the solubility, α the rate of shear over the membrane, and r the radius of the circular membrane. The rate of permeation, R, written as dM/dt elsewhere in this chapter, was considered the dependent variable, using the radius of the membrane as the independent variable. The equation obtained by least-squares regression predicts a straight line in a plot of log R versus log r, holding the other parameters constant.

(a) Prepare the graph of log R versus log r, compute the slope and intercept, and determine how well they compare with comparable quantities predicted by equation (13–115). The values of the known parameters are $D_a = 6 \times 10^{-6}$ cm^2 sec^{-1} = 3.60×10^{-4} cm^2 min^{-1}; $C_s = 9.4 \times 10^{-4}$ mole/liter = 9.4×10^{-7} mole cm^{-3}; and $\alpha = 35.006$ min^{-1}; the experimental R and r values for the plot are:

Data for *Problem 13–6*

R (mole/min)	1.325×10^{-8}	2.712×10^{-8}	3.881×10^{-8}
r (cm)	0.65	1	1.25

(b) Choose one of the three values of r from the above table and the known parameters given above; substitute these into the least-squares regression equation and into the CD equation (equation (13–115)). Compare your results from these two methods for calculating R. What is the percentage error in these two methods relative to the experimental value of R?

(c) This system is under aqueous diffusion layer control. Compute the thickness h_a of the static aqueous layer, using $r = 1.25$ cm and $R = 3.881 \times 10^{-8}$ mole min^{-1} = 6.47×10^{-10} mole sec^{-1}.

Notes: In preparation for graphing, be sure to first convert R and r to logarithms. Recall that when converted to logarithmic form in equation (13–115) quantities multiplied together are added. Therefore equation (13–115), written as log R versus r, becomes log (2.157) + 2/3 log D_a + log C_s + 1/3 log α + 5/3 log r, and for D_a, C_s, and α held constant:

$$\log R = \log(2.157 \, D_a^{2/3} C_s \alpha^{1/3}) + 5/3 \log r \qquad (13\text{–}116)$$

with the first log term on the right side as the intercept and 5/3 = 1.667 in the second log term as the slope.

Partial Answer: **(a)** The equation of the linear regression line is log $R = -7.569 + 1.646$ log r. The slope, 1.646, and intercept, -7.569, compare well with the values 1.667 and -7.4739 predicted by the convective diffusion (CD) equation (13–115). **(b)** For $r = 1.25$ cm substituted into equation (13–116) for the linear regression line:

$$\log R = -7.569 + 1.646 \log(1.25) = -7.4095$$

$R = 3.90 \times 10^{-8}$ mole/min. From the CD equation, $R = 4.87 \times 10^{-8}$ mole/min. The regression equation (13–116) has an error of about 0.5% and the CD equation, (13–115), an error of about 26% in relation to the experimental value of $R = 3.881 \times 10^{-8}$ mole/min. **(c)** Under aqueous diffusion layer control, p. 338, equation (13–58),

$$J = \frac{dM}{dt} \frac{1}{S} = \left(\frac{D_a}{2 \, h_a}\right) C_s; \quad R = \frac{dM}{dt} = \left(\frac{S \, D_a}{2 \, h_a}\right) C_s = \left(\frac{\pi \, r^2 \, D_a}{2 \, h_a}\right) C_s;$$

$h_a = 0.0214$ cm. The actual dimethicone membrane thickness is about 0.025 cm.

13–7. Shah and Nelson[77] studied the dissolution rate of alkyl *p*-aminobenzoates using a convective diffusion model (see p. 334 and *Example 13–6*), where for a circular shaped tablet of surface radius r, the equation is

$$R = 2.157 \, D^{2/3} C_s \alpha^{1/3} r^{5/3} \qquad (13\text{–}115)$$

D is the diffusivity, C_s the solubility of the drug, and α the rate of shear over the dissolving surface of the tablet. R is the tablet dissolution rate.

(a) If C_s is 9.33×10^{-7} mole/cm^3, α is 255 min^{-1}, r is 0.5012 cm, and R, the measured dissolution rate, 1.553×10^{-8} mole min^{-1}, what is the numerical value of the diffusion coefficient?

(b) One may wish to study the change in the dissolution rate R with a change in the radius r, or regarding the change of another parameter, such as the solubility C_s or the rate of shear α. Because of the exponents in equation (13–115) this is best done by plotting the logarithm of R versus the logarithm of r, holding D, C_s, and α constant. The equation becomes:

$$\log R = \log(2.157 + \tfrac{2}{3}\log D + \log C_s + \tfrac{1}{3}\log \alpha) + \tfrac{5}{3}\log r \qquad (13\text{–}117)$$

Using the data from table (a) below, plot log R versus log r on rectangular coordinate graph paper. If the plot is linear with a slope of 5/3 = 1.667, or approximately so, you have a good indication that the convective diffusion approach is a satisfactory model for the dissolution kinetic study under investigation. Next, one can plot log R versus log C_s, for example, using the data in table (b), while holding D, α, and r constant. What should be the slope of this line?

Data (a) for *Problem 13–7*

R (cm^2/min)	log R	r (cm)	log r
1.26×10^{-7}	-6.90	0.398	-0.40
2.34×10^{-7}	-6.63	0.575	-0.24
4.17×10^{-7}	-6.38	0.794	-0.10

Data (b) for *Problem 13–7*

R (cm^2/min)	log R	C_s (mole/cm^3)	log C_s
1.82×10^{-7}	-6.74	6.31×10^{-6}	-2.20
2.82×10^{-7}	-7.55	9.33×10^{-7}	-3.03
7.94×10^{-9}	-8.10	2.9×10^{-7}	-3.57

The authors show that other properties such as viscosity of the solution may also be tested by the convective diffusion model for their effects on the system.

Answers: **(a)** $D = 2.39 \times 10^{-4}$ cm^2/min; **(b)** in a plot of log R versus log r, the slope obtained from regression analysis is 1.732. The theoretical slope is 5/3 = 1.667 because of the final term in equation (13–117). In a plot of log R versus log C_s the slope should be 1.00 since the exponent on C_s in equation (13–115) or (13–116) is unity. The least-square equation obtained is log $R = -4.556 + 0.991$ log C_s. The squared correlation coefficient, r^2, = 0.999.

13–8. The release of ethynodiol diacetate through a silicone dosage form may be calculated using the Higuchi equation,

$$Q/t^{1/2} = [D(2A - C_s)C_s]^{1/2}$$

since diffusion is found in this case to be the rate-limiting factor for drug release. A, the amount of drug per unit volume of the silicone matrix, is 100 g/(10^3 cm^3), the solubility C_s of the drug in the silicone polymer is 1.50 g/(10^3 cm^3), and D, the diffusivity of the drug in the silicone matrix, is 3.4×10^{-2} cm^2/day. Calculate the rate of drug release from the silicone dosage form in units of g/(10^3 cm^2) per day$^{1/2}$.

Answer: 3.182 g/(10^3 cm^2) per day$^{1/2}$

13–9. When C_s is small relative to A, as found in *Problem 13–8*, the Higuchi equation reduces to $Q/t^{1/2} = \sqrt{2DAC_s}$. Recalculate the results of *Problem 13–8* using this abbreviated equation.

Answer: 3.194 g/(10^3 cm^2) per day$^{1/2}$. A value of about 3.1 g/(10^3 cm^2) per day$^{1/2}$ is obtained experimentally.[78]

13–10. The permeation of methyl *p*-aminobenzoate through a dimethicone membrane of thickness $h_m = 0.0254$ cm was conducted in a laminar flow cell at 25° C.[79] At high flow rates the membrane D_m and aqueous solvent D_a diffusivities are $D_m = 2.72 \times 10^{-6}$ cm^2 sec^{-1} and $D_a = 6 \times 10^{-6}$ cm^2 sec^{-1}. The thickness of the aqueous layer h_a is 0.003 cm, the solubility C of the drug is 1.04×10^{-2} mole/liter, and the partition coefficient K across the drug–membrane interface is 0.26.

(a) By appropriate calculations, suggest whether the flux is controlled by the aqueous diffusion layer or by the membrane.

(b) Compute the flux, J (mole cm^{-2} min^{-1}). See page 338 for membrane and diffusion layer control.

Answers: **(a)** $2h_aKD_m < h_mD_a$; the process is one of membrane control. Show this to be true by calculating these two quantities. **(b)** The flux $J = (KD_m/h_m)C$ for membrane control is 1.74×10^{-8} mole cm^{-2} min^{-1}. Using the entire equation (13–59), page 339, we obtain $J = 1.69 \times 10^{-8}$ mole cm^{-2} min^{-1}, which compares favorably with $J = 1.74 \times 10^{-8}$ mole cm^{-2} min^{-1}, the membrane control result.

13–11. A cell contains a silastic membrane with diffusion layers of identical thickness on either side and butyl-aminobenzoate at concentration $C = 1.72$ mmole/liter or 1.72×10^{-3} mmole/cm^3 in the donor compartment. Calculate the steady-state flux, J, through the membrane in millimoles per cm^2 per hour. The equation that represents the process in which both membrane and diffusion-layer control obtain is

$$J = \left[\frac{D_mKD_a}{h_mD_a + 2h_aKD_m}\right]C$$

The data obtained from an experiment at 37° C are as follows: $D_m = 2.7 \times 10^{-6}$ cm^2/sec or 0.00972 cm^2/hr, $D_a = 6.0 \times 10^{-6}$ cm^2/sec = 0.02160 cm^2/hr, $h_m = 0.006$ cm, $h_a = 0.0188$ cm, and $K = 10.3$.

Answer: $J = 9.55 \times 10^{-4}$ mmole/(cm^2 hr)

13–12. Borodkin and Tucker[80] studied the diffusion of salicylic acid from a polymer film containing dispersed drug. The kinetics was made linear with time, i.e., zero order, by laminating a second film, consisting of a hydroxypropylcellulose-polyvinyl acetate membrane of thickness $h_m = 0.0164$ cm to the releasing side of the film with the drug as a reservoir layer.

The drug layer controlled the duration of release, while the nondrug layer consisting of the cellulose membrane served as a rate-controlling membrane. Diffusion through the film is the limiting factor in a drug release, so that equation (13–72) on page 341 applies. Q, the amount of drug released per unit surface area, is given for various times:

Data for *Problem 13–12*

Q (mg/cm²)	0.46	1.00	1.54	2.19	2.69	3.23	3.54
time (hr)	1	2	3	4	5	6	7

Equation (13–72) may also be written as

$$\frac{dQ}{dt} = \frac{D_m C_p}{h_m} \qquad (13-118)$$

the instantaneous rate of release of drug at time t. Integration of this equation and evaluation of the integration constants yields a term for the lag time, t_{lag}:

$$Q = \frac{D_m C_p}{h_m} t - \frac{D_m C_p}{h_m} t_{lag} \qquad (13-119)$$

Equation (13–119) shows that a plot of Q against t yields a straight line of slope $= D_m C_p / h_m = k_o$, the apparent zero-order rate constant. The intercept of equation (13–119) is $(D_m C_p / h_m) t_{lag} = k_o t_{lag}$, from which t_{lag} can be computed.

(a) Plot Q versus time, t, from the data given in the table. (b) Regress Q against t and obtain $k_o = D_m C_p / h_m$ (mg cm⁻²) from the slope and t_{lag} from the intercept. (c) Knowing the lag time and the thickness h_m of the nondrug layer, compute the diffusion coefficient, D_m. You will need the lag time equation (13–14a) from page 328. (d) From the slope obtained in part (b) and the diffusion coefficient D_m calculated in part (c), compute the value of C_p, the concentration of the drug, salicylic acid, in the reservoir layer of the base film.

Answer: (b) $k_o = D_m C_p / h_m - 0.530$ mg cm⁻² hr⁻¹; $t_{lag} - 0.0539$ hr or 3.23 min; (c) $D_m = 2.31 \times 10^{-7}$ cm² sec⁻¹ using $h_m = 0.0164$ cm; (d) $C_p = 10.46$ mg cm⁻³

13–13. Farng and Nelson[81] studied the effect of polyelectrolytes, such as carboxymethylcellulose (CMC), on the permeation rate of sodium salicylate across a cellulose membrane at 37° C. Fick's law may be written to cover this case, assuming the existence of three barriers in series: the membrane and an unstirred liquid diffusion layer on either side. The reciprocal of the permeation coefficient for the three layers is

$$1/P = h_1/D_1 + h_m/\phi D_m K + h_2/D_2 K$$

in which $h_1 = h_2 = 82 \times 10^{-4}$ cm for the two static diffusion layers; $h_m = 46.6 \times 10^{-4}$ cm for the cellulose membrane thickness, $D_1 = 1.33 \times 10^{-5}$ cm²/sec, $D_2 = 1.11 \times 10^{-5}$/cm² sec, and $D_m = 1.69 \times 10^{-6}$ cm²/sec for the three diffusion coefficients. The partition coefficient K for the salicylate between the solution in compartment 1 (left-hand reservoir) and water in the membrane is 1.16. The volume fraction ϕ of water in the membrane is 0.667. Calculate the permeability P for the salicylate and compare it with $P_{(obs)} = 1.86 \times 10^{-4}$ cm/sec.

Answer: $P_{(calc)} = 2.08 \times 10^{-4}$ cm/sec

13–14. Sulfadiazine, pK_a 6.50 at 25° C, as with all weak acids, shows a variable-percent dissociation as a function of pH. (a) Prepare a table showing the percent dissociated and percent undissociated sulfadiazine at pH 2, 4, 6.5, 7, 8, 10, and 12. (b) Plot the results on rectangular graph paper. (c) Predict the absorption of sulfadiazine from the gut and from the small intestine in terms of the pH–partition hypothesis and from the results obtained in parts (a) and (b)

Partial Answer: Percent dissociation at pH 4 = 0.32%; at pH 8 = 96.93%

13–15. Bile acids are transported across the ileum by active and passive processes.[47] For dilute nonmicellar bile acid solutions, the absorption rate constant is given by equation (13–93):

$$K_u = \frac{S}{V} \frac{P_{aq}}{1 + \dfrac{P_{aq}}{P_o X_s° + P_m^* X_s^-}}$$

in which P_m^* is the permeability constant for the active transport of bile acid anions; P_o the permeability constant of undissociated species undergoing passive diffusion; P_{aq} the permeability constant of the aqueous diffusion layer; and $X_s°$ and X_s^- the fraction of undissociated and anionic species, respectively.

For taurocholic acid, pK_a 2.0, the bile acid is essentially all in the ionic form at pH 6 to 7. Therefore, $X_s° \approx 0$, $X_s^- \approx 1.0$, and K_u becomes

$$K_u = \frac{S}{V} \frac{P_{aq}}{1 + \dfrac{P_{aq}}{P_m^*}}$$

If S/V, the ratio of effective surface area to solution volume, is 10 cm⁻¹, P_{aq} is 2×10^{-4} cm/sec, and P_m^* is 1×10^{-3} cm/sec, what is K_u, the rate constant for the absorption of taurocholic acid across the ileum?

Answer: $K_u = 1.67 \times 10^{-3}$ sec⁻¹

13–16. In situ rat gut permeation experiments were performed at 37° C to determine the influence of the Hildebrand solubility parameter, δ. The rat intestinal preparation is shown in Figure 13–18 and the solubility parameter is defined on page 224. The drug theophylline, with a solubility parameter or delta value, δ_2, of 14 (cal/cm³)$^{1/2}$ and a molar volume, V_2, of 124 cm³/mole, was dissolved in the solvent mixtures of polyethylene glycol 400 and water of various polarities as expressed by their solubility parameters, δ_1.

It is postulated that the more alike are the delta values of the drug δ_2 and the solvent mixture δ_1 the greater would be the attraction of solvent and drug and the poorer the release of the drug for absorption. Conversely, when δ_1 and δ_2 are quite different and also when the solubility parameters of the drug δ_2 and the intestinal mucosa δ_o are similar, the drug is readily released from the solvent for bioabsorption.

A partition parameter K_p is obtained in the rat gut experiment from drug absorption k_1 and desorption k_2 rate constants, in which $K_p = k_1/k_2$. The experimental data for this problem are found in the table:

Data for *Problem 13–16*

% PGE 400 in water	Solvent delta value δ_1(cal/cm³)$^{1/2}$	$(\delta_1-\delta_2)$ $(\delta_2 = 14)$	k_1 min⁻¹	k_2 min⁻¹	$K_p = k_1/k_2$	$\ln K_p$
90	11.8	−2.2	0.041	0.028	1.464	0.381
80	13.1	−0.9	0.040	0.039	1.026	0.026
75	13.7	−0.3	0.054	0.083	0.651	−0.429
70	14.4	0.4	0.048	0.075	0.640	−0.446
65	15.0	1.0	0.036	0.064	0.0563	−0.574
60	15.7	1.7	0.037	0.036	1.028	0.028

(a) Plot $\ln K_p$ versus $(\delta_1 - \delta_2)$ and note from the curve obtained how the partition parameter varies with the delta value difference $(\delta_1 - \delta_2)$.

(b) Regress $\ln K_p$ against $(\delta_1 - \delta_2)$ using a parabolic (quadratic) or better, a cubic least-squares regression procedure. Plot a sufficient number of points, obtained from either the quadratic or the cubic equation, on the graph prepared for (a). This statistical regression analysis should give a smooth line approximating the rough angular plot obtained from drawing straight lines joining the experimental points in (a).

(c) Calculate a theoretical partition parameter (ln K_p) using the empirical equation suggested by Davis[82]:

$$\ln K_p \approx \frac{V_2 \, \phi_1^2}{RT} [(\delta_1 - \delta_2)^2 - (\delta_0 - \delta_2)^2] \qquad (13-120)$$

where V_2, the molar volume of theophylline, is 124 cm³/mole and δ_0 is the solubility parameter of the rat gut membrane, 12.6 (cal/cm³)$^{1/2}$ as determined in the work of Adjei et al.[83], R is the gas constant, and T the absolute temperature (37° C or 310° K). The volume fraction (p. 224), ϕ_1, of the solvent mixture is approximately unity in this problem and may be disregarded in equation (13–120). Are the experimental ln K_p values fit better with the ln K_p obtained from solving equation (13–120) or by the ln K_p from the quadratic or cubic regression equation? Observe the points on the graph or the data in your summary table (see below) to answer this part.

Partial Answer: (b) The squared correlation coefficient r^2 had a value of only 0.784 when carrying out parabolic (quadratic) regression, so the quadratic equation was dropped from further consideration. The cubic equation is

$$\ln K_p = -0.4541 - 0.3689 \, x + 0.2166 \, x^2 + 0.0960 \, x^3 \quad (13-121)$$

and has a satisfactory r^2 of 0.957. The term x in the equation stands for $(\delta_1 - \delta_2)$. (c) The results of calculating ln K_p from equation (13–120) are shown in the following summary table, together with ln K_p (experimental) and ln K_p calculated by carrying out cubic regression (equation 13–121).

Answers for *Problem 13–16*

% PGE 400 in water	Solvent δ_1(cal/cm³)$^{1/2}$	$(\delta_1-\delta_2)$	ln K_p (exp.)	ln K_p (cubic eq.) (13–121)	ln K_p (Eq. (13–120))
90	11.8	−2.2	0.381	0.384	0.579
80	13.1	−0.9	0.026	0.017	−0.231
75	13.7	−0.3	−0.429	−0.327	−0.376
70	14.4	0.4	−0.446	−0.561	−0.362
65	15.0	1.0	−0.574	−0.510	−0.193
60	15.7	1.7	0.028	0.017	0.187

It is seen in the summary table, column 5, that the ln K_p values obtained by cubic regression correspond satisfactorily to the ln K_p (experimental) and the cubic equation, (13–121), can be used to calculate ln K_p and therefore K_p.

The calculated ln K_p values from equation (13–120) (column 6 in the summary table) differ from the experimental ln K_p values, but the principle remains that the largest $(\delta_1 - \delta_2)$, i.e., the largest differences between δ_1 and δ_2, correspond to the greatest ln K_p (experimental) and through the expression $K_p = k_1/k_2$ to the largest absorption rate constants. Conversely, the smallest ln K_p (equation (13–120)) occurs at δ_1 of 13.7 to 14.4 in which region is found the drug's delta value, namely 14.0. Here the solubility parameter of the mixed solvent, PGE 400–water, is sufficiently close to that of the drug, theophylline, to interact with it and hinder the bioabsorption of the drug.

13–17. (a) As a continuation of work on transcorneal permeation of pilocarpine (see *Example 13–14*, p. 346), you are asked to plot the experimentally determined corneal membrane permeability P versus pH (Table 13–5, p. 346) on ordinary rectangular graph paper.

(b) Calculate P(theoretical) (see *Example 13–14*, equation (13–98)) using the values $P_B = 9.733 \times 10^{-6}$ cm/sec and $P_{BH^+} = 4.836 \times 10^{-6}$ cm/sec. The nonionized fraction f_B of pilocarpine at each pH value is calculated from equation (13–96), page 345. Plot P(theoret-

ical) versus pH on the graph prepared under (a). Note that the pH at the inflection point of the sigmoidal line is equal roughly to $pK_a = 6.67$ for the conjugate acid of pilocarpine at 34° C.

(c) Does this sigmoidal curve suggest any relationship to the titration curve of a weak acid, Figure 8–1, page 175, where, at half neutralization, pH = pK_a?

Partial Answer: (b) at pH 4.67, P(theoretical) = 4.885 × 10^{-6} cm/sec, and at pH 6.67, P(theoretical) = 7.285 × 10^{-6} cm/sec. (c) The Henderson–Hasselbalch equation is used on page 176 to arrive at the relationship pH = pK_a at the half neutralization point, and the Henderson–Hasselbalch equation is also used on page 342 to obtain an equation for the percent ionization of a weak acid at various pH values. These remarks should assist you in arriving at your answer.

13–18. The steady-state penetration of progesterone and its hydroxyl derivatives across the intact skin was found to be related to the solubility of the drug in the stratum corneum. The solubility in the stratum corneum and the rate of permeation decrease as the hydrophilicity of the progesterone derivatives increases.[84] The data are found in the following table for the progesterone derivatives numbered 1 through 7:

Data for *Problem 13–18*

Drug no.	1	2	3	4	5	6	7
Solubility (mg/mL)	1.09	2.46	7.97	2.82	12.5	32.4	47.7
Permeability rate (µg/(cm² hr))	0.15	0.31	0.97	0.29	0.57	4.73	2.37

(a) Plot the permeability rates dQ/dt, (µg/(cm² hr)), on the vertical axis against the solubility of the progesterone derivatives on the horizontal axis of three-cycle log–log paper. One may postulate a linear relationship between the steady-state rates of permeation of progesterone and its solubility in the stratum corneum. However, it is found that a linear relationship is obtained only when the data are plotted on a log–log graph, which suggests that the true relationship is a power curve. Let permeability rate dQ/dt be y and the solubility in the stratum corneum be x, and write the power curve relationship:

$$y = ax^b \qquad (13-122)$$

in which a and b are arbitrary constants.

(b) Use a hand calculator or a personal computer to obtain the values of a and b using the data given above.

(c) Now assume a relationship between y and x in the linear form

$$y = a'x + b' \qquad (13-123)$$

and compute a' and b'. Which equation, (13–122) or (13–123), better fits the data?

(d) Why did a log–log fit of the data suggest using the power equation $y = ax^b$?

(e) Do you believe it would be possible to extrapolate results such as these to the transdermal absorption of progesterone derivatives from various ointment bases into intact and damaged or diseased human skin? What factors would need to be taken into consideration?

Partial Answers: (b) $y = 0.111 \, x^{1.005}$; (c) $y = 0.0724 \, x + 0.2355$

13–19. The percutaneous absorption of chloramphenicol through mouse skin was investigated at various temperatures. Permeability coefficients were recorded together with temperatures as follows:

Data for *Problem 13–19*

Temperature, °C	25	31	37	45
P (cm/min) × 10^4	1.12	1.87	3.01	6.20

Plot the Arrhenius curve and calculate the energy of activation for permeation. Compare your results with those of Aguiar and Weiner,[85] who, in a similar study, found E_a to be 15,000 cal/mole.

Answer: 15,945 cal/mole, or 16 kcal/mole. The answer varies depending on the number of significant figures retained.

13-20. Liron and Cohen[86]* studied the percutaneous absorption of the straight chain fatty acid, propionic acid, through porcine skin. They found that the permeability coefficient, $P = KD/h$ (equation (13–11), p. 327) increased with elevation of the temperature as shown in the table:

Data for *Problem 13–20*

Temperature, °C	15	25	30	37	50
$P \times 10^3$ cm/min	0.81	1.25	1.64	3.00	6.72

Prepare an Arrhenius-like plot of $\ln P$ against reciprocal temperature $(1/T, °K^{-1})$. Obtain the activation energy, E_p, in kcal/mole, and P_o, which is proportional to the number of molecules entering the film and to the probability that these molecules have sufficient energy to engage in the diffusion process. P_o is comparable to the frequency factor A in the field of kinetics (equation (12–72), p. 295).

Answer: $E_p = 11.38$ kcal/mole; $\ln P_o = 12.62$; $P_o = 3.0 \times 10^5$

13-21. Liron and Cohen[86] applied Fick's law of diffusion to the percutaneous absorption of a drug. The delivery of valeric (pentanoic) acid from n-heptane solution (1 molar) into excised porcine skin was studied in a diffusion cell having a 1 cm² cross-sectional area. The following results were obtained:

Data for *Problem 13–21*

Time (hr)	0	0.5	1	2	3	4	5	6
Q, μmole/cm²	0	1.4	7.6	19.1	34.1	49.1	64.1	79.1

(a) Plot Q, the cumulative penetrated mass per unit area of valeric acid, against time.

(b) Find the flux at the steady state, J_s, from the slope of the linear segment of the cumulative penetrant mass per unit area Q versus time, i.e., for time 2 through 6 hours.

(c) Use J_s and the concentration of valeric acid in the donor phase, C_d, 1000 μmole/cm³, to calculate the permeability coefficient, P.

(d) Find the lag time t_L from the penetration curve by extrapolating the linear segment to zero penetration per unit cross-section.

(e) Find the diffusion coefficient D from t_L and thickness h of the skin barrier (stratum corneum); $h = 15$ micrometers (μm).

(f) From the results obtained, calculate the partition coefficient, using equation (13–11), page 327 of this chapter.

(g) Calculate the partition coefficient K using the equation of Davis.[82]

$$\ln K_p \approx \frac{V_2 \, \phi_1^2}{RT}[(\delta_1 - \delta_2)^2 - (\delta_0 - \delta_2)^2 + (V_d/V_m)] \quad (13-124)$$

in which V_2 is the molar volume of the solute, R and T have their usual meaning, δ_1 and δ_2 are the solubility parameters for the solute (drug) and solvent, respectively, V_d is the volume of the donor phase, equal to 300 μL, and V_m is the volume of the skin barrier, equal to 1 cm² × 0.015 cm = 0.015 cm³ = 15 μL. In *Problem 13–16*, the approximate equation (13–120) was used, disregarding the final term, $\ln (V_d/V_m)$; in the present case it is sufficiently important and cannot be eliminated.

---

*These authors are thanked for providing *Problems 13–20* and *13–21*.

Partial Answers: **(b)** $J_s = 15$ μmole/(cm² hr); **(c)** $P = 0.25 \times 10^{-3}$ cm/min; **(d)** $t_L = 40$ min; **(e)** from equation (13–14a), p. 328, $D = 1.6 \times 10^{-10}$ cm² sec⁻¹; **(f)** $K = 39.1$; **(g)** $K = 43.4$

13-22. Hydrocortisone was released from a silicone matrix implanted in the vaginal tract of a rabbit (see pp. 350–351). Calculate the amount of hydrocortisone (mg) released from the vaginal implant in 2.5, 5, 10, 15, 20, 25, 30, and 40 days. Plot the amount released, m (mg), versus time in days. The following data are taken from the work of Ho et al.[87] The solubility of the drug in the polymer matrix, C_s, was 0.014 mg/cm³; the diffusion coefficient in the matrix, D_e, was 4.5×10^{-7} cm²/sec; the partition coefficient for silicone/water, K_s, was 0.05; the permeability coefficient of the rabbit vaginal membrane, P_m, was 5.8×10^{-5} cm/sec; P_{aq} was 7×10^{-4} cm/sec; the loading concentration (initial amount of drug per unit volume of plastic cylinder), A, was 100 mg/cm³; the length h of the silicone cylinder was 6.0 cm, and its radius, a_o, was 1.1 cm.

Partial Answer: 36.63 mg released in 15 days

13-23. The rate at which a solute diffuses out of a single open-boundary cell, Figure 13–30, at time t is equal to the concentration gradient $\partial u/\partial x$ at the open boundary multiplied by $(D \times A)$, the diffusion coefficient of the solute multiplied by the area A of the cell.

The rate R of solute escape is given by

$$R \text{ (g/sec)} = \frac{\partial u}{\partial x}(D \cdot A)$$

$$= \frac{2 \, u_o}{h}\left[exp\left(-\frac{\pi^2 Dt}{4h^2}\right) + exp\left(-\frac{9\pi^2 Dt}{4h^2}\right) + \cdots\right](D \cdot A) \quad (13-125)$$

The area A of the cell is 6.78 cm², the cell height h is 3.92 cm, the initial concentration u_o of solute in aqueous solution at 25° C is 0.0628 g/cm³, the solute's diffusion coefficient in this medium is $D = 9.81 \times 10^{-6}$ cm²/sec, and the time of diffusion is $t = 8560$ sec (2.38 hr). Calculate the rate of escape from the cell.

Answer: $R = 3.99 \times 10^{-6}$ g/sec $= 2.39 \times 10^{-4}$ g/min

13-24. A new drug is placed in a Graham closed boundary diffusion cell (see Fig. 13–29) to determine the drug's diffusion coefficient, D. The initial concentration of the drug u_o is 0.0273 g/cm³ in water at 25° C. The total height of the cell is $H = 3.86$ cm and the height of the drug solution in the cell is $h = 1.93$ cm. A sample is taken at a depth of $x = H/6$ at time $t = 10,523$ sec (2.923 hr) and analyzed for the drug; its concentration u is found to be 0.0173 g/cm³. Rearrange equation (13–113) so as to calculate D, the drug's diffusion coefficient. (See *Example 13–16*.)

Answer: $D = 12.4 \times 10^{-5}$ cm²/sec

13-25. Diffusion through the skin may be considered as a multilayer diffusion where the main layers are the stratum corneum, epidermis, and dermis. The stratum corneum is the major diffusional barrier, and epidermis may be significantly less permeable than dermis. Yu et al.[88] performed experiments of permeation of a prodrug of vidarabine to study the diffusional characteristics of the different layers of the skin. Using dermis membranes of mice (average thickness, 350 μm), the lag time t_L for the permeation of the drug was 152.3 sec.

In a second experiment, the stratum corneum was removed with Scotch tape. The permeability coefficient of the stripped skin (P^{ss}) (without stratum corneum) was determined to be 3.74×10^{-6} cm/sec. Finally, the permeability coefficient of the whole skin (stratum corneum, epidermis, and dermis) was 2.98×10^{-8} cm/sec.

(a) Compute the permeability coefficient of the dermis. You will need equation (13–14b), page 328, for this part.

(b) Compute the permeability coefficients of the stratum corneum and the dermis. *Hint:* Use equation (13–51b), page 337, as a model.

Answers: **(a)** P (dermis) $= 3.8 \times 10^{-5}$ cm/sec; **(b)** P (stratum corneum) $= 3.0 \times 10^{-8}$ cm/sec; P (epidermis) $= 4.2 \times 10^{-6}$ cm/sec

14
Interfacial Phenomena

Liquid Interfaces
Adsorption at Liquid Interfaces
Adsorption at Solid Interfaces

Applications of Surface Active Agents
Electric Properties of Interfaces

When phases exist together, the boundary between two of them is termed an *interface*. The properties of the molecules forming the interface are often sufficiently different from those in the bulk of each phase that they are referred to as forming an "interfacial phase." Although this terminology is not correct in terms of the phase rule, it is a useful concept. For example, molecules at the liquid–gas interface may exist in a two-dimensional gaseous, liquid, or solid state depending on the prevailing conditions of temperature and pressure in the interface. Their phase-like behavior is therefore apparent.

Several types of interface can exist, depending on whether the two adjacent phases are in the solid, liquid, or gaseous state (Table 14–1). For convenience, we shall divide these various combinations into two groups, namely *liquid interfaces* and *solid interfaces*. In the former group, the association of a liquid phase with a gaseous or another liquid phase will be discussed. The section on solid interfaces will deal with systems containing solid–gas and solid–liquid interfaces. While solid–solid interfaces have practical significance in pharmacy (for example, the adhesion between granules, the preparation of layered tablets, and the flow of particles), little information is available to quantify these interactions. This is due, at least in part, to the fact that the surface region of materials in the solid

state is quiescent, in sharp contrast to the turbulence that exists at the surfaces of liquids and gases. Accordingly, solid–solid systems will not be discussed here. A final section will outline the electric properties of interfaces.

The term *surface* is customarily used when referring to either a gas–solid or a gas–liquid interface. Although this terminology will be used in the present chapter, the reader should appreciate that every surface is an interface. Thus, a table top forms a gas–solid interface with the atmosphere above it, and the surface of a rain drop constitutes a gas–liquid interface.

The symbols for the various interfacial tensions are shown in the second column of Table 14–1, where the subscript L stands for liquid, V for vapor or gas, and S for solid. Surface and interfacial tensions are defined on p. 363.

Since every particle of matter, be it cell, bacterium, colloid, granule, or man, possesses an interface at the boundary of its surroundings, the importance of the present topic is self-evident. Interfacial phenomena in pharmacy and medicine are significant factors that affect absorption of drugs onto solid adjuncts in dosage forms, penetration of molecules through biologic membranes, emulsion formation and stability, and the dispersion of insoluble particles in liquid media to form suspensions. The interfacial properties of a surface-

TABLE 14–1. *Classification of Interfaces*

Phase	Interfacial Tension	Types and Examples of Interfaces
Gas–gas	—	No interface possible
Gas–liquid	γ_{LV}	Liquid surface, body of water exposed to atmosphere
Gas–solid	γ_{SV}	Solid surface, table top
Liquid–liquid	γ_{LL}	Liquid–liquid interface, emulsion
Liquid–solid	γ_{LS}	Liquid–solid interface, suspension
Solid–solid	γ_{SS}	Solid–solid interface, powder particles in contact

active agent found lining the alveoli of the lung are responsible for the efficient operation of this organ.[1] Felmeister[2] and Seeman[3] reviewed the relationship between surface properties of drugs and their biologic activity.

LIQUID INTERFACES

Surface and Interfacial Tensions. In the liquid state, the cohesive forces between adjacent molecules are well developed. Molecules in the bulk of the liquid are surrounded in all directions by other molecules for which they have an equal attraction, as shown in Figure 14–1. On the other hand, molecules at the surface (i.e., at the liquid–air interface) can only develop attractive cohesive forces with other liquid molecules that are situated below and adjacent to them. They can develop adhesive forces of attraction with the molecules constituting the other phase involved in the interface, although, in the case of the liquid–gas interface, this adhesive force of attraction is small. The net effect is that the molecules at the surface of the liquid experience an inward force towards the bulk, as shown in Figure 14–1. Such a force pulls the molecules of the interface together and, as a result, contracts the surface, resulting in a *surface tension*. Liquid droplets tend to assume a spherical shape, since a sphere has the smallest surface area per unit volume.

This "tension" in the surface is the force per unit length that must be applied *parallel* to the surface so as to counterbalance the net inward pull. This force, the surface tension, has the units of dyne/cm in the cgs system. It is similar to the situation that exists when an object dangling over the edge of a cliff on a length of rope is pulled upward by a man holding the rope and walking away from the edge of the top of the cliff. This analogy to surface tension is sketched in Figure 14–2.

Interfacial tension is the force per unit length existing at the interface between two immiscible liquid phases and, like surface tension, has the units of dyne/cm. Although in the general sense all tensions may be referred to as *interfacial tensions*, this term is most often used for the attractive force between immiscible liquids. Later we will use the term *interfacial tension* for the force between two liquids, γ_{LL}, two solids, γ_{SS}, and for a liquid–solid interface, γ_{LS}. The term *surface tension* is reserved for liquid–vapor, γ_{LV}, and solid–vapor, γ_{SV}, tensions. These are often written simply as γ_L and γ_S. Ordinarily, interfacial tensions are less than surface tensions because the adhesive forces between two liquid phases forming an interface are greater than when a liquid and a gas phase exist together. It follows that if two liquids are completely miscible, no interfacial tension exists between them. Some representatives of surface and interfacial tensions are listed in Table 14–2.

That surface tension is a force per unit length may also be illustrated by means of a three-sided wire frame across which a movable bar is placed (Fig. 14–3). A soap film is formed over the area ABCD and can be stretched by applying a force *f* (such as a hanging mass) to the movable bar, length *L*, which acts against the surface tension of the soap film. When the mass is removed, the film will contract owing to its surface

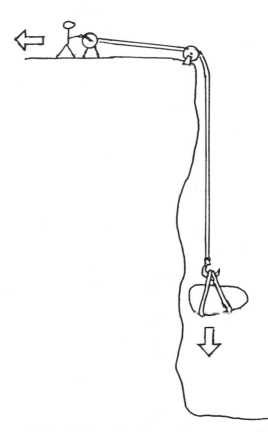

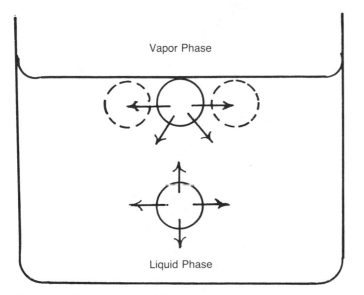

Fig. 14–1. Representation of the unequal attractive forces acting on molecules at the surface of a liquid, as compared with molecular forces in the bulk of the liquid.

Fig. 14–2. Visualization of surface tension as a person lifting a rock up the side of a cliff by pulling the rope in a horizontal direction.

TABLE 14–2. *Surface Tension and Interfacial Tension (Against Water) at 20° C**

Substance	Surface Tension (dyne/cm)	Substance	Interfacial Tension Against Water (dyne/cm)
Water	72.8	Mercury	375
Glycerin	63.4	n-Hexane	51.1
Oleic acid	32.5	Benzene	35.0
Benzene	28.9	Chloroform	32.8
Chloroform	27.1	Oleic acid	15.6
Carbon tetrachloride	26.7	n-Octyl alcohol	8.52
Castor oil	39.0	Caprylic acid	8.22
Olive oil	35.8	Olive oil	22.9
Cottonseed oil	35.4	Ethyl ether	10.7
Liquid petrolatum	33.1		

*From P. Becher, *Emulsions: Theory and Practice,* 2nd Edition, Reinhold, New York, 1962, and other sources.

tension. The surface tension, γ, of the solution forming the film is then a function of the force that must be applied to break the film over the length of the movable bar in contact with the film. Since the soap film has two liquid–gas interfaces (one above and one below the plane of the paper), the total length of contact is in fact equal to twice the length of the bar.

Thus

$$\gamma = f_b/2L \qquad (14\text{–}1)$$

in which f_b is the force required to break the film and L is the length of the movable bar.

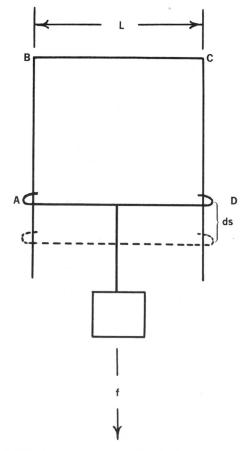

Fig. 14–3. Wireframe apparatus used to demonstrate the principle of surface tension.

Example 14–1. If the length of the bar L is 5 cm and the mass required to break a soap film is 0.50 g, what is the surface tension of the soap solution?

Recall that the downward force is equal to the mass multiplied by the acceleration due to gravity. Then

$$\gamma = \frac{0.50 \text{ g} \times 981 \text{ cm/sec}^2}{10 \text{ cm}} = 49 \text{ dynes/cm}$$

Surface Free Energy. To evaluate the work done (energy) in increasing the surface area, equation (14–1) may be written as $\gamma \times 2L = f$. When the bar is at a position AD in Figure 14–3 and a mass is added to extend the surface by a distance ds, the work dW (force multiplied by distance) is

$$dW = f \times ds = \gamma \times 2L \times ds$$

and, since $2L \times ds$ is equal to the increase in surface area dA produced by extending the soap film,

$$dW = \gamma \, dA$$

For a finite change,

$$W = \gamma \, \Delta A \qquad (14\text{–}2)$$

in which W is the work done or *surface free energy* increase expressed in ergs, γ is the surface tension in dynes/cm, and ΔA is the increase in area in cm^2. Any form of energy can be divided into an intensity factor and a capacity factor (p. 53). Surface tension is the intensity factor, and a change in area is the capacity factor of surface free energy. Surface tension may thus be defined as the *surface free energy change per unit area increase* in conformity with equation (14–2).

Example 14–2. What is the work required in *Example 14–1* to pull the wire down 1 cm as shown in Figure 14–3?

Since the area is increased by 10 cm^2, the work done is given by the equation

$$W = 49 \text{ dynes/cm} \times 10 \text{ cm}^2 = 490 \text{ ergs}$$

Repeat the calculations using SI units.

$$1 \, dyne = 10^{-5} \text{ N, or } 49 \text{ dyne} = 49 \times 10^{-5} \text{ N}$$
$$49 \text{ dyne/cm} = 49 \times 10^{-3} \text{ N/m} = 49 \times 10^{-3} \text{ Nm/m}^2$$

Also 1 Nm = 1 J (Table 1–3, p 3), and 1 J = 10^7 erg. Therefore, $W = 49 \times 10^{-3}$ Nm/m$^2 \times 10^{-3}$ m$^2 = 490 \times 10^{-7}$ J = 490 erg.

Equation 14–2 defines surface tension as the work per unit area required to produce a new surface. From thermodynamics, at T and P constant, the surface tension can also be viewed as the increment in Gibbs free energy per unit area (see Hiemenz,[4] pp. 293–296). Thus, equation (14–2) can be written as

$$\gamma = \left(\frac{\partial G}{\partial A}\right)_{T,P} \qquad (14-3)$$

This definition has the advantage that the path-dependent variable W is replaced by a thermodynamic function G, which is independent of the path. Many of the general relationships that apply to G also serve for γ. This fact enables us to compute the enthalpy and entropy of a surface:

$$G^s = \gamma = H^s - TS^s \qquad (14-4)$$

and

$$\left(\frac{\partial G^s}{\partial T}\right)_p = \left(\frac{\partial \gamma}{\partial T}\right)_p = -S^s \qquad (14-5)$$

Combining equations (14–4) and (14–5),

$$\gamma = H^s + T\left(\frac{\partial \gamma}{\partial T}\right)_p \qquad (14-6)$$

Thus from a plot of surface tension against absolute temperature, one may obtain the slope of the line $(\partial \gamma / \partial T)$ and thus has $-S^s$ from equation (14–5). If H^s does not change appreciably over the temperature range considered, the intercept gives the H^s value. It should be noted that the units on S^s and H^s are given in two dimensions, ergs cm^{-2} deg^{-1} for S^s and ergs cm^{-2} for H^s in the cgs system. In the SI system S^s is given in units of joule m^{-2}deg^{-1} and H^s in units of joule m^{-2}, where m stands for meters.

Example 14–3. The surface tension of methanol in water (10% by volume) at 20, 30, and 50° C (293.15, 303.15, and 323.15° K) is 59.04, 57.27, and 55.01 dyne/cm (or erg/cm^2) (see *CRC Handbook of Chemistry and Physics*, 63rd Edition, p. F-35 for the data). Compute S^s and H^s over this temperature range.

Using linear regression of γ versus T according to equation (14–6),

the slope is found to be -0.131 erg cm^{-2}deg$^{-1} = \left(\frac{\partial \gamma}{\partial T}\right)_p = -S^s$; hence,

$S^s = 0.131$ and the intercept is 97.34 erg cm$^{-2} = H^s$. The equation is therefore

$$G^s = \gamma = 97.34 + 0.131\, T$$

If we compute H^s at each temperature from equation (14–6) and if S^s remains constant at -0.131:

At 20° C, $H^s = 59.04 + (0.131 \times 293.15) = 97.44$ erg cm^{-2}

At 30° C, $H^s = 57.27 + (0.131 \times 303.15) = 96.98$ erg cm^{-2}

At 50° C, $H^s = 55.01 + (0.131 \times 323.15) = 97.34$ erg cm^{-2}

H^s appears to be practically constant, very similar to the intercept from the regression equation, $H^s = 97.34$ erg cm$^{-2} = 97.34$ mJ/m^{-2}. Note that the numerical value of surface tension in the cgs system, like that for H^s in the cgs system, is the same as that in the SI system when the units mJ are used. Thus one can convert surface tension readily from cgs to SI units.[4] For example, if the surface tension of methanol in water (10% by volume) at 20° C is 59.04 erg/cm^2 in the cgs system, we can write without carrying out the conversion calculation that γ for the methanol-in-water mixture at 20° C is 59.04 mJ/m^2 in SI units.

Pressure Differences Across Curved Interfaces. Another way of expressing surface tension is in terms of the pressure difference that exists across a curved interface. Consider a soap bubble (Fig. 14–4) having a radius r. The total surface free energy W is equal to $4\pi r^2 \gamma$, where $4\pi r^2$ is the area of the spherical bubble. (See the formulas, bottom, inside front cover.) Suppose that the bubble is caused to shrink so that its radius decreases by dr. The final surface free energy is now

$$W = 4\pi\gamma(r - dr)^2 \qquad (14-7)$$

$$W = 4\pi\gamma r^2 - 8\pi\gamma r\, dr + 4\pi\gamma(dr)^2 \qquad (14-8)$$

Since dr is small compared to r, the term containing $(dr)^2$ in equation (14–8) may be disregarded.

The *change* in surface free energy is therefore $-8\pi\gamma r\, dr$, where the minus sign appears because the surface area has shrunk. Opposing this change is an equal and opposite energy term that depends on the pressure difference, ΔP, across the wall of the bubble. Since pressure is a force per unit area, or force = pressure × area, the work change brought about by a decrease in radius dr is

$$W = \Delta P \times 4\pi r^2 \times -dr \qquad (14-9)$$

At equilibrium, this must equal the change in surface free energy, and so

$$-8\pi\gamma r dr = -4\Delta P\pi r^2 dr \qquad (14-10)$$

or

$$\Delta P = 2\gamma/r \qquad (14-11)$$

Therefore, as the radius of a bubble decreases, the pressure of the air inside increases relative to that outside. Equation (14–11) is a simplification of the Young–Laplace equation and can be used to explain capillary rise, as seen in the following section.

Measurement of Surface and Interfacial Tensions. Of the several methods that exist for obtaining surface and interfacial tensions, only the *capillary rise* and the *DuNoüy ring* methods will be described here. For details of the other methods, such as drop weight,

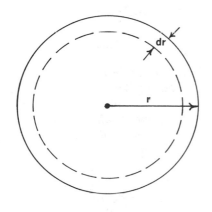

Fig. 14–4. Schematic representation of pressure difference across the curved surface of a soap bubble.

bubble pressure, pendent drop, sessile drop, and Wilhelmy plate, refer to the treatises by Adamson,[5] Harkins and Alexander,[6] Drost-Hansen,[7] and Hiemenz.[4] It is worth noting, however, that the choice of a particular method often depends on whether surface or interfacial tension is to be determined, the accuracy and convenience desired, the size of sample available, and whether or not the effect of time on surface tension is to be studied. In reality, there is no one best method for all systems.

The surface tensions of most liquids decrease almost linearly with an increase in temperature, that is, with an increase in the kinetic energy of the molecules. In the region of its critical temperature, the surface tension of a liquid becomes zero. The surface tension of water at 0° C is 75.6, at 20° C it is 72.8, and at 75° C it is 63.5 dynes/cm. It is therefore necessary to control the temperature of the system when carrying out surface and interfacial tension determinations.

Capillary Rise Method. When a capillary tube is placed in a liquid contained in a beaker, the liquid generally rises up the tube a certain distance. This is because when the force of adhesion between the liquid molecules and the capillary wall is greater than the cohesion between the liquid molecules, the liquid is said to *wet* the capillary wall, spreading over it, and rising in the tube (spreading is discussed in some detail on page 369). By measuring this rise in a capillary, it is possible to determine the surface tension of the liquid. It is not possible, however, to obtain interfacial tensions using the capillary rise method.

Consider a capillary tube of inside radius r immersed in a liquid that wets its surface, as seen in Figure 14–5a. The liquid continues to rise in the tube due to the surface tension, until the upward movement is just balanced by the downward force of gravity due to the weight of the liquid.

The upward vertical component of the force resulting from the surface tension of the liquid at any point on the circumference is given by

$$a = \gamma \cos \theta$$

as seen in the enlarged sketch (Fig. 14–5b). The total upward force around the inside circumference of the tube is

$$2\pi r \gamma \cos \theta$$

in which θ is the *contact angle* between the surface of the liquid and the capillary wall, and $2\pi r$ is the inside circumference of the capillary. For water and other commonly used liquids, the angle θ is insignificant, that is, the liquid wets the capillary wall so that $\cos \theta$ is taken as unity for practical purposes (see left side of Fig. 14–5b).

The counteracting force of gravity (mass × acceleration) is given by the product of the cross-sectional area πr^2, the height h of the liquid column to the lowest point

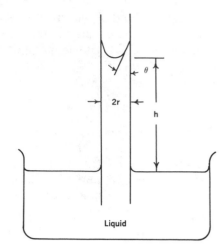

Fig. 14–5a. Measuring surface tension by means of the capillary rise principle.

of the meniscus, the difference in the density of the liquid ρ and its vapor ρ_0, and the acceleration of gravity: $\pi r^2 h(\rho - \rho_0)g + w$. The last term w is added to account for the weight of liquid above h in the meniscus. When the liquid has risen to its maximum height, which may be read from the calibrations on the capillary tube, the opposing forces are in equilibrium, and accordingly the surface tension can be calculated. The density of the vapor, the contact angle, and w can usually be disregarded; hence,

$$2\pi r \gamma = \pi r^2 h \rho g$$

and finally

$$\gamma = \tfrac{1}{2} r h \rho g \qquad (14–12)$$

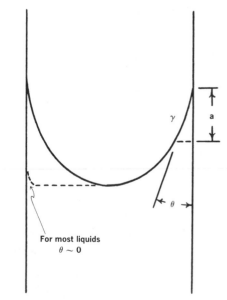

Fig. 14–5b. Enlarged view of the force components and contact angle at the meniscus of a liquid. For many liquids the contact angle θ (exaggerated in figure) is nearly zero as shown on the left-hand side of the diagram.

Example 14–4. A sample of chloroform rose to a height of 3.67 cm at 20° C in a capillary tube having an inside radius of 0.01 cm. What is the surface tension of chloroform at this temperature? The density of chloroform is 1.476 g/cm³.

$$\gamma = \tfrac{1}{2} \times 0.01 \text{ cm} \times 3.67 \text{ cm} \times 1.476 \text{ g/cm}^3 \times 981 \text{ cm/sec}^2$$

$$\gamma = 26.6 \text{ g cm(sec}^2\text{cm)} = 26.6 \text{ dynes/cm}$$

Capillary rise may also be explained as being due to the pressure difference across the curved meniscus of the liquid in the capillary. We have already seen in equation (14–11) that the pressure on the concave side of a curved surface is greater than that on the convex side. This means that the pressure in the liquid immediately below the meniscus will be less than that outside the tube at the same height. As a result, the liquid will move up the capillary until the hydrostatic head produced equals the pressure drop across the curved meniscus. Using the same symbols as before and neglecting contact angles,

$$\Delta P = 2\gamma/r = \rho g h \qquad (14\text{--}13)$$

in which $\rho g h$ is the hydrostatic head. Rearranging equation (14–13) gives

$$\gamma = r\rho g h/2$$

which is identical with equation (14–12) derived on the basis of adhesive forces versus cohesive forces.

The DuNoüy Ring Method. The *DuNoüy tensiometer*, illustrated in Figure 14–6, is widely used for measuring surface and interfacial tensions. The principle of the instrument depends on the fact that the force necessary to detach a platinum-iridium ring immersed at the surface or interface is proportional to the surface or interfacial tension. The force required to detach the ring in this manner is provided by a torsion wire and is recorded in dynes on a calibrated dial. The

surface tension is given by the formula (compare with equation [14–1])

$$\gamma = \frac{\text{dial reading in dynes}}{2 \times \text{ring circumference}} \times \text{correction factor, } \beta$$

$$(14\text{--}14)$$

In effect, the instrument measures the weight of liquid pulled out of the plane of the interface immediately before the ring becomes detached (Fig. 14–7). A correction factor is necessary in equation (14–14) because the simple theory does not take into account certain variables such as the radius of the ring, the radius of the wire used to form the ring, and the volume of liquid raised out of the surface. Errors as large as 25% may occur if the correction factor is not calculated and applied. The method of calculating the correction factor has been described by Harkins and Jordan[8] and, with care, a precision of about 0.25% can be obtained.

Example 14–5. The published surface tension of water at 18° C is 73.05 dyne/cm and the density ρ_1 of water at this temperature is 0.99860 g/cm³. The density ρ_2 of moist air—that is, air saturated with the vapor of the liquid, water, at 18° C—is 0.0012130. Therefore, $\rho_1 - \rho_2$, the density of water overlayed with air, is 0.99739 g/cm³. The dial reading in dynes or newtons on the tensiometer is equal to the mass M of the liquid lifted by the ring, multiplied by the gravity constant, 980.665 cm/sec²; that is,

$$\text{dial reading} = M \text{ (grams)} \times 980.665 \text{ cm/sec}^2$$

It is thus possible to obtain the mass M of liquid lifted with the ring, $M = 0.7866$ gram, before it breaks away from the water surface. The ring must be kept absolutely horizontal for accurate measurement. The volume V of water lifted above the free surface of water is calculated from the mass of water lifted and the density at 18° C, or

$$V = \frac{M}{\rho_1 - \rho_2} = \frac{0.7866}{0.99739} = 0.78866 \text{ cm}^3$$

The ring of the tensiometer has a radius R of 0.8078 cm, and $R^3 = 0.527122$ cm³. The radius r of the wire that forms the ring is 0.01877 cm. Two values, R^3/V and R/r, are needed to enter the tables of Harkins and Jordan[8] to obtain the correction factor, β, by interpolation.

An abbreviated table of R^3/V and R/r values needed to obtain β is given in Table 14–3. In this example $R^3/V = 0.52712/0.78866 = 0.66838$, and $R/r = 0.8078/0.01877 = 43.0368$. Introducing these

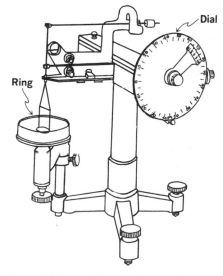

Fig. 14–6. Cenco DuNoüy tensiometer.

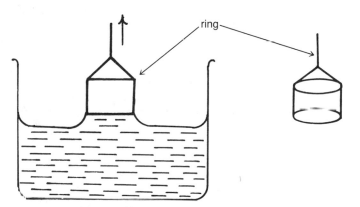

Fig. 14–7. Schematic of the tensiometer ring pulling a column of water above the surface before it breaks away.

TABLE 14–3. *Some Harkins and Jordan β Values**

R^3V $\downarrow$ $\rightarrow$ R/r	30	40	50	60
0.50	0.9402	0.9687	0.9876	0.9984
1.00	0.8734	0.9047	0.9290	0.9438
2.00	0.8098	0.8539	0.8798	0.9016
3.00	0.7716	0.8200	0.8520	0.8770
3.50	0.7542	0.8057	0.8404	0.8668

*From W. D. Harkins and H. F. Jordan, J. Am. Chem. Soc. **52**, 1751, 1930; H. L. Cupples, J. Phys. Chem. **51**, 1341, 1947.

values into Table VIII-C of Harkins and Jordan[8] and by interpolation, one obtains β = 0.9471 (18° C).

Finally, using equation (14–14), the surface tension for water at 18° C is obtained:

$$\gamma = \frac{M \times g}{4\pi R} \times \beta = \frac{(0.7866 \text{ g})(980.665 \text{ cm/sec}^2)}{4\pi(0.8078 \text{ cm})} \times 0.9471$$

$$= 71.97 \text{ dyne/cm or } 71.97 \text{ erg/cm}^2$$

Without the correction factor, β, γ is calculated here to be 75.99. The values of γ for water at 18° C are recorded in handbooks as approximately 73.05 dyne/cm. The error relative to the published value at 18° C is $\frac{73.05 - 71.97}{73.05} \times 100 = 1.48\%$.

The correction factor β may be calculated from an equation rather than obtaining it from tabulated values of R/r and R^3/V as done in *Example 14–4*. Zuidema and Waters[9] suggested an equation to calculate β, as discussed by Shaw:[10]

$$(\beta - a)^2 = \frac{4b}{\pi^2} \cdot \frac{1}{R^2} \cdot \frac{M \times g}{4\pi R \,(\rho_1 - \rho_2)} + c \quad (14–15)$$

Example 14–6. Use equation (14–15) to calculate β, the surface tension correction at 20° C where $a = 0.7250$, $b = 0.09075$ m^{-1}s^2 for all tensiometer rings, and $c = 0.04534 - 1.679°$ r/R. R is the radius of the ring in meters, r is the radius of the wire from which the ring is constructed, M is the mass in kg of the liquid lifted above the liquid surface as the ring breaks away from the surface, g is the acceleration due to gravity in meters · sec^{-2}, ρ_1 is the density of the liquid in kg meter^{-3}, and ρ_2 is the density of the air saturated with the liquid; that is, the upper phase of an interfacial system. With the following data, which must be expressed in SI units for use in equation (14–15), β is calculated and used in equation (14–14) to obtain the corrected surface tension. The terms of equation (14–15) in SI units are $R = 0.012185$ meter; $r = 0.0002008$ meter, $M = 0.0012196$ kg, $g = 9.80665$ ms^{-2}, $\rho_1 = 998.207$ kg/m^3, and $\rho_2 = 1.2047$ kg/m^3. Finally, $c = 0.04534 - 1.6790$ $r/R = 0.017671$.

Substituting into equation (15) we have

$$(\beta - a)^2 = \frac{4(0.09075 \text{ m}^{-1}\text{s}^2)}{9.869604} \cdot \frac{1}{0.00014847 \text{ m}^2} \cdot$$

$$\frac{(0.0012196 \text{ kg})(9.80665 \text{ ms}^{-2})}{4(3.14159)(0.012185 \text{ m})(998.207 - 1.2047 \text{ kg/m}^3)}$$

$$+ 0.04534 - (1.6790)(0.0002008 \text{ m})/0.012185 \text{ m}$$

$$(\beta - a)^2 = 0.0194077 + 0.0176713 = 0.0370790$$

$$\beta - 0.7250 = (0.0370790)^{1/2};$$

$$\beta = 0.7250 + 0.192559 = 0.918 \text{ (dimensionless) at } 20° \text{ C}$$

The literature value of γ for water at 20° C is 72.8 dyne/cm (or erg/cm^2) in cgs units. Using the uncorrected equation $\gamma = M \times g/(4\pi R)$ and in SI units, we obtain for water at 20° C

$$\gamma = \frac{0.0012196 \text{ kg} \times 9.80665 \text{ ms}^{-2}}{4 \times \pi \times 0.012185 \text{ m}} = 0.078109 \text{ kg s}^{-2}. \text{ Multiplying}$$

numerator and denominator by meter^2 yields the result 0.07811 Jm^{-2}, and expressing the value in mJ/m^2 we have 78.11 mJ/m^2. This is a useful way to express surface tension in SI units, for the value 78.11 is numerically the same as that in the cgs system; namely, 78.11 erg/cm^2 (see *Example 14–3*). To correct the value, $\gamma = M \times g/(4\pi R)$, expressed either in cgs or SI units, we multiply by the Harkins and Jordan or the Zuidema and Waters value for β at a given liquid density and temperature, M value, and ring dimensions.

For the particular case in this example,

$$\gamma = \frac{M \times g}{4\pi R} \times \beta = 78.11 \text{ erg/cm}^2 \text{ (or mJ/m}^2) \times 0.918$$

$$= 71.7 \text{ erg/cm}^2$$

The error in the Zuidema and Waters value of 71.7 mJ/m^2 relative to the literature value, 72.8 mJ/m^2 at 20° C, is $\frac{72.8 - 71.7}{72.8} \times 100 = 1.51\%$.

Spreading Coefficient. When a substance such as oleic acid is placed on the surface of water, it will spread as a film if the force of adhesion between the oleic acid molecules and the water molecules is greater than the cohesive forces between the oleic acid molecules themselves. The term *film* used here applies to a *duplex film*, as opposed to a monomolecular film. Duplex films are sufficiently thick (100 Å or more) so that the surface (boundary between oleic acid and air) and interface (boundary between water and oleic acid) are independent of one another.

The *work of adhesion*, which is the energy required to break the attraction between the unlike molecules, is obtained by reference to Figure 14–8. Here in (a) we see a hypothetical cylinder (cross-section area, 1 cm^2) of the sublayer liquid S overlaid with a similar section of the spreading liquid L.

By equation (14–2), surface or interfacial work is equal to surface tension multiplied by the area increment. The work required to separate the two sections of liquid in Figure 14–8, each with a cross-sectional area of 1 cm^2, is therefore numerically related to the surface or interfacial tension involved, the area increment being unity:

Work = Surface tension × unit area change

Accordingly, it is seen in Figure 14–8b that the work done is equal to the newly created surface tensions, γ_L and γ_S minus the interfacial tension γ_{LS} that has been

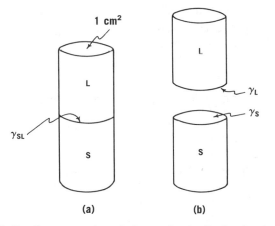

Fig. 14-8. Representation of the work of adhesion involved in separating a substrate and an overlying liquid.

destroyed in the process. The work of adhesion is thus

$$W_a = \gamma_L + \gamma_S - \gamma_{LS} \qquad (14-16)$$

The *work of cohesion*, required to separate the molecules of the spreading liquid so that it can flow over the sublayer, is obtained by reference to Figure 14-9. Obviously, no interfacial tension exists between the like molecules of the liquid, and when the hypothetical 1 cm^2 cylinder in (a) is divided, two new surfaces are created in (b), each with a surface tension of γ_L. Therefore the work of cohesion is

$$W_c = 2\gamma_L \qquad (14-17)$$

With reference to the spreading of an oil on a water surface, spreading occurs if the work of adhesion (a measure of the force of attraction between the oil and water) is greater than the work of cohesion. The term $(W_a - W_c)$ is known as the *spreading coefficient (S)*; if positive, the oil will spread over a water surface. Equations (14-16) and (14-17) may be written

$$S = W_a - W_c = (\gamma_L + \gamma_S - \gamma_{LS}) - 2\gamma_L \qquad (14-18)$$

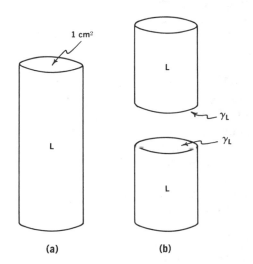

Fig. 14-9. Representation of the work of cohesion involved in separating like molecules in a liquid.

in which γ_S is the surface tension of the sublayer liquid, γ_L is the surface tension of the spreading liquid, and γ_{LS} is the interfacial tension between the two liquids. Rearranging equation (14-18) gives

$$S = \gamma_S - \gamma_L - \gamma_{LS} \qquad (14-19)$$

or

$$S = \gamma_S - (\gamma_L + \gamma_{LS}) \qquad (14-20)$$

Figure 14-10 shows a lens of material placed on a liquid surface (e.g., oleic acid on water). From equation (14-20), one sees that spreading occurs (S is positive) when the surface tension of the sublayer liquid is greater than the sum of the surface tension of the spreading liquid and the interfacial tension between the sublayer and the spreading liquid. If $(\gamma_L + \gamma_{LS})$ is larger than γ_S, the substance forms globules or a floating lens and fails to spread over the surface. An example of such a case is mineral oil on water.

Spreading may also be thought of in terms of surface free energy. Thus, the added substance will spread if, by so doing, the surface free energy of the system is reduced. Put another way, if the surface free energy of the new surface and the new interface is less than the free energy of the old surface, spreading will take place.

Up to this point, the discussion has been restricted to *initial* spreading. Before equilibrium is reached, however, the water surface becomes saturated with the spreading material, which in turn becomes saturated with water. If we use a prime (') to denote the values following equilibration (i.e., final rather than initial values), then the new surface tensions are $\gamma_{S'}$ and $\gamma_{L'}$. When mutual saturation has taken place, the spreading coefficient may be reduced or may even become negative. This means that although initial spreading of the material may occur on the liquid substrate, it can be followed by coalescence of the excess material into a lens if S' becomes negative in value. This reversal of spreading takes place when $\gamma_{S'}$ becomes less than $(\gamma_{LS} + \gamma_{L'})$. Note that the value of γ_{LS} does not change since the interfacial tension is determined under conditions of mutual saturation.

Example 14-7. If the surface tension of water γ_S is 72.8 dynes/cm at 20° C, the surface tension of benzene γ_L is 28.9, and the interfacial tension between benzene and water γ_{LS} is 35.0, what is the initial

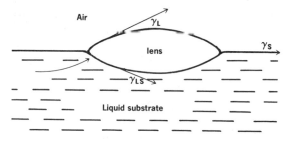

Fig. 14-10. Forces existing at the surfaces of a lens floating in a substrate liquid.

spreading coefficient? Following equilibration, $\gamma_{S'}$ is 62.2 dynes/cm and $\gamma_{L'}$ is 28.8. What is the final spreading coefficient?

$$S = 72.8 - (28.9 + 35.0) = 8.9 \text{ dynes/cm (or 8.9 ergs/cm}^2)$$

$$S' = 62.2 - (28.8 + 35.0) = -1.6 \text{ dynes/cm}$$

Therefore, while benzene spreads initially on water, at equilibrium there is formed a saturated monolayer with the excess benzene (saturated with water) forming a lens.

In the case of organic liquids spread on water, it is found that while the initial spreading coefficient may be positive or negative, the final spreading coefficient always has a negative value. Duplex films of this type are unstable and form monolayers with the excess material remaining as a lens on the surface. The initial spreading coefficients of some organic liquids on water at 20° C are listed in Table 14–4.

It is important to consider the types of molecular structures that lead to high spreading coefficients. An oil spreads over water because it contains polar groups such as COOH or OH. Hence, propionic acid and ethyl alcohol should have high values of *S*, as seen in Table 14–4. As the carbon chain of an acid, oleic acid for example, increases, the ratio of polar–nonpolar character decreases and the spreading coefficient on water decreases. Many nonpolar substances such as liquid petrolatum ($S = -13.4$) fail to spread on water. Benzene spreads on water not because it is polar but because the cohesive forces between its molecules are much weaker than the adhesion for water.

The applications of spreading coefficients in pharmacy should be fairly evident. The surface of the skin is bathed in an aqueous-oily layer having a polar–nonpolar character similar to that of a mixture of fatty acids. For a lotion with a mineral oil base to spread freely and evenly on the skin, its polarity and hence its spreading coefficient should be increased by the addition of a surfactant. The relation between spreading, HLB (*hydrophile–lipophile balance*), and emulsion stability has been studied.[11] Surfactant blends of varying HLBs were added to an oil, a drop of which was then placed on water. The HLB of the surfactant blend that caused the

oil drop to spread was related to the required HLB of the oil when used in emulsification. See pages 371 and 373 for a discussion of HLB.

ADSORPTION AT LIQUID INTERFACES

Surface free energy was defined previously as the work that must be done to increase the surface by unit area. As a result of such expansion, more molecules must be brought from the bulk to the interface. The more work that has to be expended to achieve this, the greater the surface free energy.

Certain molecules and ions, when dispersed in the liquid, move of their own accord to the interface. Their concentration at the interface then exceeds their concentration in the bulk of the liquid. Obviously, the surface free energy and the surface tension of the system is automatically reduced. Such a phenomenon, where the added molecules are partitioned in favor of the interface, is termed *adsorption*, or more correctly, *positive adsorption*. Other materials (e.g., inorganic electrolytes) are partitioned in favor of the bulk, leading to *negative adsorption* and a corresponding increase in surface free energy and surface tension. Adsorption, as will be seen later, can also occur at solid interfaces. Adsorption should not be confused with *absorption*. The former is solely a surface effect, whereas in absorption, the liquid or gas being absorbed penetrates into the capillary spaces of the absorbing medium. The taking up of water by a sponge is absorption; the concentrating of alkaloid molecules on the surface of clay is adsorption.

Surface-Active Agents. Molecules and ions that are adsorbed at interfaces are termed *surface-active agents*, or *surfactants*. An alternative expression is *amphiphile*, which suggests that the molecule or ion has a certain affinity for both polar and nonpolar solvents. Depending on the number and nature of the polar and nonpolar groups present, the amphiphile may be predominantly *hydrophilic* (water-loving), *lipophilic* (oil-loving), or reasonably well balanced between these two extremes. For example, straight-chain alcohols, amines, and acids are amphiphiles that change from being predominantly hydrophilic to lipophilic as the number of carbon atoms in the alkyl chain is increased. Thus, ethyl alcohol is miscible with water in all proportions. In comparison, the aqueous solubility of amyl alcohol, $C_5H_{11}OH$, is much reduced, while cetyl alcohol, $C_{16}H_{33}OH$, may be said to be strongly lipophilic and insoluble in water.

It is the amphiphilic nature of surface-active agents that causes them to be absorbed at interfaces, whether these be liquid–gas or liquid–liquid. Thus, in an aqueous dispersion of amyl alcohol, the polar alcoholic group is able to associate with the water molecules. The nonpolar portion is rejected, however, because the adhesive forces it can develop with water are small in

TABLE 14–4. *Initial Spreading Coefficients, S, at 20° C**

Substance	S (dynes/cm)
Ethyl alcohol	50.4
Propionic acid	45.8
Ethyl ether	45.5
Acetic acid	45.2
Acetone	42.4
Undecylenic acid	32 (25°)
Oleic acid	24.6
Chloroform	13
Benzene	8.9
Hexane	3.4
Octane	0.22
Ethylene dibromide	−3.19
Liquid petrolatum	−13.4

*From W. D. Harkins, The Physical Chemistry of Surface Films, Reinhold, New York, 1952, pp. 44, 45.

comparison to the cohesive forces between adjacent water molecules. As a result, the amphiphile is adsorbed at the interface. The situation for a fatty acid at the air–water and oil–water interface is shown in Figure 14–11. At the air–water interface, the lipophilic chains are directed upward into the air; at the oil–water interface, they are associated with the oil phase. In order for the amphiphile to be concentrated at the interface, it must be balanced with the proper amount of water- and oil-soluble groups. If the molecule is too hydrophilic, it remains within the body of the aqueous phase and exerts no effect at the interface. Likewise, if it is too lipophilic, it dissolves completely in the oil phase and little appears at the interface.

Systems of Hydrophile–Lipophile Classification. Griffin[12] devised an arbitrary scale of values to serve as a measure of the hydrophilic–lipophilic balance (HLB) of surface-active agents. By means of this number system, it is possible to establish an HLB range of optimum efficiency for each class of surfactant, as seen in Figure 14–12. The higher the HLB of an agent, the more hydrophilic it is. The Spans, sorbitan esters manufactured by ICI Americas Inc., are lipophilic and have low HLB values (1.8 to 8.6); the Tweens, polyoxyethylene derivatives of the Spans, are hydrophilic and have high HLB values (9.6 to 16.7).

The HLB of a nonionic surfactant whose only hydro-

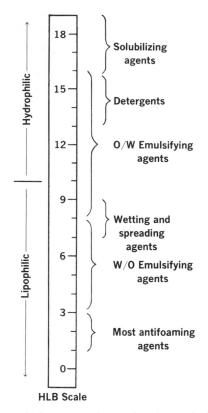

Fig. 14–12. A scale showing surfactant function on the basis of HLB values.

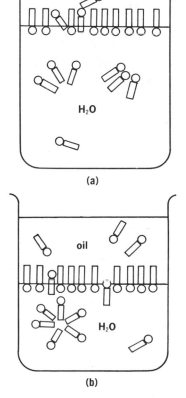

Fig. 14–11. Adsorption of fatty acid molecules (a) at a water–air interface and (b) at a water–oil interface.

philic portion is polyoxyethylene is calculated using the formula

$$HLB = E/5 \qquad (14-21)$$

in which E is the percent by weight of ethylene oxide. A number of polyhydric alcohol fatty acid esters, such as glyceryl monostearate, may be estimated by using the formula

$$HLB = 20\left(1 - \frac{S}{A}\right) \qquad (14-22)$$

in which S is the saponification number of the ester and A the acid number of the fatty acid. The HLB of polyoxyethylene sorbitan monolaurate (Tween 20), for which $S = 45.5$ and $A = 276$, is

$$HLB = 20\left(1 - \frac{45.5}{276}\right) = 16.7$$

The HLB values of some commonly used amphiphilic agents are given in Table 14–5.

The oil phase of an oil-in-water (O/W) emulsion requires a specific HLB, called the *required hydrophile–lipophile balance*, RHLB. A different RHLB is required to form a water-in-oil (W/O) emulsion from the same oil phase. The RHLB values for both O/W and W/O emulsions have been determined empirically for a number of oils and oil-like substances, some of which are listed in Table 14–6.

TABLE 14–5. *HLB Values of Some Amphiphilic Agents*

Substance	HLB
Oleic acid	1
Polyoxyethylene sorbitol beeswax derivative (G-1706)	2.0
Sorbitan tristearate	2.1
Glyceryl monostearate	3.8
Sorbitan mono-oleate (Span 80)	4.3
Diethylene glycol monostearate	4.7
Glyceryl monostearate, self-emulsifying (Tegin)	5.5
Diethylene glycol monolaurate	6.1
Sorbitan monolaurate (Span 20)	8.6
Polyethylene lauryl ether (Brij 30)	9.5
Gelatin (Pharmagel B)	9.8
Methyl cellulose (Methocel 15 cps)	10.5
Polyoxyethylene lauryl ether (G-3705)	10.8
Polyoxyethylene monostearate (Myrj 45)	11.1
Triethanolamine oleate	12.0
Polyoxyethylene alkyl phenol (Igepal Ca-630)	12.8
Polyethylene glycol 400 monolaurate	13.1
Polyoxyethylene sorbitan mono-oleate (Tween 80)	15.0
Polyoxyethylene sorbitan monolaurate (Tween 20)	16.7
Polyoxyethylene lauryl ether (Brij 35)	16.9
Sodium oleate	18.0
Potassium oleate	20
Sodium lauryl sulfate	40

TABLE 14–6. *Required HLB for Some Oil Phase Ingredients, for Both O/W and W/O Emulsions* *

	O/W	W/O
Cottonseed oil	6–7	—
Petrolatum	8	—
Beeswax	9–11	5
Paraffin wax	10	4
Mineral oil	10–12	5–6
Methyl silicone	11	—
Lanolin, anhydrous	12–14	8
Carnauba wax	12–14	—
Lauryl alcohol	14	—
Castor oil	14	—
Kerosene	12–14	—
Cetyl alcohol	13–16	—
Stearyl alcohol	15–16	—
Carbon tetrachloride	16	—
Lauric acid	16	—
Oleic acid	17	—
Stearic acid	17	—

*From Atlas HLB System, ICI Americas; P. Becher, *Emulsions, Theory and Practice,* 2nd Edition, Reinhold, New York, 1966, p. 249.

Example 14–8. For the oil-in-water emulsion:

Ingredient	Amount	RHLB (O/W)
1. Beeswax	15 g	9
2. Lanolin	10 g	12
3. Paraffin wax	20 g	10
4. Cetyl alcohol	5 g	15
5. Emulsifier	2 g	
6. Preservative	0.2 g	
7. Color	as required	
8. Water, purified q.s.	100 g	

One first calculates the overall RHLB of the emulsion by multiplying the RHLB of each oil-like component (items 1 through 4) by the weight fraction that each oil-like component contributes to the oil phase. The total weight of the oil phase is 50 g. Therefore,

Beeswax	$15/50 \times 9$	$= 2.70$
Lanolin	$10/50 \times 12$	$= 2.40$
Paraffin	$20/50 \times 10$	$= 4.00$
Cetyl alcohol	$5/50 \times 15$	$= 1.50$
Total RHLB for the emulsion		$= 10.60$

Next, a blend of two emulsifying agents is chosen, one with an HLB above and the other with an HLB below the required HLB of the emulsion (RHLB = 10.6 in this example). From Table 14–5, we choose Tween 80 with an HLB of 15 and Span 80 with an HLB of 4.3.

The formula to calculate the weight percentage of Tween 80 (surfactant with the higher HLB) is

$$\% \text{ Tween 80} = \frac{\text{RHLB} - \text{HLB low}}{\text{HLB high} - \text{HLB low}} \quad (14\text{–}23)$$

where HLB high is for the higher value, 15, and HLB low is for the lower value, 4.3.

$$\% \text{ Tween 80} = \frac{10.6 - 4.3}{15.0 - 4.3} = 0.59$$

Two grams of emulsifier has been estimated as proper protection for the O/W emulsion. Therefore, 2.0 g × 0.59 = 1.18 grams of Tween 80 is needed and the remainder, 0.82 gram, must be supplied by Span 80 for the 100-gram emulsion.

The choice of the mixture of emulsifiers and the total amount of the emulsifier phase is left to the formulator, who determines these unknowns over time by preparation and observation of the several formulas chosen.

A mathematical formula for determining the minimum amount of surfactant mixture has been suggested by Bonadeo:[13]

$$Q_s = \frac{6(\rho_s/\rho)}{10 - 0.5 \text{ RHLB}} + 4Q/1000 \quad (14\text{–}24)$$

where ρ_s is the density of the surfactant mixture, ρ is the density of the dispersed (internal) phase, and Q is the percent of the dispersant (continuous phase) of the emulsion. The required HLB, written RHLB, is the HLB of the oil phase needed to form an O/W or W/O emulsion.

Example 14–9. We wish to formulate two products, (a) a W/O and (b) an O/W emulsion containing 40 g of a mixed oil phase and 60 g of water.

(a) The oil phase consists of 70% paraffin and 30% beeswax. The density of the oil phase is 0.85 g/cm^3 and the density of the aqueous phase is about 1 g/cm^3 at room temperature. The density of the mixture of surfactants for the W/O emulsion is 0.87 g/cm^3. The required HLB values of paraffin and of beeswax for a W/O emulsion are 4.0 and 5.0, respectively.

The amount Q_s in grams of a mixture of sorbitan tristearate (HLB = 2.1) and diethylene glycol monostearate (HLB = 4.7) to obtain a *water-in-oil emulsion* is obtained by the use of equation (14–24), first calculating the RHLB of the oil phase:

$$\text{RHLB} = (4 \times 0.70) + (5 \times 0.30) = 4.3$$

$$Q_s = \frac{6(0.87/1)}{10 - (0.5 \times 4.3)} + \frac{4 \times 40}{1000} = 0.82 \text{ g}$$

Note that for a W/O emulsion we used the density of the internal phase, $\rho_{\text{water}} \cong 1$, and the percent of dispersant, oil = 40%.

(b) The RHLB of the oil phase, 70% paraffin and 30% beeswax, for an O/W emulsion is

$$\text{RHLB} = (0.70 \times 10) + (0.3 \times 9) = 9.7$$

and the total amount of surfactant mixture is

$$Q_s + \frac{6(1.05/0.85)}{10 - (0.5 \times 9.7)} + \frac{4 \times 60}{1000} = 1.68 \text{ g}$$

For an O/W emulsion, we used the density ρ of the oil as the internal phase and the percent of dispersant as the aqueous phase.

For the amount of surfactant mixture in the W/O emulsion we can raise the value Q_s roughly to 1.0 g and for the O/W emulsion to about 2.0 g. We can then calculate the weights of the two emulsifying agents for each emulsion, using the equation

$$\begin{array}{c} \text{\% surfactant of} \\ \text{higher HLB} \end{array} = \frac{\text{RHLB} - \text{HLB low}}{\text{HLB high} - \text{HLB low}} \qquad (14\text{--}25)$$

For the W/O emulsion, the percent by weight of diethylene glycol monostearate (HLB = 4.7) combined with sorbitan tristearate (HLB = 2.1) is

$$\begin{array}{c} \text{\% diethylene glycol} \\ \text{monostearate} \end{array} = \frac{4.3 - 2.1}{4.7 - 2.1} = 0.85 \text{ g or } 85\% \text{ of 1 gram}$$

The fraction or percentage of sorbitan monostearate is therefore 0.15 g or 15% of the 1 gram of mixed emulsifier.

For the O/W emulsion the percent by weight of Tween 80 (HLB = 15) combined with diethylene glycol monolaurate (HLB = 6.1) is

$$\text{\% Tween 80} = \frac{9.7 - 6.1}{15 - 6.1} = 0.40 \text{ or } 40\%$$

The fraction or percentage of diethylene glycol monolaurate is therefore 0.60 or 60%. And 0.40 or 40% of a 2-gram mixture of emulsifier phase = 0.8 gram of Tween 80. The remainder, 1.2 grams, is the amount of diethylene glycol monolaurate in the 2-gram emulsifier phase.

Other scales of hydrophile–lipophile balance have been developed, although none of these have gained the acceptance afforded the HLB system of Griffin. A titration method, as well as other techniques, for determining the hydrophile–lipophile character of surfactants, have been proposed.[14]

Types of Monolayer at Liquid Surfaces. For convenience of discussion, adsorbed materials are divided into two groups: those that form "soluble" monolayers and those that form "insoluble" films. The distinction is made on the basis of the solubility of the adsorbate in the liquid subphase. Thus, amyl alcohol may be said to form a soluble monolayer on water, while cetyl alcohol would form an insoluble film on the same sublayer. It must be emphasized that this is really only an arbitrary distinction, for the insoluble films are, in effect, the limiting case of those compounds that form soluble monolayers at liquid interfaces. There are, however, important practical reasons why such a classification is made.

It will become apparent to the student in the following sections that three interrelated parameters are important in studying liquid interfaces. These are (1) surface tension, γ; (2) surface excess, Γ, which is the amount of amphiphile per unit area of surface in excess of that in the bulk of the liquid; and (3) c, the concentration of amphiphile in the bulk of the liquid. As we shall see, it is relatively easy with soluble monolayers to measure surface tension and c and from these data to compute the surface excess. With insoluble monolayers, c is taken to be zero, while surface tension and surface excess can be obtained directly. Materials that lie on the borderline between soluble and insoluble systems

can be studied by either approach and, invariably, similar results are obtained.

Data obtained from such studies are of increasing biologic and pharmaceutical interest. For example, emulsions are stabilized by the presence of an interfacial film between the oil and water phases. A knowledge of the area occupied by each amphiphilic molecule at the interface is important in achieving optimum stability of the emulsion. The efficiency of wetting and detergent processes depends on the concentration of material adsorbed. Monolayers of adsorbed amphiphiles may be used as in vitro models for biologic membranes that are thought to consist of two monolayers placed back-to-back with the hydrocarbon chains intermeshed. Consequently, these model systems are finding increasing application for in vitro studies of drug absorption across biologic membranes. Studies of interfacial adsorption also provide valuable information on the dimensions of molecules, since it is possible to calculate the areas occupied by amphiphilic molecules.

Soluble Monolayers and the Gibbs Adsorption Equation. The addition of amphiphiles to a liquid system leads to a reduction in surface tension owing to these molecules or ions being adsorbed as a monolayer. Adsorption of amphiphiles in these binary systems was first expressed quantitatively by Gibbs in 1878 as follows:

$$\Gamma = \frac{c}{RT} \frac{d\gamma}{dc} \qquad (14\text{--}26)$$

in which Γ is the surface excess or surface concentration, that is, the amount of the amphiphile per unit area of surface in excess of that in the bulk of the liquid, c is the concentration of amphiphile in the liquid bulk, R is the gas constant, T is the absolute temperature, and $d\gamma/dc$ is the change in surface tension of the solution with change of bulk concentration of the substance. The derivation of equation (14–26) is given in the following paragraphs.

Recall (equation (3–70), p. 67) that the free energy change of a bulk phase containing two components is written

$$dG = -S\,dT + V\,dp + \mu_1\,dn_1 + \mu_2\,dn_2$$

Two immiscible bulk phases may be considered to be separated by an interface or "surface phase" in which the contribution to the volume is ignored, and a new energy term $\gamma\,dA$ (see equation (14–2)) is introduced to account for the work involved in altering the surface area A. The surface tension γ is the work done at a constant temperature and pressure per unit increase of surface area. The new work done on the surface phase is equal to the surface free energy increase, dG^s. Therefore, we can write

$$dG^s = -S^s\,dT + \gamma\,dA + \mu_1{}^s\,dn_1{}^s + \mu_2{}^s\,dn_2{}^s \qquad (14\text{--}27)$$

At equilibrium, the free energy of the entire system is zero under the conditions of constant temperature, pressure, and surface area. Since no matter passes in or out of the system as a whole, the chemical potential of a component i is the same in the two bulk phases as it is in the surface phase s:

$$\mu_{i\alpha} = \mu_{i\beta} = \mu_{is} \qquad (14\text{--}28)$$

Such a system consisting of two immiscible liquids, water α and oleic acid β, separated by the surface phase s is shown in Figure 14–13a. Equation (14–27) may be integrated at constant temperature and composition to give the surface free energy,

$$G^s = \gamma A + n_1{}^s \mu_1{}^s + n_2{}^s \mu_2{}^s \qquad (14\text{--}29)$$

Since the surface free energy depends only on the state of the system, dG^s is an exact differential and may be obtained by general differentiation of (14–29) under the condition of variable composition.

$$dG^s = \gamma\, dA + A\, d\gamma + n_1{}^s\, d\mu_1{}^s$$
$$+ n_2{}^s\, d\mu_2{}^s + \mu_1{}^s\, dn_1{}^s + \mu_2{}^s\, dn_2{}^s \quad (14\text{--}30)$$

Comparing this result with equation (14–27) shows that

$$A\, d\gamma + S^s\, dT + n_1{}^s\, d\mu_1{}^s + n_2{}^s\, d\mu_2{}^s = 0 \qquad (14\text{--}31)$$

and at constant temperature

$$A\, d\gamma + n_1{}^s\, d\mu_1{}^s + n_2{}^s\, d\mu_2{}^s = 0 \qquad (14\text{--}32)$$

When equation (14–32) is divided through by the surface area A, and $n_1{}^s/A$ and $n_2{}^s/A$ are given the symbols Γ_1 and Γ_2, respectively,

$$d\gamma + \Gamma_1\, d\mu_1{}^s + \Gamma_2\, d\mu_2{}^s = 0 \qquad (14\text{--}33)$$

As expressed by equation (14–33), the chemical potentials of the components in the surface are equal to those in the bulk phases provided that the system is in equilibrium at constant temperature, pressure, and surface area.

Now consider a single-phase solution of oleic acid (solute or component 2) in water (solvent or component 1) as shown in Figure 14–13b. Under these circumstances, it is possible to drop the superscripts on the chemical potentials and write

$$d\gamma + \Gamma_1\, d\mu_1 + \Gamma_2\, d\mu_2 = 0 \qquad (14\text{--}34)$$

in which Γ_1 and Γ_2 are the number of moles of the components per unit area in the surface and μ_1 and μ_2 are the chemical potentials of the two components in the solution.

It is possible to make an arbitrary choice of the surface, and we do so in a manner that makes Γ_1 equal to zero, that is, we arrange the boundary so that none of the solvent is present in the surface (cf. Fig. 14–13b). Then equation (14–34) becomes

$$d\gamma + \Gamma_2\, d\mu_2 = 0 \qquad (14\text{--}35)$$

and

$$\Gamma_2 = -\left(\frac{\partial \gamma}{\partial \mu_2}\right)_T \qquad (14\text{--}36)$$

The chemical potential of the solute can be expressed in terms of the activity using the equation

$$\mu_2 = \mu^\circ + RT \ln a_2$$

and by differentiating at constant temperature, one obtains

$$\partial \mu_2 = RT\, \partial \ln a_2 \qquad (14\text{--}37)$$

Substituting this value in equation (14–36) produces the result

$$\Gamma_2 = -\frac{1}{RT}\left(\frac{\partial \gamma}{\partial \ln a_2}\right)_T \qquad (14\text{--}38)$$

From differential calculus, if $y = \ln a_2$, then $d \ln a_2 = da_2/a_2$. Substituting this result in equation (14–38), results in the *Gibbs adsorption equation*,

$$\Gamma_2 = -\frac{a_2}{RT}\left(\frac{\partial \gamma}{\partial a_2}\right)_T \qquad (14\text{--}39)$$

This is equation (14–26), which was given on page 373 in terms of concentration c instead of activity. If the solution is dilute, a_2 may be replaced by c without introducing a significant error.

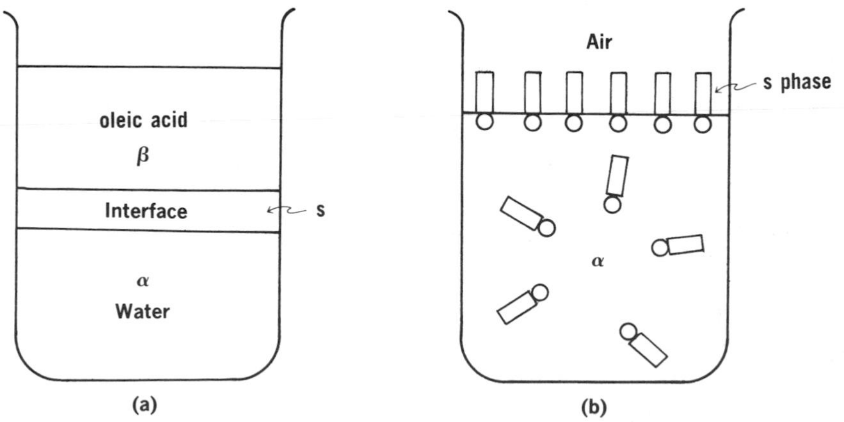

Fig. 14–13. A system consisting of oleic acid and water. (*a*) Graphic description of the two bulk phases, α and β, and the interface s. (*b*) Condition under which only the α phase and the surface or s phase need be considered.

When the surface tension γ of a surfactant is plotted against the logarithm of the surfactant activity or concentration, log c_2, the plot takes on the shape shown in Figure 14–14. The initial curved segment A–B is followed by a linear segment, B–D, along which there is a sharp decrease in surface tension as log c_2 increases. The point D corresponds to the critical micelle concentration, cmc, the concentration at which micelles form in the solution (p. 396). Beyond the cmc the line becomes horizontal, further additions of surfactant no longer being accompanied by a decrease in surface tension. Along the linear segment B–D, the surface excess Γ is constant because from equation (14–38), replacing activity with concentration,

$$\Gamma_2 = -\frac{1}{RT}\left(\frac{\partial \gamma}{\partial \ln c_2}\right) \qquad (14\text{–}40)$$

the slope $\partial\gamma/\partial \ln c_2$ reaches a limiting value and remains constant. Saturation adsorption of the surfactant has been reached at point B; that is, Γ_2 does not increase further as the bulk concentration increases. However, the surface tension decreases greatly until point D is reached. Within the segment B–D of the curve the surfactant molecules are closely packed at the surface and the surface area occupied per molecule is constant. Both the surface excess Γ_2 and the area per surfactant molecule may be calculated using equation (14–40).

Example 14–10. The limiting slope of a plot of γ versus $\ln c_2$ for a nonionic surfactant, $C_{12}H_{25}O(CH_2CH_2O)_{12}H$,[15] is $\partial\gamma/\partial \ln c_2 = -5.2937$ dyne/cm at 23.0° C. Calculate Γ_2 and the area per molecule of this surfactant.

From the Gibbs adsorption equation (14–40),

$$\Gamma_2 = -\left(\frac{1}{8.3143 \times 10^7 \text{ erg deg}^{-1} \text{ mole}^{-1} \times 296.15° \text{ K}}\right)(-5.2937 \text{ dyne/cm})$$

$\Gamma_2 = 2.15 \times 10^{-10}$ mole/cm^2

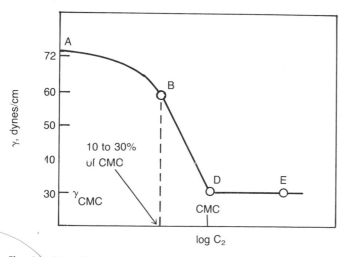

Fig. 14–14. Decrease in the surface tension of water when a straight-chain amphiphile is added. (From H. Schott, J. Pharm. Sci. **69**, 852, 1980, reproduced with permission of the copyright owner.)

The surface excess, 2.15×10^{-10} mole/cm^2, is multiplied by 6.0221×10^{23} mole^{-1}, Avogadro's number, to obtain molecules/cm^2. The reciprocal then gives the area per molecule:

$$\text{Area/molecule} = \frac{1}{6.0221 \times 10^{23} \text{ molecule mole}^{-1} \times 2.15 \times 10^{-10} \text{ mole/cm}^2}$$

$$= 7.72 \times 10^{-15} \text{ cm}^2/\text{molecule} = 77 \text{ Å}^2/\text{molecule}$$

The validity of the Gibbs equation has been verified experimentally. One of the more ingenious methods is due to McBain,[16] who literally fired a small microtome blade across a liquid surface so as to collect the surface layer. Analysis of the liquid scooped up and collected by the speeding blade agreed closely with that predicted by the Gibbs equation. More recently, radioactive techniques using weak beta emitters have been used successfully.[17]

Insoluble Monolayers and the Film Balance. Insoluble monolayers have a fascinating history that goes back to before the American Revolution. During a voyage to England in 1757, Benjamin Franklin observed, as had seamen for centuries before him, that when cooking grease was thrown from the ship's galley onto the water, the waves were calmed by the film that formed on the surface of the sea. In 1765, Franklin followed up this observation with an experiment on a half-acre pond in England and found that the application of 1 teaspoonful of oil was just sufficient to cover the pond and calm the waves. In 1899, Lord Rayleigh showed that when small amounts of certain slightly soluble oils were placed on a clean surface of water contained in a trough, they spread to form a layer one molecule thick (monomolecular layer). Prior to Rayleigh's work, a woman named Agnes Pockels, from Lower Saxony, Germany, who had no formal scientific training, developed a "film balance" for studying insoluble monolayers. She carried out a series of experiments, which she summarized in a letter to Lord Rayleigh in January, 1881. In fact, she invented the film balance in 1883, over 30 years before Langmuir, whose name is normally associated with this type of apparatus. These and other early contributions in the area of surface phenomena are described in a series of papers by Giles and Forrester.[18]

Knowing the area of the film and the volume of the spreading liquid, it should be possible to compute the thickness of such films. The film thickness is equal to the length of the molecules standing in a vertical position on the surface when the molecules are packed in closest arrangement. Furthermore, if the molecular weight and the density of the spreading oil are known, the cross-sectional area available to the molecules should be easily computed.

Example 14–11. We have noted that Benjamin Franklin placed 1 teaspoonful ($\cong 5$ cm^3) of a fatty acid "oil" on a half-acre ($\cong 2 \times 10^7$ cm^2) pond. Assume that the acid, having a molecular weight of 300 and a density of 0.90 g/cm^3, was just sufficient to form a condensed monomolecular film over the entire surface. What was the length and the cross-sectional area of the fatty acid molecule?

(*a*) Thickness of oil on the pond ≅ length of the vertically oriented fatty acid molecule.

$$\frac{5 \text{ cm}^3}{2 \times 10^7 \text{ cm}^2} = 25 \times 10^{-8} \text{ cm} = 25 \text{ Å}$$

(*b*)

$$5 \text{ cm}^3 \times 0.9 \text{ g/cm}^3 = 4.5 \text{ g}$$

$$\frac{4.5 \text{ g}}{300 \text{ g/mole}} = 0.015 \text{ mole}$$

$$0.015 \text{ mole} \times 6.02 \times 10^{23} \text{ molecules/mole} = 9 \times 10^{21} \text{ molecules}$$

$$\frac{2 \times 10^7 \text{ cm}^2, \text{ pond area}}{9 \times 10^{21} \text{ molecules}} = 22 \times 10^{-16} \text{ cm}^2/\text{molecule}$$

$$= 22 A^2/\text{molecule}$$

We can readily see from this example that the area of cross section per molecule is given by

$$\text{Cross-sectional area/molecule} = \frac{MS}{V \rho N} \qquad (14\text{--}41)$$

in which M is molecular weight of the spreading liquid, S the surface area covered by the film, V the volume of the spreading liquid, ρ its density, and N Avogadro's number.

Langmuir, Adam, Harkins, and others have made quantitative studies of the properties of films that are spread over a clear surface of the substrate liquid (usually water) contained in a trough. The film can be compressed against a horizontal float by means of a movable barrier. The force exerted on the float is measured by a torsion wire arrangement similar to that employed in the ring tensiometer. The apparatus, called a *film balance*, is shown in Figure 14–15. The compressive force per unit area on the float is known as the *surface* or *film pressure*, π; it is the difference in surface tension between the pure substrate, γ_0, and that with a film spread on it, γ, and is written

$$\pi = (\gamma_0 - \gamma) \qquad (14\text{--}42)$$

Surface tension (interfacial tension) is resistance of the surface (interface) to an expansion in area, and film pressure, π, is the lowering of this resistance to expansion, as expressed quantitatively in equation (14–42). Schott[15] states that the film pressure, π, is an expansion pressure exerted on the monolayer that opposes the surface tension, γ_o, or contraction of the clean (water) surface. The surface active molecules of the monolayer are thought to insert themselves into the surface of the water molecules of a film balance to reduce the resistance of the water surface to expansion. The presence of the surfactant molecules increases the ease of expansion, presumably by breaking or interfering with hydrogen bonding, van der Waals interaction, and other cohesive forces among the water molecules. These attractive forces produce the "spring-like" action in the water surface, as measured by the surface tension, γ_o, and the introduction of surfactant molecules into the clean water surface reduces the springiness of

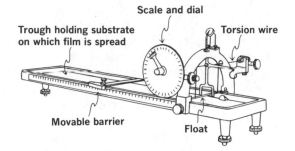

Fig. 14–15. Film balance, Cenco model.

the interacting water molecules and decreases the surface tension γ_o to ($\gamma_o - \gamma$) or π (equation (14–42)).

In carrying out an experiment with the film balance, the substance under study is dissolved in a volatile solvent (e.g., hexane) and is placed on the surface of the substrate, which has previously been swept clean by means of a paraffined or Teflon strip. The liquid spreads as a film, and the volatile solvent is permitted to evaporate. A cross-sectional view of the interface after spreading is shown in Figure 14–16. The movable barrier is then moved to various positions in the direction of the float. The area of the trough available to the film at each position is measured, and the corresponding film pressure is read from the torsion dial. The film pressure is then plotted against the area of the film or, more conveniently, against the cross-sectional area per molecule in A^2 (cf. *Example 14–11* and equation [14–41] for computing the molecule's cross-sectional area from the area of the film). The results for stearic acid and lecithin may be represented as shown in Figure 14–17.

Frequently, a variety of phase changes are observed when an insoluble film is spread at an interface and then compressed. A representation of what can occur with a straight-chain saturated aliphatic compound at the air–water interface is shown in Figure 14–18. When the film is spread over an area greater than 50 to 60 A^2/molecule (region G), it exerts little pressure on the floating barrier. The film acts like a gas in two dimensions. As the film begins to be compressed (region L_1-G), a liquid phase L_1 appears that coexists in

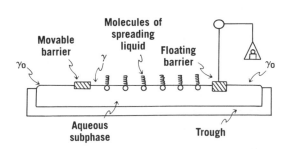

Fig. 14–16. Cross-section view of spreading liquid on the surface of a film balance.

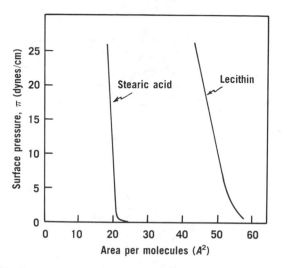

Fig. 14–17. Surface film pressure π for stearic acid and lecithin plotted as a function of cross-sectional area per molecule.

equilibrium with the gas phase. This occurs at a low surface pressure (e.g., 0.2 dyne/cm or less.) The liquid expanded state (region L_1) may be thought of as a bulk liquid state, but in two dimensions. Further compression of the film often leads to the appearance of an intermediate phase (region I) and then a less compressible condensed liquid state, region L_2. This then gives way to the least compressible state (region S), where the film can be regarded as being in a two-dimensional solid state. In these latter stages of film compression,

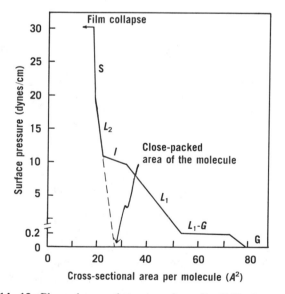

Fig. 14–18. Phase changes that occur when a liquid film is spread at an interface and then compressed. Key: G, two-dimensional gas; $L_1 - G$, liquid phase in equilibrium with two-dimensional gas; L_1, liquid expanded or two-dimensional bulk liquid state; I, intermediate state; L_2, condensed liquid state; S, two-dimensional solid state. When compressed by a force greater than required to form a solid surface, the film collapses, as shown by the arrow at the top of this figure. (From P. C. Heimenz, *Principles of Colloid and Surface Chemistry,* 2nd Edition, Dekker, NY 1986, p. 364, with permission of the copyright owner.)

the film or surface pressure, $\pi = \gamma_0 - \gamma_1$ rises rapidly as the curve passes through the regions L_2 and S in Figure 14–18. This increase in π with compression of the surfactant film results from surface active molecules being forcibly inserted and crowded into the surface. This process opposes the natural tendency of the water surface to contract, and the surface tension decreases from γ_0 to γ. Finally the molecules slip over one another, and the film breaks when it is greatly compressed. The regions marked along the plot in Figure 14–18 can be represented schematically in terms of the positioning of the spreading molecules in the surface, as shown in Figure 14–19. In region G in Figure 14–18 the molecules in the monolayer lie on the surface with great distances between them, as in a three-dimensional gas. In the part of the curve marked L_1 and L_2 (see Fig. 14–18), the molecules are forced closer together, and, as shown schematically in Figure 14–19b, are beginning to stand erect and interact with one another, analogous to a three-dimensional liquid. In region S of Figure 14–18, the spreading molecules are held together by strong forces; and this condition, analogous to the solid state in three-dimensional chemistry, shows little compressibility relative to that of a gas or a liquid. The S state is shown schematically in Figure 14–19c where the molecules on the surface of the film balance are compressed together as far as possible. Further compression of the film (by a movement from right to left on the horizontal axis of the graph in Figure 14–18—that is, a movement from left to right of the movable barrier shown in Fig. 14–15) brings about a collapse of the monolayer film, one part sliding over the other, as depicted in Figure 14–19d.

The cross-sectional area per molecule of the close-packed film at zero surface pressure is obtained by extrapolating the linear portion of the curve to the horizontal axis, as seen in Figure 14–18. The values for some organic molecules, determined in this way by Langmuir,[19] are listed in Table 14–7. It is seen that myricyl alcohol with 30 carbons in the chain has a length almost twice that of the other molecules. Its cross-sectional area at the interface is not markedly different from other single-chain molecules, however, confirming that it is the cross-sectional area of the alkyl chain, rather than the length, that is being measured. Tristearin, with three fatty acid chains, has a cross-sectional area about three times that of the molecules with only one aliphatic chain.

The electrical potential and viscosity of monomolecular films may be studied by means of the film balance, and the molecular weight of high polymers such as proteins can be estimated by its use. The film-balance technique also has considerable significance in the study of biologic systems. Some protein molecules unfold from a spherical configuration into a flat film when spread on the surface of the film trough, and the relationship between unfolding and biologic activity can be studied.

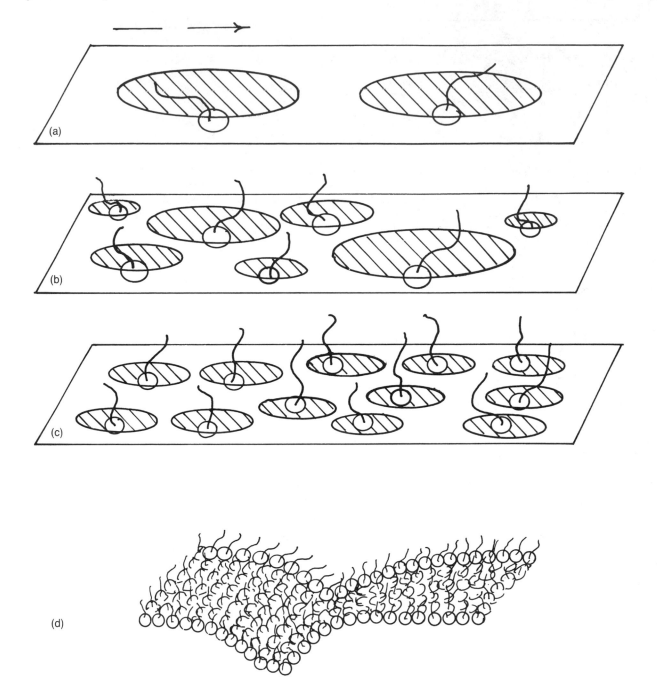

Fig. 14–19. Effective areas (cross-hatched ellipses) per molecule at the various degrees of monolayer compression. *(a)* gaseous state; *(b)* expanded liquid state; *(c)* condensed liquid and two-dimensional solid state; *(d)* film collapse. (From P. C. Hiemenz, *Principles of Colloid and Surface Chemistry*, 2nd Edition, Dekker, New York, 1986, p. 366, reproduced with permission of the copyright owner.)

The sizes and shapes of molecules of steroids, hormones, and enzymes and their interaction with drugs at interfaces can also be investigated by means of the film balance. The interaction between insulin injected under the surface layer and several lipids spread at constant surface pressure on a film balance were studied by Schwinke et al.[20] The film balance and its applications are discussed in the books of Adam,[21] Harkins,[22] Sobotka,[23] and Gaines.[24]

Mention has been made of the fact that materials forming an insoluble monolayer may be thought of as being in the gaseous, liquid, or solid state, depending on the degree of compression to which the film is subjected. Thus, the surface presssure for molecules in the gaseous state at an interface is comparable to the pressure P that molecules in three-dimensional gaseous systems exert on the walls of their containers. Just as the equation of state for an ideal gas in three dimensions is $PV = nRT$ (p. 25), that for a monolayer is

$$\pi A = nRT \qquad (14\text{--}43)$$

in which π is the surface pressure in dynes/cm and A is the area that each mole of amphiphile occupies at the interface.

TABLE 14-7. *Dimensions of Organic Molecules Determined by Means of the Film Balance*

Substance	Formula	Length of Molecule (angstroms, Å)	Cross-Sectional Area (sq. angstroms, Å²)
Stearic acid	$C_{17}H_{35}COOH$	25	22
Tristearin	$(C_{128}H_{35}O_2)_3C_3H_5$	25	66
Cetyl alcohol	$C_{16}H_{33}OH$	22	21
Myricyl alcohol	$C_{30}H_{61}OH$	41	27

Equation (14–43), the two-dimensional ideal gas law, may be derived as follows. When the concentration of amphiphile at the interface is small, solute–solute interactions are unimportant. Under these conditions, surface tension decreases in a linear fashion with concentration. We may therefore write that

$$\gamma = bc + \gamma_0 \qquad (14-44)$$

in which γ_0 is the surface tension of the pure substrate, γ is the surface tension produced by the addition of c moles/liter of adsorbate, and b is the slope of the line. Since the slope of such a plot is negative, and since $\pi = \gamma_0 - \gamma$, equation (14–44) may be rewritten as

$$\pi = -bc \qquad (14-45)$$

The Gibbs adsorption equation (14–26) can be expressed in the following form:

$$-(d\gamma/dc) = -b = \Gamma RT/c \qquad (14-46)$$

since $(d\gamma/dc)$ is the slope of the line.

Substituting for equation (14–45) in equation (14–46) and cancelling c, which is common to both sides, we obtain

$$\pi = \Gamma RT \qquad (14-47)$$

Surface excess has the dimensions of moles/cm² and can be represented by n/A, in which n is the number of moles and A is the area in cm². Thus:

$$\pi = nRT/A$$

or

$$\pi A = nRT$$

which is equation (14–43).

As with the three-dimensional gas law, equation (14–43) can be used to compute the molecular weights of materials adsorbed as gaseous films at an interface. (See *Problems 14–24* and *14–25*.). Nonideal behavior also occurs, and plots of πA versus π for monolayers give results comparable to those in three-dimensional systems when PV is plotted against P. Equations similar to van der Waal's equation (p. 26) for nonideal behavior have been developed.

The relation between the Gibbs adsorption equation and equation (14–43) emphasizes the point made earlier that the distinction between soluble and insoluble films is an arbitrary one, made on the basis of the experi-mental techniques used rather than any fundamental differences in physical properties.

The variation of the surface pressure π with temperature at the several "phase changes" observed in the two-dimensional isotherm, π-area, (see Fig. 14–18) may be analyzed by a relationship analogous to the Clapeyron equation (p. 68):

$$\frac{d\pi}{dT} = \frac{\Delta H}{T(A_1 - A_2)} \qquad (14-48)$$

where A_1 and A_2 are the molar areas (cm² mol⁻¹) of the two phases and T and ΔH are the temperature and enthalpy for the phase change.[25] Note that π, ΔH, and $(A_1 - A_2)$ are the two-dimensional equivalents of pressure, enthalpy, and change of volume in the Clapeyron equation.

Example 14-12. Monolayers of insoluble amphiphilic compounds with a polymerizable group serve to investigate the polymerization behavior at the gas–water interface. The π-A isotherms resulting from film balance experiments with *n*-hexadecyl acrylate monolayers in the temperature range 13° to 28° C showed two breaks corresponding to phase transitions (changes in state).

Compute ΔH, the enthalpy change of transition from the condensed liquid state L_2 to the liquid expanded state L_1. The areas per molecule at L_1 and L_2 are 0.357 and 0.265 nm²/molecule. The change of surface pressure with temperature, $d\pi/dt = 0.91$ mN m⁻¹ °K⁻¹, and the temperature of transition is 24.2° C.[25]

From equation (14–48):

$$\Delta H = T(A_1 - A_2)\frac{d\pi}{dT}$$

$$\Delta H = 297.2°\ K\ (0.357 - 0.265) \times 10^{-18}\ m^2/molecule \times$$

$$0.91 \times 10^{-3}\ \frac{N}{m\ °K} = 2.49 \times 10^{-20}\ J/molecule$$

$$2.49 \times 10^{-20} \times 6.022 \times 10^{23} = 14{,}995\ J/mol \cong 15\ kJ/mole$$

ADSORPTION AT SOLID INTERFACES

Adsorption of material at solid interfaces may take place from either an adjacent liquid or gas phase. The study of adsorption of gases is concerned in such diverse applications as the removal of objectionable odors from rooms and food, the operation of gas masks, and the measurement of the dimensions of particles in a powder. The principles of solid–liquid adsorption are utilized in decolorizing solutions, adsorption chromatography, detergency, and wetting.

In many ways, the adsorption of materials from a gas or liquid onto a solid surface is similar to that discussed under liquid surfaces. Thus, adsorption of this type may be considered as an attempt to reduce the surface free energy of the solid. The surface tensions of solids are invariably more difficult to obtain, however, than those of liquids. In addition, the solid interface is immobile in comparison to the turbulent liquid interface. The average lifetime of a molecule at the water–gas interface is about 1 microsecond, whereas an atom in the surface of a nonvolatile metallic solid may have an average lifetime of 10^{37} seconds.[26] Frequently, the surface of a solid may not be homogeneous, in contrast to liquid interfaces.

The Solid–Gas Interface. The degree of adsorption of a gas by a solid depends on the chemical nature of the *adsorbent* (the material used to adsorb the gas) and the *adsorbate* (the substance being adsorbed), the surface area of the adsorbent, the temperature, and the partial pressure of the adsorbed gas. The types of adsorption are generally recognized as physical or van der Waals' adsorption, and chemical adsorption or chemisorption. *Physical adsorption*, associated with van der Waals' forces, is reversible, the removal of the adsorbate from the adsorbent being known as *desorption*. A physically adsorbed gas may be desorbed from a solid by increasing the temperature and reducing the pressure. *Chemisorption*, in which the adsorbate is attached to the adsorbent by primary chemical bonds, is irreversible.

The relationship between the amount of gas physically adsorbed on a solid and the equilibrium pressure or concentration at constant temperature yields an *adsorption isotherm* when plotted as shown in Figure 14–20. The term *isotherm* refers to a plot at constant temperature. The number of moles, grams, or milliliters x of gas adsorbed on m grams of adsorbent at STP (standard temperature and pressure) is plotted on the vertical axis against the equilibrium pressure of the gas in mm Hg on the horizontal axis, as seen in Figure 14–20a.

One method of obtaining adsorption data is by the use of an apparatus similar to that shown in Figure 14–21, which consists essentially of a balance contained within a vacuum system. The solid, previously degassed, is placed on the pan, and known amounts of gas are allowed to enter. The increase in weight at the corresponding equilibrium gas pressures is recorded. This may be achieved by noting the extension of a calibrated quartz spring used to suspend the pan containing the sample. The data are then used to construct an isotherm based on one or more of the following equations.

Freundlich[27] suggested a relationship, the *Freundlich isotherm*,

$$y = \frac{x}{m} = kp^{1/n} \qquad (14\text{--}49)$$

in which y is the mass of gas x adsorbed per unit mass m of adsorbent, and k and n are constants that can be evaluated from the results of the experiment. The equation is handled more conveniently when written in the logarithmic form,

$$\log \frac{x}{m} = \log k + \frac{1}{n} \log p \qquad (14\text{--}50)$$

which yields a straight line when plotted as seen in Figure 14–20b. The constant, $\log k$, is the intercept on the ordinate, and $1/n$ is the slope of the line.

Langmuir[28] developed an equation based on the theory that the molecules or atoms of gas are adsorbed on active sites of the solid to form a layer one molecule thick (monolayer). The fraction of centers occupied by gas molecules at pressure p is represented by θ, and the fraction of sites not occupied is $1 - \theta$. The rate r_1 of adsorption or condensation of gas molecules on the surface is proportional to the unoccupied spots $1 - \theta$ and to the pressure p, or

$$r_1 = k_1(1 - \theta)p \qquad (14\text{--}51)$$

The rate r_2 of evaporation of molecules bound on the surface is proportional to the fraction of surface occupied, θ, or

$$r_2 = k_2\theta \qquad (14\text{--}52)$$

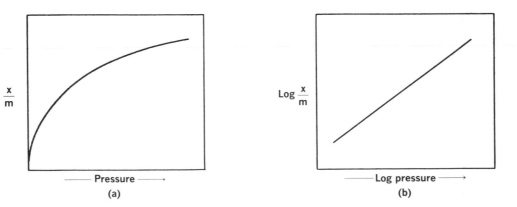

Fig. 14–20. Adsorption isotherms for a gas on a solid. (*a*) Amount x of gas adsorbed per unit mass m of adsorbent plotted against the equilibrium pressure. (*b*) Log of the amount of gas adsorbed per unit mass of adsorbent plotted against the log of the pressure.

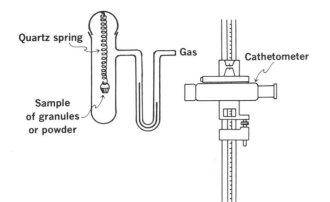

Fig. 14-21. Schematic of apparatus used to measure adsorption of gases on solids.

and at equilibrium $r_1 = r_2$ or

$$k_1(1 - \theta)p = k_2\theta \qquad (14-53)$$

By rearrangement, we obtain

$$\theta = \frac{k_1 p}{k_2 + k_1 p} = \frac{(k_1/k_2)p}{1 + (k_1/k_2)p} \qquad (14-54)$$

We can replace k_1/k_2 by b and θ by y/y_m, in which y is the mass of gas adsorbed per gram of adsorbent at pressure p and at constant temperature, and y_m is the mass of gas that 1 gram of the adsorbent can adsorb when the monolayer is complete. Inserting these terms into equation (14-54) produces the formula

$$y = \frac{y_m b p}{1 + bp} \qquad (14-55)$$

which is known as the *Langmuir isotherm*. By inverting equation (14-55) and multiplying through by p, it may be written for plotting as

$$\frac{p}{y} = \frac{1}{by_m} + \frac{p}{y_m} \qquad (14-56)$$

A plot of p/y against p should yield a straight line, and y_m and b can be obtained from the slope and intercept.

Equations (14-49), (14-50), (14-55), and (14-56) are adequate for the description of curves only of the type shown in Figure 14-20a. This is known as the Type I isotherm. Extensive experimentation, however,

has shown that there are four other types of isotherms, as seen in Figure 14-22, that are not described by these equations. Type II isotherms are sigmoidal in shape and occur when gases undergo physical adsorption onto nonporous solids to form a monolayer followed by multilayer formation. The first inflection point represents the formation of a monolayer; the continued adsorption with increasing pressure indicates subsequent multilayer formation. Type II isotherms are best described by an expression derived by Brunauer, Emmett, and Teller and termed for convenience the *BET equation*. This equation may be written as

$$\frac{p}{y(p_0 - p)} = \frac{1}{y_m b} + \frac{b - 1}{y_m b} \frac{p}{p_0} \qquad (14-57)$$

in which p is the pressure of the adsorbate in mm Hg at which the mass y of vapor per gram of adsorbent is adsorbed, p_0 is the vapor pressure when the adsorbent is saturated with adsorbate vapor, y_m is the quantity of vapor adsorbed per unit mass of adsorbent when the surface is covered with a monomolecular layer, and b is a constant proportional to the difference between the heat of adsorption of the gas in the first layer and the latent heat of condensation of successive layers. The saturated vapor pressure p_0 is obtained by bringing excess adsorbate in contact with the adsorbent. For the case of simple monolayer adsorption, the BET equation reduces to the Langmuir isotherm.

Isotherms of the shape shown as IV in Figure 14-22 are typical of adsorption onto porous solids. The first point of inflection, when extrapolated to zero pressure, again represents the amount of gas required to form a monolayer on the surface of the solid. Multilayer formation and condensation within the pores of the solid are thought to be responsible for the further adsorption shown, which reaches a limiting value before the saturation vapor pressure, p_0 is attained. Type III and Type V isotherms are produced in a relatively few instances in which the heat of adsorption of the gas in the first layer is *less* than the latent heat of condensation of successive layers. As with Type IV isotherms, those of Type V show capillary condensation, and adsorption reaches a limiting value before p_0 is attained. The Type II isotherm results when b is greater than 2.0 and Type III when b is smaller than 2.0 in the

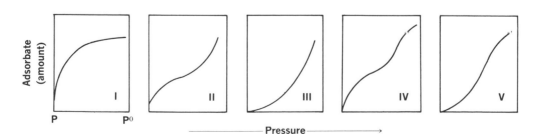

Fig. 14-22. Various types of adsorption isotherms.

BET expression, equation (14–57). Types IV and V frequently involve hysteresis and appear as shown in Figures 14–23 and 14–24, respectively.

The total surface area of the solid can be determined from those isotherms in which formation of a monolayer can be detected, that is, Types I, II, and IV. This information is obtained by multiplying the total number of molecules in the volume of gas adsorbed by the cross-sectional area of each molecule. The surface area per unit weight of adsorbent, known as the *specific surface*, is important in pharmacy since the dissolution rates of drug particles depend, in part, on their surface area (see p. 331). Other techniques for determining specific surface are discussed in Chapter 16.

The Solid–Liquid Interface. Drugs such as dyes, alkaloids, fatty acids, and even inorganic acids and bases may be absorbed from solution onto solids such as charcoal and alumina. The adsorption of solute molecules from solution may be treated in a manner analogous to the adsorption of molecules at the solid–gas interface. Isotherms, which fit one or more of the equations mentioned previously, may be obtained by substituting solute concentration for the vapor pressure term used for solid–gas systems. For example, the adsorption of strychnine, atropine, and quinine from aqueous solutions by six different clays[29] was capable of being expressed by the Langmuir equation in the form

$$\frac{c}{y} = \frac{1}{b y_m} + \frac{c}{y_m} \qquad (14\text{–}58)$$

in which c is the equilibrium concentration in milligrams of alkaloidal base per 100 mL of solution, y is the amount of alkaloidal base x in milligrams adsorbed per gram m of clay (i.e., $y = x/m$), and b and y_m are constants defined earlier. In later studies, Barr and

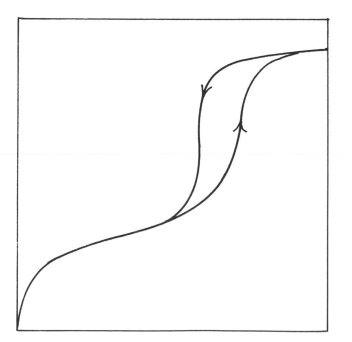

Fig. 14–23. Type IV isotherm showing hysteresis.

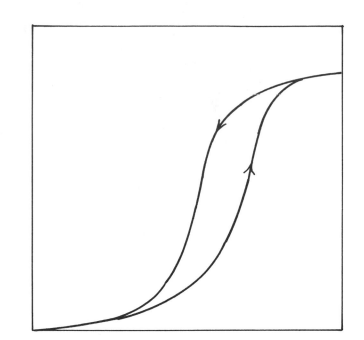

Fig. 14–24. Type V isotherm showing hysteresis.

Arnista[30] investigated the adsorption of diphtheria toxin and several bacteria by various clays. They concluded that attapulgite, a hydrous magnesium aluminum silicate, was superior to kaolin as an intestinal adsorbent. The results of the adsorption of strychnine on activated attapulgite, halloysite (similar to kaolinite) and kaolin, all washed with gastric juice, are shown in Figure 14–25.

The smaller the slope, the better the adsorption. Thus, it can be calculated from Figure 14–25 that an equilibrium concentration of, say, 400 mg strychnine/ 100 mL of solution, x/m for the three adsorbents is approximately 40, 20, and 6.7 mg/g for attapulgite, halloysite, and kaolin, respectively. When an orally administered drug causes gastrointestinal disturbances, commercial adsorbent, antacid, or antidiarrheal preparations are often taken by the patient, and these preparations may interact with the drug to reduce its bioabsorption. The absorption of quinidine salts (an antiarrhythmic agent), for example, is impaired by combining with kaolin, pectin, montmorillonite, and similar adsorbents. Moustafa et al.[31] found that the adsorption of quinidine sulfate by antacid and antidiarrheal preparations, Kaopectate, Simeco, magnesium trisilicate, and bismuth subnitrate, were well expressed by both Freundlich and Langmuir adsorption isotherms.

Nikolakakis and Newton[32] studied the solid–solid adsorption of a fine cohesive powder onto the surface of coarse free-flowing particles to form what is called an "ordered" mixture. These systems provide very homogeneous mixtures of powders ordinarily having good physical stability. Examples of "ordered" mixtures are dry blends of sucrose and antibiotics that can be reconstituted with water to provide antibiotic syrup formulations. Sorbitol can replace sucrose to prepare

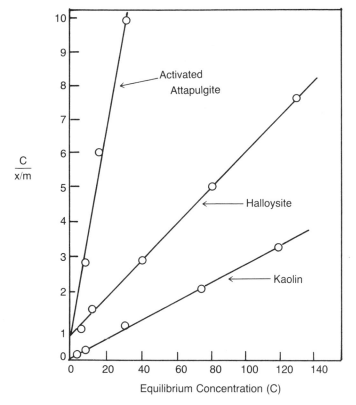

Fig. 14–25. Adsorption of strychnine on various clays. (Modified from M. Barr and S. Arnista, J. Am. Pharm. Assoc., Sci. Ed. **46**, 486, 488, 1957.)

sucrose-free formulations for diabetic patients. During blending, a fine powder of an antibiotic is adsorbed onto the surface of coarse particles of sorbitol. Nikolakakis and Newton obtained an apparent Langmuir or Type I isotherm when the weight of drug adsorbed per unit weight of sorbitol (x/m) was plotted against the concentration c of nonadsorbed drug at equilibrium. Thus, using the linear form, equation (14–58), the b and y_m values can be computed. The y_m value is the amount of antibiotic per unit weight of sorbitol required to form a monolayer on the surface of sorbitol particles. This can be considered as a measure of the adsorption capacity or number of binding sites of sorbitol for the antibiotic. The quantity b is an empirical affinity or binding constant that is given thermodynamic significance by some workers (see Hiemenz,[4] pp. 398–407).

Example 14–13. The values of c/y against c for the solid–solid adsorption of cephalexin monohydrate onto sorbitol are

c (% (w/w))*	5	10	15	20
c/y (%(w/w)) (g (adsorbate)/g (adsorbent))	54.85	84.5	114.15	143.8

Calculate b and y_m.

*Note that we express c as percent w/w on both the x- and the y axes. We express $y = (x/m)$ as gram (adsorbate)/gram (adsorbent), which is dimensionless. Therefore, the units on c/y on the x/axis are simply, %(w/w). Like y, y_m is dimensionless and b has the units, $1/\%$(w/w).

Using a regression analysis of c/y (y-axis) against c (x-axis), the equation is $c/y = 25.2 + 5.93c$.

$$\text{Slope} = \frac{1}{y_m} = 5.93; \qquad y_m = 0.169 \text{ g/g (dimensionless)}$$

$$\text{Intercept} = \frac{1}{by_m} = 25.2 \text{ \%(w/w)};$$

$$b = \frac{1}{25.2 \text{ \%(w/w)} \times 0.169 \text{ g/g}} = 0.235 \text{ \%(w/w)}^{-1}$$

Activated Charcoal. In an investigation of the adsorption of drugs on activated charcoal and its effects on the bioabsorption of drugs in man, Tsuchiya and Levy[33] concluded that reasonable in vivo predictions could be made from in vitro studies concerning the antidotal effectiveness of activated charcoal.

Activated charcoal is used as an antidote in poisonings by sulfonylureas such as tolbutamide, acetohexamide, and other drug and nondrug compounds. Contrary to earlier reports, Kannisto and Neuvonen[34] reported that charcoal effectively adsorbs sulfonylureas and can prevent their gastrointestinal absorption and subsequent toxicity in cases of overdose. The data were analyzed by the authors using the Langmuir adsorption isotherm.

In large overdosage, the analgesic acetaminophen (paracetamol) may cause liver damage, renal failure, and death owing to hepatotoxicity and sometimes renal tubular necrosis (15 grams may be fatal). Activated charcoal has been used to adsorb acetaminophen, and acetylcysteine to neutralize the toxic metabolites that deplete hepatic glutathione. However, there has been concern that activated charcoal will absorb the acetylcysteine as well as the acetaminophen and reduce or nullify the effectiveness of acetylcysteine in preventing liver damage and kidney failure. Rybolt et al.[35] have shown, however, that acetylcysteine is adsorbed by charcoal in sufficiently small amounts that the concurrent use of acetylcysteine and activated charcoal is a useful treatment for acetaminophen poisoning.

The adsorption of drugs by activated charcoal not only prevents bioabsorption from the gastrointestinal tract but also may increase the diffusion of the drug from the tissues into the gastrointestinal tract and elimination from the body by a process called *gastrointestinal dialysis*. In this process the adsorbing charcoal establishes a gradient between the systemic circulation in the body and the fluids in the gastrointestinal tract.[36] A rather thorough list of references to the systemic removal of drugs by charcoal adsorption is given in the 1988 paper by Huang and Tzou.[36]

Gessner and Hasan[37] studied the adsorption of solutes from aqueous solution onto activated charcoal. The adsorption data gave a good fit to the Freundlich isotherm and a poor fit to the Langmuir isotherm, even for published data that were considered earlier to adhere well to the Langmuir isotherm. Furthermore, the Freundlich isotherm accounted better for the effectiveness of activated charcoal to serve as an in vivo antidote against drug overdosing and poisoning.

Kleeman and Bailey[38] developed an in vitro approach for quantitatively ranking the affinity of drugs, toxicants, and suspended materials used in the treatment of public water supplies, to activated charcoal using high-performance liquid chromatography as the analytic tool. The authors provide an excellent review of the literature.

The adsorption of phenobarbital from simulated intestinal and gastric fluids by two activated charcoals of different pore size and specific surface area (pp. 440, 393) was investigated by Wurster et al.,[39] fitting the data to the linearized Langmuir expression (see equation [14-58]) and to a least-squares regression equation. A new activated charcoal with a specific surface of nearly 3000 m^2/g was found to adsorb about three times as much phenobarbital as the charcoal with a specific surface of 1500 m^2/g. It was concluded that the poorer adsorption by the older charcoal occurred because the site spacings on its surface were not sufficient for optimum arrangement of the phenobarbital molecules.

Hajratwala[40] referred to adsorption of drugs on charcoal, talc, and other adsorbents and discussed the manner of obtaining Langmuir and Freundlich constants from adsorption isotherms.

Wetting. Adsorption at solid surfaces is involved in the phenomena of wetting and detergency.

A *wetting agent* is a surfactant that, when dissolved in water, lowers the advancing contact angle and aids in displacing an air phase at the surface and replacing it with a liquid phase. Examples of the application of wetting to pharmacy and medicine include the displacement of air from the surface of sulfur, charcoal, and other powders for the purpose of dispersing these drugs in liquid vehicles; the displacement of air from the matrix of cotton pads and bandages so that medicinal solutions may be absorbed for application to various body areas; the displacement of dirt and debris by the use of detergents in the washing of wounds; and the application of medicinal lotions and sprays to the surface of the skin and mucous membranes.

The most important action of a wetting agent is to lower the *contact angle* between the surface and the wetting liquid. The contact angle is the angle between a liquid droplet and the surface over which it spreads. As shown in Figure 14-26, the contact angle between a liquid and a solid may be 0°, signifying complete wetting, or it may approach 180°, at which wetting is insignificant. The contact angle may also have any value between these limits, as illustrated in the sketches. At equilibrium, the surface and interfacial tensions can be resolved into

$$\gamma_s = \gamma_{SL} + \gamma_L \cos \theta \qquad (14\text{-}59)$$

which is known as Young's equation.

When γ_s of equation (14-59) is substituted into equation (14-19), we have

$$S = \gamma_L (\cos \theta - 1) \qquad (14\text{-}60)$$

and combining equation (14-59) with equation (14-16) results in

$$W_a = W_{SL} = \gamma_L (1 + \cos \theta) \qquad (14\text{-}61)$$

which is an alternative form of Young's equation. Equations (14-60) and (14-61) are useful expressions since they do not include γ_S or γ_{SL}, neither of which can be easily or accurately measured. The contact angle between a water droplet and a greasy surface results when the applied liquid, water, wets the greasy surface incompletely. When a drop of water is placed on a scrupulously clean glass surface, it spreads spontaneously and no contact angle exists. This result can be described by assigning to water a high spreading coefficient on clean glass, or by stating that the contact angle between water and glass is zero. If the appropriate wetting agent is added to water, the solution will spread spontaneously on a greasy surface. For a wetting agent to function efficiently, in other words, to exhibit a low contact angle, it should have an HLB of about 6 to 9 (see p. 371).

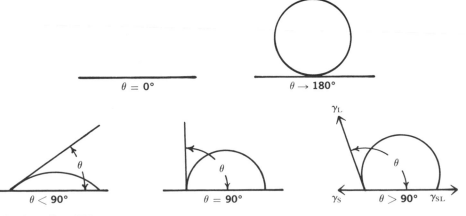

Fig. 14-26. Contact angles from 0° to 180°.

Example 14–14. Wettability of tablet surfaces influences disintegration and dissolution, and the subsequent release of the active ingredient(s) from the tablet.

A *tablet binder* is a material that contributes cohesiveness to a tablet so that the tablet remains intact after compression. The influence of tablet binders on wettability of acetaminophen tablets was studied by Esezobo et al.[41] The contact angle of water on the acetaminophen tablets, the surface tension of the liquid, and the disintegration time of the tablets are found in the following table. The water on the tablet surface is saturated with the basic formulation ingredients excluding the binder. The concentration of the tablet binders, povidone (polyvinylpyrrolidone, PVP), gelatin, and tapioca, is constant at 5% w/w.

Binder	$\gamma (Nm^{-1})$*	Cos θ	t (min)
Povidone (PVP)	71.23	0.7455	17.0
Gelatin	71.23	0.7230	23.5
Tapioca	71.33	0.7570	2.0

*The surface tension γ is given in Jm^{-1} or newtons, the SI force unit, divided by meters. In the cgs system γ is expressed in the force unit of dyne divided by cm, or in erg/cm^2.

Using equations (14–60) and (14–61), compute S, the spreading coefficient, and W_{SL}, the work of adhesion, for water on the tablet surface, comparing the influence of the three binders in the formulation. Observe the disintegration times found in the table and use them to refute or corroborate the S and W_{SL} results.

	Spreading Coefficient $S = \gamma (\cos \theta - 1)$
PVP	$S = 71.23 (0.7455 - 1) = -18.13$
Gelatin	$S = 71.23 (0.7230 - 1) = -19.73$
Tapioca	$S = 71.33 (0.7570 - 1) = -17.33$

	Work of Adhesion $W_{SL} = \gamma (1 + \cos \theta)$
PVP	$W_{SL} = 71.23 (1 + 0.7455) = 124.33$ Nm^{-1}
Gelatin	$W_{SL} = 71.23 (1 + 0.7230) = 122.73$ Nm^{-1}
Tapioca	$W_{SL} = 71.33 (1 + 0.7570) = 125.33$ Nm^{-1}

The spreading coefficient is negative, but the values are small. Tapioca shows the smallest negative value, $S = -17.33$, followed by PVP and finally gelatin. These results agree with the work of adhesion, tapioca > PVP > gelatin. The higher the work of adhesion the stronger is the bond between water and the tablet surface and the better is the wetting.

From the table, we observe the tablet disintegration times to be in the order tapioca < PVP < gelatin, which agrees qualitatively with the S and W_{SL} values. That is, the better the wetting, reflected in a larger work of adhesion and a smaller negative spreading coefficient, the shorter is the tablet disintegration time. Other factors, such as tablet porosity, which were not considered in the study, cause the relationship to be only qualitative.

Zisman and his associates[42] found that when the cosine of the contact angle, cos θ, was plotted versus the surface tension for a homologous series of liquids spread on a surface such as Teflon (polytetrafluoroethylene), a straight line resulted. The line may be extrapolated to cos θ = 1; that is, to a contact angle of zero, signifying complete wetting. The surface tension at cos θ = 1 was given the term *critical surface tension*

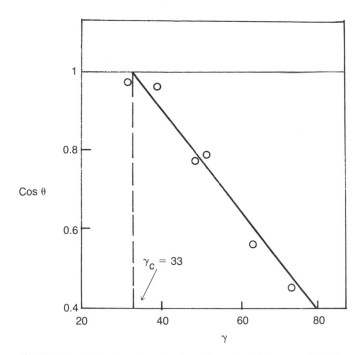

Fig. 14–27. Critical surface tension (Zisman) plot for a model skin. (From J. C. Charkoudian, J. Soc. Cosmet. Chem. **39**, 225, 1988, reproduced with permission of the copyright owner.)

and the symbol γ_c. Various series of liquids on a given solid surface were all found to have about the same value of γ_c, as observed in Figure 14–27. Zisman concluded that γ_c was characteristic for each solid, Teflon, for example, having a value of about 18 erg/cm^2. Since the surface of Teflon consists of —CF_2— groups, Zisman reasoned that all surfaces of this nature would have critical surface tensions of about 18 erg/cm^2, and any liquid with a surface tension less than 18 erg/cm^2 would wet a surface composed of —CF_2— groups.[43,44]

Example 14–15. Charkoudian[45] designed a model skin surface with physical and chemical properties approximating those reported for human skin. The model skin consisted of a protein (cross-linked gelatin), a synthetic lipid-like substance, and water, with the protein and lipid in a ratio of 3 to 1. To further characterize the artificial skin, the surface tensions of several liquids and their contact angles on the model skin surface were determined at 20° C, as given in the following table.

Plot the cos θ versus γ and compute the critical surface tension γ_c for complete wetting of the artificial skin surface. The values of γ_c for in vivo human skin are about 26 to 28 dyne/cm.

From the results obtained, which liquid in the table below would be expected to best wet the model skin surface?

The plot is shown in Figure 14–27. Although the liquids in the table do not constitute a homologous series, they appear to fit nicely the Zisman principle, producing a straight line that extrapolates to cos θ corresponding to a critical surface tension of $\gamma_c = 33$ dyne/cm.

Mineral oil, with a surface tension of 31.9 dyne/cm, most closely approximates the critical surface tension $\gamma_c = 33$ dyne/cm of the

Liquid	Water	Glycerin	Diiodomethane	Ethylene glycol	Benzyl alcohol	Mineral oil
γ (dyne/cm)	72.8	63.4	50.8	48.3	39.2	31.9
cos θ	0.45	0.56	0.79	0.77	0.96	0.97

model skin surface. For a more exact calculation of γ_c, least-squares linear regression analysis may be applied to yield

$$\cos \theta = -0.0137 \, \gamma + 1.450, \quad r^2 = 0.972$$

For the specific value of $\cos \theta = 1$, we obtain $\gamma_c = 33.0$ dyne/cm. It is noted that the critical surface tension γ_c for the artificial skin used in this study is somewhat higher ($\gamma_c = 33.0$ dyne/cm) than values reported elsewhere in the literature for human skin ($\gamma_c = 26-28$ dyne/cm). According to the author, this is due in part to the absence of sweat and sebaceous secretions, which lower the γ_c value of viable human skin.

Although one frequently desires to determine the relative efficiencies of wetting agents, it is difficult to measure the contact angle. Nor are spreading coefficients usually available, since no convenient method is known for directly measuring the surface tension of a solid surface. As a result of these difficulties, empiric tests are used in industry, one of the best known wetting tests being that of Draves. The *Draves test* involves measuring the time for a weighted skein of cotton yarn to sink through the wetting solution contained in a 500-mL graduate. No method has yet been suggested for estimating the ability of a wetting agent to promote spreading of a lotion on the surface of the skin, and the application properties of such products are ordinarily determined by subjective evaluation. However, see *Problems 14–11* and *14–14*.

Detergents are surfactants that are used for the removal of dirt. Detergency is a complex process involving the removal of foreign matter from surfaces. The process includes many of the actions characteristic of specific surfactants: initial wetting of the dirt and of the surface to be cleaned; deflocculation and suspension, emulsification or solubilization of the dirt particles; and sometimes foaming of the agent for entrainment and washing away of the particles. Since the detergent must possess a combination of properties; its efficiency is best ascertained by actual tests with the material to be cleaned.

Other dispersion stabilizers, including deflocculating, suspending, and emulsifying agents, are considered in Chapter 18.

APPLICATIONS OF SURFACE ACTIVE AGENTS

In addition to the use of surfactants as emulsifying agents, detergents, wetting agents, and solubilizing agents, they find application as antibacterial and other protective agents and as aids to the absorption of drugs in the body.

A surfactant may affect the activity of a drug or may itself exert drug action. As an example of the first case, the penetration of hexylresorcinol into the pinworm *Ascaris* is increased by the presence of a low concentration of surfactant. This potentiation of activity is due to a reduction in interfacial tension between the liquid phase and the cell wall of the organism. As a result, the adsorption and spreading of hexylresorcinol over the surface of the organism is facilitated. When the concentration of surface-active agent present exceeds that required to form micelles, however, the rate of penetration of the anthelmintic decreases nearly to zero. This is because the drug is now partitioned between the micelles and the aqueous phase, resulting in a reduction in the effective concentration. Quaternary ammonium compounds are examples of surface-active agents that in themselves possess antibacterial activity. This may depend in part on interfacial phenomena, but other factors are also important. The agents are adsorbed on the cell surface and supposedly bring about destruction by increasing the permeability or "leakiness" of the lipid cell membrane. Death then occurs through a loss of essential materials from the cell. Both gram-negative and gram-positive organisms are susceptible to the action of the cationic quaternary compounds, whereas gram-positive organisms are attacked more easily by anionic agents than are gram-negative bacteria. Nonionic surfactants are least effective as antibacterial agents. In fact, they often aid rather than inhibit the growth of bacteria, presumably by providing long-chain fatty acids in a form that is easily metabolized by the organism.

Miyamoto et al.[46] studied the effects of surfactants and bile salts on the gastrointestinal absorption of antibiotics using an in situ rat gut perfusion technique. Polyoxyethylene lauryl ether reduced the absorption of propicillin in the stomach and increased it in the small intestine. It is a well-known fact that some surfactants increase the rate of intestinal absorption, while others decrease it. Some of these effects may result from alteration of the membrane by the surfactant. The effects of surfactants on the solubility of drugs and their bioabsorption has been reviewed by Mulley[47] and by Gibaldi and Feldman.[48]

Foams and Antifoaming Agents. Any solutions containing surface-active materials produce stable foams when mixed intimately with air. A foam is a relatively stable structure consisting of air pockets enclosed within thin films of liquid, the gas-in-liquid dispersion being stabilized by a *foaming agent*. The foam dissipates as the liquid drains away from the area surrounding the air globules, and the film finally collapses. *Agents* such as alcohol, ether, castor oil, and some surfactants may be used to break the foam and are known as *antifoaming agents*. Foams are sometimes useful in pharmacy but are usually a nuisance and are prevented or destroyed when possible. The undesirable foaming of solubilized liquid preparations poses a problem in formulation.

ELECTRIC PROPERTIES OF INTERFACES

This section deals with some of the principles involved with surfaces that are charged in relation to their surrounding liquid environment. Discussion of the applications arising from this phenomenon will be reserved for the chapters dealing with colloidal systems (Chapter 15) and suspensions (Chapter 18).

Particles dispersed in liquid media may become

charged mainly in one of two ways. The first involves the selective adsorption of a particular ionic species present in solution. This may be an ion added to the solution or, in the case of pure water, it may be the hydronium or hydroxyl ion. The majority of particles dispersed in water acquire a negative charge due to preferential adsorption of the hydroxyl ion. Secondly, charges on particles arise from ionization of groups (such as COOH) that may be situated at the surface of the particle. In these cases, the charge is a function of pK and pH. A third, less common, origin for the charge on a particle surface is thought to arise when there is a difference in dielectric constant between the particle and its dispersion medium.

The Electric Double Layer. Consider a solid surface in contact with a polar solution containing ions, for example, an aqueous solution of an electrolyte. Further, let us suppose that some of the cations are adsorbed onto the surface, giving it a positive charge. Remaining in solution are the rest of the cations plus the total number of anions added. These anions are attracted to the positively charged surface by electric forces that also serve to repel the approach of any further cations once the initial adsorption is complete. In addition to these electric forces, thermal motion tends to produce an equal distribution of all the ions in solution. As a result, an equilibrium situation is set up in which *some* of the excess anions approach the surface, while the remainder are distributed in decreasing amounts as one proceeds away from the charged surface. At a particular distance from the surface, the concentration of anions and cations are equal, that is, conditions of electric neutrality prevail. It is important to remember that the system *as a whole* is electrically neutral, even though there are regions of unequal distribution of anions and cations.

Such a situation is shown in Figure 14–28, where *aa'* is the surface of the solid. The adsorbed ions that gave the surface its positive charge are referred to as the *potential-determining ions.* Immediately adjacent to this surface layer is a region of tightly bound solvent molecules, together with some negative ions, also tightly bound to the surface. The limit of this region is given by the line *bb'* in Figure 14–28. These ions, having a charge opposite to the potential-determining

ions, are known as *counterions* or *gegenions.* The degree of attraction of the solvent molecules and counterions is such that if the surface is moved relative to the liquid, the shear plane is *bb'* rather than *aa'*, the true surface. In the region bounded by the lines *bb'* and *cc'*, there is an excess of negative ions. The potential at *bb'* is still positive, since, as previously mentioned, there are fewer anions in the tightly bound layer than cations adsorbed onto the surface of the solid. Beyond *cc'*, the distribution of ions is uniform and electric neutrality is obtained.

Thus, the electric distribution at the interface is equivalent to a double layer of charge, the first layer (extending from *aa'* to *bb'*) tightly bound, and a second layer (from *bb'* to *cc'*) that is more diffuse. The so-called diffuse double layer therefore extends from *aa'* to *cc'*.

Two situations other than that represented by Figure 14–28 are possible. (1) If the counterions in the tightly bound, solvated layer equal the positive charge on the solid surface, then electric neutrality occurs at the plane *bb'* rather than *cc'*. (2) Should the total charge of the counterions in the region *aa'–bb'* exceed the charge due to the potential-determining ions, then the net charge at *bb'* will be negative, rather than less positive as shown in Figure 14–28. This means that, in this instance, for electric neutrality to be obtained at *cc'*, an excess of positive ions must be present in the region *bb'–cc'*.

The student should appreciate that if the potential-determining ion is negative, the arguments just given still apply, although now positive ions will be present in the tightly bound layer.

Nernst and Zeta Potentials. The changes in potential with distance from the surface for the various situations discussed in the previous section may be represented as shown in Figure 14–29. The potential at the solid surface *aa'*, due to the potential-determining ion, is the *electrothermodynamic (Nernst) potential,* E, and is defined as the difference in potential between the actual surface and the electroneutral region of the solution. The potential located at the shear plane *bb'* is known as the *electrokinetic,* or *zeta, potential,* ζ. The zeta potential is defined as the difference in potential between the surface of the tightly bound layer (shear plane) and the electroneutral region of the solution. As shown in Figure 14–29, the potential drops off rapidly initially, followed by a more gradual decrease as the distance from the surface increases. This is because the counterions close to the surface act as a screen that reduces the electrostatic attraction between the charged surface and those counterions further away from the surface.

Zeta potential has practical application in the stability of systems containing dispersed particles since this potential, rather than the Nernst potential, governs the degree of repulsion between adjacent, similarly charged, dispersed particles. If the zeta potential is reduced below a certain value (which depends on the particular system being used), the attractive forces

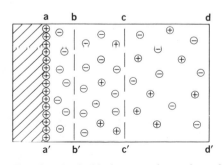

Fig. 14–28. The electric double layer at the surface of separation between two phases, showing distribution of ions. The system as a whole is electrically neutral.

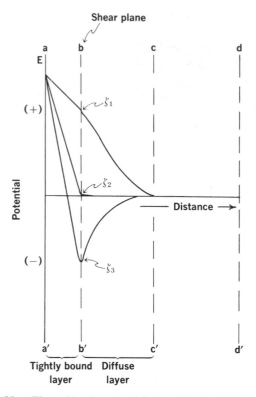

Fig. 14–29. Electrokinetic potential at solid–liquid boundaries. Curves are shown for three cases characteristic of the ions or molecules in the liquid phase. Note that although E is the same in all three cases, the zeta potentials are positive (ζ_1), zero (ζ_2), and negative (ζ_3).

exceed the repulsive forces, and the particles come together. This phenomenon is known as *flocculation* and is discussed in the chapters dealing with colloidal and coarse dispersions (see Chapters 15 and 18).

Effect of Electrolytes. As the concentration of electrolyte present in the system is increased, the screening effect of the counterions is also increased. As a result, the potential falls off more rapidly with distance because the thickness of the double layer shrinks. A similar situation occurs when the valency of the counterion is increased while the total concentration of electrolyte is held constant. The overall effect frequently causes a reduction in zeta potential.

References and Notes

1. S. I. Said, Med. Clin. North Am. **51**, 391, 1967.
2. A. Felmeister, J. Pharm. Sci. **61**, 151, 1972.
3. P. Seeman, Pharmacol. Rev. **24**, 583, 1972.
4. P. C. Hiemenz, *Principles of Colloid and Surface Chemistry*, 2nd Edition, Dekker, New York, 1986.
5. A. W. Adamson, *Physical Chemistry of Surfaces*, 4th Edition, Wiley, New York, 1982, Chapter 2.
6. W. D. Harkins and A. E. Alexander, in *Physical Methods of Organic Chemistry*, Vol. 1, A. Weissberger, Ed., 3rd Edition, Interscience, New York, 1959, Chapter 14.
7. W. Drost-Hansen, in *Chemistry and Physics of Interfaces*, Am. Chem. Soc., Washington, D.C., 1965, Chapters 2 and 3.
8. W. D. Harkins and H. F. Jordan, J. Am. Chem. Soc. **52**, 1751, 1930; H. L. Cupples, J. Phys. Chem. **51**, 1341, 1947.
9. H. H. Zuidema and G. W. Waters, Ind. Eng. Chem. (Anal.) **13**, 312, 1941.
10. D. J. Shaw, *Introduction to Colloid and Surface Chemistry*, 2nd Edition, Butterworths, Boston, 1970, p. 62.
11. P. Becher, J. Soc. Cosmetic Chem. **11**, 325, 1960.
12. W. C. Griffin, J. Soc. Cosmetic Chem. **1**, 311, 1949.
13. I. Bonadeo, *Cosmética, Ciencia y Technología*, Editorial Ciencia, Madrid, 1988, p. 123.
14. H. L. Greenwald, G. L. Brown and M. N. Fineman, Anal. Chem. **28**, 1693, 1956; P. Becher, *Emulsions: Theory and Practice*, 2nd Editions, Reinhold, New York, 1965.
15. H. Schott, J. Pharm. Sci. **69**, 852, 1980.
16. J. W. McBain and R. C. Swain, Proc. Royal Soc. **A154**, 608, 1936.
17. J. K. Dixon, A. J. Weith, A. A. Argyle and D. J. Salby, Nature, **163**, 845, 1949.
18. C. H. Giles and S. D. Forrester, *Chemistry and Industry*, November 8, 1969; January 17, 1970; January 9, 1971.
19. I. Langmuir, J. Am. Chem. Soc. **40**, 1361, 1918.
20. D. L. Schwinke, M. G. Ganesan and N. D. Weiner, J. Pharm. Sci. **72**, 244, 1983.
21. N. K. Adam, *The Physics and Chemistry of Surfaces*, Oxford University Press, London, 1941, Chapter 2.
22. W. D. Harkins, *The Physical Chemistry of Surface Films*, Reinhold, New York, 1952, p. 119.
23. H. Sobotka, *Monomolecular Layers*, Am. Assoc. Adv. Sci. Washington, D.C., 1954.
24. G. L. Gaines, Jr., *Insoluble Monolayers at Gas-Liquid Interfaces*, Interscience, New York, 1966.
25. W. Rettig and F. Kuschel, Colloid and Polym. Sci. **267**, 151, 1989.
26. A. W. Adamson, *Physical Chemistry of Surfaces*, 1st Edition, 1960, p. 231.
27. H. Freundlich, *Colloid and Capillary Chemistry*, Methuen, London, 1926.
28. I. Langmuir, J. Am. Chem. Soc. **39**, 1855, 1917.
29. N. Evcim and M. Barr, J. Am. Pharm. Assoc., Sci. Ed. **44**, 570, 1955.
30. M. Barr and S. Arnista, J. Am. Pharm. Assoc., Sci. Ed. **46**, 486, 490, 493, 1957.
31. M. A. Moustafa, H. I. Al-Shora, M. Gaber and M. W. Gouda, Int. J. Pharm. **34**, 207, 1987.
32. I. Nikolakakis and J. M. Newton, J. Pharm. Pharmacol. **41**, 145, 1989.
33. T. Tsuchiya and G. Levy, J. Pharm. Sci. **61**, 586, 624, 1972.
34. H. Kannisto and P. J. Neuvonen, J. Pharm. Sci. **73**, 253, 1984.
35. T. R. Rybolt, D. E. Burrell, J. M. Shults and A. K. Kelly, J. Pharm. Sci. **75**, 904, 1986.
36. J.-D. Huang and M.-C. Tzou, J. Pharm. Sci. **75**, 923, 1986; J.-D. Huang, ibid. **77**, 959, 1988.
37. P. K. Gessner and M. M. Hasan, J. Pharm Sci. **76**, 319, 707, 1987.
38. W. P. Kleeman and L. C. Bailey, J. Pharm. Sci. **77**, 506, 1988.
39. D. E. Wurster, G. M. Burke, M. J. Berg, P. Veng-Pedersen and D. D. Schottelius, Pharm. Res. **5**, 183, 1988.
40. B. R. Hajratwala, J. Pharm. Sci. **71**, 125, 1982.
41. S. Esezobo, S. Zubair and N. Pilben, J. Pharm. Pharmacol. **41**, 7, 1989.
42. W. Z. Zisman, in *Contact Angle Wettability and Adhesion*, F. M. Fowkes, Editor (Adv. Chem. Ser. No. 43) Washington, D.C., 1964, pp. 1–27; H. W. Fox and W. A. Zisman, J. Colloid Sci. **7**, 428, 1952; E. G. Shafrin and W. A. Zisman, J. Phys. Chem. **64** 519, 1960.
43. A. W. Adamson, *Physical Chemistry of Surfaces*, 4th Edition, Wiley, New York, 1982, pp. 350, 351.
44. D. Attwood and A. T. Florence, *Surfactant Systems*, Chapman and Hall, London, New York, 1983, pp. 32, 33.
45. J. C. Charkoudian, J. Soc. Cosmet. Chem. **39**, 225, 1988.
46. E. Miyamoto, A. Tsuji and T. Yamana, J. Pharm. Sci. **72**, 651, 1983.
47. B. A. Mulley, in *Advances in Pharmaceutical Sciences*, H. S. Bean, A. H. Beckett and J. E. Carless, Eds. Vol. 1. Academic Press, New York, 1964, pp. 87–194.
48. M. Gibaldi and S. Feldman, J. Pharm. Sci. **59**, 579, 1970.
49. P. C. Hiemenz, *Principles of Colloid and Surface Chemistry*, 2nd Edition, Dekker, New York, 1986, p. 296; ibid., 1st Edition, 1977, p. 213.
50. P. C. Hiemenz, *Principles of Colloid and Surface Chemistry*, 2nd Edition, Dekker, New York, 1986, pp. 333–334.
51. A. N. Paruta and J. M. Cross, Am. Perfumer **76**, 43, 1961.
52. C. F. Lerk, A. J. M. Schoonen and J. T. Fell, J. Pharm. Sci. **65**, 843, 1976.
53. K. P. Das and D. K. Chattoraj, J. Colloid Interface Sci. **78**, 422, 1980.
54. Tanford et al., J. Am. Chem. Soc. **77**, 6421, 1955.

55. Z. Korazac, A. Dhathathreyan and D. Möbius, Colloid Polym. Sci. **267**, 722, 1989.
56. E. M. Sellers, V. Khouw and L. Dolman, J. Pharm. Sci. **66**, 1640, 1977.
57. R. J. Sturgeon, C. Flanagan, D. V. Naik and S. G. Schulman, J. Pharm. Sci. **66**, 1346, 1977.
58. O. Al-Gohary, J. Lyal and J. B. Murray, Pharm. Acta Helv. **63**, 13, 1988.
59. W. D. Harkins, *Physical Chemistry of Surface Films*, Reinhold, New York, 1952, pp. 80–83.
60. A. Sharma and E. Ruckenstein, J. Colloid Interface Sci. **133**, 358, 1989.
61. G. Strom, M. Fredrickson and P. Stenius, J. Colloid Interface Sci. **134**, 117, 1990.

Problems*

14–1. Water has an unusually high surface tension, and like other liquids, its surface tension decreases with increasing temperature. What is your explanation for these two phenomena?

Hint: What kind of intermolecular forces do you believe might contribute to these observations?

14–2. You wish to formulate a sunscreen product that lowers surface tension and thus spreads easily on the skin. You choose *p*-aminobenzoic acid, a powerful sunscreen.

(a) Calculate the surface tension of a 12.35 weight percent of *p*-aminobenzoic acid solution in water at 25° C. The DuNoüy tensiometer ring circumference is 12.47 cm and the correction factor β according to Harkins and Jordan is 0.920. The dial reading in dynes was obtained experimentally as 1989.

(b) What agent might you add to improve the spreading qualities of this product?

Answer: **(a)** $\gamma = 73.37$ dyne/cm

14–3. Equation (14–1), page 364, considers γ as a force per unit length (dyne/cm) in the surface, while equation (14–2), page 364, views γ as an energy per unit area (erg/cm^2) of the surface. Show the dimensional equivalency in both cgs and SI units for these two interpretations of the surface tension.

Answer: Check your answer with Hiemenz[19]

14–4. What is the pressure difference ΔP in dyne/cm^2 across a soap bubble formed from the soap solution of *Example 14–1*, page 364? The radius of the soap bubble is 2.50 cm.

Answer: 39.2 dyne/cm^2

14–5. A soap bubble is blown up at the bowl opening of a clay pipe; the pressure of air inside the bubble decreases as the radius of the bubble increases according to the equation

$$\Delta P = \frac{2\gamma}{r}$$

where ΔP is the pressure difference across the soap film, γ is the surface free energy or surface tension of the soap solution, and r is the radius of the bubble. If the soap solution has a surface tension of 3.2 dyne/cm and the radius of the bubble expands to 7.6 cm, what is the pressure difference in dyne/cm^2 across the surface film of the soap bubble? Express the result both in dyne/cm^2 and in atmospheres.

Answer: $\Delta P = 0.84$ dyne/cm^2 or 8.3×10^{-7} atm

14–6. Calculate the surface tension of a 2%(w/v) solution of a wetting agent that has a density of 1.008 g/cm^3 and that rises 6.60 cm in a capillary tube having an inside radius of 0.02 cm.

Answer: 65.2 dyne/cm

14–7. The surface tension of benzene at 20° C is 28.85 dyne/cm. In a capillary apparatus, the liquid rose to a height of 1.832 cm. The density of benzene is 0.8765 g/cm^3 at 20° C. Using the capillary-rise equation, calculate the diameter of the capillary tube. The acceleration of gravity is 981 cm/sec.^2

Answer: 0.073 cm diameter. The answer is not exact since the equation is an approximate one. An iteration procedure is required to

obtain accurate results for the capillary rise problem, as discussed by Hiemenz.[50]

14–8. Water has a surface tension of 71.97 dyne/cm at 25° C, and its density at 25° C is 0.9971 g/cm^3.

(a) How high will the water rise in a very fine capillary tube of radius 0.0023 cm?

(b) If water rises by capillary action only 64 cm in a narrow tube equivalent to a xylem tube in a living plant, how is it possible to lift aqueous nutrients to the top-most leaves in the tall trees in a forest?

Answer: 64.0 cm. The important process is not capillary action but rather appears to be osmosis.

14–9. (a) How high will the liquid carbon tetrachloride rise in a capillary tube of radius 0.015 cm at 20° C? The density of carbon tetrachloride is 1.595 g/cm^3 and its surface tension is 26.99 dyne/cm at 20° C.

(b) Could one use this experiment to estimate the acceleration, g., caused by gravity on the earth?

Answer: **(a)** 2.30 cm

14–10. Pure ethyl alcohol rises 2.48 cm in a capillary rise apparatus at 30° C. The capillary tube has a radius of 0.0230 cm, and the density of ethyl alcohol at 30° C is 0.781 g/cm^3. What is the surface tension of ethyl alcohol at 30° C?

Answer: 21.85 dyne/cm

14–11. (a) Paruta and Cross[51] studied the spreading on water of a number of surfactants (spreading promoters) added to mineral oil as a laboratory test in the design of cosmetic creams and lotions. The surface tension of water at 25° C is ~72.0 dyne/cm. the surface tension of a test lotion consisting of 5 g/dL (5% w/v) solution of sorbitan monooleate in mineral oil was found to be 31.2 dyne/cm and the interfacial tension γ_{it} of the oil–surfactant solution measured against water was 5.7 dyne/cm. Calculate the initial spreading coefficient $S_{initial}$ of the oil–surfactant solution (the oil phase) on water.

(b) What is the significance of the positive spreading coefficient? Could you suggest a better substrate than water to test the spreadability of a cosmetic lotion? See Paruta and Cross for another approach.[51]

Answer: **(a)** the spreading coefficient $S_{initial} = 35.10$ dyne/cm

14–12. The surface tension of an organic liquid is 25 erg/cm^2, the surface tension of water is 72.8 erg/cm^2, and the interfacial tension between the two liquids is 30 erg/cm^2 at 20° C. What is the work of cohesion of the organic liquid, the work of adhesion between the liquid and water, and the initial spreading coefficient of the liquid on the water surface at 20° C?

Answer: $W_c = 50$ erg/cm^2; $W_a = 67.8$ erg/cm^2; $S_{initial} = 17.8$ erg/cm^2

14–13. The surface tension of *n*-heptyl alcohol is 27.0 erg/cm^2, the surface tension of water is 72.8 erg/cm^2, and the interfacial tension between the two liquids is 8.0 erg/cm^2 at 20° C. Calculate W_c, W_a, and $S_{initial}$.

Answer: $W_c = 54$ erg/cm^2; $W_a = 91.8$ erg/cm^2; $S_{initial} = 37.8$ erg/cm^2

14–14. The contact angle θ for a skin lotion when applied to the back of the hand of a number of subjects was found to have an average value of 103° at 24° C. the surface tension γ_L of the lotion measured at 24° C in a capillary rise experiment was 63.2 dyne/cm, or 63.2 mN m^{-1} in SI units (The symbol m stands for both *milli* and *meters;* 63.2 mN m^{-1} is read "63.2 millinewtons per meter.") What is the work of adhesion W_{SL} and the initial spreading coefficient $S_{initial}$ for this lotion on the skin?

Answer: $W_{SL} = 48.98$ erg/cm^2 or 0.049 N/m; $S_{initial} = -77.42$ erg/cm^2 or -0.077 N/m

14–15. Magnesium stearate and lactose are excipients commonly used in tablet formulation. The measured contact angles of water or of a saturated aqueous solution on the surfaces of compacts of these two powders are $\theta = 121°$ and $\theta = 30°$. Their surface tensions (against air) are 72.3 and 71.6 dyne/cm. The surface tension of water (against air) at 20° C is 72.8 dyne/cm.

(a) Compute the interfacial tension between water and each of these compacted powders. You will need equation 14–59.

---

*Problems 14–26 through 14–29 were prepared by B. Hajratwala, Wayne State University, Detroit.

(b) Compute the spreading of water on the solid surfaces. (Data from Lerk et al.[52])

(c) How do you explain the quite different spreading results on these two powder compacts?

Partial Answers: **(a)** Magnesium stearate: $\gamma_{SL} = 109.8$ dyne/cm; lactose: $\gamma_{SL} = 8.55$ dyne/cm; **(b)** for magnesium stearate, $S_{initial} = -110.3$ dyne/cm; for lactose, $S_{initial} = -9.76$ dyne/cm

14–16. p-Toluidine, a yellow liquid used in the manufacture of dyes is only slightly soluble in water. The surface tension of para-toluidine was measured at various concentrations at 25° C (298° K) and the results were plotted. The slope $d\gamma/dc$ of the line at $c = 5 \times 10^{-3}$ g/cm³ was found to be $-32,800$ cm³/sec². Using the Gibb's adsorption equation, compute the excess surface concentration in mole/cm² and in g/cm². The molecular weight of p-toluidine is 107.15 g/mole.

Answer: $\Gamma = 6.6 \times 10^{-9}$ mole/cm²; 7.1×10^{-7} g/cm²

14–17. The surface tension of aminobutyric acid in water at 25° C is given as a function of concentration (weight per cent of aminobutyric acid) in the following table:

Data for *Problem 14–17*

Weight % w/w	4.96	9.34	13.43
γ (dyne/cm)	71.91	71.67	71.40

(a) Plot the data and obtain the slope $\partial\gamma/\partial(\text{wt}\%)$ from the two-point formula or from regression analysis. (If you use regression analysis, the intercept should be close to the surface tension value of water at 25° C, 71.97 dyne/cm.)

(b) Calculate the surface excess (the Gibb's adsorption coefficient Γ) for aminobutyric acid at the surface of water for each of these three concentrations (weight %).

(c) What is the area occupied by each molecule of aminobutyric acid at the water surface?

(d) Regarding your results, do you think that aminobutyric acid acts as a surfactant within this concentration range?

Answers: **(a)** $\partial\gamma/\partial(\text{wt}\%) = -0.06015$ erg cm^{-2} (wt%)$^{-1}$; **(b)** $\Gamma = 1.2 \times 10^{-11}$, 2.27×10^{-11}, and 3.26×10^{-11} mole cm^{-2}; **(c)** the areas per molecule are 1383, 730, and 510 Å²; **(d)** Does aminobutyric acid significantly lower the surface tension of water?

14–18. The adsorption of proteins at the oil–water interfaces are of biologic interest because in cell membranes various proteins attached to polar lipid-bilayer regions control cellular aggregation and cellular growth.

The adsorption of bovine serum albumin (BSA) to a polar peanut oil–water interface varies with ionic strength and pH. At 30° C and ionic strength $\mu = 0.1$, the maximum adsorption (surface excess values) are $\Gamma = 2.54$ mg m^{-2} at pH 5, and $\Gamma = 0.70$ mg m^{-2} at pH 4. The isoelectric point of BSA is near 5.[53] Compute the area per molecule of BSA at the two different pH values and the limiting slope $(d\gamma/d\ln c)$. Why does A, the area per molecule of BSA, differ at these two pH values? *Hint:* Does protein conformation vary with pH? The molecular weight of BSA is about 69,000 daltons. You will need the Gibbs adsorption equation, $\Gamma = -\dfrac{1}{RT}\left(\dfrac{d\gamma}{d\ln c}\right)$, and for the area per molecule, A, you will need the equation $A = 1/(N\Gamma)$, where N is Avogadro's number and Γ is the surface excess. You will want to convert Γ (g/m²) into mole/m² using the molecular weight (g/mole) of BSA.

Answer: At pH 5, $(d\gamma/d\ln c) = 9.28 \times 10^{-5}$ N/m; $A = 45$ (nm)²/molecule. At pH 4, $(d\gamma/d\ln c) = 2.5 \times 10^{-5}$ N/m; $A = 160$ (nm)²/molecule = 16,400 Å²/molecule. Tanford et al.[54] calculated the area of bovine serum albumin at pH 4 using intrinsic viscosity and obtained 16,286 Å²/molecule.

14–19. The surface excess Γ in the limiting concentration range, B–D in Figure 14–14, page 375, for a nonionic surface active drug is 5.45×10^{-10} mole cm^{-2} at 25° C. Compute the limiting slope, $(d\gamma/d\ln c_2)$ and the area per molecule for the drug. The relevant

equations are $(d\gamma/d\ln\text{ c}) = -\Gamma RT$ and for the area per molecule, $A = 1/(N\Gamma)$, where N is Avogadro's number.

Answer: $(d\gamma/d\ln c_2) = -13.51$ dyne/cm; area per molecule = 30.48×10^{-16} cm²/molecule = 30.48 Å²/molecule

14–20. Korazac et al.[55] studied the isotherms of surface pressure π versus area per molecule A for insoluble monolayers of dipalmitoylphosphatidyl choline on an aqueous substrate of pH 5.2. They obtained the following results (read from Figure 1 of their article):

Data for *Problem 14–20*

π (mN/m)	60	40	20	6	4	2	1	0
$A \times 10^{-20}$ m²	40	44	50	52	68	94	95	96

Plot π against A as in Figure 14–18. For the several segments of the curve, extrapolate the line to the x-axis to obtain the limiting areas of the phase changes observed. Identify the phase changes that occur. Express the areas in nm² and in Å².

Answer: Check your answers against Figure 1 of the article by Korazac et al.[55] Extrapolating to the lower end of the curve yields an area/molecule $A \cong 52 \times 10^{-20}$ m² = 52 Å². Extrapolating to the end of the curve yields $A \cong 96 \times 10^{20}$ m² = 96 Å².

14–21. When 1×10^{-4} cm³ of stearic acid, dissolved in benzene, is placed on the surface of water in a trough, the stearic acid spreads over the surface and the benzene evaporates off. The monomolecular layer of acid that is formed covers an area of 400 cm². Calculate the length in angstroms of the stearic acid molecules.

Answer: 25 Å

14–22. Stearic acid has a molecular weight of 284.3 g/mole and a density of 0.85 g/cm³. Using the data of *Problem 14–21*, compute the cross-sectional area of the acid molecule in square angstroms.

Answer: 22 Å

14–23. When 1×10^{-4} cm³ of myricyl alcohol dissolved in benzene was spread on the surface of water in a trough, the monomolecular layer of alcohol that formed when the benzene had evaporated covered an area of 250 cm². Calculate the length in angstroms of the myricyl alcohol molecule and the cross-sectional area per molecule in square angstroms. Myricyl alcohol has a molecular weight of 453 and a density of 0.70 g/cm³.

Answer: 40 Å²; 27 Å²

14–24. By analogy of monomolecular films to a two-dimensional gas, the molecular weight of a substance can be obtained with the film balance using the equation $\pi A = (w/M)RT$. By plotting the product of the film pressure π and the area A against π and extrapolating to $\pi = 0$, a value of $\pi A/w = 2.4 \times 10^6$ erg/g at 292.15° K was obtained for w grams of a synthetic gum. Compute the molecular weight M of the gum. (*Note:* $R = 8.314 \times 10^7$ erg/mole deg.)

Answer: M = 10,121 g/mole

14–25. Insulin was spread as a film on the surface of an aqueous solution having a pH of 2.05 and an ionic strength of 0.01. The value of $\pi A/w$ extrapolated to $\pi = 0$ was obtained as 4.02×10^6 erg/g at 292.15° K. Compute the molecular weight of insulin using the equation given in *Problem 14–24*.

Answer: 6042 g/mole

14–26. From the logarithmic form of the Freundlich isotherm, equation (14–50), page 380, using concentration, c, instead of pressure, p, a plot of log (x/m) (y-axis) against log c (x-axis), gives a straight line. When the value of c equals 1.0, log $c = 0$, the y-intercept is log $(x/m) = \log k$, from which the value of k is obtained. The n value is computed from the slope. The use of log–log graph paper allows one to read directly the k value from the y-intercept axis where the x-axis is $c = 1$. Caution: one cannot obtain the slope n from a direct reading on a log–log plot.

A newly synthesized steroid is adsorbed on activated charcoal at 37° C. Data are obtained for adsorption from a phosphate buffer solution at pH 7.4:

Data for *Problem 14-26*

Amount (mole) of steroid adsorbed per gram of charcoal, x/m	Equilibrium concentration, c, of steroid (mole/liter)
1.585×10^{-4}	3.162×10^{-5}
2.310×10^{-4}	5.012×10^{-5}
3.162×10^{-4}	7.079×10^{-5}
5.012×10^{-4}	1.122×10^{-4}
7.943×10^{-4}	1.995×10^{-4}
1.259×10^{-3}	3.162×10^{-4}

(a) Plot x/m against c using log–log graph paper, and obtain k and n. *Hint:* Use *6 cycle × 6 cycle* log–log graph paper because you will need to extrapolate the line to read the y-intercept at $c = 1$.

(b) Regress $\log (x/m)$ against $\log c$ and compute k and n from the intercept and the slope, respectively.

Answers: **(a)** $n = 1.1$, $k = 1.76$ liter/g; **(b)** $n = 1.1$, $k = 1.76$ liter/g

14-27. The following data are obtained for the adsorption of timolol, an antihypertensive agent, from aqueous solution onto kaolin at $37°$ C.

Data for *Problem 14-27**

x/m (mg adsorbed per g adsorbent)	c (mg/100 mL)	$c/(x/m)$ (g/100 mL)
3.1	20	6.45
2.8	17	6.07
1.8	9	5.00
0.84	3.0	3.57

*Data from B. C. Walker, B. Pharm. Thesis, University of Otago, New Zealand, 1978.

(a) Plot the data on log–log paper according to the Freundlich isotherm and evaluate n and k (equation (14–50), using concentration, c, instead of pressure, p.

(b) Plot $c/(x/m)$ (y-axis) against c (x-axis) according to the Langmuir plot as shown in Figure 14–25. Compute b and y_m according to the Langmuir equation (equation (14–58)). (The y_m value is calculated from the slope, and b is computed from the intercept.)

(c) What are the units on n, k, y_m, and b?

Answer: **(a)** Using the 2-point formula and the Freundlich isotherm for slope, $1/n$; and reading directly from the y-intercept on the log-log plot for k, one obtains $1/n = 0.688$ (dimensionless) and $k = 0.4$ mg/g.

The units on k are taken as mg/g because at the intercept the Freundlich equation requires that $c = 1$ mg/mL or in logarithmic form $\log c = \log 1 = 0$. Then $\log (x/m) = \log k + (1/n) \log c = \log k + 0$ and $\log (x/m) = \log k$. Therefore $(x/m) = k$ and k has the same units, mg/g, as has x/m.

Using regression analysis on the Freundlich log-log equation, $\log (x/m) = -0.4048 + 0.6906 \log c$; $r^2 = 0.9999$. The slope $= 1/n = 0.6906$ (dimensionless) and from the intercept, $\log k = -0.4048$; $k = $ antilog $(-0.4048) = 0.394$ mg/g.

(b) Using the 2-point formula and the Langmuir isotherm for $1/y_m$, the slope:

$$1/y_m = \frac{(c/y)_1 - (c/y)_2}{(c)_1 - (c)_2} = \frac{6.45 - 3.57}{20 - 3} = 0.1694 \text{ g/mg}$$

$$y_m = 1/0.1694 = 5.903 \text{ mg/g}$$

For the intercept, one reads directly from the graph to obtain $1/(by_m) = 3.35$ g/dl. $1/b =$ Intercept $\times y_m = 3.35$ g/dl $\times 5.903$ mg/g $1/b = 19.78$ mg/dl; $b = 0.051$ dl/mg.

Using regression analysis on the Langmuir equation:

$$c/y = 1/(by_m) + (1/y_m) c;$$

$$c/y = 3.247 + 0.1653\, c; \; r^2 = 0.978$$

$$\text{Slope} = 0.1653 \text{ g/mg} = 1/y_m; \; y_m = 6.0496 \text{ mg/g}$$

$$\text{Intercept} = 1/(by_m) = 3.247 \text{ g/dl}$$

$$1/b = 3.247 \times 6.0496 = 19.643 \text{ mg/dl}$$

$$b = 0.051 \text{ dl/mg}$$

14-28. Sellers et al.[56] reported the following constants for adsorption of various drugs by activated charcoal at $37°$ C:

Data for *Problem 14-28*

Drug	y_m	b	Tablet strength (mg)
Aspirin	262	0.012	300
Chlordiazepoxide	157	0.010	25
Diazepam	136	0.010	5

In cases of drug overdose and poisoning, one practice is to administer an aqueous slurry (suspension) of 1 g activated charcoal/kg body weight as an antidote. If the patient weighs 72 kg, how many tablets overdose of each type is such a slurry capable of handling?

Answer: Aspirin, 63 tablets; chlordiazepoxide, 452 tablets; and diazepam, 1958 tablets.

14-29. Sturgeon et al.[57] studied the adsorption of doxorubicin, an anthracycline antibiotic, on tribasic calcium phosphate where c is the concentration of doxorubicin and x is its amount in mg adsorbed on m mg of the adsorbent.

Data for *Problem 14-29*

$c/(x/m) \times 10^3$ (g/mL)	$c \times 10^3$, mg/mL
1.25	2.0
2.25	3.5
2.90	4.5
3.40	5.3

(a) Plot the Langmuir isotherm and evaluate y_m, the maximum binding capacity in mg/g, and b, the affinity or binding constant, in mL/mg.

(b) Tribasic calcium phosphate is not used as an antidote in poisoning. Why did the authors choose to study the adsorption of doxorubicin on tribasic calcium phosphate?

Answers: **(a)** $y_m = 1.56$ mg/g, $b = $ infinite; **(b)** bone tissue from patients receiving extended doxorubicin therapy were found to be stained by long-term therapy with this drug; the authors used solid tribasic calcium phosphate as a model to approximate adsorption of the drug by bone tissues samples

14-30. From the affinity or binding constant, b, obtained from the Langmuir isotherms, the standard free energy of adsorption can be computed as

$$\Delta G° = -RT \ln b$$

because the affinity b is an equilibrium constant.[58] The Langmuir constants for the adsorption of nadolol, an adrenergic drug, onto magnesium trisilicate were determined at two temperatures:

Data for *Problem 14-30*

T (°C)	y_m (mg/g)	b (liter/g)	b (liter/mole)
$37°$ C	58.2	0.33227	102.14
$50°$ C	53.8	0.34168	105.457

(a) Compute $\Delta G°$ at the two temperatures; (b) use the integrated form of the van't Hoff equation and compute $\Delta H°$. (c) Compute $\Delta S°$ at 37° and 50° C. (d) Using the nonlinear form of the Langmuir equation, i.e., $x/m = \dfrac{y_m bc}{1 + bc}$, together with the parameters y_m mg/g and b (liter/g) given in the table at the two temperatures, compute x/m for the following concentrations, c: 0.5, 5, 20, 50 mg/100 mL. Plot the Langmuir isotherms at the two temperatures on the same graph.

Answers: (a) $\Delta G° = -2.9$ kcal/mole at 37° C and -3.0 kcal/mole at 50° C; (b) $\Delta H° = 490$ cal/mole; (c) $\Delta S°$ (37°) = 10.8 u.e. and $\Delta S°$(50°) = 10.8 u.e.; (d) x/m (37° C) = 8.3 mg/g; at 50° C, x/m = 7.9 mg/g at c (mg/100 mL) = 0.5

14–31. Use the data for the surface tension, γ, of glycerol at three temperatures, 20°, 90° and 150° C from a handbook of physics and chemistry,* viz: 63.4, 58.6, and 51.9 erg/cm². (a) Plot γ versus temperature (°K on the horizontal axis). Use regression analysis or a tangent drawn at each temperature to obtain the slope $(\partial\gamma/\partial T)_p = -S^s$. (b) Knowing γ and the entropy of the surface, S^s, calculate the surface enthalpy H^s at each of the three temperatures using the appropriate equation, page 365. Does H^s appear to remain constant over this temperature range? (c) What is the meaning of H^s in surface chemistry? How do you interpret (explain) the entropy value obtained?

Partial Answers: (b) $S^s = 0.0879$ erg cm^{-2} deg^{-1}; $H^s = 89.17$, 90.52, and 89.09 erg cm^{-2} at 20°, 90°, and 150° C, respectively. (c) See Harkins[59] for an interpretation of H^s and S^s.

14–32. Use the following data to obtain the entropy of formation of a surface and the surface enthalpy at 20°, 100°, and 200° C for carbon tetrachloride.

Data for *Problem 14–32*

T (°K)	293.15	373.15	473.15
γ (dyne/cm)	26.95	17.26	6.53

Calculate S^s from the slope of a plot of γ against T and using this value, compute H^s at the three temperatures.

Partial Answer: $S^s = 0.113$ erg cm^2 deg^{-1}; H^s at 20° C = 60.08 erg cm^2.

14–33. Provided that the enthalpy of a surface H^s does not appreciably vary over the temperature range under study, H^s can be computed from the intercept of a plot of γ against T, according to the equation

$$\gamma = H^s + T\left(\frac{\partial\gamma}{\partial T}\right) = H^s - TS^s$$

where S^s, the surface entropy, is the slope of the line.

Use the data for the surface tension of water found between $-8°$ C (265.15° K) and 100° C (373.15° K) from CRC* or a comparable table of data, together with linear regression analysis to obtain H^o and S^s.

Answer: $S^s = 0.1647$ erg cm^{-2} deg^{-1}; $H^s = 120.9$ erg cm^{-2}

14–34. The contact angle θ of a liquid on a solid surface can be evaluated from the Girifalco–Good–Fowkes–Young equation[60] and Hiemenz,[4] pages 339 to 345:

$$(1 + \cos\theta)\gamma_L = 2\sqrt{\gamma_s^d\,\gamma_L^d}$$

where γ_L is the total (dispersion + polar) surface tension of the liquid and γ_s^d and γ_L^d are the surface tension of the solid and the liquid due to the dispersion (weak electrostatic or London force) components, d. For relatively nonpolar liquids $\gamma_L \approx \gamma_L^d$.

(a) Compute the contact angles, θ, of water, ethylene glycol, and benzene on teflon. The surface tensions of water, ethylene glycol, and benzene are 72.8, 49, and 29 dyne/cm, respectively, and the corresponding γ_L^d are 21.8, 28.6, and 29 dyne/cm; γ_s^d for teflon is 19.5 dyne/cm at 25° C.

(b) What significance do these values have? See Sharma and Ruckenstein[60] and Hiemenz[4] for the meaning of these values.

Answer: (a) θ (water) = 115.7°, θ (ethylene glycol) = 92°, θ (benzene) = 50.2°

14–35. The interfacial tension between oil and water or an aqueous solution can be computed from the surface tension of the pure components by means of the Girifalco–Fowkes equation:

$$\gamma_{o,aq} = \gamma_o + \gamma_{aq} - 2\sqrt{\gamma_o^d\,\gamma_{aq}^d}$$

where the subscripts o and aq stand for the oil and aqueous phases and the superscript d signifies the dispersion or weak electrostatic interaction part of the surface tension of the aqueous phase.[61]

Compute the interfacial tension between a 10% by volume aqueous solution of ethylene glycol monomethyl ether ($\gamma_{aq} = 56.9$ mJ/m² and $\gamma_{aq}^d = 22$ mJ/m²) and paraffin oil ($\gamma_o = 30.8$ mJ/m²). *Note:* mJ/m² is read, "millijoules per square meter." Also note that for a paraffin oil $\gamma_o^d = \gamma_o$ because the paraffin oil is a nonpolar substance.

Answer: 35.6 mJ/m². (Note that the numerical value 35.6 for the surface tension in the SI units of mJ/m² is the same as the numerical value for surface tension in the cgs system, namely 35.6 erg/cm².)

---

*The values are found using the data from the CRC *Handbook of Physics and Chemistry*, 63rd Edition, 1982, pp. F-35–37.

15
Colloids

INTRODUCTION

Dispersed Systems. It is important that the pharmacist understand the theory and technology of disperse systems. Although the quantitative aspects of this subject are not as well developed as are those of micromolecular chemistry, the theories that can be proposed in the field of colloidal chemistry are quite helpful in approaching the puzzling problems that arise in the preparation and dispensing of emulsions, suspensions, ointments, powders, and compressed dosage forms. A knowledge of interfacial phenomena and a familiarity with the characteristics of colloids and small particles are fundamental to an understanding of the behavior of pharmaceutical dispersions.

Dispersed systems consist of particulate matter, known as the *dispersed phase*, distributed throughout a *continuous*, or *dispersion*, *medium*. The dispersed material may range in size from particles of atomic and molecular dimensions to particles whose size is measured in millimeters. Accordingly, a convenient means of classifying dispersed systems is on the basis of the mean particle diameter of the dispersed material. Three size classifications are generally used, namely *molecular* dispersions, *colloidal* dispersions, and *coarse* dispersions. The size ranges assigned to these classes, together with some of the associated characteristics, are shown in Table 15–1. The size limits are somewhat arbitrary, there being no distinct transition between either molecular and colloidal dispersions or colloidal and coarse dispersions. For example, certain *macro-* (i.e., large) molecules, such as the polysaccharides, proteins, and polymers in general, are of sufficient size that they may be classified as forming both molecular and colloidal dispersions. Some suspensions and emulsions may contain a range of particle sizes such that the smaller particles lie within the colloidal range while the larger ones are classified as coarse particles.

Molecular dispersions are homogeneous in character and form true solutions. The properties of these systems have been discussed in the previous section of this text. Colloidal dispersions will be considered in the present chapter, powders and granules in Chapter 16, and coarse dispersions in Chapter 18; all are examples of heterogeneous systems.

Size and Shape of Colloidal Particles. Particles lying in the colloidal size range possess a surface area that is enormous compared with the surface area of an equal volume of larger particles. Thus, a cube having a 1-cm edge and a volume of 1 cm^3 has a total surface area of 6 cm^2. If the same cube is subdivided into smaller cubes, each having an edge of 100 μm, the total volume remains the same, but the total surface area increases to 600,000 cm^2. This represents a 10^5-fold increase in surface area. To compare quantitatively the surface areas of different materials, the term *specific surface* is used. This is defined as the surface area per unit weight or volume of material. In the example just given, the first sample had a specific surface of 6 cm^2/cm^3, while the second sample had a specific surface of 600,000 cm^2/cm^3. The possession of a large specific surface results in many of the unique properties of colloidal dispersions. For example, platinum is effective as a catalyst only when in the colloidal form as platinum black. This is because catalysts act by adsorbing the reactants onto their surface. Hence, their catalytic activity is related to their specific surface. The color of colloidal dispersions is related to the size of the particles present. Thus, as the particles in a red gold sol increase in size, the dispersion takes on a blue color. Antimony

TABLE 15–1. *Classification of Dispersed Systems on the Basis of Particle Size**

Class	Range of Particle Size†	Characteristics of System	Examples
Molecular dispersion	Less than 1.0 nm (mμ)	Particles invisible in electron microscope; pass through ultrafilter and semipermeable membrane; undergo rapid diffusion.	Oxygen molecules, ordinary ions, glucose
Colloidal dispersion	1.0 nm to 0.5 μm	Particles not resolved by ordinary microscope although they may be detected under ultramicroscope; visible in electron microscope; pass through filter paper but do not pass semipermeable membrane; diffuse very slowly.	Colloidal silver sols, natural and synthetic polymers
Coarse dispersion	Greater than 0.5 μm (μ)	Particles visible under microscope; do not pass through normal filter paper or dialyze through semipermeable membrane; particles do not diffuse.	Grains of sand, most pharmaceutical emulsions and suspensions, red blood cells

*Modified from Oswald: Kuhn's Kolloid chemisches Taschenbuch, as quoted in part from H. B. Weiser, *Colloid Chemistry*, 2nd Edition, Wiley, New York, 1949.
†A micrometer (μm), formerly called a micron (μ), is a unit of length equal to one thousandth of a millimeter or 10^{-3} mm. A nanometer (nm), formerly called a millimicron (mμ), is one thousandth of a micron or 10^{-6} mm. It follows that 1 cm is equal to 10^4 μm or 10^7 nm.

and arsenic trisulfides change from red to yellow as the particle size is reduced from that of a coarse powder to that within the colloidal size range.

Because of their size, colloidal particles may be separated from molecular particles with relative ease. The technique of separation, known as *dialysis*, uses a semipermeable membrane of collodion or cellophane, the pore size of which will prevent the passage of colloidal particles, yet will permit small molecules and ions, such as urea, glucose, and sodium chloride, to pass through. The principle is illustrated in Figure 15–1, which shows that, at equilibrium, the colloidal material is retained in compartment A, while the subcolloidal material is distributed equally on both sides of the membrane. By continually removing the liquid in compartment B, it is possible to obtain colloidal material in A that is free from subcolloidal contaminants.

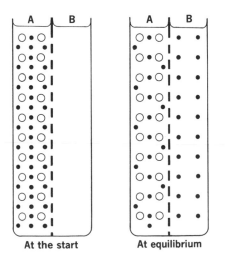

At the start   **At equilibrium**

Fig. 15–1. Sketch showing the removal of electrolytes from colloidal material by diffusion through a semipermeable membrane. Conditions on the two sides, A and B, of the membrane are shown at the start and at equilibrium. The open circles are the colloidal particles that are too large to pass through the membrane. The solid dots are the electrolyte particles that pass through the pores of the membrane.

Dialysis may also be used to obtain subcolloidal material that is free from colloidal contamination—in this case, one simply collects the effluent. *Ultrafiltration* has also been used to separate and purify colloidal material. According to one variation of the method, filtration is conducted under negative pressure (suction) through a dialysis membrane supported in a Büchner funnel. When dialysis and ultrafiltration are used to remove charged impurities, such as ionic contaminants, the process may be hastened by the use of an electric potential across the membrane. This process is called *electrodialysis*.

Dialysis has been used increasingly in recent years to study the binding of materials of pharmaceutical significance to colloidal particles. Dialysis occurs in vivo. Thus, ions and small molecules pass readily from the blood, through a natural semipermeable membrane, to the tissue fluids; the colloidal components of the blood remain within the capillary system. The principle of dialysis is utilized in the artificial kidney, which removes small-molecular-weight impurities from the body by passage through a semipermeable membrane.

The shape adopted by colloidal particles in dispersion is important, since the more extended the particle, the greater its specific surface and the greater the opportunity for attractive forces to develop between the particles of the dispersed phase and the dispersion medium. A colloidal particle is something like a hedgehog—in a friendly environment, it unrolls and exposes maximum surface area. Under adverse conditions, it rolls up and reduces its exposed area. Some representative shapes of spherocolloids and fibrous colloids are shown in Figure 15–2. As will be seen in later discussions, such properties as flow, sedimentation, and osmotic pressure are affected by changes in the shape of colloidal particles. Particle shape may also influence pharmacologic action. Cromoglycic acid, an agent administered by inhalation to control asthmatic attacks, was found by Chan and Gonda[1] to be suitably deposited

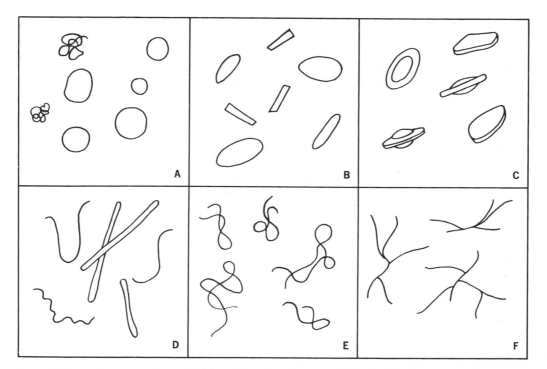

Fig. 15–2. Some shapes that may be assumed by colloidal particles: *(a)* spheres and globules; *(b)* short rods and prolate ellipsoids; *(c)* oblate ellipsoids and flakes; *(d)* long rods and threads; *(e)* loosely coiled threads; *(f)* branched threads.

in the respiratory tract when prepared as well-formed rod-shaped crystals.

Pharmaceutical Applications of Colloids. Certain medicinals have been found to possess unusual or increased therapeutic properties when formulated in the colloidal state. Colloidal silver chloride, silver iodide, and silver protein are effective germicides and do not cause the irritation that is characteristic of ionic silver salts. Coarsely powdered sulfur is poorly absorbed when administered orally, yet the same dose of colloidal sulfur may be absorbed so completely as to cause a toxic reaction and even death. Colloidal copper has been used in the treatment of cancer, colloidal gold as a diagnostic agent for paresis, and colloidal mercury for syphilis.

Many natural and synthetic polymers are important in contemporary pharmaceutical practice. Polymers are macromolecules formed by the polymerization or condensation of smaller, noncolloidal, molecules. Proteins are important natural colloids and are found in the body as components of muscle, bone, and skin. The plasma proteins are responsible for binding certain drug molecules to such an extent that the pharmacologic activity of the drug is affected. Naturally occurring plant macromolecules such as starch and cellulose that are used as pharmaceutical adjuncts are capable of existing in the colloidal state. Hydroxyethyl starch (HES) is a macromolecule used as a plasma substitute. Other synthetic polymers are applied as coatings to solid dosage forms to protect drugs that are susceptible to atmospheric moisture or degradation under the acid conditions of the stomach. Colloidal electrolytes (surface-active agents) are sometimes used to increase the

solubility, stability, and taste of certain compounds in aqueous and oily pharmaceutical preparations.

TYPES OF COLLOIDAL SYSTEMS

Colloidal systems are best classified into three groups—lyophilic, lyophobic, and association— on the basis of the interaction of the particles, molecules, or ions of the dispersed phase with the molecules of the dispersion medium.

Lyophilic Colloids. Systems containing colloidal particles that interact to an appreciable extent with the dispersion medium are referred to as *lyophilic* (solvent-loving) colloids. Owing to their affinity for the dispersion medium, such materials form colloidal dispersions, or *sols*, with relative ease. Thus, lyophilic colloidal sols are usually obtained simply by dissolving the material in the solvent being used. For example, the dissolution of acacia or gelatin in water or celluloid in amyl acetate leads to the formation of a sol.

The various properties of this class of colloids are due to the attraction between the dispersed phase and the dispersion medium, which leads to *solvation*, the attachment of solvent molecules to the mlecules of the dispersed phase. In the case of hydrophilic colloids, in which water is the dispersion medium, that is termed *hydration*. Most lyophilic colloids are organic molecules, for example, gelatin, acacia, insulin, albumin, rubber, and polystyrene. Of these, the first four produce lyophilic colloids in aqueous dispersion media (hydrophilic sols). Rubber and polystyrene form lyophilic colloids in nonaqueous, organic, solvents. These materials accordingly are referred to as *lipophilic* colloids. These examples illustrate the important point that the term *lyophilic* has meaning only when applied to the material dispersed in a specific dispersion medium. A material that forms a lyophilic colloidal system in one liquid (e.g., water) may not do so in another liquid (e.g., benzene).

Lyophobic Colloids. The second class of colloids is composed of materials that have little attraction, if any, for the dispersion medium. These are the *lyophobic* (solvent-hating) colloids and, predictably, their properties differ from those of the lyophilic colloids. This is due primarily to the absence of a solvent sheath around the particle. Lyophobic colloids are generally composed of inorganic particles dispersed in water. Examples of such materials are gold, silver, sulfur, arsenous sulfide, and silver iodide.

In contrast to lyophilic colloids, it is necessary to use special methods to prepare lyophobic colloids. These are (a) dispersion methods, in which coarse particles are reduced in size, and (b) condensation methods, in which materials of subcolloidal dimensions are caused to aggregate into particles within the colloidal size range. Dispersion may be achieved by the use of high-intensity ultrasonic generators operating at frequencies in excess of 20,000 cycles per second. A second dispersion method involves the production of an electric arc within a liquid. Owing to the intense heat generated by the arc, some of the metal of the electrodes is dispersed as vapor, which condenses to form colloidal particles. Milling and grinding processes may be used, although their efficiency is low. So-called colloid mills, in which the material is sheared between two rapidly rotating plates set close together, reduce only a small amount of the total particles to the colloidal size range.

The required conditions for the formation of lyophobic colloids by condensation or aggregation involve a high degree of initial supersaturation followed by the formation and growth of nuclei. Supersaturation may be brought about by change in solvent or reduction in temperature. For example, if sulfur is dissolved in alcohol and the concentrated solution is then poured into an excess of water, many small nuclei form in the supersaturated solution. These grow rapidly to form a colloidal sol. Other condensation methods depend on a chemical reaction, such as reduction, oxidation, hydrolysis, or double decomposition. Thus, neutral or slightly alkaline solutions of the noble metal salts, when treated with a reducing agent such as formaldehyde or pyrogallol, form atoms that combine to form charged aggregates. The oxidation of hydrogen sulfide leads to the formation of sulfur atoms and the production of a sulfur sol. If a solution of ferric chloride is added to a large volume of water, hydrolysis occurs with the formation of a red sol of hydrated ferric oxide. Chromium and aluminum salts also hydrolyze in this manner. Finally, the double decomposition between hydrogen sulfide and arsenous acid results in an arsenous

sulfide sol. If an excess of hydrogen sulfide is used, HS^- ions are adsorbed onto the particles. This creates a large negative charge on the particles, leading to the formation of a stable sol.

Association Colloids: Micelles and the CMC. *Association*, or *amphiphilic*, colloids form the third group in this classification. As we have seen in Chapter 14, which dealt with interfacial phenomena (p. 370), certain molecules or ions, termed *amphiphiles* or *surface-active agents*, are characterized by having two distinct regions of opposing solution affinities within the same molecule or ion. When present in a liquid medium at low concentrations, the amphiphiles exist separately and are of such a size as to be subcolloidal. As the concentration is increased, aggregation occurs over a narrow concentration range. These aggregates, which may contain 50 or more monomers, are called *micelles*. Since the diameter of each micelle is of the order of 50 Å, micelles lie within the size range we have designated as colloidal. The concentration of monomer at which micelles form is termed the *critical micelle concentration*, or *cmc*. The number of monomers that aggregate to form a micelle is known as the *aggregation number* of the micelle.

The phenomenon of micelle formation can be explained as follows. Below the cmc, the concentration of amphiphile undergoing adsorption at the air–water interface increases as the total concentration of amphiphile is raised. Eventually a point is reached at which both the interface and the bulk phase become saturated with monomers. This is the cmc. Any further amphiphile added in excess of this concentration aggregates to form micelles in the bulk phase and, in this manner, the free energy of the system is reduced. The effect of micellization on some of the physical properties of solutions containing surface-active agents is shown in Figure 15–3. Note particularly that surface tension decreases up to the cmc. From Gibbs' adsorption equation (p. 370), this means increasing interfacial adsorption. Above the cmc, the surface tension remains essentially constant, showing that the interface is saturated and micelle formation has taken place in the bulk phase.

In the case of amphiphiles in water, the hydrocarbon chains face inward into the micelle to form, in effect, their own hydrocarbon environment. Surrounding this hydrocarbon core are the polar portions of the amphiphiles associated with the water molecules of the continuous phase. Aggregation also occurs in nonpolar liquids. The orientation of the molecules is now reversed, however, with the polar heads facing inward while the hydrocarbon chains are associated with the continuous nonpolar phase. These situations are shown in Figure 15–4, which also shows some of the shapes postulated for micelles. It seems likely that spherical micelles exist at concentrations relatively close to the cmc. At higher concentrations, laminar micelles have an increasing tendency to form and exist in equilbrium with sperical micelles. The student is cautioned against

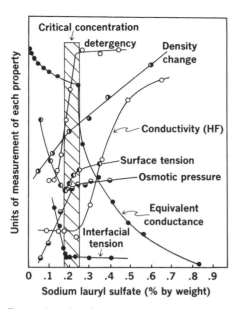

Fig. 15–3. Properties of surface-active agents showing changes that occur sharply at the critical micelle concentration. (Modified from Preston, W. J. Phys. Coll. Chem. **52**, 85, 1948. Copyright © 1948, The Williams & Wilkins Co., Baltimore.)

regarding micelles as solid particles. The individual molecules forming the micelle are in dynamic equilibrium with those monomers in the bulk and at the interface.

As with lyophilic sols, formation of association colloids is spontaneous, provided that the concentration of the amphiphile in solution exceeds the cmc.

Amphiphiles may be anionic, cationic, nonionic, or ampholytic (zwitterionic), and this provides a convenient means of classifying association colloids. A typical example of each type is given in Table 15–2. Thus, Figure 15–4a represents the micelle of an anionic association colloid. A certain number of the sodium ions are attracted to the surface of the micelle, reducing the overall negative charge somewhat. These bound ions are termed *gegenions*.

Mixtures of two or more amphiphiles are usual in pharmaceutical formulations. Assuming an ideal mixture, the cmc of the mixture can be predicted from the cmc values of the pure amphiphiles and their mole fractions x in the mixture, according to the expresssion[2]

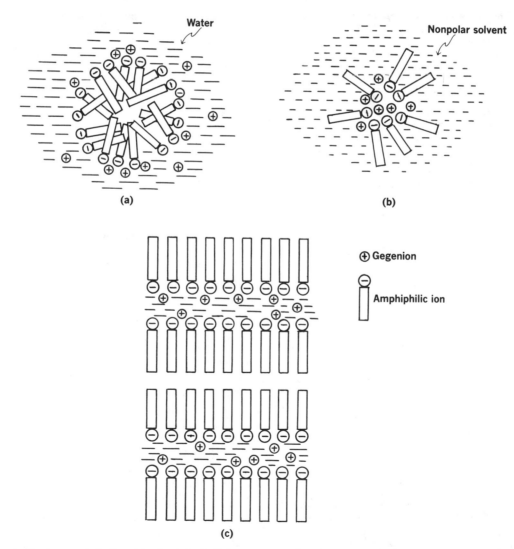

Fig. 15–4. Some probable shapes of micelles: *(a)* spherical micelle in aqueous media; *(b)* reversed micelle in nonaqueous media; *(c)* laminar micelle, formed at higher amphiphile concentration, in aqueous media.

TABLE 15–2. *Classification of Association Colloids*

Type	Compound	Amphiphile	Gegenions
Anionic	Sodium lauryl sulfate	$CH_3(CH_2)_{11}OSO_3^-$	Na+
Cationic	Cetyl trimethylammonium bromide	$CH_3(CH_2)_{15}N^+(CH_3)_3$	Br$^-$
Nonionic	Polyoxyethylene lauryl ether	$CH_3(CH_2)_{10}CH_2O(CH_2OCH_2)_{23}H$	—
Ampholytic	Dimethyldodecylammonio-propane sulfonate	$CH_3(CH_2)_{11}N^+(CH_3)_2(CH_2)_3OSO_2^-$	—

TABLE 15–3. *Comparison of Properties of Colloidal Sols**

Lyophilic	Association (Amphiphilic)	Lyophobic
Dispersed phase consists generally of large organic *molecules* lying within colloidal size range.	Dispersed phase consists of aggregates *(micelles)* of small organic molecules or ions whose size *individually* is below the colloidal range.	Dispersed phase ordinarily consists of inorganic particles, such as gold or silver.
Molecules of the dispersed phase are solvated, i.e., they are associated with the molecules comprising the dispersion medium.	Hydrophilic or lipophilic portion of the molecule is solvated, depending on whether the dispersion medium is aqueous or nonaqueous.	Little, if any, interaction (solvation) occurs between particles and dispersion medium.
Molecules disperse spontaneously to form colloidal solution.	Colloidal aggregates are formed spontaneously when the concentration of amphiphile exceeds the critical micelle concentration (cmc).	Material does not disperse spontaneously, and special procedures therefore must be adopted to produce colloidal dispersion.
Viscosity of the dispersion medium ordinarily is increased greatly by the presence of the dispersed phase. At sufficiently high concentrations, the sol may become a gel. Viscosity and gel formation are related to solvation effects and to the shape of the molecules, which are usually highly asymmetric.	Viscosity of the system increases as the concentration of the amphiphile increases, as micelles increase in number and become asymmetric.	Viscosity of the dispersion medium is not greatly increased by the presence of lyophobic colloidal particles, which tend to be unsolvated and symmetric.
Dispersions are stable generally in the presence of electrolytes. They may be salted out by high concentrations of very soluble electrolytes. Effect is due primarily to desolvation of lyophilic molecules.	In aqueous solutions, the critical micelle concentration is reduced by the addition of electrolytes. Salting-out may occur at higher salt concentrations.	Lyophobic dispersions are unstable in the presence of even small concentrations of electrolytes. Effect is due to neutralization of the charge on the particles. Lyophilic colloids exert a protective effect.

*From J. Swarbrick and A. Martin, *American Pharmacy*, 6th Edition, Lippincott, Philadelphia, 1966, p. 161.

$$\frac{1}{cmc} = \frac{x_1}{cmc_1} + \frac{x_2}{cmc_2} \qquad (15-1)$$

Example 15–1. Compute the cmc of a mixture of *n*-dodecyl octaoxyethylene glycol monoether ($C_{12}E_8$) and *n*-dodecyl β-D-maltoside (DM). The cmc of $C_{12}E_8$ is $cmc_1 = 8.1 \times 10^{-5}$ mole/liter and its mole fraction is $x_1 = 0.75$; the cmc of DM is $cmc_2 = 15 \times 10^{-5}$ mole/liter.

$$x_2 = (1 - x_1) = (1 - 0.75) = 0.25$$

From equation (15–1),

$$\frac{1}{cmc} = \frac{0.75}{8.1 \times 10^{-5}} + \frac{(1 - 0.75)}{15 \times 10^{-5}} = 10926$$

$$cmc = \frac{1}{10926} = 9.15 \times 10^{-5} \text{ mole/liter}$$

The experimental value is 9.3×10^{-5} mole/liter.

The properties of lyophilic, lyophobic, and association colloids are outlined in Table 15–3. These properties, together with the relevant methods, will be discussed in the following sections.

OPTICAL PROPERTIES OF COLLOIDS

The Faraday–Tyndall Effect. When a strong beam of light is passed through a colloidal sol, a visible cone, resulting from the scattering of light by the colloidal particles, is formed. This is the *Faraday–Tyndall effect.*

The *ultramicroscope*, developed by Zsigmondy, allows one to examine the light points responsible for the *Tyndall cone.* An intense light beam is passed through the sol against a dark background at right angles to the plane of observation, and, although the particles cannot be seen directly, the bright spots corresponding to particles can be observed and counted.

Electron Microscope. The use of the ultramicroscope has declined in recent years since it frequently does not resolve lyophilic colloids. The *electron microscope,* capable of yielding pictures of the actual particles, even those approaching molecular dimensions, is now widely used to observe the size, shape, and structure of colloidal particles.

The success of the electron microscope is due to its high resolving power, which may be defined in terms of d, the smallest distance by which two objects are separated and yet remain distinguishable. The smaller the wavelength of the radiation used, the smaller is d and the greater the resolving power. The optical microscope uses visible light as its radiation source and is only able to resolve two particles separated by about 200 Å. The radiation source of the electron microscope is a beam of high-energy electrons having wavelengths in the region of 0.1 Å. With current instrumentation, this results in d being approximately 5 Å, a much increased power of resolution over the optical microscope.

Light Scattering. This property depends on the Faraday–Tyndall effect and is a widely used method for determining the molecular weight of colloids. It may also be used to obtain information as to the shape and size of these particles. Scattering may be described in terms of the turbidity, τ, the fractional decrease in intensity due to scattering as the incident light passes through 1 cm of solution. It may be expressed as the intensity of light scattered in all directions, I_s, divided by the intensity of the incident light, I. At a given concentration of dispersed phase, the turbidity is proportional to the molecular weight of the lyophilic colloid. Because of the low turbidities of most lyophilic colloids, it is more convenient to measure the scattered light (at a particular angle relative to the incident beam) rather than the transmitted light.

The turbidity can then be calculated from the intensity of the scattered light provided that the dimensions of the particle are small compared with the wavelength of the light used. The molecular weight of the colloid may be obtained from the following equation:

$$Hc/\tau = 1/M + 2Bc \qquad (15–2)$$

in which τ is the turbidity in cm^{-1}, c the concentration of solute in g/cm^3 of solution, M the weight average molecular weight in g/mole or daltons, and B an interaction constant (see osmotic pressure, pp. 401–402). H is constant for a particular system and is written

$$H = \frac{32\pi^3 n^2 (dn/dc)^2}{3\lambda^4 N}$$

in which n (dimensionless) is the refractive index of the solution of concentration c (g/cm^3) at a wavelength λ in cm^{-1}, (dn/dc) is the change in refractive index with concentration at c, and N is Avogadro's number. A plot of Hc/τ against concentration, Figure 15–5, results in a straight line with a slope of $2B$. The intercept on the Hc/τ axis is $1/M$, the reciprocal of which yields the molecular weight of the colloid (see Problem 15–2).

When the molecule is asymmetric, the intensity of the scattered light varies with the angle of observation. Data of this kind permit an estimation of the shape and size of the particles. Light scattering has been used to

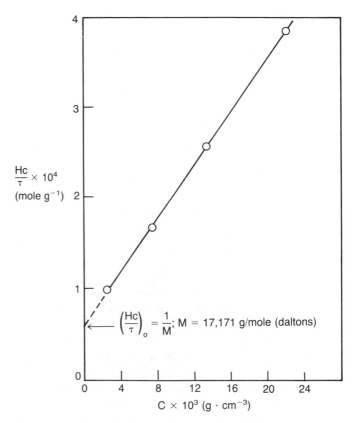

Fig. 15–5. A plot of Hc/τ against the concentration of a polymer (colloid) (see Problem 15–2).

study proteins, synthetic polymers, association colloids, and lyophobic sols.

Chang and Cardinal[3] used light scattering to study the pattern of self-association in aqueous solution of the bile salts sodium deoxycholate and sodium taurodeoxycholate. Analysis of the data showed that the bile salts associate to form dimers, trimers, and tetramers, and a larger aggregate of variable size.

Racey et al.[4] used quasi-elastic light scattering (QELS), a new light-scattering technique that uses laser light and may determine diffusion coefficients and particle sizes (Stokes' diameter, p. 425) of macromolecules in solution. Quasi-elastic light scattering allowed the examination of heparin aggregates in commercial preparations stored for various times and at various temperatures. Both storage time and refrigeration caused an increase in the aggregation state of heparin solutions. It has not yet been determined whether the change in aggregation has any effect on the biologic activity of commercial preparations.

Light Scattering and Micelle Molecular Weight. Equation (15–2) can be applied after suitable modification to compute the molecular weight of colloidal aggregates and micelles. When amphiphilic molecules associate to form micelles, the turbidity of the micellar dispersion differs from the turbidity of the solution of the amphiphilic molecules because micelles are now also present in equilibrium with the monomeric species. Below the cmc, the concentration of monomers increases linearly with the total concentration, c; above the cmc the monomer concentration remains nearly constant; that is, $c_{monomer} \cong$ cmc. The concentration of micelles may therefore be written

$$c_{micelle} = c - c_{monomer} \div c - c_{cmc} \quad (15\text{-}3)$$

The corresponding turbidity of the solution due to the presence of micelles is obtained by subtracting the turbidity due to monomers, $\tau_{monomer} = \tau_{cmc}$, from the total turbidity of the solution:

$$\tau_{micelle} = \tau - \tau_{cmc} \quad (15\text{-}4)$$

Accordingly, equation (15-2) is modified to

$$\frac{H(c - c_{cmc})}{(\tau - \tau_{cmc})} = \frac{1}{M} + 2B(c - c_{cmc}) \quad (15\text{-}5)$$

where the subscript cmc stands for turbidity or concentration at the critical micelle concentration, and B and H have the same meaning as in equation (15-2). Thus, the molecular weight M of the micelle and the second virial coefficient B (p. 401) are obtained from the intercept and the slope, respectively, of a plot of $H(c - c_{cmc})/(\tau - \tau_{cmc})$ versus $(c - c_{cmc})$. Equation (15-5) is valid for two-component systems, that is, for a micelle and a molecular surfactant in this instance.

When the micelles interact neither among themselves nor with the molecules of the medium, the slope of a plot of equation (15-5) is zero; that is, the second virial coefficient B is zero and the line is parallel to the horizontal axis, as seen in Figure 15-6. This behavior is typical of nonionic and zwitterionic micellar systems in which the size distribution is narrow. However, as the concentration of micelles increases, intermicellar interactions lead to positive values of B, the slope of the line having a positive value. For ionic micelles the plots are linear with positive slopes, owing to repulsive intermicellar interactions that result in positive values of the interaction coefficient, B. A negative second virial coefficient is usually an indication that the micellar system is polydisperse.[5,6]

Example 15-2. Using the following data compute the molecular weight of micelles of dimethylalkylammoniopropane sulfonate, a zwitterionic surfactant investigated by Herrmann[6]:

$(c - c_{cmc}) \times 10^3$ (g/mL)	0.98	1.98	2.98	3.98	4.98
$\left[\dfrac{H(c - c_{cmc})}{\tau - \tau_{cmc}}\right] \times 10^5$ (mole/g)	1.66	1.65	1.66	1.69	1.65

Using equation (15-5), the micellar molecular weight is obtained from a plot of $\dfrac{H(c - c_{cmc})}{\tau - \tau_{cmc}}$ versus $(c - c_{cmc})$ (see Fig. 15-6); the intercept is $\dfrac{1}{M} = 1.66 \times 10^{-5}$ mole/g; therefore, $M = 60{,}241$ g/mole. The slope is zero; that is, $2B$ in equation (15-5) is zero.

KINETIC PROPERTIES OF COLLOIDS

Grouped under this heading are several properties of colloidal systems that relate to the motion of particles with respect to the dispersion medium. The motion may be thermally induced (Brownian movement, diffusion, osmosis), gravitationally induced (sedimentation), or applied externally (viscosity). Electrically induced motion is considered in the section on electric properties of colloids.

Brownian Motion. Long before Zsigmondy had described the random movement of colloidal particles in the microscopic field, Robert Brown (1827) studied this phenomenon. The erratic motion, which may be observed with particles as large as about 5 μm, was later explained as resulting from the bombardment of the particles by the molecules of the dispersion medium. The motion of the molecules cannot be observed, of course, since the molecules are too small to see. The velocity of the particles increases with decreasing particle size. Increasing the viscosity of the medium, which may be accomplished by the addition of glycerin or a similar agent, decreases and finally stops the Brownian movement.

Diffusion. Particles diffuse spontaneously from a region of higher concentration to one of lower concentration until the concentration of the system is uniform throughout. Diffusion is a direct result of Brownian movement.

According to *Fick's first law* (p. 325), the amount dq of substance diffusing in time dt across a plane of area S is directly proportional to the change of concentration dc with distance traveled dx.

Fick's law is written

$$dq = -DS \frac{dc}{dx} dt \quad (15\text{-}6)$$

D is the *diffusion coefficient*, the amount of material diffusing per unit time across a unit area when dc/dx, called the *concentration gradient*, is unity. D thus has the dimensions of area per unit time. The coefficient may be obtained in colloidal chemistry by diffusion experiments in which the material is allowed to pass through a porous disc, and samples are removed and

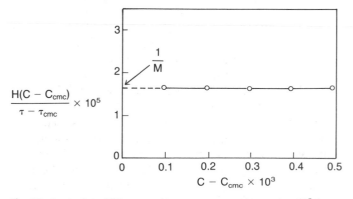

Fig. 15-6. A plot of $H(c - c_{cmc})/\tau - \tau_{cmc}$ versus $(c-c_{cmc}) \times 10^3$ for a zwitterionic surfactant in which B is zero.[6]

analyzed periodically. Another method involves measuring the change in the concentration or refractive index gradient of the free boundary that is formed when the solvent and colloidal solution are brought together and allowed to diffuse.

If the colloidal particles can be assumed to be approximately spherical, the following equation, suggested by Sutherland and Einstein, can be used to obtain the radius of the particle and the particle weight or molecular weight:

$$D = \frac{kT}{6\pi\eta r}$$

or

$$D = \frac{RT}{6\pi\eta r N} \qquad (15-7)$$

in which D is the diffusion coefficient obtained from Fick's law as already explained, k is the Boltzmann constant, R is the molar gas constant, T is the absolute temperature, η is the viscosity of the solvent, r is the radius of the spherical particle, and N is Avogadro's number. Equation (15-7) is called the *Sutherland–Einstein* or the *Stokes–Einstein* equation. The measured diffusion coefficient may be used to obtain the molecular weight of approximately spherical molecules, such as egg albumin and hemoglobin, by use of the equation,

$$D = \frac{RT}{6\pi\eta N} \sqrt[3]{\frac{4\pi N}{3 M \bar{v}}} \qquad (15-8)$$

in which M is molecular weight and $\bar{v}$ is the partial specific volume (approximately equal to the volume in cm^3 of 1 gram of the solute, obtained from density mesurements).

Example 15–3. The diffusion coefficient for a spherical protein at 20° C is 7.0×10^{-7} cm²/sec and the partial specific volume is 0.75 cm³/g. The viscosity of the solvent is 0.01 poise (0.01 g/cm sec). Compute (a) the molecular weight and (b) the radius of the protein particle.

(a) By rearranging equation (15–8), we obtain

$$M = \frac{1}{162\bar{v}} \left(\frac{1}{\pi N}\right)^2 \left(\frac{RT}{D\eta}\right)^3$$

$$M = \frac{1}{162 \times 0.75} \left(\frac{1}{3.14 \times (6.02 \times 10^{23})}\right)^2 \cdot \left(\frac{(8.31 \times 10^7) \times 293}{(7.0 \times 10^{-7}) \times 0.01}\right)^3$$

$$\cong 100,000 \text{ g/mole}$$

(b) From equation (15–7):

$$r = \frac{RT}{6\pi\eta N D}$$

$$= \frac{(8.31 \times 10^7) \times 293}{6 \times 3.14 \times 0.01 \times (6.02 \times 10^{23}) \times (7.0 \times 10^{-7})}$$

$$= 31 \times 10^{-8} \text{ cm} = 31 \text{ Å}$$

Osmotic Pressure. The van't Hoff equation

$$\pi = cRT \qquad (15-9)$$

can be used to calculate the molecular weight of a colloid in a dilute solution. Replacing c with c_g/M in equation

(15–9), in which c_g is the grams of solute per liter of solution and M is the molecular weight, we obtain

$$\pi = \frac{c_g}{M} RT \qquad (15-10)$$

Then,

$$\frac{\pi}{c_g} = \frac{RT}{M} \qquad (15-11)$$

which applies in a very dilute solution. The quantity π/c_g for a polymer having a molecular weight of, say, 50,000 is often a linear function of the concentration c_g, and the following equation can be written:

$$\frac{\pi}{c_g} = RT\left(\frac{1}{M} + Bc_g\right) \qquad (15-12)$$

in which B is a constant for any particular solvent/solute system and depends on the degree of interaction between the solvent and the solute molecules. The term Bc_g in equation (15–12) is needed because equation (15–11) holds only for ideal solutions, namely, those containing low concentrations of spherocolloids. With linear lyophilic molecules, deviations occur because the solute molecules become solvated, leading to a reduction in the concentration of "free" solvent and an apparent increase in solute concentration. The role of B in estimating the asymmetry of particles and their interactions with solute has been discussed by Hiemenz.[7]

A plot of π/c_g against c_g generally results in one of three lines (Fig. 15–7), depending on whether the system is ideal (line I) or real (lines II and III). Equation (15–11) applies to line I, and equation (15–12)

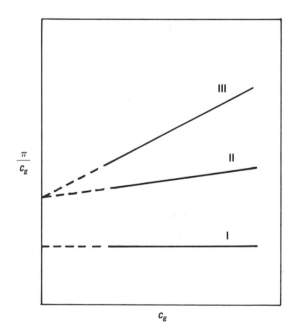

Fig. 15–7. Determination of molecular weight by means of the osmotic pressure method. Extrapolation of the line to the vertical axis where $c_g = 0$ gives RT/M, from which M is obtained. Refer to text for significance of lines I, II, and III. Lines II and III are taken to represent two samples of a species of hemoglobin.

describes lines II and III. The intercept is RT/M, and if the temperature at which the determination was carried out is known, the molecular weight of the solute can be calculated. In lines II and III, the slope of the line is B, the interaction constant. In line I, B equals zero and is typical of a dilute spherocolloidal system. Line III is typical of a linear colloid in a solvent having a high affinity for the dispersed particles. Such a solvent is referred to as a "good" solvent for that particular colloid. There is a marked deviation from ideality as the concentration is increased and B is large. At higher concentrations, or where interaction is marked, type III lines can become nonlinear, requiring that equation (15–12) be expanded and written as a power series:

$$\frac{\pi}{c_g} = RT\left(\frac{1}{M} + Bc_g + Cc_g^2 + \cdots\right) \quad (15\text{–}13)$$

in which C is another interaction constant. Line II depicts the situation in which the same colloid is present in a relatively poor solvent having a reduced affinity for the dispersed material. Note, however, that the extrapolated intercept on the π/c_g axis is identical for both lines II and III, showing that the calculated molecular weight is independent of the solvent used.

Example 15–4. Let us assume that the intercept $(\pi/c_g)_o$ for line III in Figure 15–7 has the value 3.623×10^{-4} liter atm/gram, and the slope of the line is 1.80×10^{-6} liter^2 atm g^{-2}. What is the molecular weight and the second virial coefficient B for a sample of hemoglobin using the data given here?

In Figure 15–7, line III crosses the vertical intercept at the same point as line II. These two samples of hemoglobin have the same *limiting reduced osmotic pressure*, as $(\pi/c_g)_o$ is called, and therefore have the same molecular weight. The B values, and therefore the shape of the two samples and their interaction with the medium, differ as evidenced by the different slopes of lines II and III.

At the intercept $(\pi/c_g)_o = RT/M$. Therefore,

$$M = RT/(\pi/c_g)_o = \frac{(0.08206 \text{ liter atm/deg mole})(298° \text{ K})}{3.623 \times 10^{-4} \text{ liter atm g}^{-1}}$$

$M = 67,496$ g/mole (daltons) for both hemoglobins.

The slope of line III, representing one of the hemoglobin samples, is divided by RT to obtain B, as observed in equation (15–12):

$B = 1.80 \times 10^{-6}$ liter^2 atm g^{-2}/(0.08206 liter atm/mole deg)(298° K)

$\quad = 7.36 \times 10^{-8}$ liter mole g^{-2}

The other hemoglobin sample, represented by line II, has a slope of 4.75×10^{-9} liter^2 atm g^{-2}, and its B value is therefore calculated as follows:

$B = 4.75 \times 10^{-9}$ liter^2 atm g^{-2}/(0.08206 liter atm/mole deg)(298° K)

$\quad = 1.94 \times 10^{-10}$ liter mole g^{-2}

What would you estimate the B value to be for the protein represented by line I? Would you assume its molecular weight to be larger or smaller than that of samples II and III? Referring to equations (15–11) and (15–12) will assist you in arriving at your answers.

Sedimentation. The velocity v of sedimentation of spherical particles having a density ρ in a medium of density ρ_o and a viscosity η_0 is given by *Stokes' law:*

$$v = \frac{2r^2(\rho - \rho_o)g}{9\eta_0} \quad (15\text{–}14)$$

in which g is the acceleration due to gravity. If the particles are subjected only to the force of gravity, then the lower size limit of particles obeying Stokes' equation is about 0.5 μm. This is because Brownian movement becomes significant and tends to offset sedimentation due to gravity and promotes mixing instead. Consequently, a stronger force must be applied to bring about the sedimentation of colloidal particles in a quantitative and measurable manner. This is accomplished by use of the *ultracentrifuge*, developed by Svedberg in 1925, which can produce a force a million times that of gravity.

In a centrifuge, the acceleration of gravity is replaced by $\omega^2 x$, in which ω is the angular velocity and x is the distance of the particle from the center of rotation. Equation (15–14) is accordingly modified to

$$v = \frac{dx}{dt} = \frac{2r^2(\rho - \rho_o)\omega^2 x}{9\eta_0}$$

The speed at which a centrifuge is operated is commonly expressed in terms of the number of revolutions per minute (rpm) of the rotor. It is frequently more desirable to express the rpm as angular acceleration ($\omega^2 x$) or the number of times that the force of gravity is exceeded.

Example 15–5. A centrifuge is rotating at 1500 rpm. The midpoint of the cell containing the sample is located 7.5 cm from the center of the rotor (i.e., $x = 7.5$ cm). What is the average angular acceleration and the number of "g"s on the suspended particles?

$$\text{Angular acceleration} = \omega^2 x$$

$$= \left(\frac{1500 \text{ revolutions}}{\text{minute}} \times \frac{2\pi}{60}\right)^2 \times 7.5 \text{ cm}$$

$$= 1.851 \times 10^5 \text{ cm/sec}^2$$

$$\text{Number of "g"s} = \frac{1.851 \times 10^5 \text{ cm/sec}^2}{981 \text{ cm/sec}^2}$$

$$= 188.7 \text{ "g"s}$$

that is, the force produced is 188.7 times that due to gravity.

The instantaneous velocity $v = dx/dt$ of a particle in a unit centrifugal field is expressed in terms of the *Svedberg sedimentation coefficient s,*

$$s = \frac{dx/dt}{\omega^2 x} \quad (15\text{–}15)$$

Owing to the centrifugal force, particles having a high molecular weight pass from position x_1 at time t_1 to position x_2 at time t_2, and the sedimentation coefficient is obtained by integrating equation (15–15) to give

$$s = \frac{\ln (x_2/x_1)}{\omega^2(t_2 - t_1)} \quad (15\text{–}16)$$

The distances x_1 and x_2 refer to positions of the boundary between the solvent and the high-molecular-weight component in the centrifuge cell. The boundary is located by the change of refractive index, which may be attained at any time during the run and translated into a peak on a photographic plate. Photographs are taken at definite intervals, and the peaks of the *schlieren patterns*, as they are called, give the position x of the boundary at each time, t. If the sample consists of a component of a definite molecular weight, the schlieren pattern will have a single sharp peak at any moment during the run. If components with different molecular weights are present in the sample, the particles of greater weight will settle faster, and several peaks will appear on the schlieren patterns. Therefore, ultracentrifugation is useful not only for determining the molecular weight of polymers, particularly proteins, but also may be used to ascertain the degree of homogeneity of the sample. Gelatin, for example, is found to be a polydisperse protein with fractions of molecular weight 10,000 to 100,000. (This accounts in part for the fact that gelatin from various sources is observed to have variable properties when used in pharmaceutical preparations.) Insulin, on the other hand, is a monodisperse protein composed of two polypeptide chains, each made up of a number of amino acid molecules. The two chains are attached together by disulfide—S—S— bridges to form a definite unit having a molecular weight of about 6000.

The sedimentation coefficient s may be computed from equation (15–16) after the two distances x_1 and x_2 are measured on the schlieren photographs obtained at times t_1 and t_2; the angular velocity ω is equal to 2π times the speed of the rotor in revolutions per second. Knowing s and obtaining D from diffusion data, it is possible to determine the molecular weight of a polymer, such as a protein, by use of the expression

$$M = \frac{RTs}{D(1 - \bar{v}\rho_o)} \qquad (15–17)$$

in which R is the molar gas constant, T is the absolute temperature, $\bar{v}$ is the partial specific volume of the protein, and ρ_o is the density of the solvent. Both s and D must be obtained at, or corrected to, 20° C for use in equation (15–17).

Example 15–6. The sedimentation coefficient s for a particular fraction of methylcellulose at 20° C (293° K) is 1.7×10^{-13} sec, the diffusion coefficient D is 15×10^{-7} cm²/sec, the partial specific volume $\bar{v}$ of the gum is 0.72cm³/g, and the density of water at 20° C is 0.998 g/cm³. Compute the molecular weight of methylcellulose. The gas constant R is 8.31×10^7 erg/(deg mole).

$$M = \frac{(8.31 \times 10^7) \times 293 \times (1.7 \times 10^{-13})}{15 \times 10^{-7}[1 - (0.72 \times 0.998)]}$$

$$= 9800 \text{ g/mole}$$

Kirschbaum[8] has reviewed the usefulness of the analytic ultracentrifuge and has used it to study the micellar properties of drugs (Fig. 15–8a, b). Richard [9] determined the apparent micellar molecular weight of the antibiotic fusidate sodium by ultracentrifugation. He concluded the primary micelles composed of five monomer units are formed, followed by aggregation of these pentamers into larger micelles at higher salt concentrations.

The sedimentation method already described is known as the *sedimentation velocity* technique. A

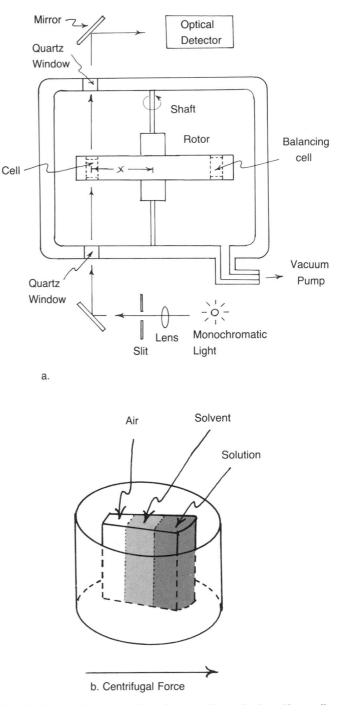

Fig. 15–8. (*a*) Schematic of the ultracentrifuge. (*b*) Centrifuge cell. (From H. R. Allcock and F. W. Lampe, *Contemporary Polymer Chemistry*, Prentice-Hall, Englewood Cliffs, N.J., 1981, pp. 366, 367, reproduced with permission of the copyright owner.)

second method, involving *sedimentation equilibrium*, may also be used. Equilibrium is established when the sedimentation force is just balanced by the counteracting diffusional force and the boundary is therefore stationary. In this method, the diffusion coefficient need not be determined; however, the centrifuge may have to be run for several weeks to attain equilibrium throughout the cell. Newer methods of calculation have been developed recently for obtaining molecular weights by the equilibrium method without requiring these long periods of centrifugation, enabling the protein chemist to obtain molecular weights rapidly and accurately.

Molecular weights determined by sedimentation velocity, sedimentation equilibrium, and osmotic pressure determinations are in good agreement, as may be seen from Table 15–4.

Viscosity. Viscosity is an expression of the resistance to flow of a system under an applied stress. The more viscous a liquid, the greater the applied force required to make it flow at a particular rate. The fundamental principles and applications of viscosity are discussed in detail in Chapter 17. The present section is concerned with the flow properties of dilute colloidal systems and the manner in which viscosity data can be used to obtain the molecular weight of material comprising the disperse phase. Viscosity studies also provide information regarding the shape of the particles in solution.

Einstein developed an equation of flow applicable to dilute colloidal dispersions of spherical particles, namely,

$$\eta = \eta_o(1 + 2.5\phi) \qquad (15\text{--}18)$$

In equation (15–18), which is based on hydrodynamic theory, η_o is the viscosity of the dispersion medium and η is the viscosity of the dispersion when the volume fraction of colloidal particles present is ϕ. The volume fraction is defined as the volume of the particles divided by the total volume of the dispersion; it is therefore equivalent to a concentration term. Both η_o and η may be determined using a capillary viscometer, described on pp. 461–462.

Several viscosity coefficients may be defined with respect to this equation. These include *relative viscosity*, *specific viscosity* (η_{sp}), and *intrinsic viscosity* $[\eta]$. From equation (15–18),

$$\eta_{rel} = \frac{\eta}{\eta_o} = 1 + 2.5\phi \qquad (15\text{--}19)$$

and

$$\eta_{sp} = \frac{\eta}{\eta_o} - 1 = \frac{\eta - \eta_o}{\eta_o} = 2.5\phi \qquad (15\text{--}20)$$

or

$$\frac{\eta_{sp}}{\phi} = 2.5 \qquad (15\text{--}21)$$

Since volume fraction is directly related to concentration, equation (15–21) may be written as

$$\frac{\eta_{sp}}{c} = k \qquad (15\text{--}22)$$

in which c is expressed in grams of colloidal particles per 100 mL of total dispersion. For highly polymeric materials dispersed in the medium at moderate concentrations, the equation is best expressed as a power series:

$$\frac{\eta_{sp}}{c} = k_1 + k_2 c + k_3 c^2 \qquad (15\text{--}23)$$

By determining η at various concentrations and knowing η_o, η_{sp} can be calculated from equation (15–20). If η_{sp}/c is plotted against c (see Fig. 15–9, and the line extrapolated to infinite dilution, the intercept is k_1 (equation [15–23]). This constant, commonly known as the intrinsic viscosity, $[\eta]$, is used to calculate the approximate molecular weights of polymers. According to the Mark–Houwink equation,

$$[\eta] = KM^a \qquad (15\text{--}24)$$

in which K and a are constants characteristic of the particular polymer–solvent system. These constants, which are virtually independent of molecular weight, are obtained initially by determining $[\eta]$ experimentally for polymer fractions whose molecular weights have been determined by other methods such as light scattering, osmotic pressure, or sedimentation. Once K and a are known, measurement of $[\eta]$ provides a simple yet accurate means of obtaining molecular weights for fractions not yet subjected to other methods. The details of the calculation are brought out by working through Problem 15–19. Intrinsic viscosity $[\eta]$, together with an interaction constant k', provides an equation, $\eta_{sp}/c = [\eta] + k'[\eta]^2 c$, for use to choose solvent

TABLE 15–4. *Molecular Weights of Proteins in Aqueous Solution**

Material	Molecular Weight		
	Sedimentation Velocity	Sedimentation Equilibrium	Osmotic Pressure
Ribonuclease	12,700	13,000	—
Myoglobin	16,900	17,500	17,000
Ovalbumin	44,000	40,500	45,000
Hemoglobin (horse)	68,000	68,000	67,000
Serum albumin (horse)	70,000	68,000	73,000
Serum globulin (horse)	167,000	150,000	175,000
Tobacco mosaic virus	59,000,000	—	—

*From D. J. Shaw, *Introduction to Colloid and Surface Chemistry*, Butterworths, London, 1970, p. 32. For an extensive listing of molecular weights of macromolecules, see C. Tanford, *Physical Chemistry of Macromolecules*, Wiley, New York, 1961.

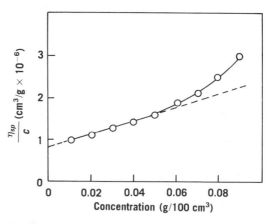

Fig. 15–9. Determination of molecular weight using viscosity data. (D. R. Powell J. Swarbrick and G. S. Banker, J. Pharm. Sci. **55**, 601, 1966, reproduced with permission of copyright owner.)

mixtures for tablet film coating polymers such as ethyl cellulose.[10]

The viscosity of colloidal dispersions is affected by the shapes of particles of the disperse phase. Spherocolloids form dispersions of relatively low viscosity, while systems containing linear particles are more viscous. As we have seen in previous sections, the relationship of shape and viscosity reflects the degree of solvation of the particles. If a linear colloid is placed in a solvent for which it has a low affinity, it tends to "ball up," that is, to assume a spherical shape, and the viscosity falls. This provides a means of detecting changes in the shape of flexible colloidal particles and macromolecules.

The characteristics of polymers used as substitutes for blood plasma (plasma extenders) depend in part on the molecular weight of the material. These characteristics include the size and shape of the macromolecules and the ability of the polymers to impart the proper viscosity and osmotic pressure to the blood. The methods described in this chapter are used to determine the average molecular weights of hydroxyethyl starch, dextran, and gelatin preparations used as plasma extenders. Ultracentrifugation, light scatter-

ing, x-ray analysis (small-angle x-ray scattering[11]), and other analytic tools[12] were used by Paradies to determine the structural properties of tyrothricin, a mixture of the peptide antibiotics gramicidine and tyrocidine B. The antibiotic aggregate has a molecular weight of 28,600 daltons and was determined to be a rod of 170 Å in length and 30 Å in diameter.

ELECTRIC PROPERTIES OF COLLOIDS

The properties of colloids that depend on, or are affected by, the presence of a charge on the surface of a particle are discussed under this heading. The various ways in which the surface of particles dispersed in a liquid medium acquire a charge has already been outlined in Chapter 14 (which treated interfacial phenomena) (p. 386). Mention was also made of the *zeta (electrokinetic)* potential and how it is related to the *Nernst (electrothermodynamic)* potential. The potential versus distance diagram for a spherical colloidal particle may be represented as shown in Figure 15–10. Such a system may be formed, for example, by adding

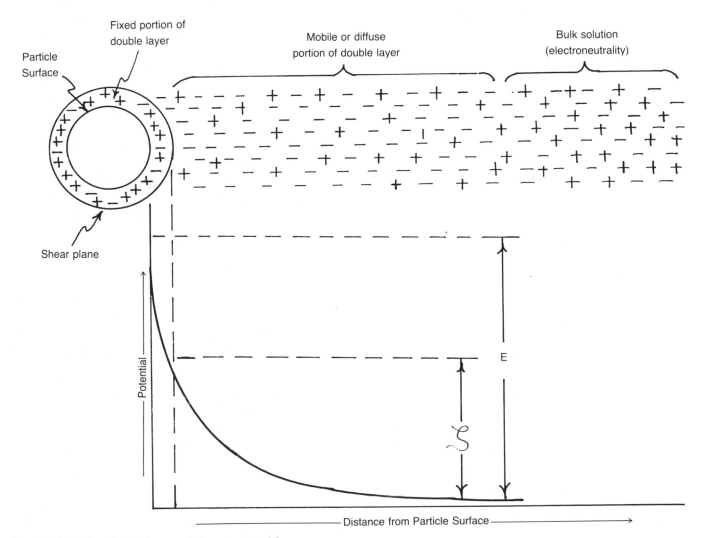

Fig. 15–10. Diffuse double layer and the zeta potential.

a dilute solution of potassium iodide to an equimolar solution of silver nitrate. A colloidal precipitate of silver iodide particles is produced and, because the silver ions are in excess and are adsorbed, a positively charged particle is produced. If the reverse procedure is adopted, that is, if silver nitrate is added to the potassium iodide solution, iodide ions are adsorbed on the particles as the potential-determining ion and result in the formation of a negatively charged sol.

Electrokinetic Phenomena. The movement of a charged surface with respect to an adjacent liquid phase is the basic principle underlying four electrokinetic phenomena: *electrophoresis, electroosmosis, sedimentation potential,* and *streaming potential.*

Electrophoresis involves the movement of a charged particle through a liquid under the influence of an applied potential difference. An electrophoresis cell, fitted with two electrodes, contains the dispersion. When a potential is applied across the electrodes, the particles migrate to the oppositely charged electrode. Figure 15–11 illustrates the design of a commercially available instrument. The rate of particle migration is observed by means of an ultramicroscope and is a function of the charge on the particle. As the shear plane of the particle is located at the periphery of the tightly bound layer, the rate-determining potential is the zeta potential. From a knowledge of the direction and rate of migration, the sign and magnitude of the zeta potential in a colloidal system may be determined. The relevant equation

$$\zeta = \frac{v}{E} \times \frac{4\pi\eta}{\epsilon} \times (9 \times 10^4) \qquad (15\text{–}25)$$

which yields the zeta potential (ζ) in volts, requires a knowledge of the velocity of migration v of the sol in cm/sec in an electrophoresis tube of a definite length in

cm, the viscosity of the medium η in poises (dyne sec/cm^2), the dielectric constant of the medium ϵ, and the potential gradient E in volts/cm. The term v/E is known as the *mobility.*

It is instructive to carry out the dimensional analysis of equation (15–25). In one system of fundamental electric units, E, the electric field strength, can be expressed in electrostatic units of statvolt/cm (a coulomb is equal to 3×10^9 statcoulombs, and 1 statvolt equals 300 practical volts). The dielectric constant is not dimensionless here, but rather from Coulomb's law may be assigned the units of statcoulomb^2/(dyne cm^2). The equation

$$\zeta = \frac{v}{E} \frac{4\pi\eta}{\epsilon} \qquad (15\text{–}26)$$

may then be written dimensionally, recognizing that statvolts $\times$ statcoulombs = dyne cm, as

$$\zeta = \frac{\text{cm/sec}}{\text{statvolts/cm}}$$

$$\times \frac{\text{dyne sec/cm}^2}{\text{statcoulomb}^2/(\text{dyne cm}^2)} = \text{statvolts} \qquad (15\text{–}27)$$

It is more convenient to express zeta potential in practical volts that in statvolts. Since 1 statvolt is equal to 300 practical volts, equation (15–27) is multiplied by 300 to make this conversion, that is, statvolts $\times$ 300 practical volts/statvolt = 300 practical volts. Furthermore, E is ordinarily measured in practical volts/cm and not in statvolt/cm, and this conversion is made by again multiplying the right-hand side of equation (15–27) by 300. The final expression is equation (15–25), in which the factor, $300 \times 300 = 9 \times 10^4$, converts electrostatic units to volts.

For a colloidal system at 20° C in which the dispersion medium is water, equation (15–25) reduces approximately to

$$\zeta \cong 141 \frac{v}{E} \qquad (15\text{–}28)$$

The coefficient, 141, at 20° C becomes 128 at 25° C.

Example 15–7. The velocity of migration of an aqueous ferric hydroxide sol was determined at 20° C using the apparatus shown in Figure 15–11 and was found to be 16.5×10^{-4} cm/sec. The distance between the electrodes in the cell was 20 cm, and the applied emf was 110 volts. What is (a) the zeta potential of the sol and (b) the sign of the charge on the particles?

(a)
$$\frac{v}{E} = \frac{16.5 \times 10^{-4} \text{ cm/sec}}{110/20 \text{ volts/cm}} = 3 \times 10^{-4} \text{ cm}^2 \text{ volt}^{-1} \text{ sec}^{-1}$$

$$\zeta = 141 \times (3 \times 10^{-4}) = 0.042 \text{ volt}$$

(b) The particles were seen to migrate toward the negative electrode of the electrophoresis cell; therefore, the colloid is positively charged. The zeta potential is often used to estimate the stability of colloids, as discussed in a later section.

Electroosmosis is essentially the opposite in principle to that of electrophoresis. In the latter, the

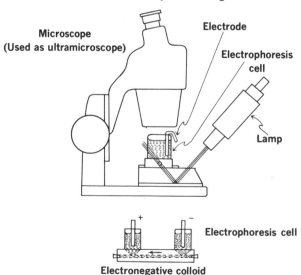

Particles viewed by reflected light

Microscope (Used as ultramicroscope)

Electrode

Electrophoresis cell

Lamp

+ −

Electrophoresis cell

Electronegative colloid

Fig. 15–11. Principle of zeta potential measurement (based on Zeta Meter) showing ultramicrocope and flow cell.

application of a potential causes a charged particle to move relative to the liquid, which is stationary. If the solid is rendered immobile (i.e., by forming a capillary or making the particles into a porous plug), however, the liquid now moves relative to the charged surface. This is electroosmosis, so called because liquid moves through a plug or membrane across which a potential is applied. Electroosmosis provides another method for obtaining zeta potential by determining the rate of flow of liquid through the plug under standard conditions.

Sedimentation potential, the reverse of electrophoresis, is the creation of a potential when particles undergo sedimentation. *Streaming potential* differs from electroosmosis in that the potential is created by forcing a liquid to flow through a plug or bed of particles.

Schott[13] studied the electrokinetic properties of magnesium hydroxide suspensions that are used as antacids and laxatives. The zero point of charge occurred at pH $\cong 10.8$, the zeta potential, ζ, of magnesium hydroxide being positive below this pH value. Increasing the pH or hydroxide ion concentration produced a change in the sign of ζ from positive to negative, with the largest negative ζ value occurring at pH 11.5.

Takenaka and associates[14] studied the electrophoretic properties of *microcapsules* (pp. 516–517) of sulfamethoxazole in droplets of a gelatin–acacia coacervate as part of a study to stabilize such drugs in microcapsules.

Crommelin[15] determined the effect of adding charge-inducing agents such as stearylamine or phosphatidylserine on the zeta potential of liposomes (p. 513) of phosphatidylcholine and cholesterol in aqueous media. The physical stability of the liposomes was predicted on the basis of the Derjaguin–Landau–Verwey–Overbeek (DLVO) theory (p. 408). The physical stability predicted from the theory did not, however, correlate with the experimentally obtained stability.

Schott and Young [16] determined the electrophoretic mobility of the gram-positive *Streptococcus faecalis* and the gram-negative *Escherichia coli* as a function of ionic strength and pH. An increase in concentration of buffer electrolytes (increased ionic strength) reduced the mobility, v/E, of *S. faecalis*. Both *E. coli* and *S. faecalis* were negatively charged over the pH range studied. The chemical group responsible for the charge at the surface of both bacteria presumably is the carboxyl group.

The magnitude and sign of the electric charge of ampholytic drugs (p. 149) at physiologic pH influences their absorption from the gastrointestinal tract and their passage through bacterial membranes. Schott and Astigarrabia[17] determined the isoelectric points (p. 149) of four very slightly soluble sulfonamides by electrophoresis of their suspensions as a function of pH. The isoelectric points of all four sulfonamides were between 3.5 and 4.6, indicating that the sulfonamides are weak acids rather than zwitterions at the normal physiologic pH of 7.4.

Donnan Membrane Equilibrium. If sodium chloride is placed in solution on one side of a semipermeable membrane, and a negatively charged colloid, together with its counterions R^-Na^+, is placed on the other side, the sodium and chloride ions can pass freely across the barrier but not the colloidal anionic particles. The system at equilibrium is represented in the following diagram, in which R^- is the nondiffusible colloidal anion and the vertical line separating the various species represents the semipermeable membrane. The volumes of solution on the two sides of the membrane are considered to be equal.

outside (o)	inside (i)
	R^-
Na^+	Na^+
Cl^-	Cl^-

After equilibrium has been established, the concentration in dilute solutions (more correctly the activity) of sodium chloride must be the same on both sides of the membrane, according to the principle of escaping tendencies (p. 106). Therefore,

$$[Na^+]_o[Cl^-]_o = [Na^+]_i[Cl^-]_i \qquad (15\text{–}29)$$

The condition of electroneutrality must also apply. That is, the concentration of positively charged ions in the solutions on either side of the membrane must balance the concentration of negatively charged ions. Therefore, on the outside,

$$[Na^+]_o = [Cl^-]_o \qquad (15\text{–}30)$$

and inside,

$$[Na^+]_i = [R^-]_i + [Cl^-]_i \qquad (15\text{–}31)$$

Equations (15–30) and (15–31) may be substituted into (15–29) to give

$$[Cl^-]_o^2 = ([Cl^-]_i + [R^-]_i)[Cl^-]_i$$
$$= [Cl^-]_i^2 \left(1 + \frac{[R^-]_i}{[Cl^-]_i}\right) \qquad (15\text{–}32)$$

$$\frac{[Cl^-]_o}{[Cl^-]_i} = \sqrt{1 + \frac{[R^-]_i}{[Cl^-]_i}} \qquad (15\text{–}33)$$

Equation (15–33), the *Donnan membrane equilibrium*, gives the ratio of concentrations of the diffusible anion outside and inside the membrane at equilibrium. The equation shows that a negatively charged polyelectrolyte inside a semipermeable sac would influence the equilibrium concentration ratio of a diffusible anion. It tends to drive the ion of like charge out through the membrane. When $[R^-]_i$ is large compared with $[Cl^-]_i$, the ratio roughly equals $\sqrt{[R^-]_i}$. If, on the other hand, $[Cl^-]_i$ is quite large with respect to $[R^-]_i$, the ratio in equation (15–33) becomes equal to unity, and the concentration of the salt is thus equal on both sides of the membrane.

The unequal distribution of diffusible electrolyte ions on the two sides of the membrane will obviously result in erroneous values for osmotic pressures of polyelectrolyte solutions. If, however, the concentration of salt in the solution is made large, the Donnan equilibrium effect can be practically eliminated in the determination of molecular weights of proteins involving the osmotic pressure method.

Higuchi et al.[18] modified the Donnan membrane equilibrium, equation (15–33), to demonstrate the use of the polyelectrolyte sodium carboxymethylcellulose for enhancing the absorption of drugs such as sodium salicylate and potassium benzylpenicillin. If $[Cl^-]$ in equation (15–33) is replaced by the concentration of the diffusible drug, anion $[D^-]$ at equilibrium, and $[R^-]$ is used to represent the concentration of sodium carboxymethylcellulose at equilibrium, we have a modification of the *Donnan membrane equilibrium* for a diffusible drug anion, $[D^-]$:

$$\frac{[D^-]_o}{[D^-]_i} = \sqrt{1 + \frac{[R^-]_i}{[D^-]_i}} \qquad (15\text{--}34)$$

It will be observed that when $[R^-]_i/[D^-]_i = 8$, the ratio $[D^-]_o/[D^-]_i = 3$, and when $[R^-]_i/[D^-]_i = 99$, the ratio $[D^-]_o/[D^-]_i = 10$. Therefore, the addition of an anionic polyelectrolyte to a diffusible drug anion should enhance the diffusion of the drug out of the chamber. By kinetic studies, Higuchi et al.[18] showed that the presence of sodium carboxymethylcellulose more than doubled the rate of transfer of the negatively charged dye, scarlet red sulfonate.

Other investigators have found by in vivo experiments that ion-exchange resins and even sulfate and phosphate ions that do not diffuse readily through the intestinal wall, tend to drive anions from the intestinal tract into the bloodstream. The opposite effect, that of retardation of drug absorption, may occur if the drug complexes with the macromolecule.

Example 15–8. A solution of dissociated nondiffusible carboxymethylcellulose is equilibrated across a semipermeable membrane with a solution of sodium salicylate. The membrane allows free passage of the salicylate ion. Compute the ratio of salicylate on the two sides of the membrane at equilibrium, assuming that the equilibrium concentration of carboxymethylcellulose is 1.2×10^{-2} gram equivalent/liter and the equilibrium concentration of sodium salicylate is 6.0×10^{-3} gram equivalent/liter. The modified Donnan membrane expression, equation (15–34), is used:

$$\frac{[D^-]_o}{[D^-]_i} = \sqrt{1 + \frac{[R^-]_i}{[D^-]_i}}$$

$$= \sqrt{1 + \frac{12 \times 10^{-3}}{6 \times 10^{-3}}} = 1.73$$

Stability of Colloid Systems. The presence and magnitude, or absence, of a charge on a colloidal particle is an important factor in the stability of colloidal systems. Stabilization is accomplished essentially by two means: providing the dispersed particles with an electric charge, and surrounding each particle with a protective solvent sheath that prevents mutual adherence when the particles collide as a result of Brownian movement. This second effect is significant only in the case of lyophilic sols.

A lyophobic sol is thermodynamically unstable. The particles in such sols are stabilized only by the presence of electric charges on their surfaces. The like charges produce a repulsion that prevents coagulation of the particles. If the last traces of ions are removed from the system by dialysis, the particles can agglomerate and reduce the total surface area, and, owing to their increased size, they may settle rapidly from suspension. Hence, addition of a small amount of electrolyte to a lyophobic sol tends to stabilize the system by imparting a charge to the particles. Addition of electrolyte beyond that necessary for maximum adsorption on the particles, however, sometimes results in the accumulation of opposite ions and reduces the zeta potential below its *critical value.* The critical potential for finely dispersed oil droplets in water (oil hydrosol) is about 40 millivolts, this high value signifying relatively great instability. The critical zeta potential of a gold sol, on the other hand, is nearly zero, which suggests that the particles require only a minute charge for stabilization; hence, they exhibit marked stability against added electrolytes. The valence of the ions having a charge opposite to that of the particles appears to determine the effectiveness of the electrolyte in coagulating the colloid. The precipitating power increases rapidly with the valence or charge of the ions, and a statement of this fact is known as the *Schulze–Hardy rule.*

These observations permitted Verwey and Overbeek[19] and Derjaguin and Landau[20] to independently develop a theory that describes the stability of lyophobic colloids. According to this approach, known as the DLVO theory, the forces on colloidal particles in a dispersion are due to electrostatic repulsion and London-type van der Waal's attraction. These forces result in potential energies of repulsion, V_R, and attraction, V_A, between particles. These are shown in Figure 15–12 together with the curve for the composite potential energy, V_T. There is a deep potential "well" of attraction near the origin and a high potential barrier of repulsion at moderate distances. A shallow secondary trough of attraction (or minimum) is sometimes observed at longer distances of separation. The presence of a secondary minimum is significant in the controlled flocculation of coarse dispersions (see Chapter 18). Following this principle, one can determine somewhat quantitatively the amount of electrolyte of a particular valence type required to precipitate a colloid.

Not only do electrolytes bring about coagulation of colloidal particles; the mixing of oppositely charged colloids can also result in mutual agglomeration.

Lyophilic and association colloids are thermodynamically stable and exist in true solution so that the system constitutes a single phase. The addition of an electrolyte to a lyophilic colloid in moderate amounts does not

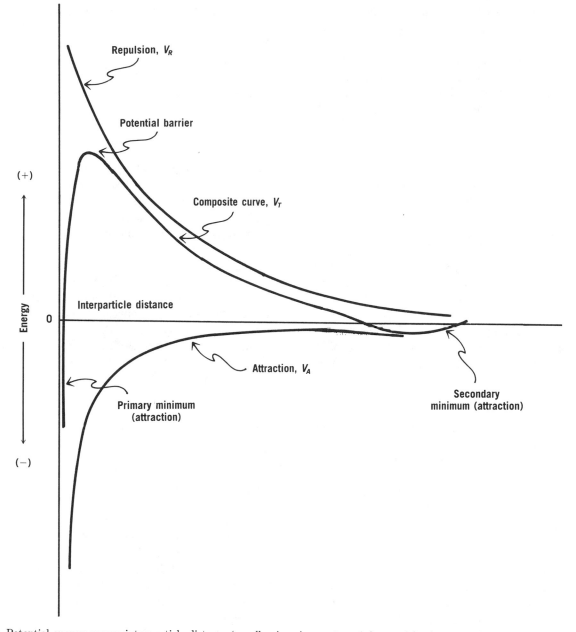

Fig. 15–12. Potential energy versus interparticle distance (usually given in angstroms) for particles in suspension.

result in coagulation, as was evident with lyophobic colloids. If sufficient salt is added, however, agglomeration and sedimentation of the particles may result. This phenomenon, referred to as "salting-out," was discussed in the chapter on solubility.

Just as the Schulze–Hardy rule arranges ions in the order of their capacity to coagulate hydrophobic colloids, the *Hofmeister* or *lyotropic series* ranks cations and anions in order of coagulation of hydrophilic sols. Several anions of the Hofmeister series in decreasing order of precipitating power are citrate, tartrate, sulfate, acetate, chloride, nitrate, bromide, and iodide. The precipitating power is directly related to the hydration of the ion and hence to its ability to separate water molecules from the colloidal particles.

Alcohol and acetone can also decrease the solubility of hydrophilic colloids so that the addition of a small

amount of electrolytes may then bring about coagulation. The addition of the less polar solvent renders the solvent mixture unfavorable for the colloid, and electrolytes can then salt out the colloid with relative ease. We may thus regard flocculation on the addition of alcohol, followed by salts, as a gradual transformation from a sol of a lyophilic nature to one of a more lyophobic character.

When negatively and positively charged hydrophilic colloids are mixed, the particles may separate from the dispersion to form a layer rich in the colloidal aggregates. The colloid-rich layer is known as a *coacervate*, and the phenomenon in which macromolecular solutions separate into two liquid layers is referred to as *coacervation*. As an example, consider the mixing of gelatin and acacia. Gelatin at a pH below 4.7 (its isoelectric point) is positively charged; acacia carries a negative charge that is relatively unaffected by pH in the acid range. When solutions of these colloids are mixed in a certain proportion, coacervation results. The viscosity of the upper layer, now poor in colloid, is markedly decreased below that of the coacervate, and in pharmacy this is considered to represent a physical incompatibility. Coacervation need not involve the interaction of charged particles; the coacervation of gelatin may also be brought about by the addition of alcohol, sodium sulfate, or a macromolecular substance such as starch.

Takenaka et al.[21] microencapsulated (p. 516) sulfamethoxazole in a gelatin–acacia coacervate, and reported on the particle size, wall thickness, and porosity of the microcapsules.

Badawi and El-Sayed[22] investigated the equilibrium solubility and dissolution rate of a coacervate of sulfathiazole complexed with povidone. They found the dissolution rate to be enhanced by coacervation. In forming the coacervate, an amorphous precipitate is formed when the sulfonamide is treated by acid or base in aqueous solution or when an alcoholic solution of the drug is diluted with water. In the presence of povidone a complex is formed with the partially precipitated sulfathiazole, resulting in a coacervate. The addition of resorcinol, a coacervating agent for povidone, to an aqueous mixture of sulfathiazole sodium and povidone also resulted in coacervation.

Sensitization and Protective Colloidal Action. The addition of a small amount of hydrophilic or hydrophobic colloid to a hydrophobic colloid of opposite charge tends to sensitize or even coagulate the particles. This is considered by some workers to be due to a reduction of the zeta potential below the critical value (usually about 20 to 50 millivolts). Others attribute the instability of the hydrophobic particles to a reduction in the thickness of the ionic layer surrounding the particles and a decrease in the coulombic repulsion between the particles. The addition of large amounts of the *hydrophile* (hydrophilic colloid), however, stabilizes the system, the hydrophile being adsorbed on the hydrophobic particles. This phenomenon is known as *protection*, and the added hydrophilic sol is known as a *protective colloid*. The several ways in which stabilization of hydrophobic colloids can be achieved (i.e., protective action) have been reviewed by Schott.[23]

The protective property is expressed most frequently in terms of the *gold number*. The gold number is the minimum weight in milligrams of the protective colloid (dry weight of dispersed phase) required to prevent a color change from red to violet in 10 mL of a gold sol on the addition of 1 mL of a 10% solution of sodium chloride. The gold numbers for some common protective colloids are given in Table 15–5.

A pharmaceutical example of sensitization and protective action is provided when bismuth subnitrate is suspended in a tragacanth dispersion; the mixture forms a gel that sets to a hard mass in the bottom of the

TABLE 15–5. *The Gold Number of Protective Colloids*

Protective Colloid	Gold Number
Gelatin	0.005–0.01
Albumin	0.1
Acacia	0.1–0.2
Sodium oleate	1–5
Tragacanth	2

container. Bismuth subcarbonate, a compound that does not dissociate sufficiently to liberate the bismuth ions, is compatible with tragacanth.

These phenomena probably involve a sensitization and coagulation of the gum by the Bi^{3+} ions. The flocculated gum then aggregates with the bismuth subnitrate particles to form a gel or a hard cake. If phosphate, citrate, or tartrate are added, they protect the gums from the coagulating influence of the Bi^{3+} ions, and, no doubt, by reducing the zeta potential on the bismuth particles, partially flocculate the insoluble material. Partially flocculated systems tend to cake considerably less than deflocculated systems, and this effect is significant in the formulation of suspensions[24] (Chapter 18).

SOLUBILIZATION

An important property of association colloids in solution is the ability of the micelles to increase the solubility of materials that are normally insoluble, or only slightly soluble, in the dispersion medium used. This phenomenon, known as *solubilization*, has been reviewed by many authors including Mulley,[25] Nakagawa,[26] Elworthy and coauthors,[27] and Attwood and Florence.[28] Solubilization has been used with advantage in pharmacy for many years; as early as 1892, Engler and Dieckhoff[29] solubilized a number of compounds in soap solutions.

Knowing the location, distribution, and orientation of solubilized drugs in the micelle is important to understanding the kinetic aspect of the solubilization process and the interaction of drugs with the different elements that constitute the micelle. These factors may also affect the stability and bioavailability of the drug. The location of the molecule undergoing solubilization in a micelle is related to the balance between the polar and nonpolar properties of the molecule. Lawrence[30] was the first to distinguish between the various sites. He proposed that nonpolar molecules in aqueous systems of ionic surface-active agents would be located in the hydrocarbon core of the micelle, while polar solubilizates would tend to be adsorbed onto the micelle surface. Polar–nonpolar molecules would tend to align themselves in an intermediate position within the surfactant molecules forming the micelle. Nonionic surfactants are of most pharmaceutical interest as solubilizing agents because of their lower toxicity.

Their micelles show a gradient of increased polarity from the core to the polyoxyethylene–water surface. The extended interfacial region between the core and the aqueous solution, that is, the polar mantle, is greatly hydrated. The anisotropic distribution of water molecules within the polar mantle favors the inclusion (solubilization) of a wide variety of molecules.[31] Solubilization may therefore occur in both the core and the mantle, also called the *palisade layer*. Thus, certain compounds (e.g., phenols and related compounds with a hydroxy group capable of bonding with the ether oxygen of the polyoxyethylene group) are held between the polyoxyethylene chains. Under these conditions, such compounds may be considered as undergoing inclusion within the polyoxyethylene exterior of the micelle rather than adsorption onto the micelle surface. Figure 15–13 depicts a spherical micelle of a nonionic, polyoxyethylene monostearate, surfactant in water. The figure is drawn in conformity with Reich's suggestion[32] that such a micelle may be regarded as a hydrocarbon core, made up of the hydrocarbon chains of the surfactant molecules, surrounded by the polyoxyethylene chains protruding into the continuous aqueous phase. Benzene and toluene, nonpolar molecules, are shown solubilized in the hydrocarbon interior of the micelle. Salicylic acid, a more polar molecule, is oriented with the nonpolar part of the molecule directed toward the central region of the micelle and the polar group toward the hydrophilic chains that spiral outward into the aqueous medium. Parahydroxybenzoic acid, a predominantly polar molecule, is found completely between the hydrophilic chains.

Nuclear magnetic resonance (NMR) and spectroscopic imaging techniques employing the visible and ultraviolet regions of the spectrum are used to establish the site of solubilization. Some ultraviolet spectroscopic

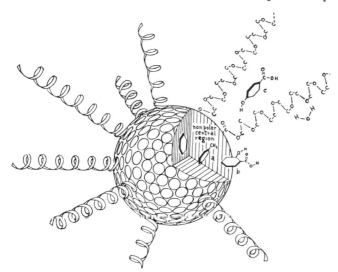

Fig. 15–13. Artist's conception of a spherical micelle of nonionic surfactant molecules. (*a*) A nonpolar molecule solubilized in the nonpolar region of the micelle. (*b*) A more polar molecule found partly embedded in the central region and partly extending into the palisade region. (*c*) A polar molecule found lying well out in the palisade layer attracted by dipolar forces to the polyoxyethylene chains.

characteristics are sensitive to the polarity of the medium. Thus the spectral shifts of compounds solubilized in micelles are used to determine the microenvironmental polarity of their sites of solubilization. Mukerjee and coworkers[33,34] determined the dielectric constant D of the microenvironment of benzene solubilized both in sodium dodecyl sulfate, an anionic surfactant, and in cetyltrimethylammonium chloride, a cationic surfactant. The results of the dielectric constant study show quite polar and similar microenvironments ($D = 40$) in the two micelles of different charge type, suggesting that benzene is mainly located at the surface, that is, in the polar part of the micelle rather than in the core.

These researchers[33,34] proposed a *two-state model* of solubilization. The less polar state involves the hydrocarbon core and is called the *dissolved state*. The other region is the micelle–water interface, the *adsorbed state*, where the environment is more polar. In this model, the total solubilizing power of a micelle is the sum of the "adsorbed" fraction and the "dissolved" fraction of solubilizate. When adsorption occurs, the solubilization is increased beyond that can be attributed alone to the solvent power of the core. Another interesting finding predicted by the model is that the microenvironmental polarity of solubilizate shows little dependence on the kind of charge on the micelle. The equilibrium between the "adsorbed" and "dissolved" states can be assumed to be similar to that in bulk systems such as in the immiscible liquid pair dodecane–water. Thus, a quantitative estimate of the solvent power of the hydrocarbon core for the solubilizate can be obtained from the dodecane–water partition coefficient of the solubilizate.

However, for a more detailed picture, the core is subjected to a substantial *Laplace pressure*, which reduces its solvent power as compared with dodecane. The Laplace pressure P is due to the curved interface and is given by the relation (p. 365)

$$P = 2\gamma/r \qquad (15-35)$$

where γ is the interfacial tension and r is the radius of the micelle. The pressure P opposes the entry of all guest molecules to be solubilized. The factor χ by which the solubility is reduced is related to the partial molar volume of the solubilizate according to the relationship[33,34]

$$P\bar{v} = RT \ln \chi \qquad (15-36)$$

Equation (15–36) indicates that χ varies exponentially with P and therefore with $1/r$ when surface tension, γ, is constant. Using equation (15–36) and knowing K, the dodecane–water distribution coefficient, it is possible to estimate the partitioning of a solubilizate between the hydrocarbon core and the aqueous medium—that is, the solubilizing power of the core.

Example 15–9. (*a*) Compute the factor χ in reducing the solubility of a new anesthetic that is solubilized in the core of sodium dodecyl sulfate micelles. The partial molar volume of the anesthetic drug, $\bar{v}$, is 173 cm^3/mole. The micelle–water interfacial tension is 31.3 erg/cm^2, and the radius r of the micelle is 18 Å.

(b) If the partition coefficient, dodecane–water, of the drug compound is $K = 21.9$, what is the partition coefficient of the anesthetic solubilizate in the core–water system?

(a) First, we compute the Laplace pressure P for the micelles of the surfactant, sodium dodecyl sulfate. Using equation (15–35),

$$P = 2\,\gamma/r = (2 \times 31.3 \text{ erg/cm}^2)/(18 \times 10^{-8} \text{ cm})$$

$$P = 3.48 \times 10^8 \text{ dyne/cm}^2 \text{ or } 343 \text{ atm}$$

$$(1 \text{ dyne/cm}^2 = 9.869 \times 10^{-7} \text{ atm})$$

Notice how great is the pressure (343 atm) inside the micelle core when its radius is small ($r = 18$ Å)! From equation (15–36),

$$\ln \chi = \frac{P\bar{v}}{RT} = \frac{(3.48 \times 10^8 \text{ dyne/cm}^2) \times (173 \text{ cm}^3/\text{mole})}{8.3143 \times 10^7 \text{ erg deg}^{-1} \text{ mole}^{-1} \times 298° \text{ K}}$$

$$\ln \chi = 2.43; \chi = 11.36$$

Thus the solubility of the new anesthetic drug in the hydrocarbon core of the surfactant is reduced by a factor of 11.36 relative to its solubility in dodecane, due to the Laplace pressure on the micelle.

(b) The partition coefficient of the new compound in the micellar core–water system is obtained by dividing the partition coefficient K in dodecane–water by the χ value obtained in part (a):

Partition coefficient (core–water) = 21.9/11.36 = 1.93

That is to say, the distribution of the drug compound in the core of the micelle is roughly twice that in the water phase.

The fraction of drug located at the surface of the micelle in the "adsorbed" state is related to the surface activity of the drug. Benzene is moderately surface-active at the heptane–water interface. However, its surface activity is greatly magnified in micellar solution owing to the extremely high surface-to-volume ratio of the micelles. Thus, the surface activity of benzene in micelles provides an explanation of its location mainly at the surface, that is, in the "adsorbed" state.

The pharmacist must give due attention to several factors when attempting to formulate solubilized systems successfully. It is essential that, at the concentration employed, the surface-active agent, if taken internally, be nontoxic, miscible with the solvent (usually water), compatible with the material to be solubilized, free from disagreeable odor and taste, and relatively nonvolatile. Toxicity is of paramount importance, and, for this reason, most solubilized systems are based on nonionic surfactants. The amount of surfactant used is important: a large excess is undesirable, from the point of view of both possible toxicity and reduced absorption and activity; an insufficient amount can lead to precipitation of the solubilized material. The amount of material that can be solubilized by a given amount of surfactant is a function of the polar–nonpolar characteristics of the surfactant (commonly termed the *hydrophile–lipophile balance*, or HLB; see p. 371) and of the molecule being solubilized.

It should be appreciated that changes in absorption and biologic availability and activity may occur when the material is formulated in a solubilized system. Drastic changes in the bactericidal activity of certain compounds take place when they are solubilized, and

the pharmacist must ensure that the concentration of surface-active agent present is optimum for that particular system. The stability of materials against oxidation and hydrolysis may be modified by solubilization.

Solubilization has been used in pharmacy to bring into solution a wide range of materials including volatile oils, coal tar and resinous materials, phenobarbital, sulfonamides, vitamins, hormones, and dyes.[27,35]

A new antimalarial drug, β-arteether, isolated in China from the plant *Artemesia annua L.*, is highly active against both chloroquine-sensitive and chloroquine-resistant forms of *Plasmodium falciparum*, the protozoa that spends part of its life cycle in the *Anopheles* mosquito. The drug is very insoluble (17 mg/L) in water but quite soluble (>200 g/L) in various organic solvents. Krishna and Flanagan[36] studied the solubilization of β-arteether in a number of anionic, cationic, and nonionic surfactant solutions above their critical micelle concentrations. They found that anionic and cationic surfactants increased the solubility dramatically by micellar solubilization, while nonionic surfactants showed little effect in enhancing the solubility of the drug. The increase in solubility of β-arteether with increasing micellar concentration of two anionic surfactants and one cationic surfactant is shown in Figure 15–14. On the vertical axis is given the relative solubility of the drug, expressed as S_t/S_o, where S_t is the total solubility of β-arteether in micellar solution and S_o is the solubility of the drug in water alone.

O'Malley et al.[37] investigated the solubilizing action of Tween 20 on peppermint oil in water and presented their results in the form of a tenary diagram as shown in Figure 15–15. They found that on the gradual addition of water to a 50:50 mixture of peppermint oil and Tween 20, polysorbate 20, the system changed from a homogeneous mixture (region I) to a viscous gel

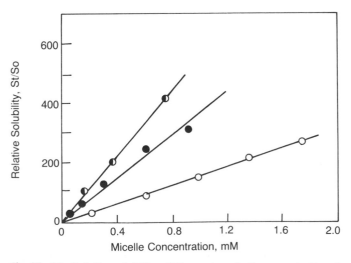

Fig. 15–14. Relative solubility, S_t/S_o, versus micelle concentration of β-arteether. Key: ○ = decyl sodium sulfate; ◐ = tetradecyl sodium sulfate; ● = hexadecyl trimethylammonium bromide. (From A. K. Krishna and D. R. Flanagan, J. Pharm. Sci. **78,** 574, 1989, reproduced with permission of the copyright owner.)

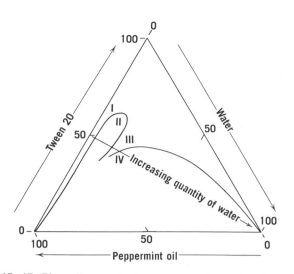

Fig. 15–15. Phase diagram for the ternary system water, Tween 20, and peppermint oil.

(region II). On the further addition of water, a clear solution (region III) again formed, which then separated into two layers (region IV). This sequence of changes corresponds to the results one would obtain by diluting a peppermint oil concentrate in compounding and manufacturing processes. Analyses such as this therefore can provide important clues for the research pharmacist in the formulation of solubilized drug systems.

Determination of a phase diagram was also carried out by Boon and co-workers[38] in order to formulate a clear, single-phase liquid vitamin A preparation containing the minimum quantity of surfactant needed to solubilize the vitamin. Phase equlibrium diagrams are particularly useful when the formulator wishes to predict the effect on the phase equilibria of the system of dilution with one or all of the components in any desired combination or concentration.

Factors Affecting Solubilization. The solubilization capacity of surfactants for drugs varies greatly with the chemistry of the surfactants and with the location of the drug in the micelle. If a hydrophobic drug is solubilized in the micelle core, an increase of the lipophilic alkyl chain length of the surfactant should enhance solubilization. At the same time, an increase in the micellar radius by increasing the alkyl chain length reduces the Laplace pressure, thus favoring the entry of drug molecules into the micelle (see *Example 15–9*).

For micelles consisting of ionic surfactants, an increase in the radius of the hydrocarbon core is the principal method of enhancing solubilization,[39] whereas for micelles built up from nonionic surfactants, evidence of this effect is not well-grounded. Attwood et al.[40] have shown that an increase of carbon atoms above 16 in an *n*-polyoxyethylene glycol monoether—a nonionic surfactant—increases the size of the micelle but, for a number of drugs, does not enhance solubilization. Results from NMR imaging, viscosity and density testing[41] suggested that some of the polar groups of the micelle, that is, some polyoxyethylene groups outside

the hydrocarbon core of the micelle, double back and intrude on the core depressing its melting point and producing a fluid micellar core (Fig. 15–16). However, this movement of polyethylene groups into the hydrocarbon core disrupts the palisade layer and tends to destroy the region of solubilization for polar–nonpolar compounds (semipolar drugs).

Patel et al.[42] suggested that the solubilizing nature of the core be increased with a more polar surfactant that would not disrupt the palisade region. Attwood et al.[40] investigated the manner in which an ether or keto group introduced into the hydrophobic region of a surfactant, octadecylpolyoxyethylene glycol monoether, affects the solubilization and micellar character of the surfactant. It was observed that the ether group lowered the melting point of the hydrocarbon and thus was able to create a liquid core without the intrusion phenomenon, which reduced the solubilizing nature of the surfactant for semipolar drugs.

The principal effect of pH on the solubilizing power of nonionic surfactants is to alter the equilbrium between the ionized and un-ionized drug (solubilizate). This affects the solubility in water (pp. 233–234) and modifies the partitioning of the drug between the micellar and the aqueous phases. As an example, the more lipophilic un-ionized form of benzoic acid is solubilized to a greater extent in polysorbate 80[43] than the more hydrophilic ionized form. However, solubilization of drugs having hydrophobic parts in the molecule and more than one dissociation constant may not correlate with lipophilicity of the drug. Ikeda et al.[44] studied the solubilization of tetracycline by nonionic, anionic, and cationic surfactants. Tetracycline derivatives may exist in solution as positively and/or negatively charged species (zwitterions, p. 149) as a function of pH. At the pH range of 2.1 to 5.6 the species present are the cationic form and the zwitterionic form, and both contribute to the apparent partition coefficient in a micelle–water system. The equilibrium can be represented as[44]

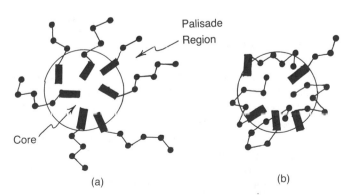

(a)   (b)

Fig. 15–16. Schematic of nonionic micelle of *n*-polyoxyethylene glycol monoether showing intrusion of polyoxyethylene chains into the micelle core. (*a*) Micelle with palisade environment intact. (*b*) Palisade layer partially destroyed by loss of polyoxyethylene groups into the hydrophobic core.

$$C_m^+ \overset{K_c}{\rightleftharpoons} C_w^+ \overset{K_1}{\rightleftharpoons} C_w^\pm \overset{K_z}{\rightleftharpoons} C_m^\pm$$

where K_1 is the first dissociation constant of tetracycline derivatives and K_c and K_z are the partition coefficients for the system, micelle–water, for the cationic (+) and zwitterionic (±) species. C_m and C_w denote the drug concentration in the micellar and aqueous phases, respectively. The apparent partition coefficient K_{app} is related to pH as follows[44]:

$$K_{app} ([H^+]_w + K_1) = K_c[H^+]_w + K_z K_1 \quad (15\text{--}37)$$

where $[H^+]$ is the hydrogen ion concentration in the aqueous phase. Using this equation, K_c and K_z can be estimated from the slope and the intercept of a linear plot or a regression of $K_{app} ([H^+]_w + K_1)$ against $[H^+]_w$.

Example 15–10. The apparent partition coefficient K_{app} (micelle–water) of tetracycline solubilized in micelles of the nonionic surfactant polyoxyethylene lauryl ether, at 25° C and at several pH values, is given in the following table:

pH	2.1	3.0	3.9	5.6
K_{app}	8.05	7.61	6.54	5.68

Compute the partition coefficients of the zwitterionic, K_z, and cationic, K_c, species. The dissociation constant given by Ikeda et al.[44] for tetracycline is $K_1 = 4.68 \times 10^{-4}$.

First, we compute the term $K_{app} ([H^+]_w + K_1)$ at the several pH values. For example, at pH = 2.1, $[H^+]_w = 7.943 \times 10^{-3}$ and $K_{app} ([H^+]_w + K_1) = 8.05 [(7.943 \times 10^{-3}) + (4.68 \times 10^{-4})] = 0.068$. Analogous calculations give the results in the table below, where pH is converted into $[H^+]_w$ concentration:

$[H^+]_w \times 10^3$	7.94	1.00	0.126	0.0025
$K_{app} ([H^+]_w + K_1)$	0.068	0.011	0.0039	0.0027

Now we regress $K_{app} ([H^+]_w + K_1)$ against $[H^+]_w$ from the values given in the table to obtain the slope, $K_c = 8.21$ and the intercept, $K_1 K_z = 2.776 \times 10^{-3}$. Solving for K_z, we have

$$K_z = \frac{2.776 \times 10^{-3}}{4.68 \times 10^{-4}} = 5.93$$

The results indicate that the cationic form is more solubilized than the zwitterionic form, that is, $K_c > K_z$. Ikeda et al. suggested that the greater solubilization of the cationic form of tetracycline is due to the formation of hydrogen bonds between an acidic proton of the cationic species of tetracycline and the oxygen atom of the polyoxyethylene chain of the nonionic surfactant. Since the zwitterionic form of tetracycline has lost its acidic proton it cannot hydrogen-bond; thus, it is solubilized to a lesser extent.

Tetracycline is solubilized much more in micelles of an anionic surfactant, sodium lauryl sulfate, than in micelles of cationic surfactants, such as trimethyl ammonium, particularly at pH 2.1. The cationic form of tetracycline predominates at pH 2.1. At this pH value, Ikeda et al.[44] found that $K_{app} = 2860$ in the anionic surfactant. This is due to the greatest inter-action occurring at pH 2.1 between the protonated species of the drug and the anionic micelles of sodium lauryl sulfate. On the other hand, the electrostatic repulsion between the cationic form of the drug and dodecyltrimethyl ammonium, the cationic micelle, does not result in solubilization at pH 2.1; thus, at this pH value $K_{app} = 0$. The repulsion is reduced as the pH increases since the cationic nature of the drug decreases. Consequently, solubilization of tetracycline in the cationic surfactant micelles becomes greater with an increase of pH.

Thermodynamics of Solubilization.[45] Solubilization may be considered as a partitioning of the drug between the micellar phase and the aqueous environment. Thus, the standard free energy of solubilization, ΔG_s^o, can be computed from the partition coefficient K of the micelle/aqueous medium:

$$\Delta G_s^o = -RT \ln K \quad (15\text{--}38)$$

The standard free enthalpy and entropy of solubilization can be computed from the usual relationships:

$$\ln K = \frac{-\Delta H_s^o}{R} \frac{1}{T} + \text{constant} \quad (15\text{--}39)$$

and

$$\Delta G_s^o = \Delta H_s^o - T\Delta S_s^o \quad (15\text{--}40)$$

The sign and magnitude of the thermodynamic functions ΔH_s^o and ΔS_s^o may be related to the location of the solubilized drug in the micelle as follows. The solubilization of a hydrocarbon in the hydrophobic core is similar to hydrocarbon transfer from water to an organic medium. In both cases the thermodynamic functions are of the same order of magnitude. The standard free enthalpy is approximately zero or a small positive number; and ΔG_s^o ordinarily is negative. The main contribution to the negative ΔG_s^o is a strongly positive entropy change. Due to their hydrophobicity, hydrocarbons dissolve mainly in the core of the micelle.

For a polar solute, ΔG_s^o of transfer from an aqueous to an organic medium is positive and ΔS_s^o is negative. These unfavorable terms may be associated with poor penetration of the solute into the organic phase. This argument can be applied to the penetration of a polar solute into the core of a micelle. The thermodynamic functions for transfer of various solutes of different polarity from water to micellar solutions and to organic solvents at 25° C are given in Table 15–6. Benzoic acid is considered to be mainly adsorbed on the micellar surface of nonionic surfactants; the thermodynamic functions ΔG_s^o, ΔH_s^o, and ΔS_s^o for benzoic acid solubilization are negative (see Table 15–6). Barbituric acid derivatives solubilized in sodium alkyl sulfonate, an anionic surfactant, show ΔG_s^o, ΔH_s^o, and ΔS_s^o values similar to those of benzoic acid. Barbiturates must be distributed in the most exterior part of the micelle—the polyoxyethylene region—rather than the hydrocar-

TABLE 15–6. *Transfer of Solutes from Water to Organic Solvents or Micelles at 25° C*[45]

Solute	Organic Medium	ΔG^o (cal/mole)	ΔH^o (cal/mole)	ΔS^o [cal/(mole deg)]
Ammonium chloride	Ethanol	+5010	−2830	−26.3
Methane	Cyclohexane	−2280	+2380	+15.6
Amobarbital	Micellar solution*	−2340	−1700	+2.1
Barbital	Micellar solution*	−790	−2600	−6.0
Benzoic acid	Micellar solution†	−2320	−3700	−4.7
Ethane	Micellar solution	−3450	+2000	+18.3
Phenobarbital	Micellar solution*	−1850	−3800	−6.5
Propane	Micellar solution*	−4230	+1000	+17.5

*Sodium lauryl sulfate, 0.06 mole/liter.
†n-Alkylpolyoxyethylene, $E_{16}H_{16}$.

bon core owing to their negative ΔS_s^o value. These results with benzoic acid and barbiturates can perhaps be explained by the reasoning given in Table 11–11, p. 276, where it is shown that the thermodynamic functions ΔH^o and ΔS_o are due to several kinds of interactions. In Table 11–11, donor–acceptor and hydrogen bonding are associated with both negative ΔH^o and ΔS^o, the large negative ΔH^o values overcoming the unfavorable entropy change. Thus, $\Delta G_s{}^o$ is negative and the solubilization process is spontaneous.

Example 15–11. The apparent partition coefficients, K, for the transfer of barbital between water and sodium alkyl sulfonate at several temperatures are[45]

Temperature (°C)	25	35	45	55
Partition coefficient, K	3.8	3.5	3.2	2.5

Compute $\Delta G_s{}^o$, $\Delta H_s{}^o$, and $\Delta S_s{}^o$.

From equation (15–39), a regression of ln K against $1/T$ (Kelvin degrees) gives $\Delta H_s{}^o$ from the slope. The values needed for the regression are shown as

$1/T \times 10^3$	3.36	3.25	3.14	3.05
ln K	1.335	1.253	1.163	0.916

The equation obtained is ln $K = 1274.35 \ 1/T − 2.91$.

$\Delta H_s{}^o = −(\text{slope}) \times (R) = −(1274.35)(1.9872) = −2.5$ kcal/mole

$\Delta G_s{}^o$ is obtained from equation (15–38):

at 25° C, $\Delta G_s{}^o = −(1.9872)(298)(1.335) = −790.57$ cal/mole

Analogous calculations give $\Delta G_s{}^o = −766.91$, −734.93, and −597.05 cal/mole at 35°, 45°, and 55° C.

The $\Delta S_s{}^o$ value is obtained using equation (15–40) at each temperature; at 25° C,

$$\Delta S_s{}^o = \frac{\Delta H_s{}^o - \Delta G_s{}^o}{T} = \frac{-2500 - (-790.57) \text{ cal/mole}}{298° \text{ K}}$$

$$= -5.7 \text{ cal/(mole deg)}$$

$\Delta S_s{}^o$ is −5.6, −5.6, and −5.8 cal/(mole deg) at 35°, 45°, and 55° C, respectively. Notice that the constant in equation (15–39) is $\Delta S^o/R$ (see equation [11–52]). Therefore, ΔS^o can also be obtained from the intercept of the regression line on a plot of ln K versus $1/T$; that is, $\Delta S_s{}^o = (\text{intercept}) \times (R) = (−2.91)(1.9872) = −5.8$ cal/(mole deg), a value very similar to the values obtained by the use of equation (15–40) at several temperatures. The $\Delta G_s{}^o$ values obtained are not strongly negative owing to the unfavorable negative value of $\Delta S_s{}^o$. The negative $\Delta H_s{}^o$ and $\Delta S_s{}^o$ may be related to hydrogen bonding (see

Table 11–11) of the barbiturates within the polyoxyethylene palisade of the micelles.

Krafft Point and Cloud Point. Another feature of micelle-forming surfactants is the rapid increase in solubility above a definite temperature, known as the *Krafft point*, K_t. The Krafft point is the temperature at which the solubility of the surfactant equals the cmc. Below K_t, an increase in the concentration of the surface-active agent leads to precipitation rather than micelle formation. The surfactant has a limited solubility, and below the Krafft point, the solubility is insufficient for micellization. As the temperature is elevated, the solubility increases slowly. At the Krafft point, corresponding to the critical micelle concentration, the surfactant crystals melt and are incorporated into the micelles. The micelles are highly soluble; therefore, a rapid increase in solubility occurs with increasing temperature above K_t. Not all surfactants show a rapid increase in solubility above a certain temperature. Only certain ionic and nonionic surface-active agents, for example, have been reported to show a Krafft temperature.[46]

The Krafft point, K_t, can be obtained by plotting the logarithm of molar solubility for a surface active carboxylic acid at several pH values against the inverse of the absolute temperature, as seen in Figure 15–17.[47] For a surfactant solution that has a Krafft point the log solubility–reciprocal temperature profile exhibits a break, that is, a change in slope; the temperature at which the break in the curve occurs at a definite pH is the Krafft point. Actually, a curvature rather than a sharp break occurs in the slope, suggesting that K_t is a temperature range rather than a definite point on the temperature scale. The Krafft point at each pH value is estimated from the intersection of the tangents to the two line segments of different slope shown in Figure 15–17 (see *Problem 15–25* for the calculation of K_t for a surface active benzoic acid derivative at pH 7.0). For ionic surfactants, pH has a definite effect on the Krafft point, as observed in Figure 15–17.

A lower consolute temperature, as discussed on page 41, is also observed for many nonionic, polyoxyethylated surfactants in solution. This temperature, above

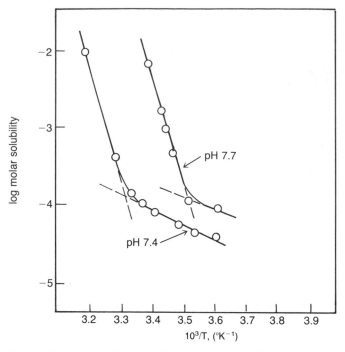

Fig. 15–17. A plot of log solubility against reciprocal temperature to obtain the Krafft point for a surface-active carboxylic acid at two pH values. (From N. K. Pandit and J. M. Strykowski, J. Pharm. Sci. **78**, 768, 1989, reproduced with permission of the copyright owner.)

which cloudiness suddenly appears, is known as the *cloud point*. The surfactant separates as a precipitate, or when in high concentration as a gel, from aqueous solution at an elevated temperature because of self-association and loss of water of hydration of the individual molecules. Schott and Han[46] have reported on the effects of various salts on the Krafft and cloud points of nonionic surfactants, and Schott[48] has compared HLB to the cloud points of a large number of nonionic surfactants.

Coacervation and Cloud Point Phenomena. Solubilization may change certain properties of micelles such as the cloud point and the size of the micelles. Organic solubilizates generally decrease the cloud point of nonionic surfactants. Aliphatic hydrocarbons tend to raise the cloud point, whereas aromatic hydrocarbons and alkanols may lower or raise the cloud point of the surfactant, depending on its concentration. For example, both indomethacin, an antiinflammatory drug, and sorbitol lower the cloud point of 2% aqueous solutions of the nonionic surfactant polysorbate 80. The effect is more pronounced for sorbitol and increases linearly with sorbitol concentration.[49] Indomethacin, a drug of very low aqueous solubility, can be considered to be entirely located within the micellar phase of polysorbate 80 in aqueous solution. Solubilized indomethacin increases the micellar size due not only to incorporation of drug molecules in the polysorbate micelles but also to an increase in the number of polysorbate monomers per micelle, that is, the *aggregation number*. The increase in micellar size suggests a restructuring of the micelle to accommodate the indomethacin molecules, the larger

size producing a more symmetrical micelle with greater hydration.

That solubilizates may favor the transition from rodlike to globular micelles has been recently investigated.[50] Rod-shaped micelles are found in nonionic as well as ionic surfactant solutions in which the charge on the micelle is shielded by salt ions or by strongly binding counterions. The solubilizing capacity of these systems is particularly large when near to coacervate formation. An example is the phase separation of nonionic surfactants above the cloud point. The long rods are transformed into globular micelles after a certain amount of aliphatic or aromatic hydrocarbon is solubilized. The difference between the solubilization of aliphatic and aromatic hydrocarbons by rod-shaped micelles is that the aromatic compounds can lead to coacervate formation before the aggregates shrink and are transformed into spherical micelles. This process is explained as follows. After solubilization of the aromatic hydrocarbon by rodlike aggregates the system separates into two phases with formation of a coacervate. Coacervation can be described as a transition from a solution with rodlike micelles in the gaseous state into two solutions, one of which is in a more condensed state and the other in a more dilute state. The condensed micellar aggregates can still accommodate more hydrocarbon; and after further addition of hydrocarbon the transition from rods to globules takes place. The attractive forces between the small globules are weak and the system cannot simultaneously be in a condensed and a gaseous state. It reverts back to the isotropic single-phase state. Thus, these systems show the interesting phenomenon that a two-phase binary surfactant system (a coacervate) can be transformed into a single-phase solution by solubilization of hydrocarbons[50] in the micelles.

The fact that rodlike micelles can be changed into globular micelles has considerable interest in the practical application of surfactants. Surfactant systems with rodlike micelles may have high viscosities. If highly viscous systems are not desired, one can solubilize enough hydrocarbon to break the rods. When the long rods are transformed into globular micelles the attractive forces between the micelles become smaller and the cloud point of nonionic surfactants is increased. That is, the solubility of the surfactant in the medium becomes greater. Thus, rod–sphere transitions provide an explanation for the rather unusual increase of the cloud point by solubilization of hydrocarbons in the micelles. Alcohols stabilize the rods and for this reason lower the cloud point.[50] That is to say, alcohols decrease the solubility of the surfactant.

ADDENDUM: THERMODYNAMICS OF MICELLIZATION

Two models can be used to explain the properties of micellar solutions.[51] According to the *phase-separation model*, micellization can be considered as the formation of a separate phase in a bulk aqueous medium. Below the cmc, the system contains surfactant molecules (monomers) molecularly dispersed in water. Above the cmc, the system contains two phases in equilibrium: one consisting of monomers of the surfactant in aqueous solution and the other represented by micelles of the surfactant. In this model, micellization is not a progressive association of the surfactant monomer but rather a one-step process.[52]

The second approach is provided by the *mass-action model*. According to this view, micellization can be considered as a stepwise association of monomers to form an aggregate. This model is appropriate when micelles are relatively small. Thoma and Christian[51] have shown that the phase-separation model is a special case of the mass-action model when the aggregation number of the micelles is large. (The *aggregation number* is simply the number of surfactant molecules that come together to form a single micelle.) Both models can be combined to derive an expression for the *standard free energy of micellization*.

In the formation of an ionic micelle from an anionic surfactant, such as sodium lauryl sulfate ($C_{12}H_{25}SO_4^- Na^+$, abbreviated $R^- X^+$) n amphiphilic ions R^-, together with m counterions X^+, form a negatively charged micelle:

$$nR^- + mX^+ \rightleftharpoons [R_nX_m]^Q \qquad (15-A1)$$

where Q^- is the net charge on the micelle, $Q^- = n - m$, n is the aggregation number, and m is the number of counterions bound to the micelle (see Fig. 15–18). For example, for a micelle of $C_{12}H_{25}SO_4^- Na^+$, the aggregation number[53] $n = 50$ ($C_{12}H_{25}SO_4^-$), or 50 negatively charged lauryl sulfate ions, and $m = 45$ Na^+, or 45 positively charged sodium ions. Therefore, the charge on the micelle is $Q = n - m = 5$ negative charges.

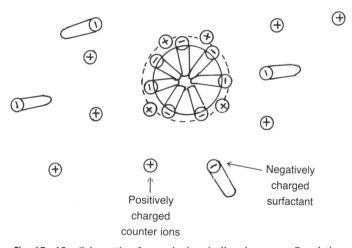

Positively charged counter ions

Negatively charged surfactant

Fig. 15–18. Schematic of an anionic micelle where $n = 7$ and the charge $Q = 7 - 4 = 3^-$. The four positive ions needed for electroneutrality are immediately outside the micelle. The figure shows monomers of the dissociated surfactant in equilibrium with the micelle, as expressed in equation (15–A1). A more realistic example is given in the text where $n = 58$.

To give electroneutrality, five positively charged Na^+ ions must also be present in solution in the outside palisade region of the micelle; they are not considered in equation (15–A1). From the mass-action law, the equilibrium constant is

$$K = \frac{[R_nX_m]^{Q-}}{[R^-]^n[X^+]^m} \qquad (15-A2)$$

or, as for the example above,

$$K = \frac{[(C_{12}H_{25}SO_4^-)_{50}\,(Na^+)_{45}]^5}{[C_{12}H_{25}SO_4^-]^{50} \cdot [Na^+]^{45}} \qquad (15-A3)$$

The standard free energy of micellization, $\Delta G^o{}_{mic}$, that is, the standard free energy per mole of surfactant monomer, $\Delta G^o/n$, is

$$\Delta G^o{}_{mic} = \frac{\Delta G^o}{n} = -\frac{RT}{n} \ln K \qquad (15-A4)$$

Notice that each term is divided by the aggregation number n to give the *free energy per individual monomer*. From equations (15–A3) and (15–A4),

$$\Delta G^o{}_{mic} = -\frac{RT}{n} \ln \frac{[R_nX_m]^{Q-}}{[R^-]^n[X^+]^m} \qquad (15-A5)$$

According to the phase-separation model, at the cmc the concentration of monomers is $[R^-] = [X^+] = $ cmc. Rearranging equation (15–A5), we have

$$\Delta G^o{}_{mic} = -RT\left[\frac{1}{n} \ln [R_nX_m]^{Q-}\right.$$
$$\left. - \ln (\text{cmc}) - \frac{m}{n} \ln (\text{cmc})\right] \qquad (15-A6)$$

At the cmc, the term $1/n \ln [R_nX_m]^{Q-}$ may be neglected.[54] Thus, equation (15–A6) reduces to

$$\Delta G^o{}_{mic} = RT\left(1 + \frac{m}{n}\right) \ln (\text{cmc}) \qquad (15-A7)$$

or, since $m = n - Q^-$, equation (15–A7) can also be written

$$\Delta G^o{}_{mic} = RT\left(2 - \frac{Q^-}{n}\right) \ln (\text{cmc}) \qquad (15-A8)$$

Knowing the cmc, the aggregation number n, and the charge on the micelle, one can calculate $\Delta G^o{}_{mic}$ for an anionic micelle. The same equation can be applied to a cationic micelle, substituting Q^- in equation (15–A8) with the positive charge Q^+ on the micelle (see Problem 15–29). Q^+ and Q^- are determined from the degree of ionization (p. 130) of the surfactant, which in turn is obtained by light scattering, EMF, or conductivity measurements.

For nonionic micelles, $m = 0$ and equation (15–A8) becomes

$$\Delta G^o{}_{mic} = RT \ln (\text{cmc}) \qquad (15-A9)$$

The standard enthalpy and entropy changes of micellization can be computed from the expressions

$$\ln(\text{cmc}) = -\frac{\Delta H^{o}_{\text{mic}}}{R}\frac{1}{T} + \frac{\Delta S^{o}_{\text{mic}}}{R} \quad (15\text{-}A10)$$

and

$$\Delta G^{o}_{\text{mic}} = \Delta H^{o}_{\text{mic}} - T\Delta S^{o}_{\text{mic}} \quad (15\text{-}A11)$$

The standard free energy for a nonionic micelle is calculted in Problem 15–31.

References and Notes

1. H. K. Chan and I. Gonda, J. Pharm. Sci. **78**, 176, 1989.
2. C. J. Drummond, G. G. Warr, F. Grieser, B. W. Nihaen and D. F. Evans, J. Phys. Chem. **89**, 2103, 1985.
3. Y. Chang and J. R. Cardinal, J. Pharm Sci. **67**, 994, 1978.
4. T. J. Racey, P. Rochon, D. V. C. Awang and G. A. Neville, J. Pharm. Sci. **76**, 314, 1987; T. J. Racey, P. Rochon, F. Mori and G. A. Neville, J. Pharm. Sci. **78**, 214, 1989.
5. P. Mukerjee, J. Phys. Chem. **76**, 565, 1972.
6. K. W. Herrmann, J. Colloid Interface Sci. **22**, 352, 1966.
7. P. C. Hiemenz, *Principles of Colloid and Surface Chemistry*, 2nd. Edition, Dekker, New York, 1986, pp. 127, 133, 148.
8. J. Kirschbaum, J. Pharm. Sci. **63**, 981, 1974.
9. A. J. Richard, J. Pharm. Sci. **64**, 873, 1975.
10. H. Arwidsson and M. Nicklasson, Int. J. Pharm. **58**, 73, 1990.
11. H. H. Paradies, Eur. J. Biochem. **118**, 187, 1981.
12. H. H. Paradies, J. Pharm. Sci. **78**, 230, 1989.
13. H. Schott, J. Pharm. Sci. **70**, 486, 1981.
14. H. Takenaka, Y. Kawashima and S. Y. Lin, J. Pharm. Sci. **70**, 302, 1981.
15. D. J. A. Crommelin, J. Pharm. Sci. **73**, 1559, 1984.
16. H. Schott and C. Y. Young, J. Pharm. Sci. **61**, 182, 1972.
17. H. Schott and E. Astigarrabia, J. Pharm. Sci. **77**, 918, 1988.
18. T. Higuchi, R. Kuramoto, L. Kennon, T. L. Flanagan and A. Polk, J. Am. Pharm. Assoc., Sci. Ed. **43**, 646, 1954.
19. E. J. W. Verwey and J. Th. G. Overbeek, *Theory of the Stability of Lyophobic Colloids*, Elsevier, Amsterdam, 1948.
20. B. Derjaguin and L. Landau, Acta Physica. Chim., USSR, *14*, 663, 1941; J. Exp. Theor. Physics, USSR, **11**, 802, 1941.
21. H. Takenaka, Y. Kawashima and S. Y. Lin, J. Pharm. Sci. **69**, 513, 1980.
22. A. A. Badawi and A. A. El-Sayed, J. Pharm. Sci. **69**, 492, 1980.
23. H. Schott, in *Remington's Pharmaceutical Sciences*, 16th Edition, Mack Publishing, Easton, Pa., 1980, Chapter 20.
24. B. Haines and A. N. Martin, J. Pharm. Sci. **50**, 228, 753, 756, 1961.
25. B. A. Mulley, in *Advances in Pharmaceutical Sciences*, Academic Press, New York, 1964, Vol. 1, pp. 87–194.
26. T. Nakagawa, in *Nonionic Surfactants*, M. J. Schick, Dekker, New York, 1967.
27. P. H. Elworthy, A. T. Florence and C. B. Macfarlane, *Solubilization by Surface-Active Agents*, Chapman & Hall, London, 1968.
28. D. Attwood and A. T. Florence, *Surfactant Systems*, Chapman & Hall, London and New York, 1983.
29. C. Engler and E. Dieckhoff, Arch. Pharm. **230**, 561, 1892.
30. A. S. C. Lawrence, Trans. Faraday Soc. **33**, 815, 1937.
31. E. Keh, S. Partyka and S. Zaini, J. Colloid Interface Sci. **129**, 363, 1989.
32. I. Reich, J. Phys. Chem. **60**, 260, 1956.
33. P. Mukerjee and J. Cardinal, J. Phys. Chem. **82**, 1620, 1978.
34. C. Ramachandran, R. A. Pyter and P. Mukerjee, J. Phys. Chem. **86**, 3198, 1982.
35. B. W. Barry and D. I. El Eini, J. Pharm. Pharmacol. **28**, 210, 1976.
36. A. K. Krishna and D. R. Flanagan, J. Pharm. Sci. **78**, 574, 1989.
37. W. J. O'Malley, L. Pennati and A. Martin, J. Am. Pharm. Assoc., Sci. Ed. **47**, 334, 1958.
38. P. F. G. Boon, C. L. J. Coles and M. Tait, J. Pharm. Pharmacol. **13**, 200T, 1961.
39. T. Anarson and P. H. Elworthy, J. Pharm. Pharmacol. **32**, 381, 1980.
40. D. Attwood, P. H. Elworthy and M. J. Lawrence, J. Pharm. Pharmacol. **41**, 585, 1989.
41. P. H. Elworthy and M. S. Patel, J. Pharm. Pharmacol. **36**, 565; ibid. **36**, 116, 1984.
42. M. S. Patel, P. H. Elworthy and A. K. Dewsnup, ibid, **33**, 64P, 1981.
43. J. H. Collett and L. Koo, J. Pharm. Sci. **64**, 1253, 1975.
44. K. Ikeda, H. Tomida and T. Yotsuyanagi, Chem. Pharm. Bull. **25**, 1067, 1977.
45. V. Vaution, C. Treiner, F. Puisieux and J. T. Carstensen, J. Pharm. Sci. **70**, 1238, 1981.
46. H. Schott and S. K. Han, J. Pharm. Sci. **65**, 979, 1976; ibid, **66**, 165, 1977.
47. N. K. Pandit and J. M. Strykowski, J. Pharm. Sci. **78**, 767, 1989.
48. H. Schott, J. Pharm. Sci. **58**, 1443, 1969.
49. D. Attwood, G. Ktistis, Y. McCormick and M. J. Story, J. Pharm. Pharmacol. **41**, 83, 1989.
50. H. Hoffmann and W. Ulbricht, J. Colloid Interface Sci. **129**, 388, 1989.
51. D. C. Thomas and S. D. Christian, J. Colloid Interface Sci. **78**, 466, 1980.
52. W. Binana-Limbele and R. Zana, Colloid Polymer Sci. **267** 440, 1989.
53. D. Attwood and A. T. Florence, *Surfactant Systems*, Chapman & Hall, London and New York, 1983, p. 93.
54. P. C. Hiemenz, *Principles of Colloid and Surface Chemistry*, 2nd Edition, Dekker, New York, 1986, pp. 441–448.
55. D. Attwood and O. K. Udeala, J. Pharm. Pharmacol. **26**, 854, 1974.
56. H. V. Tartar and A. L. M. Lelong, J. Phys. Chem. **59**, 1185, 1956.
57. A. Einstein, *Investigations on the Theory of Brownian Movement*, Dover, New York, 1956.
58. D. J. Shaw, *Introduction to Colloid and Surface Chemistry*, Butterworths, Boston, 1970, pp. 20, 21.
59. L. J. Ravin, E. G. Shami and E. S. Rattie, J. Pharm. Sci. **64**, 1830, 1975.
60. S. Chibowski, J. Colloid Interface Sci. **134**, 1, 174, 1990.
61. H. Schott, J. Pharm. Sci. **65**, 855, 1976.
62. K. A. Johnson, G. B. Westermann-Clark and D. O. Shah, J. Colloid Interface Sci. **130**, 480, 1989.
63. M. J. Rosen et al., J. Phys. Chem. **86**, 541, 1982; ibid., Colloids Surf. **3**, 201, 1981.

Problems

15–1. The equivalent conductivity Λ of a solution containing a surface active agent decreases sharply at the critical micelle concentration owing to the lower mobility of micelles. A plot of Λ (vertical axis) against the concentration or the square root of the concentration of the surface active agent shows an inflection point at the critical micelle concentration. (See Figure 15–3)

Chlorcyclizine hydrochloride, an antihistamine used for the

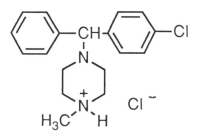

Chlorcyclizine Hydrochloride

relief of urticaria and hay fever, is surface active and forms micelles in aqueous solution. The dependence of Λ in mho m^2 mole^{-1} (see p. 127 for the unit, mho) on $\sqrt{c}$ is given below (partially based on the data of Attwood and Udeala[55]):

Data for Problem 15–1

$\Lambda \times 10^3$ mho m^2 mole^{-1}	4.7	5.1	6.0	6.6	7.0	7.5	8.0	8.7
$\sqrt{c}$ $(\text{mole/liter})^{1/2}$	0.33	0.30	0.26	0.24	0.23	0.20	0.17	0.14

Plot Λ versus $\sqrt{c}$ and estimate the cmc.

Answer: cmc = 0.053 mole/liter

15–2. The turbidity τ of an aqueous sodium dodecylbenzene sulfonate (SDBS) solution was determined in a light-scattering photometer at various concentrations above its cmc (modified from data in Tartar and Lelong[56]).

Data for Problem 15–2

$c \times 10^3$ (g/cm^3)	2.68	7.58	13.30	22.15
$\tau \times 10^4$ (cm^{-1})	1.09	1.80	2.08	2.31

The turbidity τ increases with concentration because the surfactant molecules aggregate to form structures with molecular weights much greater than the molecular weight of the monomer SDBS, namely, 349 g/mole. The value of H in equation (15–2), page 399, is 4.00×10^{-6} mole cm^2 g^{-2}. Plot Hc/τ versus c and using equation (15–2) obtain the molecular weight of the aggregate in the aqueous solution. Also give the value of the solute–solvent interaction constant B. The degree of aggregation is obtained by dividing the molecular weight of the aggregate by the molecular weight of the SDBS monomer. What is the degree of aggregation?

Answer: M = 17,170 g/mole; slope = $2B$ = 0.0147; B = 7.35×10^{-3} mole cm^3 g^{-2}. Degree of aggregation = 49, that is, each micelle contains an average of 49 molecules of SDBS.

15–3. The average displacement, $\bar{x}$ in meters, of a microscopic particle is related to its diffusion D (m^2/sec) and the time t of movement. The relation according to Einstein[57] is $\bar{x} = \sqrt{2Dt}$. If a particle moves in a fluid medium with a diffusion coefficient of D = 2.72×10^{-10} meter^2/sec, what is its average Brownian displacement over a time interval of 2.30 sec?

Answer: $\bar{x}$ = 3.54×10^{-5} meter = 3.54×10^{-3} cm.

15–4. For spherical particles we may express the diffusion in terms of their radii r, the viscosity η of the medium, and the absolute temperature T (equation (15–7), p. 401). In 1908 Perrin used this equation and a suspension of gamboge particles of accurately determined size to calculate Avogadro's constant N_A. He obtained values lying between 5.5×10^{23} particles/mole and 8×10^{23} particles/mole. Currently[58] the accepted value of N_A is 6.022×10^{23} mole^{-1}.

Using equation (15–7) in the expression $\bar{x} = \sqrt{2Dt}$ we obtain an equation, $\bar{x} = \sqrt{\dfrac{RTt}{3\pi\eta r N_A}}$, for the calculation of the mean Brownian displacement of a particle.

For a particle of radius r = 10^{-6} meter (10^{-4} cm) in water (η = 0.01 poise) at a temperature of 20° C, T = 293.15° K, its displacement $\bar{x}$ is to be observed over a period of 1 hour (t = 3600 sec). R is the gas constant, expressed in units of 8.3143×10^7 erg deg^{-1} mole^{-1}. The poise is expressed as dyne sec/cm^2 or erg sec/cm^3. Calculate the mean Brownian displacement to be expected. How might you use this equation to determine Avogadro's number?

Answer: $\bar{x}$ = 3.93×10^{-3} cm = 39.3 μm or 3.93×10^{-5} meter displacement in 1 hour.

15–5. When insulin solutions are stored at room temperature, a process of self-association occurs and the molecules aggregate. The degree of aggregation is affected by pH, ionic strength, and temperature. The aggregation process was studied in the temperature range of room temperature (20° C) to human body temperature (~35° C) at pH 7.5 and ionic strength μ = 0.1. The diffusion coefficients of aggregates at the various temperatures and viscosities of the solvent are found at the top of the next column.

Compute the hydrodynamic radii of the aggregates at the various temperatures. See the Stokes–Einstein equation. The poise is equal to 1 g cm^{-1} sec^{-1}

Answer: equation (15–7) may be used. It gives 28.4, 54.5, 78.9, and 104 Å at the four temperatures.

Data for Problem 15–5*

T (°C)	20	25	30	35
$D \times 10^7$ (cm^2 sec^{-1})	7.8	4.6	3.7	3.0
η (poises)	0.0097	0.0087	0.0076	0.0072

*Data from H. B. Bohidar, Colloid Polym. Sci. **267**, 159, 1989.

15–6. A sample of horse albumin in an aqueous solution at a concentration of c_g = 3.20 grams per liter was placed in an osmometer at 28° C. Its osmotic pressure π was measured and found to be 0.00112 atm. What is the molecular weight of the serum albumin, assuming the solution is sufficiently dilute for the use of equation (15–11)? The gas constant R = 0.0821 liter atm/mole deg.

Answer: 70,641 gram/mole

15–7. The osmotic pressure π of a fraction of polystyrene was determined at 25° C at various concentrations c_g as recorded here:

Data for Problem 15–7

$\pi/c_g \times 10^5$ (1 atm g^{-1})	12.5	16.3	20.0	23.8
c_g (g/liter)	6.0	12	18	24

Calculate the molecular weight and the second virial coefficient, B, for the polystyrene fraction. Use equation (15–13) disregarding the $C \times c_g^2$ and higher terms. Can this large molecular weight be determined by the osmotic pressure method? What other methods are available to obtain the molecular weight of such a large molecule?

Answer: M = 2.797×10^5 or 279,700 daltons; B = 2.56×10^{-7} liter mole g^{-2}.

15–8. An ultracentrifuge is operated at 6000 rpm. The mid-point of the cell with the sample in place is 1.2 cm from the center of the rotor. What is the angular acceleration and the number of "g's" acting on the sample?

Answer: Angular acceleration = 4.737×10^5 rad/sec^2, and the number of "g's" is 483 or a force 483 times that of gravity acting on the sample.

15–9. What is the angular velocity ω of an ultracentrifuge such that a micelle moves from a position in the centrifuge cell of x_1 = 5.957 cm to x_2 = 6.026 cm in 15 minutes? (15 × 60 sec per min = 900 sec.) The sedimentation coefficient s is 7.756×10^{-13} sec.[59] Express the result in rpm.

Answer: 38,787 rpm. More realistically it is rounded to 38,800 rpm.

15–10. Find the angular acceleration in rad/sec^2 for an ultracentrifuge with a rotor of radius 6.5 cm rotating at 1200 rpm. Convert this angular acceleration into "g's," assuming that the acceleration due to gravity is 981 cm/sec^2.

Answer: 10.26×10^4 rad/sec^2, or 105 "g's"

15–11. Determine the molecular weight of egg albumin from the following ultracentrifuge data obtained at 20° C: the Svedberg constant, s = 3.6×10^{-13} sec, D = 7.8×10^{-7} cm^2/sec, the partial specific volume, $\bar{v}$ = 0.75 cm^3/g, and the density of water at 20° C is 0.998 g/cm^3.

Answer: 44,727 g/mole $\cong$ 45,000 g/mole

15–12. The sedimentation coefficient s at 20° C of saramycetin, an antifungal antibiotic, is 5.3 svedberg (1 svedberg = 10^{-13} sec), the diffusion coefficient is D = 6×10^{-7} cm^2 sec^{-1}, and the partial specific volume is $\bar{v}$ = 0.607 cm^3 g^{-1} ($\bar{v}$ is obtained by use of an accurate pycnometer and a microbalance) (selected data from Kirschbaum[8]).

(a) Compute the molecular weight of saramycetin. The density of the solvent is 0.998 g/cm^3.

(b) Compute the radius of the saramycetin particle. Assume that the particles are spherical. The viscosity of the solvent is 1.002×10^{-2} poise.

Answers: **(a)** 54,613 or 54,600 dalton; **(b)** radius, r = 36. Å

15-13. Compute the molecular weight of a cellulose nitrate fraction using equation (15-24) where $K = 4.0 \times 10^{-5}$ and $a = 0.990$ at 27° C. The intrinsic viscosity of the fraction is 2.40 cm³ g⁻¹.

Answer: 67,053 g/mole or 67,000 dalton

15-14. (a) Use the Mark-Houwink expression, equation (15-24), to calculate the intrinsic viscosity [η] in dL/g of a methylcellulose polymer having a number average molecular weight of 15,200 g/mole. The constant K is equal to 1.1×10^{-3} dL mole g⁻¹, where dL stands for deciliters, which equals 100 cm³. The exponent, a, of equation (15-24) is 0.983 and is dimensionless.

(b) The units of dL mole g⁻² on K are not quite correct in the problem. Can you suggest the exact units?

Answers: **(a)** 14.2 dL/g; **(b)** dL mole⁰·⁹⁸³ gram⁻¹·⁹⁸³. These units would differ, however, for each polymer having a different a value. Since the Mark-Houwink equation is an empiric one, in practice, the units on K are obtained disregarding altogether the M^a units. The units on K then become the same as those on intrinsic viscosity, dL/g.

15-15. The variation of reduced viscosity η_{sp}/c with concentration for a new nonionic surfactant is given in the table below.

Data for Problem 15-15*

η_{sp}/c	8.96	9.39	9.82	10.25	10.69
c (mole/kg)	0.005	0.01	0.015	0.02	0.025

*Data from D. Attwood, P. H. Elworthy and M. J. Lawrence, J. Pharm. Pharmacol. **41**, 585, 1989.

Compute the intrinsic viscosity, [η], of the surfactant.

Answer: [η] = 8.53 kg/mole of solvent = 8.53 molality⁻¹

15-16. It requires 40 seconds for a volume of water, density 1.0 g/cm³, to flow through a capillary viscometer and 614 seconds for an equal volume of a glycerin solution having a density of 1.12 g/cm³. What is the viscosity at 25° C and the relative viscosity of this solution? The viscosity of water at 25° C is 0.01 poise or 1.0 cp. See pages 454-455 and 461-462.

Answer: Viscosity of the solution is 0.172 poise. Relative viscosity $n_1/n_2 = 17.2$ (dimensionless).

15-17. The molecular weight of a spherical protein is 20,000 g/mole and the partial specific volume $\bar{v}$ is 0.80 cm³/g at 20° C. The viscosity of the solvent is 0.01 poise. Calculate the value of D, the diffusion coefficient at this temperature. (See equation (15-8).) Notice that one is dealing with a *cube root*.

Answer: $D = 11.15 \times 10^{-7}$ cm²/sec

15-18. Polyvinyl alcohol was separated into four fractions of various molecular weights by means of a column packed with the chromatographic gel, Sephadex G-150. Compute the molecular weight of these fractions from the intrinsic viscosities using the Mark-Houwink equation. The value of a is 0.71 (dimensionless) and K is 2.7×10^{-4} cm³ g⁻¹. The experimental intrinsic viscosities are 0.463, 0.875, 1.09, and 1.15 cm³/g.[60]

Answer: 36,000, 88,000, 120,000, and 129,000 g/mole

15-19. The intrinsic viscosities [η] of several molecular weight fractions M of a new cellulose plasma extender were obtained by plotting η_{sp}/c for each fraction versus the concentration c in g/dL (where 1 dL = 100 cm³) as seen in Figure 15-9. The resulting intrinsic viscosities, together with the molecular weights M determined separately by osmotic pressure (equation (15-12) at 25° C, are given as:

Data for Problem 15-19

M (g/mole)	67,820	153,756	206,200	329,150
[η] (dL/g)	1.21	2.65	3.54	5.56

(a) Plot ln[η] as the dependent variable versus ln M (M = molecular weight) to obtain the constants K and a of the Mark-Houwink equation.

(b) Use the values of K and a in the Mark-Houwink expression (equation (15-24)) to calculate the molecular weight of a newly synthesized cellulose plasma extender, the experimentally determined intrinsic viscosity of which is 7.83 dL/g.

Answers: $K = 2.60 \times 10^{-5}$ dL g⁻¹, $a = 0.966$. Using the Mark-Houwink equation in logarithmic form, the molecular weight of the newly synthesized sample is found to be 469,583, or 470,000 daltons.

15-20. The mobility v/E of a silver iodide sol at 20° C in a Burton electrophoresis cell was observed to be 25×10^{-5} cm² volt⁻¹ sec⁻¹. Compute the zeta potential of the colloid.

Answer: $\zeta = 35.3$ millivolts

15-21. The zeta potential ζ for a colloidal system in an aqueous electrolyte solution is given by the formula

$$\zeta = \frac{4\pi\eta}{\epsilon} \frac{v}{E} (9 \times 10^4)$$

where 9×10^4 converts electrostatic units into volts.

(a) The term $\frac{4\pi\eta}{\epsilon} (9 \times 10^4)$ is given on page 406 as equal approximately to 128 at 25° C and 141 at 20° C. Refer to a handbook of chemistry and physics for the viscosity in poise (dyne sec/cm²) or g/(cm sec) and the dielectric constant ϵ at 20° C and 25° C and verify the values 128 and 141 for this term in equation (15-28).

(b) The electrophoretic mobility, v/E (in cm/sec per volt/cm) for bentonite in water is given by Schott[61] as -3.39 (± 0.07) $\times 10^{-4}$ at 24° C. The quantity ± 0.07 in parentheses indicates that the value -3.39 was measured experimentally to within a precision of $-3.39 - 0.07 \times 10^{-4}$ to $-3.39 + 0.07 \times 10^{-4}$. The electrophoretic mobility of bismuth subnitrate particles (13.18% w/w) in water at 24° to 25° C is $+2.20$ $\pm(0.09) \times 10^{-4}$ cm/sec per volt/cm. Calculate the zeta potential of bentonite and of bismuth subnitrate at 25° C. Why do we find both positive and negative zeta potential values in this problem?

Partial Answer: Bentonite, $\zeta = -43.4$ millivolts; bismuth subnitrate, $\zeta = +28.2$ millivolts. The reader should see the paper by Schott for the reason for the positive and negative ζ values.

15-22. Compute the ratio of concentrations at equilibrium of diffusible benzylpenicillin ions *outside* to those *inside* a semipermeable membrane when the concentration of an anionic polyelectrolyte inside the sac is 12.5×10^{-3} gram equivalent per liter and that of benzylpenicillin inside the sac is 3.20×10^{-3} mole/liter at equilibrium. Set up the Donnan membrane equilibrium (see equation (15-34)) and solve the equation for the ratio of diffusible benzylpenicillin ions outside to those inside the membrane.

Answer: 2.22 to 1

15-23. The Donnan effect is important in concentrating ions in various body fluid compartments. The interstitial fluid of the body lies between the vascular system with its plasma and erythrocytes and the tissue cells of the body. The plasma and the cells contain nondiffusible protein anions, whereas the interstitial fluid contains only diffusible ions such as K^+, Na^+, and Cl^-. Therefore the Donnan membrane effect in the body is to influence the distribution of the diffusible ions. The protein anions tend to attract and retain small cations (K^+ and Na^+) in the tissue cells and blood vessels, and repel small anions (Cl^-) into the surrounding interstitial fluid.

In the normal body the concentration of plasma protein is 16 mEq/liter and that of the chloride ions is 113 mEq/liter. What is the ratio of chloride ions across the interstitial (fluid$_{(outside)}$ − plasma$_{(inside)}$) membrane? *Hint:* The Donnan membrane principle (equation (15-33)) is used to calculate the ratio of chloride ions.

Answer: $[Cl^-]_o/[Cl^-]_i = 1.07$ to 1

15-24. The diffusion of a drug compound, solubilized in a micelle and hindered by passage through microporous membranes, provides a method to control the release of the drug.

The ratio of the diffusion coefficient of a spherical particle in a cylindrical pore (D_p) relative to the diffusion coefficient of the same particle in free solution (D) is given by the following equation[62]:

$$D_p/D = (1 - \xi)^2[1 - 2.1044 \xi^2 + 2.089 \xi^3 - 0.948\xi^5] \quad (15-41)$$

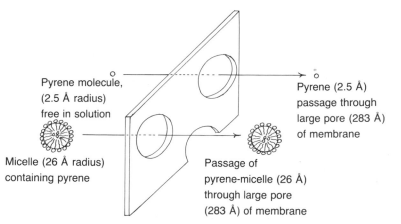

Fig. 15–19. Passage of pyrene, both free in solution and enclosed in a micelle, through large pores of a membrane.

where ξ is r/r_p, the ratio of the particle-to-pore radii, and D_p is the intrapore diffusion coefficient. When the radius of the particle is much smaller than the radius of the pore, the intrapore diffusion coefficient is practically the same as the diffusion coefficient in free solution.

The diffusion of pyrene, solubilized in micelles of the surfactant sodium dodecyl sulfate, across microporous membranes at 25° C was studied by Johnson et al.[62] The radius of the micelle is 26 Å and the viscosity of the solvent 0.089 poise. The pore radius of the membrane is 283 Å.

(a) Compute the diffusion coefficient D of the micelle in the free solution (see equation (15–7), p. 401).

(b) Compute the diffusion coefficient, D_p, of the micelle particle in the pore. Compare this value to the diffusion coefficient of free pyrene (not present in micellar form), which is determined in a separate experiment, $D_{\text{free}} = 5.6 \times 10^{-6}$ cm²/sec. The radius of the pyrene molecule is approximately 2.5 Å.

(c) Comment on your results. Figure 15–19 is helpful in viewing the problem more clearly.

Answers: (a) $D = 9.4 \times 10^{-8}$ cm²/sec; (b) $D_p = 7.6 \times 10^{-8}$ cm²/sec; (c) *Hint:* Is the radius of the pyrene "particle" larger in the micelle or in free solution? Are the diffusion coefficients directly or inversely proportional to the radii? How can this information be used to design a drug for passage through the membrane pores of a new dosage form?

15–25. The change in molar solubility S with temperature of a surface active carboxylic acid, 3-(4-heptobenzyl) benzoic acid (HBB), in aqueous solution at pH 7.0 is given in the table below (data read from Figure 2 of Pandit and Strykowski[47]).

Plot log S (vertical axis) against $1/T$ (see Fig. 15–17) and estimate the Krafft point K_t of the surfactant. See page 415 for an understanding of the Krafft point.

Answer: $K_t = 43.5°$ C

15–26. According to Pandit and Strykowski[47] the Krafft point can be estimated from a plot of the surface pressure π of saturated solutions of the surfactant as a function of temperature (°C). The surface pressure π is the difference between the surface tensions of the solvent and solution at a fixed temperature, $\pi = \gamma_{\text{solvent}} - \gamma_{\text{solution}}$. The surface pressure increases with temperature usually because the concentration of surfactant in the saturated solution (the solubility) also increases with temperature. When the Krafft point is reached, any further increase in temperature (and consequently, any increase in concentration of surfactant) causes no additional change in surface pressure. Therefore, the profile of surface pressure versus temperature reaches a plateau above the Krafft point. The K_f value can be

estimated from the intersection point of the two segments of the plot.

The surface pressure values π (dyne/cm) of saturated solutions of a surfactant at several temperatures are as follows (data read at pH 7 from Figure 3 of Pandit and Strykowski[47]).

Data for Problem 15–26

π (dyne/cm)	40	40	40	28	21.3	13.8	4.4	1.6	0.3
T (°C)	54	52	50	42	38	25	18	12	4

Plot the π values (vertical axis) against T (°C) and estimate the Krafft point of the surfactant.

Answer: $K_t = 49°$ C at pH 7

15–27. Cloud points of nonionic surfactants have been related to properties of micelles such as the critical micelle concentration (cmc) and the weight of the micelle. The effect of various concentrations of alcohol and sodium sulfate in solutions of a nonionic surfactant on the cloud point, the cmc, and the aggregation number is shown in the table.

Data for Problem 15–27

Additive	Na₂SO₄			None	Ethyl alcohol	
Concentration	0.5 N	0.3 N	0.1 N	0	5% v/v	15% v/v
Cloud point (°C)	42.7	49.7	58.0	64.0	75.9	107.0
cmc × 10³ (wt%)	4.6	5.4	6.0	6.8	7.5	11.0
Aggregation no. (n)	301	192	142	128	106	78

Plot on a single graph both the cmc and the aggregation number, n, along the vertical axis against the cloud point (horizontal axis). Find a linear relationship between aggregation number and cloud point and between cmc and cloud point. Use any transformation of the dependent variable (the variable on the vertical axis), to the logarithm, the square root, or the reciprocal as necessary to produce straight lines. Then, compute the slope and the intercept. Comment on your results; for example, note the sign of the slope obtained, and

Data for Problem 15–25

log S	−1.208	−2.542	−2.854	−3.833	−4.0	−4.167	−4.375	−4.708
$1/T \times 10^3$(°K⁻¹)	3.05	3.08	3.10	3.19	3.22	3.29	3.37	3.51

the fact that the aggregation number n is related to the size of the micelle.

15–28. The standard free energy of micellization ΔG°_m is related to the standard free energy of adsorption ΔG°_{ad} at the (air–saturated monolayer) interface through the following relationship:

$$\Delta G^\circ_{ad} = \Delta G^\circ_m - (\pi_{cmc}/\Gamma_{max}) \qquad (15\text{--}42)$$

where π_{cmc} is the surface pressure at the critical micelle concentration; and the surface excess Γ_{max} (pp. 373–375) is the maximum adsorption (in number of moles per unit area) at the air–saturated monolayer interface.

The standard free energy of micellization of n-dodecyl β-D-maltoside (DDM) in aqueous solution at 25° C is $\Delta G^\circ_m = -31.8$ kJ mole^{-1}. The surface tension of the solution at the critical micelle concentration, measured by the Du Noüy ring method, is $\gamma_{cmc} = 36.22$ mN m^{-1} at 25° C, and the surface tension of water at 25° C is 71.97 mN m^{-1} (millinewton per meter). The minimum area per molecule A_{min} at the air–saturated monolayer interface was found by Drummond et al.[2] to be 49.9 Å^2. (1 Å $= 10^{-10}$ meter, therefore 1 Å$^2 = 10^{-20}$ meter^2.) The maximum value of Γ, the surface excess, corresponds to the minimum area per molecule of DDM, $\Gamma_{max} = \dfrac{1}{N_A}\dfrac{1}{A_{min}}$, where N_A is Avogadro's number. Γ_{max} is expressed in mole/m^2.

Compute the standard free energy of adsorption of n-dodecyl β-D-maltoside at the air–solution interface. You will need the expressions, $\pi_{cmc} = \gamma_{water} - \gamma_{cmc}$ and $\Gamma_{max} = \dfrac{1}{N_A}\dfrac{1}{A_{min}}$.

Answer: $\Delta G^\circ_{ad} = -42.6$ kJ mole$^{-1} = -4.26 \times 10^{11}$ erg mole$^{-1} = -10,182$ cal/mole. For an explanation of the terms in equation (15–42) and its applications, see Rosen et al.[63]

15–29. Bromodiphenhydramine, an antihistaminic drug, shows surface activity and forms micelles of aggregation number $n = 11$ at 303° K. The degree of ionization α and the critical micelle concentration, obtained from light-scattering experiments, are $\alpha = Q/n = 0.20$ and cmc $= 9.5 \times 10^{-4}$ expressed as mole fraction.[55] Compute the free energy of micellization per mole of monomeric drug. Express the

results in kJ/mole. *Hint:* You will need equation (15–A8), Appendix at the end of this chapter.

Answer: $\Delta G^\circ = -31.6$ kJ/mole

15–30. Compute ΔG°, ΔH°, and ΔS° of micellization of an alkyl dimethylaminopropane sulfonate (a zwitterionic surfactant). ΔH° and ΔS° can be computed from a regression of $\ln(cmc)$ versus $1/T$. The cmc varies with temperature as follows:

Data for Problem 15–30*

cmc $\times 10^3$ (mole fraction)	3	2.9	2.7
T (°C)	15	25	35

*Data based on B. Sesta and C. La Mesa, Colloid Polym. Sci. **267**, 748, 1989.

Answer: (*Hint:* $\Delta G^\circ = RT \ln(cmc) = \Delta H^\circ - T\Delta S^\circ$.) $\Delta H^\circ = 932$ cal/mole, $\Delta S^\circ = 14.76$ e.u.; $\Delta G^\circ = -3326$ cal/mole, -3462 cal/mole, and -3622 cal/mole at 15°, 25°, and 35° C, respectively.

15–31. (**a**) Compute ΔG°_{mic} for the nonionic surfactant of formula $C_{12}H_{25}(OC_2H_4)_7OH$ in aqueous solution at 10°, 25°, and 40° C, knowing that the cmc in mole/liter $\cong$ mole/kg water (molality units) in this dilute solution. Therefore, the cmc values at these 3 temperatures are given as 12.1×10^{-5} m, 8.2×10^{-5} m, and 7.3×10^{-5} m, respectively.[63]

(**b**) Compute ΔG°_{mic}, first changing the cmc values of part (a) into mole fraction units. The molecular weight of the solvent medium (water) is 18.015 g/mole. Does the value of ΔG° depend on the units used for cmc?

(**c**) Compute ΔH°_{mic} and ΔS°_{mic} using mole fraction units for the cmc in equation (15–A10) (Appendix at the end of this chapter).

(**d**) Discuss the magnitude and sign of the thermodynamic quantities obtained for the micellization process in terms of the several kinds of interactions shown in Table 11–11, page 276.

Partial Answer: (**a**) Using molality units on cmc, ΔG°_{mic} (10° C) $= -5.0$ kcal/mole; (**b**) using mole fraction units on cmc, ΔG°_{mic} (10° C) $= -7.3$ kcal/mole and ΔG°_{mic} (40° C) $= -8.4$ kcal/mole; (**c**) over this temperature range $\Delta H^\circ_{mic} = +3.2$ kcal/mole; $\Delta S^\circ_{mic} = +37.16$ cal/(deg mole)

16
Micromeritics

Particle Size and Size Distribution
Methods for Determining Particle Size
Particle Shape and Surface Area

Methods for Determining Surface Area
Pore Size
Derived Properties of Powders

The science and technology of small particles have been given the name *micromeritics* by Dalla Valle.[1] Colloidal dispersions are characterized by particles that are too small to be seen in the ordinary microscope, whereas the particles of pharmaceutical emulsions and suspensions and the "fines" of powders fall in the range of the optical microscope. Particles having the size of coarser powders, tablet granulations, and granular salts fall within the sieve range. The approximate size ranges of particles in pharmaceutical dispersions are listed in Table 16–1a. The sizes of other materials, including microorganisms, are found in Tables 16–1b and c. The unit of particle size used most frequently in micromeritics is the micrometer, μm, also called the micron, μ, and equal to 10^{-6} m, 10^{-4} cm, or 10^{-3} mm. One must not confuse μm with mμ, the latter being the symbol for a millimicron or 10^{-9} m. The millimicron now is most commonly referred to as the nanometer (nm).

Knowledge and control of the size, and the size range, of particles is of profound importance in pharmacy. Thus, size, and hence surface area, of a particle can be related in a significant way to the physical, chemical, and pharmacologic properties of a drug. Clinically, the particle size of a drug can affect its release from dosage forms that are administered orally, parenterally, rec-

tally, and topically. The successful formulation of suspensions, emulsions, and tablets, from the viewpoints of both physical stability and pharmacologic response, also depends on the particle size achieved in the product. In the area of tablet and capsule manufacture, control of the particle size is essential in achieving the necessary flow properties and proper mixing of granules and powders. These and other factors reviewed by Lees[2] make it apparent that a pharmacist today must possess a sound knowledge of micromeritics.

PARTICLE SIZE AND SIZE DISTRIBUTION

In a collection of particles of more than one size (i.e., in a polydisperse sample), two properties are important, namely (1) the shape and surface area of the individual particles, and (2) the size range and number or weight of particles present and, hence, the total surface area. Particle size and size distributions will be considered in this section; shape and surface area will be discussed subsequently.

The size of a sphere is readily expressed in terms of its diameter. As the degree of assymmetry of particles

TABLE 16–1a. *Particle Dimensions in Pharmaceutical Disperse Systems*

Particle Size, Diameter			
Micrometers (μm)	Millimeters	Approximate Sieve Size	Examples
0.5–10	0.0005–0.010	—	Suspensions, fine emulsions
10–50	0.010–0.050	—	Upper limit of subsieve range, coarse emulsion particles; flocculated suspension particles
50–100	0.050–0.100	325–140	Lower limit of sieve range, fine powder range
150–1000	0.150–1.000	100–18	Coarse powder range
1000–3360	1.000–3.360	18–6	Average granule size

TABLE 16–1*b***.** *A scale of the Ranges of Various Small Particles, together with the Wavelength of Light and Other Electromagnetic Waves That Illuminate Materials Found in These Size Ranges. From Gelman* Science, *1980, p. 4.*

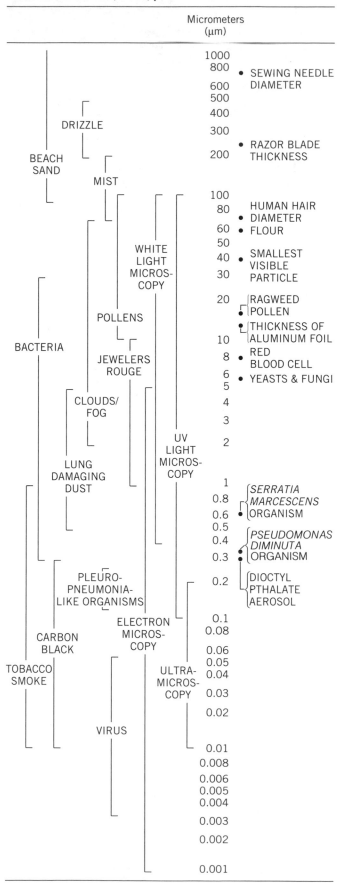

TABLE 16−1c. *A Table of Rod Length and Diameter of Various Microorganisms From* **Gelman Science,** *1980, p. 4.*

Organism	Rod Length (μm)	Rod or Coccus Diameter (μm)	Significance
Acetobacter melanogenus	1.0−2.0	0.4−0.8	Strong beer/vinegar bacterium
Alcaligenes viscolactis	0.8−2.6	0.6−1.0	Causes ropiness in milk
Bacillus anthracis	3.0−10.0	1.0−1.3	Causes anthrax in mammals
B. stearothermophilus	2.0−5.0	0.6−1.0	Biologic indicator for steam sterilization
B. subtilis	2.0−3.0	0.7−0.8	Biologic indicator for ethylene oxide sterilization
Clostridium botulinum (B)	3.0−8.0	0.5−0.8	Produces exotoxin causing botulism
C. perfringens	4.0−8.0	1.0−1.5	Produces toxin causing food poisoning
C. tetani	4.0−8.0	0.4−0.6	Produces exotoxin causing tetanus
Diplococcus pneumoniae		0.5−1.25	Causes lobar pneumonia
Erwinia aroideae	2.0−3.0	0.5	Causes soft rot in vegetables
Escherichia coli	1.0−3.0	0.5	Indicator of fecal contamination in water
Haemophilus influenzae	0.5−2.0	0.2−0.3	Causes influenza and acute respiratory infections
Klebsiella pneumoniae	5.0	0.3−0.5	Causes pneumonia and other respiratory inflammations
Lactobacillus delbrueckii	2.0−9.0	0.5−0.8	Causes souring of grain mashes
Leuconostoc mesenteroides		0.9−1.2	Causes slime in sugar solutions
Mycoplasma pneumoniae (PPLO)		0.3−0.5	Smallest known free-living organism
Pediococcus acidilactici		0.6−1.0	Causes mash spoilage in brewing
P. cerevisiae		1.0−1.3	Causes deterioration in beer
Pseudomonas diminuta	1.0	0.3	Test organism for retention of 0.2-μm membranes
Salmonella enteritidis	2.0−3.0	0.6−0.7	Causes food poisoning
S. hirschfeldii	1.0−2.5	0.3−0.5	Causes enteric fever
S. typhimurium	1.0−1.5	0.5	Causes food poisoning in man
S. typhosa	2.0−3.0	0.6−0.7	causes typhoid fever
Sarcina maxima		4.0−4.5	Isolated from fermenting malt mash
Serratia marcescens	0.5−1.0	0.5	Test organism for retention of 0.45-μm membranes
Shigella dysenteriae	1.0−3.0	0.4−0.6	Causes dysentery in man
Staphylococcus aureus		0.8−1.0	Causes pus-forming infections
Streptococcus lactis		0.5−1.0	Contaminant in milk
S. pyogenes		0.6−1.0	Causes pus-forming infections
Vibrio percolans	1.5−1.8	0.3 0.4	Test organism for retention of 0.2-μm membranes

increases, however, so does the difficulty of expressing size in terms of a meaningful diameter. Under these conditions, there is no one unique diameter for a particle. Recourse must be made to the use of an *equivalent spherical diameter*, which relates the size of the particle to the diameter of a sphere having the same surface area, volume, or diameter. Thus, the surface diameter, d_s, is the diameter of a sphere having the same surface area as the particle in question. The diameter of a sphere having the same volume as the particle is the volume diameter, d_v, while the projected diameter, d_p, is the diameter of a sphere having the same observed area as the particle when viewed normal to its most stable plane. The size may also be expressed as the Stokes' diameter, d_{st}, which describes an equivalent sphere undergoing sedimentation at the same rate as the asymmetric particle. Invariably, the type of diameter used reflects the method employed to obtain the diameter. As will be seen later, the projected diameter is obtained by microscopic techniques, while the Stokes' diameter is determined from sedimentation studies on the suspended particles.

Any collection of particles is usually polydisperse. It is therefore necessary to know not only the size of a certain particle, but also how many particles of the same size exist in the sample. Thus, we need an estimate of the size range present and the number or weight fraction of each particle size. This is the particle size distribution, and from it we may calculate an average particle size for the sample.

If a drug product formulator desires to work with particles of approximately uniform size (i.e., *monodisperse* rather than *polydisperse*) he or she may obtain batches of latex particles as small as 0.060 μm (60 nm) in diameter with a standard deviation σ of ±0.012 μm and particles as large as 920 μm (0.920 nm) with σ = ±32.50. Such particles of uniform size[3] are used in science, medicine, and technology for various diagnostic tests; as particle size standards for particle analyzers; for the accurate determination of pore sizes in filters; and as uniformly sized surfaces upon which antigens may be coated for effective immunization. Nanosphere Size Standards[4] are available in 22 sizes, from 21 nm (0.021 μm) to 900 nm (0.9 μm or 0.0009 mm) in diameter for instrument calibration and quality control in the manufacture of submicron-sized products such as liposomes, nanoparticles, and microemulsions, described in Chapters 18 and 19.

Average Particle Size. Suppose we have conducted a microscopic examination of a sample of a powder and recorded the number of particles lying within various size ranges. Data from such a determination are shown in Table 16−2. To compare these values with those from, say, a second batch of the same material, we usually compute an average or mean diameter as our basis for comparison.

TABLE 16—2. *Calculation of Statistical Diameters from Data Obtained by Use of the Microscopic Method (Normal Distribution)*

Size Range in Micrometers	Mean of Size Range (d) in Micrometers	Number of Particles in Each Size Range (n)	(nd)	(nd^2)	(nd^3)	(nd^4)
0.50–1.00	0.75	2	1.50	1.13	0.85	0.64
1.00–1.50	1.25	10	12.50	15.63	19.54	24.43
1.50–2.00	1.75	22	38.50	67.38	117.92	206.36
2.00–2.50	2.25	54	121.50	273.38	615.11	1384.00
2.50–3.00	2.75	17	46.75	128.56	353.54	972.24
3.00–3.50	3.25	8	26.00	84.50	274.63	892.55
3.50–4.00	3.75	5	18.75	70.31	263.66	988.73
		$\Sigma n = 118$	$\Sigma nd = 265.50$	$\Sigma nd^2 = 640.89$	$\Sigma nd^3 = 1645.25$	$\Sigma nd^4 = 4468.95$

Edmundson[5] has derived a general equation for the average particle size, whether it be an arithmetic, geometric, or harmonic mean diameter.

$$d_{\text{mean}} = \left(\frac{\Sigma nd^{p+f}}{\Sigma nd^f}\right)^{1/p} \qquad (16\text{–}1)$$

In equation (16–1), n is the number of particles in a size range whose midpoint, d, is one of the equivalent diameters mentioned previously. The term p is an index related to the size of an individual particle, since d raised to the power $p = 1$, $p = 2$, or $p = 3$ is an expression of the particle length, surface, or volume, respectively. The value of the index p also decides whether the mean is arithmetic (p is positive), geometric (p is zero), or harmonic (p is negative). For a collection of particles, the frequency with which a particle in a certain size range occurs is expressed by nd^f. When the frequency index, f, has values of 0, 1, 2, or 3, then the size frequency distribution is expressed in terms of the total number, length, surface, or volume of the particles, respectively.

Some of the more significant arithmetic (p is positive) mean diameters are shown in Table 16–3. These are based on the values of p and f used in equation (16–1). The diameters calculated from the data in Table 16–2 are also included. For a more complete description of these diameters, refer to the work of Edmundson.[5]

Particle Size Distribution. When the number, or weight, of particles lying within a certain size range is plotted against the size range or mean particle size, a so-called *frequency distribution curve* is obtained. Typical examples are shown in Figure 16–1 (based on Table 16–2) and Figure 16–2 (based on Table 16–4).

TABLE 16—3. *Statistical Diameters**

$\left(\dfrac{\Sigma nd^{p+f}}{\Sigma nd^f}\right)^{1/p}$	p	f	Type of Mean	Size Parameter	Frequency	Mean Diameter	Value for Data in Table 16—2 (micrometers)	Comments
$\dfrac{\Sigma nd}{\Sigma n}$	1	0	Arithmetic	Length	Number	Length–number mean d_{ln}	2.25	Satisfactory if size range is narrow and distribution is normal. These conditions are rarely found in pharmaceutical powders.
$\sqrt{\dfrac{\Sigma nd^2}{\Sigma n}}$	2	0	Arithmetic	Surface	Number	Surface–number mean d_{sn}	2.33	Refers to particle having average surface area.
$\sqrt[3]{\dfrac{\Sigma nd^3}{\Sigma n}}$	3	0	Arithmetic	Volume	Number	Volume–number mean d_{vn}	2.41	Refers to particle having average weight and is related inversely to N, the number of particles per gram of material (p. 430).
$\dfrac{\Sigma nd^2}{\Sigma nd}$	1	1	Arithmetic	Length	Length	Surface–length or length–weighted mean, d_{sl}	2.41	No practical significance
$\dfrac{\Sigma nd^3}{\Sigma nd^2}$	1	2	Arithmetic	Length	Surface	Volume–surface or surface–weighted mean, d_{vs}	2.57	Important pharmaceutically because inversely related to S_w, the specific surface (p. 436).
$\dfrac{\Sigma nd^4}{\Sigma nd^3}$	1	3	Arithmetic	Length	Weight	Weight–moment or volume–weighted mean, d_{wm}	2.72	Limited pharmaceutical significance.

*Modified with permission from I. C. Edmundson, *Advances in Pharmaceutical Sciences*, Vol. 2, Edited by H. S. Bean, J. E. Carless and A. H. Beckett, Academic Press, London, 1967, p. 950, copyright Academic Press Inc. (London) Ltd.

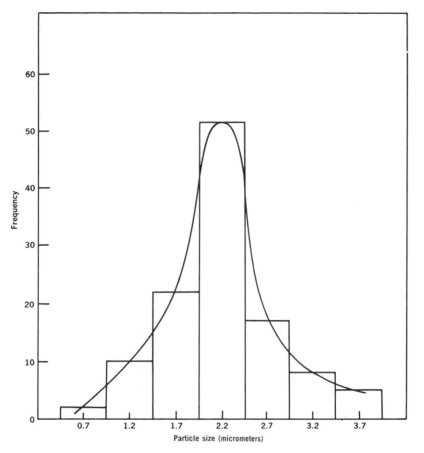

Fig. 16–1. A plot of the data of Table 16–2 so as to yield a size-frequency distribution. The data are plotted as a bar graph or *histogram*, and a superimposed smooth line or frequency curve is shown drawn through the histogram.

Such plots give a visible representation of the distribution that an average diameter cannot achieve. This is important, for it is possible to have two samples with the same average diameter but different distributions. Also, it is immediately apparent from a frequency distribution curve what particle size occurs most frequently within the sample. This is termed the *mode*.

An alternative method of representing the data is to plot either the cumulative percentage over or under a particular size versus particle size. This has been done in Figure 16–3 using the cumulative percent undersize (column 5, Table 16–4). A sigmoidal curve results, with the mode being that particle size at the greatest slope.

The reader should be familiar with the concept of a *normal* distribution, introduced in Chapter 1. As the name implies, the distribution is symmetric around the mean, which is also the mode.

The standard deviation, σ, is an indication of the distribution about the mean.* In a normal distribution,

68% of the population lie ±1σ from the mean, 95.5% lie within the mean ±2σ, and 99.7% lie within the mean ±3σ. The normal distribution, shown in Figure 16–1, is not commonly found in pharmaceutical powders, which are frequently processed by milling or precipitation.[6] Rather, these systems tend to have an unsymmetric, or skewed, distribution of the type depicted in Figure 16–2. When the data in Figure 16–2 (taken from Table 16–4) are plotted as frequency versus the *logarithm* of the particle diameter, a typical bell-shaped curve is frequently obtained. This is depicted in Figure 16–4. A size distribution fitting this pattern is spoken of as a *log-normal distribution*, in contrast to the normal distribution shown in Figure 16–1.

A log-normal distribution has several properties of interest. When the logarithm of the particle size is plotted against the cumulative percent frequency on a probability scale, a linear relationship is observed (Fig. 16–5). Such a linear plot has the distinct advantage that we can now characterize a log-normal distribution *curve* by means of two parameters—the slope of the line and a reference point. Knowing these two parameters, one can reproduce Figure 16–5 and, by working back, can come up with a good approximation of Figures 16–2, 16–3, or 16–4. The reference point used is the logarithm of the particle size equivalent to 50% on the probability scale, that is, the 50% size. This is known as the *geometric mean diameter* and is given the symbol

---

*The statistic, σ, is the standard deviation of a very large number of measurements approximating the total population or universe of particles. Since the particle sample measured in pharmaceutical systems ordinarily is small relative to the universe, the statistic used to express the variability of a sample is usually written as *s* rather than σ. Authors of works on particle size analysis frequently do not make a distinction between σ and *s*, a practice that is followed in this chapter.

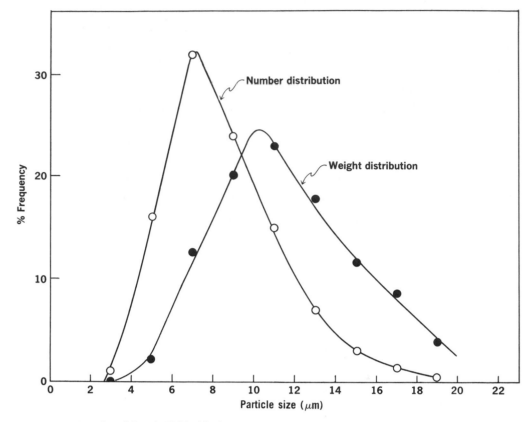

Fig. 16–2. Frequency distribution plot of data in Table 16–4.

d_g. The slope is given by the geometric standard deviation, σ_g, which is the quotient of the ratio (84% undersize or 16% oversize)/(50% size) or (50% size)/(16% undersize or 84% oversize). This is simply the slope of the straight line. In Figure 16–5, for the number distribution data, $d_g = 7.1$ μm and $\sigma_g = 1.43$. Sano et al.[7] used a spherical agglomeration technique with soluble polymers and surfactants to increase the dissolution rate of the poorly soluble crystals of tolbutamide. The spherical particles were free-flowing and yielded log probability plots as shown in Figure 16–5. The dissolution of the tolbutamide agglomerates followed the Hixon–Crowell cube root equation, as did the

dissolution rate of tolbutamide crystals alone (see pp. 333–334 for Table 13–3 and *Example 13–4;* and *Problem 13–5* on p. 357).

Number and Weight Distributions. The data in Table 16–4 are shown as a number distribution, implying that they were collected by a counting technique such as microscopy. Frequently, we are interested in obtaining data based on a weight, rather than a number, distribution. Although this can be achieved by using a technique such as sedimentation or sieving, it will be more convenient, if the number data are already at hand, to convert the number distribution to a weight distribution, and vice versa.

TABLE 16–4. *Conversion of Number Distribution to Weight Distribution (Log-Normal Distribution)*

(1) Size Range in Micrometers	(2) Mean of Size Range (d) in Micrometers	(3) Number of Particles in Each Size Range (n)	(4) Percent n	(5) Cumulative Percent Frequency Undersize (Number)	(6) nd	(7) nd^2	(8) nd^3	(0) Percent nd^3 (Weight)	(10) Cumulative Percent Frequency Undersize (Weight)
2.0–4.0	3.0	2	1.0	1.0	6	18	54	0.03	0.03
4.0–6.0	5.0	32	16.0	17.0	160	800	4000	2.31	2.34
6.0–8.0	7.0	64	32.0	49.0	448	3136	21952	12.65	14.99
8.0–10.0	9.0	48	24.0	73.0	432	3888	34992	20.16	35.15
10.0–12.0	11.0	30	15.0	88.0	330	3630	39930	23.01	58.16
12.0–14.0	13.0	14	7.0	95.0	182	2366	30758	17.72	75.88
14.0–16.0	15.0	6	3.0	98.0	90	1350	20250	11.67	87.55
16.0–18.0	17.0	3	1.5	99.5	51	867	14739	8.49	96.04
18.0–20.0	19.0	1	0.5	100.0	19	361	6859	3.95	99.99
		$\Sigma n = 200$							

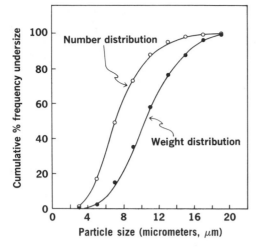

Fig. 16–3. Cumulative frequency plot of data in Table 16–4.

Two approaches are available. Provided the general shape and density of the particles are independent of the size range present in the sample, an estimate of the weight distribution of the data in Table 16–4 may be obtained by calculating the values shown in columns 9 and 10. These are based on nd^3 in column 8. These data have been plotted alongside the number distribution data in Figures 16–2 and 16–3, respectively.

The significant differences in the two distributions is apparent, even though they relate to the same sample. For example, in Figure 16–3, only 12% of the sample by number is greater than 11 μm, yet these same particles account for 42% of the total weight of the particles. For this reason, it is important to distinguish

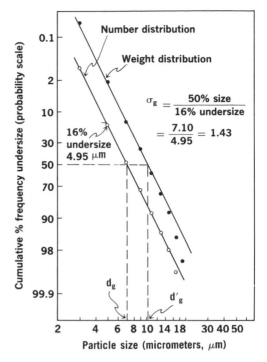

Fig. 16–5. Log-probability plots of data in Table 16–4.

carefully between size distributions on a weight and number basis. Weight distributions may also be plotted in the same manner as the number distribution data, as seen in Figures 16–4 and 16–5. Note that in Figure 16–5 the slope of the line for the weight distribution is identical with that for the number distribution. Thus, the geometric standard deviation on a weight basis, σ'_g,

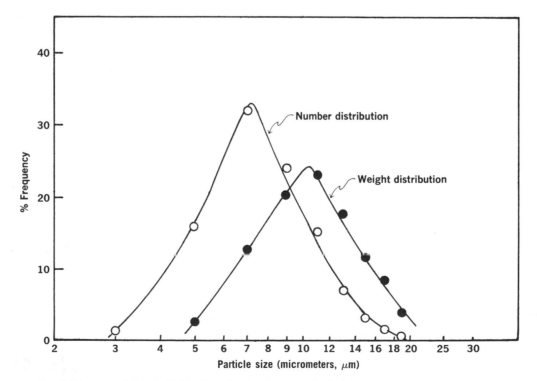

Fig. 16–4. Frequency distribution plot of data in Table 16–4 showing log-normal relation.

also equals 1.43. Customarily, the prime is dropped since the value is independent of the type of distribution. The geometric mean diameter (the particle size at the 50% probability level) on a weight basis, d'_g, is 10.4 μm, whereas $d_y = 7.1$ μm.

Provided the distribution is log-normal, the second approach is to use one of the equations developed by Hatch and Choate.[8] By this means, it is possible to convert number distributions to weight distributions with a minimum of calculation. In addition, a particular average can be readily computed by use of the relevant equation. The Hatch–Choate equations are listed in Table 16–5.

Example 16–1. From the number distribution data in Table 16–4 and Figure 16–5, it is found that $d_g = 7.1$ μm and $\sigma_g = 1.43$, or log $\sigma_g = 0.1553$. Using the relevant Hatch–Choate equation, calculate d_{ln} and d'_g.

The equation for the length–number mean, d_{ln}, is

$$log\ d_{ln} = log\ d_g + 1.151\ log^2 \sigma_g$$
$$= 0.8513 + 1.151(0.1553)^2$$
$$= 0.8513 + 0.0278$$
$$= 0.8791$$
$$d_{ln} = 7.57\ \mu m$$

To calculate d'_g, we must substitute into the following Hatch–Choate equation:

$$log\ d_{ln} = log\ d'_g - 5.757\ log^2 \sigma_g$$
$$0.8791 = log\ d'_g - 5.757(0.1553)^2$$

or

$$log\ d'_g = 0.8791 + 0.1388$$
$$= 1.0179$$
$$d'_g = 10.4\ \mu m$$

One can also use an equation suggested by Rao,[9]

$$d'_g = d_g\ \sigma_g^{(3\ ln\ \sigma_g)} \qquad (16-2)$$

to readily obtain d'_g, knowing d_g and σ_g. In the present example,

$$d'_g = 7.1(1.43)^{(3\ ln\ 1.43)}$$
$$- 10.42$$

The student should confirm that substitution of the relevant data into the remaining Hatch–Choate equations in Table 16–5 yields the following statistical diameters:

$$d_{sn} = 8.07\ \mu m; \qquad d_{vn} = 8.60\ \mu m;$$
$$d_{vs} = 9.78\ \mu m; \qquad d_{wm} = 11.11\ \mu m$$

Particle Number. A significant expression in particle technology is the *number of particles per unit weight N*, which is expressed in terms of d_{vn}.

The number of particles per unit weight is obtained as follows. Assuming that the particles are spheres, the volume of a single particle is $\pi d_{vn}^3/6$, and the mass

(volume × density) is $\pi d_{vn}^3 \rho/6$ g per particle. The number of particles per gram is then obtained from the proportion

$$\frac{(\pi d_{vn}^3 \rho)/6\ g}{1\ particle} = \frac{1\ g}{N} \qquad (16-3)$$

and

$$N = \frac{6}{\pi d_{vn}^3 \rho} \qquad (16-4)$$

Example 16–2. The mean volume number diameter of the powder, the data for which are given in Table 16–2, is 2.41 μm or 2.41×10^{-4} cm. If the density of the powder is 3.0 g/cm³, what is the number of particles per gram?

$$N = \frac{6}{3.14 \times (2.41 \times 10^{-4})^3 \times 3.0} = 4.55 \times 10^{10}$$

METHODS FOR DETERMINING PARTICLE SIZE

Many methods are available for determining particle size. Only those that are widely used in pharmaceutical practice and are typical of a particular principle are presented. For a detailed discussion of the numerous methods of particle size analysis, the reader should consult the texts by Edmundson[5] and by Allen,[10] and the references given there to other sources. The methods available to determine the size characteristics of submicrometer particles have been reviewed by Groves.[11] Such methods apply to colloidal dispersions (see Chapter 15).

Microscopy, sieving, sedimentation, and the determination of particle volume are discussed in the following section. None of the measurements are truly direct methods. Although the microscope allows the observer to view the actual particles, the results obtained are probably no more "direct" than those resulting from other methods since only two of the three particle dimensions are ordinarily seen. The sedimentation methods yield a particle size relative to the rate at which particles settle through a suspending medium, a measurement important in the development of emulsions and suspensions. The measurement of particle volume, using an apparatus called the Coulter counter, allows one to calculate an equivalent volume diameter. However, the technique gives no information as to the shape of the particles. Thus, in all these cases, the size may or may not compare with that obtained by the microscope or by other methods; the size is most

TABLE 16–5. *Hatch–Choate Equations for Computing Statistical Diameters from Number and Weight Distributions*

Diameter	Number Distribution	Weight Distribution
Length–number mean	$log\ d_{ln} = log\ d_g + 1.151\ log^2 \sigma_g$	$log\ d_{ln} = log\ d'_g - 5.757\ log^2 \sigma_g$
Surface–number mean	$log\ d_{sn} = log\ d_g + 2.303\ log^2 \sigma_g$	$log\ d_{sn} = log\ d'_g - 4.606\ log^2 \sigma_g$
Volume–number mean	$log\ d_{vn} = log\ d_g + 3.454\ log^2 \sigma_g$	$log\ d_{vn} = log\ d'_g - 3.454\ log^2 \sigma_g$
Volume–surface mean	$log\ d_{vs} = log\ d_g + 5.757\ log^2 \sigma_g$	$log\ d_{vs} = log\ d'_g - 1.151\ log^2 \sigma_g$
Weight–moment mean	$log\ d_{wm} = log\ d_g + 8.059\ log^2 \sigma_g$	$log\ d_{wm} = log\ d'_g + 1.151\ log^2 \sigma_g$

directly applicable to the analysis for which it is intended. A guide to the range of particle sizes applicable to each method is given in Figure 16–6.

Optical Microscopy. It should be possible to use the ordinary microscope for particle-size measurement in the range of 0.2 μm to about 100 μm. According to the microscopic method, an emulsion or suspension, diluted or undiluted, is mounted on a slide or ruled cell and placed on a mechanical stage. The microscope eyepiece is fitted with a micrometer by which the size of the particles may be estimated. The field can be projected onto a screen where the particles are measured more easily, or a photograph can be taken from which a slide is prepared and projected on a screen for measurement.

The particles are measured along an arbitrarily chosen fixed line, generally made horizontally across the center of the particle. Popular measurements are the *Feret diameter*, the *Martin diameter*,[12] and the *projected area diameter*, all of which may be defined by reference to Figure 16–7, as suggested by Allen.[13] Martin's diameter is the length of a line that bisects the particle image. The line may be drawn in any direction but must be in the same direction for all particles measured. The Martin diameter is identified by the number 1 in Figure 16–7. Feret's diameter, corresponding to the number 2 in the figure, is the distance between two tangents on opposite sides of the particle parallel to some fixed direction, the *y*-direction in the figure. The third measurement, number 3 in Figure 16–7, is the projected area diameter. It is the diameter of a circle with the same area as that of the particle observed perpendicular to the surface on which the particle rests.

A size-frequency distribution curve may be plotted as was seen in Figure 16–1 for the determination of the statistical diameters of the distribution. Electronic scanners have been developed to remove the necessity of measuring the particles by visual observation.

Prasad and Wan[14] used video recording equipment to observe, record, store, and retrieve particle-size data from a microscopic examination of tablet excipients, including microcrystalline cellulose, sodium carboxymethylcellulose, sodium starch glycolate, and methylcellulose. The projected area of the particle profile, Feret's diameter (p. 432), and various shape factors (elongation, bulkiness, and surface factor) were determined. The video recording technique was found to be simple and convenient for microscopic examination of excipients.

A disadvantage of the microscopic method is that the diameter is obtained from only two dimensions of the particle: length and breadth. No estimation of the depth (thickness) of the particle is ordinarily available. In addition, the number of particles that must be counted (300 to 500) to obtain a good estimation of the distribution makes the method somewhat slow and tedious. But, microscopic examination (photomicrographs) of a sample should be undertaken, even when other methods of particle-size analysis are being used, since the presence of agglomerates and particles of more than one component may often be detected.

Sieving. This method uses a series of standard sieves calibrated by the National Bureau of Standards. Sieves are generally used for grading coarser particles; if extreme care is used, however, they may be employed for screening material as fine as 44 μm (No. 325 sieve). Sieves produced by photoetching and electroforming techniques are now available with apertures from 90 μm down to as low as 5 μm. According to the method of the U.S. Pharmacopeia for testing powder fineness, a definite mass of sample is placed on the proper sieve in a mechanical shaker. The powder is shaken for a

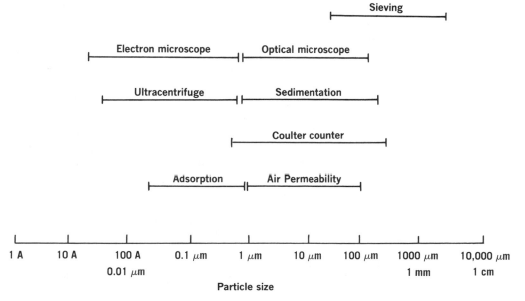

Fig. 16–6. Approximate size ranges of methods used for particle size and specific surface analysis.

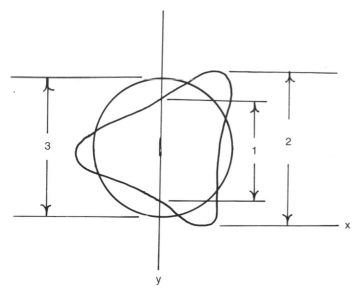

Fig. 16–7. A general diagram providing definitions of the Feret, Martin, and projected diameters. (From T. Allen, *Particle Size measurements*, 2nd Edition, Chapman & Hall, London, 1974, p. 131, reproduced with permission of the copyright owner.)

definite period of time, and the material that passes through one sieve and is retained on the next finer sieve is collected and weighed.

Another custom is to assign the particles on the lower sieve the arithmetic or geometric mean size of the two screens. Arambulo and Deardorff[15] used this method of size classification in their analysis of the average weight of compressed tablets. Frequently the powder is assigned the mesh number of the screen through which it passes or on which it is retained. King and Becker[16] expressed the size ranges of calamine samples in this way in their study of calamine lotion.

When a detailed analysis is desired, the sieves may be arranged in a nest of about five with the coarsest at the top. A carefully weighed sample of the powder is placed on the top sieve, and after the sieves are shaken for a predetermined period of time, the powder retained on each sieve is weighed. Assuming a log-normal distribution, the cumulative percent by weight of powder retained on the sieves is plotted on the probability scale against the logarithm of the arithmetic mean size of the openings of each of two successive screens. As illustrated in Figure 16–5, the geometric mean weight diameter d'_g and the geometric standard deviation σ_g can be obtained directly from the straight line.

According to Herdan,[17] sieving errors can arise from a number of variables including sieve loading and duration and intensity of agitation. Fonner et al.[18] demonstrated that sieving can cause attrition of granular pharmaceutical materials. Care must be taken, therefore, to ensure that reproducible techniques are employed so that different particle size distributions between batches of material are not due simply to different sieving conditions.

Sedimentation. The application of ultracentrifugation to the determination of the molecular weight of high polymers has already been discussed (p. 403). The particle size in the subsieve range may be obtained by gravity sedimentation as expressed in Stokes' law,

$$v = \frac{h}{t} = \frac{d_{st}^2(\rho_s - \rho_o)g}{18\eta_o} \tag{16–5}$$

or

$$d_{st} = \sqrt{\frac{18\eta_o h}{(\rho_s - \rho_o)gt}} \tag{16–6}$$

in which v is the rate of settling, h is the distance of fall in time t, d_{st} is the mean diameter of the particles based on the velocity of sedimentation, ρ_s is the density of the particles and ρ_o that of the dispersion medium, g is the acceleration due to gravity, and η_o is the viscosity of the medium. The equation holds exactly only for spheres falling freely without hindrance and at a constant rate. The law is applicable to irregularly shaped particles of various sizes as long as one realizes that the diameter obtained is a relative particle size equivalent to that of sphere falling at the same velocity as that of the particles under consideration. The particles must not be aggregated or clumped together in the suspension since such clumps would fall more rapidly than the individual particles, and erroneous results would be obtained. The proper deflocculating agent must be found for each sample that will keep the particles free and separate as they fall through the medium.

Example 16–3. A sample of powdered zinc oxide, density 5.60 g/cm³, is allowed to settle under the acceleration of gravity, 981 cm sec⁻², at 25° C. The rate of settling, v, is 7.30×10^{-3} cm/sec; the density of the medium is 1.01 g/cm³, and its viscosity is 1 cp = 0.01 poise or 0.01 g cm⁻¹ sec⁻¹. Calculate the Stokes' diameter of the zinc oxide powder.

$$d_{st} = \sqrt{\frac{18 \times 0.01 \text{ g cm}^{-1} \text{ sec}^{-1} \times 7.30 \times 10^{-3} \text{ cm sec}^{-1}}{(5.60 - 1.01) \text{ g cm}^{-3} \times 981 \text{ cm sec}^{-2}}}$$

$$= 5.40 \times 10^{-4} \text{ cm or } 5.40 \text{ μm}$$

For Stokes' law to apply, a further requirement is that the flow of dispersion medium around the particle as it sediments is *laminar* or *streamline*. In other words, the rate of sedimentation of a particle must not be so rapid that turbulence is set up, since this in turn will affect the sedimentation of the particle. Whether the flow is turbulent or laminar is indicated by the dimensionless *Reynolds number*, R_e, which is defined as

$$R_e = \frac{v \, d\rho_o}{\eta_o} \tag{16–7}$$

in which the symbols have the same meaning as in equation (16–5). According to Heywood,[19] Stokes' law cannot be used if R_e is greater than 0.2, since turbulence appears at this value. On this basis, the limiting particle size under a given set of conditions may be calculated as follows:

Rearranging equation (16–7) and combining it with equation (16–5) gives

$$v = \frac{R_e\eta}{d\rho_o} = \frac{d^2(\rho_s - \rho_o)g}{18\eta} \qquad (16\text{–}8)$$

and thus

$$d^3 = \frac{18R_e\eta^2}{(\rho_s - \rho_o)\rho_o g} \qquad (16\text{–}9)$$

Under a given set of density and viscosity conditions, equation (16–9) allows calculation of the maximum particle diameter whose sedimentation will be governed by Stokes' law, that is, when R_e does not exceed 0.2.

Example 16–4. A powdered material, density 2.7 g/cm³, is suspended in water at 20° C. What is the size of the largest particle that will settle without causing turbulence? The viscosity of water at 20° C is 0.01 poise, or g/(cm sec) and the density is 1.0 g/cm³.

From equation (16–9):

$$d^3 = \frac{(18)(0.2)(0.01)^2}{(2.7 - 1.0)1.0 \times 981}$$

$$d = 6 \times 10^{-3} \text{ cm} = 60 \text{ μm}$$

Example 16–5. If the material used in *Example 16–4* is now suspended in a syrup containing 60% by weight of sucrose, what will be the critical diameter, that is, the maximum diameter for which R_e does not exceed 0.2? The viscosity of the syrup is 0.567 poise that is, and the density 1.3 g/cm³.

$$d^3 = \frac{(18)(0.2)(0.567)^2}{(2.7 - 1.3)1.3 \times 981}$$

$$d = 8.65 \times 10^{-2} \text{ cm} = 865 \text{ μm}$$

Several methods based on sedimentation are used. Principal among these are the pipette method, the balance method, and the hydrometer method. Only the first technique is discussed here since it combines ease of analysis, accuracy, and economy of equipment.

The Andreasen apparatus is shown in Figure 16–8. It usually consists of a 550-mL vessel containing a 10-mL pipette sealed into a ground-glass stopper. When the pipette is in place in the cylinder, its lower tip is 20 cm below the surface of the suspension.

The analysis is carried out in the following manner. A 1 or 2% suspension of the particles in a medium containing a suitable deflocculating agent is introduced into the vessel and brought to the 550-mL mark. The stoppered vessel is shaken to distribute the particles uniformly throughout the suspension and the apparatus, with pipette in place, is clamped securely in a constant-temperature bath. At various time intervals, 10-mL samples are withdrawn and discharged by means of the two-way stopcock. The samples are evaporated and weighed or analyzed by other appropriate means, correcting for the deflocculating agent that has been added.

The particle diameter corresponding to the various time periods is calculated from Stokes' law, with h in equation (16–6) being the height of the liquid above the lower end of the pipette at the time each sample is removed. The residue or dried sample obtained at a

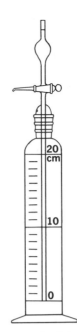

Fig. 16–8. Andreasen apparatus for determining particle size by the gravity sedimentation method.

particular time is the weight fraction having particles of sizes less than the size obtained by the Stokes' law calculation for that time period of settling. The weight of each sample residue is therefore called the *weight undersize*, and the sum of the successive weights is known as the *cumulative weight undersize*. It may be expressed directly in weight units or as percent of the total weight of the final sediment. Such data are plotted in Figures 16–2, 16–3, and 16–4. The cumulative percent by weight undersize may then be plotted on a probability scale against the particle diameter on a log scale, as in Figure 16–5, and the statistical diameters obtained as explained previously. Data that illustrate the sedimentation method employing the Andreasen apparatus are found in *Problem 16–4*, p. 450.

The Micromeritics Instrument Co., Norcross, Ga., offers the SediGraph 5100 for particle-size analysis based on the sedimentation principle. Since particles are not usually of uniform shape, the particle size is expressed as equivalent spherical diameter or Stokes' diameter.

A low-energy x-ray beam passes through the suspension and is collected at the detector. Which x-ray pulses reach the detector is determined by the distribution of settling particles in the cell; and from the x-ray pulse count the particle size distribution and the mass of particles for each particle diameter are derived. The operation is completely automatic, the apparatus is temperature-controlled, and the data are analyzed under computer software control. Particle diameters are measured from 0.1 to 300 μm at temperatures from 10° to 40° C. The Micromeritics Co. also manufactures equipment for the measurement of powder density, surface area, adsorption and desorption, pore volume, pore size, and pore size distribution (see pp. 440–442 for a discussion of pore size).

MATEC Applied Sciences, Hopkinton, Mass., has developed a particle-size measurement system for *submicron* particles in the range of 0.015 to 1.1 μm. The particles in suspension are caused to pass through capillary tubes, the larger particles attaining greater average velocities than the smaller ones. The instrument applies this principle to the determination of average particle size and size distribution by number or volume of particles. The operation, from the time of sample injection to graphics output, requires a maximum of 8 minutes. The liquid medium consists of 1 mL of water containing a surfactant and the suspended particles in the concentration of 2 to 4% solids. The particles to be analyzed are prefiltered through a 5-μm or smaller pore size filter. A computer terminal and program, printer, and plotter are available to calculate and display the size and size distribution data.

Particle Volume Measurement. A popular instrument to measure the volume of particles is the Coulter counter (Fig. 16–9). This instrument operates on the principle that when a particle suspended in a conducting liquid passes through a small orifice, on either side of which are electrodes, a change in electric resistance occurs. In practice, a known volume of a dilute suspension is pumped through the orifice. Provided the suspension is sufficiently dilute, the particles pass through essentially one at a time. A constant voltage is applied across the electrodes to produce a current. As the particle travels through the orifice, it displaces its own volume of electrolyte, and this results in an increased resistance between the two electrodes. The change in resistance, which is related to the particle volume, causes a voltage pulse that is amplified and fed to a pulse height analyzer calibrated in terms of particle size. The instrument records electronically all those particles producing pulses that are within two threshold values of the analyzer. By systematically varying the threshold settings and counting the number of particles in a constant sample size, it is possible to obtain a particle size distribution. The instrument is capable of counting particles at the rate of approximately 4000 per second, and so both gross counts and particle size distributions are obtained in a relatively short period of time. The data may be readily converted from a volume distribution to a weight distribution.

The Coulter counter has been used to advantage in the pharmaceutical sciences to study particle growth and dissolution[20,21] and the effect of antibacterial agents on the growth of microorganisms.[22]

The use of the Coulter particle-size analyzer together with a digital computer was reported by Beaubien and Vanderwielen[23] for the automated particle counting of milled and micronized drugs. Samples of spectinomycin hydrochloride and a micronized steroid were subjected to particle-size analysis, together with polystyrene spheres of 2.0 to 80.0 μm diameter which were used to calibrate the apparatus. The powders showed log-normal distributions and were well characterized by geometric volume mean diameters and geometric standard deviations. Accurate particle sizes were obtained between 2 and 80 μm diameter with a precision of about 0.5 μm. The authors concluded that the automated

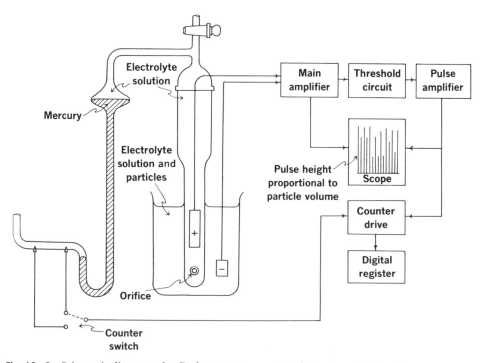

Fig. 16–9. Schematic diagram of a Coulter counter, used to determine particle volume.

Coulter counter was quite satisfactory for quality control of pharmaceutical powders. The Coulter particle counter was used by Ismail and Tawashi[24] to obtain size distributions of the mineral part of human kidney (urinary) stones and to determine whether there is a critical size range for stone formation. The study provided a better understanding of the clustering process and the packing of the mineral components of renal stones.

Limits for allowable particulates in small-volume parenterals are given in the United States Pharmacopeia XXII, pp. 1596–1597, based on results obtained using the HIAC/Royco light blockage instrument. Groves et al.[25] made a comparative study of the Coulter counter and the HIAC instrument to measure particulate contamination in parenteral solutions. The two methods measure different parameters, the Coulter instrument giving the diameter of a sphere of equivalent volume to that of the particle. The measurement is not greatly affected by the shape and orientation of the particle.

The HIAC/Royco instrument for particle size and particle contamination analysis is designed on the principle of light blockage. The particles interrupt a light beam and decrease the amount of light that reaches a photodetector. This decrease in light transmission produces a voltage pulse proportional to the projected area of each particle. The results are highly correlated with National Bureau of Standards reference particles. Particle size may be measured in viscous, aqueous, or nonaqueous liquids and can be analyzed in gas or atmospheric samples in the HIAC/Royco instrument. Cham and associates[26] counted the microspheres in 20 parenteral test solutions using two Coulter and two HIAC/Royco particle analyzers. Earlier comparative studies showed that the Coulter counter gave a higher particle count in parenteral solutions than did the HIAC instrument. The discrepancy has been attributed to particle shape, and the refractive index of the particles and the medium in which they are suspended. Uniformly sized and shaped latex microspheres 5.96 μm in diameter were chosen by Cham et al. to study these effects. Two Coulter counters and two HIAC counters were used to determine the variability for a particular type of instrument and possible differences between the two kinds of counters, the Coulter counter being based on an electrical resistance principle and the HIAC/Royco on light blockage.

The workers found that in all 20 suspensions of microspheres, lower counts were obtained using the HIAC/Royco analyzer. According to the authors, the Coulter counter appeared in this study to be quite reliable for obtaining the absolute count of particulate matter in large-volume parenteral (LVP) solutions and for comparing results from various laboratories.

Coulter Electronics also manufactures a *submicron* particle sizing instrument, the Coulter Model N4, for analyzing particles in the size range of 0.003 to 0.3 μm. By the use of photon correlation spectroscopy (PCS), the instrument senses the Brownian motion (p. 400) of the particles in suspension. The smaller a particle, the faster it moves by Brownian motion. A laser beam passes through the sample and a sensor detects the light scattered by the particles undergoing Brownian motion. The Coulter Model N4 instrument provides not only particle size and size distribution data but also molecular weights and diffusion coefficients. Submicron size determination is important in pharmacy in the analysis of microemulsions, pigments and dyes, colloids, micelles and solubilized systems, liposomes, and microparticles.

An investigation of contaminant particulate matter in parenteral solutions for adherence to the standards set by the Italian Pharmacopóeia, 1986, was conducted by Signoretti et al.[27] They studied the number and nature of the particulates in 36 large-volume injectable solutions using scanning electron microscopy (SEM) and x-ray analysis. About one fifth of the samples showed a considerable number of particles of sizes greater than 20 μm diameter. The particles were identified as textile fibers, cellulose, plastic material, and contaminants from the manufacturing and packaging processes, such as pieces of rubber and bits of metal. Because of their number, size, shape, surface properties, and chemical nature, these contaminants can cause vascular occlusions and inflammatory, neoplastic, and allergic reactions. Embolisms may occur with particles larger than 5 μm.

According to the standards of the Italian Pharmacopóeia for parenteral solutions of greater than 100 mL, no more than 100 particles 5 μm and larger and no more than four particles 20 μm in diameter and larger may be present in each milliliter of solution. These workers found that a considerable number of the manufacturers failed to produce parenteral preparations within the limits of the Pharmacopóeia, the contaminants probably occurring in most cases from filters, clothing, and container seals.

In the preparation of indomethacin sustained-release pellets, Li et al.[28] used a Microtrac particle-size analyzer (Leeds and Northrup Instruments) to determine the particle size of indomethacin as obtained from the manufacturer and as two types of micronized powder. The powders were also examined under a microscope with a magnification of 400×, and photomicrographs were taken with a Polaroid SX-70 camera. Pellets (referred to as IS pellets) containing indomethacin and Eudragit S-100 were prepared using a fluid bed granulator or a Wurster column apparatus. Eudragit® (Röhm Pharma) is an acrylic polymer for the enteric coating of tablets, capsules, and pellets. Its surface properties and chemical structure as a film coating polymer have been reviewed by Davies et al.[29] Sieve analysis with U.S. standard sieves nos. 12, 14, 16, 18, 20, 25, and 35 was used to determine the particle size distribution of the IS pellets. The yield of IS pellets depended greatly on the particle size of the indomethacin powder. Batches using two micronized powders (average diameter of 3.3 and 6.4 μm, respectively) produced a higher yield of the IS pellets than did the original indomethacin powder (40.6 μm) obtained directly from the drug manufacturer. The workers[29] concluded that both the average particle diameter and the particle size distribution of the indomethacin powder must be considered for maximum yield of the sustained-release pellets.

Carli and Motta[30] investigated the use of microcomputerized mercury porosimetry to obtain particle size and surface area distributions of pharmaceutical powders. Mercury porosimetry gives the volume of the pores of a powder, which is penetrated by mercury at each successive pressure; the pore volume is converted into a pore size distribution. The total surface area and particle size of the powder may also be obtained from the mercury porosimetry data.

PARTICLE SHAPE AND SURFACE AREA

A knowledge of the shape and surface area of a particle is desirable. The shape affects the flow and packing properties of a powder, as well as having some influence on the surface area. The surface area per unit weight or volume is an important characteristic of a powder when one is undertaking surface adsorption and dissolution rate studies.

Particle Shape. A sphere has minimum surface area per unit volume. The more asymmetric a particle, the greater the surface area per unit volume. As discussed previously, a spherical particle is characterized completely by its diameter. As the particle becomes more asymmetric, it becomes increasingly difficult to assign a meaningful diameter to the particle. Hence, as we have seen, the need for equivalent spherical diameters. It is a simple matter to obtain the surface area or volume of a sphere, since for such a particle

$$\text{Surface area} = \pi d^2 \qquad (16-10)$$

and

$$\text{Volume} = \frac{\pi d^3}{6} \qquad (16-11)$$

in which d is the diameter of the particle. The surface area and volume of a spherical particle are therefore proportional to the square and cube, respectively, of the diameter. To obtain an estimate of the surface or volume of a particle (or collection of particles) whose shape is not spherical, however, one must choose a diameter that is characteristic of the particle and relate this to the surface area or volume through a correction factor. Suppose the particles are viewed microscopically, and it is desired to compute the surface area and

volume from the projected diameter, d_p, of the particles. The square and cube of the chosen dimension (in this case, d_p) are proportional to the surface area and volume, respectively. By means of proportionality constants, we can then write

$$\text{Surface area} = \alpha_s d_p^2 = \pi d_s^2 \qquad (16-12)$$

in which α_s is the surface area factor and d_s is the equivalent surface diameter. For volume we write

$$\text{Volume} = \alpha_v d_p^3 = \frac{\pi d_v^3}{6} \qquad (16-13)$$

in which α_v is the volume factor and d_v is the equivalent volume diameter. The surface area and volume "shape factors" are, in reality, the ratio of one diameter to another. Thus, for a sphere, $\alpha_s = \frac{\pi d_s^2}{d_p^2} = 3.142$ and $\alpha_v = \frac{\pi d_v^3}{6 d_p^3} = 0.524$. There are as many of these volume and shape factors as there are pairs of equivalent diameters. The ratio α_s/α_v is also used to characterize particle shape. When the particle is spherical, α_s/α_v equals 6.0. The more asymmetric the particle, the more this ratio exceeds the minimum value of 6.

Specific Surface. The specific surface is the surface area per unit volume (S_v) or per unit weight (S_w) and may be derived from equations (16–12) and (16–13). Taking the general case, for asymmetric particles where the characteristic dimension is not yet defined,

$$S_v = \frac{\text{surface area of particles}}{\text{volume of particles}}$$
$$= \frac{n\alpha_s d^2}{n\alpha_v d^3} = \frac{\alpha_s}{\alpha_v d} \qquad (16-14)$$

in which n is the number of particles. The surface area per unit weight is therefore

$$S_w = \frac{S_v}{\rho} \qquad (16-15)$$

in which ρ = true density of the particles. Substituting for equation (16–14) in (16–15) leads to the general equation

$$S_w = \frac{\alpha_s}{\rho d_{vs} \alpha_v} \qquad (16-16)$$

in which the dimension is now defined as d_{vs}, the volume–surface diameter characteristic of specific surface. When the particles are spherical (or nearly so), equation (16–16) simplifies to

$$S_w = \frac{6}{\rho d_{vs}} \qquad (16-17)$$

since $\alpha_s/\alpha_v = 6.0$ for a sphere.

Example 16–6. What are the specific surfaces, S_w and S_v, of particles assumed to be spherical in which $\rho = 3.0$ g/cm^3, and d_{vs} from Table 16–3 is 2.57 μm?

$$S_w = \frac{6}{3.0 \times 2.57 \times 10^{-4}} = 7.78 \times 10^3 \text{ cm}^2/\text{g}$$

$$S_v = \frac{6}{2.57 \times 10^{-4}} = 2.33 \times 10^4 \text{ cm}^2/\text{cm}^3$$

METHODS FOR DETERMINING SURFACE AREA

The surface area of a powder sample can be computed from a knowledge of the particle size distribution obtained using one of the methods outlined previously. Two methods are commonly available that permit direct calculation of surface area. In the first, the amount of a gas or liquid solute that is *adsorbed* onto the sample of powder to form a monolayer is a direct function of the surface area of the sample. The second method depends on the fact that the rate at which a gas or liquid *permeates* a bed of powder is related, among other factors, to the surface area exposed to the permeant.

Adsorption Method. Particles with a large specific surface are good adsorbents for the adsorption of gases and of solutes from solution. In determining the surface of the adsorbent, the volume in cubic centimeters of gas adsorbed per gram of adsorbent may be plotted against the pressure of the gas at constant temperature to give a Type II *isotherm* (p. 381) as shown in Figure 16–10.

The adsorbed layer is monomolecular at low pressures and becomes multimolecular at higher pressures. The completion of the monolayer of nitrogen on a powder is shown as point B in Figure 16–10. The volume of nitrogen gas V_m in cm^3 that 1 gram of the powder can adsorb when the monolayer is complete is more accurately given by using the BET equation (p. 381), however, which may be written as

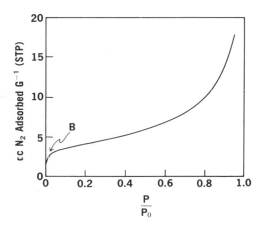

Fig. 16–10. Isotherm showing the volume of nitrogen adsorbed on a powder at increasing pressure ratios. Point B represents the volume of adsorbed gas corresponding to the completion of a monomolecular film.

$$\frac{p}{V(p_o - p)} = \frac{1}{V_m b} + \frac{(b-1)p}{V_m b p_o} \quad (16\text{–}18)$$

V is the volume of gas in cm^3 adsorbed per gram of powder at pressure p, p_o is the saturation vapor pressure (see p. 381 for a definition of p_o) of liquefied nitrogen at the temperature of the experiment, and b is a constant that expresses the difference between the heat of adsorption and heat of liquefaction of the adsorbate (nitrogen). Note that at $p/p_o = 1$, the vapor pressure p is equal to the saturation vapor pressure.

An instrument used to obtain the data needed to calculate surface area and pore structure of pharmaceutical powders is the Quantasorb, manufactured by the Quantachrome Corporation of Greenvale, N.J. Absorption and desorption of nitrogen gas on the powder sample is measured with a thermal conductivity detector when a mixture of helium and nitrogen is passed through a cell containing the powder. Nitrogen is the absorbate gas; helium is inert and is not adsorbed on the powder surface. A Gaussian or bell-shaped curve is plotted on a strip-chart recorder, the signal height being proportional to the rate of absorption or desorption of nitrogen and the area under the curve being proportional to the gas adsorbed on the particles. Quantasorb and similar instruments have replaced the older vacuum systems constructed of networks of glass tubing. These required long periods of time to equilibrate and were subject to leakage at valves and breaks in the glass lines. The sensitivity of the new instrument is such that small powder samples may be analyzed. Quantasorb's versatility allows the use of a number of individual gases or mixture of gases as adsorbates over a range of temperatures. The instrument may be used to measure the true density of powdered material and to obtain pore size and pore volume distributions. The characteristics of porous materials and the method of analysis are discussed in the following sections.

Instead of drawing the graph shown in Figure 16–10, a plot of $p/V(p_o - p)$ against p/p_o, as shown in Figure 16–11, is ordinarily used to obtain a straight line, the slope and intercept of which yield the values b and V_m. The specific surface of the particles is then obtained by application of the equation

$$S_w = \frac{A_m N}{M/\rho} \times V_m \text{ cm}^3/\text{g}$$

$$S_w = \frac{(16.2 \times 10^{-16})(6.02 \times 10^{23})}{22{,}414 \times 10^4} \times V_m$$

$$S_w = 4.35 \text{ m}^2/\text{cm}^3 \times V_m \text{ cm}^3/\text{g}$$

$$(16\text{–}19)$$

in which M/ρ is the molar volume of the gas, 22,414 cm^3/mole at STP, and the factor 10^4 is included in the denominator to convert square centimeters to square meters. N is Avogadro's number, 6.02×10^{23} molecules/mole, and A_m is the area of a single close-packed

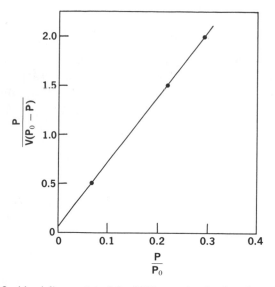

Fig. 16–11. A linear plot of the BET equation for the adsorption of nitrogen on a powder.

nitrogen molecule adsorbed as a monolayer on the surface of the particles. Emmett and Brunauer[31] suggested that the value, A_m, for nitrogen be calculated from the formula

$$A_m = 1.091 \left(\frac{M}{\rho N}\right)^{2/3} \quad (16-20)$$

in which M is the molecular weight, 28.01 g/mole, of N_2, ρ is the density, 0.81 g/cm³, of N_2 at its boiling point, 77° K (−196° C), and N is Avogadro's number. The quantity 1.091 is a packing factor for the nitrogen molecules on the surface of the adsorbent.

$$A_m = 1.091 \left(\frac{28.01 \text{ g/mole}}{(0.81 \text{ g/cm}^3)(6.02 \times 10^{23} \text{ molecule/mole})}\right)^{2/3}$$
$$= 16.2 \times 10^{-16} \text{ cm}^2 = 16.2 \text{ Å}^2$$

A_m for liquid nitrogen has been obtained by several methods and is generally accepted as 16.2 Å² or 16.2 × 10^{-16} cm². The specific surface is calculated from equation (16–19) and is exessed in square meters per gram.

Experimentally, the volume of nitrogen that is adsorbed by the powder contained in the evacuated glass bulb of the Quantasorb or similar surface-area apparatus is determined at various pressures and the results are plotted as shown in Figure 16–11. The procedure was developed by Brunauer, Emmett, and Teller[32] and is commonly known as the *BET method*. It is discussed in some detail by Hiemenz and by Allen[33]. Swintosky et al.[34] used the procedure to determine the surface area of pharmaceutical powders. They found the specific surface of zinc oxide to be about 3.5 m²/g; the value for barium sulfate was about 2.4 m²/g.

Example 16–7. Using the Quantasorb apparatus, a plot of $p/V(p_o - p)$ versus p/p_o was obtained as shown in Figure 16–11 for a new antibiotic powder. Calculate S_w, the specific surface of the powder in

m²/g. The data may be read from the graph to obtain the following values:

| $p/V (p_o - p)$ | 0.05 | 0.150 | 0.20 |
| p/p_o | 0.07 | 0.220 | 0.290 |

Following the BET equation (equation [16–18]) and using linear regression, the intercept, $1/(V_m b)$, is $I = 0.00198$ and the slope, $(b - 1)/(V_m b)$, is $S = 0.67942$. by rearranging equation (16–18), V_m is obtained:

$$V_m = \frac{1}{I + S} = \frac{1}{0.00198 + 0.67942}$$
$$= 1.46757 \text{ cm}^3/\text{g}$$

The specific surface S_w is obtained using equation 16–19:

$$S_w = 4.35 \text{ m}^2/\text{cm}^3 \times V_m \text{ cm}^3/\text{g} = 6.38 \text{ m}^2\text{g}^{-1}$$

Assuming that the particles are spherical, the mean volume–surface diameter can be calculated by use of equation (16–17):

$$d_{vs} = \frac{6}{\rho S_w}$$

in which ρ is the density of the adsorbent and S_w is the specific surface in square centimeters per gram of adsorbent. Employing this method, Swintosky et al. found the mean volume–surface diameter of zinc oxide particles to be 0.3 µm.

Air Permeability Method. The principle resistance to the flow of a fluid, such as air, through a plug of compacted powder is the surface area of the powder. The greater the surface area per gram of powder, S_w, the greater the resistance to flow. Hence permeability, for a given pressure drop across the plug, is inversely proportional to specific surface; measurement of the former provides a means of estimating this parameter. From equation (16–16) or (16–17), it is then possible to compute d_{vs}.

A plug of powder may be regarded as a series of capillaries whose diameter is related to the average particle size. The internal surface of the capillaries is a function of the surface area of the particles. According to Poiseuille's equation,

$$V = \frac{\pi d^4 \, \Delta Pt}{128 \, l\eta} \quad (16-21)$$

where V is the volume of air flowing through a capillary of internal diameter d and length l in t seconds under a pressure difference of ΔP. The viscosity of the fluid (air) is η poise.

In practice, the flow rate through the plug, or bed, is also affected by (1) the degree of compression of the particles and (2) the irregularity of the capillaries. The more compact the plug, the lower the *porosity*, which is the ratio of the total space between the particles to the total volume of the plug. Porosity is discussed in more detail on pages 442–446. The irregularity of the capillaries means that they are longer than the length of the plug and are not circular.

The Kozeny–Carman equation, derived from the Poiseuille equation, is the basis of most air permeability methods. Stated in one form it is

$$V = \frac{A}{\eta S_w^2} \cdot \frac{\Delta P t}{Kl} \cdot \frac{\epsilon^3}{(1 - \epsilon)^2} \qquad (16\text{-}22)$$

in which A is the cross-sectional area of the plug, K is a constant (usually 5.0 ± 0.5) that takes account of the irregular capillaries, and ϵ is the porosity. The other terms are as defined previously.

A commercially available instrument is the Fisher subsieve sizer. The principle of its operation is illustrated in Figure 16–12. This instrument has been modified by Edmundson[35] to improve its accuracy and precision.

Equation (16–22) apparently takes account of the effect of porosity on S_w or d_{vs}. It is frequently observed, however, that d_{vs} decreases with decreasing porosity. This is especially true of pharmaceutical powders that have diameters of a few micrometers. It is customary, therefore, in these cases to quote the minimum value obtained over a range of porosities as the diameter of the sample. This noncompliance with equation (16–22) probably arises from initial bridging of the particles in the plug to produce a nonhomogeneous powder bed.[5] It is only when the particles are compacted firmly that the bed becomes uniform and d_{vs} reaches a minimum value.

Because of the simple instrumentation and the speed with which determinations can be made, permeability methods are widely used pharmaceutically for specific surface determinations, especially when the aim is to control batch-to-batch variations. When using this technique for more fundamental studies, it would seem prudent to calibrate the instrument.

Bephenium hydroxynaphthoate, official in the British Pharmaceutical Codex, 1973, is standardized by means of an air permeability method. The drug, used as an anthelmintic and administered as a suspension, must possess a surface area of not less than 7000 cm^2/g. As the specific surface of the material is reduced, the activity of the drug also falls.

Seth et al.[36] studied the air permeability method of the U.S. Pharmacopeia XX, which used a Fisher subsieve sizer for determining the specific surface area of griseofulvin (see also U.S.P. XXII, p. 616). The authors suggested improvements in the method, principal among which was the use of a defined porosity, such as 0.50. This specified value is used in the ASTM Standard, C-204-79, 1979, for measuring the fineness of Portland cement.

The volume surface diameter, d_{vs}, and therefore the specific surface, S_w, or surface area per unit weight in grams (equation [16–19]) of a powder may be obtained by use of this instrument (see Fig. 16–12). It is based on measuring the flow rate of air through the powder sample. If the sample weight is made exactly equal to the density of the powder sample, a more elaborate equation[37,38] for the average particle diameter, d_{vs}, is reduced to the simple expression

$$d_{vs} = \frac{c \cdot L}{[(A \cdot L) - 1]^{3/2}} \cdot \sqrt{\frac{F}{P - F}} \qquad (16\text{-}23)$$

where c is an instrument constant, L the sample height in cm, A the cross-sectional area of the sample holder in cm^2, F the pressure drop across a flow-meter resistance built into the instrument, and P the air pressure as it enters the sample. The pressure (in cm of water) is measured with a water manometer rather than the better known mercury manometer. Problem 16–13 illustrates the use of equation (16–23) to obtain d_{vs} and consequently S_w for a sample of griseofulvin.

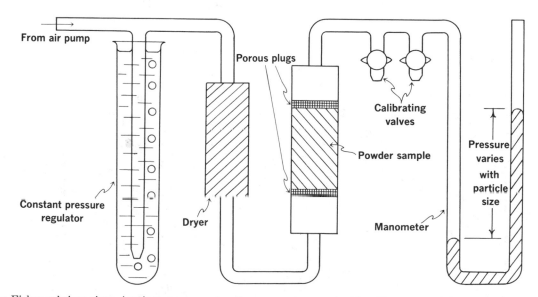

Fig. 16–12. The Fisher subsieve sizer. An air pump generates air pressure to a constant head by means of the pressure regulator. Under this head, the air is dried and conducted to the powder sample packed in the tube. The flow of air through the powder bed is measured by means of a calibrated manometer and is proportional to the surface area or the average particle diameter.

PORE SIZE

Materials of high specific area may have cracks and pores that adsorb gases and vapors, such as water, into their interstices. Relatively insoluble powdered drugs may dissolve more or less rapidly in aqueous medium depending upon their adsorption of moisture or air. Other properties of pharmaceutical importance, such as the dissolution rate of drug from tablets, may also depend on the adsorption characteristics of drug powders. The adsorption isotherms for porous solids display hysteresis, as seen in Figures 16–13 and 16–14, in which the desorption or down-curve branch lies above and to the left of the adsorption or up-curve. In Figure 16–13, the open hysteresis loop is due to a narrow-neck or "ink-bottle" type of pore (see the insert in Fig. 16–13) that traps adsorbate, or to irreversible changes in the pore when adsorption of the gas has occurred so that desorption follows a different pattern than adsorption. The curve of Figure 16–14 with its closed hysteresis loop is more difficult to account for. One will notice in Figures 16–13 and 16–14 that at each relative pressure p/p_o, there are two volumes (at points a and b in Figure 16–14) corresponding to a relative pressure c.

The up-curves of Figures 16–13 and 16–14 correspond to gas adsorption into the capillaries and the down-curve to desorption of the gas. A smaller volume of gas is adsorbed during adsorption (point a of Figure 16–14) than is lost during desorption (point b). Vapor condenses to a liquid in small capillaries at a value less than p_o, the saturation vapor pressure, which may be taken as the vapor pressure at a flat surface. If the radius of the pore is r and the radius of the meniscus is R (Fig. 16–15 point a), p/p_o may be calculated using an expression known as the *Kelvin equation*:

$$NkT \ln p/p_o = -\frac{2M\gamma}{\rho R} \qquad (16\text{–}24)^*$$

in which M is molecular weight of the condensing gas and ρ is its density at a particular temperature, M/ρ is the molar volume of the fluid and γ is its surface tension, N is Avogadro's number, and k is the Boltzmann constant, 1.381×10^{-16} erg deg^{-1} molecule^{-1}. If the condensing vapor is water with a density of 0.998 at 20° C and a surface tension of 72.8 ergs/cm^2, and if the radius of the meniscus in the capillary R is 1.67×10^{-7} cm, p/p_o is calculated to be

$$\ln \frac{p}{p_o} = -\frac{2(18.015 \text{ g/mole})(72.8 \text{ erg/cm}^2)}{(6.022 \times 10^{23} \text{ molecule/mole})}$$
$$\times\ 1/[(1.381 \times 10^{-16} \text{ erg/deg molecule})]$$
$$\times\ 1/[(0.998 \text{ g/cm}^3)(1.67 \times 10^{-7} \text{ cm})(293.15° \text{ K})]$$

---

*Note that the solubility-of-solids equation on page 236 has essentially the same form as equation (16–24), modified as necessary to deal with liquid or solid particles. Note further that R in equation (16–24) is not the gas constant but rather the radius of a meniscus.

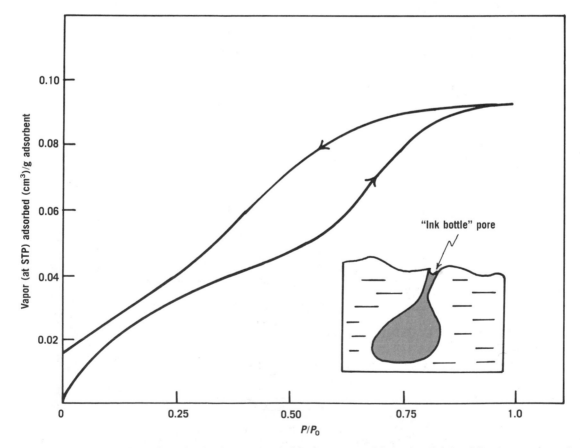

Fig. 16–13. Open hysteresis loop of an adsorption isotherm, presumably due to materials having "ink-bottle" pores, as shown in the insert.

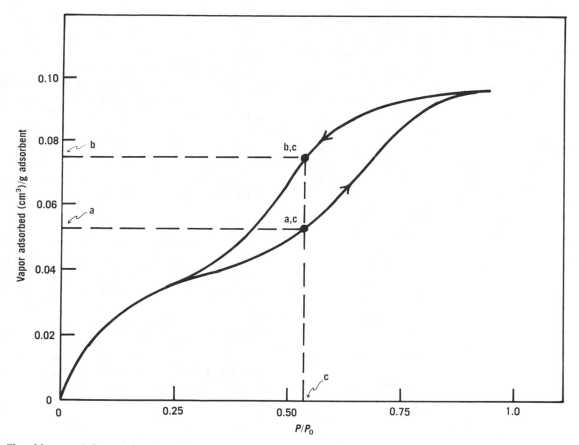

Fig. 16-14. Closed hysteresis loop of the adsorption isotherm of a porous material. At $p/p_o = c$ on the up-curve of the loop, the volume of the pore is given by point a. At relative pressure c on the down-curve the pore, volume is given by point b.

$$\ln \frac{p}{p_o} = -0.6455$$

$$\frac{p}{p_o} = 0.5244$$

During adsorption, the capillary is filling (point a,c in Figure 16–14) and the contact angle θ_a (advancing contact angle) is greater than that during desorption θ_d at which time the capillary is emptying. The radius of the meniscus will be smaller in the receding stage than in the advancing stage, because the capillary is partly filled with fluid from multilayer adsorption. This smaller receding contact angle means a smaller radius of the meniscus, as seen in Figure 16–15b, and p/p_o will decrease, since R is in the denominator of the Kelvin equation, the right-hand side of which is negative.

The Kelvin equation gives a reasonable explanation for the differences of p/p_o on adsorption and desorption and consequently provides for the existence of the

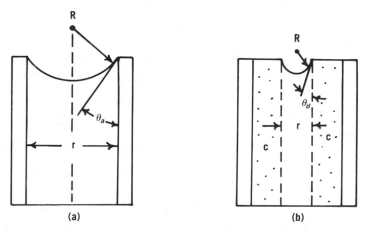

Fig. 16-15. (a) Pore into which vapor is condensing, corresponding to point a,c on the up-curve of Figure 16–14. Key: θ_a, advancing contact angle; r, pore radius; R, radius of meniscus. (b) Pore from which the liquid is vaporizing, corresponding to point b,c on the down-curve of Figure 16–14. Key: θ_d, receding or desorption contact angle; R and r defined as in (a); c, condensed vapor on walls of the capillary.

hysteresis loop. The Kelvin equation, together with the hysteresis loops in adsorption–desorption isotherms (Fig. 16–14), can be used to compute the pore size distribution.[39] During desorption, at a given p/p_o value, water will *condense* only in pores of radius equal to or below the value given by the Kelvin equation. Water will *evaporate* from pores of larger radius. Thus, from the desorption isotherm, the volume of water retained at a given pressure p/p_o corresponds to the volume of pores having radius equal to or below the radius calculated from the Kelvin equation at this p/p_o value.

Example 16–8. Yamanaka et al.[40] obtained the experimental values for a water adsorption–desorption isotherm at 20° C on a clay. These values, which are given in Table 16–6, have been selected from Figure 7 in reference 40.

(a) Compute the radius of pores corresponding to the relative pressures p/p_o given in Table 16–6.

(b) Assuming that all pores are of radius less than 265 Å, compute the cumulative percent of pore volume with radii less than those found in part *(a)*.

(c) Compute the percent of pore volume at 20° C with radii between 40 and 60 Å.

(a) Using the Kelvin equation for $p/p_o = 0.2$,

$$r = -[(2 \gamma V)/(RT \ln p/p_o)] = -\frac{2 \times 72.8 \times 18}{(8.3143 \times 10^7 \times 293)(\ln 0.2)}$$

$$= (+)6.7 \times 10^{-8} \text{ cm} = 6.7 \text{ Å}$$

The results for the several p/p_o values are shown in the fourth column of Table 16–6.

(b and c) The total cumulative pore volume is 0.224 mL/g corresponding to the intersection of the adsorption and desorption curves (row 7 in Table 16–6). It corresponds to 100% cumulative pore volume. Therefore, for, say, pores of radius <48.4 Å (see Table 16–6, column 4, row 6), the cumulative percent of pore volume is

$$\% = \frac{0.200}{0.224} \times 100 = 89.3\%$$

where the value 0.200 mL/g is taken from the desorption isotherm (see Table 16–6, column 3, row 6). The results are given in column 5 of Table 16–6.

Christian and Tucker[41] have done a careful and extensive study of pore models and concluded that a model that included a combination of cylindric and slit-shaped pores provided the best quantitative fit of the data obtained on both the adsorption and desorption branches of the pore distribution plots. A modification of the BET equation, assuming multilayer adsorption at the capillary walls, has also been found to provide a satisfactory model for the hysteresis that occurs with porous solids.[42]

The adsorption of water vapor, flavoring agents, perfumes, and other volatile substances into films, containers, and other polymeric materials used in pharmacy are important in product formulation and in the storage and use of drug products. Sadek and Olsen[43] showed that the adsorption isotherms for water vapor on methylcellulose, povidone (PVP), gelatin, and polymethylmethacrylate all exhibited hysteresis loops. Hydration of gelatin films was observed to be lowered by treatment with formaldehyde, which causes increased cross-linking in gelatin and a decrease in pore size. Povidone showed increased water adsorption by treatment with acetone, which enlarged pore size and increased the number of sites for water sorption. In a study of the action of tablet disintegrants, Lowenthal and Burress[44] measured the mean pore diameter of tablets in air permeability apparatus. A linear correlation was observed between log mean pore diameter and tablet porosity, allowing a calculation of mean pore diameter from the more easily obtained tablet porosity. Gregg and Sing[45] discussed pore size and pore size distribution in some detail.

DERIVED PROPERTIES OF POWDERS

The preceding sections of this chapter have been concerned mainly with size distribution and surface areas of powders. These are the two *fundamental* properties of any collection of particles. There are, in addition, numerous *derived* properties that are based upon these fundamental properties. Those of particular relevance to pharmacy are discussed in the remainder of this chapter. Very important properties, those of particle dissolution and dissolution rate, are subjects of separate chapters (Chapters 10 and 13).

Porosity. Suppose a powder, such as zinc oxide, is placed in a graduated cylinder and the total volume is noted. The volume occupied is known as the *bulk volume* V_b. If the powder is nonporous, that is, has no

TABLE 16–6. *Water Adsorption and Desorption on a Clay as a Function of Relative Pressure p/p_o*

Column No.	1	2	3	4	5
Row No.	p/p_o	V_1 (Adsorption) (mL/g)	V_2 (Desorption) (mL/g)	Radius (Å)	Cumulative Pore Volume (%)
1	0.20	0.079	0.123	<6.7	54.9
2	0.31	0.109	0.147	<9.2	65.6
3	0.40	0.135	0.165	<11.7	73.7
4	0.49	0.141	0.182	<15.1	81.3
5	0.66	0.152	0.191	<30	85.3
6	0.80	0.170	0.200	<48.4	89.3
7	0.96	0.224	0.224	<265	100

internal pores or capillary spaces, the bulk volume of the powder consists of the true volume of the solid particles plus the volume of the spaces between the particles. The volume of the spaces, known as the *void volume, v*, is given by the equation,

$$v = V_b - V_p \qquad (16\text{--}25)$$

in which V_p is the *true volume* of the particles. The method for determining the volume of the particles will be given later.

The *porosity* or *voids* ϵ of the powder is defined as the ratio of the void volume to the bulk volume of the packing:

$$\epsilon = \frac{V_b - V_p}{V_b} = 1 - \frac{V_p}{V_b} \qquad (16\text{--}26)$$

Porosity is frequently expressed in percent, $\epsilon \times 100$.

Example 16–9. A sample of calcium oxide powder with a true density of 3.203 and weighing 131.3 g was found to have a bulk volume of 82.0 cm³ when placed in a 100-mL graduated cylinder. Calculate the porosity.

The volume of the particles is

$$131.3 \text{ g}/(3.203 \text{ g/cm}^3) = 41.0 \text{ cm}^3$$

From equation (16–25), the volume of void space is

$$v = 82.0 \text{ cm}^3 - 41.0 \text{ cm}^3 = 41.0 \text{ cm}^3$$

and the porosity from equation (16–26) is

$$\epsilon = \frac{82 - 41}{82} = 0.5 \text{ or } 50\%$$

Packing Arrangements. Powder beds of uniform sized spheres can assume either one of two ideal packing arrangements: (1) *closest* or *rhombohedral*, and (2) *most open, loosest,* or *cubic packing*. The theoretic porosity of a powder consisting of uniform spheres in closest packing is 26% and for loosest packing is 48%. The arrangements of spherical particles in closest and loosest packing are shown in Figure 16–16.

The particles in real powders are neither spherical in shape nor uniform in size. It is to be expected that the particles of ordinary powders may have any arrangement intermediate between the two ideal packings of Figure 16–16, and most powders in practice have porosities between 30 and 50%. If the particles are of greatly different sizes, however, the smaller may sift between the larger to give porosities below the theoretic minimum of 26%. In powders containing flocculates or aggregates, which lead to the formation of

bridges and arches in the packing, the porosity may be above the theoretic maximum of 48%. In real powder systems, then, almost any degree of porosity is possible. Crystalline materials compressed under a force of 100,000 lb/in.² can have porosities of less than 1%.

Densities of Particles. Since particles may be hard and smooth in one case and rough and spongy in another, one must express densities with great care. Density is universally defined as weight per unit volume; the difficulty arises when one attempts to determine the volume of particles containing microscopic cracks, internal pores, and capillary spaces.

For convenience, three types of densities may be defined.[45,46] (1) *true density* of the material itself, exclusive of the voids and intraparticle pores larger than molecular or atomic dimensions in the crystal lattices, (2) *granule density* as determined by the displacement of mercury, which does not penetrate at ordinary pressures into pores smaller than about 10 μm, and (3) *bulk density* as determined from the bulk volume and the weight of a dry powder in a graduated cylinder.*

When a solid is nonporous, true and granule density are identical, and both can be obtained by the displacement of helium or a liquid such as mercury, benzene, or water. When the material is porous, having an internal surface, the true density is best approximated by the displacement of helium, which penetrates into the smallest pores and is not adsorbed by the material. The density obtained by liquid displacement is considered as approximately equal to true density but may differ from it somewhat when the liquid does not penetrate well into the pores.

The methods for determining the various densities are now discussed.

True density, ρ, is the density of the actual solid material. Methods for determining the density of nonporous solids by displacement in liquids in which they are insoluble are found in general pharmacy books. If the material is porous, as is the case with most powders, the true density may be determined by use of a helium densitometer, as suggested by Franklin.[47] The volume of the empty apparatus (dead space) is first determined by introducing a known quantity of helium. A weighed amount of powder is then introduced into the sample tube, adsorbed gases are removed from the powder by an out-gassing procedure, and helium, which is not adsorbed by the material, is again introduced. The pressure is read on a mercury manometer, and by application of the gas laws, the volume of helium surrounding the particles and penetrating into the small cracks and pores is calculated. The difference between the volume of helium filling the empty apparatus and

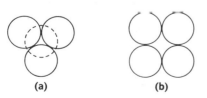

(a)   (b)

Fig. 16–16. Schematic representation of particles arranged in (*a*) closest packing and (*b*) loosest packing. The dotted circle in (*a*) shows the position taken by a particle in a plane above that of the other three particles.

---

*The term *apparent density* has been used by various authors to mean granular or bulk density, and some have used it to mean true density obtained by liquid displacement. Because of this confusion, the use of the term *apparent density* should be discouraged.

the volume of helium in the presence of the powder sample yields the volume occupied by the powder. Knowing the weight of the powder, one is then able to calculate the true density. The procedure is equivalent to the first step in the BET method for determining the specific surface area of particles.

The density of solids usually listed in handbooks is often determined by liquid displacement. It is the weight of the body divided by the weight of the liquid it displaces, in other words, the loss of weight of the body when suspended in a suitable liquid. For solids that are insoluble in the liquid and heavier than it, an ordinary pycnometer may be used for the measurement. For example, if the weight of a sample of glass beads is 5.0 grams and the weight of water required to fill a pycnometer is 50.0 grams, then the total weight would be 55.0 grams. When the beads are immersed in the water and the weight is determined at 25° C, the value is 53.0 grams or a displacement of 2.0 cm³ of water, and the density is 5.0 g/2.00 cm³ = 2.5 g/cm³. The true density determined in this manner may differ slightly depending on the ability of the liquid to enter the pores of the particles, the possible change in the density of the liquid at the interface, and other complex factors.

Since helium penetrates into the smallest pores and crevices (Fig. 16–17), it is generally conceded that the helium method gives the closest approximation to true density. Liquids such as water and alcohol are denied entrance into the smallest spaces, and liquid displacement accordingly gives a density somewhat smaller than the true value. True densities are found in Table 16–7 for some powders of pharmaceutical interest.

Granule density, ρ_g, may be determined by a method similar to the liquid displacement method. Mercury is used since it fills the void spaces but fails to penetrate into the internal pores of the particles. The volume of

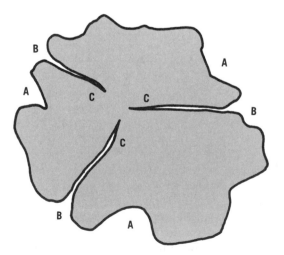

Fig. 16–17. Pores and crevices of a pharmaceutical granule. Water or mercury surrounds such a particle and rests only in the surface irregularities such as regions *A* and *B*. Helium molecules may enter deep into the cracks at points *C*, allowing calculation of true rather than granule density.

the particles together with their *intraparticle spaces* then gives the granule volume, and from a knowledge of the powder weight, the granule density is obtained. Strickland et al.[48] determined the granule density of tablet granulations by the mercury displacement method using a specially designed pycnometer. A measure of true density was obtained by highly compressing the powders. The samples were compressed to 100,000 lb/sq inch, and the resulting tablets were weighed. The volumes of the tablets were computed after measuring the tablet dimensions with calipers. The weight of the tablet divided by the volume then gave the "true" or high-compression density.

The *intraparticle porosity* of the granules may be computed from a knowledge of the true and granule density. The porosity is given by the equation

$$\epsilon_{\text{intraparticle}} = \frac{V_g - V_p}{V_g} = 1 - \frac{V_p}{V_g}$$
$$= 1 - \frac{\text{weight/true density}}{\text{weight/granule density}}$$

(16–27)

or

$$\epsilon_{\text{intraparticle}} = 1 - \frac{\text{granule density}}{\text{true density}} = 1 - \frac{\rho_g}{\rho}$$ (16–28)

in which V_p is the true volume of the solid particles and V_g is the volume of the particles together with the intraparticle pores.

Example 16–10. The granule density ρ_g of sodium bicarbonate is 1.450 and the true density ρ is 2.033. Compute the intraparticle porosity.

$$\epsilon_{\text{intraparticle}} = 1 - \frac{1.450}{2.033} = 0.286, \text{ or } 28.6\%$$

The granule densities and internal porosity or percent pore spaces in the granules, as obtained by Strickland et al.,[48] are shown in Table 16–8. The difference in porosity depends on the method of granulation, as brought out in the table.

Bulk density, ρ_b, is defined as the mass of a powder divided by the bulk volume. A standard procedure for obtaining bulk density or its reciprocal, *bulk specific volume*, has been established.[49] A sample of about 50 cm³ of powder, which has previously been passed through a U.S. Standard No. 20 sieve, is carefully introduced into a 100-mL graduated cylinder. The cylinder is dropped at 2-second intervals onto a hard wood surface three times from a height of 1 inch. The bulk density is then obtained by dividing the weight of the sample in grams by the final volume in cm³ of the sample contained in the cylinder. The bulk density does not actually reach a maximum until the container has been dropped or tapped some 500 times; however, the three-tap method has been found to give the most consistent results among various laboratories. The bulk density of some pharmaceutical powders is compared

TABLE 16–7. *True Density in g/cm³ of Solids Commonly Used in Pharmacy*

Aluminum oxide	4.0	Mercuric chloride	5.44
Benzoic acid	1.3	Mercuric iodide	6.3
Bismuth subcarbonate	6.86	Mercuric oxide	11.1
Bismuth subnitrate	4.9	Mercurous chloride	7.15
Bromoform	2.9	Paraffin	0.90
Calcium carbonate (calcite)	2.72	Potassium bromide	2.75
Calcium oxide	3.3	Potassium carbonate	2.29
Chalk	1.8–2.6	Potassium chloride	1.98
Charcoal (air free)	2.1–2.3	Potassium iodide	3.13
Clay	1.8–2.6	Sand, fine dry	1.5
Cork	0.24	Silver iodide	5.67
Cotton	1.47	Silver nitrate	4.35
Gamboge	1.19	Sodium borate, borax	1.73
Gelatin	1.27	Sodium bromide	3.2
Glass beads	2.5	Sodium chloride	2.16
Graphite	2.3–2.7	Sucrose	1.6
Kaolin	2.2–2.5	Sulfadiazine	1.50
Magnesium carbonate	3.04	Sulfur, precipitated	2.0
Magnesium oxide	3.65	Talc	2.6–2.8
Magnesium sulfate	1.68	Zinc oxide (hexagonal)	5.59

with true and apparent densities in Table 16–9. The term "light" as applied to pharmaceutical powders means low bulk density or large bulk volume, whereas "heavy" signifies a powder of high bulk density or small volume. It should be noted that these terms have no relationship to granular or true densities.

The bulk density of a powder depends primarily on particle size distribution, particle shape, and the tendency of the particles to adhere to one another. The particles may pack in such a way as to leave large gaps between their surfaces, resulting in a light powder or powder of low bulk density. On the other hand, the smaller particles may sift between the larger ones to form a heavy powder or one of high bulk density.

The *interspace* or *void porosity* of a powder of porous granules is the relative volume of interspace voids to the bulk volume of the powder, exclusive of the intraparticle pores. The interspace porosity is computed from a knowledge of the bulk density and the granule density and is expressed by the equation

$$\epsilon_{interspace} = \frac{V_b - V_g}{V_b} = 1 - \frac{V_g}{V_b}$$
$$= 1 - \frac{weight/granule\ density}{weight/bulk\ density} \quad (16-29)$$

$$\epsilon_{interspace} = 1 - \frac{bulk\ density}{granule\ density}$$
$$= 1 - \frac{\rho_b}{\rho_g} \quad (16-30)$$

in which $V_b = w/\rho_b$ is the bulk volume and $V_g = w/\rho_g$ is the granule volume, that is, the volume of the particles plus pores.

The *total porosity* of a porous powder is made up of voids between the particles as well as pores within the particles. The total porosity is defined as

$$\epsilon_{total} = \frac{V_b - V_p}{V_b} = 1 - \frac{V_p}{V_b} \quad (16-31)$$

in which V_b is the bulk volume and V_p is the volume of the solid material itself. This equation is identical with that for nonporous powders (cf. equation [16–26]). As in the previous cases, V_p and V_p may be expressed in terms of powder weights and densities:

$$V_p = \frac{w}{\rho}$$

TABLE 16–8. *Densities and Porosities of Tablet Granulations**

Granulation	"True" or High-Compression Density (g/cm³)	Granule Density by Mercury Displacement (g/cm³)	Percent Pore Space in Granules (Porosity)
Sulfathiazole[†]	1.530	1.090	29
Sodium bicarbonate[†]	2.033	1.450	29
Phenobarbital[†]	1.297	0.920	29
Aspirin[‡]	1.370	1.330	2.9

*From W. A. Strickland Jr., L. W. Busse and T. Higuchi, J. Am. Pharm. Assoc., Sci. Ed. **45**, 482, 1956, reproduced by permission of the copyright owner.
[†]Granulation prepared by wet method using starch paste.
[‡]Granulation prepared by dry method (slugging process).

TABLE 16-9. *Comparison of Bulk Densities with True Densities*

	Bulk Density (g/cm³)	True Density (g/cm³)
Bismuth subcarbonate heavy	1.01	6.9*
Bismuth subcarbonate light	0.22	6.9*
Magnesium carbonate heavy	0.39	3.0*
Magnesium carbonate light	0.07	3.0*
Phenobarbital	0.34	1.3†
Sulfathiazole	0.33	1.5†
Talc	0.48	2.7*

*Density obtained by liquid displacement.
†True density obtained by helium displacement.

and

$$V_b = \frac{w}{\rho_b}$$

in which w is the mass ("weight") of the powder, ρ is the true density, and ρ_b is the bulk density. Substituting these relationships into equation (16–31) gives

$$\text{Total porosity, } \epsilon_{total} = 1 - \frac{w/\rho}{w/\rho_b} \qquad (16\text{–}32)$$

or

$$\epsilon_{total} = 1 - \frac{\rho_b}{\rho} \qquad (16\text{–}33)$$

Example 16-11. The weight of a sodium iodide tablet was 0.3439 g and the bulk volume was measured by use of calipers and found to be 0.0963 cm³. The true density of NaI is 3.667 g/cm³. What is the bulk density and the total porosity of the tablet?

$$\text{bulk density } \rho_b = \frac{0.3439}{0.0963} = 3.571 \text{ g/cm}^3$$

$$\epsilon_{total} = 1 - \frac{3.571}{3.667}$$

$$= 0.026 \text{ or } 2.6\%$$

In addition to supplying valuable information about tablet porosity and its evident relationship to tablet hardness and disintegration time, bulk density may be used to check the uniformity of bulk chemicals and to determine the proper size of containers, mixing apparatus, and capsules for a given mass of the powder. These topics are considered in subsequent sections of this chapter.

In summary, the differences between the three densities (true, granule, and bulk) can be understood better by reference to their reciprocals: specific true volume, specific granule volume, and specific bulk volume.

The specific true volume of a powder is the volume of the solid material itself per unit mass of powder. When the liquid used to measure it does not penetrate completely into the pores, the specific volume is made up of the volume per unit weight of the solid material itself and the small part of the pore volume within the granules that is not penetrated by the liquid. When the proper liquid is chosen, however, the discrepancy should not be serious. Specific granule volume is the volume of the solid and essentially all of the pore volume within the particles. Finally, specific bulk volume constitutes the volume per unit weight of the solid, the volume of the *intra*particle pores, and the void volume or volume of *inter*particle spaces.

Example 16-12. The following data apply to a 1-g sample of a granular powder:

$$\text{volume of the solid alone} = 0.3 \text{ cm}^3/\text{g}$$

$$\text{volume of intraparticle pores} = 0.1 \text{ cm}^3/\text{g}$$

$$\text{volume of spaces between particles} = 1.6 \text{ cm}^3/\text{g}$$

(*a*) What is the specific true volume V, the specific granule volume V_g, and the specific bulk volume V_b?

$$V = 0.3 \text{ cm}^3$$

$$V_g = V + \text{intraparticle pores}$$

$$= 0.3 + 0.1 = 0.4 \text{ cm}^3/\text{g}$$

$$V_b = V + \text{intraparticle pores}$$

$$+ \text{ spaces between particles}$$

$$= 0.3 + 0.1 + 1.6$$

$$= 2.0 \text{ cm}^3/\text{g}$$

(*b*) Compute the total porosity ϵ_{total}, interspace porosity $\epsilon_{interspace}$ or void spaces between the particles, and the intraparticle porosity $\epsilon_{intraparticle}$ or pore spaces within the particles.

$$\epsilon_{total} = \frac{V_b - V_p}{V_b} = \frac{2.0 - 0.3}{2.0}$$

$$= 0.85 \text{ or } 85\%$$

$$\epsilon_{interspace} = \frac{V_b - V_g}{V_b} = \frac{2.0 - 0.4}{2.0}$$

$$= 0.80 \text{ or } 80\%$$

$$\epsilon_{intraparticle} = \frac{V_g - V_p}{V_g} = \frac{0.4 - 0.3}{0.4}$$

$$= 0.25 \text{ or } 25\%$$

Thus the solid, itself, constitutes 15% of the total bulk, and 85% is made up of void space; 80% of the bulk is contributed by the voids between the particles and 5% of the total bulk by the pores and crevices within the particles. These pores, however, contribute 25% to the volume of granules, that is, particles plus pores.

Bulkiness. Specific bulk volume, the reciprocal of bulk density, is often called *bulkiness* or *bulk*. It is an important consideration in the packaging of powders. The bulk density of calcium carbonate may vary from 0.1 to 1.3, and the lightest or bulkiest type would require a container about 13 times larger than that needed for the heaviest variety. Bulkiness increases with a decrease in particle size. In a mixture of materials of different sizes, however, the smaller particles sift between the larger ones and tend to reduce the bulkiness.

Flow Properties. A bulk powder is somewhat analogous to a non-Newtonian liquid (p. 455), which exhibits plastic flow and sometimes dilatancy, the particles being influenced by attractive forces to varying degrees. Accordingly, powders may be *free-flowing* or *cohesive* ("sticky"). Neumann[50] has discussed the factors that affect the flow properties of powders. Of special signifiance are particle size, shape, porosity and density, and surface texture. Those properties of solids that determine the magnitude of particle–particle interactions have been reviewed by Hiestand.[51]

With relatively small particles (less than 10 μm), particle flow through an orifice is restricted because the cohesive forces between particles are of the same magnitude as gravitational forces. Since these latter forces are a function of the diameter raised to the third power, they become more significant as the particle size increases and flow is facilitated. A maximum flow rate is reached, after which the flow decreases as the size of the particles approach that of the orifice.[52] If a powder contains a reasonable amount of small particles, the powder's flow properties may be improved be removing the "fines" or adsorbing them onto the larger particles. Occasionally, poor flow may result from the presence of moisture, in which case drying the particles will reduce the cohesiveness. *Cohesive Pharmaceutical Powders* is the title of a review by Pilpel[53] dealing with the various apparatus for the measurement of the properties of cohesive powders and the effects of cohesive powders of particle size, moisture, glidants, caking, and temperature.

Dahlinder et al.[54] reviewed the methods for evaluating flow properties of powders and granules, including the *Hauser ratio* or packed bulk density versus loose bulk density, the rate of tamping, the flow rate and free flow through an orifice, and a "drained" angle of respose. The Hauser ratio, the free flow, and the angle of repose correlated well with one another and were applicable even for fairly cohesive tablet granulations.

Elongated or flat particles tend to pack, albeit loosely, to give powders with a high porosity. Particles with a high density and a low internal porosity tend to possess free-flowing properties. This can be offset by surface roughness, which leads to poor flow characteristics due to friction and cohesiveness.

Free-flowing powders are characterized by "dustibility," a term meant to signify the opposite of stickiness. Lycopodium shows the greatest degree of dustibility; if it is arbitrarily assigned a dustibility of 100%, talcum powder has value of 57%, potato starch 27%, fine charcoal 23%. Finely powdered calomel has a relative dustibility of 0.7%.[50] These values should have some relation to the uniform spreading of dusting powders when applied to the skin, and stickiness, a measure of the cohesiveness of the particles of a compacted powder, should be of some importance in the flow of powders through filling machines and in the operation of automatic capsule machines.

Poorly flowing powders or granulations present many difficulties to the pharmaceutical industry. The production of uniform tablet dosage units has been shown to depend on several granular properties. Arambulo and coworkers[55] observed that as the granule size was reduced, the variation in tablet weight fell. The minimum weight variation was attained with granules having a diameter of 400 to 800 μm. As the granule size was reduced further, the granules flowed less freely and the tablet weight variation increased. The particle size distribution affects the internal flow and segregation of a granulation.

Raff et al.[56] have studied the flow of tablet granulations. They found that internal flow and granule demixing (i.e., the tendency of the powder to separate into layers of different sizes) during flow through the hopper contribute to a decrease in tablet weight during the latter portion of the compression period. Hammerness and Thompson[57] observed that the flow rate of a tablet granulation increased with an increase in the quantity of fines added. An increase in the amount of lubricant also raised the flow rate, and the combination of lubricant and fines appeared to have a synergistic action.

The frictional forces in a loose powder can be measured by the *angle of repose*, ϕ. This is the maximum angle possible between the surface of a pile of powder and the horizontal plane. If more material is added to the pile, it slides down the sides until the mutual friction of the particles, producing a surface at an angle ϕ, is in equilibrium with the gravitational force. The tangent of the angle of repose is equal to the coefficient of friction μ between the particles:

$$\tan \phi = \mu \qquad (16\text{--}34)$$

Hence, the rougher and more irregular the surface of the particles, the higher will be the angle of repose. This situation has been observed by Fonner et al.,[58] who, studying granules prepared by five different methods, found the repose angle to be primarily a function of surface roughness. Ridgeway and Rupp[59] have studied the effect of particle shape on powder properties. Using closely sized batches of sand separated into different shapes, they showed that, with increasing departure from the spherical, the angle of repose increased while bulk density and flowability decreased.

To improve flow characteristics, materials termed *glidants* are frequently added to granular powders. Examples of commonly used glidants are magnesium stearate, starch, and talc. Using a recording powder flow meter, which measured the weight of powder flowing per unit time through a hopper orifice, Gold et al.[60] found the optimum glidant concentration to be 1% or less. Above these level, a decrease in flow rate was usually observed. No correlation was found between flow rate and repose angle. By means of a shear cell and a tensile tester, York[61] was able to determine an optimum glidant concentration for lactose and calcium hydrogen phosphate powders. In agreement with Gold et al., the angle of repose was found to be unsuitable for assessing the flowability of the powders used.

Nelson[62] studied the repose angle of a sulfathiazole granulation as a function of average particle size, presence of lubricants, and admixture of fines. He found that, in general, the angle increased with decreasing particle size. The addition of talc in low concentration decreased the repose angle, but in high concentration it increased the angle. The addition of fines—particles smaller than 100 mesh—to coarse granules resulted in a marked increase of the repose angle.

The ability of a powder to flow is one of the factors involving in mixing different materials to form a powder blend. Mixing, and the prevention of unmixing, is an important pharmaceutical operation involved in the preparation of many dosage forms, including tablets and capsules.[63] Other factors affecting the mixing process are particle aggregation, size, shape, density differences, and the presence of static charge. The theory of mixing has been described by Train[64] and Fischer.[65]

Compaction: Compressed Tablets. Neumann[66] found that when powders were compacted under a pressure of about 5 kg/cm^2, the porosities of the powders composed of rigid particles (sodium carbonate, for example) were higher than the porosities of powders in closest packing, as determined by tapping experiments. Hence, these powders were *dilatant*, that is, they showed an unexpected expansion, rather than contraction, under the influence of stress. In the case of soft and spongy particles (e.g., kaolin), however, the particles deformed on compression, and the porosities were lower than after tapping the powder down to its condition of closest packing. Similar experiments might be conducted to determine the optimum condition for packing powders into capsules on the manufacturing scale.

The behavior of powders under compression is significant in pharmaceutical tableting. While basic information can be obtained from the literature on powder metallurgy and the compression of metallic powders, Train,[67] who has performed some of the fundamental work in this area, has pointed out that not all the theories developed for the behavior of metals will necessarily hold when applied to nonmetals.

Much of the early work was carried out by Higuchi and associates,[68] who studied the influence of compression force on the specific surface area, granule density, porosity, tablet hardness, and disintegration time of pharmaceutical tablets. As illustrated in Figure 16–18, the specific surface of a sulfathiazole tablet granulation, determined by the BET method, increased to a maximum and then decreased. The initial increase in surface area can be attributed to the formation of new surfaces as the primary crystalline material is fragmented, while the decrease in specific surface beyond a compression force of 2500 pounds is presumably due to cold bonding between the unit particles. It was also observed that

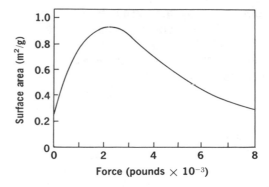

Fig. 16–18. The influence of compressional force on the specific surface of a sulfathiazole granulation. (After T. Higuchi et al.[68]).

porosity decreased and density increased as a linear function of the logarithm of the compression force, except at the higher force levels. As the compression is increased, so the tablet hardness and fracture resistance also rise. Typical results obtained using an instrumented rotary tablet machine[69] are shown in Figure 16–19.

The strength of a compressed tablet depends on a number of factors, the most important of which are compression force and particle size. The literature dealing with the effect of particle size has been outlined by Hersey et al,[70] who, as a result of their studies, concluded that, over the range 4 to 925 μm, there is no simple relationship between strength and particle size. These workers did find that for simple crystals, the strength of the tablet increasing with decreasing particle size in the range of 600 to 100 μm.

The work initiated by Higuchi and co-workers[68] involved the investigation of other tablet ingredients, the development of an instrumented tablet machine, and the evaluation of tablet lubricants. The reader who desires to follow this interesting work should consult the original reports, as well as other studies[71-75] in this area. Tableting research and technology were comprehensively reviewed in 1972 by Cooper and Rees.[76] Deformation processes during decompression may be

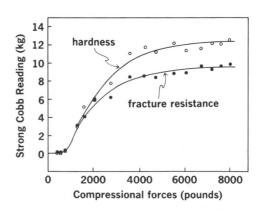

Fig. 16–19. Effect of compressional force on tablet hardness and fracture strength. (After E. L. Knoechel, C. C. Sperry and C. J. Lintner, J. Pharm. Sci. **56,** 116, 1967.)

the principal factors responsible for the success or failure of compact formation.[77]

References and Notes

1. J. M. DallaValle, *Micromeritics*, 2nd Edition, Pitman, New York, 1948, p. xiv.
2. K. A. Lees, j. Pharm. Pharmacol. **15**, 43T, 1963.
3. Seradyn, Particle Technology Division, 1200 Madison Ave., Box 1210, Indianapolis, In., 46206.
4. Duke Scientific, 1135D San Antonio Road, Palo Alto, Calif., 94303.
5. I. C. Edmundson, *Advances in Pharmaceutical Sciences*, Vol. 2, Edited by H. S. Bean, J. E. Carless and A. H. Beckett, Academic Press, New York, 1967, p. 95.
6. E. L. Parrott, J. Pharm. Sci. **63**, 813, 1974.
7. A. Sano, T. Kuriki, T. Handa, H. Takeuchi and Y. Kawashima, J. Pharm. Sci. **76**, 471, 1987.
8. T. Hatch, J. Franklin Inst. **215**, 27, 1933; T. Hatch and S. P. Choate, ibid. **207**, 369, 1929.
9. H. L. Rao, private communication. Manipal, India, May, 1986.
10. T. Allen, *Particle Size Measurement*, 2nd Edition, Chapman & Hall, London, 1974.
11. M. J. Groves, Pharm. Tech. 4(5), 781, 1980.
12. G. Martin, British Ceramic Soc. Trans. **23**, 61, 1926; **25**, 51, 1928; **27**, 285, 1930.
13. T. Allen, *Particle Size Measurement*, 2nd Edition, Chapman & Hall, London, 1974, p. 131.
14. K.P.P. Prasad and L.S.C. Wan, Pharm. Res. **4**, 504, 1987.
15. A. S. Arambulo and D. L. Deardorff, J. Am. Pharm. Assoc., Sci. Ed. **42**, 690, 1953.
16. L. D. King and C. H. Becker, Drug Standards **21**, 1, 1953.
17. G. Herdan, *Small Particle Statistics*, Elsevier, New York, 1953, p. 72.
18. D. E. Fonner, Jr., G. S. Banker and J. Swarbrick, J. Pharm. Sci. **55**, 576, 1966.
19. H. J. Heywood, J. Pharm. Pharmacol. **15**, 56T, 1963.
20. W. I. Higuchi et al., J. Pharm. Sci., **51**, 1081, 1962; ibid. **52**, 162, 1963; ibid. **53**, 405, 1964; ibid. **54**, 74, 1205, 1303, 1965.
21. S. Bisaillon and R. Tawashi, J. Pharm. Sci. **65**, 222, 1976.
22. E. R. Garrett, G. H. Miller and M. R. W. Brown, J. Pharm. Sci. **55**, 593, 1966; G. H. Miller, S. Khalil and A. Martin, J. Pharm. Sci. **60**, 33, 1971.
23. L. J. Beaubien and A. J. Vanderwielen, J. Pharm. Sci. **69**, 651, 1980.
24. S. I. Ismail and R. Tawashi, J. Pharm. Sci. **69**, 829, 1980.
25. M. J. Groves and J. Wong, Drug Dev. Ind. Pharm. **13**, 193, 1987; M. J. Groves and D. Wana, Powder Technol. **18**, 215, 1977.
26. T. M. Cham, H. M. Yu and L. C. Tung, Drug Dev. Ind. Pharm. **15**, 2441, 1989.
27. E. C. Signoretti, A. Dell'Utri, L. Paoletti, D. Bastisti and L. Montanari, Drug Dev. Ind. Pharm. **14**, 1, 1988.
28. S. P. Li, K. M. Feld and C. R. Kowarski, Drug Dev. Ind. Pharm. **15**, 1137, 1989.
29. M. C. Davies, I. R. Wilding, R. D. Short, M. A. Khan, J. F. Watts and C. D. Melia, Int. J. Pharm. **57**, 183, 1989.
30. F. Carli and A. Motta, J. Pharm. Sci. **73**, 197, 1984.
31. P. H. Emmett and S. Brunauer, J. Am. Chem. Soc. **59**, 1553, 1937; S. J. Gregg and K. S. W. Sing, *Adsorption, Surface Area and Porosity*, 2nd Edition, Academic Press, New York, 1982, p. 62.
32. S. Brunauer, P. H. Emmett and F. Teller, J. Am. Chem. Soc. **60**, 309, 1938.
33. P. C. Hiemenz, *Principles of Colloid and Surface Chemistry*, Dekker, New York, 2nd Edition, 1986, pp. 513–529; T. Allen, *Particle Size Measurement*, Chapman & Hall, London, 1975, pp. 358–366.
34. J. V. Swintosky, S. Riegelman, T. Higuchi and L. W. Busse, J. Am. Pharm. Assoc., Sci. Ed. **38**, 210, 308, 378, 1949.
35. I. C. Edmundson, Analyst, Lond. **91**, 1082, 1966.
36. P. Seth, N. Møller, J. C. Tritsch and A. Stamm, J. Pharm. Sci. **72**, 971, 1983.
37. P. C. Carman, J. Soc. Chem. Ind., London **57**, 225, 1938; F. M. Lea and R. W. Nurse, ibid. **58**, 277, 1939.
38. E. L. Gooden and C. M. Smith, Ind. Eng. Chem., Analyt. Edn. **12**, 479, 1940.
39. J. T. Carstensen, *Solid Pharmaceutics: Mechanical Properties and Rate Phenomena*, Academic Press, New York, 1980, pp. 130–131.
40. S. Yamanaka, P. B. Malla and S. Komarheni, J. Colloid. Interface Sci. **134**, 51, 1990.
41. S. D. Christian and E. E. Tucker, Am. Lab. **13**, 42, 1981; ibid. **13**, 47, 1981.
42. P. C. Hiemenz, *Principles of Colloid and Surface Chemistry*, 2nd Edition, Dekker, New York, 1986, pp. 534–539; A. W. Adamson, *Physical Chemistry of Surfaces*, 4th Edition, Wiley, New York, 1982, pp. 584, 594.
43. H. M. Sadek and J. Olsen, Pharm. Technol. **5**, 40, 1981.
44. W. Lowenthal and R. Burress, J. Pharm. Sci. **60**, 1325, 1971; W. Lowenthal, ibid. **61**, 303, 1972.
45. S. J. Gregg and K. S. W. Sing, *Adsorption, Surface Area and Porosity*, Academic Press, New York, 1982; S. J. Gregg, *The Surface Chemistry of Solids*, 2nd Edition, Reinhold, New York, 1982, pp. 132–152.
46. J. J. Kipling, Quart. Rev. **10**, 1, 1956.
47. R. E. Franklin, Trans. Faraday Soc. **45**, 274, 1949.
48. W. A. Strickland, Jr., L. W. Busse and T. Higuchi, J. Am. Pharm. Assoc., Sci. Ed. **45**, 482, 1956.
49. A. Q. Butler and J. C. Ransey, Jr., Drug Standards **20**, 217, 1952.
50. B. S. Neumann, *Advances in Pharmaceutical Sciences*, Vol. 2, Edited by H. S. Bean, J. E. Carless and A. H. Beckett, Academic Press, New York, 1967, p. 181.
51. E. N. Hiestand, J. Pharm. Sci. **55**, 1325, 1966.
52. C. F. Harwood and N. Pilpel, Chem. Process Engineering, July 1968.
53. N. Pilpel, *Advances in Pharmaceutical Sciences*, vol. 3, Edited by H. S. Bean, A. H. Beckett and J. E. Carless, Academic Press, New York, 1971, pp. 173–219.
54. L.-E. Dahlinder, M. Johansson and J. Sjögren, Drug Dev. Ind. Pharm. **8**, 455, 1982.
55. A. S. Arambulo, H. Suen Fu and D. L. Deardorff, J. Am. Pharm. Assoc., Sci. Ed. **42**, 692, 1953.
56. A. M. Raff, A. S. Arambulo, A. J. Perkins and D. L. Deardorff, J. Am. Pharm. Assoc., Sci. Ed. **44**, 290, 1955.
57. F. C. Hammerness and H. O. Thompson, J. Am. Pharm. Assoc., Sci. Ed. **47**, 58, 1958.
58. D. E. Fonner, Jr., G. S. Banker and J. Swarbrick, J. Pharm. Sci. **55**, 181, 1966.
59. K. Ridgway and R. Rupp, J. Pharm. Pharmacol. Suppl. **30S**, 1969.
60. G. Gold, R. N. Duvall, B. T. Palermo and J. G. Slater, J. Pharm. Sci. **55**, 1291, 1966.
61. P. York, J. Pharm. Sci. **64**, 1216, 1975.
62. E. Nelson, J. Am. Pharm. Assoc., Sci. Ed. **44**, 435, 1955.
63. E. L. Parrott, Drug and Cosmetic Ind. **115**(8), 42, 1974.
64. D. Train, J. Am. Pharm. Assoc., Sci. Ed. **49**, 265, 1960.
65. J. J. Fischer, Chem. Engineering, August 1960, p. 107.
66. B. S. Neumann, *Flow Properties of Disperse Systems*, Edited by J. J. Hermans, Interscience, New York, 1953, Chapter 10.
67. D. Train, J. Pharm. Pharmacol. **8**, 745, 1956; Trans. Inst. Chem. Eng. **35**, 258, 1957.
68. T. Higuchi et al., J. Am. Pharm. Assoc., Sci. Ed. **41**, 93, 1952; ibid. **42**, 194, 1953; ibid. **43**, 344, 596, 685, 718, 1954; ibid. **44**, 223, 1955; ibid. **49**, 35, 1960; J. Pharm. Sci. **52**, 767, 1963.
69. E. L. Knoechel, C. C. Sperry and C. J. Lintner, J. Pharm. Sci. **56**, 116, 1967.
70. J. A. Hersey, G. Bayraktar and E. Shotton, J. Pharm. Pharmacol. **19**, 24S, 1967.
71. E. Shotton and D. Ganderton, J. Pharm. Pharmacol. **12**, 87T, 93T, 1960; ibid. **13**, 144T, 1961.
72. J. Varsano and L. Lachman, J. Pharm. Sci. **55**, 1128, 1966.
73. S. Leigh, J. E. Carless and B. W. Burt, J. Pharm. Sci. **56**, 888, 1967.
74. J. E. Carless and S. Leigh, J. Pharm. Pharmacol. **26**, 289, 1974.
75. P. York and N. Pilpel, J. Pharm. Pharmacol. **24** (Suppl.), 47P, 1972.
76. J. Cooper and J. E. Rees, J. Pharm. Sci. **61**, 1511, 1972.
77. E. N. Hiestand, J. E. Wells, C. B. Peot and J. F. Ochs, J. Pharm. Sci. **66**, 510, 1977.
78. H. Sunada, I. Shinohara, A. Otsuka and Y. Yonezawa, Chem. Pharm. Bull. **37**, 1889, 1989.
79. C. Bloom and E. F. Livesy, Manuf. Chemist **24**, 371, 1953.

80. B. Millan-Hernandez, "Physical Chemical Properties of Pharmaceutical Suspensions," Thesis, University of Texas, 1981.

Problems

16–1. Suppose that, by means of an optical microscope, the following hypothetical data were collected:

Data for *Problem 16–1*

diameter (μm)	10	20	30
number (*n*) of particles	3	2	1

Compute the arithmetic (length-number) mean particle diameter d_{ln}, the mean volume surface diameter d_{vs}, and the specific surface in cm^2/g, assuming that the particles have a true density of 1.5 g/cm^3 and are spherical.

Answer: d_{ln} = 16.7 μm; d_{vs} = 23 μm; S_w = 1740 cm^2/g

16–2. According to the cube root law (Chapter 13, pages 333 to 334), the dissolution behavior of a powder sample is defined by the initial particle size of a monodisperse system. In a polydisperse system, if the dissolution behavior is well defined by the cube root law, a mean particle size can be evaluated. Thus, equation (13–28), page 333, can be written in terms of an apparent mean diameter *d* as follows[78]:

$$(M_o^{1/3} - M^{1/3}) = [(2kC_s/\rho f)(M_o^{1/3}/d)]t \qquad (16-35)$$

where all the symbols have the same meaning as in equations (13–28) and (13–29), page 333; *f* is a dimensionless coefficient concerned with the shape, *d* is the initial average diameter, and ρ is the particle density. Rearranging equation (16–35) to yield

$$(M/M_o)^{1/3} = 1 - \frac{(2kC_s/\rho f)}{d} t \qquad (16-36)$$

allows one to check the cube root law and to determine an apparent mean diameter *d*. In order to test the applicability of equation (16–36), Sunada et al.[78] studied the dissolution of two samples of *n*-propyl *p*-hydroxybenzoate of different average particle size. According to equation (16–36), a plot of $(M/M_o)^{1/3}$ (vertical axis) against *t* (horizontal axis) should give a straight line that intersects at a point on the vertical axis equal to unity regardless of the original surface area and particle size. The apparent mean diameter *d* can be computed from the slope.

The $(M/M_o)^{1/3}$ values for the two samples, as well as the dissolution time, are expressed in the following table:

Data for *Problem 16–2**

t (min)	Sample II $(M/M_o)^{1/3}$	Sample V $(M/M_o)^{1/3}$
0	1	1
30	0.95	0.925
60	0.875	0.850
100	0.800	0.750
130	0.725	0.675
150	0.700	0.625
180	0.600	0.550
210	0.550	0.475
240	0.500	—

*Data from Figure 4 of H. Sunada, I. Shinohara, A. Otsuka and Y. Yonezawa, Chem. Pharm. Bull. **37**, 1889, 1989.

Plot $(M/M_o)^{1/3}$ (vertical axis) against *t* (horizontal axis) for the two samples and compute the apparent mean diameters. The constants for equation (16–36) are *k* = 0.166 cm/min, ρ = 1.28 g/cm^3, C_s = 0.00033 g/cm^3, and *f* = 0.369 for the two samples.

Answer: d for sample II, 0.108 cm; for sample V, 0.093 cm

16–3. A sample of silica was analyzed by the microscope method, and the following data were collected:

Data for *Problem 16–3*

diameter (μm)	10	15	20	25
frequency (*n*)	73	77	82	37

Compute d_{ln}, d_{vs}, and d_{wm}.

Answer: d_{ln} = 16.5; d_{vs} = 19.5; d_{wm} = 20.6 μm

16–4. A sample of heavy magnesium oxide was analyzed in an Andreasen apparatus and the following data were obtained:

Data for *Problem 16–4*

h/t (cm/min)	Stokes' law diameter (μm)	Cum. percent of powder below stated size percent
15.4	96	94
5	53	81
0.70	20	32
0.20	10	12

Plot the data on log probability paper and obtain d_g' and σ_g. Then compute d_{ln}, d_{sn}, and d_{vn} using the Hatch–Choate equations.

Answer: d_g' = 27, σ_g = 2.3, d_{ln} = 4.77; d_{sn} = 6.74; d_{vn} = 9.54 μm

16–5. Using the Stokes' law equation (16–6), calculate the particle diameter, d_{St} of magnesium oxide powder, ρ = 3.65 g/cm^3 in an aqueous medium having a density, ρ_0 = 1.05 g/cm^3 at 25° C and a viscosity of 0.013 poise (i.e., 0.013 g cm^{-1} sec^{-1}). The particles settle a distance of 24.0 mm in 1.00 hour under gravity acceleration *g* of 980 cm/sec^2. *Hint:* Remember to convert 24.0 mm/hr to cm/sec for the rate of settling of the particles.

Answer: 2.47 × 10^{-4} cm = 2.47 μm

16–6. What is the specific surface S_v of the particles of a sulfathiazole powder having a particle density of 1.5 g/cm^3 and an average diameter d_{vs} of 2 μm? It is assumed that the particles are perfect spheres.

Answer: 2.0 × 10^4 cm^2/g or 2.0 m^2/g

16–7. What is the total surface in cm^2 of 4 g of a local anesthetic powder in which the particles have an average diameter d_{vs} of 2 × 10^{-4} cm and a true density of 2.0 g/cm^3. Assume that the particles are spheres.

Answer: 6 × 10^4 cm^2 or 6 m^2

16–8. An animal-feed distributor desires to add an antibiotic at the rate of 20 mg per ton (2000 lb) to a chick feed. He asks your advice with respect to the fineness of the mix. Assume that each chick eats 40 grains of food mix at a meal and that each of these 40-grain portions must contain at least 1000 particles of the antibiotic on the average to ensure even dosage of the drug among the chicks. Calculate the diameter in micrometers to which the antibiotic must be pulverized. The antibiotic has a true density of 1.2 g/cm^3 and is assumed to consist of spherical particles.[79]

Answer: 4.5 μm

16–9. Two formulations of pellets of indomethacin combined with the film coating polymer Eudragit (Rohm Pharma), see page 435, had true densities of 1.191 g/cm^3 and 1.170 g/cm^3, respectively. Li et al.[28] used the mean volume surface diameter d_{vs} to calculate the specific surface (surface area per gram, S_w). The mean diameters of the two formulations were 1284 μm and 911 μm, respectively. Obtain

S_w, the surface area per gram, for the two formulations. Express the results in m²/gram.

Answer: 39.24×10^{-4} m²/g; 56.29×10^{-4} m²/g

16–10. Millan–Hernandez[80] obtained the specific surface S_w and the mean volume surface diameter of micronized griseofulvin powder. In the experimental work using the Quantasorb apparatus, one replaces V and V_m of equation (16–18) by the mass X and X_m. At the final stage of the work, X_m is converted to V_m by dividing X_m, the mass of nitrogen, by its density:

$$\frac{X_m \text{ gram gas/gram powder}}{\rho_{N_2} = 1.250 \times 10^{-3} \text{ g/cm}^3} = V_m \text{ cm}^3/\text{gram powder}$$

Nitrogen gas is introduced into the apparatus at three pressures, p in mm Hg, and X, the grams of nitrogen gas adsorbed on the powder sample, is recorded. The saturated vapor pressure $p_o = 758.71$ mm Hg, for N_2 at its boiling point, 77.2° K, is also required for the calculations. The data p/p_o and $p[X(p_o - p)]$ are obtained for each of the three gas pressures, and $p[X(p_o - p)]$ is plotted on the vertical axis against p/p_o on the horizontal axis. See equation (16–18), page 437, and *Example 16–7*.

The data for one experiment is shown here:

Data for *Problem 16–10*

p/p_o (x axis)	0.0970	0.1970	0.2920
$p/[X(p_o - p)]$ (y axis)	815.58	1515.37	2199.58

(a) Using linear regression analysis, obtain the slope $S = (b - 1)/[X_m b]$ and the intercept $I = 1/[X_m b]$. These terms conform to the slope and intercept in equation (16–18) except that X and X_m have replaced V and V_m. By simple algebra, it can be shown that the reciprocal of the sum of the slope S and the intercept I yield the value of mass X_m of N_2 gas that 1 gram of the powder can adsorb. That is,

$$X_m = \frac{1}{S + I}$$

(b) Then, using the density of N_2, 1.250×10^{-3} g/cm³, convert X_m to V_m (cm³/g) and obtain the specific surface S_w (m²/g) and d_{vs}. The density of griseofulvin is 1.455 g/cm³.

Answers: **(a)** slope, $S = 7096.56$ gram⁻¹, intercept, $I = 123.98$ gram⁻¹; **(b)** $S_w = 0.482$ meter²/gram; $d_{vs} = 8.56$ μm

16–11. A sample of charcoal was analyzed in the BET apparatus before and after activation, and the V_m values obtained were 3.4 cm³/g and 260 cm³/g, respectively. Calculate the specific surface of the charcoal before and after activation.

Answer: S_w (before) = 14.8 meter²/g; S_w (after) = 1131 meter²/g

16–12. Using the Quantasorb apparatus and the BET expression (equation (16–18)), the following data were collected for a sample of very fine zinc oxide powder:

Data for *Problem 16–12*

$p/V(p_o - p)$	0.038	0.064	0.090	0.116
p/p_o	0.10	0.20	0.30	0.40

The particles are nearly spherical and nonporous. Calculate S_w, the specific surface, and d_{vs}, the mean volume-surface diameter for this zinc oxide powder of density 5.60 g/cm³.

Answer: $S_w = 16.0$ m²/g; $d_{sv} = 0.067$ μm

16–13. The Fisher subsieve sizer (Fig. 16–13) is used to obtain the mean volume surface diameter d_{vs} and from it the specific surface, S_w, of a sample of griseofulvin. The equation for d_{vs} using the Fisher subsieve sizer is found on page 439 (equation (16–23)):

$$d_{vs} = \frac{c \cdot L}{(A \cdot L - 1)^{3/2}} \sqrt{\frac{F}{P - F}}$$

where c is a instrument constant equal to 3.80 cm, $L = 2.19$ cm is the height of the griseofulvin powder in its sample holder, $A = 1.267$ cm² is the cross-sectional area of the sample holder, $F = 25$ cm² is the pressure drop across the flow-meter resistance, and $P = 50$ cm² is the air pressure as measured with the water manometer as the air enters and permeates the powder sample. The density of griseofulvin is $\rho = 1.455$ g/cm³. Calculate d_{vs} and S_w for the griseofulvin sample. Does this sample meet USP XXII specifications?

Answer: $d_{vs} = 3.52 \times 10^{-4}$ cm; $S_w = 1.17 \times 10^4$ cm²/g. See the USP XXII to determine whether this sample meets specifications for griseofulvin.

16–14. Water (molecular weight 18.015 g/mole, surface tension 72.8 erg/cm², and density 0.998 g/cm³ at 293.15° K) is allowed to condense in the pores of griseofulvin particles. Calculate the vapor pressure ratio p/p_o using the Kelvin expression, equation (16–24), if the radius of the griseofulvin pores is 5.30×10^{-7} cm

Answer: $p/p_o = 0.816$

16–15. The experimental values of a water adsorption/desorption isotherm at 20° C on a type of clay are given in the following table.

Data for *Problem 16–15**

p/p_0	V_1 (adsorption) (mL/g)	V_2 (desorption) (mL/g)
0.20	0.079	0.123
0.31	0.109	0.147
0.35	0.129	0.150
0.40	0.135	0.165
0.45	0.141	0.177
0.49	0.141	0.182
0.56	0.150	0.188
0.66	0.152	0.191
0.77	0.161	0.194
0.80	0.170	0.200
0.89	0.182	0.209
0.96	0.224	0.224

*Values from Figure 7 in S. Yamanaka, P. B. Malla and S. Komareni, J. Colloid Interface Sci. **134**, 51, 1990.

(a) Plot V_1 (adsorption) and V_2 (desorption) on the vertical axis against p/p_o (horizontal axis). What is the meaning of this isotherm?

(b) Using the Kelvin equation (16–24), compute the radius of the pores corresponding to the relative pressures given in the table. See *Example 16–8*.

(c) Assuming that all pores are of radius less than 265 Å, compute the cumulative per cent of pore volume with radii less than those found in part (b).

(d) Compute the percent of pore volume with radius between 40 and 60 Å.

Answers: **(a)** Check your answer with pages 440 to 442. **(b)** Partial answer: 6.7 and 9.2 Å; **(c)** Partial answer: for $p/p_o = 0.2$ and $r < 6.7$ Å, pore volume is 54.9%; **(d)** 5.5%

16–16. Calculate the porosity of a sample of aluminum oxide having a true density of 4.0 g/cm³. When 75 g of the powder was placed in a graduate cylinder, the Al_2O_3 was found to have a bulk volume of 62 cm³

Answer: 69.8%

16–17. (a) If the weight of a tablet is 0.2626 g and its bulk volume is 0.0836 mL, what is the bulk density?

(b) If the true density of the mixture of ingredients is 3.202, what is the porosity of the tablet?

Answers: **(a)** 3.14;   **(b)** 0.019 or 1.9%

16–18. Calculate the percent porosity of a sample of talc that has a true density of 2.70 g/cm³. When 324 g of the powder was placed in a graduate, the talc was found to have a bulk volume of 200 mL.

Answer: 40%

16–19. The true density of aspirin is 1.37 and the granule density is 1.33. What is the porosity or percent void spaces within the granules?

Answer: 3%

16–20. The true density of a powder mixture is 3.203. When compressed into tablet form, the granule density of the mixture is found to be 3.138. What is the porosity of the tablet?

Answer: 2%

17
Rheology

Introduction
Newtonian Systems
Non-Newtonian Systems
Thixotropy

Determination of Rheologic Properties
Viscoelasticity
Psychorheology
Applications to Pharmacy

INTRODUCTION

The term rheology, from the Greek *rheo* (to flow) and *logos* (science), was suggested by Bingham and Crawford (as reported by Fischer[1]) to describe the flow of liquids and the deformation of solids. *Viscosity* is an expression of the resistance of a fluid to flow; the higher the viscosity, the greater the resistance. As will be seen later, simple liquids can be described in terms of absolute viscosity. The rheologic properties of heterogeneous dispersions are more complex, however, and cannot be expressed by a single value.

In recent years, the fundamental principles of rheology have been used in the study of paints, inks, doughs, road building materials, cosmetics, dairy products, and other materials. The study of the viscosity of true liquids, solutions, and dilute and concentrated colloidal systems is of much practical as well as theoretic value. These points have been discussed in Chapter 15, which deals with colloids. Scott-Blair[2] recognized the importance of rheology in pharmacy and suggested its application in the formulation and analysis of such pharmaceutical products as emulsions, pastes, suppositories, and tablet coatings. The manufacturer of medicinal and cosmetic creams, pastes, and lotions must be capable of producing a product with an acceptable consistency and smoothness and must be able to reproduce these qualities each time a new batch is prepared. In many industries, the judgment of proper consistency is made by a trained person with long experience who handles the material periodically during manufacture to determine its "feel" and "body." The variability of subjective tests at different times under varying environmental conditions is, however, well recognized. A more serious objection, from a scientific standpoint, is the failure of subjective methods to distinguish the various properties that make up the total consistency of the product. If these individual physical characteristics are delineated and studied objectively according to the analytic methods of rheology, valuable information can be obtained for use in formulating better pharmaceutical products.

Rheology is involved in the mixing and flow of materials, their packaging into containers, and their removal prior to use, whether this is achieved by pouring from a bottle, extrusion from a tube, or passage through a syringe needle. The rheology of a particular product, which can range in consistency from fluid to semisolid to solid, can affect its patient acceptability, physical stability, and even biologic availability. Thus, viscosity has been shown to affect the absorption rate of drugs from the gastrointestinal tract.

The rheologic properties of a pharmaceutical system can influence the choice of processing equipment to be used in its manufacture. Furthermore, lack of appreciation for the correct choice of a piece of processing equipment can result in an undesirable product, at least in terms of its flow characteristics. These and other aspects of rheology that apply to pharmacy are discussed by Martin et al.[3]

When classifying materials according to the types of flow and deformation, it is customary to place them in one of two categories: Newtonian or non-Newtonian systems. The choice depends on whether or not their flow properties are in accord with Newton's law of flow.

NEWTONIAN SYSTEMS

Newtonian's Law of Flow. Consider a "block" of liquid consisting of parallel plates of molecules, similar to a deck of cards, as shown in Figure 17–1. The bottom layer is considered to be fixed in place. If the top plane of liquid is moved at a constant velocity, each lower layer will move with a velocity directly proportional to

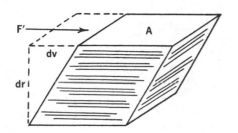

Fig. 17–1. Representation of the shearing force required to produce a definite velocity gradient between the parallel planes of a block of material.

its distance from the stationary bottom layer. The difference of velocity dv between two planes of liquid separated by an infinitesimal distance dr is the *velocity gradient* or *rate of shear*, dv/dr. The force per unit area F'/A required to bring about flow is called the *shearing stress* and is given the symbol F. Newton was the first to study the flow properties of liquids in a quantitative way. He recognized that the higher the viscosity of a liquid, the greater the force per unit area (*shearing stress*) required to produce a certain rate of shear. Rate of shear is given the symbol G. Hence, the rate of shear should be directly proportional to the shearing stress, or

$$\frac{F'}{A} = \eta \frac{dv}{dr} \qquad (17\text{–}1)$$

in which η is the *coefficient of viscosity*, usually referred to simply as *viscosity*.

Equation (17–1) is frequently written as

$$\eta = \frac{F}{G} \qquad (17\text{–}2)$$

in which $F = F'/A$ and $G = dv/dr$. A representative flow curve, or *rheogram*, obtained by plotting F versus G for a Newtonian system is shown in Figure 17–2a. As implied by equation (17–2), a straight line passing through the origin is obtained.

The unit of viscosity is the *poise*, defined with reference to Figure 17–1 as the shearing force required to produce a velocity of 1 cm/sec between two parallel planes of liquid each 1 cm^2 in area and separated by a distance of 1 cm. The cgs units for the poise are dyne sec cm^{-2} (that is, dyne sec/cm^2) or g cm^{-1} sec^{-1} (that is, g/(cm sec)). These units are readily obtained by a dimensional analysis of the viscosity coefficient. Rearranging equation (17–1) to

$$\eta = \frac{F'\ dr}{A\ dv} = \frac{\text{dynes} \times \text{cm}}{\text{cm}^2 \times \text{cm/sec}} = \frac{\text{dyne sec}}{\text{cm}^2}$$

gives the result

$$\frac{\text{dyne sec}}{\text{cm}^2} = \frac{\text{g} \times \text{cm/sec}^2 \times \text{sec}}{\text{cm}^2} = \frac{\text{g}}{\text{cm sec}}$$

A more convenient unit for most work is the *centipoise* cp (plural, *cps*), 1 cp being equal to 0.01 poise. *Fluidity*, ϕ, a term sometimes used, is defined as the reciprocal of viscosity:

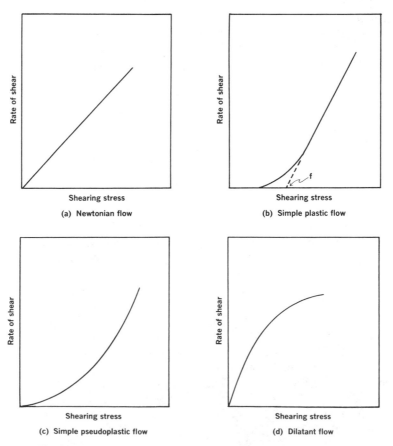

(a) Newtonian flow

(b) Simple plastic flow

(c) Simple pseudoplastic flow

(d) Dilatant flow

Fig. 17–2. Representative flow curves for various materials.

$$\phi = \frac{1}{\eta} \qquad (17-3)$$

Kinematic Viscosity. The U.S. Pharmacopeia includes an explanation of *kinematic viscosity*, which is the absolute viscosity as defined in equation (17–1) divided by the density of the liquid at a definite temperature:

$$\text{kinematic viscosity} = \frac{\eta}{\rho} \qquad (17-4)$$

The units of kinematic viscosity are the *stoke* (*s*) and the *centistoke* (*cs*). Arbitrary scales, Saybolt, Redwood, Engler, and others, for the measurement of viscosity are used in various industries; these are sometimes converted by use of tables or formulas to absolute viscosities and vice versa.

Example 17– 1. (*a*). Using an Ostwald viscometer (see Fig. 17–11), acetone was measured and found to have a viscosity of 0.313 cp at 25° C. Its density at 25° C is 0.788 g/cm³. What is the kinematic viscosity of acetone at 25° C?

(*b*) Water is ordinarily used as a standard for viscosity of liquids. Its viscosity at 25° C is 0.8904 cp. What is the viscosity of acetone relative to that of water (relative viscosity, η_{rel}) at 25° C?

(*a*) kinematic viscosity = 0.313 centipoise ÷ 0.788 g/cm³ = 0.397 poise/(g/cm³) or 0.397 centistokes.

(*b*) $\eta_{rel(acetone)}$ = 0.313 cp/0.8904 cp = 0.352 (dimensionless).

The viscosity of some liquids commonly used in pharmacy are given in Table 17–1 at 20° C. A number of viscosity–increasing agents are given in the U.S. Pharmacopeia XXII, p. 1858.

Temperature Dependence and the Theory of Viscosity. While the viscosity of a gas increases with temperature, that of a liquid decreases as the temperature is raised, and the fluidity of a liquid, the reciprocal of viscosity, increases with temperature. The dependence of the viscosity of a liquid on temperature is expressed approximately for many substances by an equation analogous to the Arrhenius equation (p. 295) of chemical kinetics:

$$\eta = Ae^{Ev/RT} \qquad (17-5)$$

in which A is a constant depending on the molecular weight and molar volume of the liquid, and E_v is an "activation energy" required to initiate flow between the molecules.

The energy of vaporization of a liquid is the energy required to remove a molecule from the liquid, leaving a "hole" behind equal in size to that of the molecule that

TABLE 17– 1. *Absolute Viscosity of Some Newtonian Liquids at 20° C*

Liquid	Viscosity (cps)
Castor oil	1000
Chloroform	0.563
Ethyl alcohol	1.19
Glycerin, 93%	400
Olive oil	100
Water	1.0019

has departed. A hole must also be made available in a liquid if one molecule is to flow past another. The activation energy for flow has been found to be about one third that of the energy of vaporization, and it can be concluded that the free space needed for flow is about one third the volume of a molecule. This is presumably because a molecule in flow can back, turn, and maneuver in a space smaller than its actual size, like a car in a crowded parking lot. More energy is required to break bonds and permit flow in liquids composed of molecules that are associated through hydrogen bonds. These bonds are broken at higher temperatures by thermal movement, however, and E_v decreases markedly. Diffusion (see Chapter 13) is similar to viscosity flow and, like fluidity, the reciprocal of viscosity, the rate of diffusion increases exponentially with temperature.

Example 17–2. The modified Arrhenius equation 17–5, is used to obtain the dependence of viscosity of liquids on temperature. Use equation (17–5) and the viscosity versus temperature data for glycerin (Table 17–2) to obtain the constant A, and E_v (the activation energy to initiate flow). What is the value of r^2, the square of the correlation coefficient?

Equation (17–5) is written in logarithmic form

$$\ln \eta = \ln A + \frac{E_v}{R}\frac{1}{T} \qquad (17-6)$$

According to equation (17–6), a regression of $\ln \eta$ against $1/T$ gives E_v from the slope and $\ln A$ from the intercept. Using the values given in Table 17–2, the equation is

$$\ln \eta = -23.4706 + 9012\frac{1}{T}$$

Slope = 9012 = E_v/R; E_v = 9012 × 1.9872 = 17,909 cal/mole

Intercept = −23.4706 = $\ln A$; A = 6.40985 × 10⁻¹¹; r^2 = 0.997

NON-NEWTONIAN SYSTEMS

The pharmacist probably deals more frequently with non-Newtonian materials than with simple liquids, and should therefore have suitable methods for the study of these complex substances. *Non-Newtonian bodies* are those substances that fail to follow Newton's equation of flow; liquid and solid heterogeneous dispersions such as colloidal solutions, emulsions, liquid suspensions, ointments, and similar products make up this class. When non-Newtonian materials are analyzed in a rotational viscometer (see pp. 463–466) and the results are plotted, various consistency curves, representing three classes of flow, are recognized: *plastic, pseudoplastic,* and *dilatant.*

Plastic Flow. In Figure 17–2*b*, the curve represents a body that exhibits plastic flow; such materials are known as *Bingham bodies* in honor of the pioneer of modern rheology and the first investigator to study plastic substances in a systematic manner.

The plastic flow curve does not pass through the origin but rather intersects the shearing stress axis (or will if the straight part of the curve is extrapolated to the axis) at a particular point referred to as the *yield*

TABLE 17-2. *Viscosity of Glycerin at Several Temperatures**

Temp. °C	-42	-20	0	6	15	20	25	30
Temp. °K	231	253	273	279	288	293	298	303
$1/T$ (°K^{-1})	0.00432	0.00395	0.00366	0.00358	0.00347	0.00341	0.00336	0.00330
η, cp	6.71×10^6	1.34×10^5	12110	6260	2330	1490	954	629
ln η	15.719	11.806	9.402	8.742	7.754	7.307	6.861	6.444

*Data from *CRC Handbook of Chemistry and Physics,* 63rd Edition, CRC Press, Boca Raton, Fla., 1982, p. F-44.

value. A Bingham body does not begin to flow until a shearing stress, corresponding to the yield value, is exceeded. At stresses below the yield value, the substance acts as an elastic material. The rheologist classifies Bingham bodies, that is, those substances that exhibit a yield value, as solids, whereas substances that begin to flow at the smallest shearing stress and show no yield value are defined as liquids. Yield value is an important property of certain dispersions.

The slope of the rheogram in Figure 17-2b is termed *mobility,* analogous to fluidity in Newtonian systems, and its reciprocal is known as the *plastic viscosity, U.* The equation describing plastic flow is

$$U = \frac{(F - f)}{G} \qquad (17-7)$$

in which *f* is the yield value, or intercept, on the shear stress axis in dynes cm^{-2}, and *F* and *G* are as previously defined.

Example 17-3. A plastic material was found to have a yield value of 5200 dynes cm^{-2}. At shearing stresses above the yield value, *F* was found to increase linearly with *G*. If the rate of shear was 150 sec^{-1} when *F* was 8000 dynes cm^{-2}, calculate *U*, the plastic viscosity of the sample.

Substituting into equation (17-7):

$$U = (8000 - 5200)/150$$
$$= 2800/150$$
$$= 18.67 \text{ poise.}$$

Plastic flow is associated with the presence of flocculated particles in concentrated suspensions. As a result, a continuous structure is set up throughout the system. The yield value is present because of the contacts between adjacent particles (brought about by van der Waals forces), which must be broken down before flow can occur. Consequently, the yield value is an indication of the force of flocculation: the more flocculated the suspension, the higher will be the yield value. Frictional forces between moving particles can also contribute to the yield value. As was shown in *Example 17-3,* once the yield value has been exceeded, any further increase in shearing stress (i.e., *F* − *f*) brings about a directly proportional increase in *G*, the rate of shear. In effect, a plastic system resembles a Newtonian system at shear stresses above the yield value.

Pseudoplastic Flow. A large number of pharmaceutical products, including natural and synthetic gums, for example, liquid dispersions of tragacanth, sodium alginate, methylcellulose, and sodium carboxymethylcellulose, exhibit *pseudoplastic flow.* As a general rule,

pseudoplastic flow is exhibited by polymers in solution, in contrast to plastic systems, which are composed of flocculated particles in suspension. As seen in Figure 17-2c the consistency curve for a pseudoplastic material begins at the origin (or at least approaches it at low rates of shear). Consequently, in contrast to Bingham bodies, there is no yield value. Since, however, no part of the curve is linear, one cannot express the viscosity of a pseudoplastic material by any single value.

The viscosity of a pseudoplastic substance decreases with increasing rate of shear. An apparent viscosity may be obtained at any rate of shear from the slope of the tangent to the curve at the specified point. The most satisfactory representation for a pseudoplastic material at the present time, however, is probably a graphic plot of the entire consistency curve.

The curved rheogram for pseudoplastic materials results from a shearing action on the long-chain molecules of materials such as linear polymers. As the shearing stress is increased, the normally disarranged molecules begin to align their long axes in the direction of flow. This orientation reduces the internal resistance of the material and allows a greater rate of shear at each successive shearing stress. In addition, some of the solvent associated with the molecules may be released, resulting in an effective lowering of the concentration and the size of the dispersed molecules. This, too, will effect a lowering of the apparent viscosity.

Obviously, objective comparisons between different pseudoplastic systems are more difficult than with either Newtonian or plastic systems. Thus, a Newtonian system is completely described by η, the viscosity. A system exhibiting plastic flow is adequately described by the yield value and the plastic viscosity. Accordingly, several approaches have been used to obtain meaningful parameters that will allow different pseudoplastic materials to be compared. Of those discussed by Martin et al.,[3] the exponential formula

$$F^N = \eta'G \qquad (17-8)$$

has been used most frequently for pseudoplastics. The exponent *N* rises as the flow becomes increasingly non-Newtonian. When *N* = 1, equation (17-8) reduces to equation (17-2) and the flow is Newtonian. The term η' is a viscosity coefficient. Following rearrangement, equation (17-8) may be written in the logarithmic form:

$$\log G = N \log F - \log \eta' \qquad (17-9)$$

This is an equation for a straight line. Many pseudoplastic systems fit this equation when log G is plotted as a function of log F.[4] Several of the more important pseudoplastic suspending agents used in pharmacy, however, do not conform to equation (17–9).[5] Modified equations have been suggested by Shangraw et al. and by Casson and Patton.[6] An analog computer has been used to characterize pseudoplastic systems, based on the assumption that the typical rheogram of a pseudoplastic substance is composed of a first-order segment and a zero-order segment.[7]

Dilatant Flow. Certain suspensions with a high percentage of dispersed solids exhibit an increase in resistance to flow with increasing rates of shear. Such systems actually increase in volume when sheared and are hence termed *dilatant;* their flow properties are illustrated by Figure 17–2d. It should be immediately obvious that this type of flow is the inverse of that possessed by pseudoplastic systems. Whereas pseudoplastic materials are frequently referred to as "shear-thinning systems," dilatant materials arc often termed "shear-thickening systems." When the stress is removed, a dilatant system returns to its original state of fluidity.

Equation (17–8) can be used to describe dilatancy in quantitative terms. In this case, N is always less than 1 and decreases as the degree of dilatancy increases. As N approaches 1, the system becomes increasingly Newtonian in behavior.

Substances possessing dilatant flow properties are invariably suspensions containing a high concentration (about 50% or greater) of small, deflocculated particles. As discussed previously, particulate systems of this type that are flocculated would be expected to possess plastic, rather than dilatant, flow characteristics. Dilatant behavior may be explained as follows. At rest, the particles are closely packed with the interparticle volume, or voids, being at a minimum. The amount of vehicle in the suspension is sufficient, however, to fill this volume and permits the particles to move relative to one another at low rates of shear. Thus, one may pour a dilatant suspension from a bottle since under these conditions it is reasonably fluid. As the shear stress is increased, the bulk of the system expands or dilates; hence the term *dilatant*. The particles, in an attempt to move quickly past each other, take on an open form of packing, as depicted in Figure 17–3. Such an arrangement leads to a significant increase in the interparticle void volume. The amount of vehicle remains constant and, at some point, becomes insufficient to fill the increased voids between the particles. Accordingly, the resistance to flow increases because the particles are no longer completely wetted, or lubricated, by the vehicle. Eventually, the suspension will set up as a firm paste. Behavior of this nature necessitates that great care be taken in processing dilatant materials. Conventionally, the processing of dispersions containing solid particles is facilitated by the use of high-speed mixers, blenders, or mills. Although this is advantageous with all other rheologic systems, dilatant materials may solidify under these conditions of high shear, thereby overloading and damaging the processing equipment.

THIXOTROPY

Previously the reader was introduced to the several types of behavior observed when the rate of shear was progressively increased and plotted against the resultant shear stress. It was tactily assumed that if the rate of shear was reduced once the desired maximum rate had been reached, the down-curve would be identical with and superimposed on the up-curve. While this is so with Newtonian systems, the down-curve for non-Newtonian systems can be displaced with regard to the up-curve. With shear-thinning systems (i.e., pseudoplastic), the down-curve is frequently displaced to the left of the up-curve (as in Fig. 17–4), showing that the material has a lower consistency at any one rate of shear on the down-curve than it had on the up-curve. This indicates a breakdown of structure (and hence shear thinning) that does not reform immediately when the stress is removed or reduced. This phenomenon,

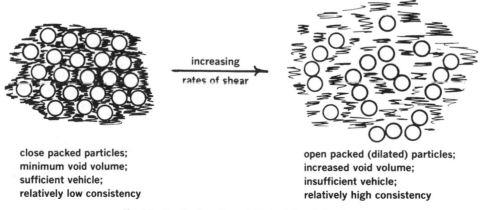

increasing
rates of shear →

close packed particles;
minimum void volume;
sufficient vehicle;
relatively low consistency

open packed (dilated) particles;
increased void volume;
insufficient vehicle;
relatively high consistency

Fig. 17–3. Explanation of dilatant flow behavior.

known as *thixotropy*, may be defined[8] as "an isothermal and comparatively slow recovery, on standing of a material, of a consistency lost through shearing." As so defined, thixotropy may be applied only to shear-thinning systems. Typical rheograms for plastic and pseudoplastic systems exhibiting this behavior are shown in Figure 17–4.

Thixotropic systems usually contain asymmetric particles that, through numerous points of contact, set up a loose three-dimensional network throughout the sample. At rest, this structure confers some degree of rigidity on the system, and it resembles a gel. As shear is applied and flow starts, this structure begins to break down as the points of contact are disrupted and the particles become aligned. The material undergoes a gel-to-sol transformation and exhibits shear thinning. Upon removal of the stress, the structure starts to reform. This process is not instantaneous; rather, it is a progressive restoration of consistency as the asymmetric particles come into contact with one another by undergoing random Brownian movement. The rheograms obtained with thixotropic materials are therefore highly dependent on the rate at which shear is increased or decreased and the length of time a sample is subjected to any one rate of shear. In other words, the previous history of the sample has a significant effect on the rheologic properties of a thixotropic system. For example, suppose that in Figure 17–5 the shear rate of a thixotropic material is increased in a constant manner from *a* to point *b* and is then decreased at the same rate back to *e*. Typically, this would result in the so-called hysteresis loop *abe*. If, however, the sample was taken to point *b* and the shear rate held constant for a certain period of time (say, t_1 seconds), the shearing stress, and hence the consistency, would decrease to an extent depending on the time of shear, the rate of shear, and the degree of structure in the sample. Decreasing the shear rate would then result in the *hysteresis loop, abce*. If the sample had been held at the same rate of shear for t_2 seconds, the loop *abcde* would have been observed. Obviously, therefore, the rheogram of a thixotropic material is not unique but will depend on the rheologic history of the sample and the approach used in obtaining the rheogram. This is an important point to

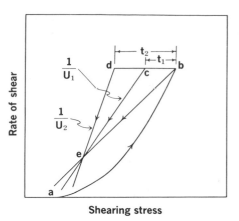

Fig. 17–5. Structural breakdown with time of a plastic system possessing thixotropy when subjected to a constant rate of shear for t_1 and t_2 seconds. See text for discussion.

bear in mind when attempting to obtain a quantitative measure of thixotropy. This will become apparent in the subsequent section.

Measurement of Thixotropy. A quantitative measurement of thixotropy can be attempted in several ways. The most apparent characteristic of a thixotropic system is the hysteresis loop, formed by the up- and down-curves of the rheogram. This *area of hysteresis* has been proposed as a measure of thixotropic breakdown; it may be obtained readily by means of a planimeter or other suitable technique.

With plastic (Bingham) bodies, two approaches are frequently used to estimate the degree of thixotropy. The first is to determine the structural breakdown with time at a *constant* rate of shear. The type of rheogram needed for this estimation is shown in Figure 17–5; the steps necessary to obtain it have already been described. Based on such a rheogram, a thixotropic coefficient *B*, the rate of breakdown with time at constant shear rate, is calculated as follows:

$$B = \frac{U_1 - U_2}{\ln \dfrac{t_2}{t_1}} \qquad (17\text{--}10)$$

in which U_1 and U_2 are the plastic viscosities of the two down-curves, calculated from equation (17–7), after shearing at a constant rate for t_1 and t_2 seconds, respectively. The choice of shear rate is arbitrary. A more meaningful, though time-consuming, method for characterizing thixotropic behavior is to measure the fall in stress with time several rates of shear.

The second approach is to determine the structural breakdown due to *increasing* shear rate. The principle involved in this approach is shown in Figure 17–6, in which two hysteresis loops are obtained having different maximum rates of shear, v_1 and v_2. In this case, a thixotropic coefficient *M*, the loss in shearing stress per unit increase in shear rate, is obtained from

$$M = \frac{(U_1 - U_2)}{\ln (v_2/v_1)} \qquad (17\text{--}11)$$

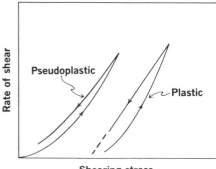

Fig. 17–4. Thixotropy in plastic and pseudoplastic flow systems.

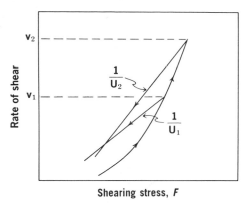

Fig. 17–6. Structural breakdown of a plastic system possessing thixotropy when subjected to increasing shear rates. See text for discussion.

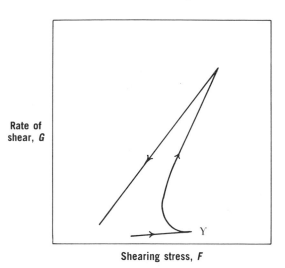

Fig. 17–8. Rheogram of a thixotropic material showing a spur value Y in the hysteresis loop.

in which M is in dynes sec/cm^2 and U_1 and U_2 are the plastic viscosities for two separate down-curves having maximum shearing rates of v_1 and v_2, respectively. A criticism of this technique is that the two rates of shear, v_1 and v_2, are chosen arbitrarily; the value of M will depend on the rate of shear chosen since these shear rates will affect the down-curves and hence the values of U that are calculated.

Bulges and Spurs. Dispersions employed in pharmacy may yield complex hysteresis loops when sheared in a viscometer in which shear rate (rather than shear stress) is increased to a point, then decreased, and the shear stress is read at each shear rate value to yield appropriate rheograms. Two such complex structures are shown in Figures 17–7 and 17–8. A concentrated aqueous bentonite gel, 10 to 15% by weight, produces a hysteresis loop with a characteristic *bulge* in the up-curve. It is presumed that the crystalline plates of bentonite form a "house-of-cards structure" that causes the swelling of bentonite magmas. This three-dimensional structure results in a bulged hysteresis loop as observed in Figure 17–7. In still more highly struc-

tured systems, such as a procaine penicillin gel formulated by Ober et al.[9] for intramuscular injection, the bulged curve may actually develop into a spur-like protrusion (Fig. 17–8). The structure demonstrates a high yield or *spur value*, Y, that traces out a bowed up-curve when the three-dimensional structure breaks in the viscometer, as observed in Figure 17–8. The spur value represents a sharp point of structural breakdown at low shear rate. It is difficult to produce the spur, and it may not be observed unless a sample of the gel is allowed to age undisturbed in the cup and bob assembly for some time before the rheologic run is made. The spur value is obtained by using an instrument in which the rate of shear can be slowly and uniformly increased, preferably automatically, and the shear stress read out or plotted on an X–Y recorder as a function of shear rate. Ober et al.[9] found that penicillin gels having definite Y values were very thixotropic, forming intramuscular depots upon injection that afforded prolonged blood levels of the drug.

Negative Thixotropy. From time to time in the measurement of supposedly thixotropic materials, one observes a phenomenon called *negative thixotropy* or *antithixotropy*, which represents an increase rather than a decrease in consistency on the down-curve. This increase in thickness or resistance to flow with increased time of shear was observed by Chong et al.[10] in the rheologic analysis of magnesia magma. It was detected at shear rates of greater than 30 sec^{-1}; below 30 sec^{-1} the magma showed normal thixotropy, the down-curve appearing to the left of the up-curve. As pointed out by Chong et al., antithixotropy had been reported by other investigators, but not in pharmaceutical systems.

It was observed that when magnesia magma was alternately sheared at increasing and then decreasing rates of shear, the magma continuously thickened (an increase in shearing stress per unit shear rate) but at a decreasing rate, and it finally reached an equilibrium

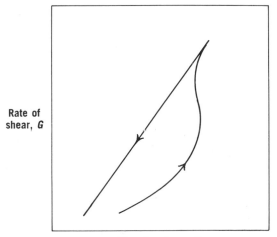

Fig. 17–7. Rheogram of a thixotropic material showing a bulge in the hysteresis loop.

state in which further cycles of increasing-decreasing shear rates no longer increased the consistency of the material. The antithixotropic character of magnesia magma is demonstrated in Figure 17–9. The equilibrium system was found to be gel-like and to provide great suspendability, yet it was readily pourable. When allowed to stand, however, the material returned to its sol-like properties.

Antithixotropy or negative thixotropy should not be confused with dilatancy or rheopexy. Dilatant systems are deflocculated and ordinarily contain greater than 50% by volume of solid dispersed phase, whereas antithixotropic systems have low solids content (1 to 10%) and are flocculated, according to Samyn and Jung.[11] *Rheopexy* is a phenomenon in which a solid forms a gel more readily when gently shaken or otherwise sheared that when allowed to form the gel while the material is kept at rest.[12] In a rheopectic system, the gel is the equilibrium form, whereas in antithixotropy, the equilibrium state is the sol. Samyn and Jung note that magnesia magma and clay suspensions may show a negative rheopexy, analogous to negative thixotropy. It is believed that antithixotropy results from an increased collision frequency of dispersed particles or polymer molecules in suspension, resulting in increased interparticle bonding with time. This changes the original state consisting of a large number of individual particles and small floccules to an eventual equilibrium state consisting of a small number of relatively large floccules. At rest, the large floccules break up and gradually return to the original state of small floccules and individual particles.

As more rheologic studies are done with pharmaceuticals, negative thixotropy no doubt will be observed in other materials.

Thixotropy in Formulation. Thixotropy is a desirable property in liquid pharmaceutical systems that ideally should have a high consistency in the container, yet pour or spread easily. For example, a well-formulated thixotropic suspension will not settle out readily in the container, will become fluid on shaking, and will remain long enough for a dose to be dispensed. Finally, it will regain consistency rapidly enough so as to maintain the particles in a suspended state. A similar pattern of behavior is desirable with emulsions, lotions, creams, ointments, and parenteral suspensions to be used for intramuscular depot therapy.

With regard to suspension stability, there is a relationship between the degree of thixotropy and the rate of sedimention; the greater the thixotropy, the lower the rate of settling. Concentrated parenteral suspensions containing from 40 to 70% *w/v* of procaine penicillin G in water were found to have a high inherent thixotropy and were shear-thinning.[13] Consequently, breakdown of the structure occurred when the suspension was caused to pass through the hypodermic needle. The consistency was then recovered as the rheologic structure reformed. This led to the formation of a depot of drug at the site of injection in the muscle, from which drug was slowly removed and made available to the body. The degree of thixotropy was shown to be related to the specific surface of the penicillin used.

The reader should also appreciate that the degree of thixotropy may change over time and result in an inadequate formulation. Thixotropic systems are complex, and it is unrealistic to expect that rheologic changes can be meaningfully followed by the use of one parameter. Thus, in a study concerned with the aging effects of thixotropic clay, Levy[14] found it necessary to follow changes in plastic viscosity, area of hysteresis, yield value, and spur value.

DETERMINATION OF RHEOLOGIC PROPERTIES

Choice of Viscometer. The successful determination and evaluation of the rheologic properties of a particular system depend, in large part, on choosing the correct instrumental method. Since the rate of shear in a Newtonian system is directly proportional to the shearing stress, one can use instruments that operate at a single rate of shear. These "one-point" instruments provide a single point on the rheogram; extrapolation of a line through this point to the origin will result in a complete rheogram. Implicit in the use of a "one-point" instrument is the prior knowledge that the flow characteristics of the material are Newtonian. Unfortunately, this is not always the case, and should the system be non-Newtonian, a "one-point" determination is virtually useless in characterizing the flow properties of the system. It is therefore essential that, with non-Newtonian systems, the instrumentation used be able to operate at a variety of rates of shear. Only by the use of "multipoint" instruments is it possible to obtain the complete rheogram for those systems. The use of a "one-point" instrument, even as a quality

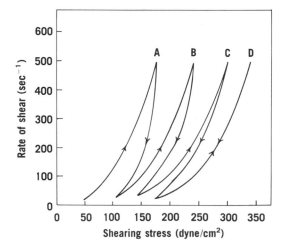

Fig. 17–9. Rheogram of magnesia magma showing antithixotropic behavior. The material is sheared at repeated increasing and then decreasing rates of shear. At stage *D*, further cycling no longer increased the consistency, and the up- and down-curves coincided. (From C. W. Chong, S. P. Eriksen, and J. W. Swintosky, J. Am. Pharm. Assoc., Sci. Ed. **49**, 547, 1960, reproduced with permission of the publisher.)

control in industry, is erroneous if the system is non-Newtonian since, as illustrated in Figure 17–10, the flow properties could vary significantly, yet will appear to be unchanged.

The important conclusion, therefore, is that while all viscometers can be used to determine the viscosity of Newtonian systems, only those with variable shear-stress controls can be used for non-Newtonian materials.

Other rheologic properties such as tackiness or stickiness, "body," "slip," and "spreadability" are difficult to measure by means of conventional apparatus and, in fact, do not have precise meanings. The individual factors, however—viscosity, yield value, thixotropy, and the other properties that contribute to the total consistency of non-Newtonian pharmaceuticals—can be analyzed to some degree of satisfaction in reliable apparatus. An attempt must be made to express these properties in meaningful terms if rheology is to aid in the development, production, and control of pharmaceutical preparations.

The many types of viscometers have been discussed in detail by Hatschek,[15] Martin et al.,[3] Sherman,[16] and Van Wazer et al.[17] The present discussion will be limited to four instruments, namely the capillary, falling sphere, cup and bob, and cone and plate viscometers. The first two are for use only with Newtonian materials, while the latter two may be used with both types of flow system.

Pseudoplastic materials should be studied with an instrument that is capable of a wide range of shearing rates. The results can then be used to represent the viscosity of a suspending agent at rest, that is, at a negligible rate of shear, and while being agitated, poured from a bottle, or applied to the skin at moderately high rates of shear. Capillary and falling ball viscometers, operating at a single rate of shear, are unable to describe these changes. Even rotational instruments, unless properly designed, will not give satisfactory results.

Capillary Viscometer. The viscosity of a Newtonian liquid may be determined by measuring the time required for the liquid to pass between two marks as it flows by gravity through a vertical capillary tube, known as an *Ostwald viscometer*. A modern adaptation of the original Ostwald viscometer is shown in Figure 17–11. The time of flow of the liquid under test is compared with the time required for a liquid of known viscosity (usually water) to pass between the two marks. If η_1 and η_2 are the viscosities of the unknown and the standard liquids, ρ_1 and ρ_2 are the densities of the liquids, and t_1 and t_2 are the respective flow times in seconds, the absolute viscosity of the unknown liquid, η_1, is determined by substituting the experimental values in the equation

$$\frac{\eta_1}{\eta_2} = \frac{\rho_1 t_1}{\rho_2 t_2} \qquad (17-12)$$

The value $\eta_1/\eta_2 = \eta_{rel}$ is known as the *relative viscosity* of the liquid under test.

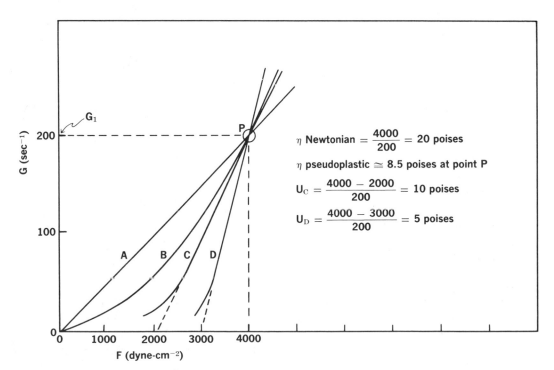

Fig. 17–10. Illustration of errors inherent in the use of a "one-point" instrument for non-Newtonian systems. Regardless of the fact that A is Newtonian, B is pseudoplastic, and C and D are two different plastic systems, a "one-point" instrument could indicate a common viscosity of 20 poises (F = 4000 dynes cm^{-2} and G = 200 sec^{-1}). Use of a "one-point" instrument is proper only in the case of the Newtonian systems. (From A. Martin, G. S. Banker, and A. H. C. Chun, in *Advances in Pharmaceutical Sciences*, H. S. Bean, A. H. Beckett and J. E. Carless, Eds., Academic Press, London, 1964, Chapter 1, reproduced with permission of the copyright owner.)

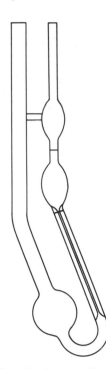

Fig. 17–11. Ostwald–Cannon–Fenske viscometer.

Example 17–4. Consider the viscosity measurement of acetone discussed in *Example 17–1*. Assume that the time required for acetone to flow between the two marks on the capillary viscometer was 45 seconds, and for water the time was 100 seconds at 25° C. The density of acetone is 0.786 g/cm³ and that of water is 0.997 g/cm³ at 25° C. The viscosity of water is 0.8904 centipoise at this temperature. The viscosity of acetone at 25° C may be calculated using equation (17–12):

$$\frac{\eta_1}{0.8904} = \frac{0.786 \times 45.0}{0.997 \times 100}$$

$$\eta_1 = 0.316 \text{ cp}$$

Equation (17–12) is based on *Poiseuille's law* for a liquid flowing through a capillary tube,

$$\eta = \frac{\pi r^4 t\, \Delta P}{8lV} \qquad (17\text{–}13)$$

in which r is the radius of the inside of the capillary, t is the time of flow, ΔP is the pressure head in dyne/cm² under which the liquid flows, l is the length of the capillary, and V is the volume of liquid flowing. Equation (17–12) is obtained from Poiseuille's law (equation (17–13)) as follows. The radius, length, and volume of a given capillary viscometer are invariants and may be combined into a constant, K. Equation (17–13) may then be written

$$\eta = Kt\, \Delta P \qquad (17\text{–}14)$$

The pressure head ΔP depends on the density ρ of the liquid being measured, the acceleration of gravity, and the difference in heights of the liquid levels in the two arms of the viscometer. The acceleration of gravity is a constant, however, and if the levels in the capillary are kept constant for all liquids, we can incorporate these terms in the constant and write for the viscosities of the unknown and the standard liquids:

$$\eta_1 = K't_1\rho_1 \qquad (17\text{–}15)$$

$$\eta_2 = K't_2\rho_2 \qquad (17\text{–}16)$$

Therefore, when the flow periods for two liquids are compared in the same capillary viscometer, the division of (17–15) by (17–16) gives equation (17–12). The U.S. Pharmacopeia XXII, p. 1619, suggested a capillary apparatus for determining the viscosity of high-viscosity types of methylcellulose solutions.

Example 17–5. The Poiseuille equation may be used to calculate the pressure difference in the arteries and capillaries: Figure 17–12 depicts blood circulation in the body.[18] The systolic pressure is normally about 120 mm Hg and the diastolic pressure about 80 mm Hg. Therefore, at rest the average blood pressure is about 100 mm Hg.

The Poiseuille equation (17–13) may be written

$$r = \left(\frac{8\eta l(V/t)}{\pi\Delta P}\right)^{1/4}$$

in which the viscosity, η, of the blood at normal body temperature is 4 cps or 0.04 poise = 0.04 dyne sec cm⁻², and l is the distance, say 1 cm, along an artery. The average rate of blood flow V/t at rest is 80 cm³ sec⁻¹, and the pressure drop ΔP over a distance of 1 cm along the artery is 3.8 mm Hg (1 dyne cm⁻² = 7.5×10^{-4} mm Hg). Calculate

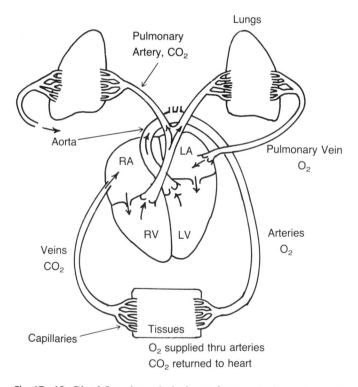

Fig. 17–12. Blood flow through the heart, lungs, arteries, veins, and capillaries. Blood with oxygen bound to hemoglobin is pumped through the left ventricle, LV, of the heart to the arteries and is released in the tissues. Carbon dioxide is taken up by the venous blood and is pumped to the right ventricle, RV, of the heart by way of the right atrium, RA. The blood then passes to the lungs, where carbon dioxide is released and oxygen is taken up. The blood, now rich in oxygen, passes from the lungs to the left atrium, LA, and through the left ventricle, LV, to complete the cycle. See problems 17–15, 17–16, and 17–17 involving the viscosity of flowing blood.

the radius r in cm of the artery. In the following equation, "s" stands for seconds.

$$r \text{ (cm)} = \left(\frac{8(0.04 \text{ dyne s cm}^{-2})(1 \text{ cm})(80 \text{ cm}^3 \text{ s}^{-1})}{\pi(3.8 \text{ mm Hg}) \times (1 \text{ dyne cm}^{-2}/7.50 \times 10^{-4} \text{ mm Hg})} \right)^{1/4}$$

The radius in cm $= (0.001608)^{1/4} = 0.200$ cm.

Falling Sphere Viscometer. In this type of viscometer, a glass or steel ball rolls down an almost vertical glass tube containing the test liquid at a known constant temperature. The rate at which a ball of a particular density and diameter falls is an inverse function of the viscosity of the sample. The Hoeppler viscometer, shown in Figure 17–13, is a commercial instrument based on this principle. The sample and ball are placed in the inner glass tube and allowed to reach temperature equilibrium with the water in the surrounding constant-temperature jacket. The tube and jacket are then inverted, which effectively places the ball at the top of the inner glass tube. The time for the ball to fall between two marks is accurately measured and repeated several times. The viscosity of a Newtonian liquid is then calculated from

$$\eta = t(S_b - S_f)B \qquad (17-17)$$

in which t is the time interval in seconds for the ball to fall between the two points, and S_b and S_f are the specific gravities of the ball and fluid under examination at the temperature being used. B is a constant for a particular ball and is supplied by the manufacturer. Since a variety of glass and steel balls of different diameters are available, this instrument can be used over the range 0.5 to 200,000 poise. For best results, a ball should be used such that t is not less than 30 seconds.

Cup and Bob Viscometer. In cup and bob viscometers, the sample is sheared in the space between the outer wall of a bob and the inner wall of a cup into which the bob fits. The principle is illustrated in Figure 17–14. The various instruments available differ mainly in whether the torque set up in the bob results from the cup or from the bob being caused to revolve. In the

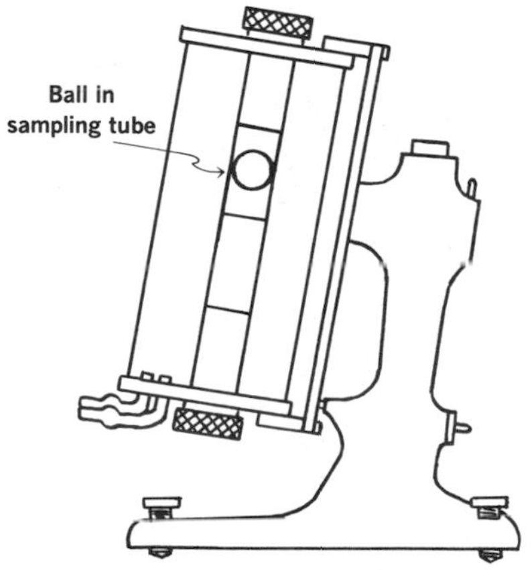

Fig. 17–13. Hoeppler falling ball viscometer.

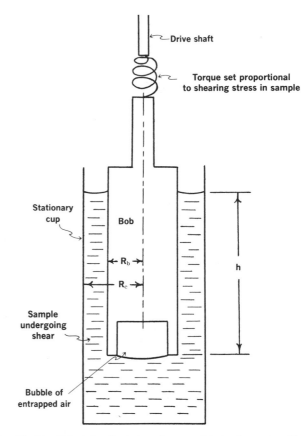

Fig. 17–14. Principle of rotational cup and bob viscometer (Searle type). See text for explanation.

Couette type of viscometer, the cup is rotated. The viscous drag on the bob due to the sample causes it to turn. The resultant torque is proportional to the viscosity of the sample. The MacMichael viscometer is an example of such an instrument. The *Searle* type of viscometer involves the principle of a stationary cup and a rotating bob. The torque resulting from the viscous drag of the system under examination is generally measured by a spring or sensor in the drive to the bob. The Rotovisco viscometer, shown in Figure 17–15, is an example of this type; it can also be modified to operate as a cone and plate instrument.

Example 17–6. The Haake Rotovisco apparatus uses interchangeable measuring heads, MK-50 and MK-500. The shear stress, F, in dyne/cm^2 is obtained from a dial reading S and is calculated using the formula

$$F(\text{dyne/cm}^2) = K_F \cdot S \qquad (17-18)$$

where K_F is a shear stress factor.

The shear rate, G, in sec^{-1}, is proportional to the adjustable speed, n, in revolutions per minute, of the rotating cylinder in the cup containing the sample. The formula for shear rate is

$$G \text{ (sec}^{-1}) = K_G \cdot n \qquad (17-19)$$

where K_G is a shear rate factor that varies with the particular rotating cylinder used. Three cups and cylinders (sensor systems) are supplied with the instrument, MVI, MVII, and MVIII. For the measuring head MK-50 and the sensor system MVI, the values for the constants K_F and K_G are $K_F = 2.95$ dyne/cm^2 and $K_G = 2.35$ min/sec.

In the analysis of a solution of a new glucose derivative, which is found to be Newtonian, the following data were obtained in a typical

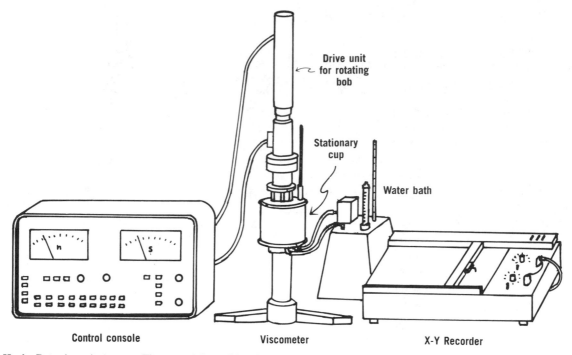

Fig. 17–15. Haake Rotovisco viscometer. The rate of shear G is selected manually or programmed for automatic plotting of up- and down-curves. Its value in $\sec^{-1}$ is proportional to the speed of the bob shaft, dialed in and read as n on the console. The shear stress is read on the scale S or obtained from the rheogram, plotted on the $X–Y$ recorder.

experimental run at 25° C using the Haake viscometer with the MK-50 head and MVI sensor system. With the cylinder rotating at 180 rpm, the dial reading S was obtained as 65.5 scale divisions.[19] Calculate the Newtonian viscosity of the new glucose derivative. What are the values of shear stress, F, and the rate of shear, G?

Using equations (17–18) and (17–19),

$$F = 2.95 \times 65.5 = 193.2 \text{ dyne/cm}^2$$

$$G = 2.35 \times 180 = 423.0 \text{ sec}^{-1}$$

Now, the Newtonian viscosity is readily obtained as

$$\eta = \frac{F}{G} = \frac{193.2}{423.0} = 0.457 \text{ poise, or 45.7 cp}$$

A popular viscometer based on the Searle principle is the Stormer instrument. This viscometer, a modification of that described by Fischer,[20] is shown in Figure 17–16. In operation, the test system is placed in the space between the cup and the bob and allowed to reach temperature equilibrium. A weight is placed on the hanger, and the time for the bob to make 100 revolutions is recorded by the operator. This data is then converted to rpm. The weight is increased and the whole procedure repeated. In this way, a rheogram can be constructed by plotting rpm *versus* weight added. By the use of appropriate constants, the rpm values can be converted to actual rates of shear in sec $^{-1}$. Similarly, the weights added can be transposed into the units of shear stress, namely, dyne cm^{-2}. According to Araujo,[21] the Stormer instrument should not be used with systems having a viscosity below 20 cps.

It can be shown that, for a rotational viscometer, equation (17–1) becomes

$$\Omega = \frac{1}{\eta}\frac{T}{4\pi h}\left(\frac{1}{R_b{}^2} - \frac{1}{R_c{}^2}\right) \qquad (17–20)$$

in which Ω is the angular velocity in radians $\sec^{-1}$ produced by T, the torque in dynes cm. The depth to which the bob is immersed in the liquids is h, while R_b and R_c are the radii of the bob and cup, respectively (see Fig. 17–14). The viscous drag of the sample on the base of the bob is not taken into account by equation (17–20). Either an "end correction" must be applied or, more usually, the base of the bob is recessed, as shown in Figure 17–14. In this case, a pocket of air is entrapped between the sample and the base of the bob, rendering the contribution from the base of the bob negligible. It is frequently more convenient to combine

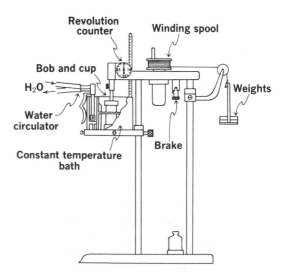

Fig. 17–16. Stormer viscometer. The falling weights cause the bob to rotate in the stationary cup. The velocity of the bob is obtained by means of a stop watch and the revolution counter.

all the constants in equation (17–20), with the result that

$$\eta = K_v \frac{T}{\Omega} \qquad (17–21)$$

in which K_v is a constant for the instrument. With the modified Stormer viscometer, Ω is a function of v, the rpm generated by the weight w, in grams, that is proportional to T. Equation (17–21) may then be written as

$$\eta = K_v \frac{w}{v} \qquad (17–22)$$

The constant K_v may be determined by analyzing an oil of known viscosity in the instrument; reference oils for this purpose are obtained from the National Bureau of Standards.

The equation for plastic viscosity when employing the Stormer viscometer is

$$U - K_v \frac{w - w_f}{v} \qquad (17–23)$$

in which U is the plastic viscosity in poises, w_f is the yield value intercept in grams, and the other symbols have the meaning previously given in equation (17–22).

The yield value of a Bingham body is obtained by use of the expression

$$f = K_f \times w_f \qquad (17–24)$$

in which K_f is equal to

$$K_v \times \frac{2\pi}{60} \times \frac{1}{2.303 \log (R_c/R_b)}$$

in which R_c is the radius of the cup and R_b is the radius of the bob.

Example 17–7. A sample of a gel was analyzed in a modified Stormer viscometer (see Fig. 17–16). A driving weight w of 450 g produced a bob velocity v of 350 rpm. A series of velocities were obtained using other driving weights, and the data were plotted as shown in curve b of Figure 17–2. The yield value intercept w_f was obtained by extrapolating the curve to the shearing stress axis where $v = 0$, and the value of w_f was found to be 225 grams. The instrumental constant K_v is 52.0, and K_f is 20.0. What is the plastic viscosity and the yield value of the sample?

$$U = 52.0 \times \frac{450 - 225}{350} = 33.4 \text{ poises}$$

$$f = 20 \times 225 = 4500 \text{ dyne/cm}^2.$$

The Brookfield Viscometer (Brookfield Engineering, Stoughton, Mass.) is a rotational viscometer of the Searle type that is popular in the quality-control laboratories of pharmaceutical manufacturers. A number of spindles (bobs) of various geometries, including cylinders, t-bars, and a cone–plate configuration, are available to provide scientific rheologic data for Newtonian and non-Newtonian liquids and for empirical viscosity measurements on pastes and other semisolid materials. Various models of the Brookfield Viscometer are available for high-, medium-, and low-viscosity

applications. Figure 17–17 depicts a cone-and-plate type of Brookfield viscometer. The cone–plate viscometer (the Ferranti–Shirley viscometer of Ferranti Ltd.) is described in some detail on pages 466–467.

Plug Flow. One potential disadvantage of the cup and bob viscometer is variable shear stress across the sample between the bob and the cup. We have seen that, in contrast to Newtonian systems, the apparent viscosity of non-Newtonian systems varies with shear stress. With plastic materials, the apparent viscosity below the yield value can be regarded as infinite. Above the yield value, the system possesses a finite viscosity U, the plastic viscosity. In a viscometer of the Searle type, the shear stress close to the rotating bob at relatively low rates of shear may be sufficiently high so as to exceed the yield value. The shear stress at the inner wall of the cup could (and frequently does), however, lie below the yield value. Material in this zone would therefore remain as a solid plug and the measured viscosity would be in error. A major factor determining whether or not *plug flow* occurs is the gap between the cup and the bob. The operator should always use the largest bob possible with a cup of a definite circumference so as to reduce the gap and minimize the chances of plug flow. In a system exhibiting plug flow in the viscometer, more and more of the sample is sheared at a stress above the yield value as

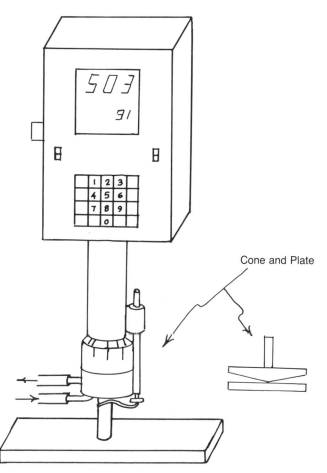

Cone and Plate

Fig. 17–17. A digital-type cone and plate viscometer, Brookfield.

the speed of rotation of the bob is increased. It is only when the shear stress at the wall of the cup exceeds the yield value, however, that the system as a whole undergoes laminar, rather than plug, flow, and the correct plastic viscosity is obtained.

The phenomenon of plug flow is important in the flow of pastes and concentrated suspensions through an orifice, for example, the extrusion of toothpaste from a tube. Thus, the high shear conditions along the inner circumference of the tube aperture cause a drop in consistency. This facilitates extrusion of the material in the core as a plug. This phenomenon is, however, undesirable when attempting to obtain the rheogram of a plastic system with a cup and bob viscometer. The next instrument to be discussed does not suffer from this drawback.

Cone and Plate Viscometer. The Ferranti–Shirley viscometer (Ferranti Ltd., England) is an example of a rotational cone and plate viscometer. The measuring unit of the apparatus is shown in Figure 17–18; the indicator unit and speed control amplifier are not shown. In operation, the sample is placed at the center of the plate, which is then raised into position under the cone, as shown in Figure 17–19.

The cone is driven by a variable-speed motor and the sample is sheared in the narrow gap between the stationary plate and the rotating cone. The rate of shear in revolutions per minute is increased and decreased by a selector dial and the viscous traction or torque (shearing stress) produced on the cone is read on the indicator scale. A plot of rpm or rate of shear versus

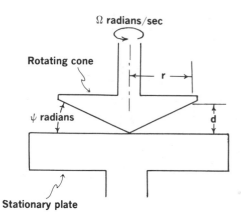

Fig. 17–19. Constant shear rate conditions in the cone and plate viscometer. The cone-to-plate angle, Ψ, is greatly exaggerated here; it is ordinarily less than 1° (< 0.02 radians).

scale reading or shearing stress may thus be constructed in the ordinary manner.

The viscosity in poises of a Newtonian liquid measured in the cone–plate viscometer is calculated by use of the equation

$$\eta = C \frac{T}{v} \qquad (17\text{--}25)$$

in which C is an instrumental constant, T is the torque reading, and v is the speed of the cone in revolutions per minute. For a material showing plastic flow, the plastic viscosity is given by the equation

$$U = C \frac{T - T_f}{v} \qquad (17\text{--}26)$$

and the yield value is given by

$$f = C_f \times T_f \qquad (17\text{--}27)$$

in which T_f is the torque at the shearing stress axis (extrapolated from the linear portion of the curve), and C_f is an instrumental constant.

Example 17–8. A new ointment base was designed and subjected to rheologic analysis at 20° C in a cone–plate viscometer with an instrumental constant C of 6.277 cm^{-3}. At a cone velocity of $v = 125$ rpm the torque reading T was 1287.0 dyne cm. The torque T_f at the shearing stress axis was found to be 63.5 dyne cm.

The plastic viscosity of the ointment base at 20° C was thus calculated using equation (17–26) to be

$$U = \frac{1287 - 63.5}{125} \times 6.277 = 61.44 \text{ poise}$$

The yield value f is obtained using equation (17–27) where $C_f = 113.6$ cm^{-3} for the medium-size cone (radius of 2.007 cm):

$$f = 113.6 \times 63.5 = 7214 \text{ dyne/cm}^2$$

A cone and plate viscometer possesses several significant advantages over the cup and bob type of instrument. Most important is the fact that the rate of shear is constant throughout the entire sample being sheared. As a result, any chance of plug flow is avoided. The principle is illustrated in Figure 17–19, from which it may be seen that G, the rate of shear at any diameter,

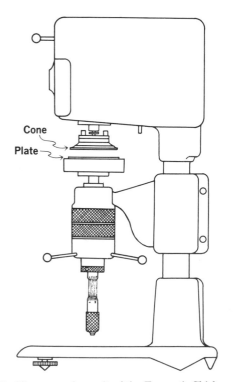

Fig. 17–18. The measuring unit of the Ferranti–Shirley cone–plate viscometer.

is the ratio of the linear velocity $\Omega\, r$ to the gap width, d. Thus,

$$G = \frac{\Omega\, r}{d}\,\frac{\text{cm/sec}}{\text{cm}} \qquad (17\text{--}28)$$

The ratio r/d is a constant and is proportional to ψ, the angle between the cone and the plate in radians. Thus,

$$G = \frac{\Omega}{\psi}\,\sec^{-1} \qquad (17\text{--}29)$$

and is independent of the radius of the cone. The cone angle generally ranges from 0.3° to 4°, with the smaller angles being preferred. Other advantages of a cone and plate viscometer are the time saved in cleaning and filling, and the temperature stabilization of the sample during a run. While a cup and bob viscometer may require 20 to 50 mL of a sample for a determination, the cone and plate viscometer requires a sample volume of only 0.1 to 0.2 mL. By means of a suitable attachment, it is also possible to increase and then decrease the rate of shear in a predetermined, reproducible manner. At the same time, the shear stress is plotted as a function of the rate of shear on an X–Y recorder. This is a valuable aid when determining the area of hysteresis or thixotropic coefficients, for it allows comparative studies to be run in a consistent manner. The use of this instrument in the rheologic evaluation of some pharmaceutical semisolids has been described by Hamlow,[22] Gerding,[23] and Boylan.[24]

VISCOELASTICITY

A number of methods have been used to measure the consistency of pharmaceutical and cosmetic semisolid products. The discussion in this chapter has centered on the fundamentals of continuous or steady shear rheometry of non-Newtonian materials. Oscillatory and creep measurements are also of considerable importance for investigating the properties of semisolid drug products, foods, and cosmetics that are classified as viscoelastic materials.

Continuous shear mainly employs the rotational viscometer and is plotted as flow curves (see Fig. 17–2), which provide useful information by which to characterize and control products in industry. Continuous shear does not keep the material being tested in its rheologic "ground state" but, rather, resorts to gross deformation and alteration of the material during measurement. Analysis of viscoelastic materials is designed instead not to destroy the structure, so that measurements can provide information on the intermolecular and interparticle forces in the material.

Viscoelastic measurements are based on the mechanical properties of materials that exhibit both viscous properties of liquids and elastic properties of solids. Many of the systems studied in pharmacy belong to this class, examples being creams, lotions, ointments, suppositories, suspensions, and the colloidal dispersing, emulsifying, and suspending agents. Biologic materials such as blood, sputum, and cervical fluid also show viscoelastic properties. Whereas steady shear in rotational viscometers and similar flow instruments yield large deformations and may produce false results, oscillatory and creep methods allow the examination of rheologic materials under nearly quiescent equilibrium conditions. Davis[25] described creep and oscillatory methods for evaluating the viscoelastic properties of pharmaceutical materials, and Barry[26] reviewed these methods for pharmaceutical and cosmetic semisolids.

A semisolid is considered to demonstrate both solid and liquid characteristics. The flow of a Newtonian fluid is expressed by using equation (17–2),

$$\eta = F/G$$

relating shear stress F and shear rate G. A solid material, on the other hand, is not characterized by flow but rather by elasticity, and its behavior is expressed by the equation for a spring (derived from Hooke's law of physics):

$$E = F/\gamma \qquad (17\text{--}30)$$

in which E is the elastic modulus (dyne cm^{-2}), F the stress (dyne cm^{-2}), and γ the strain, dimensionless. Using a mechanical model, a viscous fluid may be represented as movement of a piston in a cylinder (or *dashpot*, as it is called) filled with a liquid, as seen in Figure 17–20a. An example of a dashpot is the well-known automobile shock absorber. An elastic solid is modeled by the movement of a Hooke's spring (Fig. 17–20b). The behavior of a semisolid as a viscoelastic body may therefore be described by the combination of the dashpot and spring, as observed in Figure 17–20c. The combination of spring and shock absorber in a car, which provides a relatively smooth ride over rough roads, is analogous to the spring and dashpot of Figure 17–20c.

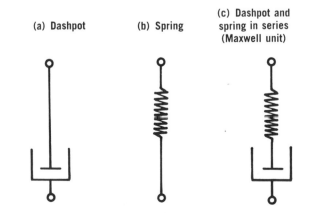

(a) Dashpot   **(b) Spring**   **(c) Dashpot and spring in series (Maxwell unit)**

Fig. 17–20. Mechanical representation of a viscoelastic material using a dashpot and spring. The dashpot and spring in series is called a *Maxwell element* or *unit*.

This mechanical model of a viscoelastic material, a non-Newtonian material showing both viscosity of the liquid state and elasticity of the solid state, and combined in *series* is called a *Maxwell element*. The spring and dashpot may also be combined in a *parallel* arrangement as seen in Figure 17–21. This second model for viscoelasticity is known as a *Voigt element*.

As a constant stress is applied to the Maxwell unit, there is a strain on the material that can be thought of as a displacement of the spring. The applied stress may be thought of as also producing a movement of the piston in the dashpot due to viscous flow. Removal of the stress leads to complete recovery of the spring, but the viscous flow shows no recovery, that is, no tendency to return to its original state. In the Voigt model, the spring and dashpot being attached in parallel rather than series, the drag of the viscous fluid in the dashpot simultaneously influence the extension and compression of the spring which characterizes the solid nature of the material, and the strain will vary in an exponential manner with time. Strain is expressed as a deformation or *compliance*, J, of the test material in which J is strain per unit stress. The compliance of a viscoelastic material following the Voigt model is given as a function of time t by the expression

$$J = J_\infty(1 - e^{-t/\tau}) \qquad (17\text{--}31)$$

in which J_∞ is the compliance or strain per unit stress at infinite time and τ is viscosity per unit modulus, η/E (dyne sec cm^{-2}/dyne cm^{-2}), which is called *retardation time* and has the unit of sec.

The mechanical models, Maxwell and Voigt, representing viscoelastic behavior in two different ways, may be combined into a generalized model to incorporate all possibilities of flow and deformation of non-Newtonian materials. One of several Voigt units may be combined with Maxwell elements to represent the changes that a pharmaceutical solid, such as an ointment or cream, undergoes as it is stressed. As observed in Figure 17–22, two Voigt elements are combined with a Maxwell element to reproduce the behavior of a sample of wool fat[25] at 30° C. The compliance J as a

function of time is measured with an instrument known as a *creep viscometer* (Fig. 17–23) and is plotted in Figure 17–22 to obtain a *creep curve*. The creep curve is observed to be constructed of three parts, first a sharply rising portion AB corresponding to the elastic movement of the uppermost spring; second, a curved portion BC, a viscoelastic region representing the action of the two Voigt units; and third, a linear portion CD corresponding to movement of the piston in the dashpot at the bottom of the Maxwell–Voigt model representing viscous flow.

The compliance equation corresponding to the observed behavior of wool fat (Fig. 17–22), as simulated by the Maxwell–Voigt model (insert (a) in Fig. 17–22), is

$$J = \frac{\gamma_0}{F} + J_m(1 - e^{-t/\tau_m})$$

$$+ J_n(1 - e^{-t/\tau_n}) + \frac{\gamma}{F} \qquad (17\text{--}32)$$

in which γ_0 is the instantaneous strain and F the constant applied shear stress.[25,26] The quantity, γ_0/F, is readily obtained from the experimental curve (region AB) in Figure 17–22. The viscoelastic region of the curve (BC) is represented by the intermediate term of equation (17–32), in which J_m and J_n are the mean compliance of bonds in the material and τ_m *and* τ_n are the mean retardation times for the two Voigt units of Figure 17–22. It is sometimes found that three or more Voigt units are needed in the model to reflect the observed behavior of the material. The final term of equation (17–32) corresponds to the linear portion, CD, of the creep curve. This section represents a condition of Newtonian compliance in which the rupture of bonds leads to the flow of the material, where F is the constant applied stress and γ is the shear strain in this region of the curve.

When stress is removed by the operator of the creep rheometer (Fig. 17–23), a recovery DEF of the sample is obtained. It is composed of an instantaneous elastic recovery, DE, equivalent to AB, followed by an elastic recovery region EF equivalent to BC. In the creep compliance curve of Figure 17–22, flow occurs in region CD, irreversibly destroying the structure, and in the recovery curve this portion is not reproduced. By such an analysis, Davis[25] obtained the elastic moduli (insert (a) of Figure 17–22) $E_0 = 2.7 \times 10^4$ dyne cm^{-1}, $E_1 = 5.4 \times 10^4$ dyne cm^{-1}, and $E_2 = 1.4 \times 10^4$ dyne cm^{-1}; and the three viscosities, $\eta_1 = 7.2 \times 10^5$ poise, $\eta_2 = 4.5 \times 10^6$ poise, and $\eta_0 = 3.1 \times 10^7$ poise for wool fat.

The creep curve used to measure the viscoelasticity of non-Newtonian pharmaceutical, dermatologic, and cosmetic materials may shed some light on the molecular structure of the materials and therefore provide information for modification and improvement of these vehicles. Creep compliance curves were used by Barry[26] to study the changes with temperature in

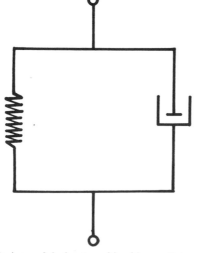

Fig. 17–21. Spring and dashpot combined in parallel as a mechanical model of a viscoelastic material, known as a *Voigt element*.

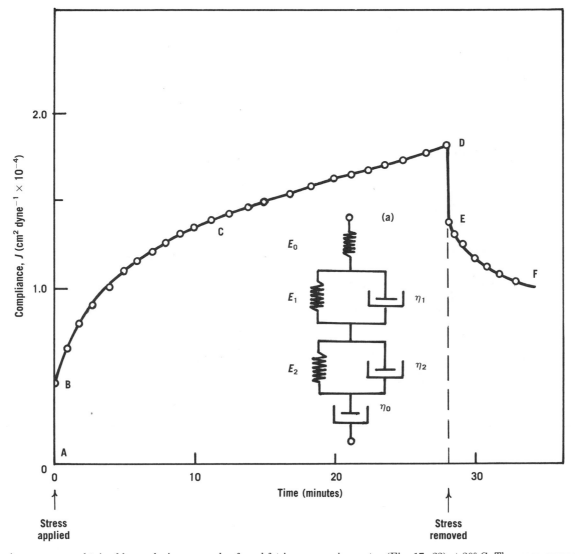

Fig. 17–22. A creep curve obtained by analyzing a sample of wool fat in a creep viscometer (Fig. 17–23) at 30° C. The creep curve results from a plot of compliance, J, equation (17–31), against the time in minutes during which a stress is applied to the sample. (*a*) The insert shows the combination of Maxwell and Voigt elements required to represent the viscoelasticity of the wool fat sample. E_0, E_1, and E_2, the spring moduli, may be calculated from the plot and by use of equation (17–32) and the three viscosities η_1, η_2, and η_0. (From S. S. Davis, Pharm. Acta Helv. **49**, 161, 1974, reproduced with permission of the copyright owner.)

samples of white petrolatum (White Soft Paraffin, British Pharmacopoeia) as observed in Figure 17–24. The behavior was complex, requiring five Voigt units and one Maxwell element to describe the observed creep compliance curves at 5° and 25° C, and three Voigt units at 45° C where some of the structure had been destroyed by melting. Three curves are characteristic of the crystalline bonding and the interaction of crystalline and amorphous material that constitute petrolatum. The curves were automatically plotted on an *X–Y* recorder as the material was stressed in the creep viscometer. The open circles plotted along the lines of Figure 17–24 were obtained by use of an equation similar to equation (17–32), showing the accuracy with which the creep curves can be reproduced by a theoretic model of Voigt and Maxwell units.

Another dynamic rheologic method that does not disturb the structure of a material is that of oscillatory testing.[25–28] A thin layer of material is subjected to an oscillatory driving force in an apparatus such as that shown in Figure 17–25. Another instrument for oscillatory analysis is the rheogoniometer (Martin Sweets Co., Louisville, Ky.). The shearing stress produced by the oscillating force in the membrane apparatus of Figure 17–25 results in a shear rate proportional to the surface velocity of the material. The viscoelastic behavior of materials obtained by oscillatory shear measurements may be analyzed by an extension of the Maxwell spring and dashpot model.

Steady shear methods involving rotational viscometers tend to break down materials under analysis, and although they yield useful data on thixotropy and yield stress, for example, they do not provide information about the original structure and bonding in pharmaceutical and cosmetic semisolids. Viscoelastic analysis performed by creep or oscillatory methods is particu-

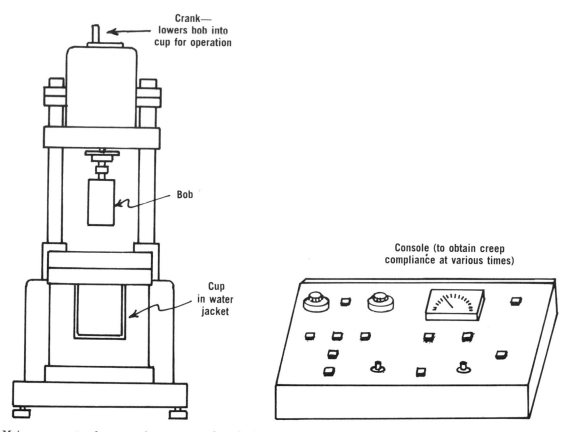

Fig. 17—23. Main components of a creep viscometer used to obtain creep compliance curves such as those found in Figures 17—22 and 17—24.

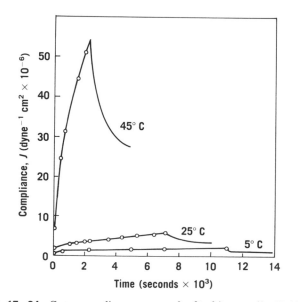

Fig. 17—24. Creep compliance curves of soft white paraffin (British. Pharmacopoeia) at three temperatures. (From B. W. Barry, in *Advances in Pharmaceutical Sciences*, H. S. Bean, A. H. Beckett and J. E. Carless, Eds., Vol. 4, Academic Press, New York, 1974, p. 36, reproduced with permission of the copyright owner.)

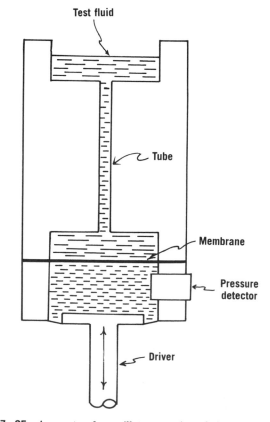

Fig. 17—25. Apparatus for oscillatory testing of viscoelastic materials. (From G. B. Thurston and A. Martin, J. Pharm. Sci. **67,** 1499, 1978, reproduced with permission of the copyright owner.)

larly useful for studying the structure of liquid and semisolid emulsions and gels.[27] Viscoelastic measurements can also be used to measure the rheologic changes occurring in a cream after it is broken down in various stages by milling, incorporation of drugs, or by spreading on the skin.

Radebaugh and Simonelli[29] studied the viscoelastic properties of anhydrous lanolin, which were found to be a function of strain, shear frequency, shear history, and temperature. The energy of activation E_v was calculated for the structural changes of the lanolin sample, which was found to undergo a major mechanical transition between 10° and 15° C. The E_v for the transition was $\cong 90$ kcal, that expected for glass transition. But rather than a sharp change from a rubbery to a glasslike state, anhydrous lanolin appeared to change to a state less ordered than glass. Glass–rubber transition and the glass transition temperature are discussed on pages 586 to 588. The viscoelastic properties were determined using a Rheometrics mechanical spectrometer (RMS 7200, Rheometrics, Inc., Union, N.J.). The rheometer introduces a definite deformation into the sample at a specified rate and at a chosen temperature.

Viscoelastic methods are also of value in the analysis of sputum, for the design of mucolytic agents in the treatment of bronchitis, asthma, and cystic fibrosis. Other biologic fluids such as blood, vaginal material, and synovial fluids may be analyzed by viscoelastic test methods. The unsteady shear to which synovial fluids are subjected in the body during the movement of leg and arm joints requires the elastic properties of these fluids, in addition to viscous properties that are observed only in steady shear. Thurston and Greiling[30] used oscillatory shear to analyze cases of noninflammatory and inflammatory joint disease associated with arthritis. The macromolecule hyaluronic acid is primarily responsible for the high viscosity and non-Newtonian character of synovial fluid and gives it simple Newtonian rather than the desired non-Newtonian properties. Changes in viscoelasticity of synovial fluids, measured in the oscillatory instrument shown in Figure 17–25, may therefore serve as sensitive indicators of joint disease.

PSYCHORHEOLOGY

In addition to desirable pharmaceutical and pharmacologic properties, topical preparations must meet criteria of feel, spreadability, color, odor, and other psychologic and sensory characteristics. Workers in the food industry have long tested products such as butter, chocolate, mayonnaise, and bread dough for proper consistency during manufacture, packaging, and end use. Sensations in the mouth, between the fingers, and on the skin are important considerations for manufacturers of foods, cosmetics, and dermatologic products.

Scott-Blair[31] discussed *psychorheology* (as this subject is called) in the food industry. Kostenbauder and Martin[32] assessed the spreadability of ointments in relation to their rheologic properties. In consultation with dermatologists, they divided the products into three classes. Class I products were soft, mainly for ophthalmic use; Class II included common medicated ointments of intermediate consistency; and Class III involved stiff protective products for use in moist ulcerative conditions. The yield values and plastic viscosity for each class of product were reported.

Boylan[24] has shown that the thixotropy, consistency, and yield value of bacitracin ointment, USP, decreased markedly as the temperature was raised from 20° to 35° C. Thus, while a product may be sufficiently thixotropic in its container, this property can be lost following application to the skin.

Barry et al.[33] carried out sensory testing on topical preparations. They used a panel to differentiate textural parameters and established rheologic methods for use in industry as control procedures to maintain uniform skin feel and spreadability of dermatologic products. Cussler et al.[34] studied the texture of non-Newtonian liquids of widely different rheologic properties applied to the skin. It was found that the consistency of a material could be accurately assessed by a panel of untrained subjects by the use of only three attributes: smoothness, thinness, and warmth. Smoothness was related to a coefficient of friction, and thinness to non-Newtonian viscous parameters that could be measured with appropriate instruments. The characteristic of warmth was found to be sufficiently complex to require further study.

APPLICATIONS TO PHARMACY

The rheologic behavior of poloxamer vehicles was studied as a function of concentration over a temperature range of 5° to 35° C using a cone–plate viscometer.[35] Poloxamers are block polymers of BASF Wyandotte Corp., having the chemical structure

$$HO(CH_2CH_2O)_a \, (CH[CH_3]CH_2O)_b \, (CH_2CH_2O)_c \, H$$

Poloxamers with a wide range of molecular weights are available as Pluronics®. Some of the poloxamers are used in the dermatologic bases or topical ophthalmic preparations because of their low toxicity and their ability to form clear water-based gels.

The aqueous solubility of the poloxamers decreases with an increase in temperature, the hydration of the polymer being reduced by breaking of hydrogen bonds at higher temperatures. The desolvation that results, together with the entanglement of the polymer chains, probability accounts for the gel formation of the poloxamers.

A linear relationship was found between shear rate and shear stress (Newtonian behavior) for the poloxamer vehicles in the sol state, which exists at low concentrations and low temperatures. As the concentration and temperature were increased, some of the poloxamers exhibited a sol–gel transformation and became non-Newtonian in their rheologic character. The addition of sodium chloride, glycerin, or propylene glycol resulted in increased apparent viscosities of the vehicles.

Polymer solutions may be used in ophthalmic preparations, as wetting solutions for contact lens, and as tear replacement solutions for the condition known as *dry eye syndrome.* Both natural (e.g., dextran) and synthetic (e.g., polyvinyl alcohol) polymers are used with the addition of various preservatives. A high-molecular-weight preparation of sodium hyaluronate at concentrations of 0.1 to 0.2% has been introduced to overcome the dry eye condition.

For high-polymer solutions, the viscosity levels off to a *zero shear viscosity* (a high viscosity) at low shear rates. The viscosity decreases as the shear rate is increased, for the normally twisted and matted polymer molecules align in the streamlined flow pattern and exhibit pseudoplasticity or shear thinning.

Bothner and colleagues[36] suggest that a suitable tear substitute should have shear thinning properties as do natural tears, to conform to the low shear rate during non-blinking and the very high shear rate during blinking. The low viscosity at high shear rates produces lubrication during blinking, and the high viscosity at zero shear rate prevents the fluid from flowing away from the cornea when the lids are not blinking. Using a computer-controlled Couette viscometer, the rheologic properties of eight commercial tear substitutes, together with 0.1% and 0.2% solutions of sodium hyaluronate, were studied. For five of the commercial products, the viscosity was independent of shear rate; thus, these products behaved as Newtonian liquids. Two products showed slight shear thinning at high shear rates. Only the commercial product Neo-Tears and the two noncommercial sodium hyaluronate solutions showed the desired pseudoplastic behavior. For Neo-Tears the viscosity at high shear rate, 1000 sec^{-1}, was threefold that at zero shear. For 0.1% sodium hyaluronate the value was fivefold and for 0.2% sodium hyaluronate it was thirtyfold. Therefore, sodium hyaluronate appears to be an excellent candidate as a tear replacement solution.

The rheologic properties of suppositories at rectal temperatures can influence the release and bioabsorption of drugs from suppositories, particularly those having a fatty base. Grant and Liversidge[37] studied the characteristics of triglyceride suppository bases at various temperatures using a rotational rheometer. Depending on the molten (melted) character of the base, it behaved either as Newtonian material or as a plastic with thixotropy.

Fong-Spaven and Hollenbeck[38] studied the rheologic properties as a function of the temperature of mineral oil–water emulsions stabilized with triethanolamine stearate (TEAS). The stress required to maintain a constant rate of shear was monitored as the temperature was raised from 25° to 75° C. Unexpected, but reproducible, discontinuities in the plots of temperature versus apparent viscosity were obtained using a Brookfield digital viscometer (see p. 465), and were attributed possibly to shifts in the liquid crystalline (pp. 36–37) structures. As seen in Figure 17–26, where apparent viscosity is plotted versus temperature for a 5% TEAS mineral oil–water emulsion, the viscosity decreases as temperature is raised to about 48° C. The viscosity reverses and increases to a small peak at 54° C, and then decreases again with increasing temperature. This unusual behavior is considered to result from gel formation, which stabilizes the internal phase. Liquid crystalline structures of TEAS exist and at higher temperatures the structures disintegrate or "melt" to form a large number of TEAS molecules in a gel-like arrangement that exhibits an increased resistance to flow. As the temperature rises above 54° C the gel structure is gradually destroyed and the viscosity again decreases, as shown in Figure 17–26.

Patterned after the manufacture and use of cosmetic sticks, solidified sodium stearate–based sticks were prepared and tested for topical application using a Ferranti–Shirley cone–plate viscometer. The sticks contained propylene glycol (PG), polyethylene glycol 400 and polyethylene glycol 600 (PEG 400 and PEG 600) as humectants, and the topically active drugs panthenol, chlorphenesin, and lignocaine. Thixotropic breakdown was much lower in these medicated sticks than in comparable bases. The addition of the three topical drugs to the stearate-based sticks caused changes in the yield values, thixotropy, and plastic viscosity; possible reasons for the changes were advanced.[39]

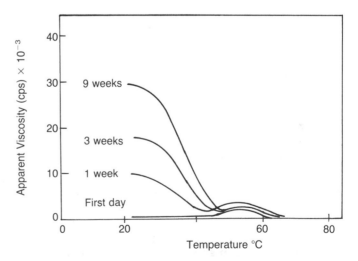

Fig. 17–26. Viscosity versus temperature plots of an oil–water emulsion over a period of 9 weeks. (From F. Fong-Spaven and R. G. Hollenbeck, Drug Dev. Ind. Pharm. **12,** 289, 1986, reproduced with permission of the copyright owner.)

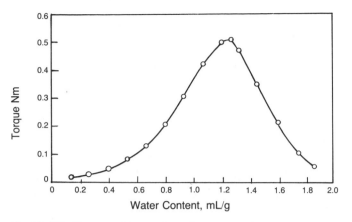

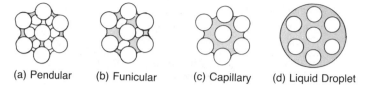

(a) Pendular   (b) Funicular   (c) Capillary   (d) Liquid Droplet

Fig. 17–28. The states of liquid saturation of a powder. (*a*) *Pendular* state with lenses of liquid at the contact points of the particles. (*b*) A mixture of liquid and air between the particles, producing the *funicular* state. (*c*) Pores filled with liquid to yield the *capillary* state. (*d*) Liquid droplets completely enveloping particles (the *liquid-droplet* state). (Modified from D. M. Newitt and J. M. Conway-Jones, Trans. Inst. Chem. Eng. **36**, 422, 1958.)

Fig. 17–27. Changes of torque in a mixer torque rheometer as water is added to a mixture of powders. (From R. C. Rowe and G. R. Sadeghnejad, Int. J. Pharm. **38**, 227, 1987, reproduced with permission of the copyright owner.)

Rowe and Sadeghnejad[40] studied the rheologic properties of microcrystalline cellulose,* an ingredient incorporated in wet powder masses to facilitate the granulation process in the manufacture of tablets and granules. The authors designed a *mixer torque rheometer* to measure the torque changes as water was added to the powder mixture. (*Torque* is the force acting to produce rotation of a body.) As the mixture became wetter the torque increased until the mass was saturated, then decreased with further addition of water as a slurry (suspension) was formed. A plot of torque in Newton meters (1 Nm = 1 joule) against increasing water content produced a bell-shaped curve, as shown in Figure 17–27. This behavior was explained, according to the authors, by the three states of liquid saturation of a powder mass, as described by Newitt and Conway-Jones.[41]

With the early addition of liquid, a *pendular state* exists (see Fig. 17–28) with lenses of liquid at the contact points of the particles. The liquid forces out some of the air originally filling all the spaces between the particles. As more liquid is added, a mixture of liquid and air exists between the particles to produce the *funicular state.* The torque on the mixer increases for these two conditions until the end of the funicular state. The pores are then filled with liquid to yield the *capillary state,* and with the addition of more liquid the torque decreases as a slurry (suspension) is produced *(liquid-droplet state).* These stages of saturation are depicted schematically in Figure 17–28.

The three microcrystalline celluloses from different sources[40] exhibited essentially the same plot of torque versus water added (see Fig. 17–27). Yet the curves, only one of three shown here, rose to slightly different heights and the maxima occurred at different amounts of water added.

*Avicel of FMC Corp., Philadelphia; Emcocel of Finnish Sugar Co., Helsinki; Unimac of Unitika Rayon, Osaka.

An account of the rheology of suspensions, emulsions, and semisolids is presented in Chapter 18, while the flow properties of powders have been dealt with in Chapter 16. Consideration has also been given in Chapter 15 to the rheology of colloid materials, which find wide application in pharmacy as suspending agents. Some of the rheologic aspects of parenteral suspensions and emulsions have been considered by Boylan.[24]

A summary of the major areas of product design and processing in which rheology is significant are listed in Table 17–3. While the effects of processing can affect the flow properties of pharmaceutical systems, a detailed discussion of this area is outside the scope of our text. For an account of this topic, as well as a comprehensive presentation of the theoretic and instrumental aspects of rheology, refer to the review by Martin et al.[3] The theory and application of viscoelasticity have been briefly reviewed in the previous section. Detailed discussions of this approach are given in the references cited.

TABLE 17–3. *Pharmaceutical Areas in which Rheology is Significant**

1. Fluids
   a. Mixing
   b. Particle-size reduction of disperse systems with shear
   c. Passage through orifices, including pouring, packaging in bottles, and passage through hypodermic needles
   d. Fluid transfer, including pumping and flow through pipes
   e. Physical stability of disperse systems
2. Quasisolids
   a. Spreading and adherence on the skin
   b. Removal from jars or extrusion from tubes
   c. Capacity of solids to mix with miscible liquids
   d. Release of the drug from the base
3. Solids
   a. Flow of powders from hoppers and into die cavities in tabletting or into capsules during encapsulation
   b. Packagability of powdered or granular solids
4. Processing
   a. Production capacity of the equipment
   b. Processing efficiency

*With permission from A. Martin, G. S. Banker and A. H. C. Chun, in *Advances in Pharmaceutical Sciences,* H. S. Bean, A. H. Beckett and J. E. Carless, Eds., Academic Press, London, 1964, Chapter 1. Copyright, Academic Press Inc. (London) Ltd.

References

1. E. K. Fischer, J. Colloid Sci. **3**, 73, 1948.
2. G. W. Scott-Blair, Pharm. J. **154**, 3, 1945.
3. A. Martin, G. S. Banker and A. H. C. Chun, in *Advances in Pharmaceutical Sciences*, H. S. Bean, A. H. Beckett and J. E. Carless, Eds., Academic Press, London, 1964, Chapter 1.
4. S. P. Kabre, H. G. DeKay and G. S. Banker, J. Pharm. Sci. **53**, 492, 1964.
5. E. E. Hamlow, Ph.D. Correlation of Rheological Methods for Measuring Newtonian and Non-Newtonian Materials. Thesis, Purdue University, 1958.
6. R. Shangraw, W. Grim and A. M. Mattocks, Trans. Soc. Rheology, **5**, 247, 1961; N. Casson, in *Rheology of Disperse Systems*, C. C. Mill, Ed., Pergamon Press, New York, 1959, pp. 84–104; T. C. Patton, *Paint Flow and Pigment Dispersion*, 2nd Edition, Wiley, 1979, Chapter 16.
7. G. J. Yakatan and O. E. Araujo, J. Pharm. Sci. **57**, 155, 1968.
8. M. Reiner and G. W. Scott-Blair, in *Rheology*, vol. 4, F. E. Eirich, Ed., Academic Press, New York, 1967, Chapter 9.
9. S. S. Ober, H. C. Vincent, D. E. Simon and K. J. Frederick, J. Am. Pharm. Assoc., Sci. Ed. **47**, 667, 1958.
10. C. W. Chong, S. P. Eriksen and J. W. Swintosky, J. Am. Pharm. Assoc., Sci. Ed. **49**, 547, 1960.
11. J. C. Samyn and W. Y. Jung, J. Pharm. Sci. **56**, 188, 1967.
12. H. Freundlich and F. Juliusburger, Trans. Faraday Soc. **31**, 920, 1935.
13. S. S. Ober, H. C. Vincent, D. E. Simon and K. J. Frederick, J. Am. Pharm. Assoc., Sci. Ed. **47**, 667, 1958.
14. G. Levy, J. Pharm. Sci. **51**, 947, 1962.
15. E. Hatschek, *Viscosity of Liquids*, Bell and Sons, London, 1928.
16. P. Sherman, in *Emulsion Science*, Academic Press, London, 1968, p. 221.
17. J. R. Van Wazer, J. W. Lyons, K. Y. Kim and R. E. Colwell, *Viscosity and Flow Measurement—A Laboratory Handbook of Rheology*, Interscience, New York, 1963.
18. R. Chang, *Physical Chemistry with Applications to Biological Systems*, 2nd Edition, Macmillan, New York, 1981, pp. 76, 77, 93.
19. B. Millan-Hernandez, *Properties and Design of Pharmaceutical Suspensions*, M. S. Thesis, University of Texas, 1981.
20. E. K. Fischer, *Colloidal Dispersions*, Wiley, New York, 1950, Chapter 5.
21. O. E. Araujo, J. Pharm. Sci. **56**, 1023, 1967.
22. E. E. Hamlow, Ph.D. Thesis, Purdue University, 1958.
23. T. G. Gerding, Ph.D. Thesis, Purdue University, 1961.
24. J. C. Boylan, Bull. Parent. Drug Assoc. **19**, 98, 1965; J. Pharm. Sci. **55**, 710, 1966.
25. S. S. Davis, Pharm. Acta Helv. **49**, 161, 1974.
26. B. W. Barry, in *Advances in Pharmaceutical Sciences*, H. S. Bean, A. H. Beckett, and J. E. Carless, Eds., Vol. 4, Academic Press, New York, 1974, pp. 1–72.
27. G. B. Thurston and S. S. Davis, J. Coll. Interface Sci. **69**, 199, 1979.
28. G. B. Thurston and A. Martin, J. Pharm. Sci. **67**, 1949, 1978.
29. G. W. Radebaugh and A. P. Simonelli, J. Pharm. Sci., **72**, 415, 422, 1983; ibid. **73**, 590, 1984.
30. G. B. Thurston and H. Greiling, Rheol. Acta **17**, 433, 1978.
31. G. W. Scott-Blair, *Elementary Rheology*, Academic Press, New York, 1969.
32. H. B. Kostenbauder and A. Martin, J. Am. Pharm. Assoc., Sci. Ed. **43**, 401, 1954.
33. B. W. Barry and A. J. Grace, J. Pharm. Sci. **60**, 1198, 1971; J. Pharm. Sci. **61**, 335, 1972; B. W. Barry and M. C. Meyer, J. Pharm. Sci. **62**, 1349, 1973.
34. E. L. Cussler, S. J. Zlolnick and M. C. Shaw, Perception and Psychophysics, **21**, 504, 1977.
35. S. C. Miller and B. R. Drabik, Int. J. Pharm. **18**, 269, 1984.
36. H. Bothner, T. Waaler and O. Wik, Drug Dev. Ind. Pharm. **16**, 755, 1990.
37. D. J. W. Grant and G. G. Liversidge, Drug Dev. Ind. Pharm. **9**, 247, 1983.
38. F. Fong-Spaven and R. G. Hollenbeck, Drug Dev. Ind. Pharm. **12**, 289, 1986.
39. A. G. Mattha, A. A. Kassem and G. K. El-Khatib, Drug Dev. Ind. Pharm. **10**, 111, 1984.
40. R. C. Rowe and G. R. Sadeghnejad, Int. J. Pharm. **38**, 227, 1987.
41. D. M. Newitt and J. M. Conway-Jones, Trans. Inst. Chem. Eng., **36**, 422, 1958.

Problems

17-1. (a) Following *Example 17-2*, compute the energy of activation, E_v, and the Arrhenius factor A using the viscosity data for water in the *CRC Handbook of Chemistry and Physics*, for example, page F-40, 63rd Edition. Use the logarithmic form of the expression (equation (17–6)) analogous to the Arrhenius equation.

(b) Utilize the values of E_v and A together with the Arrhenius-like equation to back-calculate the viscosity in units of cp for water at 29°, 45°, and 88° C. Compare your results with the data in the CRC table for water at these three temperatures.

Answer:

Temperature °C	29°	45°	88°
η (cp) (calculated)	0.8484	0.6231	0.3114
1982–83 CRC Handbook, p. F-40	0.8148	0.5960	0.3221

17-2. The following data were collected when a sample of zinc oxide in liquid petrolatum was analyzed at 25° C in a Stormer viscometer, Figure 17–16: $w = 1800$ g, $w_f = 1420$ g, $v = 500$ rpm, and $K_v = 50$. What is the plastic viscosity in poises of this sample?

Answer: 38 poises

17-3. A 1.0% solution of a high-viscosity grade of sodium carboxymethylcellulose was analyzed at 27° C in a Haake Rotovisco viscometer (Fig. 17–15). The solution was observed to be pseudoplastic; thus the exponential, $F^N = \eta'G$, was used to fit the data using the logarithmic form, equation (17–9), and the data from the following table,

Data for *Problem 17-3:*

Scale Reading S at Various Revolutions per Minute, n

n	25	50	75	100	150	200	300
S	40	52	60	72	81	89	100

(a) Plot G versus F and $\ln G$ versus $\ln F$ on separate graphs. F is calculated from equation (17–18) in which K_F, an instrumental constant, has been found using reference oils to have a value of 21.34. S is the scale reading (for shearing stress, F) of the instrument.

The revolutions per minute of the rotating bob are converted to shear rates, G by multiplying the revolutions per minute, n, for a particular cup and rotating cylinder by an instrumental constant, K_G, which has a value of 18.75. G is computed from equation (17–19). Convert the raw data of the above table into G, F, $\ln G$, and $\ln F$ so as to answer part (a).

(b) Calculate N and η' for this dispersion of high viscosity sodium carboxymethylcellulose.

(c) Describe the significance of N.

(d) Using the value of N and $\ln \eta'$ that you obtain from linear regression analysis, back-calculate F, the shear stress, when G, the rate of shear, has a value of 1875 sec^{-1}. Compare your result with the value of F obtained under (a).

Partial Answer: **(a)** For n (rpm) = 100, $G = 1875$ sec^{-1}; for S (scale reading) = 72, $F = 1536.5$ dyne/cm^2. **(b)** $N = 2.624$ (a dimensionless number); $\eta' = 106,724$ poise (dyne sec/cm^2). **(d)** When the shear rate G is 1875 sec^{-1} the shear stress F has a value, by back-calculation, of 1457 dyne cm^{-2}. *Note:* η', the antiln of $\ln \eta'$, is a rather large number. The student should not be surprised to find η' in the thousands or millions of poise.

Another approach to solving for F is as follows. One begins with the expression $\ln G = -\ln \eta' + N \ln F$ and from regression analysis using this equation one obtains $\eta' = 106{,}724$ and $N = 2.6239$. Therefore, using $F^N = \eta' G$, for $G = 1875 \text{ sec}^{-1}$,

$$F^{2.6239} = (106{,}724)(1875) = 2.00107 \times 10^8$$

Using the y^x key on a hand calculator, the student may run through the exercise, $2^3 = 8$; therefore; $2 = 8^{1/3}$. With this kind of operation applied in our problem, $F^{2.6239} = 200{,}107{,}000$, $F = 200{,}107{,}000^{1/2.6239}$ $= 200{,}107{,}000^{0.381112}$; $F = 1458 \text{ dyne/cm}^2$.

17–4. The following data were obtained at 25° C for a plastic system by means of a cup-and-bob viscometer. Calculate the yield value, f, and the plastic viscosity U of this material.

Data for *Problem 17–4*

G, rate of shear (sec^{-1})	F, shearing stress (dynes cm^{-2})
100	10,200
200	11,200
300	12,200
400	13,200
500	14,200
600	15,200

Answer: f (yield value) $= 9200 \text{ dyne cm}^{-2}$; $U = 10$ poise

17–5. Based on Figure 17–5, calculate the plastic viscosities U_1 and U_2 and the thixotropic coefficient B, given the following data obtained at 25° C:

The constant rate of shear G is 240 sec^{-1}, while t_1 and t_2 are 50 and 80 seconds, respectively. Points c and d in Figure 17–5 have shearing stresses F of 9440 and 6728 dyne cm^{-2}, respectively. The yield value f in both cases is 5000 dyne cm^{-2}, since both down-curves intersect the F-axis at this shearing stress.

Answer: $U_1 = 18.5$ poise; $U_2 = 7.2$ poise; $B = 24$ dyne sec/cm^2

17–6. A sample of petrolatum was analyzed in a Stormer viscometer at 25° C. To obtain the coefficient of thixotropic breakdown M, two upcurves were run, the upper curve having a top rate of shear of $v_1 = 543$ rpm and the lower of $v_2 = 325$ rpm. The values of the constants were $K_v = 40.5$ and $K_f = 15.9$. The driving weights in grams w_1 and w_2 for the two shear rates v_1 and v_2 were found from the flow curves to be $w_1 = 269$ g and $w_2 = 225$ g. The yield value intercepts for the two curves were $w_{f_1} = 124$ g and $w_{f_2} = 96$ g. Compute the plastic viscosities, yield values, and the coefficient of thixotropic breakdown, M.

Answer: $U_1 = 11$ poise, $U_2 = 16$ poise; $f_1 = 1972 \text{ dyne cm}^{-2}$, $f_2 = 1526 \text{ dyne cm}^{-2}$; $M = 10 \text{ dyne sec cm}^{-2}$

17–7. In calibrating the cup-and-bob combination of a Stormer viscometer, an N.B.S. Newtonian oil with a viscosity of 200.0 poise at 20° C was used. With a weight of 1600 g on the weight hanger, the bob rotated at 400 rpm. Compute the instrumental constant K_v.

Answer: 50 poise/(g min)

17–8. To calibrate rotational viscometers, viscosity data are collected[5] using a standardized Newtonian oil from the National Bureau of Standards or from other reference sources. The carefully determined viscosity of oil #4 at 25° C is 1.455 poise. The weights in grams placed on the weight hanger of a Stormer viscometer and the velocity (v) of the rotating cylinder in revolutions per minute (rpm) are recorded here at 25° C.

Data (a) for *Problem 17–8*

Mass (g)	50	100	150	200	250	300
rpm (v)	67.5	137	202	270	337	400

Plot the velocity in rpm (vertical or y-axis of the graph) versus mass in grams on the weight hanger of the Stormer viscometer (horizontal or x-axis). The equation for calculating Newtonian viscosity is

$$\eta = K_v \left(\frac{\text{mass in grams}}{\text{velocity in rpm}} \right) \qquad (17\text{--}33)$$

or

$$\text{rpm} = \frac{K_v}{\eta} (\text{mass}) \qquad (17\text{--}34)$$

The slope (y/x) of the line, using linear regression, provides the value of rpm/mass $= K_v/\eta$, and knowing the viscosity at 25° C of the oil viscosity standard, it is possible to obtain an accurate value of the instrumental constant, K_v, using the experimentally obtained data in the table above.

Once the constant K_v is found for the Stormer viscometer, it is possible to calculate the viscosity of a Newtonian oil of unknown consistency. The slopes (rpm/mass) of the plots of rpm versus mass for these N.B.S. oils at 25° C are:

Data (b) for *Problem 17–8*

Oil number	1	6	9
Slope (K_v/η)	0.2160	2.7933	18.5185

The Newtonian viscosities of these oils at 25° C have been determined by the National Bureau of Standards and have the values

Data (c) for *Problem 17–8*

Oil number	1	6	9
Viscosity (poise)	9.344	0.6725	0.09134

Using the K_v value calculated for the Stormer viscometer, compute the viscosities of the three Newtonian oils using equation (17–33). Compare these results with the accurate viscosity values obtained by the National Bureau of Standards.

Partial Answer: $K_v = 1.9376$; viscosity of oil no. 1 $= 8.970$ poise. From the table above, the N.B.S. value for oil number 1 is 9.344 poise. Our result is therefore in error by 4%.

17–9. A liquid flavoring concentrate for a cough syrup was analyzed at 25° C in a Stormer viscometer having an instrumental constant, $K_v = 8.460$ poise/(g min). The rates of shear in rpm for various weights on the weight hanger are:

Data for *Problem 17–9*

Weights (g)	160	240	320	480
rpm (v)	227	340	452	680

Plot the rpm versus weight on the weight hanger and calculate the viscosity of the flavoring agent. Is it a Newtonian or non-Newtonian liquid? The slope, (rpm/wt), may be obtained by linear regression or by the two-point formula (p. 8, 9).

Answer: $\eta = 597.7$ cps. A plot of the data shows the liquid to be Newtonian.

17–10. (a) The Ferranti–Shirley cone–plate viscometer was used to determine the viscosity of a Newtonian oil at 30° C. The torque reading T was found to be 120 at an rpm of 55. The instrument constant C is 1.168 for the large cone used. Compute the viscosity.

(b) An o/w mineral oil emulsion was found to show plastic flow when analyzed in the cone–plate viscometer. Calculate the plastic viscosity of the emulsion using the following data: torque, T = 110 at rpm – 200 and T_f = 25 at rpm = 0, C = 1.168.

(c) Calculate the yield value f for the emulsion in part (b). The yield value is obtained by the use of the equation $f = 0.122 \times T_f$ when the large cone is employed in the Ferranti–Shirley viscometer.

Answers: **(a)** 2.55 poise; **(b)** 0.50 poise; **(c)** 3.1 dyne/cm^2

17–11. To obtain the Newtonian viscosity of three oils in a cone–plate viscometer, the following cone speeds, v (rpm) were held constant and the torque values, T (dyne cm), for the oils were obtained at 25° C.

Data for *Problem 17–11*

Oil number	1	2	3
Torque, T (dyne cm)	169	95.0	49.4
Cone speed, v (rpm)	73.0	73.0	73.0

The large cone was used, having an instrumental constant $C = 1.168$. The constant, C, takes account of the dimensions such that when T is given in dyne cm and v in rpm, the viscosity is given in poise.

Partial Answer: For oil no. 1, η = 2.704 poise

17–12. The yield value f and plastic viscosity U of a gel of lithium stearate and liquid petrolatum were determined in a cone–plate viscometer at 23° C following equations (17–26) and (17–27) on page 466. T_f, the torque reading at the yield value, i.e., the torque extrapolated to the shearing stress axis, was found experimentally to have a value of 34.51 dyne cm.

The instrumental constant C_f is obtained from the equation

$$C_f = \frac{3S}{2\pi R^3}$$

in which S is a torque spring constant, a dimensionless number equal to 1923; R is the radius of the cone, 2.007 cm; and π = 3.14159, the ratio of the circumference to the diameter of a circle.

(a) What is the value of the instrumental constant, C_f?

(b) Calculate the yield value f for the gel for which T_f is 34.51 dyne cm.

(c) If T, the torque reading, is found to be 137.74 dyne cm at a rotational velocity of the cone of 73.0 rpm and C = 6.277 cm^{-3}, what is the plastic viscosity of the gel?

Answers: **(a)** C_f = 113.57 cm^{-3}; **(b)** f = 3919 dyne cm^{-2}; **(c)** U = 8.876 poise

17–13. Use an Ostwald viscometer at 20° C the time for the flow of water through the apparatus is 297.3 seconds. When the instrument was dried and filled with carbon disulfide, the time of flow was 85.1 sec. The density of water at 20° C is 0.9982 and that of CS$_2$ is 1.2632 g/mL. The viscosity of water at 20° C is 1.002 cp. What is the viscosity of carbon disulfide at 20° C.

Answer: Check your result for the viscosity of CS$_2$ at 20° C against the value in a handbook of chemistry.

17–14. (a) The time for water to flow through an Ostwald pipette at 20° C was 297.3 sec. The density of water at 20° C is 0.9982 and the density of a sample of olive oil is 0.910 g/mL. The viscosity of water at 20° C is 1.002 cp and the viscosity of the sample of olive oil is 84.0 cp. How long will it take for the olive oil to flow through the Ostwald pipette at 20° C?

(b) Would you reason that water was a good choice to use as the reference liquid in this experiment? What other liquid might you choose and on what basis would you choose it? Would it be wise to use an Ostwald pipette with a larger or smaller bore to determine the viscosity of olive oil?

Answer: 27339 sec or 7.59 hours

17–15. The radius of a vascular capillary in the body is approximately 1 to 10 μm (10^{-4} to 10^{-3} cm), the viscosity of blood at 37° C is about 0.04 dyne sec cm^{-2}, and the average rate of blood flow V/t is 1.20×10^{-6} cm^3 sec^{-1}. See Figure 17–12 for a schematic of the anatomy of the heart, capillaries, and other vessels. What is the pressure drop in mm Hg over a distance of 0.5 cm along the capillary with a radius of 8.45×10^{-4} cm? Use the Poiseuille law (equation (17–13)).

Answer: ΔP = 90 mm Hg. Now, convert to SI units: $\Delta P = 1.20 \times 10^4$ N m^{-2}

17–16. The viscosity η of whole blood at body temperature, 37° C (310° K), is 0.04 poise (dyne sec/cm^2). The pressure drop ΔP is 20 mm Hg, or 2.67×10^4 dyne/cm^2, over a distance ℓ of 3.2 mm in the capillary. The radius, r, of the capillary is 0.0012 cm. (*Note:* From a table of conversion factors 20 mm Hg × 1333.25 dyne cm^{-2}/mm Hg = 2.67×10^4 dyne cm^{-2}.) What is the volume rate, V/t, of blood flow in the capillary? The flow of blood in the body is shown in Figure 17–12.

Answer: V/t = 1.70×10^{-6} cm^3/sec

17–17. The volume rate of blood flow in the aorta (see Figure 17–12) of a patient where the radius of the artery is approximately 0.5 cm was measured and found to be V/t = 4.8 cm^3/sec. The pressure difference ΔP over a distance of ℓ = 1 cm was 0.0052 mm Hg (*Note:* 0.0052 torr (or mm Hg) × 1333.22 (dyne/cm^2)/mm Hg = 6.93 dyne/cm^2.) Calculate the viscosity of the patient's blood at 37° C using the Poiseuille equation, page 462.

Answer: The viscosity of the patient's blood was also measured in a capillary viscometer at 37° C and found to be 0.0372 poise. How does your calculated result compare with this experimentally determined viscosity of the blood?

17–18. Explain how one would set up a sensory testing panel and carry out a psychorheologic study to correlate the properties of commercial hand lotions in relation to client acceptance.

Answer: See several of the works listed under references 31 to 34.

18
Coarse Dispersions

Particulate systems have been classified previously (Table 15–1, p. 394) on the basis of size into molecular dispersions (Chapter 5), colloidal systems (Chapter 15), and coarse dispersions (this chapter). The present discussion attempts to provide the pharmacist with an insight into the role of physics and chemistry in the research and development of the several classes of coarse dispersions. The theory and technology of these important pharmaceutical classes are based on interfacial and colloidal principles, micromeritics, and rheology. These topics have been introduced in the four previous chapters.

SUSPENSIONS

A pharmaceutical suspension is a coarse dispersion in which insoluble solid particles are dispersed in a liquid medium. The particles have diameters for the most part greater than 0.1 μm, and some of the particles are observed under the microscope to exhibit Brownian movement if the dispersion has a low viscosity.

Suspensions contribute to pharmacy and medicine by supplying insoluble and often distasteful substances in a form that is pleasant to the taste, by providing a suitable form for the application of dermatologic materials to the skin and sometimes to the mucous membranes, and for the parenteral administration of insoluble drugs. Therefore, pharmaceutical suspensions may be classified into three groups: orally administered mixtures, externally applied lotions, and injectable preparations.

Examples of oral suspensions are the oral antibiotic syrups, which normally contain 125 to 500 mg per 5 mL of solid material. When formulated for use as pediatric drops, the concentration of suspended material is correspondingly greater. Antacid and radioopaque suspensions generally contain high concentrations of dispersed solids. Externally applied suspensions for topical use are legion and are designed for dermatologic, cosmetic, and protective purposes. The concentration of dispersed phase may exceed 20%. Parenteral suspensions contain from 0.5 to 30% of solid particles. Viscosity and particle size are significant factors since they affect the ease of injection and the availability of the drug in depot therapy.

An acceptable suspension possesses certain desirable qualities, including the following. The suspended material should not settle rapidly; the particles that do settle to the bottom of the container must not form a hard cake but should be readily redispersed into a uniform mixture when the container is shaken; and the suspension must not be too viscous to pour freely from the orifice of the bottle or to flow through a syringe needle. In the case of an external lotion, the product must be fluid enough to spread easily over the affected area and yet must not be so mobile that it runs off the surface to which it is applied; the lotion must dry quickly and provide an elastic protective film that will not rub off easily; and it must have an acceptable color and odor.

It is important that the characteristics of the dispersed phase are chosen with care so as to produce a suspension having optimum physical, chemical, and pharmacologic properties. Particle size distribution, specific surface area, inhibition of crystal growth, and changes in polymorphic form are of special significance, and the formulator must ensure that these and other properties[1-3] do not change sufficiently during storage to adversely affect the performance of the suspension. Finally, it is desirable that the product contain readily obtainable ingredients that can be incorporated into the mixture with relative ease by the use of standard methods and equipment.

The remainder of this section will be devoted to a discussion of some of the properties that provide the desirable characteristics just enumerated.

For pharmaceutical purposes, *physical stability* of suspensions may be defined as the condition in which the particles do not aggregate and in which they remain uniformly distributed throughout the dispersion. Since this ideal situation is seldom realized, it is appropriate to add the statement that if the particles do settle, they should be easily resuspended by a moderate amount of agitation.

INTERFACIAL PROPERTIES OF SUSPENDED PARTICLES

Little is known about energy conditions at the surfaces of solids; yet a knowledge of the thermodynamic requirements is needed for the successful stabilization of suspended particles.

Work must be done to reduce a solid to small particles and disperse them in a continuous medium. The large surface area of the particles that results from the comminution is associated with a surface free energy that makes the system *thermodynamically unstable*, by which we mean that the particles are highly energetic and tend to regroup in such a way as to decrease the total area and reduce the surface free energy. The particles in a liquid suspension therefore tend to *flocculate*, that is, to form light, fluffy conglomerates that are held together by weak van der Waals forces. Under certain conditions—in a compacted cake, for example—the particles may adhere by stronger forces to form what are termed *aggregates*. Caking often occurs by the growth and fusing together of crystals in the precipitates to produce a solid aggregate.

The formation of any type of agglomerate, either floccules or aggregates, is taken as a measure of the system's tendency to reach a more thermodynamically stable state. An increase in the work W or surface free energy ΔG brought about by dividing the solid into smaller particles and consequently increasing the total surface area ΔA is given by

$$\Delta G = \gamma_{SL} \cdot \Delta A \qquad (18-1)$$

in which γ_{SL} is the interfacial tension between the liquid medium and the solid particles.

Example 18–1. Compute the change in the surface free energy of a solid in a suspension if the total surface is increased from 10^3 cm^2 to 10^7 cm^2. Assume that the interfacial tension between the solid and the liquid medium is $\gamma_{LS} = 100$ dyne/cm.

The initial free energy is

$$G_1 = 100 \times 10^3 = 10^5 \text{ erg/cm}^2$$

When the surface area is 10^7 cm^2,

$$G_2 = 100 \times 10^7 = 10^9 \text{ erg/cm}^2$$

The change in the free energy, ΔG_{21}, is $10^9 - 10^5 \simeq 10^9$ erg/cm^2. The free energy has been increased by 10^9, which makes the system more thermodynamically unstable.

In order to approach a stable state, the system tends to reduce the surface free energy; equilibrium is reached when $\Delta G = 0$. This condition may be accomplished, as seen from equation (18–1), by a reduction of interfacial tension, or it may be approached by a decrease of the interfacial area. The latter possibility, leading to flocculation or aggregation, may be desirable or undesirable in a pharmaceutical suspension, as considered in a later section.

The interfacial tension can be reduced by the addition of a surfactant but cannot ordinarily be made equal to zero. A suspension of insoluble particles, then, usually possesses a finite positive interfacial tension, and the particles tend to flocculate. An analysis paralleling this one could also be made in the breaking of an emulsion.

The forces at the surface of a particle affect the degree of flocculation and agglomeration in a suspension. Forces of attraction are of the London–van der Waals type; the repulsive forces arise from the interaction of the electric double layers surrounding each particle. The formation of the electric double layer has been considered in detail in Chapter 14, which dealt with interfacial phenomena. The student is advised to review, at this point, the section dealing with the electrical properties of interfaces (pp. 386–388) since particle charge, electrical double layer formation, and zeta potential are all relevant to the present topic.

The potential energy of two particles is plotted in Figure 18–1 as a function of the distance of separation. Shown are the curves depicting the energy of attraction, the energy of repulsion, and the net energy, which has a peak and two minima. When the repulsion energy is high, the potential barrier is also high, and collision of the particles is opposed. The system remains deflocculated, and, when sedimentation is complete, the particles form a close-packed arrangement with the smaller particles filling the voids between the larger ones. Those particles lowest in the sediment are gradually pressed together by the weight of the ones above; the energy barrier is thus overcome, allowing the particles to come into close contact with each other. In order to resuspend and redisperse these particles, it is again necessary to overcome the high energy barrier. Since this is not easily achieved by agitation, the particles tend to remain strongly attracted to each other and form a hard cake. When the particles are flocculated, the energy barrier is still too large to be surmounted, and so the approaching particle resides in the second energy minimum, which is at a distance of separation of perhaps 1000 to 2000 Å. This distance is sufficient to

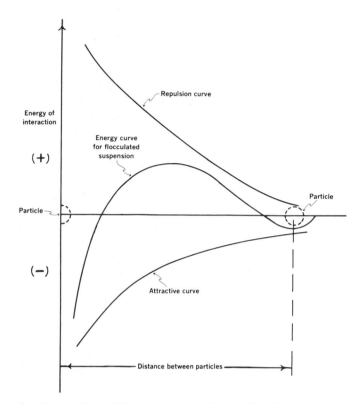

Fig. 18-1. Potential energy curves for particle interactions in suspension (from A. Martin, J. Pharm. Sci., **50**, 514, 1961, reproduced with permission of the copyright owner.)

form the loosely structural flocs. These concepts evolve from the DLVO theory for the stability of lyophobic sols (p. 408). Schneider et al.[4] prepared a computer program to calculate the repulsion and attraction energies in pharmaceutical suspensions. They showed the methods of handling the DLVO equations, and the careful consideration that must be given to the many physical units involved. Detailed examples of calculations were given.

To summarize, flocculated particles are weakly bonded, settle rapidly, do not form a cake, and are easily resuspended; deflocculated particles settle slowly and eventually form a sediment in which aggregation occurs with the resultant formation of a hard cake that is difficult to resuspend.

SETTLING IN SUSPENSIONS

As mentioned earlier, one aspect of physical stability in pharmaceutical suspensions is concerned with keeping the particles uniformly distributed throughout the dispersion. Although it is seldom possible to prevent settling completely over a prolonged period of time, it is necessary to consider the factors that influence the velocity of sedimentation.

Theory of Sedimentation. As discussed in Chapter 16, the velocity of sedimentation is expressed by Stokes' law:

$$v = \frac{d^2(\rho_s - \rho_o)g}{18\eta_o} \quad (18-2)$$

in which v is the terminal velocity in cm/sec, d is the diameter of the particle in cm, ρ_s and ρ_o are the densities of the dispersed phase and dispersion medium, respectively, g is the acceleration due to gravity, and η_o is the viscosity of the dispersion medium in poise.

Dilute pharmaceutical suspensions containing less than about 2 g of solids per 100 mL of liquid conform roughly to these conditions. (Some workers feel that the concentration must be less than 0.5 g/100 mL before Stokes' equation is valid.) In dilute suspensions, the particles do not interfere with one another during sedimentation, and *free settling* occurs. In most pharmaceutical suspensions that contain dispersed particles in concentrations of 5%, 10%, or higher percentages, the particles exhibit *hindered settling*. The particles interfere with one another as they fall, and Stokes' law no longer applies.

Under these circumstances, some estimation of physical stability may be obtained by diluting the suspension so that it contains about 0.5 to 2.0% *w/v* of dispersed phase. This is not always recommended, however, because the stability picture obtained is not necessarily that of the original suspension. The addition of a diluent may affect the degree of flocculation (or deflocculation) of the system, thereby effectively changing the particle size distribution.

To account for the nonuniformity in particle shape and size invariably encountered in real systems. Stokes' equation may be written in other forms. One of the proposed modifications is as follows:[5]

$$v' = v\epsilon^n \quad (18-3)$$

where v' is the rate of fall at the interface in cm/sec and v is the velocity of sedimentation according to Stokes' law. The term ϵ represents the initial porosity of the system, that is, the initial volume fraction of the uniformly mixed suspension, which varies from zero to unity. The exponent n is a measure of the "hindering" of the system. It is a constant for each system.

Example 18-2. The average particle diameter of calcium carbonate in aqueous suspension is 54 μm. The densities of $CaCO_3$ and water, respectively, are 2.7 and 0.997 g/cm³. The viscosity of water is 0.009 poise at 25° C. Compute the rate of fall v' for $CaCO_3$ samples at two different porosities, $\epsilon_1 = 0.95$ and $\epsilon_2 = 0.5$. The n value is 19.73.

From Stokes' law (equation (18-2)),

$$v = \frac{(54 \times 10^{-4})^2(2.7 - 0.997)981}{18 \times 0.009} = 0.30 \text{ cm/sec}$$

Taking logarithms on both sides of equation (18-3), $\ln v'$ = $\ln v + n \ln \epsilon$.

For $\epsilon_1 = 0.95$,

$$\ln v' = -1.204 + [19.73(-0.051)] = -2.210$$

$$v' = 0.11 \text{ cm/sec}$$

Analogously, for $\epsilon_2 = 0.5$, $v' = 3.5 \times 10^{-7}$ cm/sec. Note that at low porosity values (i.e., 0.5, which corresponds to a high concentration of solid in suspension), the sedimentation is hindered, leading to small v'

values. On the other hand, when the suspension becomes infinitely diluted (i.e., $\epsilon = 1$), the rate of fall $v' = v$. In the present example, if $\epsilon = 1$,

$$v' = 0.3 \times 1^{19.73} = 0.3 \text{ cm/sec}$$

which is the Stokes' law velocity.

Effect of Brownian Movement. For particles having a diameter of about 2 to 5 μm (depending on the density of the particles and the density and viscosity of the suspending medium), Brownian movement counteracts sedimentation to a measurable extent at room temperature by keeping the dispersed material in random motion. The *critical radius r* below which particles will be kept in suspension by kinetic bombardment of the particles by the molecules of the suspending medium (Brownian movement) has been worked out by Burton.[6]

It may be seen in the microscope that Brownian movement of the smallest particles in a field of particles of a pharmaceutical suspension is usually eliminated when the sample is dispersed in a 50% glycerin solution, having a viscosity of about 5 cps. Hence, it is unlikely that the particles in an ordinary pharmaceutical suspension, containing suspending agents, are in a state of vigorous Brownian motion.

Sedimentation of Flocculated Particles. When sedimentation is studied in flocculated systems, it is observed that the flocs tend to fall together, producing a distinct boundary between the sediment and the supernatant liquid. The liquid above the sediment is clear because even the small particles present in the system are associated with the flocs. Such is not the case in deflocculated suspensions having a range of particle sizes, in which, in accordance with Stokes' law, the larger particles settle more rapidly than the smaller particles. No clear boundary is formed (unless only one size particle is present), and the supernatant remains turbid for a considerably longer period of time.

Whether or not the supernatant liquid is clear or turbid during the initial stages of settling is a good indication of whether the system is flocculated or deflocculated, respectively.

According to Hiestand,[7] the initial rate of settling of flocculated particles is determined by the floc size and the porosity of the aggregated mass. Subsequently, the rate depends on compaction and rearrangement processes within the sediment. The term *subsidence* is sometimes used to describe settling in flocculated systems.

Sedimentation Parameters. Two useful parameters that may be derived from sedimentation (or more correctly, subsidence) studies are *sedimentation volume*, V, or *height*, H, and *degree of flocculation*.

The sedimentation volume, F, is defined as the ratio of the final, or ultimate, volume of the sediment, V_u, to the original volume of the suspension, V_o, before settling. Thus

$$F = V_u/V_o \qquad (18-4)$$

The sedimentation volume can have values ranging from less than 1 to greater than 1. F is normally less than 1, and in this case, the ultimate volume of sediment is smaller than the original volume of suspension, as shown in Figure 18–2a, in which $F = 0.5$. If the volume of sediment in a flocculated suspension equals the original volume of suspension, then $F = 1$ (Fig. 18–2b). Such a product is said to be in "flocculation equilibrium" and shows no clear supernatant on standing. It is therefore pharmaceutically acceptable. It is possible for F to have values greater than 1, meaning that the final volume of sediment is greater than the original suspension volume. This comes about because the network of flocs formed in the suspension are so loose and fluffy that the volume they are able to encompass is greater than the original volume of

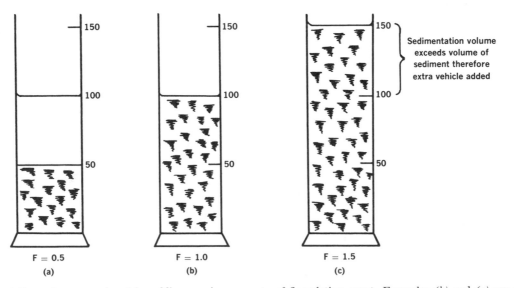

Fig. 18–2. Sedimentation volumes produced by adding varying amounts of flocculating agent. Examples *(b)* and *(c)* are pharmaceutically acceptable.

suspension. This situation is illustrated in Figure 18–2c, in which sufficient extra vehicles has been added to contain the sediment. In example shown, $F = 1.5$.

The sedimentation volume gives only a qualitative account of flocculation since it lacks a meaningful reference point.[7] A more useful parameter for flocculation is β, the *degree of flocculation*.

If we consider a suspension that is completely deflocculated, the ultimate volume of the sediment will be relatively small. Writing this volume as V_∞, based on equation (18–4), we have

$$F_\infty = V_\infty/V_o \qquad (18–5)$$

in which F_∞ is the sedimentation volume of the deflocculated, or peptized, suspension. The degree of flocculation, β, is therefore defined as the ratio of F to F_∞, or

$$\beta = F/F_\infty \qquad (18–6)$$

Substituting equations (18–4) and (18–5) in equation (18–6), we obtain

$$\beta = \frac{V_u/V_o}{V_\infty/V_o} = V_u/V_\infty \qquad (18–7)$$

The degree of flocculation is a more fundamental parameter than F since it relates the volume of flocculated sediment to that in a deflocculated system. We can therefore say that

$$\beta = \frac{\text{ultimate sediment volume of } \textit{flocculated} \text{ suspension}}{\text{ultimate sediment volume of } \textit{deflocculated} \text{ suspension}}$$

Example 18–3. Compute the sedimentation volume of a 5% (*w/v*) suspension of magnesium carbonate in water. The initial volume is $V_o = 100$ mL and the final volume of the sediment is $V_u = 30$ mL. If the degree of flocculation is β = F/F_∞ = 1.3, what is the deflocculated sedimentation volume, F_∞?

$$F = \frac{30}{100} = 0.30$$

$$F_\infty = F/\beta = 0.30/1.3 = 0.23$$

FORMULATION OF SUSPENSIONS

The approaches commonly used in the preparation of physical stable suspensions fall into two categories— the use of structured vehicle to maintain deflocculated particles in suspension, and the application of the principles of flocculation to produce flocs that, although they settle rapidly, are easily resuspended with a minimum of agitation.

Structured vehicles are pseudoplastic and plastic in nature; their rheologic properties have been discussed in Chapter 17. As we shall see in a later section, it is frequently desirable that thixotropy be associated with these two types of flow. Structured vehicles act by entrapping the particles (generally deflocculated) so that, ideally, no settling occurs. In reality, some degree of sedimentation will usually take place. The "shear-thinning" property of these vehicles does, however, facilitate the reformation of a uniform dispersion when shear is applied.

A disadvantage of deflocculated systems, mentioned earlier, is the formation of a compact cake when the particles eventually settle. It is for this reason that the formulation of flocculated suspensions has been advocated.[8] Optimum physical stability and appearance will be obtained when the suspension is formulated with flocculated particles in a structured vehicle of the hydrophilic colloid type. Consequently, most of the subsequent discussion will be concerned with this approach and the means by which controlled flocculation may be achieved. Whatever approach is used, the product must (1) flow readily from the container and (2) possess a uniform distribution of particles in each dose.

Wetting of Particles. The initial dispersion of an insoluble powder in a vehicle is an important step in the manufacturing process and requires further consideration. Powders sometimes are added to the vehicle, particularly in large-scale operations, by dusting on the surface of the liquid. It is frequently difficult to disperse the powder owing to an adsorbed layer of air, minute quantities of grease, and other contaminants. The powder is not readily wetted, and although it may have a high density, it floats on the surface of the liquid. Finely powdered substances are particularly susceptible to this effect because of entrained air, and they fail to become wetted even when forced below the surface of the suspending medium. The *wettability* of a powder may be ascertained easily by observing the contact angle (p. 384) that powder makes with the surface of the liquid. The angle is approximately 90° when the particles are floating well out of the liquid. A powder that floats low in the liquid has a lesser angle, and one that sinks obviously shows no contact angle. Powders that are not easily wetted by water and accordingly show a large contact angle, such as sulfur, charcoal, and magnesium stearate, are said to be *hydrophobic*. Powders that are readily wetted by water when free of adsorbed contaminants are called *hydrophilic*. Zinc oxide, talc, and magnesium carbonate belong to the latter class.

Surfactants are quite useful in the preparation of a suspension in reducing the interfacial tension between solid particles and a vehicle. As a result of the lowered interfacial tension, the advancing contact angle is lowered, air is displaced from the surface of particles, and wetting and deflocculation are promoted. Schott et al.[9] studied the deflocculating effect of octoxynol, a nonionic surfactant, to enhance the dissolution rate of prednisolone from tablets. The tablets break up into fine granules that are deflocculated in suspension. The deflocculating effect is proportional to the surfactant concentration. However, at very high surfactant concentration, say, 15 times the critical micelle concentration, the surfactant produces extensive flocculation. Glycerin and similar hygroscopic substances are also valuable in levigating the insoluble material. Apparently, glycerin flows into the voids between the particles to displace the air and, during the mixing operation, coats and separates the material so that water can penetrate and wet the individual particles. The dispersion of particles of colloidal gums by alcohol, glycerin, and propylene glycol, allowing water to subsequently penetrate the interstices, is a well-known practice in pharmacy.

To select suitable wetting agents that possess a well-developed ability to penetrate the powder mass, Hiestand[7] has used a narrow trough, several inches long and made of a hydrophobic material, such as Teflon, or coated with paraffin wax. At one end of the trough is placed the powder and at the other end the solution of the wetting agent. The rate of penetration of the latter into the powder can then be observed directly.

Controlled Flocculation. Assuming that the powder is properly wetted and dispersed, attention may now be given to the various means by which controlled flocculation may be produced so as to prevent formation of a compact sediment that is difficult to redisperse. The topic, described in detail by Hiestand,[7] is conveniently discussed in terms of the material used to produce flocculation in suspensions, namely electrolytes, surfactants, and polymers.

Electrolytes act as flocculating agents by reducing the electric barrier between the particles, as evidenced by a decrease in the zeta potential and the formation of a bridge between adjacent particles so as to link them together in a loosely arranged structure.

If we disperse particles of bismuth subnitrate in water, we find that, based on electrophoretic mobility studies, they possess a large positive charge, or zeta potential. Because of the strong forces of repulsion between adjacent particles, the system is peptized or deflocculated. By preparing a series of bismuth subnitrate suspensions containing increasing concentrations of monobasic potassium phosphate, Haines and Martin[10] were able to show a correlation between apparent zeta potential and sedimentation volume, caking, and flocculation. The results are summarized in Figure 18–3 and are explained in the following manner.

The addition of monobasic potassium phosphate to the suspended bismuth subnitrate particles causes the positive zeta potential to decrease owing to the adsorption of the negatively charged phosphate anion. With the continued addition of the electrolyte, the zeta potential eventually falls to zero and then increases in a negative direction, as shown in Figure 18–3. Microscopic examination of the various suspensions shows that at a certain positive zeta potential, maximum flocculation occurs and will persist until the zeta potential has become sufficiently negative for deflocculation to occur once again. The onset of flocculation coincides with the maximum sedimentation volume determined. *F* remains reasonably constant while floc-

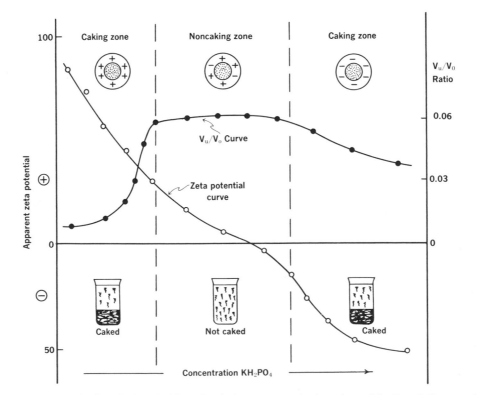

Fig. 18–3. Caking diagram, showing the flocculation of a bismuth subnitrate suspension by means of the flocculating agent, monobasic potassium phosphate. (From A. Martin and J. Swarbrick, in Sprowls, *American Pharmacy*, 6th Edition, Lippincott, Philadelphia, 1966, p. 205, reproduced with permission of the copyright owner.)

culation persists, and only when the zeta potential becomes sufficiently negative to effect repeptization does the sedimentation volume start to fall. Finally, the absence of caking in the suspensions correlates with the maximum sedimentation volume, which, as stated previously, reflects the amount of flocculation. At less than maximum values of *F*, caking becomes apparent.

These workers[10] also demonstrated a similar correlation when aluminum chloride was added to a suspension of sulfamerazine in water. In this system, the initial zeta potential of the sulfamerazine particles is negative and is progressively reduced by adsorption of the trivalent aluminum cation. When sufficient electrolyte is added, the zeta potential reaches zero and then increases in a positive direction. Colloidal and coarse dispersed particles may possess surface charges that depend on the pH of the system. An important property of the pH-dependent dispersions is the zero point of charge, that is, the pH at which the net surface charge is zero. The desired surface charge can be achieved through adjusting the pH by the addition of HCl or NaOH to produce a positive, zero, or negative surface charge. The negative zeta potential of nitrofurantoin decreases considerably when the pH values of the suspension are charged from basic to acidic.[11]

Surfactants, both ionic and nonionic, have been used to bring about flocculation of suspended particles. The concentration necessary to achieve this effect would appear to be critical since these compounds may also act as wetting and deflocculating agents to achieve dispersion.

Polymers are long-chain, high-molecular-weight compounds containing active groups spaced along their length. These agents act as flocculating agents because part of the chain is adsorbed on the particle surface, with the remaining parts projecting out into the dispersion medium. Bridging between these latter portions leads to the formation of flocs.

Felmeister and others[12] studied the influence of a xanthan gum (an anionic heteropolysaccharide) on the flocculation characteristics of sulfaguanidine, bismuth subcarbonate, and other drugs in suspension. Addition of xanthan gum resulted in increased sedimentation volume, presumably by a polymer bridging phenomenon. Hiestand[13] has reviewed the control of floc structure in coarse suspensions by the addition of polymeric materials.

Hydrophilic polymers also act as protective colloids (p. 410), and particles coated in this manner are less prone to cake than are uncoated particles. These polymers exhibit pseudoplastic flow in solution, and this property serves to promote physical stability within the suspension. Gelatin, a polyelectrolytic polymer, exhibits flocculation that depends on the pH and ionic strength of the dispersion medium. Sodium sulfathiazole, precipitated from acid solution in the presence of gelatin, was shown by Blythe[14] to be free flowing in the dry state and not to cake when suspended. Sulfa-

thiazole normally carries a negative charge in aqueous vehicles. The coated material, precipitated from acid solution in the presence of gelatin, however, was found to carry a positive charge. This is due to gelatin being positively charged at the pH at which precipitation was carried out. It has been suggested[8] that the improved properties result from the positively charged gelatin-coated particles being partially flocculated in suspension, presumably because the high negative charge has been replaced by a smaller, albeit positive, charge. Positively charged liposomes have been used as flocculating agents to prevent caking of negatively charged particles. Liposomes are vesicles of phospholipids having no toxicity and that can be prepared in various particle sizes.[15] They are adsorbed on the negatively charged particles. (See page 513 for a discussion of liposomes.)

Flocculation in Structured Vehicles. Although the controlled flocculation approach is capable of fulfilling the desired physical chemical requisites of a pharmaceutical suspension, the product can look unsightly if *F*, the sedimentation volume, is not close, or equal, to 1. Consequently, in practice, a suspending agent is frequently added to retard sedimentation of the flocs. Such agents as carboxymethylcellulose (CMC), Carbopol 934, Veegum, tragacanth, or bentonite have been employed, either alone or in combination.

This may lead to incompatibilities, depending on the initial particle charge and the charge carried by the flocculating agent and the suspending agent. For example, suppose we prepare a dispersion of positively charged particles that is then flocculated by the addition of the correct concentration of an anionic electrolyte such as monobasic potassium phosphate. We can improve the physical stability of this system by adding a minimal amount of one of the hydrocolloids mentioned above. No physical incompatibility will be observed because the majority of hydrophilic colloids are themselves negatively charged and are thus compatible with anionic flocculating agents. If, however, we flocculate a suspension of negatively charged particles with a cationic electrolyte (aluminum chloride), the subsequent addition of a hydrocolloid may result in an incompatible product, as evidenced for the formation of an unsightly stringy mass that has little or no suspending action and itself settles rapidly.

Under these circumstances, it becomes necessary to use a protective colloid to change the sign on the particle from negative to positive. This is achieved by the adsorption onto the particle surface of a fatty acid amine (which has been checked to ensure its nontoxicity) or a material such as gelatin, which is positively charged below its isoelectric point. We are then able to use an anionic electrolyte to produce flocs that are compatible with the negatively charged suspending agent.

The student should note that this approach may be used regardless of the charge on the particle. The sequence of events is depicted in Figure 18–4, which is self-explanatory.

Rheologic Considerations. The principles of rheology may be applied to a study of the following factors: the viscosity of a suspension as it affects the settling of dispersed particles, the change in flow properties of the suspension when the container is shaken and when the product is poured from the bottle, and the spreading qualities of the lotion when it is applied to an affected area. Rheologic considerations are also important in the manufacture of suspensions.

The only shear that occurs in a suspension in storage is due to a settling of the suspended particles; this force is negligible and may be disregarded. When the container is shaken and the product is poured from the bottle, however, a high shearing rate is manifested. As suggested by Mervine and Chase,[16] the ideal suspending agent should have a *high* viscosity at negligible shear, that is, during shelf storage; and it should have a *low* viscosity at high shearing rates, that is, it should be free-flowing during agitation, pouring, and spreading. As seen in Figure 18–5, pseudoplastic substances such as tragacanth, sodium alginate, and sodium carboxymethylcellulose show these desirable qualities. The Newtonian liquid, glycerin, is included in the graph for comparison. Its viscosity is suitable for suspending particles but is too high to pour easily and to spread on the skin. Furthermore, glycerin shows the undesirable property of tackiness (stickiness) and is too hygroscopic to use in undiluted form. The curves in Figure 18–5 were obtained by use of the modified Stormer viscometer described on page 464.

A suspending agent that is thixotropic as well as pseudoplastic should prove to be useful since it forms a gel on standing and becomes fluid when disturbed.

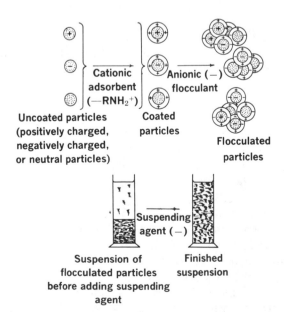

Fig. 18–4. The sequence of steps involved in the formation of a stable suspension (From A. Martin and J. Swarbrick; in Sprowls, *American Pharmacy*, 6th Edition, Lippincott, Philadelphia, 1966, p. 206, reproduced with permission of the copyright owner.)

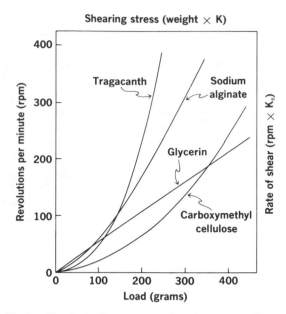

Fig. 18–5. Rheologic flow curves of various suspending agents analyzed in a modified Stormer viscometer.

Figure 18–6 shows the consistency curves for bentonite, Veegum (Vanderbilt Co.), and a combination of bentonite and sodium carboxymethylcellulose (CMC). The hysteresis loop of bentonite is quite marked. Veegum also shows considerable thixotropy, both when tested by inverting a vessel containing the dispersion and when analyzed in a rotational viscometer. When bentonite and CMC dispersions are mixed, the resulting curve shows both pseudoplastic and thixotropic characteristics. Such a combination should produce an excellent suspending medium.

Preparation of Suspensions. The factors entering into the preparation and stabilization of suspensions involve certain principles of interest to physical pharmacy and are briefly discussed here. The physical principles involved in the dispersion of solids by different types of equipment have been discussed by Oldshue.[17]

A suspension is prepared on the small scale by grinding or levigating the insoluble material in the

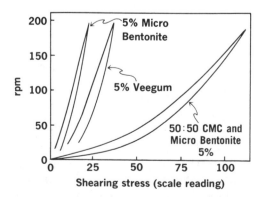

Fig. 18–6. Flow curves for 5% suspending agents in water showing thixotropy. The curves were obtained with the Ferranti–Shirley cone–plate viscometer.

mortar to a smooth paste with a vehicle containing the dispersion stabilizer and gradually adding the remainder of the liquid phase in which any soluble drugs may be dissolved. The slurry is transferred to a graduate, the mortar is rinsed with successive portions of the vehicle, and the dispersion is finally brought to the final volume.

On a large scale, dispersion of solids in liquids is accomplished by the use of ball, pebble, and colloid mills. Dough mixers, pony mixers, and similar apparatus are also employed. Only the colloid mill is described here; a discussion of the other mills can be found in the book by Fischer.[18] Dry grinding in ball mills is treated by Fischer, by Berry and Kamack and by Prasher.[18]

The colloid mill is based on the principle of a high-velocity cone-shaped rotor that is centered with respect to a stator at a small adjustable clearance. The suspension is fed to the rotor by gravity through a hopper, sheared between the rotor and stator, and forced out below the stator, where it may be recycled or drawn off.

The efficiency of the mill is based on the clearance between the disks, the peripheral velocity of the rotor, and the non-Newtonian viscosity of the suspension. The mill breaks down the large aggregates and flocs so that they may be dispersed throughout the liquid vehicle and then protected by the dispersion stabilizer. The shearing action that leads to disaggregation occurs at the surfaces of the rotating and stationary disks, and between the particles themselves in a concentrated suspension. If the yield value is too great, the material fails to flow; if the viscosity is low, a loss in effectiveness of shearing action occurs. Therefore, the yield value should be low, and the plastic or apparent viscosity of the material should be at a maximum consistent with the optimum rate of flow through the mill. If the material is highly viscous or if the plates are adjusted to a clearance that is too narrow, the temperature rises rapidly, and cooling water must be circulated around the stator to dissipate the heat that is produced. Dilatant materials—for example, deflocculated suspensions containing 50% or more of solids—are particularly troublesome. They flow freely into the mill but set up a high shearing rate and produce overheating and stalling of the motor. Beginning any milling process with the plates set at a wide clearance minimizes this danger. If this technique fails, however, the material must be milled in another type of equipment or the paste must be diluted with a vehicle until dilatancy is eliminated.

Physical Stability of Suspensions. Raising the temperature often leads to flocculation of *sterically stabilized* suspensions, that is, suspensions stabilized by nonionic surfactants. Repulsion due to steric interactions depends on the nature, thickness, and completeness of the surfactant-adsorbed layers on the particles. When the suspension is heated the energy of repulsion between the particles may be reduced owing to dehydration of the polyoxyethylene groups of the surfactant. The attractive energy is increased and the particles flocculate.[19] Zapata et al.[20] studied the mechanism of freeze–thaw instability in aluminum hydrocarbonate and magnesium hydroxide gels as model suspensions because of their well known sensitivity to temperature changes. During the freezing process, particles are able to overcome the repulsive barrier caused by ice formation, which forces the particles close enough to experience the strong attractive forces present in the primary minimum, and form aggregates according to the DLVO theory (see Fig. 15–12, p. 409). When the ice melts, the particles remain as aggregates unless work is applied to overcome the primary energy peak. Aggregate size was found to be inversely related to the freezing rate: the higher the freezing rate, the smaller the size of ice crystals formed. These small crystals do not result in the aggregation of as many suspension particles as do large ice crystals.

In addition to particle aggregation, particle growth is also a destabilizing process resulting from temperature fluctuations or *Ostwald ripening* during storage. Fluctuations of temperature may change the particle size distribution and polymorphic form of a drug, altering the absorption rate and drug bioavailability.[21] Particle growth is particularly important when the solubility of the drug is strongly dependent on the temperature. Thus, when temperature is raised, crystals of drug may dissolve and form supersaturated solutions, which favor crystal growth. This can be prevented by the addition of polymers or surfactants. Simonelli et al.[22] studied the inhibition of sulfathiazole crystal growth by polyvinylpyrrolidone. These authors suggested that the polymer forms a noncondensed netlike film over the sulfathiazole crystal, allowing the crystal to grow out only through the openings of the net. The growth is thus controlled by the pore size of the polymer network at the crystal surface. The smaller the pore size, the higher the supersaturation of the solution required for the crystals to grow. This can be shown using the Kelvin equation (p. 440), as applied to a particle suspended in a saturated solution:[22]

$$\ln \frac{c}{c_o} = \frac{2\gamma M}{NkT\rho R} \qquad (18\text{–}8)$$

where c is the solubility of a small particle of radius R in an aqueous vehicle and c_o the solubility of a very large crystalline particle; γ is the interfacial tension of the crystal, ρ is the density of the crystal, and M is the molecular weight of the solute. N is Avogadro's number, k is the Boltzmann constant and $N \times k = 8.314 \times 10^7$ erg deg^{-1} mole^{-1}. The ratio c/c_o defines the supersaturation ratio that a large crystal requires in the aqueous solution saturated with respect to the small particle. According to equation (18–8), as the radius of curvature of a protruding crystal decreases, the protrusion will require a correspondingly larger supersaturation ratio before it can grow. The radius of curvature of a protrusion must equal that of the pore of the polymer on the crystal surface.

Example 18–4. Assume that the interfacial tension of a particle of drug in an aqueous vehicle is 100 erg/cm², its molecular weight 200 g/mole, and the temperature of solution 30° C or 303° K. (*a*) Compute the supersaturation ratio c/c_o that is required for the crystal to grow. The radius R of the particle is 5 μm or 5×10^{-4} cm and its density is 1.3 g/cm³. (*b*) Compute the supersaturation ratio when the particle is covered by a polymer and the pore radius R of the polymer at the crystal surface is 6×10^{-7} cm.

Using the Kelvin equation,

(*a*)

$$\ln \frac{c}{c_o} = \frac{2 \times 100 \times 200}{8.314 \times 10^7 \times 1.3 \times 303 \times 5 \times 10^{-4}} = 0.0024$$

$$c/c_o = \text{antiln}(0.0024) = 1.002$$

(*b*)

$$\ln \frac{c}{c_o} = \frac{2 \times 100 \times 200}{8.314 \times 10^7 \times 1.3 \times 303 \times 6 \times 10^{-7}} = 2.036$$

$$c/c_o = \text{antiln}(2.036) = 7.66$$

Notice that c/c_o *in part (a)* represents slight oversaturation whereas in (*b*) the supersaturation concentration must be 7.6 times larger than the solubility of the drug molecule for the crystalline particle to grow. In other words, the addition of a polymer greatly increases the point at which supersaturation occurs and makes it more difficult for the drug crystal to grow.

Ziller and Rupprecht[23] designed a control unit to monitor crystal growth and studied the inhibition of growth by PVP in acetaminophen suspensions. According to these workers, some of the segments of the polymer PVP attach to the free spaces on the drug crystal lattice and the polymer is surrounded by a hydration shell (Fig. 18–7). The adsorbed segments of the polymer inhibit crystal growth of acetaminophen because they form a barrier that impedes the approach of the drug molecules from the solution to the crystal surface. High-molecular-weight polymers of PVP are more effective than low-molecular-weight polymers since the adsorption of the polymer on the crystal surface becomes more irreversible as the chain length increases.

The stability of suspensions may also decrease owing to interaction with excipients dissolved in the dispersion medium. Zatz and Lue[19] studied the flocculation by sorbitol in sulfamerazine suspensions containing nonionic surfactants as wetting agents. The flocculation by sorbitol depends on the cloud point of the surfactant. Thus, the lower the cloud point, the less sorbitol was needed to induce flocculation. The fact that the cloud point can be lowered by preservatives such as methylparaben shows that the choice of additives may change the resistance to caking of a suspension containing nonionic surfactants. Zatz and Lue[19] suggested that the cloud point may be used to estimate the critical flocculation concentration of sorbitol. Lucks et al.[24] studied the adsorption of preservatives such as cetylpyridinium chloride on zinc oxide particles in suspension. Increasing amounts of this preservative led to charge reversal of the suspension. Cetylpyridinium chloride, a

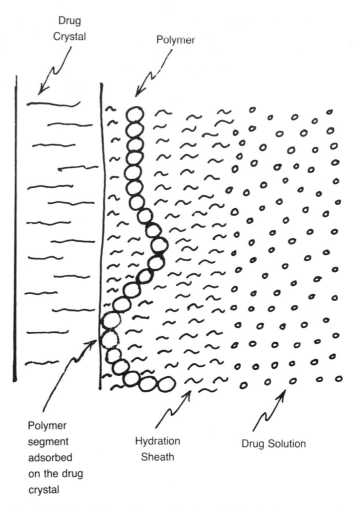

Fig. 18–7. Dissolution and crystallization of a drug in the presence of a polymer adsorbed on the drug crystal. (From K. H. Ziller and H. Rupprecht, Drug Dev. Ind. Pharm. **14**, 2341, 1988, reproduced with permission of the copyright owner.)

cationic surfactant, has a positive charge and is strongly adsorbed at the particle surface. The positive end of the preservative molecule adsorbs on the negatively charged surface of the zinc oxide particles, forming a layer with the hydrocarbon chains oriented outward toward the dispersion medium. A second layer of preservative adsorbs at this monolayer, with the positively charged groups now directed toward the dispersion medium. Thus, the physical stability of the suspension may be enhanced owing to the repulsion of like-charged particles. However, the strong adsorption of the preservative on the zinc oxide particles reduces the biologically active free fraction of preservative in the dispersion medium, and the microbiologic activity is diminished.

EMULSIONS

An emulsion is a thermodynamically unstable system consisting of at least two immiscible liquid phases, one of which is dispersed as globules (the dispersed phase) in the other liquid phase (the continuous phase), stabilized by the presence of an *emulsifying agent*. The various types of emulsifying agents are discussed later in this section. Either the dispersed phase or the continuous phase may range in consistency from that of a mobile liquid to a semisolid. Thus, emulsified systems range from lotions of relatively low viscosity to ointments and creams, which are semisolid in nature. The particle diameter of the dispersed phase generally extends from about 0.1 to 10 μm, although particle diameters as small as 0.01 μ and as large as 100 μm are not uncommon in some preparations.

Emulsion type. Invariably, one liquid phase in an emulsion is essentially polar (e.g., aqueous), while the other is relatively nonpolar (e.g., an oil). When the oil phase is dispersed as globules throughout an aqueous continuous phase, the system is referred to as an *oil-in-water* (*o/w*) emulsion. When the oil phase serves as the continuous phase, the emulsion is spoken of as a *water-in-oil* (*w/o*) product. Medicinal emulsions for oral administration are usually of the *o/w* type and require the use of an *o/w* emulsifying agent. These include synthetic nonionic surfactants, acacia, tragacanth, and gelatin. Not all emulsions that are consumed, however, belong to the *o/w* type. Certain foods such as butter and some salad dressings are *w/o* emulsions.

Externally applied emulsions may be *o/w* or *w/o*, the former employing the following emulsifiers in addition to the ones mentioned previously: sodium lauryl sulfate, triethanolamine stearate, monovalent soaps such as sodium oleate, and self-emulsifying glyceryl monostearate, that is, glyceryl monostearate mixed with a small amount of a monovalent soap or an alkyl sulfate. Pharmaceutical *w/o* emulsions are used almost exclusively for external application and may contain one or several of the following emulsifiers: polyvalent soaps such as calcium palmitate, sorbitan esters (*Spans*), cholesterol, and wool fat.

Several methods are commonly used to determine the type of an emulsion. A small quantity of a water-soluble dye such as methylene blue or brilliant blue FCF may be dusted on the surface of the emulsion. If water is the external phase (i.e., if the emulsion is of the *o/w* type), the dye will dissolve and uniformly diffuse throughout the water. If the emulsion is of the *w/o* type, the particles of dye will lie in clumps on the surface. A second method involves dilution of the emulsion with water. If the emulsion mixes freely with the water, it is of the *o/w* type. Another test uses a pair of electrodes connected to an external electric source and immersed in the emulsion. If the external phase is water, a current will pass through the emulsion and can be made to deflect a voltmeter needle or cause a light in the circuit to glow. If the oil is the continuous phase, the emulsion fails to carry the current.

Pharmaceutical Applications. An *o/w* emulsion is a convenient means of orally administering water-insoluble liquids, especially when the dispersed phase has an unpleasant taste. More significant in contemporary pharmacy is the observation that some oil-soluble compounds, such as some of the vitamins, are absorbed more completely when emulsified than when administered orally as an oily solution. The use of intravenous emulsions has been studied as a means of maintaining debilitated patients who are unable to assimilate materials administered orally. Tarr et al.[25] prepared emulsions of taxol, a compound with antimitotic properties, for intravenous administration as an alternative method to the use of cosolvents in taxol administration. Davis and Hansrani[26] studied the influence of droplet size and emulsifying agents on the phagocytosis of lipid emulsions. When the emulsion is administered intravenously, the droplets are normally rapidly taken up by the cells of the reticuloendothelial system, in particular the fixed macrophages in the liver. The rate of clearance by the macrophages increases as the droplet size becomes larger or the surface charge, either positive or negative, increases. Therefore, emulsion droplets stabilized by a nonionic surfactant (zero surface charge) were cleared much more slowly than the droplets stabilized by negatively charged phospholipids. Radiopaque emulsions have found application as diagnostic agents in x-ray examinations.

Emulsification is widely used in pharmaceutical and cosmetic products for external use. This is particularly so with dermatologic and cosmetic lotions and creams since a product that spreads easily and completely over the affected area is desired. Such products can now be formulated to be water washable and nonstaining and, as such, are obviously more acceptable to the patient and physician than some of the greasy products used a decade or more ago. Emulsification is used in aerosol products to produce foams. The propellant that forms the dispersed liquid phase within the container vaporizes when the emulsion is discharged from the container. This results in the rapid formation of a foam.

THEORIES OF EMULSIFICATION

There is no universal theory of emulsification, because emulsions can be prepared using several different types of emulsifying agent, each of which depends for its action on a different principle to achieve a stable product. For a theory to be meaningful, it should be capable of explaining (1) the stability of the product and (2) the type of emulsion formed. Let us consider what happens when two immiscible liquids are agitated together so that one of the liquids is dispersed as small droplets in the other. Except in the case of very dilute oil-in-water emulsions (oil hydrosols), which are somewhat stable, the liquids separate rapidly into two clearly defined layers. Failure of two immiscible liquids to remain mixed is explained by the fact that the *cohesive* force between the molecules of each separate liquid is greater than the *adhesive* force between the two liquids. The cohesive force of the individual phases is manifested as an interfacial energy or tension at the boundary between the liquids, as explained in Chapter 14.

When one liquid is broken into small particles, the interfacial area of the globules constitutes a surface that is enormous compared with the surface area of the original liquid. If 1 cm³ of mineral oil is dispersed into globules having a volume–surface diameter d_{vs} of 0.01 μm (10^{-6} cm) in 1 cm³ of water so as to form a fine emulsion, the surface area of the oil droplets becomes 600 square meters. The surface free energy associated with this area is about 34×10^7 ergs, or 8 calories. The total volume of the system, however, has not increased; it remains at 2 cm³. The calculations are made by use of equations (16–15) and (16–17), p. 436, from which

$$S_v = \frac{6}{d_{vs}}$$

$$S_v = \frac{6}{10^{-6}} = 6 \times 10^6 \text{ cm}^2 = 600 \text{ m}^2$$

The work input or surface free energy increase is given by the equation $W = \gamma_{ow} \times \Delta A$, and the interfacial tension γ_{ow} between mineral oil and water is 57 dyne/cm (erg/cm²).

$$W = 57 \text{ erg/cm}^2 \times (6 \times 10^6 \text{ cm}^2)$$

$$= 34 \times 10^7 \text{ ergs} = 34 \text{ joules}$$

and since

$$1 \text{ cal} = 4.184 \text{ joules}$$

$$34/4.184 = 8 \text{ calories}$$

In summary, if 1 cm³ of mineral oil is mixed with 1 cm³ of water to produce fine particles ($d_{vs} = 0.01$ μm), the total surface is equivalent to an area slightly greater than that of a basketball court, or about 600 square meters! (In real emulsions, the particles are ordinarily about 10 to 100 times larger than this, and the surface area is proportionately smaller.) The increase in energy, 8 calories, associated with this enormous surface is sufficient to make the system thermodynamically unstable, hence the droplets have a tendency to coalesce.

To prevent coalescence or at least to reduce its rate to negligible proportions, it is necessary to introduce an emulsifying agent that will form a film around the dispersed globules. Emulsifying agents may be divided into three groups, as follows:

(1) Surface-active agents, which are adsorbed at oil–water interfaces to form monomolecular films and reduce interfacial tension. These agents have been discussed in detail in Chapter 14, dealing with interfacial phenomena.

(2) Hydrophilic colloids (discussed in Chapter 15), which form a *multi*molecular film around the dispersed droplets of oil in an *o/w* emulsion.[27,28]

(3) Finely divided solid particles, which are adsorbed at the interface between two immiscible liquid phases and form what amounts to a film of particles around the dispersed globules. The factor common to all three classes of emulsifying agent is the formation of a film, whether it be monomolecular, multimolecular, or particulate.

On this basis, we can now discuss some of the more important theories relating to the stability and type of emulsion formed.

Examples of typical emulsifying agents are given in Table 18–1.

Monomolecular Adsorption. Surface-active agents, or amphiphiles, reduce interfacial tension because of their adsorption at the oil–water interface to form monomolecular films. Since the surface free energy increase W equals $\gamma_{o/w} \times \Delta A$, and since we must, of necessity, retain a high surface area for the dispersed phase, any reduction in $\gamma_{o/w}$, the interfacial tension, will reduce the surface free energy and hence the tendency for coalescence. It is not unusual for a good emulsifying agent of this type to reduce the interfacial tension to 1 dyne/cm; we can therefore reduce the surface free energy of the system to approximately one sixtieth of that calculated earlier.

The reduction in surface free energy is of itself probably not the main factor involved. Of more likely

TABLE 18–1. *Some Typical Emulsifying Agents*

Name	Class	Type of Emulsion Formed
Triethanolamine oleate	Surface-active agent (anionic)	o/w (HLB = 12)
N-cetyl N-ethyl morpholinum ethosulfate (Atlas G-263)	Surface-active agent (cationic)	o/w (HLB = 25)
Sorbitan mono-oleate (Atlas Span 80)	Surface-active-agent (nonionic)	w/o (HLB = 4.3)
Polyoxyethylene sorbitan mono-oleate (Atlas Tween 80)	Surface-active agent (nonionic)	o/w (HLB = 15)
Acacia (salts of d-glucuronic acid)	Hydrophilic colloid	o/w
Gelatin (polypeptides and aminoacids)	Hydrophilic colloid	o/w
Bentonite (hydrated aluminum silicate)	Solid particle	o/w (and w/o)
Veegum (magnesium aluminum silicate	Solid particle	o/w
Carbon black	Solid particle	w/o

significance is the fact that the dispersed droplets are surrounded by a coherent monolayer that helps to prevent coalescence between two droplets as they approach one another. Ideally, such a film should be flexible so that it is capable of reforming rapidly if broken or disturbed. An additional effect promoting stability is the presence of a surface charge (see p. 387), which will cause repulsion between adjacent particles.

In practice, combinations of emulsifiers rather than single agents are used most frequently today in the preparations of emulsions. In 1940, Schulman and Cockbain[29] first recognized the necessity of a predominantly hydrophilic emulsifier in the aqueous phase and a hydrophobic agent in the oil phase to form a complex film at the interface. Three mixtures of emulsifying agents at the oil–water interface are depicted in Figure 18–8. The combination of sodium cetyl sulfate and cholesterol leads to a complex film (Fig. 18–8a) that produces an excellent emulsion. Sodium cetyl sulfate and oleyl alcohol do not form a closely packed or condensed film (Fig. 18–8b), and consequently, their combination results in a poor emulsion. In Figure 18–8c, cetyl alcohol and sodium oleate produce a

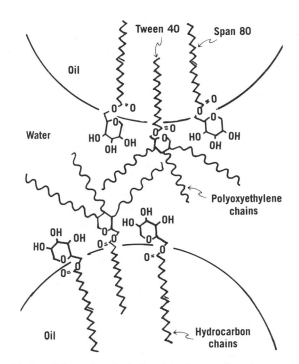

Fig. 18–9. Schematic of oil droplets in an oil–water emulsion, showing the orientation of a Tween and a Span molecule at the interface. (From J. Boyd, C. Parkinson and P. Sherman, J. Coll. Interface Sci. **41,** 359, 1972, reproduced with permission of the copyright owner.)

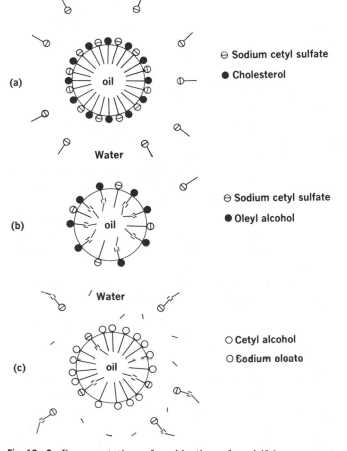

Fig. 18–8. Representations of combinations of emulsifying agents at the oil–water interface of an emulsion. (After J. H. Schulman and E. G. Cockbain, Trans. Faraday Soc. **36,** 651, 1940.)

close-packed film, but complexation is negligible, and again a poor emulsion results.

Atlas-ICI* recommends that a hydrophilic Tween be combined with a lipophilic Span, varying the proportions so as to produce the desired o/w or w/o emulsion.[30] Boyd et al.[31] discussed the molecular association of Tween 40 and Span 80 in stabilizing emulsions. In Figure 18–9, the hydrocarbon portion of the Span 80 (sorbitan mono-oleate) molecule lies in the oil globule and the sorbitan radical lies in the aqueous phase. The bulky sorbitan heads of the Span molecules prevent the hydrocarbon tails from associating closely in the oil phase. When Tween 40 (polyoxyethylene sorbitan monopalmitate) is added, it orients at the interface such that part of its hydrocarbon tail is in the oil phase, and the remainder of the chain, together with the sorbitan ring and the polyoxyethylene chains, is located in the water phase. It is observed that the hydrocarbon chain of the Tween 40 molecule is situated in the oil globule between the Span 80 chains, and this orientation results in effective van der Waals attraction. In this manner, the interfacial film is strengthened and the stability of the o/w emulsion is increased against particle coalescence. The same principle of mixed emulsifying agents may be applied in the use of combinations such as

---

*Atlas surfactants, ICI United States, Inc., Wilmington, Del.

sodium stearate and cholesterol, sodium lauryl sulfate and glyceryl monostearate, and tragacanth and Span. Chun et al.[32] determined the hydrophile–lipophile balance of some natural agents and further discussed the principle of mixed emulsifiers.

The type of emulsion that is produced, *o/w* or *w/o*, depends primarily on the property of the emulsifying agent. This characteristic is referred to as the *hydrophile–lipophile* balance, that is, the polar–nonpolar nature of the emulsifier. In fact, whether a surfactant is an emulsifier, wetting agent, detergent, or solubilizing agent may be predicted from a knowledge of the hydrophile–lipophile balance, as discussed in a previous chapter (p. 371). In an emulsifying agent, such as sodium stearate, $C_{17}H_{35}COONa$, the nonpolar hydrocarbon chain, $C_{17}H_{35}$—, is the *lipophilic* or "oil-loving" group; the carboxyl group, —COONa, is the *hydrophilic* or "water-loving" portion. The balance of the hydrophilic and lipophilic properties of an emulsifier (or combination of emulsifiers) determines whether an *o/w* or *w/o* emulsion will result. In general, *o/w* emulsions are formed when the HLB of the emulsifier is within the range of about 9 to 12, and *w/o* emulsions are formed when the range is about 3 to 6. An emulsifier with a high HLB, such as a blend of Tween 20 and Span 20, will form an *o/w* emulsion. On the other hand, Span 60 alone, having an HLB of 4.7, tends to form a *w/o* emulsion.

It would appear, therefore, that the type of emulsion is a function of the relative solubility of the surfactant, the phase in which it is more soluble being the continuous phase. This is sometimes referred to as the *rule of Bancroft*, who observed this phenomenon in 1913. Thus, an emulsifying agent with a high HLB is preferentially soluble in water and results in the formation of an *o/w* emulsion. The reverse situation is true with surfactants of low HLB, which tend to form *w/o* emulsions. Beerbower, Nixon, and Hill[33] suggested an explanation for emulsion type and stability and devised a general scheme for emulsion formulation based on the Hildebrand and Hansen solubility parameters (pp. 224, 225).

Multimolecular Adsorption and Film Formation. Hydrated lyophilic colloids have been used for many years as emulsifying agents, although their use is declining because of the large number of synthetic surfactants now available. In a sense, they may be regarded as surface active since they appear at the oil–water interface. They differ, however, from the synthetic surface-active agents in that (1) they do not cause an appreciable lowering of interfacial tension, and (2) they form a multi- rather than a monomolecular film at the interface. Their action as emulsifying agents is due mainly to the latter effect, for the films thus formed are strong and resist coalescence. An auxiliary effect promoting stability is the significant increase in the viscosity of the dispersion medium. Since the emulsifying agents that form multilayer films around the

droplets are invariably hydrophilic, they tend to promote the formation of *o/w* emulsions.

Solid Particle Adsorption. Finely divided solid particles that are wetted to some degree by both oil and water can act as emulsifying agents. This results from their being concentrated at the interface, where they produce a particulate film around the dispersed droplets so as to prevent coalescence. Powders that are wetted preferentially by water form *o/w* emulsions, whereas those more easily wetted by oil form *w/o* emulsions.

PHYSICAL STABILITY OF EMULSIONS

Probably the most important consideration with respect to pharmaceutical and cosmetic emulsions is the stability of the finished product. The stability of a pharmaceutical emulsion is characterized by the absence of coalescence of the internal phase, absence of creaming, and maintenance of elegance with respect to appearance, odor, color, and other physical properties. Some workers define instability of an emulsion only in terms of agglomeration of the internal phase and its separation from the product. Creaming, resulting from flocculation and concentration of the globules of the internal phase, sometimes is not considered as a mark of instability. An emulsion is a dynamic system, however, and flocculation and resultant creaming represent potential steps toward complete coalescence of the internal phase. Furthermore, in the case of pharmaceutical emulsions, creaming results in a lack of uniformity of drug distribution and, unless the preparation is thoroughly shaken before administration, leads to variable dosage. Certainly, the eye-appeal of an emulsion is affected by creaming, and this is just as real a problem to the pharmaceutical compounder as is separation of the internal phase.

Another phenomenon important in the preparation and stabilization of emulsions is *phase inversion*, which can be an aid or a detriment in emulsion technology. Phase inversion involves the change of emulsion type, from *o/w* to *w/o* or vice versa. Should phase inversion occur following preparation, it may logically be considered as an instance of instability.

In the light of these considerations, the instability of pharmaceutical emulsions may be classified as follows:

(*a*) flocculation and creaming
(*b*) coalescence and breaking
(*c*) miscellaneous physical and chemical changes
(*d*) phase inversion

Creaming and Stokes' Law. Those factors that find importance in the creaming of an emulsion are related by Stokes' law, equation (18–2) (p. 479). The limitations of this equation to actual systems have been discussed previously for suspensions (p. 479), and these apply equally to emulsified systems.

Analysis of the equation shows that if the dispersed phase is less dense than the continuous phase, which is generally the case in *o/w* emulsions, the velocity of sedimentation becomes negative, that is, an upward *creaming* results. If the internal phase is heavier than the external phase, the globules settle, a phenomenon customarily noted in *w/o* emulsions in which the internal aqueous phase is more dense than the continuous oil phase. This effect may be referred to as *creaming in a downward direction*. The greater the difference between the density of the two phases, the larger the oil globules and the less viscous the external phase, the greater is the rate of creaming. By increasing the force of gravity through centrifugation, the rate of creaming may also be increased. The diameter of the globules is seen to be a major factor in determining the rate of creaming. Doubling the diameter of the oil globules increases the creaming rate by a factor of four.

Example 18–5. Consider an *o/w* emulsion containing mineral oil with a specific gravity of 0.90 dispersed in an aqueous phase having a specific gravity of 1.05. If the oil particles have an average diameter of 5 μm or 5×10^{-4} cm, the external phase has a viscosity of 0.5 poise (0.5 dyne sec/cm^2 or 0.5 g/cm sec), and the gravity constant is 981 cm/sec^2, what is the velocity of creaming in cm per day?

$$v = \frac{(5 \times 10^{-4})^2 \times (0.90 - 1.05) \times 981}{18 \times 0.5}$$

$$= -4.1 \times 10^{-6} \text{ cm/sec}$$

and since a 24-hour day contains 86,400 sec, the rate of upward creaming, $-v$, is

$$-v = 4.1 \times 10^{-6} \text{ cm/sec} \times 86,400 \text{ sec/day} = 0.35 \text{ cm/day}$$

The factors in Stokes' equation may be altered to reduce the rate of creaming in an emulsion. The viscosity of the external phase can be increased without exceeding the limits of acceptable consistency by adding a *viscosity improver* or *thickening agent* such as methylcellulose, tragacanth, or sodium alginate. The particle size of the globules may be reduced by homogenization; this, in fact, is the basis for the stability against creaming of homogenized milk. If the average particle size of the emulsion in the example just given is reduced to 1 μm or one fifth of the original value, the rate of creaming is reduced to 0.014 cm per day or about 5 cm per year. Actually, when the particles are reduced to a diameter below 2 to 5 μm, Brownian motion at room temperature exerts sufficient influence so that the particles settle or cream slower than predicted by Stokes' law.

Little consideration has been given to the adjustment of densities of the two phases in an effort to reduce the rate of creaming. Theoretically, adjusting the external and internal phase densities to the same value should eliminate the tendency to cream. This condition is seldom realized, however, since temperature changes alter the densities. Some research workers have increased the density of the oil phase by the addition of oil-soluble substances, such as α-bromonaphthalene, bromoform, and carbon tetrachloride, which, however, cannot be used in medicinal products. Mullins and Becker[34] added a food grade of a brominated oil to adjust the densities in pharmaceutical emulsions.

Equation (18–2) gives the rate of creaming of a single droplet of the emulsion, whereas one is frequently interested in the rate of creaming at the center of gravity of the mass of the disperse phase. Greenwald[35] has developed an equation for the mass creaming rate, to which the interested reader is referred for details.

Coalescence and Breaking. Creaming should be considered as separate from breaking, since creaming is a reversible process, whereas breaking is irreversible. The cream floccules may be redispersed easily, and a uniform mixture is reconstituted from a creamed emulsion by agitation, since the oil globules are still surrounded by a protective sheath of emulsifying agent. When breaking occurs, simple mixing fails to resuspend the globules in a stable emulsified form, since the film surrounding the particles has been destroyed and the oil tends to coalesce. Considerable work has been devoted to the study of breaking instability. The effects of certain factors on breaking are summarized in the following paragraphs.

King[36] showed that reduction of particle size does not necessarily lead to increased stability. Rather, he concluded that an optimum degree of dispersion for each particular system exists for maximum stability. As in the case of solid particles, if the dispersion is nonuniform, the small particles wedge between larger ones, permitting stronger cohesion so that the internal phase may coalesce easily. Accordingly, a moderately coarse dispersion of uniform-sized particles should have the best stability. Viscosity alone does not produce stable emulsions; however, viscous emulsions may be more stable than mobile ones by virtue of the retardation of flocculation and coalescence. Viscous or "tacky" emulsifiers seem to facilitate shearing of the globules as the emulsion is being prepared in the mortar, but this bears little or no relationship to stability. Knoechel and Wurster[37] have shown that viscosity plays only a minor role in the gross stability of *o/w* emulsions. Probably an *optimum* rather than a *high* viscosity is needed to promote stability.

The *phase–volume ratio* of an emulsion has a secondary influence on the stability of the product. This term refers to the relative volumes of water and oil in the emulsion. As shown in the section on powders (p. 443), uniform spherical particles in loose packing have a porosity of 48% of the total bulk volume. The volume occupied by the spheres must then be 52%.

If the spheres are arranged in closest packing, theoretically they cannot exceed 74% of the total volume regardless of their size. Although these values do not consider the distortions of size and shape and the possibility of small particles lying between larger spheres, they do have some significance with respect to real emulsions. Ostwald[38] and others have shown that if one attempts to incorporate more than about 74% of oil in an *o/w* emulsion, the oil globules often coalesce and the emulsion breaks. This value, known as the *critical point*, is defined as the concentration of the internal phase above which the emulsifying agent cannot produce a stable emulsion of the desired type. In some stable emulsions, the value may be higher than 74% owing to the irregular shape and size of the globules. Generally speaking, however, a phase–volume ratio of 50:50 (which approximates loose packing) results in about the most stable emulsion. This fact was discovered empirically by pharmacists many years ago, and most medicinal emulsions are prepared with a volume ratio of 50 parts of oil to 50 parts of water.

Emulsions can be stabilized by electrostatic repulsion between the droplets, that is, by increasing their zeta potential. Magdassi and Siman-Tov[39] used lecithin to stabilize perfluocarbon emulsions, which appear to be a good blood substitute. Lecithin is a mixture of phospholipids having a negative charge at physiologic pH. The stabilizing effect is due to the adsorption of lecithin at the droplet surface, which creates a negative charge and consequently electrostatic repulsion. Lecithin produces very stable emulsions of triglyceride acids in water for intravenous administration. However, the stability of these emulsions may be poor because in clinical practice they are mixed with electrolytes, amino acids, and other compounds for total parenteral nutrition. The addition of positively charged species such as sodium and calcium ions or cationic amino acids—the charge on the latter depending on the pH—reduces the zeta potential and may cause flocculation. Johnson et al.[40] studied the effect of heparin and various electrolytes, frequently used clinically, on the stability of parenteral emulsions. Heparin, an anticoagulant, is a negatively charged polyelectrolyte that causes rapid flocculation in emulsions containing calcium and lecithin. The critical flocculation concentration occurs at a specific zeta potential. The value of this zeta potential can be determined by plotting the flocculation rate against the surface potential and extrapolating to zero flocculation rate.[41] Johnson et al.[40] explained the destabilizing effect of heparin as follows. Divalent electrolytes such as calcium bind strongly to the surface of droplets stabilized with lecithin to form 1:2 ion–lipid complexes. This causes a charge reversal on the droplets, leading to positively charged particles. The droplets are then flocculated by a bridging of the negatively charged heparin molecules across the positively charged particles, as depicted in Figure 18–10.

When the oil particles, which usually carry a negative charge, are surrounded in an o/w emulsion by a film of emulsifier, particularly a nonionic agent, the electrokinetic effects are probably less significant than they are in suspensions in maintaining the stability of the system. The effect of electrolytes in these systems has been studied by Schott and Royce.[42] Probably the most important factors in the stabilization of an emulsion are the physical properties of the emulsifier film at the interface. To be effective, an emulsifier film must be both tough and elastic and should form rapidly during emulsification. Serrallach et al.[43] have measured the strength of the film at the interface. They found that a good emulsifying agent or emulsifier combination brings about a preliminary lowering of the interfacial tension to produce small uniform globules and forms

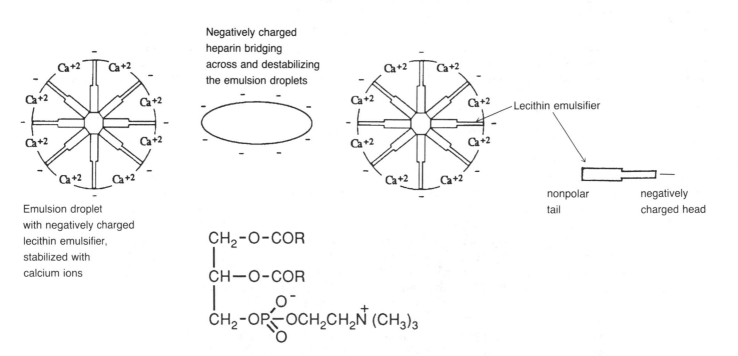

Lecithin (surfactant and emulsifier)

Fig. 18–10. Parenteral emulsion droplets in the presence of the negatively charged emulsifier lecithin, and stabilized by electrostatic repulsion by calcium ions. The emulsion may be flocculated and destabilized by the bridging effect of heparin, a negatively charged polyelectrolyte, which overcomes the stabilizing electrostatic repulsion of the Ca^{2+} ions. (From O. L. Johnson, C. Washington, S. S. Davis and K. Schaupp, Int. J. Pharm. **53**, 237, 1989, reproduced with permission of the copyright owner.)

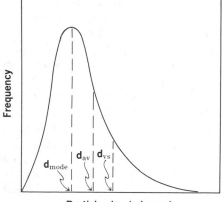

Fig. 18–11. Particle size distribution of an emulsion. Such curves ordinarily are skewed to the right as shown in the figure, and the mode diameter, i.e., the highest point on the curve or the most frequent value, is seen to occur at the lower end of the scale of diameters. The arithmetic mean diameter d_{av} will be found somewhat to the right of the mode in a right skewed distribution and the mean volume–surface diameter d_{vs} is to the right of the arithmetic mean.

rapidly to protect the globules from reaggregation during manufacture. The film then slowly increases in strength over a period of days or weeks.

Evaluation of Stability. According to King and Mukherjee,[44] the only precise method for determining stability involves a size-frequency analysis of the emulsion from time to time as the product ages. For rapidly breaking emulsions, macroscopic observation of separated internal phase is adequate, although the separation is difficult to read with any degree of accuracy. In the microscopic method, the particle diameters are measured, and a size-frequency distribution of particles ranging from 0.0 to 0.9 μm, 1.0 to 1.9 μm, 2.0 to 2.9 μm, etc., is made as shown in Figure 18–11. The particle size or diameter of the globules in micrometers is plotted on the horizontal axis against the frequency or number of globules in each size range on the vertical axis. Finkle et al.[45] were probably the first workers to use this method to determine the stability of emulsions. Since that time, many similar studies have been made. Schott and Royce[46] showed that the experimental problems involved in microscopic size determinations are Brownian motion, creaming, and field flow. Brownian motion affects the smallest droplets, causing them to move in and out of focus so that they are not consistently counted. Velocity of creaming is proportional to the square of the droplet diameter, and creaming focuses attention on the largest droplets because they move faster toward the cover glass than do smaller ones. *Field flow* is the motion of the entire volume of emulsion in the field due to the pressure exerted by the immersion objective on the cover glass, evaporation of the continuous phase, or convection currents resulting from heating by the light source. These workers[46] described an improved microscopic technique that overcomes these experimental problems and gives a more accurate measure of the droplet size.

An initial frequency distribution analysis on an emulsion is not an adequate test of stability, since stability is not related to initial particle size. Instead, one should perhaps consider the coalescence of the dispersed globules of an aging emulsion, or the separation of the internal phase from the emulsion over a period of time. Boyd et al.,[31] however, deemed this

method unsatisfactory since the globules may undergo considerable coalescence before the separation becomes visible. These workers conducted particle size analyses with a Coulter centrifugal photosedimentometer. Mean volume diameters were obtained, and these were converted to number of globules per milliliter. King and Mukherjee[44] determined the specific interfacial area, that is, the area of interface per gram of emulsified oil, of each emulsion at successive times. They chose the reciprocal of the decrease of specific interfacial area with time as a measure of the stability of an emulsion.

Other methods used to determine the stability of emulsions are based on accelerating the separation process, which normally takes place under storage conditions. These methods employ freezing, thaw–freezing cycles, and centrifugation.

Merrill[47] introduced the centrifuge method to evaluate the stability of emulsions. Garrett, Vold, and others[48] have used the ultracentrifuge as an analytic technique in emulsion technology. Coulter counting (p. 434), turbidimetric analysis, and temperature tests have also been used in an effort to evaluate new emulsifying agents and to determine the stability of pharmaceutical emulsions. Garti and Magdassi[49] developed a method to evaluate the stability of oil–water viscous emulsions (ointments and cosmetic creams) containing nonionic surfactants. The method is based on electrical conductivity changes (see pp. 127–128 for conductivity) during nondestructive short heating–cooling–heating cycles. Conductivity curves are plotted during the temperature cycling. A stability index is defined as Δ/h, where h is the change in the conductivity between 35° and 45° C and Δ is the conductivity interval within the two heating curves at 35° C, as shown in Figure 18–12. The *stability index* indicates the relative change in conductivity between two cycles. The smaller the conductivity, the greater is the stability of the emulsion. The method was applied in a series of emulsions at different HLB's, emulsifier concentrations, and oil phase concentrations. The authors reviewed earlier work on electrical conductivity of emulsions as related to stability.

Phase Inversion. When controlled properly during the preparation of an emulsion, phase inversion often results in a finer product, but when it gets out of hand during manufacturing or is brought about by other factors after the emulsion is formed, it can cause considerable trouble.

An *o/w* emulsion stabilized with sodium stearate can be inverted to the *w/o* type by adding calcium chloride to form calcium stearate. inversion may also be produced by alterations in phase–volume ratio. In the manufacture of an emulsion, one can mix an *o/w*

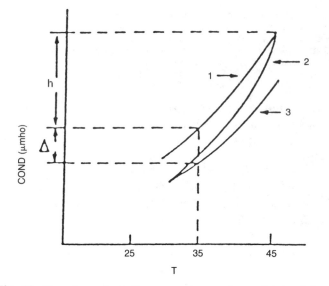

Fig. 18–12. A conductivity versus temperature plot involving successively (1) heating, (2) cooling, and (3) heating. (From N. Garti and S. Magdassi, Drug Dev. Ind. Pharm. 8, 475, 1982, reproduced with permission of the copyright owner.)

emulsifier with an oil and then add a small amount of water. Since the volume of the water is small compared with the oil, the water is dispersed by agitation in the oil even though the emulsifier preferentially forms an oil-in-water system. As more water is slowly added, the inversion point is gradually reached and the water and emulsifier envelope the oil as small globules to form the desired *o/w* emulsion. This procedure is sometimes used in the preparation of commercial emulsions, and it is the principle of the *Continental method* used in compounding practice. The preparation of emulsions is discussed in books on general pharmacy and on compounding and dispensing.

PRESERVATION OF EMULSIONS

While it is not always necessary to achieve sterile conditions in an emulsion, even if the product is for topical or oral use, certain undesirable changes in the properties of the emulsion can be brought about by the growth of microorganisms. These include physical separation of the phases, discoloration, gas and odor formation, and changes in rheologic properties.[50] Emulsions for parenteral use obviously must be sterile.

The propagation of microorganisms in emulsified products is supported by one or more of the components present in the formulation. Thus, bacteria have been shown to degrade nonionic and anionic emulsifying agents, glycerin, and vegetable gums present as thickeners, with a consequent deterioration of the emulsion. As a result, it is essential that emulsions are formulated to resist microbial attack by including an adequate concentration of preservative in the formulation. Given that the preservative has inherent activity against the type of contamination encountered, the main problem is

obtaining an *adequate* concentration of preservative in the product. Some of the factors that must be considered to achieve this end are presented here.

Emulsions are heterogeneous systems in which partitioning of the preservative will occur between the oil and water phases. In the main, bacteria grow in the aqueous phase of emulsified systems, with the result that a preservative that is partitioned strongly in favor of the oil phase may be virtually useless at normal concentration levels because of the low concentration remaining in the aqueous phase. The phase–volume ratio of the emulsion is significant in this regard. In addition, the preservative must be in an un-ionized state to penetrate the bacterial membrane. Therefore, the activity of weak acid preservatives decreases as the pH of the aqueous phase rises. Finally, the preservative molecules must not be "bound" to other components of the emulsion since the complexes are ineffective as preservatives. Only the concentration of free, or unbound, preservative is effective. These points have been discussed in some detail in earlier sections of the text. The distribution of solutes between immiscible solvents was presented in Chapter 10, and the preservative action of weak acids in oil–water systems was introduced on page 240. Binding of molecules was discussed in Chapter 12, and the student should consult that chapter for information regarding the types of interaction that are possible between preservative molecules and the components of emulsions, such as nonionic surfactants. In addition to partitioning, ionization, and binding, the efficacy of a particular preservative is also influenced by emulsion type, nutritive value of the product, degree of aeration, and type of container used. These factors are discussed by Wedderburn.[50]

RHEOLOGIC PROPERTIES OF EMULSIONS

Emulsified products may undergo a wide variety of shear stresses during either preparation or use. In many of these processes, the flow properties of the product will be vital for the proper performance of the emulsion under the conditions of usage or preparation. Thus, spreadability of dermatologic and cosmetic products must be controlled to achieve a satisfactory preparation. The flow of a parenteral emulsion through a hypodermic needle, the removal of an emulsion from a bottle or tube, and the behavior of an emulsion in the various milling operations employed in the large-scale manufacture of these products all indicate the need for correct flow characteristics. Accordingly, it is important for the pharmacist to appreciate how formulation can influence the rheologic properties of emulsions.

The fundamentals of rheology have been discussed in Chapter 17. Most emulsions, except dilute ones, exhibit non-Newtonian flow, which complicates interpretation of data and quantitative comparisons between different systems and formulations. In a comprehensive review,

Sherman[51] has discussed the principal factors that influence the flow properties of emulsions. The material of this section outlines some of the viscosity-related properties of the dispersed phase, the continuous phase, and the emulsifying agent. For a more complete discussion of these and other factors that can modify the flow properties of emulsions, the reader is referred to the original article by Sherman[51] and the book *Rheology of Emulsions*.[52]

The factors related to the dispersed phase include the phase–volume ratio, particle size distribution, and the viscosity of the internal phase itself. Thus, when volume concentration of the dispersed phase is low (less than 0.05), the system is Newtonian. As the volume concentration is increased, the system becomes more resistant to flow and exhibits pseudoplastic flow characteristics. At sufficiently high concentrations, plastic flow occurs. When the volume concentration approaches 0.74, inversion may occur with a marked change in viscosity. Reduction in mean particle size increases the viscosity; the wider the particle size distribution, the lower the viscosity when compared with a system having a similar mean particle size but a narrower particle size distribution.

The major property of the continuous phase that affects the flow properties of an emulsion is not, surprisingly, its own viscosity. The effect of the viscosity of the continuous phase may be greater, however, than that predicted by determining the bulk viscosity of the continuous phase alone. There are indications that the viscosity of a thin liquid film, of say 100 to 200 Å, is several times the viscosity of the bulk liquid. Higher viscosities may therefore exist in concentrated emulsions when the thickness of the continuous phase between adjacent droplets approaches these dimensions. Sherman points out that the reduction in viscosity with increasing shear may be due in part to a decrease in the viscosity of the continuous phase as the distance of separation between globules is increased.

Another component that may influence the viscosity of an emulsion is the emulsifying agent. The type of agent will affect particle flocculation and interparticle attractions, and these in turn will modify flow. In addition, for any one system, the greater the concentration of emulsifying agent, the higher will be the viscosity of the product. The physical properties of the film and its electric properties are also significant factors.

MICROEMULSIONS

The term *microemulsion* may be a misnomer, since microemulsions consist of large or "swollen" micelles containing the internal phase, much like that found in a solubilized solution. Unlike the common macroemulsions, they appear as clear transparent solutions, but unlike micellar solubilized systems, microemulsions

may not be thermodynamically stable. They appear to represent a state intermediate between thermodynamically stable solubilized solutions and ordinary emulsions, which are relatively unstable. Microemulsions contain droplets of oil in a water phase (*o/w*) or droplets of water in oil (*w/o*) with diameters of about 10 to 200 nm, and the volume fraction of the dispersed phase varies from 0.2 to 0.8.

As often recommended in the formation of ordinary or macroemulsions, an emulsifying adjunct or cosurfactant is used in the preparation of microemulsions. An anionic surfactant, sodium lauryl sulfate or potassium oleate, may be dispersed in an organic liquid such as benzene, a small measured amount of water is added, and the microemulsion is formed by the gradual addition of pentanol, a lipophilic cosurfactant, to form a clear solution at 30° C. The addition of pentanol temporarily reduces the surface tension to approximately zero, allowing spontaneous emulsification. The surfactant and cosurfactant molecules form an adsorbed film on the microemulsion particles to prevent coalescence.

Shinoda and Kunieda[53] showed that by choosing a surfactant and cosurfactant that have similar HLB values, solubilization of an organic liquid in water may be increased and the microemulsion droplet size enlarged without affecting stability. With ionic surfactants at normal temperatures, one expects *o/w* microemulsions to be formed when the phase volume ratio favors water, analogous to the rule for macroemulsions.

The microemulsion region is usually characterized by constructing ternary-phase diagrams, as shown in Figure 18–13, the axes representing water, mineral oil, and a mixture of surfactant and cosurfactant at differ-

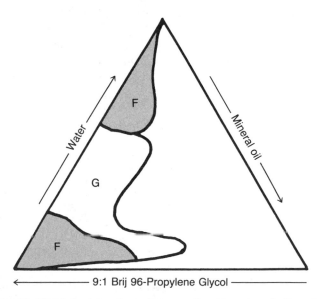

Fig. 18–13. A ternary-phase diagram of water, mineral oil, and a mixture of surfactants showing the boundary of the microemulsion region. The zones within the microemulsion region are labeled F for fluid and G for gel. (From N. J. Kale and L. V. Allen, Jr., Int. J. Pharm. **57,** 87, 1989, reproduced with permission of the copyright owner.)

ent ratios.[54] The phase diagrams allow one to determine the ratios oil:water:surfactant–cosurfactant at the boundary of the microemulsion region. The microemulsion appears by visual observation as an isotropic, optically clear liquid system. Kale and Allen[54] studied water-in-oil microemulsions consisting of the system Brij 96–cosurfactant–mineral oil–water. Brij 96 (polyoxyethylene (10) oleyl ether) is a nonionic surfactant commonly used in the preparation of macro- and microemulsions. The cosurfactants studied were ethylene glycol, propylene glycol, and glycerin. Figure 18–13 shows the phase diagram for the system upon varying the ratio Brij 96:propylene glycol. Within the microemulsion region, zones of different viscosity, labeled as fluid (F) or gel (G) can be observed. The microemulsion region becomes smaller as the cosurfactant concentration increases. According to the researchers, the transition from fluid microemulsion to gel-like microemulsion may be due to the change in the nature and shape of the internal oil phase. Thus, at low water content the internal phase consists of spherical structures, whereas at higher water concentration the interfacial film expands to form gel-like cylindrical and laminar structures. As the water content is further increased, aqueous continuous systems of low viscosity with internal phases of spherical structures (droplets) are again formed.

The droplet average molecular weight of a microemulsion can be measured by light-scattering techniques (see Chapter 15, p. 399). Since the internal phase is not usually very dilute, the droplets interact with one another, resulting in a decrease in the turbidity. Thus, the effective diameter obtained is smaller than the actual droplet diameter. The latter can be obtained from a plot of the effective diameter (obtained at various dilutions of the microemulsion) against the concentration of the internal phase. Extrapolation to zero concentration gives the actual diameter.[54] Attwood and Ktistis[55] have shown that the extrapolation procedure often cannot be applied, since many microemulsions exhibit phase separation on dilution. They described a procedure to overcome these difficulties and to obtain true particle diameter using light scattering.

Microemulsions have been studied as drug delivery systems. They can be used to increase bioavailability of drugs poorly soluble in water by incorporation of the drug into the internal phase. Halbert et al.[56] studied the incorporation of both etoposide and a methotrexate diester derivative in water-in-oil microemulsions as potential carriers for cancer chemotherapy. Etoposide was rapidly lost from the microemulsion particles, whereas 60% of the methotrexate diester remained incorporated in the internal phase of the microemulsion. The methotrexate diester microemulsions showed an in vitro cytotoxic effect against mouse leukemia cells. Microemulsions have also been considered as topical drug delivery systems. Osborne et al.[57] studied the

transdermal permeation of water from water-in-oil microemulsions formed from water, octanol, and dioctyl sodium sulfosuccinate, the latter functioning as the surfactant. These kinds of microemulsions can be used to incorporate polar drugs in the aqueous internal phase. The skin used in the experiments was fully hydrated so as to maximize the water permeability. The delivery of the internal phase was found to be highly dependent on the microemulsion water content: the diffusion of water from the internal phase increased tenfold as the water amount in the microemulsion increased from 15 to 58% by weight. Linn et al.[58] compared delivery through hairless mouse skin of cetyl alcohol and octyl dimethyl PABA from water-in-oil microemulsions and macroemulsions. The delivery of these compounds from microemulsions was faster and showed deeper penetration into the skin than delivery from the macroemulsions. The authors reviewed a number of studies on the delivery of drugs from the microemulsions. These reports, including several patents, dealt with the incorporation of fluorocarbons as blood substitutes and for the topical delivery of antihypertensive and antiinflammatory drugs. Microemulsions presently are used in cosmetic science,[59] foods, dry cleaning, and wax polishing products.[60]

SEMISOLIDS

Gels. A gel is a solid or semisolid system of at least two constituents, consisting of a condensed mass enclosing and interpenetrated by a liquid. When the coherent matrix is rich in liquid, the product is often called a *jelly*. Examples are ephedrine sulfate jelly and the common table jellies. When the liquid is removed and only the framework remains, the gel is known as a *xerogel*. Examples are gelatin sheets, tragacanth ribbons, and acacia tears.

Gels may be classified either as two-phase or as single-phase systems. The gel mass may consist of floccules of small particles rather than large molecules, as found in aluminum hydroxide gel, bentonite magma, and magnesia magma, and the gel structure in these two-phase systems is not always stable (Figure 18–14a, b). such gels may be thixotropic, forming semisolids on standing and becoming liquids on agitation.

On the other hand, a gel may consist of macromolecules existing as twisted matted strands (Figure 18–14c). The units are often bound together by stronger types of van der Waals forces so as to form crystalline and amorphous regions throughout the entire system, as shown in Figure 18–14d. Examples of such gels are tragacanth and carboxymethylcellulose. These gels are considered to be one-phase systems since no definite boundaries exist between the dispersed macromolecules and the liquid.

Gels may be classified as *inorganic* and *organic*. Most inorganic gels can be characterized as two-phase sys-

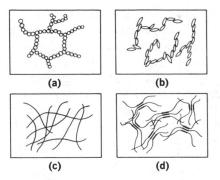

Fig. 18–14. Representations of gel structures. (*a*) Flocculated particles in a two-phase gel structure. (*b*) Network of elongated particles or rods forming a gel structure. (*c*) Matted fibers as found in soap gels. (*d*) Crystalline and amorphous regions in a gel of carboxymethylcellulose. (After H. R. Kruyt, *Colloid Science*, Vol. II, Elsevier, New York, 1949.)

tems, while organic gels belong to the single-phase class since the condensed matrix is dissolved in the liquid medium to form a homogeneous gelatinous mixture. Gels may contain water, and these are called *hydrogels*, or they may contain an organic liquid, in which case they are called *organogels*. Gelatin gel belongs to the former class, while petrolatum falls in the latter group.

Hydrogels retain significant amounts of water but remain water-insoluble and, because of these properties, are often used in topical drug design. The diffusion rate of a drug depends on the physical structure of the polymer network and its chemical nature. If the gel is highly hydrated, diffusion occurs through the pores. In gels of lower hydration, the drug dissolves in the polymer and is transported between the chains.[61] Cross-linking increases the hydrophobicity of a gel and diminishes the diffusion rate of the drug. The fractional release F of a drug from a gel at time t may be expressed in general as

$$F = \frac{M_t}{M_0} = kt^n \qquad (18\text{–}9)$$

where M_t is the amount released at time t, M_0 is the initial amount of drug, k is the rate constant, and n is a constant called the *diffusional exponent*. When $n = 0$, $t^n = 1$ and the release F is of zero order; if $n = 0.5$, Fick's law holds and the release is represented by a square root equation. Values of n greater than 0.5 indicate anomalous diffusion, due generally to the swelling of the system in the solvent before the release takes place.[62] Morimoto et al.[63] prepared a polyvinyl alcohol hydrogel for rectal administration that has a porous, tridimensional network structure with high water content. The release of indomethacin from the gel followed Fickian diffusion over a period of 10 hours.

Example 18–6. The release fraction F of indomethacin is 0.49 at $t = 240$ min. Compute* the diffusional exponent, n, knowing that $k = 3.155\%$ min^{-n}.

---

*See Problem 18–12 for calculation of the rate constant, k.

Since the rate constant k is expressed as percent, the fractional release, F, is also expressed in percentage units in equation (18–9), that is, 49%. Taking the ln on both sides of equation (18–9),

$$ln\ F = \ln k + n \ln t$$

$$n = \frac{\ln F - \ln k}{\ln t} = \frac{\ln 49 - \ln 3.155}{\ln 240}$$

$$n = \frac{3.892 - 1.149}{5.481} = 0.5$$

Therefore, with the exponent of t equal to 0.5, equation (18–9) becomes $F = kt^{1/2}$, which is a Fickian diffusion.

Syneresis and Swelling. When a gel stands for some time, it often shrinks naturally, and some of its liquid is pressed out. This phenomenon, known as *syneresis*, is thought to be due to the continued coarsening of the matrix or fibrous structure of the gel with a consequent squeezing-out effect. Syneresis is observed in table jellies and gelatin desserts. The term *"bleeding"* used in connection with the liberation of oil or water from ointment bases usually results from a deficient gel structure rather than from the contraction involved in syneresis.

The opposite of syneresis is the taking up of liquid by a gel with an increase in volume. This phenomenon is known as *swelling*. Gels may also take up a certain amount of liquid without a measurable increase in volume, and this is called *imbibition*. Only those liquids that solvate a gel can bring about swelling. The swelling of protein gels is influenced by pH and the presence of electrolytes.

Ofner and Schott[64] studied the kinetics of swelling of gelatin by measuring the increase in weight of short rectangular strips of gelatin films after immersion in buffer solutions as a function of time, t. A plot of the weight, W, in grams of aqueous buffer absorbed per gram of dry gelatin against t in hr gives the swelling isotherms (Fig. 18–15). The horizontal portions of the two isotherms correspond to equilibrium swelling. To

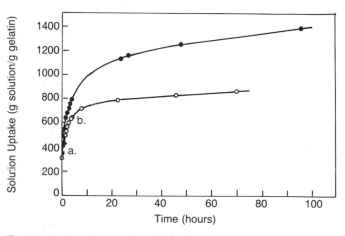

Fig. 18–15. Swelling isotherms of gelatin at two temperatures: ● at 25° C; ○ at 20° C. Swelling is measured as the increase in weight of gelatin strips in buffer solution after various times. The points **a** and **b** of this figure are discussed on p. 498. (From C. M. Ofner, III and H. Schott, J. Pharm. Sci. **75**, 790, 1986, reproduced with permission of the copyright owner.)

obtain a linear expression, t/W is plotted against t (the plot is not shown here) according to the equation

$$\frac{t}{W} = A + Bt \qquad (18-10)$$

Rearranging and differentiating equation (18–10), we obtain

$$\frac{dW}{dt} = \frac{A}{(A + Bt)^2} \qquad (18-11)$$

As $t \to 0$, equation (18–11) gives the *initial swelling rate*, $dW/dt = 1/A$, which is the reciprocal of the intercept of equation (18–10). The reciprocal of the slope, $1/B = W_\infty$, is the *equilibrium swelling*, that is, the theoretical maximum uptake of buffer solution at t_∞.

Example 18–7. The increase in weight of 330 mg for a 15% gelatin sample 0.27 mm thick was measured in 0.15 M ammonium acetate buffer at 25° C. The t/W values at several time periods are as follows:*

t (hr)	0.5	1	1.5	2	3	4
t/W $\dfrac{\text{hr}}{\text{g(buffer)/g(gelatin)}}$	0.147	0.200	0.252	0.305	0.410	0.515

Compute the initial swelling rate and the equilibrium swelling.
  A regression of t/W against t gives

$$\frac{t}{W} = 0.0946 + 0.1051\, t$$

The initial swelling rate, $1/A$, is the reciprocal of the intercept,

$$\frac{1}{A} = \frac{1}{0.0946} = 10.57 \text{ g(buffer solution)/hr g(gelatin)}$$

The equilibrium swelling

$$W_\infty = \frac{1}{B} = \frac{1}{0.1051} = 9.513 \frac{\text{g(buffer solution)}}{\text{g(gelatin)}}$$

Equation (18–10) represents a second-order process. When the constants A and B are used to back-calculate the swelling W at several times and are compared with the experimental data, the higher deviations are found in the region of maximum curvature of the isotherms (see Fig. 18–15). Ofner and Schott[64] attributed the deviations to the partially crystalline structure of gelatin. Thus, the first part of the curve (a) in Figure 18–15 corresponds to the swelling of the amorphous region, which is probably complete at times corresponding to maximum curvature, namely 6 to 10 hours at 20° C. The penetration of the solvent into the crystalline region is slower and less extensive because this region is more tightly ordered and has a higher density (part (b) in Fig. 18–15).

Gelatin is probably the most widely employed natural polymer in pharmaceutical products; it is used in the preparation of soft and hard gelatin capsules, tablet granulations and coatings, emulsions, and suppositories. Gelatin may interact with gelatin-encapsulated drugs or excipients by absorbing significant amounts of

them; and some compounds may charge the dissolution rate of soft gelatin capsules. Ofner and Schott[65] studied the effect of six cationic, anionic, and nonionic drugs or excipients on the initial swelling rate and equilibrium swelling in gelatin. The cationic compounds reduced the equilibrium swelling W_∞ substantially, while the nonionic and anionic compounds increased it. The researchers suggested that the cationic additives such as quarternary ammonium compounds may cause disintegration and dissolution problems with both hard and soft gelatin capsules.

Cross-linked hydrogels with ionizable side chains swell extensively in aqueous media. The swelling depends on the nature of the side groups and the pH of the medium. This property is important since diffusion of drugs in hydrogels depends on the water content in the hydrogel. Kou et al.[66] used phenylpropanolamine as a model compound to study its diffusion in copolymers of 2-hydroxyethyl methacrylate and methacrylic acid cross-linked with tetraethylene glycol dimethacrylate. The drug diffusivity D in the gel matrix is related to the matrix hydration by the relationship

$$\ln D = \ln D_o - K_f \left(\frac{1}{\mathbf{H}} - 1\right) \qquad (18-12)$$

where D_o is the diffusivity of the solute in water and K_f is a constant characteristic of the system. The term $\mathbf{H}$ represents the matrix hydration and is defined as

$$\mathbf{H} = \frac{\text{equilibrium swollen gel weight} - \text{dry gel weight}}{\text{equilibrium swollen gel weight}}$$

According to equation (18–12), a plot of $\ln D$ against $1/(\mathbf{H} - 1)$ should be linear with slope K_f and intercept $\ln D_o$ (see *Problem 18–14*).

Example 18–8. Compute the diffusion coefficients of phenylpropanolamine in a gel for two gel hydrations: $\mathbf{H} = 0.4$ and $\mathbf{H} = 0.9$. The diffusion coefficient of the solute in water is $D_o = 1.82 \times 10^{-6}$ cm^2/sec, and K_f, the constant of equation (18–12), $= 2.354$.
  For $\mathbf{H} = 0.4$,

$$\ln D = \ln(1.82 \times 10^{-6}) - 2.354 \left(\frac{1}{0.4} - 1\right) = -16.748$$

$$D = 5.33 \times 10^{-8} \text{ cm}^2/\text{sec}$$

For $\mathbf{H} = 0.9$,

$$\ln D = \ln(1.82 \times 10^{-6}) - 2.354 \left(\frac{1}{0.9} - 1\right) = -13.479$$

$$D = 1.4 \times 10^{-6} \text{ cm}^2/\text{sec}$$

The swelling (hydration) of the gel favors drug release, since it enhances the diffusivity of the drug, as shown in the example.

Classification of Pharmaceutical Semisolids. Semisolid preparations, with special reference to those used as bases for jellies, ointments, and suppositories, can be classified as shown in Table 18–2. The arrangement is arbitrary and suffers from certain difficulties, as do all classifications.

Some confusion of terminology has resulted in recent years, partly as a result of the rapid development of the

---

*The data are calculated from the slope and intercept given in Table III in reference 65.

TABLE 18—2. *A Classification of Semisolid Bases*

	Examples
I. Organogels	
A. Hydrocarbon type	Petrolatum, mineral oil—polyethylene gel*
B. Animal and vegetable fats	Lard, hydrogenated vegetable oils, Theobroma oil
C. Soap base greases	Aluminum stearate, mineral oil gel
D. Hydrophilic organogels	Carbowax bases, polyethylene glycol ointment
II. Hydrogels	
A. Organic hydrogels	Pectin paste, tragacanth jelly
B. Inorganic hydrogels	Bentonite gel, colloidal magnesium aluminum silicate gels
III. Emulsion-type semisolids	
A. Emulsifiable bases	
1. Water-in-oil (absorption)	Hydrophilic petrolatum, wool fat
2. Oil-in-water	Anhydrous Tween base†
B. Emulsified bases	
1. Water-in-oil	Hydrous wool fat, rose water ointment
2. Oil-in-water	Hydrophilic ointment, vanishing cream

*Plastibase (E. R. Squibb) J. Am. Pharm. Assoc., Sci. Ed. **45**, 104, 1956.
†White petrolatum, stearyl alcohol, glycerin, Tween 60 (Atlas-ICI).

newer type bases. Terms such as "emulsion-type," "water-washable," "water-soluble," "water-absorbing," "absorption base," "hydrophilic," "greaseless," and others have appeared in the literature as well as on the labels of commercial bases where the meaning is obscure and sometimes misleading. The title "greaseless" has been applied both to water-dispersible bases that contain no grease and to o/w bases because they feel greaseless to the touch and are easily removed from the skin and clothing. The terms "cream" and "paste" are also often used ambiguously. Pectin paste is a jelly, whereas zinc oxide paste is a semisolid suspension. And what does the term "absorption base" mean? Does it imply that the base is readily absorbed into the skin, that drugs incorporated in such a base are easily released and absorbed percutaneously, or that the base is capable of absorbing large quantities of water? These few examples point out the difficulties that arise when different titles are used for the same product or when different definitions are given to the same term.

Organogels. Petrolatum is a semisolid gel consisting of a liquid component together with a "protosubstance" and a crystalline waxy fraction. The crystalline fraction provides rigidity to the gel structure, while the protosubstance or gel former stabilizes the system and thickens the gel. Polar organogels include the polyethylene glycols of high molecular weight known as Carbowaxes (Union Carbide Corp., N.Y.). The Carbowaxes are soluble to about 75% in water and therefore are completely washable, although their gels look and feel like petrolatum.

Hydrogels. Bases of this class include organic and inorganic ingredients that are colloidally dispersible or soluble in water. Organic hydrogels include the natural and synthetic gums such as tragacanth, pectin, sodium alginate, methylcellulose, and sodium carboxymethylcellulose. Bentonite mucilage is an inorganic hydrogel that has been used as an ointment base in about 10 to 25% concentration.

Emulsion-Type Bases. Emulsion bases, as might be expected, have much greater affinity for water than do the oleaginous products.

The o/w bases have an advantage over the w/o bases in that the o/w products are easily removed from the skin and do not stain clothing. These bases are sometimes called *water washable*. They have the disadvantage of water loss by evaporation and of possible mold and bacterial growth, thus requiring preservation. Two classes of emulsion bases are discussed: emulsifiable and emulsified.

1. *Emulsifiable bases.* We choose to call these bases *emulsifiable* since they initially contain no water but are capable of taking it up to yield w/o and o/w emulsions. The w/o types are commonly known as *absorption bases* because of their capacity to absorb appreciable quantities of water or aqueous solutions without marked changes in consistency.

2. *Emulsified bases.* Water-in-oil bases in which water is incorporated during manufacture are referred to in this book as *emulsified w/o bases* to differentiate them from the emulsifiable w/o bases (absorption bases), which contain no water. The emulsified *oil-in-water bases* are formulated as is any emulsion with an aqueous phase, an oil phase, and an emulsifying agent. The components of emulsified ointments, however, differ in some ways from the ingredients of liquid emulsions.

The oil phase of the ointment may contain petrolatum, natural waxes, fatty acids or alcohols, solid esters, and similar substances that increase the consistency of the base and provide certain desirable application properties.

Comparison of Emulsion Bases. The absorption bases have the advantage over oleaginous products in absorption of large amounts of aqueous solution. Furthermore, they are compatible with most drugs and are stable over long periods. When compared with o/w bases, the w/o preparations are superior in that they do not lose water readily by evaporation since water is the internal phase. While emulsified *o/w* or washable bases do have the undesirable property of drying out when not stored properly and of losing some water during compounding operations, they are more acceptable than the nonwashable absorption bases because they are easily removed with water from the skin and clothing.

Hydrophilic Properties of Semisolids. Petrolatum is hydrophilic to a limited degree, taking up about 10 to 15% by weight of water through simple incorporation.

The water-absorbing capacity of oleaginous and wa-ter-in-oil bases may be expressed in terms of the *water number*, first defined in 1935 by Casparis and Meyer[67] as the maximum quantity of water that is held (partly emulsified) by 100 g of a base at 20° C. The test consists of adding increments of water to the melted base and triturating until the mixture has cooled. When no more water is absorbed, the product is placed in a refrigerator for several hours, removed, and allowed to come to room temperature. The material is then rubbed on a slab until water no longer exudes, and finally, the amount of water remaining in the base is determined. Casparis and Meyer found the water number of petrolatum to be about 9 to 15; the value for wool fat was about 185.

Rheologic Properties of Semisolids. Manufacturers of pharmaceutical ointments and cosmetic creams have recognized the desirability of controlling the consistency of non-Newtonian materials.

Probably the best instrument for determining the rheologic properties of pharmaceutical semisolids is some form of a rotational viscometer. The cone–plate viscometer (p. 466) is particularly well adapted for the analysis of semisolid emulsions and suspensions. The Stormer viscometer (p. 464), consisting of a stationary cup and rotating bob, is also satisfactory for semisolids when modified as suggested by Kostenbauder and Martin.[68]

Consistency curves for the emulsifiable bases, hydrophilic petrolatum and hydrophilic petrolatum in which water has been incorporated, are shown in Figure 18–16. It will be observed that the addition of water to hydrophilic petrolatum has lowered the yield-point (the intersection of the extrapolated down-curve and the load axis) from 520 to 340 g. The plastic viscosity (reciprocal of the slope of the downcurve) and the thixotropy (area of the hysteresis loop) are increased by the addition of water to hydrophilic petrolatum.

The effect of temperature on the consistency of an ointment base can be analyzed by use of a properly designed rotational viscometer. Figures 18–17 and 18–18 show the changes of plastic viscosity and thixot-ropy of petrolatum and Plastibase as a function of temperature.[69] The modified Stormer viscometer was used to obtain these curves. As observed in Figure 18–17, both bases show about the same temperature coefficient of plastic viscosity. These results account for the fact that the bases have about the same degree of

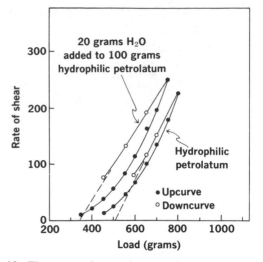

Fig. 18–16. Flow curves for hydrophilic petrolatum and hydrophilic petrolatum containing water. (After H. B. Kostenbauder and A. Martin, J. Am. Pharm. Assoc., Sci. Ed. **43**, 401, 1954.)

"softness" when rubbed between the fingers. Curves of yield value versus temperature were found to follow approximately the same relationship. The curves of Figure 18–18 suggest strongly that it is the alternation of thixotropy with temperature that differentiates the two bases. Since thixotropy is a consequence of gel structure, Figure 18–18 shows that the waxy matrix of petrolatum is probably broken down considerably as the temperature is raised, whereas the resinous structure of Plastibase withstands temperature changes over the ranges ordinarily encountered in its use.

Based on data and curves such as these, the pharmacist in the development laboratory can formulate ointments with more desirable consistency characteristics,

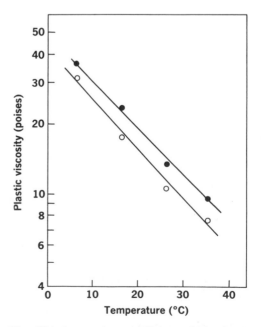

Fig. 18–17. The temperature coefficient of plastic viscosity of Plastibase, ● (E. R. Squibb and Sons) and petrolatum, ○. (After A. H. C. Chun, M. S. Thesis, Purdue University, June, 1956.)

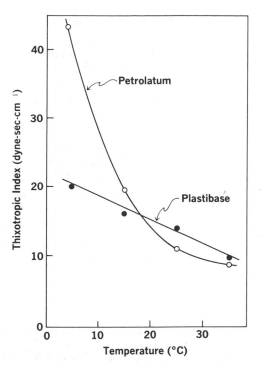

Fig. 18–18. The temperature coefficient of thixotropy of Plastibase (E. R. Squibb and Sons) and petrolatum. (After A. H. C. Chun, M. S. thesis, Purdue University, June, 1956.)

the worker in the production plant can better control the uniformity of the finished product, and the dermatologist and patient can be assured of a base that spreads evenly and smoothly in various climates, yet adheres well to the affected area and is not tacky or difficult to remove.

Rigidity and viscosity are two separate parameters used to characterize the mechanical properties of gels. Ling[70] studied the effect of temperature on rigidity and viscosity of gelatin. He used a *rigidity index, f,* which is defined as the force required to depress the gelatin surface a fixed distance. To measure rigidity, a sample of gelatin solution or gel mass is subjected to penetrative compression by a flat-ended cylindrical plunger that operates at a constant speed. In this method, the strain rate (rate of deformation of the gel) is constant and independent of stress (force applied). Ling found that thermal degradation with respect to rigidity followed second-order kinetics,

$$-df/dt = k_f f^2 \qquad (18-13)$$

The integral form of equation (18–13) is

$$\frac{1}{f} - \frac{1}{f_0} = k_f t \qquad (18-14)$$

where f is the *rigidity index* of the gelatin solution or gelatin gel at time t, f_0 is the rigidity index at time zero, k_f is the rate constant (g^{-1} hr^{-1}), and t is the heating time in hours, where g stands for gram. The quantities f_0 and k_f can be computed from the intercept and the slope of equation (18–14) at a given temperature.

Example 18–9. The rigidity degradation of a 6% pharmaceutical-grade gelatin USP was studied[70] at 65° C. The rigidity index values at several times are as follows:

t (hr)	10	20	30	40	50
$\frac{1}{f}$ (g^{-1})	0.0182	0.0197	0.0212	0.0227	0.0242

Compute the rigidity index f_0 at time zero and the rate constant k_f at 65° C.

The regression of $1/f$ versus t gives the equation

$$\frac{1}{f} = 1.5 \times 10^{-4}\, t + 0.0167$$

At $t = 0$ the intercept $1/f_0 = 0.0167$ g^{-1}; $f_0 = 59.9$ g. The slope $= k_f = 1.5 \times 10^{-4}$ g^{-1} hr^{-1}. Using the regression equation, one is able to compute the rigidity index f at time t, say 60 hr.

$$\frac{1}{f} = (1.5 \times 10^{-4} \times 60) + 0.0167 = 0.0257 \; g^{-1}$$

$$f = \frac{1}{0.0257} = 38.9 \; g$$

The force needed to depress the gelatin surface has decreased from its original value, $f_0 = 59.9$ g. Therefore, gelatin lost rigidity after heating for 60 hours.

The effect of temperature on the rate constant k_f can be expressed using the Arrhenius equation,

$$k_f = A e^{-E_a/RT} \qquad (18-15)$$

Thus, a plot of $\ln k_f$ against $1/T$ gives the Arrhenius constant A and the energy of activation E_a (see *Problem 18–15*).

Fassihi and Parker[71] measured the change in the rigidity index f of 15 to 40% gelatin gel, USP type B, before and after gamma irradiation (which is used to sterilize the gelatin). They found that the rigidity index diminished with irradiation and that the kinetics of rigidity degradation is complex. For gels containing more than 20% gelatin, the rigidity index follows a sigmoidal curve at increasing radiation doses, as shown in Figure 18–19. Gelatin is widely used in tablet manufacturing as a binder to convert fine powders into granules. The loss of rigidity index reduced the binding properties of gelatin and decreased the hardness of lactose granules prepared with irradiated gelatin. These workers suggested that doses of gamma radiation should be held to less than 2 megarad (Mrad) to obtain gelatins of acceptable quality for pharmaceutical applications.

Universe of Topical Medications. Katz[72] has devised a "universe of topical medications" (Fig. 18–20), by which one can consider the various topical medications such as pastes, absorption bases, emulsified products, lotions, and suspensions. The basic components of most dermatologic preparations are powder, water, oil, and emulsifier. Beginning at *A* on the "universal wheel" of Figure 18–20, one is confronted with the simple powder medication, used as a protective, drying agent, and lubricant and as a carrier for locally applied drugs.

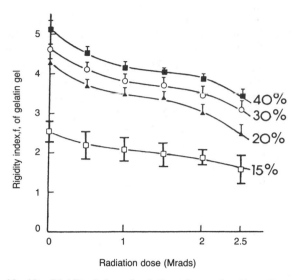

Fig. 18–19. Rigidity index of gelatin gel as a function of gamma irradiation at various concentrations (15–40%) of the gel. (From A. R. Fassihi and M. S. Parker, J. Pharm. Sci. **77**, 876, 1988, reproduced with permission of the copyright owner.)

Passing counterclockwise around the wheel, we arrive at the paste, *B*, which is a combination of powder from segment *A* and an oleaginous material such as mineral oil or petrolatum. An oleaginous ointment for lubrication and emolliency and devoid of powder is shown in segment *C*.

The next section, *D*, is a waterless absorption base, consisting of oil phase and *w/o* emulsifier and capable of absorbing aqueous solutions of drugs. At the next region of the wheel, *E*, water begins to appear along with oil and emulsifier, and a *w/o* emulsion results. The proportion of water is increased at *F* to change the ointment into a *w/o* cream. At *G*, the base is predominantly water, and an *o/w* emulsifier is used to form the

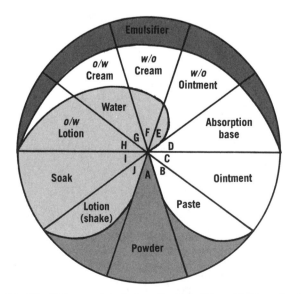

Fig. 18–20. Universe of topical medication. (From M. Katz, Design of topical drug products, in *Drug Design*, E. J. Ariens, Ed., Academic Press, New York, 1973, reproduced with permission of the copyright owner.)

opposite type of emulsion, that is, an *o/w* cream. Still more water and less oil converts the product into an *o/w* lotion at *H*. At point *I* on the universal wheel, only water remains, both oil and surfactant being eliminated, and this segment of the wheel represents an aqueous liquid preparation, a soak, or a compress.

Finally, at section *J*, the powder from *A* is incorporated, and the aqueous product becomes a shake preparation, as represented by calamine lotion. Accordingly, this ingenious wheel classifies nearly all types of topical preparations from solid pastes and ointments, through *w/o* and *o/w* emulsions, to liquid applications and shake lotions. It serves as a convenient way to discuss the various classes of dermatologic and toiletry products that are prepared by the manufacturer or practicing pharmacist and applied topically by the patient.

DRUG KINETICS IN COARSE DISPERSE SYSTEMS

The kinetics of degradation of drugs in suspension[73] can be described as a pseudo–zero-order process (see Chapter 12, p. 286).

$$M = M_0 - k_1 V C_s t \qquad (18\text{--}16)$$

where k_1 is the first-order constant of the dissolved drug, V is the volume of the suspension, and C_s is the solubility of the drug. If the solubility is very low, the kinetics may be described as found in the section on solid state kinetics (see Chapter 12, p. 313). For very viscous dispersed systems, the kinetics of degradation may be partially controlled by the dissolution rate as given by the Noyes–Whitney equation (p. 331),

$$dc/dt = KS(C_s - C) \qquad (18\text{--}17)$$

where C_s is the solubility of the drug, C the concentration of solute at time t, S the surface area of the expanded solid, and K the dissolution rate constant. It is assumed that as a molecule degrades in the liquid phase it is replaced by another molecule dissolving. The overall decrease in concentration in the liquid phase may be written as

$$dc/dt = -kC + KS(C_s - C) \qquad (18\text{--}18)$$

where $-kC$ expresses the rate of disappearance at time t due to degradation, and $KS(C_s - C)$ is the rate of appearance of the drug in the liquid phase due to dissolution of the particles. The solution of this differential equation is

$$C = [C_s KS/(k_1 + KS)]e^{-(k_1 + SK)t} \qquad (18\text{--}19)$$

At large t values, C becomes

$$C = C_s KS/(k_1 + KS) \qquad (18\text{--}20)$$

and the amount of drugs remaining in suspension at large values of t is

$$M = M_0 - [k_1 SKC_s V/(k_1 + KS)]t \quad (18\text{--}21)$$

where M_0 is the initial amount of drug in suspension. Equation (18–21) is an expression for a zero-order process, as is equation (18–16), but the slopes of the two equations are different. Since the dissolution rate constant, K, in equation (18–21) is proportional to the diffusion coefficient D (p. 331), K is inversely proportional to the viscosity of the medium; therefore, the more viscous the preparation the greater is the stability.

Example 18–10. The first-order decomposition rate of a drug in aqueous solution is 5.78×10^{-4} sec^{-1}, and the dissolution rate constant, K, is 3.35×10^{-6} cm^{-2}sec^{-1}. What is the amount of drug remaining in 25 cm^3 of a 5% *w/v* suspension after 3 days? Assume spherical particles of mean volume diameter $d_{vm} = 2 \times 10^{-4}$ cm. The density of the powder is 3 g/cm^3, and the solubility of the drug is 2.8×10^{-4} g/cm^3.

The initial amount of drug is

$$\frac{5}{100} = \frac{M_0}{25}; \; M_0 = 1.25 \text{ g/25 cm}^3$$

The number of particles N in 25 cm^3 can be computed from equation (16–4), page 430:

$$N = \frac{6}{\pi(d_{vn})^3\rho} = \frac{6}{3.1416 \times (2 \times 10^{-4})^3 \times 3}$$

$$= 7.96 \times 10^{10} \frac{\text{particles}}{\text{gram}}$$

The number of particles in 1.25 grams is $N = 7.96 \times 10^{10} \times 1.25 = 9.95 \times 10^{10}$ particles.

The total surface area is

$$S = N\pi d^2 = 9.95 \times 10^{10} \times 3.1416 \times (2 \times 10^{-4})^2 = 1.25 \times 10^4 \text{ cm}^2$$

From equation (18–21),

$$M = 1.25 -$$

$$\left[\frac{5.78 \times 10^{-4} \times 1.25 \times 10^4 \times 3.35 \times 10^{-6} \times 2.8 \times 10^{-4} \times 25}{5.78 \times 10^{-4} + (3.35 \times 10^{-6} \times 1.25 \times 10^4)} \right]$$

$$\times \, (2.6 \times 10^5 \text{ sec})$$

$$= 1.25 - [(3.99 \times 10^{-6})(2.6 \times 10^5)] = 1.25 - 1.0374 = 0.213 \text{ g}$$

Kenley et al.[74] studied the kinetics of degradation of fluocinolone acetonide incorporated into an oil-in-water cream base. The degradation followed a pseudo–first-order constant at pH values from 2 to 6 and at several temperatures. The observed rate constants increased with increasing temperature; and acid catalysis at low pH values and basic catalysis at pH above 4 were observed. The observed rate constant for the degradation process can be written as (see p. 304)

$$k = k_o + k_H[\text{H}^+] + k_{OH}[\text{OH}^-] \quad (18\text{--}22)$$

where the k_i values represent the specific rates (catalytic coefficients) associated with the various catalytic species. Figure 18–21 compares the degradation of fluocinolone acetonide from oil-in-water creams with that of triamcinolone acetonide, a related steroid, in aqueous solution. From the figure, both creams and solution share a similar log(rate)–pH profile over the pH range of 2 to 6, with a minimum rate near pH 4. This may indicate that the degradation in oil-in-water creams is confined to an aqueous environment, the

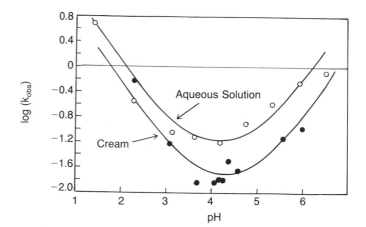

Fig. 18–21. pH–log(k_{obs}) profile for degradation of fluocinolone acetonide and triamcinolone acetonide at 50° C. Key: ● = experimentally determined k_{obs} (month^{-1}) for fluocinolone acetonide cream; ○ = triamcinolone acetonide solution. The solid lines were obtained from the calculated values of k_{obs} using equation (18–22). (From A. Kenley, M. O. Lee, L. Sukumar and M. Powell, Pharm. Res. **4**, 342, 1987, reproduced with permission of the copyright owner.)

nonaqueous components of the cream having little influence.[74]

Since $\ln k = \ln A - E_a/RT$, where A is the Arrhenius factor and E_a is the energy of activation, equation (18–22) can be rewritten in terms of activation parameters, A and E_a, for each of the catalytic coefficients, k_o, k_H, and k_{OH}:

$$k = \exp[\ln A_o - (E_{ao}/RT)]$$

$$+ \exp[\ln A_H - (E_{aH}/RT)][\text{H}^+]$$

$$+ \exp[\ln A_{OH} - (E_{aOH}/RT)][\text{OH}^-] \quad (18\text{--}23)$$

Equation (18–23) allows one to compute the degradation rate constant k at several temperatures and pH values.

Example 18–11. The natural logarithm of the Arrhenius parameters for neutral-, acid-, and base-catalyzed hydrolysis of fluocinolone acetonide in oil-in-water creams is $\ln A_O = 22.5$, $\ln A_H = 38.7$, and $\ln A_{OH} = 49.5$. The corresponding energies of activation are $E_{aO} = 17,200$, $E_{aH} = 22,200$, and $E_{aOH} = 21,100$ cal/mol. The H$^+$ and OH$^-$ concentrations in equation (18–23) are expressed, as usual, in moles per liter, and the first-order rate constant, k, is expressed in this example in month^{-1}. Compute the degradation rate constant k at 40° C and pH 4.

From equation (18–23),

$$k = \exp[22.5 - (17,200/1.9872 \times 313)] +$$

$$\exp[38.7 - (22,200/1.9872 \times 313)] \times (1 \times 10^{-4}) +$$

$$\exp[49.5 - (21,100/1.9872 \times 313)] \times (1 \times 10^{-10}) =$$

$$(5.782 \times 10^{-3}) + (2.025 \times 10^{-3}) + (5.820 \times 10^{-4})$$

$$k = 8.39 \times 10^{-3} \text{ month}^{-1}$$

Teagarden et al.[75] determined the rate constant k for the degradation of prostaglandin E$_1$ (PGE$_1$) in an oil-in-water emulsion. At acidic pH values, the degradation of PGE$_1$ showed large rate constants. This fact was attributed to the greater effective concentration of hydrogen ions at the oil–water interface, where PGE$_1$ is mainly located at low pH values.

DRUG DIFFUSION IN COARSE DISPERSE SYSTEMS

The release of drugs suspended in ointment bases can be calculated from the Higuchi equation (p. 336):

$$Q = [D(2A - C_s)C_s t]^{1/2} \qquad (18-24)$$

where Q is the amount of drug released at time t per unit area of exposure, C_s is the solubility of the drug in mass units per cm³ in the ointment, and A is the total concentration, both dissolved and undissolved, of the drug. D is the diffusion coefficient of the drug in the ointment (cm²/sec).

Iga et al.[76] studied the effect of ethyl myristate on the release rate of 4-hexylresorcinol from a petrolatum base at pH 7.4 and temperature 37° C. They found that the release rate was proportional to the square root of time, according to the Higuchi equation. Increasing concentrations of ethyl myristate enhanced the release rate of the drug owing to the increase of drug solubility, C_s, in the ointment (see equation (18–24)). This behavior was attributed to formation of 1:1 and 1:2 complexes between hexylresorcinol and ethyl myristate.

Example 18–12. The solubility of hexylresorcinol in petrolatum base is 0.680 mg/cm³. After addition of 10% ethyl myristate, the solubility C_s of the drug is 3.753 mg/cm³. Compute the amount Q of drug released after 10 hours. The diffusion coefficient D is 1.31×10^{-8} cm²/sec and the initial concentration A is 15.748 mg/cm³.

$$Q = \{1.31 \times 10^{-8} \text{ cm}^2/\text{sec } [(2 \times 15.748 \text{ mg/cm}^3) - 0.68 \text{ mg/cm}^3]\}^{\frac{1}{2}} \times$$
$$[0.68 \text{ mg/cm}^3 \times (10 \times 3600) \text{ sec}]^{\frac{1}{2}} = 0.099 \text{ mg/cm}^2$$

After addition of 10% ethyl myristate

$$Q = \{1.31 \times 10^{-8} \text{ cm}^2/\text{sec } [(2 \times 15.748 \text{ mg/cm}^3) - 3.753 \text{ mg/cm}^3]\}^{\frac{1}{2}} \times$$
$$[3.753 \text{ mg/cm}^3 \times (10 \times 3600) \text{ sec}]^{\frac{1}{2}} = 0.222 \text{ mg/cm}^2$$

The release of a solubilized drug from emulsion-type creams and ointments depends on the drug's initial concentration. It is also a function of the diffusion coefficient of the drug in the external phase, the partition coefficient between the internal and external phases, and the volume fraction of the internal phase. If the drug is completely solubilized in a minimum amount of solvent, the release from the vehicle is faster than it is from a suspension-type vehicle.

Ong and Manoukian[77] studied the delivery of lonapalene, a nonsteroidal antipsoriatic drug, from an ointment, varying the initial concentration of drug and the volume fraction of the internal phase. In the study, lonapalene was completely solubilized in the ointment systems. Most of the drug was dissolved in the internal phase, consisting of propylene carbonate–propylene glycol, but a fraction was also solubilized in the external phase of a petrolatum base consisting of glyceryl monostearate, white wax, and white petrolatum. The data were treated by the approximation of Higuchi:[78]

$$Q = 2 C_0 \sqrt{\frac{D_e t}{\pi}} \qquad (18-25)$$

in which Q is the amount of drug released per unit area of application, C_0 is the initial concentration in the ointment, D_e is the effective diffusion coefficient of the drug in the ointment, and t is the time after application. For a small volume of the internal phase,

$$D_e = \frac{D_1}{\phi_1 + K\phi_2}\left[1 + 3\,\phi_2\left(\frac{KD_2 - D_1}{KD_2 + 2D_1}\right)\right] \qquad (18-26)$$

where the subscripts 1 and 2 refer to the external and internal phases, respectively, and K is the partition coefficient between the two phases. When $D_2 \gg D_1$,

$$D_e = \frac{D_1(1 + 3\,\phi_2)}{\phi_1 + K\,\phi_2} \qquad (18-27)$$

D_e, the effective diffusion coefficient, is obtained from the release studies (equation (18–25)), and D_1 can be computed from equation (18–27) if one knows the volume fraction of the external and internal phases, ϕ_1 and ϕ_2, respectively. The drug is released according to two separate rates: an initial nonlinear and a linear diffusion-controlled rate (Fig. 18–22). The initial rates extending over a period of 30 minutes are higher than the diffusion-controlled rates owing to the larger transference of drug directly to the skin from the surface globules. The high initial rates provide immediate availability of the drug for absorption. In addition, the release of drug from the external phase contributes to the initial rates. Equation (18–25) is applicable only to the linear portion of the graph where the process becomes diffusion-controlled (see Fig. 18–22).

Example 18–13. Compute the amount of lonapalene released per cm² after $t = 24$ hours from a 0.5% *w/v* emulsified ointment. The internal phase of the ointment consists of the drug solubilized in a propylene carbonate–propylene glycol mixture and the external phase is a white petrolatum–glyceryl monostearate–white wax mixture. The volume fraction of the internal phase ϕ_2 is 0.028, the diffusion coefficient of the drug in the external phase is $D_1 = 2.60 \times 10^{-9}$ cm²/sec, and the partition coefficient K between the internal and external phases is 69.

From equation (18–27), the effective diffusion coefficient is

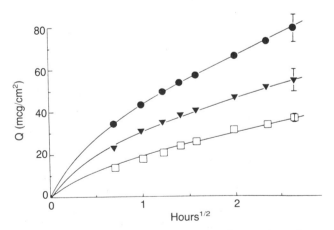

Fig. 18–22. Amount per unit area Q of lonapalene at time t from an emulsion-type ointment. Key: $\square$ = 0.5%; $\blacktriangledown$ = 1.0%; and $\bullet$ = 2.0% drug. (From J. T. H. Ong and E. Manoukian, Pharm. Res. **5,** 16, 1988, reproduced with permission of the copyright owner.)

$$D_e = \frac{2.60 \times 10^{-9} \text{ cm}^2/\text{sec } [1 + (3 \times 0.028)]}{(1 - 0.028) + (69 \times 0.028)}$$

$$= 0.97 \times 10^{-9} \text{ cm}^2/\text{sec}$$

Note that the sum of the volume fractions of internal and of external phases = 1; therefore, knowing the external volume fraction to be $\Phi_2 = 0.028$, one simply has the internal volume fraction, $\Phi_1 = (1 - 0.028)$. The initial concentration of drug is 0.5 g per 100 cm³, that is, 5 mg/mL. From equation (18–25), the amount of lonapalene released after 24 hours is

$$Q = 2 \times 5 \text{ mg/cm}^3 \sqrt{\frac{0.97 \times 10^{-9} \text{ cm}^2/\text{sec} \times (24 \times 3600) \text{ sec}}{3.1416}}$$

$$= 0.05 \text{ mg/cm}^2$$

The rate of release depends also on the solubility of the drug as influenced by the type of emulsion. Rahman et al.[79] studied the in vitro release and in vivo percutaneous absorption of naproxen from anhydrous ointments and oil-in-water and water-in-oil creams. The results fitted equation (18–25), the largest release rates being obtained when the drug was incorporated into the water phase of the creams by using the soluble sodium derivative of naproxen. After application of the formulations to rabbit skin, the absorption of the drug followed first-order kinetics, showing a good correlation with the in vitro release.

Chiang et al.[80] studied the permeation of minoxidil, an antialopecia (antibaldness) agent, through the skin from anhydrous, oil-in-water, and water-in-oil ointments. The rate of permeation was higher from water-in-oil creams.

Drug release from fatty suppositories can be characterized by the presence of an interface between the molten base and the surrounding liquid. The first step is drug diffusion into the lipid–water interface, which is influenced by the rheologic properties of the suppository. In a second step, the drug dissolves at the interface and is then transported away from the interface.[81] Since the dissolution of poorly water-soluble drugs on the aqueous side of the lipid–water interface is the rate-limiting step, the release is increased by the formation of a water-soluble complex. Arima et al.[81] found that the release of ethyl 4-biphenyl acetate, an antiinflammatory drug, from a lipid suppository base was enhanced by complexation of the drug with a hydrosoluble derivative of β-cyclodextrin. The increase in solubility and wettability as well as the decrease in crystallinity due to an inclusion-type complexation may be the cause of the enhanced release. On the other hand, complexation of flurbiprofen with methylated cyclodextrins, which are oil-soluble and surface-active, enhances the release from hydrophilic suppository bases. This is due to the decreased interaction between the drug complex and the hydrophilic base.[82] Coprecipitation of indomethacin with PVP also enhances the release from lipid suppository bases because it improves wetting, which avoids the formation of a cake at the oil–aqueous suppository interface.[83]

Nyqvist-Mayer et al.[84] studied the delivery of a eutectic mixture of lidocaine and prilocaine (two local anesthetics) from emulsions and gels. Lidocaine and prilocaine form eutectic mixtures at approximately a 1:1 ratio. The eutectic mixture has a eutectic temperature of 18° C, meaning that it is a liquid above 18° C and can therefore be emulsified at room temperature. The mechanism of release from this emulsion and transport through the skin is complex, owing to the presence of freely dissolved species, surfactant-solubilized species, and emulsified species of the local anesthetic mixture. The passage of these materials across the skin membrane is depicted in Figure 18–23. The solute lost due to transport across the membrane is replenished by dissolution of droplets as long as a substantial number of droplets are present. Micelles of surfactant with a fraction of the solubilized drug may act as carriers across the aqueous diffusion layer, diminishing the diffusion layer resistance. Droplets from the bulk are also transported to the boundary layer and supply solute, which diffuses through the membrane, thus decreasing the limiting effect of the aqueous layer to diffusion of solute. Because the oil phase of this emulsion is formed by the eutectic mixture itself, there is no transport of drug between the inert oil and water, as occurs in a conventional emulsion and which would result in a decreased thermodynamic activity, a, or "escaping tendency" (see pp. 68, 106). The system actually resembles a suspension that theoretically has high thermodynamic activity owing to the saturation of the drug in the external phase. In a suspension, the dissolution rate of the particles could be a limiting factor. In contrast, the fluid state of the eutectic mixture, lidocaine–prilocaine, may promote a higher dissolution rate. The total resistance R_T to the skin permeation of the free dissolved fraction of prilocaine is given by the sum of the resistances of the aqueous layer R_a and the resistance of the membrane R_m:

$$R_T = R_a + R_m \qquad (18\text{–}28)$$

or

$$R_T = \frac{1}{P} = \frac{h_m}{D_m K} + \frac{h_a}{D_a} \qquad (18\text{–}29)$$

where D is the diffusion coefficient of the drug, h_a is the thickness of the aqueous layer, h_m is the thickness of the membrane, and P is the permeability coefficient associated with the membrane and the aqueous layer; K

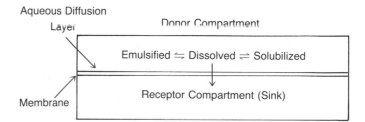

Fig. 18–23. Delivery of a eutectic mixture of lidocaine–prilocaine from an emulsion into a receptor compartment. (From A. A. Nyqvist-Mayer, A. F. Borodin and S. G. Frank, J. Pharm. Sci. **75**, 365, 1986, reproduced with permission of the copyright owner.)

is the partition coefficient between the membrane and the aqueous layer. The subscripts a and m stand for aqueous layer and membrane, respectively. Equation (18–29) is analogous to equation (13–55) (p. 338) except that the constant 2 in the denominator has been eliminated in this case because we consider only one aqueous layer (Fig. 18–24).

Example 18–14. Compute the total permeability P of a 1:1.3 ratio of lidocaine–prilocaine in the form of a eutectic mixture. The thickness of the aqueous and membrane layers are 200 μm and 127 μm, respectively. The diffusion coefficient and the partition coefficient of the drugs at the membrane–aqueous layers are as follows: lidocaine, $D_a = 8.96 \times 10^{-6}$ cm²/sec, $D_m = 2.6 \times 10^{-7}$ cm²/sec, and $K = 9.1$; prilocaine, $D_a = 9.14 \times 10^{-6}$ cm²/sec, $D_m = 3 \times 10^{-7}$ cm²/sec, and $K = 4.4$.

For lidocaine, according to equation (18–29),

$$\frac{1}{P} = \frac{127 \times 10^{-4} \text{ cm}}{2.6 \times 10^{-7} \text{ cm}^2/\text{sec} \times 9.1} + \frac{200 \times 10^{-4} \text{ cm}}{8.96 \times 10^{-6} \text{ cm}^2/\text{sec}}$$

$$= 7599.8 \text{ sec/cm}$$

$$P = 1/7599.8 = 1.32 \times 10^{-4} \text{ cm/sec}$$

For prilocaine,

$$\frac{1}{P} = \frac{127 \times 10^{-4} \text{ cm}}{3 \times 10^{-7} \text{ cm}^2/\text{sec} \times 4.4} + \frac{200 \times 10^{-4} \text{ cm}}{9.14 \times 10^{-6} \text{ cm}^2/\text{sec}}$$

$$= 11809.2 \text{ sec/cm}$$

$$P = 1/11809.2 = 8.47 \times 10^{-5} \text{ cm/sec}$$

The permeability of the mixture P_T can be calculated from the proportion of each component.[84] Since the proportion of lidocaine is 1, and that of prilocaine 1.3, the total amount is $1 + 1.3 = 2.3$. Therefore, the permeability of the mixture is

$$P_T = \frac{(1 \times 1.32 \times 10^{-4}) + (1.3 \times 8.47 \times 10^{-5})}{2.3}$$

$$= 1.05 \times 10^{-4} \text{ cm/sec}$$

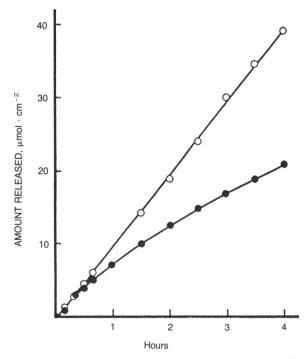

Fig. 18–24. Release of lidocaine–prilocaine from an emulsion (○) and from a gel (●). (From A. A. Nyqvist–Mayer, A. F. Borodin and S. G. Frank, J. Pharm. Sci. **75**, 365, 1986, reproduced with permission of the copyright owner.)

The total amount released from the emulsion consists of an initial steady-state portion from which the release rate can be computed. When the formulation is thickened with carbomer 934P (carbopol), a gel results. The release rate from the gel and the emulsion is compared in Figure 18–24. In the gel, the release rate continuously decreases, owing to the formation of a depletion zone in the gel. The thickness of the stagnant diffusion layer next to the membrane increases to such a degree that the release process becomes *vehicle controlled*. After 1 hour, the amount delivered is a function of the square root of time, and the apparent diffusion coefficient in the gel can be computed from the Higuchi equation (equation (18–24)). The release process is both membrane layer and aqueous layer controlled for nongelled systems (emulsions). See page 338 and 339 for a description of membrane and aqueous layer control. For gelled systems the initial release is also membrane layer and aqueous layer controlled, but later, at $t > 1$ hour, the release becomes formulation or vehicle controlled, that is, the slowest or rate-determining step in the diffusion of the drug is passage through the vehicle.

References and Notes

1. K. J. Frederick, J. Pharm. Sci. **50**, 531, 1961.
2. J. C. Samyn, J. Pharm. Sci., **50**, 517, 1961.
3. A. P. Simonelli, S. C. Mehta and W. I. Higuchi, J. Pharm. Sci. **59**, 633, 1970.
4. W. Schneider, S. Stavchansky, and A. Martin, Am. J. Pharm. Educ. **42**, 280, 1978.
5. K. S. Alexander, J. Azizi, D. Dollimore and V. Uppala, J. Pharm. Sci. **79**, 401, 1990.
6. E. F. Burton, in A. E. Alexander, *Colloid Chemistry*, Vol. I, Reinhold, New York, 1926, p. 165.
7. E. N. Hiestand, J. Pharm. Sci. **53**, 1, 1964.
8. A. Martin, J. Pharm. Sci. **50**, 513, 1961; R. A. Nash, Drug Cosmet. Ind. **97**, 843, 1965.
9. H. Schott, L. C. Kwan and S. Feldman, J. Pharm. Sci. **71**, 1038, 1982.
10. B. A. Haines and A. Martin, J. Pharm. Sci. **50**, 228, 753, 756, 1961.
11. A. Delgado, V. Gallardo, J. Salcedo and F. Gonzalez-Caballero, J. Pharm. Sci. **79**, 82, 1990.
12. A. Felmeister, G. M. Kuchtyak, S. Kozioi and C. J. Felmeister, J. Pharm. Sci., **62**, 2027, 1973; J. S. Tempio and J. L. Zaps, J. Pharm. Sci. **69**, 1209, 1980; ibid. **70**, 554, 1981; J. L. Zaps et al., Int. J. Pharm. **9**, 315, 1981.
13. E. N. Hiestand, J. Pharm. Sci. **61**, 269, 1972.
14. R. H. Blythe, U.S. Patent 2, 369, 711, 1945.
15. S.-L. Law, W.-Y. Lo and G.-W. Teh, J. Pharm. Sci. **76**, 545, 1987.
16. C. K. Mervine and G. D. Chase, Am. Pharm. Assoc. Meeting, 1952.
17. J. Y. Oldshue, J. Pharm. Sci. **50**, 523, 1961.
18. E. K. Fischer, *Colloidal Dispersions*, Wiley, New York, 1950; C. E. Berry and H. J. Kamack, *Proc. 2nd International Congress of Surface Activity*, Vol. IV, Butterworths, London, 1957, p. 196; C. L. Prasher, *Crushing and Grinding Process Handbook*, Wiley, New York, 1987, Chapter 6.
19. J. L. Zatz and R.-Y. Lue, J. Pharm. Sci. **76**, 157, 1987.
20. M. I. Zapata, J. R. Feldkamp, G. E. Peck, J. L. White and S. L. Hem, J. Pharm. Sci. **73**, 3, 1984.
21. S. C. Mehta, P. D. Bernardo, W. I. Higuchi and A. P. Simonelli, J. Pharm. Sci. **59**, 638, 1970.
22. A. P. Simonelli, S. C. Mehta and W. I. Higuchi, J. Pharm. Sci. **59**, 633, 1970.
23. K. H. Ziller and H. Rupprecht. Drug Dev. Ind. Pharm. **14**, 2341, 1988.

24. J. S. Lucks, B. W. Müller and R. H. Müller, Int. J. Pharm., **58**, 229, 1990.
25. B. D. Tarr, T. G. Sambandan and S. H. Yalkowsky, Pharm. Res. **4**, 162, 1987.
26. S. S. Davis and P. Hansrani, Int. J. Pharm. **23**, 69, 1985.
27. E. Shotton and R. F. White, in *Rheology of Emulsions*, P. Sherman, Ed., Pergamon Press, Oxford, England, 1963, p. 59.
28. J. A. Serrallach and G. Jones, Ind. Eng. Chem. **23**, 1016, 1931.
29. J. H. Schulman and E. G. Cockbain, Trans. Faraday Soc. **36**, 651, 661, 1940.
30. Atlas Booklet, A Guide to Formulation of Industrial Emulsions with Atlas Surfactants, Atlas Powder Co., Wilmington, 1953.
31. J. Boyd, C. Parkinson and P. Sherman, J. Coll. Interface Sci. **41**, 359, 1972.
32. A. H. C. Chun, R. S. Joslin and A. Martin, Drug Cosmet. Ind. **82**, 164, 1958.
33. A. Beerbower and J. Nixon, Div. Petr. Chem. Preprints, *ACS 14*, No. 1, 62, March, 1969; I & EC Prod. Res. Dev., Reprint; A. Beerbower and M. W. Hill, McCuchons Detergents and Emulsifiers, 1971, p. 223.
34. J. Mullins and C. H. Becker, J. Am. Pharm. Assoc., Sci. Ed. **45**, 110, 1956.
35. H. L. Greenwald, J. Soc. Cosmet. Chem. **6**, 164, 1955.
36. A. King, Trans. Faraday Soc. **37**, 168, 1941.
37. E. L. Knoechel and D. E. Wurster, J. Am. Pharm. Assoc., Sci. Ed. **48**, 1, 1959.
38. W. Ostwald, Kolloid Z. **6**, 103, 1910; **7**, 64, 1910.
39. S. Magdassi and A. Siman-Tov, Int. J. Pharm. **59**, 69, 1990.
40. O. L. Johnson, C. Washington, S. S. Davis and K. Schaupp, Int. J. Pharm. **53**, 237, 1989.
41. C. Washington, A. Chawla, N. Christy and S. S. Davis, Int. J. Pharm. **54**, 191, 1989.
42. H. Schott and A. E. Royce, J. Pharm. Sci. **72**, 1427, 1983.
43. J. A. Serrallach, G. Jones and R. J. Owen, Ind. Eng. Chem. **25**, 816, 1933.
44. A. King and L. N. Mukherjee, J. Soc. Chem. Ind. **58**, 243T, 1939.
45. P. Finkle, H. D. Draper and J. H. Hildebrand, J. Am. Chem. Soc. **45**, 2780, 1923.
46. H. Schott and A. E. Royce, J. Pharm. Sci. **72**, 313, 1983.
47. R. C. Merrill, Jr., Ind. Eng. Chem. Anal. Ed. **15**, 743, 1943.
48. E. R. Garrett, J. Pharm. Sci. **51**, 35, 1962; R. D. Vold and R. C. Groot, J. Phys. Chem. **66**, 1969, 1962; R. D. Vold and K. L. Mittal, J. Pharm. Sci. **61**, 869, 1972; S. J. Rehfeld, J. Coll. Interface Sci. **46**, 448, 1974.
49. N. Garti, S. Magdassi, and A. Rubenstein, Drug Dev. Ind. Pharm. **8**, 475, 1982.
50. D. L. Wedderburn, in *Advances in Pharmaceutical Sciences*, Vol. 1, Academic Press, London, 1964, p. 195.
51. P. Sherman, J. Pharm. Pharmacol. **16**, 1, 1964.
52. P. Sherman, Ed., *Rheology of Emulsions*, Pergamon Press, Oxford, 1963.
53. K. Shinoda and H. Kunieda, J. Coll. Interface Sci. **42**, 381, 1973; K. Shinoda and Friberg, Adv. Coll. Interface Sci. **44**, 281, 1975.
54. N. J. Kale and J. V. Allen, Jr., Int. J. Pharm. **57**, 87, 1989.
55. D. Attwood and G. Ktistis, Int. J. Pharm. **52**, 165, 1989.
56. G. W. Halbert, J. F. B. Stuart and A. T. Florence, Int. J. Pharm. **21**, 219, 1984.
57. D. W. Osborne, A. J. I. Ward and K. J. O'Neill, Drug Dev. Ind. Pharm. **14**, 1203, 1988.
58. E. E. Linn, R. C. Pohland and T. K. Byrd, Drug Dev. Ind. Pharm. **16**, 899, 1990.
59. H. L. Rosano, J. Soc. Cosmet. Chem. **25**, 601, 1974.
60. L. M. Prince, Ed., *Microemulsions, Theory and Practice*, Academic Press, New York, 1977.
61. J. M. Wood and J. H. Collett, Drug Dev. Ind. Pharm. **9**, 93, 1983.
62. C. Washington, Int. J. Pharm. **58**, 1, 1990.
63. K. Morimoto, A. Magayasu, S. Fukanoki, K. Morisaka, S.-H. Hyon and Y. Ikada, Pharm. Res. **6**, 338, 1989.
64. C. M. Ofner III and H. Schott, J. Pharm. Sci. **75**, 790, 1986.
65. C. M. Ofner III and H. Schott, J. Pharm. Sci. **76**, 715, 1987.
66. J. H. Kou, G. L. Amidon and P. L. Lee, Pharm. Res. **5**, 592, 1988.
67. P. Casparis and E. W. Meyer, Pharm. Acta. Helv. **10**, 163, 1935.
68. H. B. Kostenbauder and A. Martin, J. Am. Pharm. Assoc., Sci. Ed. **43**, 401, 1954.
69. A. H. C. Chun, M. S. Thesis, Purdue University, June, 1956.
70. W. C. Ling, J. Pharm. Sci. **67**, 218, 1978.
71. A. R. Fassihi and M. S. Parker, J. Pharm. Sci. **77**, 876, 1988.
72. M. Katz, Design of topical drug products, Chapter 4, in *Drug Design*, E. J. Ariens, Ed., Academic Press, New York, 1973.
73. J. T. Carstensen, Drug Dev. Ind. Pharm. **10**, 1277, 1984.
74. R. A. Kenley, M. O. Lee, L. Sukumar and M. F. Powell, Pharm. Res. **4**, 342, 1987.
75. D. L. Teagarden, B. D. Anderson and W. J. Petre, Pharm. Res. **6**, 210, 1989.
76. K. Iga, A. Hussain and T. Kashihara, J. Pharm. Sci. **70**, 939, 1981.
77. J. T. H. Ong and E. Manoukian, Pharm. Res. **5**, 16, 1988.
78. W. I. Higuchi, J. Pharm. Sci. **51**, 802, 1962; ibid. **56**, 315, 1967.
79. M. M. Rahman, A. Babar, N. K. Patel and F. M. Plakogiannis, Drug Dev. Ind. Pharm. **16**, 651, 1990.
80. C.-M. Chiang, G. L. Flynn, N. D. Weiner, W. J. Addicks and G. J. Szpunar, Int. J. Pharm. **49**, 109, 1989.
81. H. Arima, T. Irie and K. Uekama, Int. J. Pharm. **57**, 107, 1989.
82. K. Uekama, T. Imai, T. Maeda, T. Irie, F. Hirayama and M. Otagiri, J. Pharm. Sci. **74**, 841, 1985.
83. M. P. Oth and A. J. Moës, Int. J. Pharm. **24**, 275, 1985.
84. A. A. Nyqvist-Mayer, A. F. Borodin and S. G. Frank, J. Pharm. Sci. **74**, 1192, 1985; ibid. **75**, 365, 1986.
85. H. Schott, J. Pharm. Sci. **65**, 855, 1976.
86. K. Al-Khamis, S. S. Davis and J. Hadgraft, Int. J. Pharm. **40**, 111, 1987.

Problems

18-1. A hypothetical suspension contains 10^3 spherical particles of diameter $d = 10^{-3}$ cm. **(a)** Assuming that the interfacial tension between the solid and the liquid is $\gamma_{SL} = 100$ dyne/cm, compute the total surface free energy, G. **(b)** The solid particles are divided to obtain 100 particles from each initial particle. Compute the increase in the total surface area and the total surface free energy G' for the divided particles. *Hint:* Compute the volume of a particle to get its new radius and surface area. Assume that the density of the particle is unity.

Answers: **(a)** $G = 0.314$ erg; **(b)** $G' = 1.45$ erg

18-2. A coarse powder with a true density of 2.44 g/cm^3 and a mean diameter d of 100 μm was dispersed in a 2% carboxymethylcellulose dispersion having a density ρ_o of 1.010 g/cm^3. The viscosity of the medium at low shear rate was 27 poises. Using Stokes' law, calculate the average velocity of sedimentation of the powder in cm/sec.

Answer: 2.9×10^{-4} cm/sec

18-3. Using Stokes' law, compute the velocity of sedimentation in cm/sec of a sample of zinc oxide having an average diameter of 1 μm (radius of 5×10^{-5} cm) and a true density ρ of 2.5 g/cm^3 in a suspending medium having a density ρ_o of 1.1 g/cm^3 and a Newtonian viscosity of 5 poises.

Answer: 1.5×10^{-7} cm/sec

18-4. **(a)** Using the modified Stokes' expression, equation (18-3), compute the n value and v_s of a suspension of kaolin that contains tragacanth as a flocculating agent. The variation of the rate of fall v' measured at the sedimentation boundary, and the initial porosity ϵ (dimensionless) are given in the following table:

Data for *Problem 18-4**

ϵ	0.90	0.95	0.97	0.99
v' (cm/sec)	0.00164	0.038	0.127	0.415

*Data estimated from K. S. Alexander, J. Azizi, D. Dollimore and F. A. Patel, Drug Dev. Ind. Pharm. **15**, 2559, 1989.

(b) Compute the Stokes' diameter, d_{st}, of the flocs. The density of kaolin is 3.15 g/cm^3. Assume that the density and the viscosity of the aqueous medium, respectively, are 1 g/cm^3 and 0.01 poises. *Hint:* See the paper by Alexander et al. referred to in the table above. These workers obtain n as the slope and v_{st}, the Stokes velocity of sedimentation, as the intercept of a plot of log v' (y-axis) versus log ϵ

(*x*-axis). Using *v* and Stokes' law (equation (18–2)) yields the Stokes' diameter.

Answers: **(a)** n = 57.23 (dimensionless), v_{st} = 0.70 cm/sec; **(b)** d_{st} = 77 μm

18–5. Using the accompanying table, Data for Problem 18–5, and following the example shown in Figure 18–3, plot both H_u/H_o and the zeta potential, ζ, on the vertical axis against the concentration of $AlCl_3$. Note that sedimentation height is used here instead of volume. H_u is the ultimate height and H_o is the initial height of sedimentation. Draw vertical lines to separate the caking from noncaking regions of the diagram. Explain the changes in the H_u/H_o values, the changes in ζ potential, and the changes in the sign of the charge on the sulfamerazine particles as the concentration of aluminum chloride is increased. Discuss flocculation and deflocculation in relation to the caking and noncaking regions of the diagram. Graph paper with a five-cycle log scale on the horizontal axis is needed to accommodate the wide range of concentrations of the $AlCl_3$ solutions.

Answer: See pages 480 to 483 of the text.

18–6. From the data on griseofulvin given in the table below, plot both zeta potential, ζ, and V_u/V_o as shown in Figure 18–3. Draw vertical dashed lines on the graph and label each area to show: Caking Zone, Caked But Easily Dispersed Zone, Noncaking Zone, and the zone labeled Flocculated Initially but Potential Caking Later. The latter zone possibly forms caked suspensions over time. Discuss the V_u/V_o curve in relation to the ζ potential curve and their facility to differentiate the several zones of caking and noncaking. As the charge on the griseofulvin particles change with increasing concentration of $AlCl_3$, how is the caking of the suspension altered? You will

Data for *Problem 18–5:*
Sedimentation Height and Zeta Potential of Sulfamerazine in the Presence of Aluminum Chloride

$AlCl_3$ (mmole/liter)	H_u/H_o	ζ millivolts	Caking Condition
0.0	0.03	−63.4	Hard cake
0.2	0.03	−50.6	Hard cake
0.6	0.03	−38.6	Hard cake
1.0	0.08	−28.2	Slight cake
2.0	0.10	−25.4	No cake
6.0	0.10	−19.6	No cake
10.0	0.10	−14.0	No cake
20.0	0.09	−15.8	No cake
60.0	0.08	−4.0	No cake
100.0	0.08	+4.1	No cake
400.0	0.07	+3.7	No cake
600.0	0.06	−8.2	Viscous
1000	0.07	−13.5	Viscous

Data for *Problem 18–6:*
F Values and Zeta Potential of Griseofulvin Suspension in the Presence of Aluminum Chloride as Flocculating Agent*

$AlCl_3$ Sol'n (molarity)	ζ, Zeta Potential millivolts	F value V_u/V_o	Supernatant	Caking Conditions
0.0	−49.8	0.020	Opalescent	No flocculation, difficult to redisperse, caked
1×10^{-4}	−42.3	0.035	Opalescent	
5×10^{-4}	−27.9	0.140	Opalescent	Caked but easily redispersed
1×10^{-3}	−13.5	0.136	Clear	Floccule formation, easily redispersed, no caking
2×10^{-3}	−13.3	—	—	—
5×10^{-3}	−8.83	—	—	—
7.5×10^{-3}	−6.09	—	—	—
1×10^{-2}	0.0	0.144	Clear	Floccule formation, easily redispersed, no caking
1.5×10^{-2}	11.2	—	—	—
2.0×10^{-2}	11.7	0.121	Clear	Floccule formation initially but possible caking later
5.0×10^{-2}	21.1	0.123	Clear	
1×10^{-1}	24.1	0.140	Clear	

*From B. Millan-Hernandez, Thesis, University of Texas, 1981.

need graph paper with a four-cycle log scale on the horizontal axis (four-cycle semilog paper) for the concentration of the AlCl₃ solution.

18–7. Schott[85] studied the flocculation of bismuth subnitrate (diameter 3 μm) in aqueous suspension by bentonite platelets (diameter 0.2 μm). The negatively charged bentonite plates are adsorbed on and coat the much larger positively charged and lath-shaped (i.e., thin plate-like bodies) bismuth subnitrate particles. Use the data in the accompanying table to plot the sedimentation volume in milliliters and the zeta potential against the weight ratio of bentonite–bismuth subnitrate.

(a) Explain the significance of the sedimentation volume and the zeta potential curves.

(b) Show the regions of the diagram where caking and noncaking would be expected to occur.

(c) Explain how it is possible for bentonite to act as a flocculating agent similar to an electrolyte such as AlCl₃ or potassium phosphate.

Partial Answer: **(b)** See pages 482 to 483 of the text; **(c)** See J. Pharm. Sci. **65**, 855, 1976.

Data for *Problem 18–7:*
Sedimentation Volumes and Zeta Potential of Bentonite–Bismuth Subnitrate Mixtures*

Mixture number	Bentonite % (W/W)	Bismuth Subnitrate %(W/W)	Weight Ratio†	Sediment Volume (after 18 hr)	ζ milli-volts
1	0	13.18	0	5	—
2	0.00114	13.18	8.65×10^{-5}	5	+26.8
3	0.00568	13.18	4.3×10^{-4}	6	+30.2
4	0.0114	13.18	8.62×10^{-4}	6.5	+6.8
5	0.0568	13.18	4.35×10^{-3}	7	−10.4
7	0.2270	13.16	1.67×10^{-2}	12	−20.8
13	0.561	7.92	7.14×10^{-2}	43	−26.8
15	0.932	7.90	1.18×10^{-1}	59	−30.6
16	1.320	7.88	1.67×10^{-1}	85	−23.2

*The ratio, bismuth subnitrate–bentonite, has been inverted in this problem and several values in Tables I, II, and III of Schott have been eliminated. The electrophoretic mobility values of Table III have been converted to ζ values.
†Weight ratio per cent of bentonite–bismuth subnitrate.

18–8. It is possible to determine the concentration of soap present as a monomolecular layer at the surface of the oil globules in an emulsion by centrifuging the emulsion, removing the cream layer, acidifying it, and titrating with sodium hydroxide. By the use of this method, the concentration of sodium oleate at the interface of a mineral oil emulsion was found to be 0.02 mole sodium oleate per liter of oil. The particles were found by a microscopic method to have a mean diameter of 1.0 μm (1×10^{-4} cm). Calculate the mean area of a soap molecule at the surface of an oil globule in the emulsion. Explain the discrepancy between the calculated value and the value, 25 Å², for the area of a soap molecule as found by the film balance method.

Answer: 50 Å². Apparently the film of molecules at the surface of an oil globule is not as condensed as that obtained in the film balance method. See pages 376 to 378 and Figures 14–18 and 14–19.

18–9. Mineral oil was dispersed as globules in an oil–water emulsion to form a total surface area of globules of 10⁸ cm². If the presence of an emulsifying agent results in an interfacial tension between the oil and the water phase of 5 erg/cm², what is the total surface free energy of the system in calories, in SI units?

Answer: $\Delta G = 12$ cal, 5×10^{8} erg, 50.2 joule

18–10. A series of mineral oil emulsions was prepared using various combinations of Span 80 and Tween 80 (Atlas, ICI). The Span–Tween ratio of the best emulsion was found to be 40/60. Compute the HLB of this mixture. Span 80 has an HLB of 4.3 and Tween 80 an HLB of 15.0 (*Hint:* The HLB contributions of each emulsifier are obtained by multiplying the HLB of the agent by the fraction it contributes to the emulsifier phase.)

Answer: HLB = 10.7.

18–11. (a) Calculate the *required HLB*, abbreviated *RHLB*, for the oil phase in the oil-in-water lotion:

Mineral oil, light	10 g
Petrolatum	25
Stearic acid	15
Beeswax	5
Emulsifier	2
Preservative	0.2
Water	42.8
Perfume	q.s.

Hint: Multiply the percentage (actually the *fraction*, which is the percentage divided by 100) of each oil phase ingredient by its RHLB (Table 14–6) and sum to obtain the RHLB for the lotion.

(b) Calculate the amount in grams of an emulsifier pair, Tween 60 and Arlacel 60, to produce a stable oil-in-water emulsified lotion. The HLB of Tween 60 is 14.9 and that of Arlacel 60 is 4.7.

(c) State how you would combine the ingredients to produce a stable product.

Answers: **(a)** RHLB of the oil phase = 11.88; **(b)** Tween 60, 1.4 grams; Arlacel 60, 0.6 gram.

18–12. The rate constant k and the diffusional exponent n of equation (18–9) can be obtained respectively from the intercept and the slope of a plot of ln F versus ln t, where $F = (M_t/M_o) \times 100$ is the fractional release of drug from a gel (expressed as percentage), M_o being the initial amount of drug and M_t the amount released at time t. Assume the following results for the delivery of a drug from a gel:

Data for *Problem 18–12*

t (min)	10	20	50	100	200
F (%)	6.28	10.21	19.38	31.49	51.15

(a) Using regression analysis of ln F (dependent variable) versus ln t (independent variable) compute the rate constant k and diffusional exponent n. Does the release follow a Fickian model?

(b) What is the fractional release in percent at 73 minutes?

(c) Compute the time at which 100% of the drug is released from the gel.

Answers: **(a)** $n = 0.7$; $k = 1.251\%$ min$^{-0.7}$; **(b)** $(M_t/M_o) \times 100 = F = 25.2\%$; **(c)** 523 min

18–13. Ofner and Schott[65] studied the effect of cetylpyridinium chloride, a cationic compound, on the swelling of gelatin. The weight, W, in grams of an aqueous buffered solution of cetylpyridinium chloride absorbed per gram of dry gelatin as a function of time is:

Data for *Problem 18–13*

t (hr)	0.5	1	1.5	2	3	4
W (g/g)	2.84	3.98	4.60	4.99	5.44	5.71

The regression equation is:

$$t/W = A + Bt$$

in which A is the intercept and B is the slope.

(a) Plot t/W (on the y/axis) against time (on the x/axis) and compute the *initial swelling rate* given by the reciprocal of the intercept (1/A). Also, calculate the *equilibrium swelling* i.e., the maximum uptake of the solution of the cationic compound, which is given by the reciprocal of the slope (1/B). (See *example 18–7* and Figure 18–15.)

(b) Compute the percent increase or decrease in the W value for cetylpyridinium chloride in gelatin at 4 hours with respect to the increase in the W value for plain gelatin at the same time. For gelatin,

$$A = 0.0755 \frac{\text{hours} \times \text{gram gelatin}}{\text{gram solution}}$$

and $B = 0.132$ (gram gelatin)/(gram solution).

(c) Repeat part (b) for a buffered solution of an anionic compound, dicloxacillin sodium, with respect to plain gelatin. For this anionic compound,

$$A = 0.0310 \frac{\text{hour} \times \text{gram gelatin}}{\text{gram solution}}$$

and $B = 0.110$ (gram gelatin)/(gram solution). Regression analysis may be used in solving this problem.

Answers: (a) $1/A$ = initial swelling rate = 9.9 g/hr; $1/B$ = equilibrium swelling = 6.7 (g solution/g gelatin); (b) −13.7%, a decrease; (c) 28.2%, an increase

18–14. The diffusion coefficients D of phenylpropanolamine in swollen poly(hydroxyethyl methacrylate-co-methacrylic acid) hydrogels were measured at several pH values, corresponding to different gel hydration values, H[66]:

Data for *Problem 18–14*

pH	1	3	5	7
H (dimensionless hydration value)	0.352	0.337	0.639	0.880
$D \times 10^8$ cm²/sec	2.50	3.58	44.6	139.0

Compute the diffusion coefficient D_0 of phenylpropanolamine in water and the constant k_f of the system, using equation (18–12), page 498:

$$\ln D = \ln D_o - k_f \left(\frac{1}{H} - 1 \right)$$

Answer: $k_f = 2.354$; $D_o = 1.81 \times 10^{-6}$ cm²/sec

18–15. The values of the ln of the rate constant k in grams^{-1} hours^{-1} for the rigidity breakdown of a 6% gelatin solution versus the reciprocal of absolute temperature was found to be:[70]

Data for *Problem 18–15*

$(1/T) \times 10^3$ °K^{-1}	2.90	2.95	3.00	3.10	3.15
ln k	−5.978	−6.429	−6.881	−7.783	−8.235

Compute the activation energy, E_a, for rigidity degradation. Express the result in the Arrhenius exponential form.

Answer: $E_a = 17939$ cal/mole; $k = 5.938 \times 10^8 \, e^{-17939/RT}$ (gram^{-1} hour^{-1})

18–16. The results of a stability study of two brands, B and E, of ampicillin suspension at 5° C after reconstitution of the product are:

Data for *Problem 18–16**

t (days)		2	4	6	8	10
[A] (mg/5 mL)	Brand B	284.49	268.97	253.46	237.94	222.43
	Brand E	294.37	288.74	283.11	277.48	271.85

*Data calculated from rate constants given in N. A. Boraie, S. A. El-Fattah and H. M. Hassan, Drug Dev. Ind. Pharm. **14,** 831, 1988. The concentrations have been modified somewhat.

[A] is the concentration remaining at the various times, t (days). According to the labels, the products are stable for 2 weeks when refrigerated at 5° C. The USP requires that the products contain not less than 90% and not more than 120% of the label claim at this time.

(a) Compute the apparent zero-order rate constants, k_o (mg/5 mL)/day and the initial concentration in (mg/5 mL) of brands B and E at the time of reconstitution.

(b) Compute the time at which the products decompose to 90% of their original concentration (i.e., a decomposition of 10%). Do the suspensions meet the stated requirements under the storage conditions?

Answers: (a) k_o = 7.758 (mg/5 mL)/day (Brand B) and 2.815 (mg/5 mL)/day (Brand E); (b) t_{90} = 3.9 days (Brand B) and 10.6 days (Brand E) at 5° C. Product E satisfies the label claim.

18–17. Compute the energy of activation E_a for the neutral, acid-catalyzed, and base-catalyzed hydrolysis of fluocinolone acetonide in an oil–water emulsion. The rate constants are:[74]

Data for *Problem 18–17*

Temperature (°C)	80	50	40	23
k_{H+} (M^{-1} month^{-1})	759	72.5	44.7	1.32
k_{OH^-} (M^{-1} month^{-1})	168	17.0	13.6	0.372
k_o (month^{-1})	0.133	0.0116	0.00079	0.00117

Answer: 18,968 cal/mole; 22,203 cal/mole; 21,161 cal/mole

18–18. The amount per unit area, Q, of hexylresorcinol released from petrolatum ointment containing 3% of ethyl myristate at various times, t, is:

Data for *Problem 18–18*

t (hr)	2	9	16	25
$Q \times 10^3$ mg/cm²	1.45	3.07	4.10	5.12

Plot Q (vertical axis) against $t^{1/2}$. Compute the release rate (mg cm^{-2} hr$^{-1/2}$) of the drug from the slope, according to the Higuchi equation 18–24. Compute the diffusion coefficient knowing that A is 20 mg/cm³ and the apparent solubility C_s of the drug in the ointment is 2.121 mg/cm³. A is the total concentration of the drug, dissolved and undissolved.[76]

Answer: Release rate = 1.02×10^{-3} mg cm^{-2} h$^{-1/2}$; $D = 1.3 \times 10^{-8}$ cm²/hr or 3.6×10^{-12} cm²/sec

18–19. The diffusion coefficient of salicylic acid dispersed in a Plastibase vehicle was found to vary with the particle size of salicylic acid. For particles of 88 μm in diameter, $D = 1.11 \times 10^{-6}$ cm²/sec; and for particles of 5.1 μm in diameter, $D = 1.85 \times 10^{-6}$ cm²/sec, where D is the diffusion coefficient. (The diffusion coefficients and solubility are from Al-Khamis et al.[86] Compute the amount of drug released per unit area at t = 9 hr for both particle sizes using the Higuchi expression, equation (18–24). The initial amount of drug is $A = 600$ μg/cm³, and the solubility of the drug in the vehicle is $C_s = 495$ μg/cm³. Is the drug release larger or smaller when the particle size is reduced?

Answer: Q (88 μm) = 112 μg/cm²; Q (5.1 μm/cm²) = 145 μg/cm²

18–20. In an effort to determine the amount of emulsifier (a soap such as sodium stearate) required to prepare a stable mineral oil emulsion, one must ask the following questions. (Answer each question, (a) through (g), to arrive at the grams of soap for a 100 cm³ emulsion containing oil globules of 1 μm (1×10^{-4} cm) diameter. The emulsion contains 50 cm³ of oil.)

(a) The diameter of each oil globule is, on the average, 1 μm. What is the surface area of each globule? Show all calculations.

(b) If the cross-sectional area of a soap molecule is 25 Å, how many soap molecules can be placed on the surface of each oil droplet to cover it with a layer one molecule thick?

(c) If we produce an emulsion containing 50 cm³ of oil and 50 cm³ of water with the oil reduced to particles of 1 μm diameter, how many oil globules are there in the 100 cm³ emulsion? The density of the oil is 0.90 g/cm³.

(d) How many molecules of soap (sodium stearate) are required to cover all the mineral oil globules with a monolayer of soap molecules?

(e) What is the weight in grams of each of the soap molecules? *Hint:* You will need the molecular weight of sodium stearate.

(f) How many grams of soap (sodium stearate) are required to cover the 50 cm³ of oil droplets with a monolayer of soap molecules?

(g) Soap-stabilized commercial emulsions ordinarily contain 1 to 2 percent of soap. Therefore, 1 to 2 grams should be plenty for a 100 cm³ emulsion containing oil particles of 1 μm diameter. If the oil particles were larger, say 10 μm on the average, would we need more

or less soap to cover the 50 cm³ of oil globules with a layer one soap molecule thick?

Answers: **(a)** 3.14×10^{-8} cm²/oil globule. **(b)** 12.6 million soap molecules around each oil globule. **(c)** Approximately 100 trillion droplets of oil. **(d)** 1.26×10^{21} soap molecules for the 100 cm³ emulsion (which contains 50 cm³ of oil). **(e)** Approximately 50×10^{-23} gram soap/molecule. **(f)** About 0.6 grams of soap for this 100 cm³ mineral oil emulsion.

18–21. Name one commercial product or a USP-NF preparation as an example of each class of topical medication found in Figure 18–20, *A* through *J*.

Partial Answer: For *D*, absorption bases, hydrophilic petrolatum of the USP-NF is a good example.

19
Drug Product Design

Prodrugs and Drug Carriers   Routes of Administration

The principles of thermodynamics, chemical equilibria, surface and colloidal phenomena, kinetics of decomposition, diffusion of drugs through membranes, and solubility and complexation constitute the subject of previous chapters. This chapter introduces the subject of dosage form design and controlled drug delivery systems. It applies the principles of chemistry, biology, and physical pharmacy to the formulation of drug delivery systems.

Of the systems discussed some are presently approved by the U.S. FDA and are accepted in medical practice; others are in various stages of research and clinical trial. The field of new drug design and controlled delivery is developing rapidly, and limitations of space militates against the inclusion here of all new systems and devices. For example, no mention is made of new dosage forms for vaginal and intrauterine routes, delivery to the brain, erythrocyte carriers, and drugs targeted to lymph cells of the immune system.

Although the present rapid introduction into commerce of new drugs and devices makes the study of drug design and delivery somewhat difficult and confusing, the subject is simpler that it appears from a perusal of current pharmaceutical literature.

The chapter begins with a discussion of prodrugs and drug carriers. It is then organized according to routes of administration and the controlled delivery devices and absorption enhancers that have recently been developed.

The rationale for the controlled delivery of drugs is to promote therapeutic benefits while at the same time minimizing toxic effects. New drug delivery approaches to medication technology are finding use in long-term fertility control; genetically related enzyme replacement therapy; transdermal, nasal, and pulmonary administration; and treatment of glaucoma and ocular infections. Normal drug dosing may follow a "sawtooth" kinetic profile (Fig. 19–1), in which the dose first

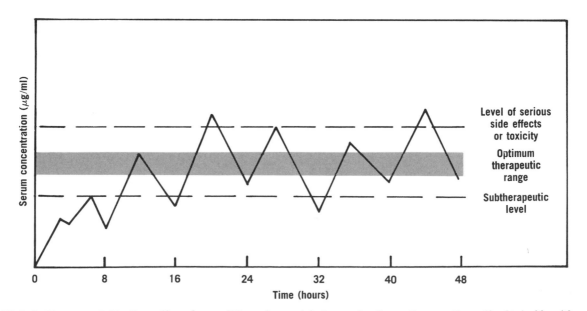

Fig. 19–1. Undesirable sawtooth kinetic profile under conditions of normal dosing, and optimum therapeutic profile obtainable with some newer delivery devices.

greatly exceeds the desired therapeutic level, then falls to a subclinical level, and on subsequent dosing rises to dangerously high values, falling again to ineffective concentrations, in continuous cycles of excessive–ineffective levels. Controlled, sustained drug delivery can reduce the undesirable fluctuation of drug levels, enhancing therapeutic action and eliminating dangerous side effects. Furthermore, the localization through preprogrammed drug delivery methods of a drug in the vicinity of its target cells can prevent systemic or side effects involving other tissues.

The most popular sustained drug delivery forms and devices used today make use of inert polymers, such as the silastics, or biodegradable polylactic acids. By the use of these materials suitable drug levels can be sustained in certain regions of the body such as the eye, vagina, the surface of the skin, or in a subcutaneous depot. Polymeric forms and recently introduced therapeutic systems will be considered in some detail following a brief discussion of chemical and biologic approaches to prolonged and intensified action of drugs in the body. The physical and chemical properties of polymers used in many of the new dosage forms are discussed in Chapter 20.

PRODRUGS AND DRUG CARRIERS

Prodrugs. According to the prodrug approach to drug delivery, a medicinal agent is chemically modified, for example, by the addition of an ester group to improve the absorption and concentration of the parent compound at the target site in the body.[1] In a prodrug, the ester group or similar carrier moiety is chemically removed in the gut or at the tissue site, usually by enzymatic action, and the parent drug is freed to produce its pharmacologic action. Prodrug formation and other chemical modifications may also facilitate pharmaceutical processing and improve the stability of the parent drug. Sparingly soluble salts of the penicillins are examples of chemical analogs that have been used for some time to promote higher blood levels and bring about better distribution in the tissues. Pivampicillin is quite lipophilic and produces high blood levels of the parent drug, ampicillin, through a prodrug mechanism. Erythromycin prodrugs are available that are tasteless and stable in aqueous suspension, the parent molecules being protected with chemical groupings that are eventually lost in the tissue.

The prodrug principle has significantly advanced the delivery of targeted drugs to selected sites in the body. Seki et al.[2] studied the effect of various esterases on the enzymatic hydrolysis of esters of p-acetylaminobenzoic acid and acetylated acetaminophen. The results showed that ester prodrugs could be formulated to hydrolyze at specific sites in the body.

Mercaptopurine together with methotrexate is used in the chemotherapy of lymphocytic leukemia. When taken orally, mercaptopurine is only about 50% absorbed. Waranis and Sloan[3] investigated the possibility of delivering mercaptopurine through hairless skin in the form of a prodrug, acyloxymethyl mercaptopurine, administered in the solvents, isopropyl myristate and propylene glycol. The solubility parameters (see pp. 224–227) of the several prodrug derivatives were found to correlate well with their permeability through the skin preparation.

Bundgaard and his associates[4,5] have studied the preparation and properties of prodrugs over the past decade. Proteins and small peptides constitute new and important classes of drugs, yet they do not pass readily through biomembranes and are easily metabolized by peptidases when given by various routes of administration. Bundgaard and Møss[5] are preparing derivatives of small peptides to yield prodrugs that show enhanced delivery and chemical stability but that break down rapidly in the body to release the biologically active parent compound. To date, prodrugs have been made from various proteins and peptides: thyrotropin-releasing hormone (TRH), luteinizing hormone–releasing hormone (LH–RH), fibrinopeptides, and collagen. Takakura et al.[6] have prepared a prodrug of mitomycin C and dextran as a delivery system in cancer chemotherapy and are studying the properties of a soybean trypsin inhibitor conjugated to dextran as a model to optimize the delivery of protein drugs. Mitomycin C is a useful antibiotic against neoplastic disease but, like other anticancer agents, it does not differentiate in its action against tumor and normal cells. Sato et al.[7] developed a polymeric prodrug— mitomycin C–dextran. They found that the prodrug liberated the parent, mitomycin C, with a greater activity against various tumors than uncomplexed mitomycin C. See Figure 11–5 for complexation of mitomycin with cyclodextrin.

Liposomes. Biologic entities, including red blood cells and liposomes, have been used as drug carriers to promote controlled release in the body. *Liposomes* are uni- or multilayered vesicles of phospholipids, first described in 1965 by Bangham et al. at Cambridge.[8] They fall in the size range of 250 Å (25 nm) to 10 μm in diameter, and may be prepared, according to one procedure, by combining a phospholipid such as phosphatidylserine, cholesterol, and cholesterol oleate in chloroform and allowing the solution to evaporate. The mixture of lipids is then dissolved in ethanol and the solution is added to isotonic saline solution containing ethylenediaminetetraacetic acid (EDTA) with stirring at pH 7.4 and 37° C. The procedure is conducted under aseptic conditions and only sterile preparations are used. In experimental work the liposome vesicles are prepared freshly each day. The finished liposomes are nearly spherical and consist of unilamellar or multilamellar lipid bilayers alternating with aqueous regions. Figure 19–2a depicts a unilamellar liposome. The lipid

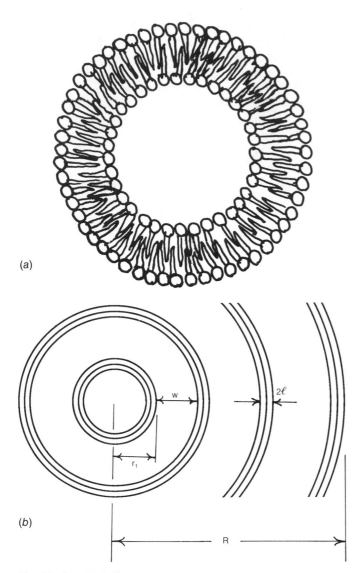

(a)

(b)

Fig. 19–2. (*a*) A liposome showing a single phospholipid bilayer (unilamellar liposome). (*b*) Drawing of a multilamellar liposome with $n = 4$ lamellae. Each lamella consists of a lipid bilayer of thickness 2ℓ and alternates with water layers of thickness w. The core is a unilamellar liposome of radius r. (From C. Pidgeon and C. A. Hunt, J. Pharm. Sci. **70**, 73, 1981, reproduced with permission of the copyright owner.)

bilayers can entrap lipid-soluble drugs and the water layers can dissolve water-soluble compounds. Drugs are introduced into liposomes by simply mixing the phospholipid and other lipid components with an aqueous solution of the drug.

Martin[9] has discussed the many factors that must be taken into consideration in the manufacture of liposomal preparations, including the choice of solvents, sterility requirements, pyrogen control, and stability of the ingredients and of the final product. One industrial-scale production method is discussed[9] with particular attention to obtaining liposomes that are of uniform size and are capable of encapsulating a maximum amount of the aqueous drug solution.

Pidgeon and Hunt[10] provide formulas to calculate the total surface area, TSA, of N liposomes; the volume of water VW_1 encapsulated in a single-layer liposome or the total volume of water, TVW, in a population of N single-layer liposomes; and the encapsulation ratio, E, or ratio of entrapped water volume to total volume of lipid. Needed for these calculations are the number N of liposome particles,* the radius R of a liposome, and the volume of lipid in the single-layer liposome. These are important quantities to know, for the distribution of liposomes in the body when injected intravenously is a function of the dose (number N of liposome particles), the size, and the surface area of the liposomes. We assume a *homogeneous population* of liposomes, in that the radius, surface area, and n, number of layers or lamellae, are the same for all particles. Shown in Figure 19–2b is a liposome of $n = 4$ lamellae. The heterogeneous case in which the radius, surface area, and number of layers differ among the vesicles in a population is discussed by the authors[10] and will not be treated here.

Example 19–1. Calculate the volume VW_1 of water entrapped in a spherical single-layer† liposome using equation (1) of Pidgeon and Hunt[10]:

$$V W_1 = \frac{4}{3} \pi R^3 - VL_1 \qquad (19-1)$$

in which $VL_1 = 1.99 \times 10^{-5}\ \mu m^3$ is the volume of phospholipid constituting the single lipid layer of the liposome and $R = 0.0225\ \mu m$ is the outside radius of the liposome.

$$V W_1 = \frac{4}{3} \pi (0.0225)^3 - 1.99 \times 10^{-5} = 2.78 \times 10^{-5}\ \mu m^3$$

This is the volume of water in the *core* of a single liposome (see Fig. 19–2a).

If the single-layer homogeneous liposome preparation is found to contain $N = 4.04 \times 10^{16}$ liposome particles, the total volume of phospholipid TVL_1 present is

$$TVL_1 = N \times VL_1 = (4.04 \times 10^{16})(1.99 \times 10^{-5}) = 8.04 \times 10^{11}\ \mu m^3$$

The total volume of entrapped water, TVW_1, in the $N = 4.04 \times 10^{16}$ liposomes is $TVW_1 = N \times VW_1 = (4.04 \times 10^{16})(2.78 \times 10^{-5}) = 1.123 \times 10^{12}\ \mu m^3$. The ratio of the total volume of enclosed water, $TVW = N_1 VW_1 = \frac{4}{3}\pi NR^3 - NVL_1 = \frac{4}{3}\pi N_1 R_1^3 - TVL$ to the total volume of phospholipid, TVL yields the *encapsulation ratio*, $E = TVW/TVL$,

$$E = \frac{\frac{4}{3}\pi N_1 R_1^3}{TVL_1} - \frac{TVL_1}{TVL_1} = \frac{\frac{4}{3}\pi N_1 R_1^3}{TVL_1} - 1 \qquad (19-2)$$

For a preparation of $N_1 = 4.04 \times 10^{16}$ liposomal particles each of radius $R_1 = 0.0225\ \mu m$, and a total phospholipid volume in the preparation of $TVL_1 = 8.04 \times 10^{11}\ \mu m^3$, the encapsulation ratio E is found to be

$$E = \frac{\frac{4}{3}\pi (4.04 \times 10^{16})(0.0225)^3}{8.04 \times 10^{11}\ \mu m^3} - 1 = 1.40$$

Thus the ratio of water to phospholipid in this preparation is 1.40 to 1.

---

*The authors describe a procedure to calculate N, the number of particles. It is assumed for our purposes that N has been obtained by an appropriate method, and in the example to follow its value is given.

†The subscript 1 on terms such as VW_1 and VL_1 indicates that we are dealing with a single-layer (unilamellar) liposome.

The total surface area TSA$_p$, that is, the area for the entire population of liposomes, is given by the equation

$$TSA_p = \sum_{i=1}^{k} 4\pi N_i R_i^2 \qquad (19-3)$$

where the summation is over the n phospholipid layers from $i = 1$ to k. Since we are dealing with a single-layer liposome, $k = 1$; therefore $N_i = N_1 = 4.04 \times 10^{16}$ and $R_i^2 = R_1^2 = (0.0225\ \mu m)^2 = 5.06 \times 10^{-4}$. And we have for the total surface area of liposomes: $TSA = 4\pi(4.04 \times 10^{16})(5.06 \times 10^{-4}) = 2.57 \times 10^{14}\ \mu m^2$

Lichtenberg and Markello[11] calculated the surface area and entrapped aqueous volume of spherical multilamellar liposomes from a knowledge of the liposome's outer radius, thickness of the interlamellar aqueous layers, and number of bilayers. From their calculations, based on an approach taken earlier by Schwartz and McConnell[12], the authors concluded that most vesicles have a definite distance between the lamellae in a given population of liposomes, with most of the aqueous medium enclosed in the internal core of the liposome. Hydrophilic drugs are encapsulated predominantly in this central aqueous cavity. *Problem 19-2*, page 551, illustrates the calculations of Lichtenberg and Markello.[11] From their results and those of Schwartz and McConnell[12], the authors concluded that liposomes consist of up to 10 lamellae, each lamella or lipid layer being about 50 Å thick. Large liposomes, fully swollen, have diameters approximately 1.5 μm with interlamellar distances of about 60 Å and a large aqueous core with a diameter somewhat greater than 1.0 μm.

Hydrophilic drugs and amphiphilic compounds such as mitomycin are not well entrapped in lipid carriers, whereas lipophilic compounds are well retained in the biologic drug carriers. When mitomycin is chemically modified to form a lipophilic prodrug it may be entrapped in liposomes and in oil-in-water emulsions.[13] Negatively and positively charged lipids can be used to produce charged liposomes. Abra et al.[14] investigated the delivery of negatively charged liposomes and the effect of vesicle size on the deposition in the lungs. Liposome preparations also have been used to administer drugs topically.[15]

Wiessner et al.,[16] studied the binding of the peptide insulin by the liposome dipalmitoyl phosphatidyl choline. Insulin, an amphiphilic molecule, may cause fusion (melting) of liposomes resulting in their aggregation; and care must be used to avoid such deleterious effects of insulin in single-layer liposomes. Guzman et al.[17] studied the entrapment of the cardiac glycosides digitoxin, digoxin, and ouabain in liposomes prepared from egg yolk phosphatidylcholine. The authors reported that drugs with high or low octanol–aqueous buffer partition coefficients are better incorporated in the vesicles than those with intermediate partition coefficients. Digoxin, with an intermediate partition coefficient, is poorly entrapped in the liposomes. Cholesterol is known to promote a close packing of the phosphatidylcholine bilayer molecules and its addition

to the liposomal preparation greatly reduced the capacity of the vesicles to entrap digoxin. When charged lipids are included in the formation of liposomes, the electrostatic repulsion between adjacent bilayers resulted in an increase in the aqueous space between the bilayer molecules. Thus the addition of diacetylphosphate, a negatively charged species, increases the incorporation of ouabain, a water-soluble cardiac glycoside.

Payne et al.[18] reviewed the limitations of liposomes as biologic carriers, including chemical and physical instability, problems of sterility, drug incompatibility, and immunologic and toxicologic difficulties. These adverse effects greatly limit aqueous suspensions of liposomes as drug carriers, and suggest the possible advantages of formulations that may be stored dry and hydrated before use to yield an aqueous suspension of liposomes. The authors refer to these formulations as *proliposomes*. They are free-flowing granular products which, when water is added, disperse to yield isotonic suspensions of liposomes for intravenous use or administration by other routes. The authors discussed the nature of the lipid drug, the suitability of carriers such as sodium chloride and sorbitol, and the amount of lipid drug deposited onto the carrier. These factors markedly influence the preparation of proliposomes and formation of an aqueous suspension of the liposomes. A stability study showed that the size distribution of the hydrated proliposomes did not change significantly over a 9-month period at 20° C. When amphotericin B was incorporated in the liposomes, its potency did not decrease over a 6-month period.

Gregoriadis[19] has prepared a comprehensive three-volume treatise on liposome technology. Other works on dosage form design and controlled delivery devices are listed on page 550.

Monolithic and Reservoir Devices.[20] The word *monolithic* refers to a single mass or block of material. In the field of controlled drug delivery, the term *monolithic device* refers to a rate-controlling polymer matrix throughout which the drug is dissolved or dispersed. In contrast to a matrix or monolithic system, a reservoir device consists of a shell-like dosage form with the drug or agent contained within a rate-controlling membrane. Systems of reservoir and matrix form are shown in Figure 19–3. The device may be spherical or cylindrical, or it may consist of layers of the drug or other agent sandwiched between layers of rate-controlling and other membranes. This third form, known as a *laminated reservoir system* (see p. 543, Fig. 19–22), is designed mainly for attachment to surfaces such as the skin, the lining of the mouth, and the cornea of the eye. If a controlled-release dosage form is introduced into the body and does not degrade with time, it must be removed surgically. For this reason biodegradable systems, such as the one shown in Figure 19–4, have been sought for the controlled release of biologically active agents. Today many polymer matrix and mem-

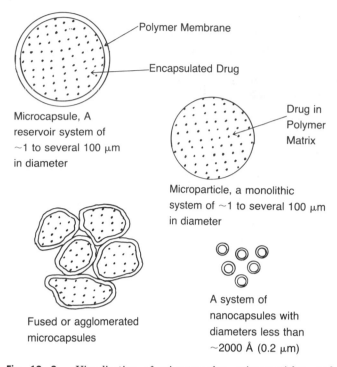

Fig. 19–3. Visualization of microcapsules, microparticles, and nanocapsules, and their approximate sizes. Nanoparticles, not shown, are approximately the same size as nanocapsules, but like microparticles they consist of a solid matrix through which the drug is dispersed.

brane materials are available that gradually degrade after the drug is released at the desired site in the body. With the use of biodegradable polymers, controlled-release implants and depot injections can be made with the assurance that the polymeric material will disappear from the body within a reasonable time. Examples of biodegradable polymers are poly(glycolic acid), poly(D,L-lactic acid), glutamic acid–ethyl glutamate copolymers, and polyacrylamides (hydrogels).

Studies on microcapsules, made from various polymers and used for different purposes, are introduced here, followed by a discussion of microparticles (microspheres), nanocapsules, and nanoparticles.

Microcapsules. In a symposium on microcapsules, Lim and Moss[21] defined microencapsulation as a process in which solids, liquids, or gases are enveloped in a membrane that may be impermeable or semipermeable. Activated charcoal, enzymes, hormones, antigens, and antisera are examples of materials that can be entrapped in microcapsules. The cells are formed by a process involving heat coagulation, by bringing an aqueous solution of the drug in contact with an organic solvent phase, or by polymerization and gelatin.

Invertase is an enzyme that catalyzes the hydrolysis of sucrose into fructose and glucose. Patients who cannot absorb sucrose are deficient in the enzyme invertase, and suffer microbial fermentation in the gut and severe diarrhea when sucrose is ingested. To overcome these digestive problems, Rambourg et al.[22] incorporated invertase into polyamide microcapsules, prepared by interfacial polymerization according to the method of Chang.[23] Interfacial polymerization is a polymerization reaction at the interface between an organic and an aqueous phase. An emulsification procedure was also tested in which the invertase was encapsulated in a cross-linked protein. In another report, Levy et al.[24] incorporated hemoglobin in microcapsules to produce a blood replacement fluid. The microcapsules were formed by linking hemoglobin, the protein, with various acylchlorides, such as terephthaloylchloride, as the cross-linking agent. Stable hemoglobin microcapsules were prepared 5 μm in diameter, that were able to carry out normal oxygen transfer but did not allow escape of the hemoglobin. A scanning electron micrograph of large, dehydrated microcapsules of hemoglobin, obtained in the early phase of the study, is shown in Figure 19–5. McGinity and associates[25] described the preparation and properties of nylon microcapsules containing three different matrices: formalized gelatin, calcium alginate, and calcium sulfate. The capsules were free-flowing and were approximately 50 to 150 μm in diameter. Various anionic, cationic, nonionic, quarternary, and amphoteric drugs were incorporated in the nylon microcapsules. Bala and

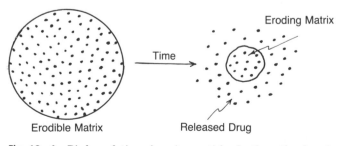

Fig. 19–4. Biodegradation of a microparticle. In time, the drug is completely released and simultaneously the degradable matrix erodes. Or the drug may be slowly released, and in a reasonable time thereafter the matrix, free of drug, gradually disappears.

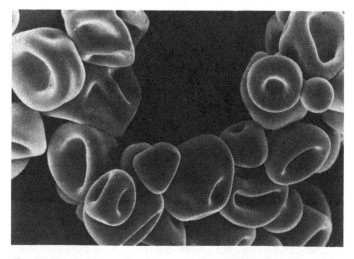

Fig. 19–5. Scanning electron micrograph of hemoglobin microcapsules. (From M.-C. Levy, P. Rambourg, J. Levy and G. Potron, J. Pharm. Sci. **71,** 759, 1982, reproduced with permission of the copyright owner.)

Vasudevan[26] designed a pH-sensitive microcapsule for the encapsulation of such agents as secretin, which is found in the upper intestinal tract and is activated when chyme, that is, the digestive secretions and partly digested food, enter the intestine. The microcapsules of polyacryloylchloride-lysine are spherical with diameters of 5 to 10 μm. The polymer dissolution and release of secretion depends on the pH of the solution in which the microcapsules are suspended. The drug is released following zero-order kinetics, which suggests the possible use of these pH-sensitive microcapsules for the delivery of drugs to the duodenum in the treatment of ulcers. The system should be useful for the delivery of drugs, in general, both under conditions of low pH and at pH values as high as 8.0, since the polymer may be eroded up to pH 8.

It has been observed that compression of microcapsules to form tablets shows the release rate and produces a sustained action. Nixon and Agyilirah[27] investigated the results of tableting microcapsules consisting of ethylcellulose shells or walls containing sodium phenobarbital in the cores. Dissolution from the capsules was found to depend on the core–wall ratio and the size of the dried microcapsule aggregates in the tablet. With a higher core-to-wall ratio the microcapsules have thinner walls so that the dissolution medium can enter the capsule more readily and the core solution can easily pass through the walls. The larger the microcapsules the greater the breakdown of the aggregates, providing additional surface for dissolution. Thus, both core-to-wall ratio and size of microcapsule aggregates increase the dissolution rate of the tableted microcapsules.

Early in the development of microcapsule technology (1966), Chang suggested the encapsulation of magnetic particles to direct entrained drug to specific sites in the body with the help of an external magnet. Povey et al.[28] suggested the addition of a suspension of magnetite, Fe_3O_4 (Ferrofluid EGM 705), to recover the magnetic microcapsules in the feces with an electromagnet for identification and study of reactive carcinogens captured from the intestinal tract. The results of their work show that magnetic polymer microcapsules are able in vitro to entrap a model carcinogen, *N*-methyl nitrosourea (NMN); and NMN can subsequently be released from the microcapsule mass by magnetic attraction for subsequent analysis. Gallo et al.[29] were able to alter the tissue distribution in the rat of adriamycin, an antineoplastic agent, by encapsulating the drug in magnetic albumin microcapsules prepared with a magnetite (Fe_2O_3) suspension and by directing the adriamycin microcapsules, following intraarterial administration, to the target site. The use of magnetic microspheres increased the drug's presence both at the target site and in the liver.

Microparticles (Microspheres). These devices differ from the reservoir system known as microcapsules in that they consist of a solid matrix throughout which the drug is distributed. Akbuga[30] prepared microspheres of furosemide, a potent diuretic, using various acrylic polymers (Eudragit, Rohm Pharma) as the microsphere matrix. These microparticles were spherical with diameters of 250 to 280 μm, and contained 75 to 80% by weight of furosemide. The release pattern of furosemide was altered by using different polymers, namely Eudragit L 100, S 100, RL 100, and RS 100. The results of dissolution experiments showed that the release of the drug followed the Higuchi[31] matrix model (p. 336). Gupta and associates[32] investigated the effects of albumin microspheres on the release rate of entrapped adriamycin (doxorubicin hydrochloride), a broad-spectrum antineoplastic agent. The behavior of albumin microspheres has been studied by a number of researchers[33] and found to be quite acceptable as polymeric carriers for the delivery of drugs in the living system.

Spenlehauer et al.[34] reported on the incorporation of cisplatin, a potent anticancer agent, into poly(D,L-lactide) microspheres by a process known simply as *solvent evaporation.* According to this method cisplatin was dispersed in methylene chloride and to this suspension was added the polymer, poly(D,L-lactide). The organic phase was emulsified in an aqueous solution of emulsifiers, namely polyvinyl alcohol and methylcellulose, and the pH was adjusted to 2 with HCl. The dispersion was stirred mechanically until the organic solvent, methylene chloride, was completely evaporated. The solid microspheres took up the cisplatin during evaporation and were collected on a filter and dried. The steps in the preparation of microspheres of cisplatin are illustrated in the flow chart shown in Figure 19–6. Cisplatin may be deposited in the polymer matrix by this process to the extent of about 45% by weight of the drug. The in vitro kinetics of cisplatin release was studied and found to depend on the amount of drug loaded into the microspheres; the greater the drug loading the faster was the drug release. Further work with microsphere entrapment of cisplatin may yield a targeted dosage form without the present side effects of nausea, vomiting, and renal disturbances.

Leucuta[35] proposed an ophthalmic drug delivery system consisting of gelatin or albumin microspheres designed to prolong the residence time of the drug in the eye and to provide improved bioavailability. Liposomes and nanoparticles have been used to obtain controlled drug delivery to the eye. Leucuta chose pilocarpine, a miotic which causes the pupil to contract and is used in the treatment of glaucoma. He prepared gelatin and albumin microspheres, containing pilocarpine nitrate, which were sufficiently large to be recognized as particles by the eye, yet not so large that they could not be readily flushed out of the eye by the natural flow of tears. The methods of preparation are described in detail in his report.[35] The release of pilocarpine from microspheres, as compared with the result with an aqueous solution of the drug, showed

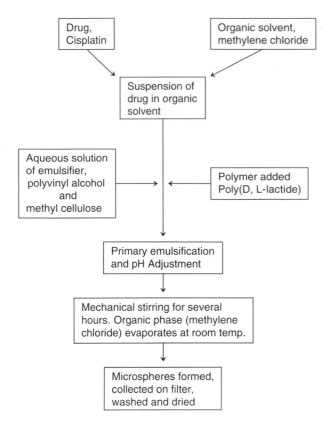

Fig. 19–6. Flow chart for the preparation of cisplatin microspheres by the solvent evaporation method.

extended contact of the microspheres at the corneal surface. Preliminary results suggested that microspheres provided a suitable dosage form to maintain water-soluble drugs such as pilocarpine nitrate in the area of the cornea.

Bodmeier and McGinity[36] evaluated the incorporation of various ionized and nonionized drugs in poly-(D,L-lactide) (PLA) microspheres. Poly(D-L-lactide) is a biodegradable polymer and its microparticles are ordinarily used as carriers for water-insoluble drugs. By adjusting the pH to minimize drug solubility, it was possible to increase the drug content in the microspheres for weakly ionizable drugs such as quinidine sulfate. The rate and amount of drug released was a strong function of the surface structure of the microspheres which, in turn, depended on the pH of the aqueous solution at the time of preparation of the microspheres. Thermal analysis (pp. 46–49) of the microspheres containing quinidine provided information regarding the glass transition temperature of the polymer and the melting and recrystallization of the drug, quinidine. The glass transition temperature T_g is a narrow temperature range over which a plastic changes on cooling from a very viscous rubbery melt to a glass state rather than from a liquid to a crystalline state (pp. 586–588).

In a second paper[37] Bodmeier and McGinity studied various methods of solvent selection in the preparation of PLA microspheres produced by the solvent evaporation method and containing the drugs quinidine and quinidine sulfate. A flow chart of the solvent evaporation method is presented in Figure 19–6. The steps in the preparation of drug-loaded microspheres as outlined in the figure should assist the reader to follow the arguments concerning the precipitation of the polymer, PLA, from the organic solvent phase, the dissolution of the drug in the aqueous phase, and concentration of the polymer in the organic phase. In the emulsification step the rate of diffusion of the organic solvent into the aqueous phase must be rapid, causing a high rate of precipitation of the polymer from the organic solvent. The use of an organic solvent of low water solubility results in slow polymer precipitation and a poor yield of microspheres. This is because the solvent solvates the polymer, PLA, and prevents its precipitation. The drug tends to escape entrapment in the microspheres, diffusing instead into the aqueous phase. Water-miscible solvents such as acetone, ethanol, and dimethyl sulfoxide should further favor precipitation of the polymer and increase the drug content in the microspheres; but this was found not to be the case. The authors found instead that the increase in the drug content with change of solvent could be explained by the effect of the solvent on the rate of precipitation of the polymer at the microdroplet interface. Rapid precipitation of PLA produced efficient entrapment of the drug in the matrix of the microspheres. The solvent methylene chloride possesses high water solubility, thus leaving the polymer to form microspheres containing the drug in its matrix. These workers[37] further found that the addition of cosolvents such as acetone or ethanol, together with the solvent methylene chloride, could increase the drug loading of the microspheres. The increased loading was attributed to the faster precipitation of PLA by the hydrophilic cosolvents, which assured the entrapment of quinidine sulfate, the drug.

Exposure to mercury compounds can result in serious poisoning, including organ damage and death. The antidote for mercury poisoning involves the administration of chelating agents such as dimercaprol, penicillamine, and polythiol resins, which bind mercury and excrete it in the feces. Margel and Hirsh[38] designed a polymercaptal microsphere that showed potential as an antidote against mercury poisoning. The microspheres were prepared by combining the mercury chelating agent pentaerythritol tetrathioglycolate with a sorbitan monolaurate surfactant to form an aqueous emulsion. Glutaraldehyde was added to the emulsion with stirring to form the microspheres, which were then separated by dialysis. By scanning electron microscopy, the diameter of the microspheres was determined to be 0.8 ± 0.02 μm and the surface area was calculated to be 8.04 (μm)^2. A suspension of the chelating microspheres was found to be free of aggregation after 1 year's storage. Both organic and inorganic mercury compounds are taken up, probably by the free thiol groups of the microspheres, over a broad range of pH. They compete strongly for mercury bound to albumin and cysteine. The effectiveness of chelating microspheres in binding mercury in vitro is demonstrated in this study.

Morimoto, Natsume, and their colleagues[39,40] have prepared mitomycin C biodegradable albumin microspheres for use in a new procedure, *chemoembolization*, against liver tumors in rats. Chemoembolization is infusion of an anticancer drug into a solid malignant tumor, using a catheter that is passed directly into an artery of the tumor. Microspheres are used in this study as the drug carrier in the embolization procedure, and can be directed to target sites in the rat liver where the anticancer drug such as mitomycin C (MMC) is released slowly over several weeks. A schematic of the procedure is shown in Figure 19–7. The antitumor effects of the MMC microspheres were considerably greater (2.5 times) than those relating from the injection of saline solution alone (the control) or from infusion of MMC in saline solution. Chemoembolization was considered to be equally as effective as surgical removal of the malignancy.

Nanocapsules and Nanoparticles. These minute particles, about 100 Å (10 nm) to 2000 Å (0.2 μm) in diameter, were introduced by Kreuter and Speiser[41] in the 1970s as controlled-release drug carriers. The *nanocapsule* is a shell-like polymeric particle, a reservoir device, in which the drug is contained in an oily solution or colloidal suspension. A *nanoparticle* consists of a solid mass of polymer, a monolithic device, from which the drug is released by a leaching process. Nanoparticles may be distinguished from nanocapsules by subjecting them to ultracentrifugation; nanoparticles form a sediment at the bottom of a centrifuge tube whereas nanocapsules rise to form a layer at the top of the tube, as do the oil globules of an *o/w* emulsion.

Two main classes of polymerization—condensation and chain (addition) polymerization—are recognized along with several others of less importance in the preparation of nanocapsules, nanoparticles, and other microvesicles.[42] In *condensation polymerization*, the monomers react chemically through their functional groups to link the monomers in a step-wise manner to generate the polymer. In *addition (chain) polymerization* an initiator reacts with the monomer to form a free radical or an appropriate ionic site. The reactive monomers combine to initiate a chain, which grows as additional monomers are added to the polymer. The active site may be blocked at any stage and polymerization terminated (see p. 558 for the chemistry of condensation and addition [chain] polymerization).

Addition polymerization is conducted by several techniques: bulk, solution, suspension, and emulsion polymerization. *Bulk* polymerization involves only a monomer and a chain initiator, whereas *solution* polymerization involves the presence of a solvent together with the monomer and initiator. *Suspension* polymerization is conducted in aqueous solution with a water-insoluble monomer and initiator suspended in the solution; whereas in *emulsion* polymerization a monomer and a polymerization initator, soluble in water but insoluble in the monomer, are added to an aqueous solution of a surfactant. For emulsion polymerization to occur the surfactant must form micelles and therefore be sufficiently concentrated to remain above its cmc. Part of the monomer dissolves in the aqueous phase, part is solubilized in the micelles of the surfactant, and the remainder forms monomer droplets in the mixture.

The free radical initiation may be formed by heating a compound such as benzoyl peroxide:

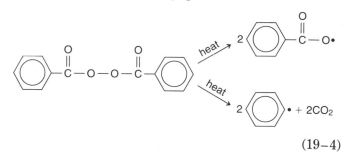

$$(19-4)$$

$$(19-5)$$

$$(19-6)$$

These steps show the *initiation, propagation,* and *termination* of the polymerization. Chain termination may occur by one of several processes, such as:

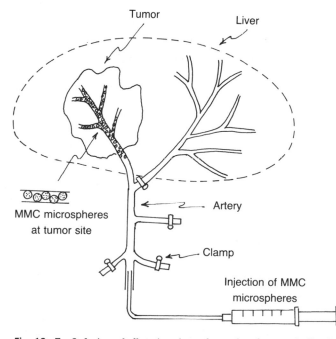

Fig. 19–7. Infusion of albumin microspheres by chemoembolization into the liver. (After Y. Morimoto et al., Int. J. Pharm. **54,** 28, 1989, reproduced with permission of the copyright owner.)

$$\underset{\text{(19–7)}}{\overset{}{}}$$

The end groups are then removed to yield the final polymer.

The polymer in its initial stage of formation enters the micelles where it grows rapidly in the presence of both solubilized monomer and free radicals R• that also enter the micelles. As more monomer is needed for continued growth of the polymer, monomer molecules leave the emulsified droplets in the aqueous medium and enter the micelles. As the process continues, the micelles are disrupted by the presence of the growing polymer molecules. The micelles essentially become "micellar swollen polymer particles," coated with surfactant and containing reacting monomer radicals.

The various species, monomers, micelles, surfactants, swollen polymer particles, and free radical initiators, together with the processes that occur in emulsion polymerization, are shown schematically in Figure 19–8.

To develop the mathematics of polymerization it is reasoned that the polymer chain reaction is begun with the formation of a free radical initiator (equations (19–4) and (19–5); the polymer is formed and grows in the propagation stage (equation 19–6) and continues until a second free radical molecule appears and terminates the chain reaction (equation (19–7)). There is a 50% chance at any moment that the $\widetilde{N}$ polymers will be terminated as in equation (19–7), and a 50% chance that the $\widetilde{N}$ micelles or swollen polymer particles are in readiness to receive another monomer and extend the polymer chains. The rate of polymerization, $\widetilde{R}_p$, is therefore proportional to one-half the number ($\frac{1}{2}\widetilde{N}$) of micelles or swollen polymer "factories." The rate of polymerization is also proportional to the concentration $[\widetilde{M}]$ of monomer present in the micelle-swollen polymer factories. Therefore, the rate of polymerization can be written

$$\widetilde{R}_p = k_p[\widetilde{M}]\left[\frac{\widetilde{N}}{2}\right] \qquad (19\text{–}8)$$

Example 19–2. Calculate the rate of polymerization $\widetilde{R}_p$ of a methyl methacrylate polymer that is undergoing emulsion polymerization with the free radical initiation provided by potassium persulfate as the initiator:

$$S_2O_8^{2-} + acid \rightarrow SO_4^-\bullet$$

The number of micelle-swollen polymer particles is $\widetilde{N} = 7.2 \times 10^{14}$ per liter, and the concentration of monomer, methyl methacrylate, in the micelle-swollen polymer "factories" is $[\widetilde{M}] = 3.5$ molar. The value k_p of the rate constant for emulsion polymerization was found experimentally to be 137.8 liters mole^{-1} sec^{-1}.

From equation (19–8):

$$\widetilde{R}_p = (137.8 \text{ liters mole}^{-1} \text{ sec}^{-1})(3.5 \text{ mole liter}^{-1})$$

$$(7.2 \times 10^{14} \text{ particles liter}^{-1})(1/2)$$

$$= 1.74 \times 10^{17} \text{ liter mole}^{-1} \text{ sec}^{-1}$$

$$\times \text{ mole liter}^{-1} \frac{\text{particle}}{\text{liter}} \times \frac{\text{mole}}{6.022 \times 10^{23} \text{ particles}}$$

$$\widetilde{R}_p = 2.89 \times 10^{-7} \text{ (mole/liter)sec}^{-1}$$

The *kinetic chain length* $\widetilde{\nu}$ in a polymerization reaction is the rate of polymerization in the propagation stage divided by the rate of initiation, or $\widetilde{\nu} = \widetilde{R}_p/\widetilde{R}_i$. It is also the number of monomer molecules polymerized to produce a finished polymer chain and is therefore referred to in polymer science as the *degree of polymerization*, *DP* (see p. 558).

Example 19–3. Calculate the kinetic chain length $\widetilde{\nu}$ or degree of polymerization, *DP*, for the emulsion polymerization of methyl methacrylate of *Example 19–2*. The rate of initiation, $\widetilde{R}_i$ is 9.43×10^{-10} (mole/liter)sec^{-1}.

$$\widetilde{\nu} = DP = \frac{\widetilde{R}_p}{\widetilde{R}_i} = \frac{2.89 \times 10^{-7}(\text{mole/liter})\text{sec}^{-1}}{9.43 \times 10^{-10}(\text{mole/liter})\text{sec}^{-1}} = 306$$

It may appear that the number, 306, of monomers in the polymer is big, but the degree of polymerization for large polymer is big, but the degree of polymeriation for large polymers may actually be in the thousands or tens of thousands.

The preparation of new polymeric drug carriers has allowed the targeting of drugs to specific cells, tissues, and organs in the body, and has minimized toxic effects in healthy tissue. Rolland et al.[43] designed a new

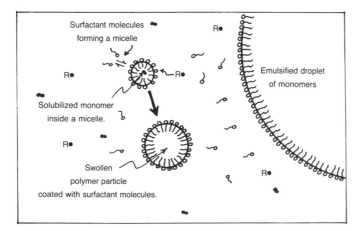

Fig. 19–8. A schematic of emulsion polymerization showing surfactant molecules, ⌇, and monomer molecules, •, in the aqueous phase; surfactant molecules on the surfaces of the monomer and the polymer droplets; surfactant molecules in the process of forming the micelle; monomer molecules solubilized in the core of the micelle; and free radical initiator molecules R• in the aqueous phase and entering the micelle. The dark arrow signifies conversion with time from the micelle containing solubilized monomer to the polymer droplet swollen with monomer and covered with surfactant molecules. (Modified from J. W. Vanderhof, E. B. Bradford, H. L. Tarkowski, J. B. Shaffer and R. M. Wiley, Adv. Chem. **34**, 32, 1962.)

site-specific drug delivery system consisting of poly-methacrylic nanoparticles (nanospheres) prepared by the addition (chain) polymerization technique. The nanoparticles themselves have been found to show very low acute and subacute toxicities. Nanoparticles loaded with the antineoplastic agent doxorubicin, formerly known as adriamycin, are under clinical trials in human patients with liver carcinomas.

Nanoparticles and nanocapsules were prepared by N. Al Khouri Fallouh et al.[44] by interfacial polymerization with stirring of isobutyl cyanoacrylate in an aqueous medium containing dextran 70 and glucose in 0.001 molar HCl. The two different structures—nanocapsules and nanoparticles—were produced by varying the polymerization procedure. Nanocapsules may be used to enclose poorly water-soluble drugs that cannot be enclosed in nanoparticles. Drugs are liberated from nanocapsules by diffusion and passage through the thin wall of the capsule, whereas nanoparticles liberate the enclosed drug by erosion and leaching from the solid polymer mass. The authors[44] also considered the possibility of adsorbing drugs on the surface of nanoparticles as a possible carrier mechanism.

Gipps et al.[45] labeled polyhexylcyanoacrylate nanoparticles with carbon-14 and injected them into mice to ascertain the distribution of the particles in the body, using liquid scintillation counting. Following a single intravenous injection of 0.2 mL of the labeled nanoparticle preparation, 45% of the radioactive carbon remained in the body after 28 days. A large amount of the label was detected in the liver, with smaller amounts retained in the spleen and lungs. On repeated injection at intervals of 28 days, larger proportions of the nanoparticles accumulated in the spleen and lungs.

Studies have shown that improved anticancer activity and longer insulin response can be realized by entrapment of the active agent in polyalkylcyanoacrylate nanoparticles. It is therefore important to know the toxicity level of carriers such as nanoparticles, nanocapsules, microparticles, and liposomes. Kante et al.[46] found that the nanoparticles did not cause cellular damage until administered in high concentration in a cell culture medium. Neither nanoparticles nor their degradation products showed mutagenicity. Couvreur et al.[47] found that doxorubicin, an antineoplastic agent, when absorbed on nanoparticles reduced the weight loss and death rate of mice. Cardiotoxicity was also reduced because of the limited uptake of the drug-loaded nanoparticles by the myocardium.

A number of studies have been reported on the use of liposomes, microcapsules, and nanoparticles for the delivery of drugs to specific sites in the body. In addition to the investigations already mentioned—both research and applied—the references at the end of this chapter will be of assistance to workers entering the rapidly expanding field of controlled-delivery systems.

ROUTES OF ADMINISTRATION

Ocular Administration. Topical instillation is used in the treatment of local diseases affecting the eye. The absorption of drugs takes place through either the conjunctival sac or the corneal membrane (Fig. 19–9),

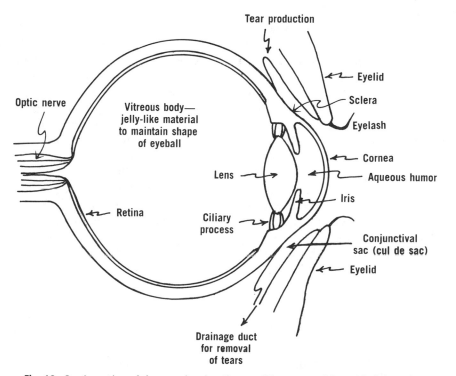

Fig. 19–9. A section of the eye showing the possible routes of drug administration.

the latter being a more effective barrier for drug absorption. The bioavailability of aqueous ophthalmic solutions is usually low owing not only to the barrier properties of the conjunctiva and cornea but also to the loss of drug by several processes. Precorneal loss of drug is due to tear turnover, drainage, systemic absorption, and in situ metabolism.[48] Tear turnover dilutes the drug, thus reducing the gradient of transport through the cornea. The difference between the pH of ophthalmic solutions of pilocarpine, between 4 and 5, and the pH of tears, about 7.47, causes increased lacrimation and loss of drug. An acidic pH is needed to increase the stability of pilocarpine. This drug is used as a topical miotic to reduce the intraocular pressure associated with glaucoma. Its ocular bioavailability is very low. About 1 to 3% of the instilled dose is absorbed into the eye; 50% of the dose is lost by systemic absorption from the conjunctiva.[49] The topical administration of beta-blocking agents such as propranolol is effective in the control of glaucoma.[50] The loss of levobunolol, also a beta-blocking agent, by systemic absorption is about 46%, and 12% is converted to dihydrolevobunolol in the ocular tissues.[51] The conjunctival and nasal mucosae play a role in the systemic absorption of ocularly applied drugs. The conjunctival mucosa has proteases capable of metabolizing peptides administered by the ocular route.[52]

Transport Through the Cornea. The corneal membrane is permselective, that is, it is able to discriminate between the transport of molecules having different charges. The electrical potential of this membrane, about 25 mV, is due to inward active Na^+ transport. At the isoelectric point (pH 3.2), the corneal membrane is electrically neutral and there is no ionic selectivity of positive or negative ions. At the tear pH of 7.47, the cornea is negatively charged and selectively permeable to cations, whereas at pH below 3.2 it is selectively permeable to anions.[53] Drug transport through the cornea is mainly a passive process. The corneal barrier can be considered as a laminated membrane consisting of the epithelial, stromal, and endothelial layers. Figure 19–10 shows the rate-limiting steps for the transport of hydrophilic and lipophilic drugs. For hydrophobic drugs, the stroma is the limiting region, whereas for hydrophilic drugs the epithelium gives the most resistance.

Grass and Robinson[54] used an in vitro perfusion technique to study the permeation of drugs through albino rabbit cornea. The total resistance to the drug transport, R, from the donor phase in the perfusion apparatus can be written as the summation of the resistance of the individual layers:

$$R = R_{a(d)} + \frac{R_m}{K} + R_{a(r)} \qquad (19-9)$$

where $R_{a(d)}$ and $R_{a(r)}$ represent the resistances of the aqueous diffusion layers on the donor side and the

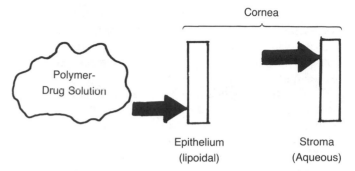

Fig. 19–10. Rate-limiting effect of corneal epithelium (lipid) and stroma (aqueous) for drugs with low *o/w* partition coefficients (arrow located low on the epithelium) and for drugs with high *o/w* partition coefficients (arrow located high on the stroma). (After G. M. Grass and J. R. Robinson, J. Pharm. Sci. **73**, 1021, 1984, reproduced with permission of the copyright owner.)

receptor side, respectively. The resistance of the stromal layer (aqueous) is included in the term, $R_{a(r)}$. R_m represents the resistance of the lipid membrane, that is, the corneal epithelial layer. Substituting resistances by the ratio of the thicknesses to the diffusion coefficients, in other words, h_i/D_i, equation (19–9) becomes

$$R = \frac{h_{a(d)}}{D_a} + \frac{h_m}{KD_m} + \frac{h_{a(r)}}{D_a} \qquad (19-10)$$

where $h_{a(d)}$ and $h_{a(r)}$ represent the thickness of the aqueous layer in the donor and receptor phase, respectively, and h_m is the thickness of the epithelial layer. Therefore, the flux of the drug is defined as a combination of membrane control and diffusion layer control (Chapter 13, p. 338):

$$J = \frac{D_m K D_a C}{h_m D_a + h_a K D_m} \qquad (19-11)$$

From equation (19–11), when the diffusion through the aqueous medium is much faster than through the membrane (i.e., $h_m D_a \gg h_a K D_m$), the diffusion is controlled by the membrane. On the other hand, when diffusion through the aqueous medium is much slower than that of the membrane (i.e., $h_m D_a \ll h_a K D_m$), the diffusion is controlled by the aqueous layer. These two limiting situations reduce equation (19–11) to equations (13–57) and (13–58) page 338. The lipophilic epithelial tissue can be viewed as a sieve in which the transport of drugs is hindered at a certain molecular size. Grass and Robinson[55] used transmission electron microscopy to visualize the actual pathway of drug transport through the cornea. The results indicated that hydrophilic compounds are preferentially located in the intercellular spaces, whereas hydrophobic compounds are present in the lipid structures of the tissue. The size of the intercellular space for diffusion of drugs was estimated to be smaller than 5 nm. Thus, the pore pathway is the main transport route for small hydrophilic molecules, as contrasted to the partition mechanism for large or lipophilic molecules.

The energy of activation E_a (pp. 295, 351, and 352) can be related to the transport mechanism.[54] This term is computed from the slope of a plot of $\ln P$ against $1/T$, where P is the permeability coefficient of the drug and T is the absolute temperature:

$$\ln P = -\frac{E_a}{R}\frac{1}{T} + \ln A \qquad (19\text{--}12)$$

The E_a values for hydrophilic molecules, such as ethanol, butanol and glycerol, ranged from 4.5 to 6.5 kcal/mole. These values are of the order of magnitude corresponding to the diffusion through an aqueous medium only. In contrast, hydrophobic molecules such as triamcinolone acetonide and hydrocortisone showed much larger E_a values, about 25 kcal/mole. These higher values result from drug transport by a partitioning mechanism.

Example 19–4. The permeability of hydrocortisone across rabbit cornea was determined at several temperatures:

$\frac{1}{T}$ (° K^{-1})	0.0032	0.0033	0.0034	0.0035
$\ln P$	-11.630	-12.911	-14.196	-15.481

Compute the energy of activation E_a for the transport of hydrocortisone.

Using linear regression, one obtains

$$\ln P = -12838\,\frac{1}{T} + 29.45 \quad (r^2 = 0.999)$$

$$\frac{E_a}{R} = -\text{slope} = -12838°\ \text{K}; \ E_a = 12838°\ \text{K} \times 1.9872\ \text{cal °K}^{-1}\ \text{mole}^{-1}$$

$$E_a = 25511\ \text{cal/mole} = 25.5\ \text{kcal/mole}$$

Schoenwald and Huang[56] found empirical correlations between the log of the permeability coefficient and the molecular weight, partition coefficient, and degree of ionization for beta-blocking agents (propranolol and related drugs). The expression is

$$\log P = 0.972 \log K - 0.112\,(\log K)^2 - 2.71 \log MW -$$
$$9.26 \log \alpha + 0.219 \qquad (19\text{--}13)$$

where K is the octanol–water partition coefficient, MW is the molecular weight of the penetrant, and α is the degree or fraction of ionization. For weakly basic compounds,

$$\alpha = \frac{1}{1 + \text{antilog}(pH - pK_a)} \qquad (19\text{--}14)$$

Equation (13–78) on page 342 gives the fraction of ionization α multiplied by 100 to convert to percentage ionization.

Example 19–5. Compute the permeability coefficient, P (cm/sec) of the hypertensive agent propranolol across rabbit cornea at pH 7.65. The octanol–water partition coefficient K is 1640, the molecular weight of propranolol is 257, and the pK_a is 9.23.

The degree of ionization at pH 7.65 is

$$\alpha = \frac{1}{1 + \text{antilog}(7.65 - 9.23)} = 0.974$$

$$\log \alpha = -0.011$$

The permeability coefficient is

$$\log P = (0.972 \times 3.215) - (0.112 \times 10.34) - (2.71 \times 2.41)$$
$$- [9.26(-0.011)] + 0.219$$
$$= -4.243$$

$$P = 5.7 \times 10^{-5}\ \text{cm/sec}$$

Controlled Ocular Drug Delivery. The action of a drug for ocular delivery can be prolonged (1) by reducing drainage by the use of viscosity-enhancing agents, suspensions, emulsions, erodible, and non-erodible matrices and (2) by enhancing the corneal penetration by using prodrugs and liposomes (see pp. 513 to 515). The optimal viscosity range to reduce drainage loss is between 12 and 15 cps when polyvinyl alcohol[57] or methyl cellulose[58] is used as a viscosity enhancer. To minimize potential irritation, ophthalmic suspensions are prepared by micronization techniques. The dissolution rate of the large particles is smaller than that of small particles, so that the large particles may drain away before dissolution takes place, thus decreasing bioavailability.[59] Hui and Robinson[60] studied the effect of dissolution rate on ocular drug bioavailability. After instillation of a suspension, the drug penetrates into the cornea or conjunctiva from the saturated solution. Additional particles dissolve to maintain a reservoir of saturated solution. To obtain the desired bioavailability, the dissolution rate of the drug must be greater than the clearance of the dose from the conjunctival sac and approximately equal to the absorption rate. Many drugs cannot satisfy these requirements.

Precorneal retention and duration of action can be increased by using water-soluble matrices in which the drug is either dispersed or dissolved. The delivery of drugs from hydrophilic matrices is fast because the tear fluid rapidly penetrates into the matrix. The prolonged action is not controlled by the vehicle but is caused by the precorneal retention of the drug. The penetration of water into the matrix can be reduced using hydrophobic polymers such as alkyl half-esters of poly(methyl vinyl ether–maleic anhydride) (PVM–MA). The surface of the matrix is water-soluble above certain pH values, owing to the ionizable carboxylic groups. However, the hydrophobic alkyl ester groups avoid the penetration of water into the matrix. The diffusion of drug from the matrix is impeded so that it is released at the rate at which the polymer surface is dissolved. In one study, pilocarpine was released from PVM–MA polymers according to zero-order kinetics and was controlled by the erosion of the polymer surface.[49] Grass let al.[61] prepared erodible and nonerodible dry films for sustained delivery of pilocarpine. The polymers used in both cases were polyvinyl alcohol and carboxyl copolymer (Carbomer 934). The release of drug from the films fitted either the Hixon–Crowell dissolution cube root equation (Chapter 13, pp. 333, 334) or the diffusion-controlled dissolution equation proposed by Cobby et al.[62,103], the latter providing the best fit. The in vivo miotic response was delayed longer than that of pilocarpine solutions.

The ocular delivery of drugs from matrices can be improved by the use of bioadhesive polymers. Johnson and Zografi[63] measured the adhesion (adhesive strength) of hydroxypropyl cellulose to solid substrates as a function of dry film thickness. A "butt adhesion test" used by these workers provided a constant slow rate of film detachment to maintain the viscoelastic contribution of the film relative to the adhesion measurements as a constant. For thickness less than 20 μm, there is a linear relationship between the adhesive strength, Y (in g/cm^2) and the film thickness, h (in μm). The adhesive failure, Y_0, can be obtained by extrapolating the adhesive strength to zero film thickness.

Example 19–6. The adhesion, Y, of hydroxypropyl cellulose to polyethylene surfaces as a function of the film thickness (h) of the adhesive is

Y (g/cm^2)	3850	2800	1750	700
h (μm)	5	10	15	20

Compute the adhesive failure, Y_0. A regression of Y (dependent variable) against h (independent variable) gives

$$Y = -210\,h + 4900$$

The adhesive failure is given by the intercept, $Y_0 = 4900$ g/cm^2.

The *work of adhesion W_a* (pp. 368–369) of the dry film on the solid surface can be computed from the surface tension of the polymer and the solid surface[63]:

$$W_a = \frac{4\gamma_s^d\gamma_p^d}{\gamma_s^d + \gamma_p^d} + \frac{4\gamma_s^p\gamma_p^p}{\gamma_s^p + \gamma_p^p} \qquad (19-15)$$

where γ_s and γ_p are the surface tensions of the solid and the polymer, respectively. The superscripts d and p represent the contribution to the total surface tension from nonpolar and polar portions of the molecule.

Example 19–7. Compute the work of adhesion of hydroxypropyl cellulose films to a solid surface of polyethylene from the following data: $\gamma_s^d = 34.2$ erg/cm^2; $\gamma_s^p = 3.4$ erg/cm^2; $\gamma_p^d = 24.7$ erg/cm^2; $\gamma_p^p = 16.3$ erg/cm^2.

$$W_a = \frac{4 \times 34.2 \times 24.7}{34.2 + 24.7} + \frac{4 \times 3.4 \times 16.3}{3.4 + 16.3}$$

$$W_a = 68.6 \text{ erg/cm}^2$$

Ocusert System. The pilocarpine-containing device Ocusert, introduced in 1975 by Alza Corporation, was the first controlled topical dosage form marketed for use in the eye. The device (Fig. 19–11a) consists of a central core or reservoir of pilocarpine between two membrane surfaces, made of an ethylene–vinyl acetate copolymer, that control the rate of release of the drug. The oval device, slightly larger than a contact lens, is

placed in the cul-de-sac under the upper or lower lid (Fig. 19–11b), where pilocarpine is released at a zero-order rate and is absorbed into the cornea of the eye. Two products are available: Ocusert P-20, which delivers a dose of 20 μg/hr, and Ocusert P-40, which delivers a dose of 40 μg/hr.

The ocular delivery system was designed to overcome the inefficient delivery of pilocarpine from ophthalmic drops. Because of the close contact with the eye and continuous release of drug from the Ocusert over a period of a week, only about one fourth as much pilocarpine must be administered as compared with the dropper technique, and this reduction in dose overcomes toxicity and side effects. The specialized medication system is expensive, however, and probably will be used only in patients who need continuous medication, can tolerate the presence of the disk in the eye, and can afford the therapy.

With drugs that are only sparingly soluble in water, such as chloramphenicol, release in the eye may be calculated from a form of Fick's law (Chapter 13):

$$M = \frac{SDKC_s}{h} t \qquad (19-16)$$

in which M is the accumulated amount released and t is the time. S is the surface area of the device in contact with the eye, D is the diffusion coefficient of the Ocusert membrane, K is a liquid–liquid partition coefficient between the Ocusert and the eye fluids, C_s is the solubility of the drug in water, and h is the Ocusert membrane thickness. As observed in Figure 19–12, a plot of accumulated drug release against time is linear, showing a break at point A (130 hr), then becoming horizontal, indicating that chloramphenicol is depleted and no more is released after 130 hours. A plot of *release rate*, rather than amount, versus time results in a straight horizontal line to point A, then tends toward zero (Fig. 19–12, inset). The curve does not fall vertically following point A, but descends parabolically as observed in the inset of Figure 19–12. These plots indicate that the release rate of a sparingly soluble drug is almost constant, that is, a zero-order release rate over most of the lifetime of the device, rather than a first-order release, which would represent a continuously decreasing rate with time.

Example 19–8. The diffusion coefficient of a new chloramphenicol derivative in the Ocusert device is 3.77×10^{-5} cm^2/hr. The surface area S of the Ocusert is 0.80 cm^2, the partition coefficient K between the Ocusert and ocular fluids is 1.03, the thickness of the membrane h is 0.007 cm, and the solubility C_s in water (25° C) of the new compound is 3.93 mg/cm^3. By use of equation (19–16), calculate the cumulative amount of drug released in 125 hours.

$$M = \frac{(0.80 \text{ cm}^2)(3.77 \times 10^{-5} \text{ cm}^2/\text{hr})(1.03)(3.93 \text{ mg/cm}^3)(125 \text{ hr})}{0.007 \text{ cm}}$$

$M = 2.18$ mg released in 125 hours

Pilocarpine is water soluble, and equation (19–16) is not an exact representation of the profile of the release

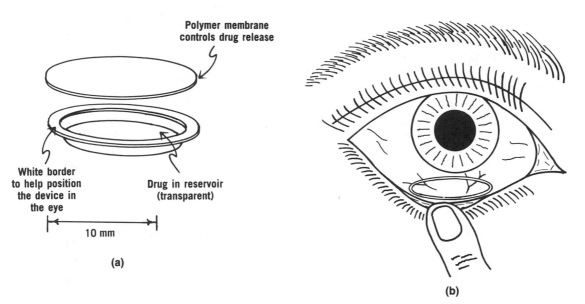

Fig. 19–11. (*a*) Schematic of Ocusert (Alza). (After K. Heilmann, *Therapeutic Systems*, Georg Thieme, Stuttgart, 1978, p. 67.) (*b*) Insertion of the Ocusert into the cul-de-sac of the eye. (ibid. p. 69: reproduced with permission of the copyright owner.)

rate with time for such a compound. The flux or rate per unit time for a water-soluble compound is not horizontal (Fig. 19–12 inset) but rather declines slowly as the release proceeds. By the proper choice of membranes for the Ocusert, however, the release rate of pilocarpine can be held essentially constant (near zero-order drug release) for up to 7 days of delivery.

Nasal Administration. The nose, Figure 19–13, consists of two openings (nostrils) that are separated by a median septum. The vestibule at the entrance of each nostril is covered with hairs, which prevent entrance of air-suspended particles. The nose cavity is divided by the septum into two chambers called *fossae*. They form passages for air movement from the nostrils to the nasopharyngeal space at the back of the nose. Each

fossa consists of two parts, an olfactory region at the front of the nose and a respiratory region that accounts for the remainder of the fossae.

The nasal cavity is lined with a mucous membrane, called the *membrana mucosa nasi*, which is continuous with the skin of the nostrils. The respiratory portion of the nasal cavity contains ciliated (hair-like) projections consisting of columnar epithelial cells.

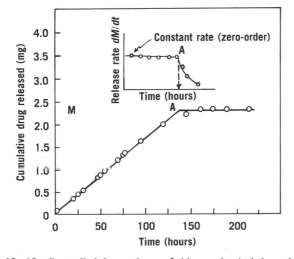

Fig. 19–12. Controlled drug release of chloramphenicol through the Ocusert membrane. The inset shows the relationship of the *release rate* rather than the cumulative amount released (main curve), versus time.

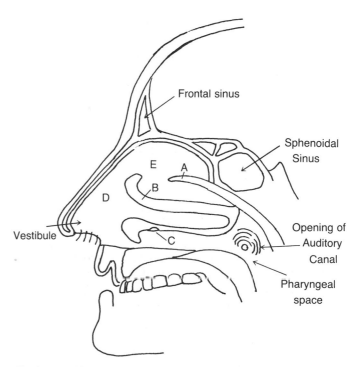

Fig. 19–13. Nasal anatomy. Modified from references 64 and 65. Key: A, upper meatus; B, middle meatus; C, opening of nasolacrimal duct on lower meatus; D, left fossa, olfactory region; E, left fossa, respiratory region.

The nasal cavity consists of three passageways or meatuses: upper, middle, and lower meatus. As observed in Figure 19–13 the nasolacrimal duct drains into the lower meatus. The nose is connected to the middle ear through the nasopharynx or postnasal space and through the auditory canal. The compartments of the nose are connected to the conjunctiva of the eye by way of the nasolacrimal and lacrimal ducts, and through several sinuses that drain into the nose. A portion of a drug administered into the conjunctiva of the eye may enter the nose through these ducts and sinuses, and may also pass into the esophagus.[64,65]

Nasal administration is widely used for local effects, but it is also a potential site for systemic drug absorption owing to its large surface area. The vascular bed of the nasal mucosa favors the rapid passage of fluids and dissolved compounds from the mucosa to the systemic circulation. The nasal route avoids the first-pass effect (that is, possible decomposition as the drug passes through the liver) and gastrointestinal degradation, providing an alternative route for oral administration. Most drug absorption occurs at the sinuses, where the mucous membrane is very thin and widely vascularized.[66] Lipophilic drugs such as propranolol produce blood levels similar to those observed after intravenous administration. Sustained nasal release formulations of propranolol result in prolonged drug levels.[67] Rapid absorption has been found for progesterone and testosterone.[68] Hydromorphone, a semisynthetic analgesic used for the relief of postoperative pain or severe chronic pain, is well absorbed by the nasal route.[69]

Huang et al.[70] developed an in situ rat technique to study nasal absorption. The drug solution is perfused at a constant rate through the nasal cavity of the rat. The extent of absorption is obtained by subtracting the initial amount of drug from that remaining in the perfusing solution. The nasal absorption of benzoic acid was found to depend on pH and followed first-order kinetics. At low pH values,

$$k_{obs} = k_{HA} \frac{[H^+]}{[H^+] + K_a} \qquad (19\text{–}17)$$

and at high pH values,

$$k_{obs} = k_{A^-} \frac{K_a}{[H^+] + K_a} \qquad (19\text{–}18)$$

where k_{obs} is the overall first-order absorption constant, and k_{HA} and k_{A^-} are the first-order absorption constants for the un-ionized and ionized species of benzoic acid, HA and A^-, respectively.

Example 19–9. (a) Compute the k_{obs} value at pH 2.4 and pH 7.19, where benzoic acid is predominantly in its nonionized and ionized forms, respectively. K_a is equal to 6.30×10^{-5}, k_{HA} is 9.75×10^{-3} min^{-1}, and k_{A^-} is 2.40×10^{-3} min^{-1}. (b) Compute the half-life for nasal absorption of benzoic acid in its nonionized form (pH 2.4) and ionized form (pH 7.19).

(a) From equation (19–17), at pH = 2.4

$$k_{obs} = 9.75 \times 10^{-3} \frac{3.98 \times 10^{-3}}{3.98 \times 10^{-3} + 6.3 \times 10^{-5}}$$

$$k_{obs} = 9.60 \times 10^{-3} \text{ min}^{-1}$$

From equation (19–18) at pH 7.19

$$k_{obs} = 2.40 \times 10^{-3} \frac{6.30 \times 10^{-5}}{6.46 \times 10^{-8} + 6.3 \times 10^{-5}}$$

$$k_{obs} = 2.40 \times 10^{-3} \text{ min}^{-1}$$

(b) From equation (12–18), page 288, the half-life for nasal absorption at 25° C is

(at pH 2.4) $\quad t_{1/2} = \dfrac{0.693}{k_{obs}} = \dfrac{0.693}{9.60 \times 10^{-3}} = 72$ min for the nonionized form

(at pH 7.19) $\quad t_{1/2} = \dfrac{0.693}{2.40 \times 10^{-3}} = 289$ min for the ionized form

Nasal administration is one of the most investigated routes for absorption of peptides and proteins. However, the bioavailability of these compounds is low due to their high molecular weight. Maitani et al.[71] studied the influence of molecular weight and charge on nasal absorption of neutral and positively charged (polycation) dextran derivatives in rabbits. These compounds were chosen as macromolecular models of water-soluble drugs. The plasma concentration resulting from nasal absorption of both neutral and charged dextrans decreased as the molecular weight of the compound increased. Additional information on nasal absorption of peptides and proteins is found in the two treatises by Chien et al.[72,73] Unfortunately, peptides are degraded at the site of administration by proteolytic enzymes, mainly aminopeptidases. Thus, the nasal dose needed for insulin is considerably greater than the parenteral dose required to produce a similar effect. Hussain et al.[74] found that even in concentrations as small as nanomolar (i.e., on the order of 10^{-9} molar), α-aminoboronic acid derivatives, which are potent inhibitors of aminopeptidases, greatly increase the absorption of leucine–enkephalin, a model peptide.

To improve the nasal absorption of peptides, various *permeability enhancers* have been investigated. Permeability enhancers are compounds that promote or enhance the absorption of drugs through the skin or mucosae, usually by reversibly altering the permeability of the membrane. Bile salts and other biologic agents have been shown to enhance drug permeability of the nasal mucosa. Thus, nasal absorption of enkephalin analogs increases from about 59% to 94% of the subcutaneous dose in the presence of 1% sodium glycholate.[75] The local antibiotic bacitracin, and sodium taurodihydrofusidate,[76] a derivative of the antibiotic fusidic acid but without antibiotic activity, markedly enhance the nasal absorption of peptides such as gonadorenin, a luteinizing hormone–releasing hormone and its agonist, buserelin. The properties of sodium salts of fusidic acid resemble those of the bile salts. It has been reported that bile salts may damage the epithelial layer, which serves as a defense against infecting organisms. In addition to mucosal damage, some drugs for local and systemic use and some additives affect ciliary movement, which is the most important process in nasal mucociliary clearance. Some beta-adrenergic and cholinergic drugs stimulate ciliary movement and increase mucociliary clearance. On the other hand, local anesthetics, propranolol, and antihistamines, as well as some enhancers such as the bile salts, suppress ciliary movement. Thus, enhancers must be chosen carefully in the design of nasal drug formulation for systemic effects, particularly in drugs meant for use in long-term treatment.[77]

Dosage forms for nasal absorption must deposit and remain in the nasal cavity long enough to allow effective absorption. The standard methods of administration are sprays and drops. The particle size in aerosols is important in determining the site of deposition. Particles less than 0.5 μm in diameter may pass through the nose and reach the terminal bronchi and alveoli of the lungs. A nasal spray requires that the particles have a diameter larger than 4 μm to be retained in the nose and to minimize passage into the lungs. Harris et al.[78] studied the influence of the delivery system on drug deposition. The nasal spray deposits drug in the forward part of the nasal atrium, whereas nasal drops are dispersed throughout the nasal cavity. A spray clears more slowly than the drops since the spray is deposited in nonciliated regions. The bioavailability of desmopressin, a peptide derivative of 8-D-arginine vasopressin, is improved by administering it with a metered-dose inhaler* rather than by nasal drops.[79] (See Figure 19–14.)

Buccal Administration. The absorption of drugs through the oral mucosa improves bioavailability of drugs that might otherwise be metabolized during their passage through the gastrointestinal tract or the liver, where the undesired first-pass effect occurs. The oral mucosa consists of stratified squamous epithelium; its thickness and degree of keratinization vary from one region to another and may affect the permeability of a drug.[80] Absorption is mainly a passive process that occurs through the buccal, sublingual, or gingival mucosa, the palatal and tongue mucosae being less permeable. In addition to circumventing first-pass metabolism, an advantage of the buccal route is its accessibility. A dosage form can easily be placed in and removed from the site of application,[81] and the buccal route is therefore used locally to administer antimicrobial and antiinflammatory agents, local anesthetics, and conventional pharmaceuticals including mouthwashes, oral gels or pastes, lozenges, and sublingual tablets. Buccal administration has been studied for the systemic

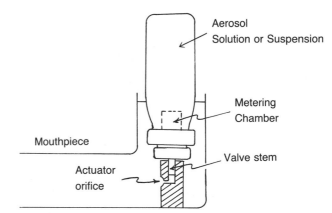

Fig. 19–14. Metered-dose device for drug administration to nasal and pulmonary regions. (From P. R. Byron, Ed., *Respiratory Drug Delivery*, CRC, Boca Raton, Fla., 1990, p. 171, reproduced with permission of the copyright owner.)

delivery of peptides, polypeptides such as insulin, and nifedipine.[82]

The dosage forms should remain in contact with the oral mucosa to allow absorption of the drug. Therefore, taste is an important factor to be considered in the design of the product. Bitter taste can be masked by using an insoluble derivative of the drug so that the threshold taste concentration is not reached. Another approach is the use of prodrugs with acceptable organoleptic characteristics. Hussain et al.[83] prepared bitterness prodrugs of several opioid antagonists by esterification of their phenolic groups. The bitter taste of these compounds is due to the interaction of the phenolic groups with a taste receptor on the tongue. The rate of absorption of the prodrugs was greater than the rate of hydrolysis, so that the bitter taste did not develop.

Conventional dosage forms do not remain in contact with the oral mucosa long enough for controlled release to be achieved. Bioadhesive polymers that bind to mucin or the epithelial surface may be used to place the drug at a specific site on the mucosa, allowing prolonged delivery. Sodium carboxymethylcellulose, Carbopol 934, and hydroxypropylcellulose are examples of polymers for use in buccal dosage forms to produce adhesiveness. When the polymer is hydrated, it adheres to the oral mucosa and inhibits salivation, tongue movements, and swallowing for a period of time. Hydrophilic functional groups such as —OH, —COOH, and NH_3 on the polymers provide good wet adhesion.[82] The adhesiveness can be evaluated in vitro by tensile testing and other methods using isolated tissues of the gastrointestinal tract or mucous membrane. Park[84] used mucin molecules adsorbed on red colloidal gold. When the mucin–gold conjugates interact with the bioadhesive polymer, a red color is developed on the surface, and the adhesiveness can be quantitatively compared by measuring the intensity of the color. Rao and Buri[85] used an in situ method in the rat jejunum

---

*A metered-dose inhaler is a device which, when manually compressed, delivers an accurate and reproducible dose of the nasal (or bronchial) medication.

and stomach to evaluate the adhesiveness of drug particles coated with several polymers. Carboxymethylcellulose adhered more strongly to the mucus than hydroxypropylmethylcellulose (HPC). These authors suggested that the adhesion was promoted by relaxation of the polymer chains, which facilitated their interlinking with the glycoproteins of the mucus.

Adhesive patches are used to achieve sustained release. Anders and Merkle[81] prepared adhesive-laminated patches for buccal administration of oligopeptides. The device consists of an impermeable backing layer and a mucoadhesive polymer layer containing the drug. The shape and size can vary depending on the site of administration; whether at the buccal, sublingual, or gingival mucosa. The duration of mucosal adhesion, as determined in humans, depended on the polymer type and the amount and viscosity of the polymer used. The release of a model drug, sodium salicylate, from the patch was controlled by the dissolution kinetics of the polymer carrier rather than the drug diffusion out of the polymer. Collins and Deasy[82] prepared three-layer devices. The upper layer consisted of a nonadhesive and flavored waxy material containing the drug, and the middle layer was prepared from magnesium stearate (antiadhesive). The lower layer, made of a mixture of HPC and carbopol, was designed to adhere to the oral mucosa. The three-layered device showed constant salivary levels of the antiinfective agent cetylpyridinium chloride in human volunteers over the 3-hour period studied.

Pulmonary Administration.[86,87] The respiratory tract has a large surface area and is easily accessible for the treatment of respiratory diseases. The surface increases from the most exterior region (nasopharyngeal) to the tracheobronchial and pulmonary regions, the latter consisting of bronchioles and alveoli. The elements of the pulmonary route are illustrated in Figure 19–15. Aerosols are widely used to deliver drugs in the respiratory tract. The deposition mechanism of the particles depends on many factors, such as the inhalation regime and particle size, shape, density, charge, and hygroscopicity. The size of solid particles or liquid droplets in aerosols normally ranges from 1 to 10 μm, and is expressed as the *aerodynamic diameter*, $d_{ae} = \rho^{1/2}d$, where ρ is the density of the particle and d the observed diameter. Generally, the particles are delivered via mouth inhalation, to bypass the nasopharyngeal cavity. However, the total retention of particles is usually only 50 to 60% of the administered dose.

Larger particles (>5 μm) are usually deposited via inertial impaction in the upper airways. Moderate size particles (1–5 μm) can settle out from the airstream under gravitational influence. Submicron particles deposit as a result of Brownian movement (see p. 400) mainly in the lower airways (bronchial and alveolar regions).[88] The inhaled particles can be transported from one region to another within the respiratory tract. The duration of local therapeutic activity is

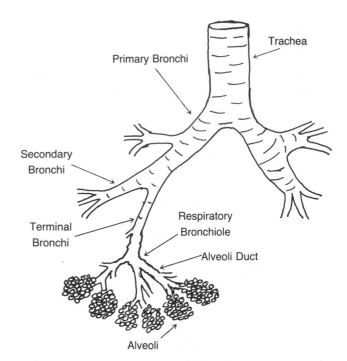

Fig. 19–15. Regions of the bronchial and pulmonary routes.

a complex function of particle deposition, mucociliary clearance, drug dissolution or release (for solid aerosols), absorption, tissue sequestration, and metabolism kinetics.

Byron[89] proposed a mathematical model to calculate drug residence times and dose fractions in the three functional portions of the respiratory tract: the nasopharyngeal region and the tracheobronchial and pulmonary (alveolar) regions. The deposition in the ciliated airways was largely unaffected by breath-holding, and the particles showed a maximum d_{ae} between 5 and 9 μm (slow inhalation) and 3 and 6 μm (fast inhalation). Alveolar deposition was dependent on the mode of inhalation and the breath-holding. The latter is a common practice and allows deposition of small particles which otherwise would be exhaled. To determine the effect of breath-holding on the deposition of particles, the *sedimentation efficiency*, S, was defined as

$$S = \frac{\text{distance the particle falls during breath-holding}}{\text{mean regional airway diameter}} \quad (19\text{–}19)$$

The mean regional diameters for the three areas considered are 5 cm for the mouth, 0.2 cm for the tracheobronchial region, and 0.073 cm for the alveoli (pulmonary region). In cases where the sedimentation efficiency was >1, S was assigned a value of unity. A total lung volume after inhalation, V_t, of 3000 cm³ was divided into 30, 170, and 2800 cm³ for the mouth (M), tracheobronchial (TB) region, and alveolary (P) region, respectively. For each particle size, the *exhaled dose fraction E* is given by

$$E = 1 - (f_M + f_{TB} + f_P) \quad (19\text{–}20)$$

where the terms f_M, f_{TB}, and f_P stand for the fractional deposition in each of the three regions. During breath-holding, additional fractions will sediment, depending on the sedimentation efficiency and the ratio of the regional volume to the total volume of the lungs. The *sedimentation dose fraction*, *SDF*, after breath-holding is calculated from the expression

$$SDF = E \left(\frac{SV_r}{V_t} \right) \qquad (19\text{--}21)$$

where V_r is the regional volume of the *M*, *TB*, or *P* regions and V_t the total volume after inhalation (3000 cm³).

Example 19–10. For a 3-μm monodisperse aerosol inhaled at 22.5 L/min, the fractional depositions were found to be $f_M = 0.04$, $f_{TB} = 0.14$ and $f_P = 0.55$. Compute the undeposited or exhaled fraction E, and the additional sedimentation of the undeposited fraction in the mouth and tracheobronchial and alveolarly regions after 10 seconds of breath-holding. The velocity of sedimentation of the particles is 0.027 cm/sec.

From equation (19–20) the undeposited (exhaled) fraction is

$$E = 1 - (0.04 + 0.14 + 0.55) = 0.27$$

After 10 seconds of breath-holding, the distance of particle fall was 10 sec × 0.027 cm/sec = 0.27 cm. Substitution of this value and the mean diameter of the alveolary (*P*) region in equation (19–19) gives the sedimentation efficiency in the pulmonary region, S_P:

$$S_P = \frac{0.27}{0.073} = 3.70$$

since $S_P > 1$, a value of $S_P = 1$ is taken. From equation (19–21) the sedimentation dose fraction becomes

$$SDF_P = (0.27)(1) \frac{2800}{3000} = 0.252$$

Analogously, for the tracheobronchial zone (mean diameter 0.2 cm), a value of $S_{TB} > 1$ is obtained, so S_{TB} is taken equal to unity, and for the sedimentation dose fraction, one obtains

$$SDF_{TB} = (0.27)(1) \frac{170}{3000} = 0.0153$$

For the mouth region, *M*, the mean diameter is 5 cm,

$$S_M = \frac{0.27}{5} = 0.054$$

and

$$SDF_M = (0.054) \frac{30}{3000} = 5.4 \times 10^{-4}$$

Thus, the total additional dose deposited after 10 seconds of breath-holding is
$SDF = SDF_P + SDF_{TB} + SDF_M = 0.252 + 0.0153 + (5.4 \times 10^{-4}) = 0.268$.

These results show that for 3-μm particles breath-holding is adequate to deposit particles in the alveolar region ($SDF_P = 0.252$); whereas breath-holding is inadequate to deposit these particles in the mouth ($SDF_M = 0.00054$) and in the tracheobronchial region ($SDF_{TB} = 0.0153$).

Byron et al.[90] used an isolated perfused rat lung preparation to study the deposition and absorption of disodium fluorescein from solid aerosols having an aerodynamic diameter of 3 to 4 μm. The aerosols were administered for 20 minutes under different inhalation regimes (respiration frequency RF, in cycles min⁻¹). The total dose administered D can be divided into a transferable amount A that diffuses into the perfusate according to a first-order rate constant k, and an untransferable amount U according to the scheme:

$$D \overset{\nearrow U}{\underset{\searrow A \overset{k}{\to} B}{}}$$

assuming instantaneous dissolution of A and first-order k. The amount in the perfusate, B, at any time, t, is given by the product of perfusate concentration and volume. The amount transferred to B can be computed from*

$$B = \frac{A}{20\,RF} \left[n - \frac{(1 - e^{-\frac{nk}{RF}}) e^{-\frac{k}{RF}}}{1 - e^{-\frac{k}{RF}}} \right] \text{ for } t \leq 20 \quad (19\text{--}22)$$

and

$$B = B_{20} + A_{20} \left[1 - e^{-k(t-20)} \right] \text{ for } t > 20 \qquad (19\text{--}23)$$

where B_{20} is computed from equation (19–22) at time $t = 20$ min, and A_{20} is calculated using the following expression:

$$A_{20} = \left[\left(\frac{A}{20\,RF} \right) (1 - e^{-20k}) e^{-\frac{k}{RF}} \right] \left(1 - e^{-\frac{k}{RF}} \right) \qquad (19\text{--}24)$$

The term, $A/20\,RF$, found in equations (19–22) and (19–24), is the transferable amount deposited after each inhalation. The inhalation or dose number, n, is equal to $t \times RF$ for $t \leq 20$, where RF is the respiratory frequency.

The ratio (transferable amount/amount deposited) increased at high respiratory frequency RF, large tidal volume, and decreasing aerosol particle size. *Tidal volume* is the amount of air that enters the lungs with each inspiration or leaves the lungs with each expiration during normal breathing.

Example 19–11. Compute the transfer B of 3-μm particles at $t = 20$ min, knowing that the transferable amount A is 37.7 μg, the respiratory frequency RF is 28, and $k = 0.049$ min⁻¹.

The inhalation or dose number is $n = 20$ min × 28 cycles/min = 560 cycles; from equation (19–22)

$$B = \frac{37.7}{560} \left\{ 560 - \frac{\left[1 - \text{ex}\left(\frac{-560 \times 0.049}{28} \right) \right] \times \text{ex}\left(\frac{-0.049}{28} \right)}{1 - \text{ex}\left(\frac{-0.049}{28} \right)} \right\}$$

$$B = 13.69 \text{ μg}$$

The pulmonary route provides effective administration of beta-adrenergic agonists in asthma treatment.

---

*In personal correspondence, Byron has noted that n is incorrectly placed in equation (2) of the paper, J. Pharm. Sci. **75**, 168, 1986. Equation (19–22) above is the correct expression.

Corticosteroids have been added to the therapeutic regime, in particular triamcinolone acetonide and beclomethasone, which are safe and effective in aerosol formulations.[91] However, this route has shown to be of limited usefulness for antimicrobial drugs. The pulmonary route is useful for controlled delivery of drugs to the respiratory tract, depending on the characteristics of the drug and the aerosol device. It is unlikely that this route will substitute for the administration of more conventional oral or parenteral drugs.

Gastrointestinal Administration. The Oral Route. Oral administration is perhaps the most widely used route for the delivery of drugs. Absorption from the gut depends on a number of factors, such as gastric emptying, intestinal motility, mucosal surface area, degradation of the drug in the stomach, and first-pass effect in the liver. The absorption varies from the stomach to the intestines owing to the increased surface area (about 4500 m^2) of the intestinal mucosa and to the greater velocity of blood (1000 mL/min) through the intestinal capillaries relative to the gastric capillaries.[92] The transport of drugs through the cellular barrier of the epithelia can be achieved through passive and carrier-mediated mechanisms. The former is mainly a diffusion process, while the latter requires the presence of a transport agent to ferry the drug across the membranes.

Sinko and Amidon[93] used a single-pass intestinal perfusion technique in rats to study the oral absorption of drugs via passive absorption and carrier-mediated mechanisms. For a passive process, the intrinsic permeability of the intestinal wall, $P_w^\star$, is calculated as

$$P_w^\star = \frac{P_{eff}^\star}{\left(1 - \dfrac{P_{eff}^\star}{P_{aq}^\star}\right)} \qquad (19\text{--}25)$$

where $P_{eff}^\star$ is the effective permeability (see equation (19–27)) and $P_{aq}^\star$ is the aqueous permeability (see equation (19–28)). Solid stars, $\star$, indicate dimensionless permeabilities.* For example, $P^\star$ is defined as

$$P^\star = \frac{PR}{D} \qquad (19\text{--}26)$$

in which $P^\star$ has the units of (cm/sec)cm(sec/cm^2) in which all units cancel. R is the radius of the intestine and D the aqueous diffusion coefficient. The values of $P_{eff}^\star$ and $P_{aq}^\star$, respectively, are calculated from

$$P_{eff}^\star = \frac{1 - (C_m/C_o)}{4\,Gz} \qquad (19\text{--}27)$$

and

$$P_{aq}^\star = (A\,G_z^{1/3})^{-1} \qquad (19\text{--}28)$$

---

*See equation (13–11), page 327, for the definition of *permeability*.

C_o and C_m are the inlet and outlet perfusate concentrations and A is a constant. The *Graetz number*, G_z, is a dimensionless quantity that expresses the ratio of axial convection to radial diffusion times,

$$G_z = \frac{\pi DL}{2Q} \qquad (19\text{--}29)$$

D is the diffusion coefficient, L is the length of the intestine, and Q is the flow rate.

The constant A in equation (19–28) depends on the Graetz number as calculated from a film model approximation (see p. 648 in reference 93):

$$A = 10.00\,G_z + 1.01 \quad \text{for } 0.004 \le G_z \ge 0.01 \quad (19\text{--}30)$$

$$A = 4.50\,G_z + 1.07 \quad \text{for } 0.01 \le G_z \ge 0.03 \quad (19\text{--}31)$$

$$A = 2.5\,G_z + 1.13 \quad \text{for } 0.03 \le G_z \quad (19\text{--}32)$$

Example 19–12. Compute the aqueous, effective, and intrinsic wall permeabilities for the passive transport of a drug in the rat jejunum from the following data: $L = 10$ cm, $D = 5 \times 10^{-6}$ cm^2/sec, and $Q = 0.25$ cm^3/min. The ratio C_m/C_o is 0.97.

The Graetz number for the experimental condition (equation 19–29)) is

$$G_z = \frac{3.1416 \times 5 \times 10^{-6} \text{ cm}^2/\text{sec} \times 10 \text{ cm}}{2(0.25/60) \text{ cm}^3/\text{sec}} = 0.0188$$

The A value is computed from equation (19–31):

$$A = (4.50 \times 0.0188) + 1.07 = 1.155$$

The aqueous permeability from equation (19–28) is

$$P_{aq}^\star = [1.155(0.0188)^{1/3}]^{-1} = 3.25$$

The effective wall permeability from equation (19–27) is

$$P_{eff}^\star = \frac{1 - 0.97}{4 \times 0.0188} = 0.399$$

and the intrinsic wall permeability, according to equation (19–25), is

$$P_w^\star = \frac{0.399}{\left(1 - \dfrac{0.399}{3.256}\right)} = 0.455$$

For a carrier-mediated mechanism, the wall permeability $P_w^\star$ may be written in terms of the carrier uptake, $\dfrac{J_{max}^\star}{K_m + C_w}$, and the passive membrane permeability, $P_m^\star$, giving

$$P_w^\star = \frac{J_{max}^\star}{K_m + C_w} + P_m^\star \qquad (19\text{--}33)$$

where $J_{max}^\star$ is the maximum flux (pp. 325–328), K_m is the intrinsic Michaelis constant (pp. 293–294), $P_m^\star$ is the intrinsic passive membrane permeability, and C_w is the concentration at the intestinal wall, calculated from

$$C_w = C_o \left(1 - \frac{P_{eff}^\star}{P_{aq}^\star}\right) \qquad (19\text{--}34)$$

where all the symbols have been defined previously. Note that the star on the P terms shows them to be dimensionless quantities. The carrier permeability, $P_c^\star$, is defined as

$$P_c^\star = \frac{J_{\max}^\star}{K_m} \qquad (19\text{--}35)$$

Substituting equation (19–35) into equation (19–33) yields

$$P_w^\star = \frac{P_c^\star}{1 + \left(\dfrac{C_w}{K_m}\right)} + P_m^\star \qquad (19\text{--}36)$$

Sinko and Amidon[93] found that the jejunal absorption of several cephalosporins fitted equation (19–36) and the term $P_m^\star$ was negligible or zero. This indicates that the transport mechanism for these antibiotics is mainly a carrier-mediated process. The absorption of captopril in the rat intestine is also mediated by a carrier peptide with a small contribution of passive transport. Captopril is an angiotensin-converting enzyme inhibitor used in the treatment of hypertension and congestive heart failure.[94] Amidon et al.[95] found that the dose fraction, F, absorbed in humans correlated well with the effective permeability of the intestinal wall $P_w^\star$ in rats according to the expression,

$$F = 1 - e^{-2P_w^\star} \qquad (19\text{--}37)$$

In equation (19–37) it is assumed that the aqueous permeability $P_{aq}^\star$ is not rate limiting, since its value is usually larger than unity (see example (19–12)). The authors were able to correlate F and $P_w^\star$ for a number of drugs (see *problem 19–18*).

An important factor in gastrointestinal (GI) absorption for ionizable drugs is the pH of the GI environment. The pH–partition theory (p. 343) states that the absorption is favored when the drug is nonionized and has an *o/w* partition coefficient larger than unity. Prieto et al.[96] studied the influence of the pH of beta-lactam antibiotics on their absorption through the rat intestinal tract using an in vivo perfusion technique. The absorption is due to a passive mechanism (diffusion) and a nonspecific carrier. The apparent rate constant, K_{app}, is transformed to metabolic weight units for the rat by introducing the term V_{app}, defined as

$$V_{app} = \frac{K_{app}}{(\text{living body weight})^{0.75}} \qquad (19\text{--}38)$$

where V_{app} is the apparent absorption rate constant per metabolic weight. The effect of pH on V_{app} was estimated from

$$V_{app} = \frac{V_o + V_{-1}\left(\dfrac{K_a}{[H^+]}\right)}{1 + \left(\dfrac{K_a}{[H^+]}\right)} \qquad (19\text{--}39)$$

where V_o and V_{-1} are the rate constant contributions of the nonionized and ionized forms, respectively, to the apparent absorption rate constant, V_{app}; and K_a is the dissociation constant of the drug.

Example 19–13. Compute V_{app} and K_{app} for a cephalosporin[96] in aqueous solution at pH 4.9 given that the drug's pK_a is 3.49, V_o is 25.072×10^{-3} mini^{-1} g^{-1}, and V_{-1} is 2.946×10^{-3} min^{-1} g^{-1}. The mean weight of the rats is 246 g.

$$V_{app} = \frac{(25.072 \times 10^{-3}) + \left[(2.946 \times 10^{-3})\left(\dfrac{3.236 \times 10^{-4}}{1.259 \times 10^{-5}}\right)\right]}{1 + \left(\dfrac{3.236 \times 10^{-4}}{1.259 \times 10^{-5}}\right)}$$

$V_{app} = 3.77 \times 10^{-3}$ min^{-1} g^{-1}

$K_{app} = (3.77 \times 10^{-3}$ min^{-1} g$^{-1})(246$ g$)^{0.75} = 0.234$ min^{-1}

Figure 19–16 shows the values of V_{app} against pH for several antibiotics. At pH values much higher than the drug's pK_a, these three antibiotics are fully ionized, and absorption takes place through aqueous channels on the membrane. Below pH 6.0 the absorption rate constant is increased significantly, the absorption rate of the nonionized fraction V_o depending for the most part on lipid solubility of the drug. The curves of Figure 19–16 show inflection points where the pH is equal to the pK_a of each drug. It should be noted from Figure 19–16 that the rate of absorption becomes constant for each of these three drugs at higher pH values.

The bioavailability of drugs administered by the oral route is greatly influenced by the physicochemical

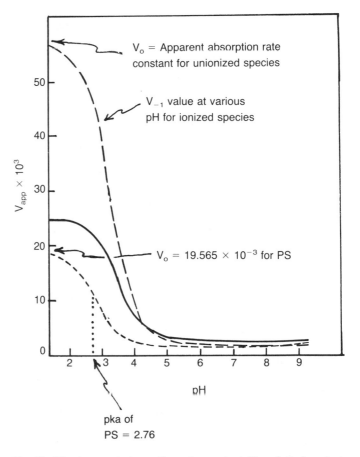

Fig. 19–16. Apparent absorption rate constant V_{app} plotted against pH using experimental data fitted to equation (19–39). Key: — —NPADC; ——7FADCK; – – –PS. The antibiotic, abbreviated PS, is benzylpenicillin sodium, pK_a 2.76. (From J. G. Prieto et al., J. Pharm. Sci. **76**, 596, 1987, reproduced with permission of the copyright owner.)

properties of the drug and the dosage form. One method to increase the oral bioavailability is to use prodrugs (p. 513). By this approach the functional group of the drug that could easily be metabolized during its passage through the liver is protected in the prodrug. The blocking or protecting substituent is then cleaved by enzymes in the blood to restore the parent compound. Hussain et al.[97] prepared prodrugs of estradiol in which the 3-phenolic hydroxyl group is protected. Use of the prodrug derivatives β-estradiol-3 acetylsalicylate and β-estradiol-3 anthranilate increased by 17-fold and by fivefold, respectively, the oral bioavailability of estradiol in dogs. Another approach to improve bioavailability is the use of *permeability enhancers* (see p. 541). Permeability enhancement is particularly useful for macromolecules and peptides against which the intestinal mucosa is largely impermeable. EDTA, bile salts, and ionic and nonionic surfactants have been studied as enhancers.

Peters et al.[98] found that 5-methoxysalicylate increased the absorption of several peptides in a rat gut preparation. (For a description of the rat gut preparation, see page 344). 5-Methoxysalicylate also enhances the gastrointestinal absorption of insulin and antibiotics. The authors suggested, however, that this adjuvant effect may occur as a result of undesirable damage that allows the peptidases of the lumen to penetrate the epithelial barrier. Mucosal damage by this and other mechanisms may discourage the search for appropriate enhancers for orally administered drugs.

Most of the oral extended-drug delivery systems are solid dosage forms: tablets, capsules, and granules. However, some extended-release liquid formulations, particularly suspensions, have also been formulated. Diffusion, dissolution, or a combination of both is the principal mechanism to achieve controlled delivery by the oral route. Several techniques for prolonging drug release are possible, based on the behavior of the dosage form in the GI tract and the properties of the excipients. The three basic approaches are (1) chemical or physicochemical bonding, (2) film coating, and (3) embedding.[99] A fourth class involves the principle of osmotic pressure.

Bonded Drug Systems. Extended release can be obtained by the use of salts or complexes of drugs (see Chapter 11) which are only slightly soluble in the GI fluids. The release occurs by slow dissolution of the salt or dissociation of the complex. The kinetics of drug delivery is usually first order, but under certain conditions may be zero order.

Another kind of physicochemical bonding is achieved when ionizable drugs are bound to water-insoluble polymers containing groups capable of exchanging ions (called *ion exchange resins*). Cation exchange resins have acidic groups such as phenolic, carboxylic, or sulfonic, whereas anion exchange resins contain basic groups such as amino or quaternary ammonium groups.

A displacement reaction in the intestinal fluid involving a resin–drug complex ($R—SO_3^-·NH_3^+—R'$) and a single acid–base species is illustrated in the equation[99]:

$$(R—SO_3^-·NH_3^+—R') + (X^+Y^-) \rightleftarrows (R—SO_3^-\ X^+) + (NH_3^+—R'Y^-) \quad (19–40)$$

where $R—SO_3^-$ is a sulfonic acid exchange resin, $NH_3^+—R'$ is a cationic (basic drug), X^+ is a cation such as H^+ or Na^+, and Y^- is an anion such as Cl^- in the GI fluids. The drug molecule is exchanged for the free cation, H^+ or Na^+ in solution, and the drug diffuses out of the resin into the bulk solution. The resins are characterized by the type of functional groups, degree of cross-linking, binding capacity, and particle size. The release rate can be further controlled by coating the drug–resin complex using microencapsulation techniques (p. 516). The dosage forms that serve as carriers for drug–resin complexes are tablets, capsules, suspensions, and microparticles. Hussain et al.[100] encapsulated phenylpropanolamine bound to a cross-linked sulfonated polystyrene ion-exchange resin in hollow fibers of polyurethane. Ion exchange resins have been used to deliver antitussives, antihistamines, central nervous system stimulants, antiarrhythmics, and other drugs.

Film-coated Dosage Forms. In the second procedure, a film surrounds the drug particles to allow delayed release. The mechanism and kinetics of drug delivery depend on the nature of the film. For insoluble membranes made of ethyl cellulose the principal mechanisms are diffusion and partitioning of the drug into the membrane. The release rate is controlled by the membrane and can be regulated by its porosity and thickness. The kinetics of delivery is usually zero order. Granules, pellets, microcapsules, and film-coated tablets are examples of coated dosage forms.

Soluble membranes such as cellulose acetate phthalate polymers of methacrylic acid are often used as enteric coating. The polymers are weak acids containing carboxyl groups and require pH values much higher than the acid values of the stomach for rapid dissolution. Ionizable drugs are frequently coated with acidic polymers. Thus, the dissolution of both the drug and the polymer becomes pH-dependent. Ozturk et al.[101] proposed a model to describe the dissolution kinetics of ionizable drugs. The method assumes that dissolution and ionization are limited to the stagnant film adjacent to the solid phase (drug surface), and that the overall process is diffusion limited. The dissolution rate, v, of a drug may be expressed (pp. 330–331) as:

$$v = S \cdot J = s \left[\frac{D}{h} (C_{T,s} - C_{T,b}) \right] \quad (19–41)$$

where J is the flux, S is the surface area, and $C_{T,s} - C_{T,b}$ are, respectively, the total solubility at the surface and the concentration of drug in the bulk. D is the diffusion coefficient and h is the thickness of the diffusion layer. If the drug ionizes, the total solubility at the surface, $C_{T,s}$, is

$$C_{T,s} = [AH]_o \left(1 + \frac{K_a}{[H^+]_s}\right) \quad \text{for acidic drugs} \quad (19\text{--}42)$$

$$C_{T,s} = [B]_o \left(1 + \frac{[H^+]_s}{K_a}\right) \quad \text{for basic drugs} \quad (19\text{--}43)$$

where $C_{T,s}$ is the solubility at the solid–liquid surface at a particular pH value and $[H^+]_s$ is the concentration of hydrogen ions at the surface. $[AH]_o$ and $[B]_o$ are the intrinsic solubilities (i.e., solubilities independent of pH) of acidic and basic drugs, respectively. Equations (19–42) and (19–43) use the pH at the surface, which differs from the pH of the bulk phase. For a weakly acidic drug in unbuffered solution, the ionization reactions at the stagnant adjacent film are

$$HA \rightleftharpoons A^- + H^+ \quad (19\text{--}44)$$

$$H_2O \rightleftharpoons OH^- + H^+ \quad (19\text{--}45)$$

$$HA + OH^- \rightleftharpoons A^- + H_2O \quad (19\text{--}46)$$

According to the authors,[101] the concentration of HA at the solid–fluid interface is the *intrinsic solubility*, $[HA]_o$. The drug diffuses from the solid–fluid interface and is simultaneously ionized to give the conjugate base A^- and hydrogen ions (equation (19–44)). The bulk liquid at the outer surface of the stagnant layer is assumed to be well mixed, and the ionic species are assumed to be completely dissolved. The solution of the mass transfer equations gives an analytic form to calculate the surface pH and subsequently the surface concentrations driving the drug dissolution. For an acidic drug,

$$[H^+]_s = \frac{-b + \sqrt{b^2 + 4c}}{2} \quad (19\text{--}47)$$

For a basic drug,

$$[H^+]_s = \frac{-b + \sqrt{b^2 + 4ac}}{2a} \quad (19\text{--}48)$$

The expressions to compute the coefficients a, b, and c are given in Table 19–1.

Example 19–14. Compute the in vitro pH of a compact of benzoic acid at the solid–liquid interface and at pH 12 in unbuffered medium.[101] The ionization constant K_a of benzoic acid is 9.33×10^{-5} M (pK_a = 4.03); the intrinsic solubility $[HA]_o$ is 0.0216 M; and the diffusivities of the species are $D_{HA} = D_{A^-} = 9.6 \times 10^{-6}$ cm^2 sec^{-1} and $D_{H^+} = D_{OH^-} = 2.7 \times 10^{-5}$ cm^2 sec^{-1}. Assume sink conditions in the bulk, that is, $[HA]_b = [A^-]_b = 0$. The surface area, S, is 0.79 cm^2; h = 0.01.

(a) If the hydrogen ion concentration in the bulk is $[H^+]_b = 10^{-12}$ mole/liter, the $[OH^-]_b$ concentration is

$$[OH^-]_b = \frac{K_w}{[H^+]_b} = \frac{1 \times 10^{-14}}{1 \times 10^{-12}} = 1 \times 10^{-2} \text{ mole/liter}$$

The coefficients γ in Table 19–1 are

$$\gamma_1 = \frac{D_{OH^-}}{D_{H^+}} = 1.0$$

$$\gamma_2 = \frac{D_{A^-}}{D_{H^+}} = \frac{9.6 \times 10^{-6}}{2.7 \times 10^{-5}} = 0.36$$

The constants b and c for acidic drugs, from Table 19–1, are

$$b = -(1 \times 10^{-12}) + (1)(1 \times 10^{-2}) + (0.36 \times 0) = 0.01 \text{ mole/liter}$$

$$c = (1)(1 \times 10^{-14}) + (0.36 \times 9.33 \times 10^{-5} \times 0.0216)$$

$$= 7.26 \times 10^{-7} \text{ (mole/liter)}^2$$

Therefore, from equation (19–48),

$$[H^+]_s = \frac{-0.01 + \sqrt{(-0.01)^2 + (4 \times 7.26 \times 10^{-7})}}{2}$$

$$= 7.20 \times 10^{-5} \text{ mole/liter}$$

The pH at the surface of the membrane is

$$(pH)_s = -\log(7.20 \times 10^{-5}) = 4.14$$

(b) Compute the dissolution rate, v, and the solubility of the drug at the surface. It is observed that the pH, 4.14, at the surface of the solid drug is much lower than the pH within the bulk solution (pH = 12). The pH at the surface controls the dissolution rate, and the drug solubilities at pH 4.14 are used in equation (19–41) to compute v.

From equation (19–42),

$$C_{T,s} = 0.0216 \left(1 + \frac{9.33 \times 10^{-5}}{7.20 \times 10^{-5}}\right) = 0.0496$$

$$C_{T,b} = 0 = \text{sink conditions}$$

From equation (19–41) for sink conditions $C_b = 0$ and

$$v = (0.79 \text{ cm}^2)\left(\frac{9.6 \times 10^{-6} \text{ cm}^2/\text{sec}}{0.01 \text{ cm}}\right)(4.96 \times 10^{-2}) \text{ mole/cm}^3$$

$$= 3.76 \times 10^{-5} \text{ mole/sec}$$

Embedded Dosage Forms. In the third procedure, the drug may be mixed with a carrier that acts as a release-rate controlling agent. Hydrophilic carriers

TABLE 19–1. *Equations for Surface pH Calculation and Related Constants (Unbuffered Medium)**

	Acidic Drug	Basic Drug
$[H^+]_s$	$(-b + \sqrt{b^2 + 4c})/2$	$(-b + \sqrt{b^2 + 4ac})/2a$
a		$K_a + \gamma_2[B]_0$
b	$-[H^+]_b + \gamma_1[OH^-]_b + \gamma_2[A^-]_b$	$(-[H^+]_b + \gamma_1[OH^-]_b - \gamma_2[BH^+]_b)K_a$
c	$\gamma_1 K_w + \gamma_2 K_a[HA]_0$	$\gamma_1 K_w K_a$
γ_1	D_{OH^-}/D_{H^+}	D_{OH^-}/D_{H^+}
γ_2	D_{A^-}/D_{H^+}	D_{BH^+}/D_{H^+}

*From S. S. Ozturk, B. O. Palsson and J. B. Dressman, Pharm. Res. **5**, 272, 1988, reproduced with permission of the copyright owner.

include methylcellulose, sodium alginate, and other gel-forming materials. The drug diffuses from the viscous gel, and the release rate can be controlled by the degree of polymerization of the carrier and the ratio of drug to carrier. Wilson and Cuff[102] found that the optimum hydrogel concentration for sustained release of isomazole, an orally active cardiotonic, was 40 to 42%. Hydrophobic and digestible carriers include glycerides, waxes, fatty alcohols, and fatty acids. They constitute eroding tablets in which the release is achieved when the surface layer is continuously eroded by the GI fluids. Matrix tablets consist of insoluble and nondigestible materials, such as polyethylene, some waxes, and polyvinylchloride. The diffusion of a drug through this kind of matrix has been discussed in Chapter 13, pages 335 to 337. The kinetics of release is a function of the square root of time, and the release rate can be controlled by the tablet porosity, addition of soluble solids, and the ratio of drug to carrier.

Jambhekar and Cobby[103] prepared slow-release tablets using a polyvinylchloride–polyoxyethylene (PVC–PE) matrix and sodium salicylate as a model drug. The in vitro release of drug from a cylindrical PVC–PE matrix when all surfaces of the tablet are exposed to the dissolution fluid is described in the following equation:

$$f_t = (q + 2)K_r(t^{1/2} - t_o^{1/2}) - (2q + 1)[K_r(t^{1/2} - t_o^{1/2})]^2 + q[K_r(t^{1/2} - t_o^{1/2})]^3 \quad (19\text{–}49)$$

where f_t is the fraction of drug released at time t, q is the ratio of tablet diameter to thickness, K_r is the rate constant, and t_o is the lag time. The rate constant, as well as the lag time, can be computed by fitting the fraction of drug released f_t to the cubic expression, equation (19–49), using a NONLIN program. Once k_r and t_o are known, the values of f_t at any time can be estimated.

Example 19–15. Compute the fraction released at 25° C of salicylate from insoluble matrices at 4:1 and 9:1 matrix-drug ratios and at $t =$ 9 hours. The dissolution rate constants are $K_r = 0.116$ *hr.*$^{-1/2}$ and 0.101 *hr.*$^{-1/2}$; the lag times are $t_o^{1/2} = 0.341$ *hr.*$^{1/2}$ and = 0.276 hr.$^{1/2}$. The ratio of tablet diameter to thickness in both cases is $q = 2.84$. For a matrix:drug ratio of 4:1, the fractional drug release is

$$f_t = (2.84 + 2)0.116(9.0^{1/2} - 0.341)$$
$$- (2 \times 2.84 + 1)[0.116(9^{1/2} - 0.341)]^2$$
$$+ 2.84[0.116(9^{1/2} - 0.341)]^3 = 0.941$$

For the matrix:drug ratio of 9:1,

$$f_t = (2.84 + 2)0.101(9.0^{1/2} - 0.276)$$
$$- (2 \times 2.84 + 1)[0.101(9^{1/2} - 0.276)]^2$$
$$+ 2.84[0.101(9^{1/2} - 0.276)]^3 = 0.885$$

Note that the fraction released depends on the matrix:drug ratio. The larger the ratio, the smaller the fraction released. Jambhekar and Cobby[103] showed that the release constant from this type of matrix was independent of the pH of the dissolution fluid and the flow rate of the fluid past the tablet, so that the in vivo behavior may be less subject to variations in the GI tract.

Osmotic Pump. The *elementary osmotic pump*, also known as Oros or Gastrointestinal Therapeutic System, was first described by Theeuwes and Yum and was introduced by Alza Corporation.[104] The dosage form has a semipermeable membrane on one surface to bring water by osmosis into the drug reservoir in the tablet. The device is shown in Figure 19–17(a). The hydrostatic pressure generated by the influx of water forces the release of a saturated solution of the drug through an opening in the tablet, as seen in Figure 19–17(b). The rate of drug release is constant (zero-order) until the excess undissolved drug is depleted. The release rate then decreases parabolically to zero (Fig. 19–18). Earlier sustained-release forms were markedly affected by physiologic pH changes. With the Oros system, the rates of release of phenobarbital, placed in both artificial gastric fluid at pH 2 and intestinal fluid at pH 7.5, were found to be independent of pH. The release rate of the device may be altered by changing the nature of the semipermeable membrane.

Sample Calculations. Theeuwes[105] first tested the elementary osmotic pump for drug delivery using potassium chloride to serve as both the osmotic agent and the drug model. In a later report, Theeuwes et al.[106] designed a therapeutic system, based on the principle of the osmotic pump, to deliver indomethacin

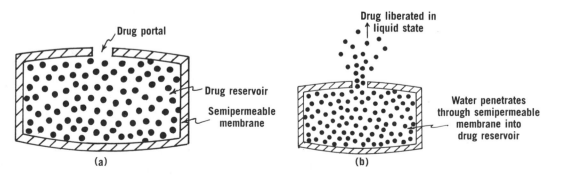

Fig. 19–17. The elementary osmotic pump, Oros (Alza), used as a gastrointestinal therapeutic system. The figure shows the liberation of the drug through the small orifice owing to osmosis of fluids through the semipermeable membrane and into the drug reservoir. (After K. Heilmann, *Therapeutic Systems*, Georg Thieme, Stuttgart, 1978, p. 49.; reproduced with permission of the copyright owner.)

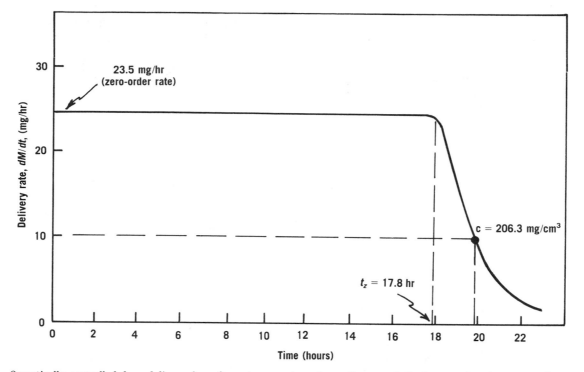

Fig. 19–18. Osmotically controlled drug delivery from Oros at zero-order release, then parabolic decrease in release rate. See the section on *Sample Calculations.*

at a constant zero-order rate. For zero-order delivery rate, these workers used the equation

$$\left(\frac{dM}{dt}\right)_z = \frac{S}{h} k' \pi_s C_s \qquad (19\text{–}50)$$

in which $(dM/dt)_z$ is the rate of delivery of the solute under zero-order conditions, S is the semipermeable membrane area (2.2 cm²); h is the membrane thickness (0.025 cm); k' is a permeability coefficient, 2.8×10^{-6} cm²/(atm hr), and π_s is the osmotic pressure, 245 atm, of the formulation under zero-order conditions (saturated solution) ($k'\pi_s = 0.686 \times 10^{-3}$ cm²/hr). The concentration of the saturated solution, C_s, at 37° C is 330 mg/cm³. The zero-order delivery rate for this system is calculated as follows.

$$\left(\frac{dM}{dt}\right)_z = \left(\frac{2.2 \text{ cm}^2}{0.025 \text{ cm}}\right)(0.686 \times 10^{-3} \text{ cm}^2/\text{hr})(330 \text{ mg/cm}^3)$$

$$\left(\frac{dM}{dt}\right)_z = 19.9 \text{ mg/hr}$$

Some of the drug is released from the device by simple diffusion through the membrane. Equation (19–50) therefore should be modified as follows:

$$\left(\frac{dM}{dt}\right)_z = \frac{S}{h} k' \pi_s C_s + \frac{S}{h} P C_s$$

or

$$\left(\frac{dM}{dt}\right)_z = \frac{S}{h} (k' \pi_s + P) C_s \qquad (19\text{–}51)$$

in which P is the permeability coefficient for passage of KCl across the semipermeable membrane (0.122×10^{-3} cm²/hr). (See the footnote on page 327 for P given as cm²/sec.)

$$\left(\frac{dM}{dt}\right)_z = \left(\frac{2.2 \text{ cm}^2}{0.025 \text{ cm}}\right)(330 \text{ mg/cm}^3)(0.686 \times 10^{-3} \text{ cm}^2/\text{hr} + 0.122 \times 10^{-3} \text{ cm}^2/\text{hr})$$

$$\left(\frac{dM}{dt}\right)_z = 23.5 \text{ mg/hr}$$

The time t_z in which the mass of the drug M_z is delivered (disregarding the start-up time required to reach equilibrium) is

$$t_z = M_t \left(1 - \frac{C_s}{\rho}\right) \frac{1}{(dM/dt)_z} \qquad (19\text{–}52)$$

in which M_t is the total mass of drug in the core (500 mg KCl) and ρ is the density of the drug (2 g/cm³ or 2000 mg/cm³):

$$t_z = (500 \text{ mg})\left(1 - \frac{330 \text{ mg/cm}^3}{2000 \text{ mg/cm}^3}\right) \frac{1}{23.5 \text{ mg/hr}}$$

$$t_z = 17.8 \text{ hr}$$

The zero-order delivery rate, $(dM/dt)_z = 23.5$ mg/hr, and the time, t_z, during which the drug is being delivered are shown in Figure 19–18.

Beyond t_z, the drug is delivered under non-zero conditions. For a drug that is released by both osmotic pumping action and passive diffusion through the membrane, the rate beyond t_z is given by

$$\frac{dM}{dt} = \frac{F_s}{S} C^2 + \left(\frac{S}{h} P\right) C \qquad (19\text{--}53)$$

in which F_s is a volume flux (cm^3/hr) used to represent the quantity $(S/h)k'\pi_s = (2.2 \text{ cm}^2/0.025 \text{ cm})(0.686 \times 10^{-3} \text{ cm}^2/\text{hr})$, or 0.0604 cm^3/hr. C is the concentration of drug in the dispensing fluid (mg/cm^3). At t values beyond t_z, the saturation concentration, C_s, has fallen to a subsaturation concentration. Let us calculate C when dM/dt in Figure 19–18 has fallen to 10 mg/hr on the parabolic descending curve. Equation (19–53) is written in the quadratic form:

$$\frac{F_s}{C_s} C^2 + \left(\frac{S}{h} P\right) C - \left(\frac{dM}{dt}\right) = 0 \qquad (19\text{--}54)$$

$$C = \frac{-b \pm \sqrt{b^2 - 4ac}}{2a} \qquad (19\text{--}55)$$

in which $a = F_s/C_s = 1.829 \times 10^{-4} \text{ cm}^6/(\text{mg hr})$; $b = SP/h = 0.0107 \text{ cm}^3/\text{hr}$; and $c = -dM/dt = -10 \text{ mg/hr}$ as shown at point C in the figure. (Only the positive root of the quadratic equation is applicable.)

$$C = \frac{-0.0107 + \sqrt{(0.0107)^2 - 4(1.829 \times 10^{-4})(-10)}}{2(1.829 \times 10^{-4})}$$

$$C = 206.4 \text{ mg/cm}^3$$

To plot the calculated line of Figure 19–18 to the right of t_z, one needs the values of t for each value of dM/dt. For $dM/dt = 10$ mg/hr used previously in this example, we obtain t using the expression[105]

$$t - t_z = \left(\frac{Vh}{SP}\right) \ln \frac{\left(\frac{F_s C}{C_s}\right) + \frac{SP}{h}}{\left(F_s + \frac{SP}{h}\right) \frac{C}{C_s}} \qquad (19\text{--}56)$$

in which V is the volume of the drug and is obtained from mass and density as

$$V = \frac{500 \text{ mg}}{2000 \text{ mg/cm}^3} = 0.250 \text{ cm}^3$$

$$t - t_z = \left(\frac{(0.250 \text{ cm}^3)(0.025 \text{ cm})}{(2.2 \text{ cm}^2)(0.122 \times 10^{-3} \text{ cm}^2/\text{hr})}\right) \times$$

$$\ln \frac{(0.0377 \text{ cm}^3/\text{hr}) + (0.0107 \text{ cm}^3/\text{hr})}{(0.0604 \text{ cm}^3/\text{hr} + 0.0107 \text{ cm}^3/\text{hr})\left(\frac{206.3 \text{ mg/cm}^3}{330 \text{ mg/cm}^3}\right)}$$

$$t - t_z = (23.286 \text{ hr}) (\ln 1.0889) = 1.98 \text{ hr}$$

$$t = 1.98 \text{ hr} + t_z = 19.8 \text{ hr}$$

This point ($dM/dt = 10$ mg/hr, $t = 19.8$ hr) is shown as a black circle on the downward-sloping curve of Figure 19–18. By calculating a sufficient number of such points, the parabolic portion of the curve is plotted.

Another interesting quantity is the maximum size of the orifice or portal (Fig. 19–17) for delivery of the drug from the osmotic pumping system. The maximum cross-sectional area is given by

$$S_{\max} = \frac{L}{f} \left(\frac{dM}{dt}\right)_z \frac{1}{DC_s} \qquad (19\text{--}57)$$

in which D is the diffusivity (see Chapter 13) of the drug delivered through the orifice ($D = 2 \times 10^{-5} \text{ cm}^2/\text{sec}$ or 0.072 cm^2/hr), L the path length of this opening (25×10^{-4} cm), and f a dimensionless sizing factor, taken to have a value of 50. The sizing factor specifies how many times greater is the zero-order pumping rate than the free diffusion rate.

We use equation (19–57) to estimate the port size for drug delivery and to convert D to cm^2/hr:

$$S_{\max} = \frac{25 \times 10^{-4} \text{ cm}}{50} (23.5 \text{ mg/hr}) \cdot \frac{1}{(0.072 \text{ cm}^2/\text{hr})(330 \text{ mg/cm}^3)}$$

$$S_{\max} = 4.945 \times 10^{-5} \text{ cm}^2 \text{ or } 4945 \text{ } \mu\text{m}^2 \text{ area}$$

(*Note:* 1 cm $= 10^4$ μm; therefore, 1 cm$^2 = 10^4 \times 10^4 = 10^8$ μm^2.) The area is equal to πr^2, and the radius of the orifice is obtained as follows:

$$4945 \text{ } \mu\text{m}^2 = 3.14159 \text{ } r^2$$

$$r = 39.675 \text{ } \mu\text{m}$$

$$\text{orifice diameter} = 79 \text{ } \mu\text{m}$$

Advancements in drug design centered on the osmotic pump principle continues to be reported in the pharmaceutical literature; examples are the work of Amidon et al.[107] and Haslam et al.[108] dealing with a lipid osmotic pump and Lindstedt et al.[109] on osmotic pumping and membrane-coated dosage forms. To release a drug from its dosage form at a constant rate, soluble tablet cores have been coated with microporous membranes to control the diffusion. Bodmeier and Paeratakul[110] used a latex consisting of poly(ethacrylate-methylmethacrylate) and containing a *pore-forming agent* insoluble in the latex but which leaches out of the membrane to form minute holes in the tablet surface when it comes in contact with the gastrointestinal fluids. (A *latex* is an aqueous dispersion of a polymer produced by emulsion polymerization.) Dicalcium phosphate, CaHPO$_4$, is insoluble in the latex but soluble in the acidic gastric fluid, and was found to yield the desired microporous tablet coating. Release of the test drug, theophylline, was linear with time and the rate could be adjusted by varying the concentration of the pore-forming agent, CaHPO$_4$, and the thickness of the latex coating.

Rectal Administration. Rectal delivery is an alternative to the oral route to avoid the gastric irritation caused by some drugs and to minimize hepatic first-pass metabolism. The mechanism of absorption is similar to that of the gastrointestinal tract—mainly by passive diffusion.[111] However, the absorption is less extensive and slower because the surface area of the rectal mucosa available for absorption is limited, being about 1/10,000 the surface area of the small intestine.

The bioavailability of a drug depends on the site of absorption in the rectal mucosa. The upper rectal (hemorrhoidal) veins drain into the portal system and the lower veins drain into the inferior vena cava.[111] Generally, drugs administered rectally are considered to be absorbed mainly in the lower hemorrhoidal veins, thus avoiding the first pass through the liver. de Boer et al.[112] showed that rectal absorption of lidocaine is greater than oral absorption, supporting the hypothesis that the rectal route can result in a bypass of the liver. This route can be useful for drugs that, like lidocaine, undergo first-pass metabolism where they are substantially decomposed by liver and/or gut wall metabolism. The bioavailability of poorly absorbable drugs can be increased by the use of enhancers in the rectal formulations. As in the case of the nasal route, rectal administration may be an alternative to the parenteral route for peptides and proteins. A number of workers have investigated enhancers and dosage formulations to promote the absorption of these macromolecules. Liversidge et al.[113] found that sodium salicylate enhances the absorption of insulin suppositories. Nishihata et al.[114] studied the promoting effect of glyceryl esters of acetoacetic acid on the rectal absorption of insulin. A decrease in the glucose level was observed in rabbits after the administration of suppositories containing the adjuvant. The addition of calcium gluconate or magnesium chloride to the suppositories markedly diminished the efficacy of the enhancer. This suggested that the promoting effect is related to the interaction of the enhancers with calcium and magnesium ions located in the rectal membrane. Calcium ions are important to preserve a tight intercellular structure. The interaction of the enhancer with calcium may cause temporary change in the integrity of the rectal barrier, increasing the permeability of the drug. This mechanism was also suggested by Morimoto et al.[115] for the rectal absorption of calcitonin, a hypocalcemic peptide hormone, from a polyacrylic acid aqueous gel. The absorption was larger at lower pH values of the gel base and was concentration-dependent in the range of 0.01 to 0.1% *w/v* polyacrylic acid. This acid has chelating properties toward calcium and was found not to damage the surface of the rectal mucosa. Permeability enhancers for the rectal absorption of ampicillin, such as bile salts, fatty acids, saponines, *N*-acyl derivatives of collagen peptide, and *N*-acyl derivatives of amino acids, also have the capacity to sequester calcium ions.[116]

Using an in situ perfusion of rat rectum, Nishihata et al.[117] found that salicylate and 5-methoxysalicylate enhanced the disappearance of phenylalanine and phenylalanylglycine from the perfusate. Nishihata et al.[118] reported that the rectal absorption of theophylline was increased in the presence of salicylate. These authors compared the enhancer effects of a surfactant, sodium lauryl sulfate, and salicylate in perfused rat rectum. The effect of salicylate was eliminated by washing out the rectum, whereas the effect of the surfactant was not eliminated. This suggested that the action of salicylate does not produce a permanent change in the membrane, whereas the surfactant seems to damage the barrier.[119] Sodium salicylate also enhances the rectal absorption of the antibiotics gentamicin sulfate[120] and ampicillin.[121] Other enhancers for rectal administration of cephalosporins include medium-chain monoglycerides and fatty acids.[122] Fatty acids may increase the transcellular permeability by perturbing membrane lipids. The intercellular enhancing effect may be due to the affinity of the fatty acids for calcium, which results in widening of closely connected conjunctions.

Fix et al.[123] investigated the use of short-chain alkyl esters of levodopa (L-dopa) as prodrugs for rectal administration. L-dopa is the drug of choice in Parkinson's disease, and significant bioavailability was obtained by these workers in dogs and rats using short-chain alkyl ester prodrugs such as L-dopa methyl ester, L-dopa isopropyl ester, and L-dopa 4-hydroxybutyl ester. When the prodrug enters the systemic circulation, the ester group is removed by enzymatic hydrolysis to yield the parent compound, L-dopa. Most of the esters enhanced rectal absorption considerably. The 4-hydroxybutyl ester produced a slower absorption rate, which the workers considered a possible advantage in the design of a sustained release L-dopa product, free of elevated plasma concentration and untoward side effects.

Buur and Bundgaard[124] prepared lipophilic derivatives of 5-fluorouracil, an antitumor agent, to avoid the first-pass metabolism in the GI tract and liver and to facilitate membrane permeability of the drug in its passage to the target site in the body. The prodrugs, 1-methoxy and 1-butoxy 5-fluorouracil, showed rapid and extensive absorption, and their conversion in plasma to the active parent 5-fluorouracil was rapid and complete. Tomita et al.[125] found that the colonic absorption of cefmetazole was greatly increased by 1% sodium caprate, sodium laurate, and mixed micelles composed of sodium oleate and sodium taurocholate. The increased absorption of cefmetazole across the intercellular route was considered to be a result of the increase in the pore size of the membrane produced by the enhancers. The colonic pore radius r may be computed from the following expression:

$$r = -a_w + (2a_w^2 + \lambda)^{\frac{1}{2}} \qquad (19\text{–}58)$$

where a_w, the radius of the water molecule, is 1.5 Å and λ (cm^2) is defined by the following equation:

$$\lambda = \left[\frac{8\eta_w D_w}{(RT/V_w)}\right]\left[\left(\frac{P_f}{P_d}\right) - 1\right] \qquad (19\text{–}59)$$

D_w is the diffusion coefficient of water, η_w is the water viscosity, R is the gas constant, V_w is the molar volume of water, and T is the absolute temperature. The term P_f/P_d represents the ratio of the osmotic water permeability coefficient, P_f, to the permeability coefficient P_d of tritiated water through the colonic membrane. The osmotic water permeability is calculated from a plot of the osmotically induced water flux J_o through the colonic membrane against the osmotic difference, $\Delta\pi$, between the two sides of the membrane as seen in the expression:

$$J_o = \frac{V_n}{A} = - (P_f \cdot \Delta\pi) \qquad (19-60)$$

in which it is assumed that the area A of the colonic membrane is known. J_o (equation (19–60)) is the osmotically induced water flux (mole min^{-1} cm^{-2}), V_n is the volume rate in mole min^{-1}, A is the area of the membrane in cm^2, P_f is the osmotic water permeability coefficient (cm min^{-1}), and $\Delta\pi$ is the osmotic difference in mOsm/kg.

Example 19–16. Compute the percent increase in pore radius of the colonic membrane at 37° C after treatment with mixed micelles of sodium oleate and sodium taurocholate. The ratio P_f/P_d is 26.48 and the water viscosity is 6.915×10^{-3} dyne sec cm^{-2} (poise). The diffusion coefficient of water is 3.24×10^{-5} cm^2 sec^{-1} and the molar volume of water is 18.14 cm^3 $mole^{-1}$ at 37° C. The initial radius of the mucosal pores is 7.9 Å.

From equation (19–59),

$$\lambda = \left[\frac{8 \times 6.915 \times 10^{-3} \text{ dyne sec/cm}^2 \times 3.24 \times 10^{-5} \text{ cm}^2/\text{sec}}{(8.3143 \times 10^7 \text{ g cm}^2/\text{sec}^2 \text{ deg mole} \times (310°\text{K}/18.14 \text{ cm}^3/\text{mole})}\right]$$
$$\times (26.48 - 1)$$

$$\lambda = 3.21 \times 10^{-14} \text{ cm}^2$$

From equation (19–58), in which $a_w = 1.5 \times 10^{-8}$ cm,

$$r = -1.5 \times 10^{-8} \text{ cm} + [2(1.5 \times 10^{-8} \text{ cm})^2 + (3.21 \times 10^{-14} \text{ cm}^2)]^{1/2}$$
$$= 16.5 \times 10^{-8} \text{ cm} = 16.5 \text{ Å}$$

The percent increase in the radius is

$$\frac{16.5 - 7.9}{7.9} \times 100 = 109\%$$

owing to the action of the enhancer, composed of mixed micelles of sodium oleate and sodium taurocholate.

Transdermal Administration. The skin has been used for centuries as the administration site of drugs in local treatment, but only recently has it been used as a pathway for systemic effects. The barrier function of the skin prevents both water loss and the entrance of external agents; however, some drugs are able to penetrate the skin layers in sufficient concentration to produce systemic action. The transdermal route is of particular interest for drugs that have a short elimination half-life and undergo extensive first-pass metabolism, therefore requiring frequent dosing.

The most exterior layer of the skin, the epidermis, consists of three main layers, the stratum corneum, the granular layer, and the basal layer. The stratum corneum is considered the most important barrier to drug transport. It is a heterogeneous nonliving structure, formed by keratinized cells, protein-rich cells, and intercellular lipid layers. The lipid composition among the epidermal layers is very different. Polar phospholipids, which are usual components of the membrane of living cells, are absent in the stratum corneum. These lipids form bilayers and their acyl chains can exist as "gel" and as "liquid crystalline" states. The transition between these two states occurs at certain temperatures without loss of the bilayer structure.[126] The principal lipids of the stratum corneum are ceramide (50%) and fatty acids (25%). Although the stratum corneum does not contain phospholipids, the mixture of ceramides, cholesterol, and fatty acids is capable of forming bilayers. These lipid bilayers are considered to provide the barrier function of the stratum corneum.[126]

To study the percutaneous transport of drugs the skin can be considered as a bilaminate membrane consisting of the dead stratum corneum (lipophilic layer) and the viable tissue (aqueous layer) which comprises the granular and basal layers of the epidermis, and the dermis, Figure 19–19. Diffusion of polar drugs is much faster through the viable tissue than across the stratum corneum.[127] The permeability coefficient through the skin, P, can be expressed as[128]

$$P = \frac{D_v D_s}{K\ell_v D_s + \ell_s D_v} \qquad (19-61)$$

where K is the partition coefficient of the drug between the stratum corneum (s) and the viable tissue (v), and ℓ_v, ℓ_s, D_v, and D_s are the diffusion path lengths and diffusion coefficients, respectively. The subscripts s and v refer to the stratum corneum and the viable tissue, respectively. If the drug diffuses slowly through the stratum corneum, $K\ell_v D_s < \ell_s D_v$, and equation (19–61) becomes

$$P = \frac{D_s}{\ell_s} \qquad (19-62)$$

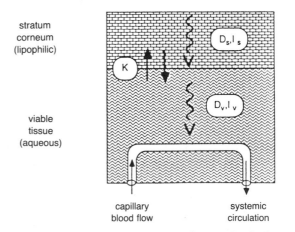

Fig. 19–19. The skin represented as two layers: the dead stratum corneum, s, and the viable or living tissue, v, (dermis and part of epidermis). The diffusion coefficients and the diffusion path lengths, ℓ_s and ℓ_v, together with the partition coefficient, K, control the transport of the penetrant through the two layers. (From R. H. Guy and J. Hadgraft, Pharm. Res. **5**, 753, 1988, reproduced with permission of the copyright owner.)

In this case the skin permeability is controlled by the stratum corneum alone. If the diffusion through the stratum corneum is fast, $K\ell_v D_s > \ell_s D_v$, and equation (19–61) becomes

$$P = \frac{D_v}{\ell_v K} \qquad (19\text{–}63)$$

In this case, the partition coefficient may be influential in the permeability. As K increases, the transport from the stratum corneum to viable epidermis becomes less favorable and slower. At large K values, partitioning of the drug is the rate-limiting step.[128]

Example 19–17. Compute the permeability of a drug across the skin assuming that D_s is 10^{-10} cm² sec⁻¹ and D_v is 10^{-7} cm² sec⁻¹. The path lengths are $\ell_s = 350$ μm and $\ell_v = 150$ μm. The large value for ℓ_s is due to the fact that the molecules follow a tortuous pathway through the intercellular spaces. The value for ℓ_v is the distance from the underside of the stratum corneum to the upper capillary region of the dermis. The partition coefficient is taken to be $K = 1$.

Since diffusion through the stratum corneum is very slow ($D_s = 10^{-10}$ cm² sec⁻¹), and the product $K\ell_v D_s = 1.0 \times 150 \times 10^{-4} \times 10^{-10} < \ell_s D_v = 350 \times 10^{-4} \times 10^{-7}$, therefore, $1.5 \times 10^{-4} \ll 3.5 \times 10^{-9}$ from equation (19–62),

$$P = \frac{10^{-10} \text{ cm}^2/\text{sec}}{350 \times 10^{-4} \text{ cm}} = 2.86 \times 10^{-9} \text{ cm/sec}$$

Using equation (19–61), we arrive at a similar order of magnitude:

$$P = \frac{(10^{-7} \text{ cm}^2/\text{sec})(10^{-10} \text{ cm}^2/\text{sec})}{(1.0 \times 150 \times 10^{-4} \times 10^{-10}) + (10^{-7} \times 350 \times 10^{-4})}$$
$$= 2.86 \times 10^{-9} \text{ cm/sec}$$

Tojo[129] proposed a random brick model for the transport of drugs across the stratum corneum. As shown in Figure 19–20, the stratum corneum is represented by the cells rich in proteins separated from one another by thin-layer intercellular lipids. The side length of the cells varies, but the total average surface area is constant. The thickness of the cells and the lipid layer are also assumed to be constant. According to this model, the transport of a drug is divided into three parallel pathways: (1) across the cellular–intercellular regions in series, (2) across the lipid intercellular spaces, and (3) across thin lipid layers sandwiched between flattened protein cells of the stratum corneum.

According to the brick model, the effective diffusion coefficient, $\overline{D}$, across the skin is

$$\overline{D} = 2\,\epsilon(1 - \epsilon)D_1 + \epsilon^2 D_2 + (1 - \epsilon)^2\, D_3 \qquad (19\text{–}64)$$

The first, second, and third right-hand terms represent the three possible routes (1), (2), and (3) (Fig. 19–20), D_1, D_2, and D_3 being the difusivities across routes (1), (2), and (3); ϵ and $(1 - \epsilon)$ are the average fraction of diffusion area of the lipid and protein on the skin surface, respectively. Substituting D_1, D_2, and D_3 by their corresponding expressions, equation (19–64) becomes

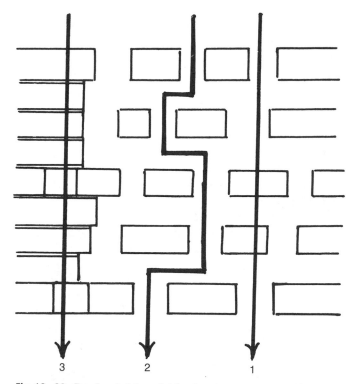

Fig. 19–20. Random brick model for the stratum corneum. Arrows 1, 2, and 3 show three possible routes of drug diffusion. (From K. Tojo, J. Pharm. Sci. **76**, 889, 1987, reproduced with permission of the copyright owner.)

$$\overline{D} = \frac{2\epsilon(1 - \epsilon)(2n + 4)}{\left(\dfrac{n}{D_p} + \dfrac{n + 4}{K D_\ell}\right)} + \epsilon^2 K D_\ell + \frac{(1 - \epsilon)^2(2n + 4)}{\left(\dfrac{2n}{D_p} + \dfrac{4}{KD_\ell}\right)}$$
$$(19\text{–}65)$$

The term n is related to the volume fraction of lipids in the skin and the average fraction of diffusion area of the lipids, ϵ; K is the lipid–protein partition coefficient and D_p and D_ℓ are the diffusion coefficients across the protein layer and the lipid layer, respectively.

The flux across the skin is given by the following expression:

$$J = \frac{dQ}{dt} = \frac{\overline{D}\, C_p}{h} \qquad (19\text{–}66)$$

where C_p is the concentration of drug in the protein cell layer, h the thickness of the skin, and $\overline{D}$ is defined by equation (19–65).

*Example 19–18.** Compute the flux at the steady state, dQ/dt, of a new drug from the following data: $D_\ell = 1 \times 10^{-10}$ cm²/sec, $D_p = 1 \times 10^{-7}$ cm²/sec, $C_p = 10$ mg/cm³, $\epsilon = 0.02$, $h = 0.0020$ cm, $K = 0.1$, and $n = 14.3$. Use the random brick model.

$$\overline{D} = \frac{(2)(0.02)(1 - 0.02)[(2 \times 14.3) + 4]}{\left[\left(\dfrac{14.3}{1 \times 10^{-7}}\right) + \dfrac{(14.3 + 4)}{(0.1)(10^{-10})}\right]} + (0.02)^2(0.1)(10^{-10}) +$$

*This example was kindly provided by K. Tojo, Kyushu Institute of Technology, Japan.

$$\frac{(1 - 0.02)^2[(2 \times 14.3) + 4]}{\left[\frac{(2 \times 14.3)}{1 \times 10^{-7}} + \frac{4}{(0.1)(1 \times 10^{-10})}\right]} = 7.89 \times 10^{-11} \text{ cm}^2\text{sec}$$

The flux is

$$J = \frac{(7.89 \times 10^{-11} \text{ cm}^2/\text{sec})(10 \text{ mg/cm}^3)}{0.0020 \text{ cm}} = 3.95 \times 10^{-7} \text{ mg/(cm}^2 \text{ sec)}$$
$$= 3.95 \times 10^{-4} \text{ μg/(cm}^2 \text{ sec)}.$$

Factors Affecting Permeability: Hydration. The permeability of a drug depends on the hydration of the stratum corneum; the higher the hydration the greater the permeability. The dermal tissue is fully hydrated, while the concentration of water in the stratum corneum is much lower, depending on ambient conditions. Hydration may promote the passage of drugs in the following way. Water associates through hydrogen bonding with the polar head groups of the lipid bilayers present in the intercellular spaces. The formation of a hydration shell loosens the lipid packing so that the bilayer region becomes more fluid.[130] This facilitates the migration of drugs across the stratum corneum. From the rate of transpiration (passage of water from inner layers to the stratum corneum) and diffusivity of water in the stratum corneum, the amount of water in the tissue can be obtained.[131]

Solubility of the Drug in the Stratum Corneum. Using the experimental results obtained from intact skin and stripped skin (layers of stratum corneum removed using Scotch tape), the solubility C of a drug in the stratum corneum was calculated from the following expression:[132]

$$C = \frac{1 - 3\tau + 2\eta\tau}{(1 + 2\eta)(1 - \eta)} \cdot \frac{6t_2}{h_2}\left(\frac{dQ}{dt}\right)_2 \quad (19\text{-}67)$$

where $(dQ/dt)_2$ is the steady-state permeation across the intact skin, τ is the ratio of the two time lags, (t_1/t_2), and η is the ratio $(dQ/dt)_2/(dQ/dt)_1$. The subscripts 1 and 2 refer to the stripped and intact skin, respectively; h_2 is the thickness of the stratum corneum.

Example 19–19. Compute the solubility of progesterone in the stratum corneum. The lag times across the intact and stripped skin are $t_2 = 5.49$ and $t_1 = 1.55$ hr, and the permeation rates across the intact and stripped skin are $(dQ/dt)_2 = 2.37$ μg/(cm² hr) and $(dQ/dt)_1 = 3.62$ μg/(cm² hr). The thickness of the stratum corneum is 10 μm (10×10^{-4} cm).

$$\tau = \frac{t_1}{t_2} = \frac{1.55}{5.49} = 0.28$$

$$\eta = \frac{(dQ/dt)_2}{(dQ/dt)_1} = \frac{2.37}{3.62} = 0.65$$

From equation (19–67),

$$C = \frac{1 - (3 \times 0.28) + (2 \times 0.65 \times 0.28)}{[1 + (2 \times 0.65)](1 - 0.65)} \cdot \frac{6 \times 5.49}{10 \times 10^{-4}} \cdot 2.37$$

$$C = 50816.8 \text{ μg/mL} = 50.8 \text{ mg/mL}$$

Excipients. Common solvents and surfactants can affect penetration of drugs though the skin. Sarpotdar and Zatz[133] studied the penetration of lidocaine through hairless mouse skin in vitro from vehicles containing various proportions of propylene glycol and polysorbate

20. Propylene glycol is a good solvent for lidocaine and reduces its partitioning into the stratum corneum, lowering the penetration rate. In this study, the effect of the surfactants depended on the concentration of propylene glycol in the vehicle. The decrease of flux for 40% *w/w* propylene glycol concentration may be explained by micellar solubilization of lidocaine. It is generally assumed that only the free form of the drug is able to penetrate the skin. Thus, the micellar solubilization of lidocaine reduces its thermodynamic activity in the vehicle and retards its penetration. At higher propylene glycol concentrations, 60% and 80%, an increase in flux was observed, possibly owing to an interaction of the surfactant with propylene glycol.

Influence of pH. According to the pH–partition hypothesis (p. 343) only the un-ionized form of the drug is able to cross the lipoidal membranes in significant amounts. However, in studies of isolated intestinal membranes, both the ionized and un-ionized forms of sulfonamides permeated the membrane. The diffusion of ionized drug through the skin may be nonnegligible, particularly at pH values at which a large number of ionized molecules are present.[134] Fleeker et al.[135] studied the influence of pH on the transport of clonidine, a basic drug, through hydrated shed snakeskin. The contribution to the total flux, J, in μg cm^{-2} hr^{-1} of the nonionized and ionized species for a basic drug can be written as

$$J = J_B + J_{BH^+} \quad (19\text{-}68)$$

where B and BH$^+$ represent the basic (nonionized) and protonated forms, respectively. The dissociation of the protonated form is represented as

$$[BH^+] \overset{K_a}{\rightleftharpoons} [B] + [H^+] \quad (19\text{-}69)$$

and

$$K_a = \frac{[B][H^+]}{[BH^+]} \quad (19\text{-}70)$$

Taking the logarithm of both sides of equation (19–70), and rearranging it, the concentration of the protonated form is

$$[BH^+] = \frac{10^{(pK_a - pH)}}{1 + 10^{(pK_a - pH)}}[T] \quad (19\text{-}71)$$

where [T] represents the total concentration of both the charged and uncharged species,

$$[T] = [B] + [BH^+] \quad (19\text{-}72)$$

The concentration of nonionized form, [B], can be computed from equation (19–72). The total flux (equation (19–68)) can also be written in terms of the permeability coefficients times the concentrations of each species:

$$J = P_B[B] + P_{BH^+}[BH^+] \quad (19\text{-}73)$$

From equations (19–71) and (19–73), provided $P_B \cong P_{BH^+}$,

(a) when pK_a = pH, [B] = [BH$^+$] and both species B and BH$^+$ will contribute to the total flux.

(b) When pH $\gg$ pK_a, [B] $\gg$ [BH$^+$] and the total flux, $J \cong P_B[B]$, and

(c) When pH $\ll$ pK_a, [B] $\ll$ [BH$^+$] and $J \cong P_{BH^+}[BH^+]$

Equation (19–73) allows one to compute the permeabilities of both species from the total experimental flux and the values of [B] and [BH$^+$] from equations (19–71) and (19–72).

Example 19–20. Compute the permeability coefficients P_B and P_{BH^+} corresponding to the nonionized and protonated forms of clonidine. The total fluxes at pH 4.6 and pH 7 are 0.208 and 0.563 $\mu g/(cm^2\ hr)$, respectively. The pK_a of the protonated form is 7.69. The total concentration* of the two species [T] = 4×10^3 μg./uv where μg/uv stands for microgram/unit volume.

At pH 4.6,

$$[BH^+] = \frac{10^{(7.69-4.6)}}{1 + 10^{(7.69-4.6)}}(4 \times 10^3) = 3.996 \times 10^3\ \mu g/uv$$

$$[B] = (4 \times 10^3) - (3.996 \times 10^3) = 4.0\ \mu g/uv$$

At pH 7,

$$[BH^+] = \frac{10^{(7.69-7)}}{1 + 10^{(7.69-7)}}(4 \times 10^3) = 3.322 \times 10^3\ \mu g/uv$$

$$[B] = (4 \times 10^3) - (3.322 \times 10^3) = 678\ \mu g/uv.$$

From equation (19–73) with the flux, J, expressed in $\mu g\ cm^{-2}\ hr^{-1}$ and the permeability coefficient, P, in units of cm hr^{-1}, at pH 4.6:

$$0.208\ \mu g\ cm^{-2}\ hr^{-1} = P_B\ (4\ \mu g\ cm^{-3}) + P_{BH^+}(3996\ \mu g\ cm^{-3})$$

At pH 7,

$$0.563\ \mu g\ cm^{-2}\ hr^{-1} = P_B\ (678\ \mu g\ cm^{-3}) + P_{BH^+}\ (3322\ \mu g\ cm^{-3})$$

P_B and P_{BH^+} are calculated by solving the two equations simultaneously:

$$P_B = (0.208 - 3996\ P_{BH^+})/4$$

$$0.563 = 678\left(\frac{0.208 - 3996\ P_{BH^+}}{4}\right) + 3322\ P_{BH^+}$$

$$P_{BH^+} = \frac{-34.693}{-674000} = 5.15 \times 10^{-5}\ cm\ hr^{-1}$$

$$P_B = (0.208 - (5.15 \times 10^{-5} \times 3996)/4 = 5.5 \times 10^{-4}\ cm\ hr^{-1}$$

It will be noted that the values found for P_{BH+} and P_B do not change with pH, whereas the fluxes, J, are markedly different at pH 4.6 and pH 7.0.

Equations (19–70) and (19–73) can be combined to give

$$\frac{J}{[B]} = \frac{P_{BH^+}}{K_a}[H^+] + P_B \qquad (19-74)$$

From equation (19–74), the permeability coefficients of the ionized [BH$^+$] and nonionized [B] forms can be computed from the slope and intercept of a plot of J/[B] against [H$^+$]. The corresponding equation for acids is

$$\frac{J}{[A^-]} = \frac{P_{HA}}{K_a}[H^+] + P_{A^-} \qquad (19-75)$$

From equation (19–75), the permeability coefficients of the nonionized [HA] and ionized [A$^-$] forms are computed from the slope and the intercept of a plot of J/[A$^-$] against [H$^+$] (see *Problem 19–24*). Swarbrick et al.[134] found that both the ionized and nonionized forms of four chromone-2 carboxylic acids permeated skin, although the permeability of the nonionized form was about 10^4 times greater.

Binding of Drug to the the Skin. The skin may act as a reservoir for some drugs that are able to bind to macromolecules. The drug fraction bound is not able to diffuse, and binding hinders the initial permeation rate of molecules, resulting in larger lag times. Banerjee and Ritschel[136] studied the binding of vasopressin and corticotropin to rat skin. Penetration of large molecules such as collagen, used in cosmetic formulations, is questionable, but partial hydrolysates of collagen are able to reach the deeper skin layers. The sorption process can be represented by the Langmuir equation (pp. 380–383):

$$\frac{c}{(x/m)} = \frac{1}{bY_m} + \frac{c}{Y_m} \qquad (19-76)$$

where c represents the equilibrium concentration of the drug, x is the amount of drug adsorbed per amount of adsorbent, m (the skin proteins in this case), b is the affinity constant, and Y_m is the maximum adsorption capacity, $(x/m)_{max}$. The sorption isotherm was obtained by Banerjee and Ritschel by equilibration of a measured weight of rat epidermis with a known concentration of radiolabeled vasopressin solution and was analyzed by scintillation counting (measured radioactivity). The small value for the adsorption constant in equation (19–76), $b = 6.44 \times 10^{-4}$ mL/μg, suggests low affinity of vasopressin for the binding sites in the skin.

Drug Metabolism in the Skin. The metabolism of drugs during transport through the skin affects bioavailability and can produce significant differences between in vivo and in vitro results. Oxidation, reduction, hydrolysis, and conjugation are kinetic processes that compete with the transport of drugs across the skin. Guzek et al.[137] and Potts et al.[138] found differences in the in vitro and the in vivo extent of enzymatic cleavage in the skin and in the distribution of the metabolites of a diester derivative of salicylic acid. The authors suggested that the in vitro measurements overestimated the metabolism because of the increased enzymatic activity and/or decreased removal of the drug in the absence of capillaries. The fact that the skin contains esterases and other enzymes is useful for the administration of prodrugs. The solubility and absorption can be improved and the prodrug can be cleaved by the enzymes to give the active parent compound in the skin.[139]

Enhancers for Percutaneous Absorption. The transport of molecules through the skin can be increased by the use of certain adjuvants known as *enhancers*. Ionic surfactants enhance transdermal absorption by disordering the lipid layer of the stratum corneum and by

---

*"Concentration," expressed in μg/uv was obtained by using four-tenths milliliter of an appropriate concentration of clonidine solution.

denaturation of the keratin. Enhancers may increase penetration by causing the stratum corneum to swell and/or leach out some of the structural components, thus reducing the diffusional resistance and increasing the permeability of the skin.[140]

Nishihata et al.[141] proposed a mechanism for the enhancing effect of reducing agents such as ascorbate and dithiothreitol. The poor permeability of the skin is due to the ordered layer of intercellular lipids and to the low water content. Proteins in keratinized tissue are rich in cysteine residues, and the strong disulfide bonds may be the reason for the insoluble nature of this protein. The reducing agents cause a decrease in the number of disulfide bridges, thus increasing the hydration of the proteins, which results in increased permeability.

Azone or laurocapram (1-dodecyl-azacycloheptan-2-one) is one of the most efficient enhancers of percuta-

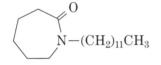

Azone (1-Dodecyl-azacycloheptan-2-one)

neous absorption. It greatly improves the penetration of hydrophilic and hydrophobic compounds, the latter to a smaller degree. Wiechers et al.[142] studied the absorption and elimination of azone in healthy volunteers. Azone is an oily liquid, insoluble in water but freely soluble in organic solvents. Most of the azone applied remains on the skin surface; the small fraction absorbed is located mainly in the stratum corneum. Azone does not form reservoirs in the skin and is rapidly cleared from the circulation by the kidneys. This fact, together with the nontoxicity of this compound in animals, indicates that azone is probably safe for human use. The compound has been found to be the most effective enhancer in the percutaneous absorption of dihydroergotamine, a drug widely used in the prevention and/or treatment of migraine.[140] Azone can be incorporated into a drug formulation, or the skin can be treated previously with the enhancer. The effect of azone increases in the presence of propylene glycol.[143] A possible mechanism of azone is its fluidization of the intercellular lipid lamellar region of the stratum corneum. As shown in Figure 19–21, azone, a very nonpolar molecule, enters the lipid bilayers and disrupts their structure. In contrast, a strongly dipolar solvent, dimethyl sulfoxide (DMSO), enters the aqueous region and interacts with the lipid polar heads to form a large solvation shell and to expand the hydrophilic region between the polar heads. As a result, both azone and DMSO increase the lipid fluidity, thus reducing the resistance of the lipid barrier to the diffusion of drugs. From differential scanning calorimetry experiments, the lipid transition temperature from an ordered structure to a fluid state is lowered.[130] Alcohol derivatives of *N,N*-disubstituted amino acids

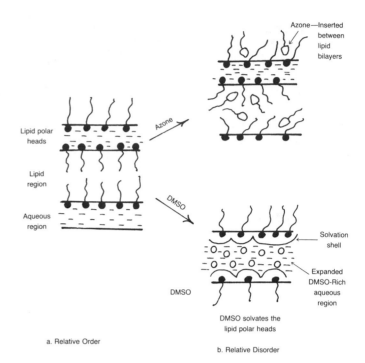

Fig. 19–21. Schematic diagram of the interaction of the enhancers, azone and DMSO, with the intercellular lipids of the stratum corneum. (*a*) Relatively ordered structure of the lipid bilayers. (*b*) Relative disorder of the lipid array due to the action of azone and DMSO. (Modified from B. W. Barry, *Int. J. Cosmet. Sci.* **10,** 281, 1988, reproduced with permission of the copyright owner.)

and hexamethylene lauramine also enhance the permeability of drugs.[144]

Membrane-Controlled Systems for the Percutaneous Absorption Route. A transdermal device is a laminated structure consisting of four layers, as shown in Figure 19–22. It consists of (1) an impermeable backing membrane, which is the mechanical support of the system; (2) an adjacent polymer layer, which serves as the drug reservoir; (3) a microporous membrane filled with a nonpolar material (e.g., paraffin); and (4) an adhesive film to make close contact with the skin and maintain the device in the desired position. Gienger et al.[145] used a computer program to calculate the drug transport through a laminated device and across the skin. In this model, all the layers except the backing membrane allow drug diffusion and transport. The authors give a description of the drug transport together with the concentration profiles of drug within each layer, as computed by the program.

Guy and Hadgraft[146] proposed a model for the transport of clonidine across the skin (Fig. 19–23) from a membrane-controlled adhesive system. The constant k_0 represents the zero-order rate constant for the membrane-controlled leaching of the drug, and k_R represents the partition between the patch and the skin surface. The system should be designed so that the partitioning favors the skin, and k_R remains negligibly small. The first-order constants k_1 and k_2 in Figure 19–23 are for drug transport across the stratum corneum and the living part of the epidermis. These constants are directly proportional to the diffusion

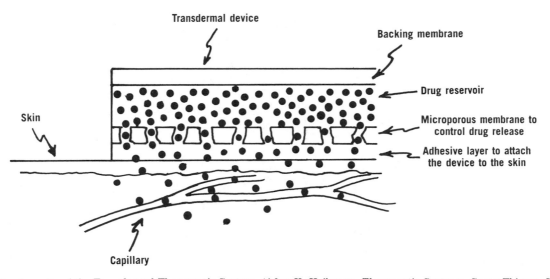

Fig. 19–22. A schematic of the Transdermal Therapeutic System. (After K. Heilmann, *Therapeutic Systems*, Georg Thieme, Stuttgart, 1978, p. 53.)

coefficients for passage through the layers of the skin, and therefore inversely proportional to the penetrant molecular weight as observed from the Stokes–Einstein equation (p. 401):

$$D = \frac{RT}{6\pi\eta N} \sqrt[3]{\frac{4\pi N}{3M\bar{v}}} \tag{19–77}$$

The rate constant k_3 of Figure 19–23 is included to express any tendency for reverse drug transport from epidermis to the stratum corneum and, in conjunction with k_2, may be considered as a partition coefficient. The authors computed the values of k_1 and k_2 for benzoic acid and used them to compute these rate constants for other drug molecules using the appropriate molecular weights. The expressions are

$$k_1 = k_1^{BA}\left(\frac{M^{BA}}{M}\right)^{\frac{1}{3}} \tag{19–78}$$

$$k_2 = k_2^{BA}\left(\frac{M^{BA}}{M}\right)^{\frac{1}{3}} \tag{19–79}$$

where k_1^{BA}, k_2^{BA}, and M^{BA} are the rate constants and molecular weight of benzoic acid, and M is the molecular weight of the drug for which the constants k_1 and k_2 are calculated. The ratio k_3/k_2 was found to be a function of the octanol–water partition coefficient, K:

$$K \cong 5(k_3/k_2) \tag{19–80}$$

Using this model, the constants k_1, k_2, and k_3 can be predicted from the physicochemical properties of the drug. The rate constant k_4 in Figure 19–23 represents the first-order elimination of the drug from the blood, and cannot be predicted. It must be measured experimentally.

Example 19–21. (a) Compute the rate constants k_1, k_2, and k_3 for the transport of clonidine from a membrane-controlled patch. The first-order rate constants k_1^{BA} and k_2^{BA} are 5.11×10^{-5} sec^{-1} and 80×10^{-5} sec^{-1}, respectively. The octanol–water partition coefficient of clonidine is $K = 6.7$. The molecular weight of benzoic acid is 122.12 g/mole, and the molecular weight of clonidine is 230.10 g/mole.

$$k_1 = 5.11 \times 10^{-5}(122.12/230.10)^{1/3} = 4.14 \times 10^{-5} \text{ sec}^{-1}$$

$$k_2 = 80 \times 10^{-5}(122.12/230.10)^{1/3} = 64.77 \times 10^{-5} \text{ sec}^{-1}$$

From equation (19–80)

$$k_3 = \frac{K\,k_2}{5} = \frac{6.7 \times 64.77 \times 10^{-5} \text{ sec}^{-1}}{5} = 8.68 \times 10^{-4} \text{ sec}^{-1}$$

(b) The steady-state plasma concentration of clonidine, C^{ss}, can be computed from

$$C^{ss} = Ak_0/V_dk_4 \tag{19–81}$$

where A is the area of the patch, k_0 is the zero-order rate constant for the delivery of clonidine from the patch, and V_d is the *volume of distribution*,* that is, the amount of drug in the body divided by the plasma concentration. For the most efficient membrane-controlled patch, which contains 2.5 mg of clonidine, A, the area of the patch, is 5 cm^2, and k_0 is 1.6 µg/(cm^2 hr). The volume of distribution V_d for

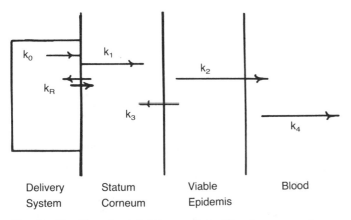

Fig. 19–23. Transdermal delivery of clonidine from a membrane-controlled patch. (From R. H. Guy and J. Hadgraft, J. Pharm. Sci. 74, 1016, 1985, reproduced with permission of the copyright owner.)

---

*To understand V_d, the volume of distribution, consider the following: If an amount of drug, say 1.5 µg, is distributed in the body plasma to give a drug concentration of 9.38×10^{-6} µg/mL, the volume of plasma containing this amount (1.5 µg) of drug is 1.5 µg/(9.38×10^{-6} µg/mL) = 160,000 mL, or V_d = 160 liters.

clonidine is 147 liters and the first-order constant, k_4, is 0.08 hr^{-1}. From equation (19–81),

$$C^{ss} = \frac{5 \text{ cm}^2 \times 1.6 \text{ µg cm}^{-2} \text{ hr}^{-1}}{147,000 \text{ cm}^3 \times 0.08 \text{ hr}^{-1}} = 6.8 \times 10^{-4} \text{ µg/mL}$$

Examples of membrane-controlled systems are the Transderm-Nitro (Ciba and Alza) for the delivery of nitroglycerin, Transderm-Scōp (Alza and Ciba-Geigy) for scopolamine,[147] and Catapress TTS (Alza/Boehringer Ingelheim) for clonidine.[148]

Adhesive Diffusion-Controlled Systems. The basic difference between this system and the previously described one is that the microporous membrane is absent. Figure 19–24 is a schematic of the adhesive system. The device consists of an impermeable plastic barrier on the top, a drug reservoir in the middle, and several rate-controlling adhesive layers next to the skin. The rate of drug release dQ/dt depends on the partition coefficient K of the drug between the reservoir (r) and the adhesive layers (a), the diffusion coefficient, D_a, the sum of the thicknesses of the adhesive layers, h_a, and the concentration C_r of the drug in the reservoir layer[147]:

$$\frac{dQ}{dt} = \frac{KD_a C_r}{h_a} \qquad (19–82)$$

Examples of these devices are the Nitrodisc (Searle) and Deponit (Pharma-Swartz) for the delivery of nitroglycerin. The in vitro release of drug as well as the in vivo permeation are zero-order processes.

Matrix-Controlled Devices. In a matrix-controlled device, the drug reservoir consists of a hydrophilic or hydrophobic polymer containing the dispersed drug, attached to a plastic backing that is impermeable to the drug. The drug reservoir is in direct contact with the skin, and the release of drug is matrix-controlled, that is, it is a function of the square root of time (see p. 336, equation (13–43). To obtain zero-order release of the drug across the skin using a matrix-controlled system, the stratum corneum must control the rate of drug delivery. This can be achieved if the release rate of the drug from the device is much greater than the rate of skin uptake. Noonan et al.[149] studied the transdermal penetration of 2% nitroglycerin formulated in a polymer gel matrix (Nitro-Dur system; Key and Schering Co's). The pharmacokinetics of delivery from these matrix systems has been studied by Berner.[150]

Iontophoresis. This technique is used to enhance the transdermal transport of drugs by applying a small current through a reservoir that contains ionized species of the drug. Positive or negative electrodes are placed between the drug reservoir and the skin. Positive ions are introduced in the skin from a positive electrode, and negative ions from a negative electrode. Figure 19–25 shows an iontophoresis circuit with the active electrode being negative. A second electrode, positive in this case, is placed a short distance away on the body to complete the circuit, and the electrodes are connected to a power supply. When the current flows, the negatively charged ions are transported across the skin, mainly through the pores (see Fig. 13–22, p. 347, for a discussion of pores). Pore transport during iontophoresis can be visualized by using a microscope and a fluorescein probe as the dye.[151] The use of this method in various diseases has been reviewed by Tyle.[152]

The isoelectric point of the skin is between 3 and 4 pH units; below pH 3 the pores are positively charged and above pH 4 they have a negative charge. Owing to the negative charge in the upper skin layers, basic drugs are relatively easy to introduce. In vitro systems designed to study iontophoretic transport involve the use of diffusion cells in which a skin membrane is placed vertically between the two halves of the cell. The "active" electrode, say the positive electrode for the transport of positive ions, is placed on the epidermal side. The other side of the cell contains a passive (oppositely charged) electrode in a conductive fluid. Glikfeld et al.[153] described an improved diffusion cell and reported iontophoretic enhancement of clonidine and morphine delivery across full-thickness hairless mouse skin. Iontophoresis enhances the transdermal absorption of insulin. At a pH below the isoelectric point of insulin (pH 5.3) the drug acts as a positive electrode, while at a pH above the isoelectric point the drug reservoir acts as a negative electrode. The greatest transport of insulin was found at pH 3.68 rather than at 7 or 8 owing possibly to low aggregation and a high charge density of insulin at pH 3.68.[154] The rate of skin permeation depends on the drug concentra-

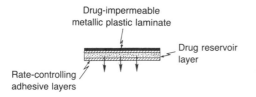

Fig. 19–24. Schematic of an adhesive diffusion-controlled transdermal drug delivery system. (From Y. W. Chien, in *Controlled Drug Delivery*, 2nd Edition, J. R. Robinson and V. H. L. Lee, Eds., Marcel Dekker, N.Y., 1987, p. 534, reproduced with permission of the copyright owner.)

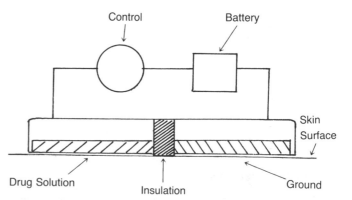

Fig. 19–25. A schematic of the iontophoresis apparatus in place on the skin.

tion, the ionic strength of the buffer solution, the magnitude of current applied, and the duration of iontophoresis.[154] Del Terzo et al.[155] found that in a series of *n*-alkanols, the iontophoretic transport of the more hydrophobic derivatives was decreased as compared with passive diffusion. These authors suggested that the transport of both nonionized and ionized molecules through the skin pores may be enhanced by iontophoresis, whereas the lipoidal pathway is inhibited by the use of this technique. Iontophoresis is a promising method to deliver peptides through the skin. Burnette and Marrero[156] showed that the flux of both ionized and nonionized species of thyrotropin releasing hormone were greater than the flux obtained by passive diffusion alone. The increased flux was proportional to the applied current density. Transport through the pores is favored for positive ions whereas transport of negative ions is probably smaller owing to electrostatic repulsion across the negatively charged skin membrane.

Faraday's law states that equal quantities of electricity will deposit equivalent quantities of ions at either electrode. However, the correlation between that predicted by Faraday's law and the experimental values is not good, owing to the many factors involved in iontophoretic transport. Kasting et al.[157] used an electrodiffusion model to study the transport of etidronate disodium, a negatively charged bone resorption agent, through excised human skin. At steady state, the flux J_i of drug through the membrane is given by the Nernst–Planck flux equation[158]:

$$J_i = -D_i \frac{dc_i}{dx} + \frac{D_i z_i e E c_i}{kT} \qquad (19\text{–}83)$$

where D_i is the diffusion coefficient for the ion i (in the x direction), z_i its charge, and c_i its concentration. The term kT is the thermal energy of the system where k is the Boltzmann constant and T is the absolute temperature. The Goldman approximation[158] provides a solution of equation (19–83):

$$J_i = \frac{-D_i K \nu}{h} \frac{c_i - c_o e^{-\nu}}{1 - e^{-\nu}} \qquad (19\text{–}84)$$

where K is the partition coefficient, h the thickness of the membrane, and c_i and c_o the concentrations at both sides of the membrane. Assuming that the concentration $c_o = 0$, in the limit as $\nu \to 0$, equation (19–84) becomes the flux passive diffusion, J_o (see equation (13–57), p. 338):

$$J_i = \frac{-D_i K c_i}{h} \qquad (19\text{–}85)$$

The term ν is a dimensionless driving force, defined as

$$\nu = \frac{z_i e V}{kT} \qquad (19\text{–}86)$$

where e is the electronic charge, z is the charge on the drug, k the Boltzmann constant, T the absolute tem-

perature, and V the applied voltage across the membrane. The *iontophoretic enhancement factor*, J_i/J_o, is

$$\frac{J_i}{J_o} = \frac{\nu}{1 - e^{-\nu}} \qquad (19\text{–}87)$$

That is, equation (19–87) measures the increase in transport of a drug relative to the passive diffusion, due to the electrical current applied. For positive values (z_i and V of the same sign in equation (19–86),), equation (19–84) predicts that the enhancement in flux is proportional to ν. For negative ν values, the flux will fall exponentially with increasing magnitude of ν.

Example 19–22. (*a*) Compute the iontophoretic enhancement factor, J_i/J_o, across human excised skin for a 10% etidronate solution. The voltage applied is 0.25 V, the average number of charges, z, per ion is 2.7. The charge on the electron is 1 eV. The value kT at 25° C is 0.025 eV.

From equation (19–86),

$$\nu = \frac{2.7 \times 1 \times 0.25}{0.025} = 27$$

Using equation (19–87) the iontophoretic enhancement factor is

$$\frac{J_i}{J_o} = \frac{27}{1 - e^{-27}} = 27$$

Thus we see that the flux for the drug promoted by iontophoresis is 27 times that expected for passive diffusion.

(*b*) Compute the flux, under the driving force of iontophoresis, knowing that the passive permeability coefficient P of the drug is 4.9×10^{-6} cm/hr and the concentration, c, is 1.02×10^5 μg/cm³.

Since $P = DK/h$ cm/hr from equation (19–85),

$$J_o = 4.9 \times 10^{-6} \times 1.02 \times 10^5 = 0.5 \ \mu g/(cm^2 \ hr)$$

From equation (19–87), using the value, 27, obtained in part (*a*) for J_i/J_o,

$$J_i = 0.5 \times 27 = 13.5 \ \mu g/(cm^2 \ hr)$$

Kasting et al.[157] found that equation (19–84) applies up to 0.25 V. At higher voltages, the flux of etidronate disodium rises much faster than the predicted values, owing to alteration of the membrane and because the diffusion coefficient is no longer a constant value, as assumed in equation (19–84). Burnette and Bagniefski[159] determined the skin electrochemical resistance R after iontophoresis. The decrease in resistance suggested that the current may alter the ion-conducting pathways of the skin even at the clinically acceptable current densities, leading to tissue damage.[151] (For electrochemical resistance R, see page 127.)

Topical Administration in Cattle. Pitman and Rostas[160] reviewed the topical administration of drugs to cattle and sheep with emphasis on a description of the absorption barriers and the mechanism of absorption, and they described the drug delivery studies on cattle and sheep that have appeared in the literature.

Parenteral Administration. The intravenous, intramuscular, subcutaneous, and intraperitoneal routes are the common avenues for parenteral administration of a drug. Advances in genetic engineering have provided a number of peptide drugs and proteins such as insulin that are orally inactive and must be given by the parenteral route. Although other routes have been investigated, such as the nasal, gastrointestinal, rectal and transdermal routes (see these sections in this chapter), parenteral administration remains the more viable route for peptides and some other drugs.[161] Controlled release can be achieved by continuous intravenous infusion, the amount of drug administered being equal to the amount of drug eliminated from the body. However, this method requires hospitalization during treatment.[162] The intravenous route is used occasionally to deliver sustained or controlled dosage forms such as liposomes, erythrocytes, nanoparticles, and small microcapsules (see pp. 513–521). Of the parenteral avenues, the subcutaneous and intramuscular routes are preferred for the controlled delivery of a drug. A number of physicochemical and physiologic factors affect the rate of release from the dosage form, as enumerated in Table 19–2. The absorption rate can be limited by the release rate from the delivery system. Figure 19–26 illustrates the rate-limiting step using several approaches such as complexation, dispersion, dissolution, adsorption, and partitioning to retard drug delivery.[163]

The drug release from aqueous solution can be prolonged by adding viscosity-increasing agents. These agents consist of water-soluble materials such as methylcellulose, sodium carboxymethylcellulose, and povidone. The increased viscosity of the medium reduces the diffusion of the drug (see the Stokes–Einstein equation, p. 401). Complex formation (Chapter 11) may prolong the delivery as long as the dissociation of the complex is slow. These same macromolecules employed as viscosity-promoting agents are used to prepare

TABLE 19–2. *Factors Influencing Parenteral Drug Absorption**

A. Drug and dosage form related factors
   1. Drug's pK_a, molecular size, solubility, dissolution rate, diffusivity, partition coefficient, etc.
   2. Type of dosage form, i.e., solution (type of solvent), suspension, etc.
   3. Physical-chemical properties of dosage form (pH, osmotic pressure, viscosity, etc.)
   4. Volume of injection
   5. Initial drug concentration in dosage form
B. Physiologic factors
   1. Site of administration
     a. Local circulation
     b. Local temperature
   2. Body movement
   3. Tissue injury

*From L. Krowczynski, *Extended-Release Dosage Forms*, CRC, Boca Raton, Fla., 1987, p. 60, reproduced with permission of the copyright owner.

complexes with drugs for intramuscular injection. The release of drugs from oily solutions depends on the partition coefficient of the drug between oil and aqueous fluids of the body and also depends on the viscosity of the vehicle. Depo-Estradiol (Upjohn) is an example of an oleaginous injectable, the active principle being dissolved in a mixture of benzyl alcohol and vegetable oil.

Suspensions usually produce a more extended release in comparison with solutions. A drug in aqueous suspension injected subcutaneously must first dissolve in the tissue fluids surrounding the particle agglomerate, diffuse into the intercellular spaces or intracellular regions of the connective tissues, then permeate the vascular membranes of the bloodstream. By mixing particles of different size, the rate of dissolution can be

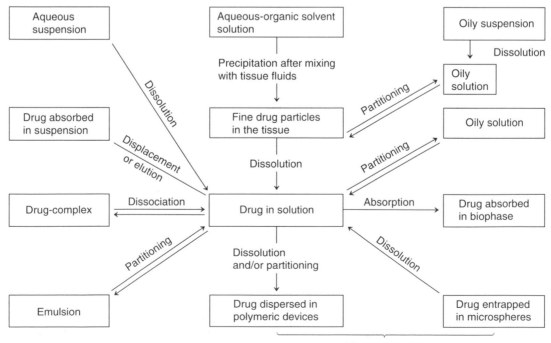

Fig. 19–26. Various approaches to achieving sustained drug action with parenteral medication. (From L. Krowczynski, *Extended-Release Dosage Forms*. CRC, Boca Raton, Fla., 1987, p. 60, reproduced with permission of the copyright owner.)

varied. Commercial zinc insulin suspensions use this approach to modulate the action of the drug. Hirano and Yamada[164] proposed a cube root expression relating the fraction of dose remaining at the subcutaneous injection site to the time,

$$\left(\frac{W}{W_o}\right)^{\frac{1}{3}} = 1 - kt \qquad (19\text{--}88)$$

where W_o is the initial amount and W is the amount of drug at time t; k is a rate constant for absorption from the depot site. The authors found that for suspensions having particle sizes between 3 and 4 μm the in vitro solubility C_s was related to the absorption constant k according to

$$\log k = 0.525 \log C_s - 0.578 \qquad (19\text{--}89)$$

where C_s is the aqueous solubility (see *Problem 19–28*). Microcapsules and microspheres, including magnetic microspheres, have been investigated as carrier suspensions for controlled delivery (see the earlier Section on microcapsules). Parenteral oil-in-water and water-in-oil emulsions can also be used as delivery systems. Examples of drug release from emulsions have been considered in Chapter 18, pages 504–506. Implants are placed subcutaneously to bring about drug delivery by way of drug diffusion, polymer dissolution, or a combination of both mechanisms. Sterile disks or cylinders (pellets) containing the drug are prepared by fusion (melting) or compression. Silicone capsules (see Chapter 13, pp. 341–342) have been used for the delivery of contraceptive hormones, L-dopa, and tranquilizers.[165] The rate of delivery is controlled by the thickness of the wall (membrane-controlled release), and produces zero-order release. The kinetics of drug delivery from matrix-type devices, on the other hand, is not zero-order, as desired. The release is proportional to the square root of time (see pp. 335, 336). The hydrophobic polymers used in the matrix-type (monolithic) devices are derived from the co-(ethylene/vinyl acetate) (EVA) polymers. The mechanism of release is not concerned with dissolution or swelling of the polymer, but rather involves diffusion of the drug through narrow channels (Fig. 19–27). Although zero-order kinetics is not usually obtained with the matrix-type systems, nearly zero-order release can be achieved by changing the geometry of the device. For example, in vitro release of bovine serum albumin is zero-order from an inward-releasing hemisphere.[161] The release from hydrogels, as contrasted to hydrophobic polymers, depends on the swelling and the degree of hydration of the polymer (pp. 497–498). Hydrogels of hydroxyethyl methacrylate (HEMA) are used as membranes for diffusion-controlled delivery of water-soluble drugs, glucose, insulin, cytochrome, and albumin.[166]

Self-regulating delivery systems have been studied for the controlled release of insulin.[167] The system is based on the competitive binding between glucose and glycosylated insulin to the specific sites of concanavalin A (Con A). Glycosylated insulin is an insulin derivative,

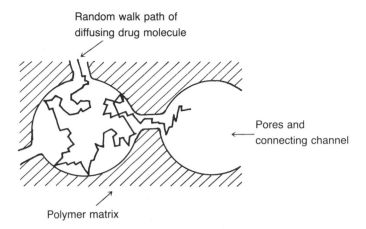

Fig. 19–27. Release of a macromolecular drug from a polymer matrix based on diffusion through narrow channels connecting larger pores. (From R. A. Siegel and R. Langer, Pharm. Res. **1**, 1, 1984, reproduced with permission of the copyright owner.)

succinyl amido phenyl-α-D glucopyranoside insulin, (SAPG-insulin). Con A is a plant protein capable of binding erythrocytes, carbohydrates, insulin, and other large biologic agents. The competitive reaction is written:

glucose + SAPG-insulin–Con A $\rightleftarrows$ glucose–Con A

$$+ \text{ SAPG-insulin} \qquad (19\text{--}90)$$

Under conditions of hyperglycemia, glucose enters the insulin delivery device, Figure 19–28, implanted in the body and releases SAPG-insulin from its Con A binding

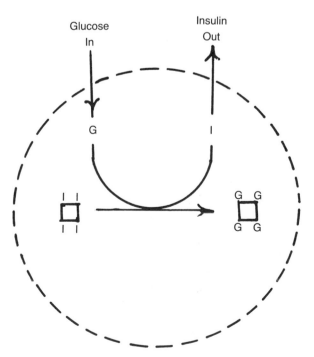

Fig. 19–28. Visualization of the insulin delivery process. Glucose, G, enters the device during bouts of hyperglycemia, displacing SAPG-insulin from the binding sites on Con A, □, forming the complex, glucose–Con A. (After S. Y. Jeong, S. W. Kim, M. J. D. Eenink and J. Feijen, J. Controlled Release **1**, 57, 1984, reproduced with permission of the copyright owner.)

sites in accordance with equation (19–90). The SAPG-insulin escapes through the membrane of the delivery system to counteract the hyperglycemia. Because of its high molecular weight (~110,000 daltons), Con A cannot pass through the membrane and is retained in the device. Similar self-regulating systems under development are based on the reaction

$$\text{glucose} + \text{glucose oxidase} \rightarrow$$

$$\text{gluconic acid} + H_2O \quad (19\text{--}91)$$

In these systems, the formation of gluconic acid is accompanied by a reduction of pH, promoting the permeability of the membrane and increasing the delivery of insulin in response to an increase in glucose concentration.[168] Additional reference sources dealing with drug product design and controlled delivery are listed following the section on **References and Notes.**

References and Notes

1. T. Higuchi and V. Stella, Eds., *Prodrugs as Novel Drug Delivery Systems*, American Chemical Society, Washington, D.C., 1975.
2. H. Seki, T. Kawaguchi and T. Higuchi, J. Pharm. Sci. **77**, 855, 1988.
3. R. P. Waranis and K. B. Sloan, J. Pharm. Sci. **77**, 210, 1988.
4. H. Bundgaard, M. Johansen, V. Stella and M. Cortese, Int. J. Pharm. **10**, 181, 1982.
5. H. Bundgaard and J. Møss, J. Pharm. Sci. **78**, 122, 1989.
6. Y. Takakura, Y. Kaneko, T. Fujita, M. Hashida, H. Maeda and H. Sezaki, J. Pharm. Sci. **78**, 117, 1989; Y. Takakura, M. Kitajima, S. Matsumoto, M. Hashida and H. Sezaki, Int. J. Pharm. **37**, 135, 1987.
7. K. Sato, K. Itakura, K. Nishida, K. Takakura, M. Hashida and H. Sezaki, J. Pharm. Sci. **78**, 11, 1989.
8. A. D. Bangham and R. W. Horne, J. Mol. Biol. **8**, 660, 1964; A. D. Bangham, M. M. Standish and J. C. Watkins, J. Mol. Biol. **13**, 238, 1965.
9. F. J. Martin, in *Specialized Drug Delivery Systems*, P. Tyle, Ed., Marcel Dekker, N.Y., 1990, Chapter 6.
10. C. Pidgeon and C. A. Hunt, J. Pharm. Sci. **70**, 173, 1981.
11. D. Lichtenberg and T. Markello, J. Pharm. Sci. **73**, 122, 1984.
12. M. A. Schwartz and H. M. McConnell, Biochemistry **17**, 837, 1978.
13. H. Sasaki, T. Kakutani, M. Hashida and H. Sezaki, J. Pharm. Sci. **75**, 1166, 1986.
14. R. M. Abra, C. A. Hunt and D. T. Lau, J. Pharm. Sci. **73**, 203, 1984.
15. R. Mezei and V. Gulasekharam, Life Sci. **26**, 1473, 1980.
16. J. H. Wiessner, H. Mar, D. G. Baskin and K. J. Hwang, J. Pharm. Sci. **75**, 259, 1986.
17. M. Guzman, A. Abeger and E. Sellés, Pharm. Acta Helv. **62**, 163, 1987.
18. N. I. Payne, P. Timmins, C. V. Ambrose, M. D. Ward and F. Ridgway, J. Pharm. Sci. **75**, 325, 1986; N. I. Payne, I. Browning and C. A. Haynes, J. Pharm. Sci. **75**, 330, 1986.
19. G. Gregoriadis, Ed., *Liposome Technology*, Vol. I, II, III, CRC, Boca Raton, Fla., 1984.
20. R. Baker, *Controlled Release of Biologically Active Agents*, Wiley, N.Y., 1987, pp. 14, 15.
21. F. Lim and R. D. Moss, J. Pharm. Sci. **70**, 351, 1981.
22. P. Rambourg, J. Lévy and M.-C. Lévy, J. Pharm. Sci. **71**, 753, 1982.
23. T. M. S. Chang, Science **146**, 524, 1964.
24. M.-C. Lévy, P. Rambourg, J. Lévy and G. Potron, J. Pharm. Sci. **71**, 759, 1982.
25. J. W. McGinity, A. Martin, G. W. Cuff and A. B. Combs, J. Pharm. Sci. **70**, 372, 1981.
26. K. Bala and P. Vasudevan, J. Pharm. Sci. **71**, 960, 1982.
27. J. R. Nixon and G. A. Agyilirah, J. Pharm. Sci. **73**, 52, 1984.
28. A. C. Povey, H. Bartsch, J. R. Nixon and I. K. O'Neill, J. Pharm. Sci. **75**, 831, 1986.
29. J. M. Gallo, P. K. Gupta, C. T. Hung and D. G. Perrier, J. Pharm. Sci. **78**, 190, 1989; P. K. Gupta, C. T. Hung and N. S. Rao, J. Pharm. Sci. **78**, 290, 1989.
30. J. Akbuğa, Int. J. Pharm. **53**, 99, 1989.
31. T. Higuchi, J. Pharm. Sci. **52**, 1145, 1963; R. W. Baker and H. K. Lonsdale, in *Controlled Release of Biologically Active Agents*, A. C. Tanquary and R. E. Lacey, Eds., Plenum, N.Y. 1974, pp. 15–71.
32. P. K. Gupta, F. C. Lam and C. T. Hung, Int. J. Pharm. **51**, 253, 1989.
33. J. M. Gallo, C. T. Hung and D. C. Perrier, Int. J. Pharm. **22**, 63, 1984.
34. G. Spenlehauer, M. Veillard and J.-P. Benoit, J. Pharm. Sci. **75**, 750, 1986.
35. S. E. Leucuta, Int. J. Pharm. **54**, 71, 1989.
36. R. Bodmeier and J. W. McGinity, Pharm. Res. **4**, 465, 1987.
37. R. Bodmeier and J. W. McGinity, Int. J. Pharm. **43**, 179, 1988.
38. S. Margel and J. Hirsh, J. Pharm. Sci. **71**, 1030, 1982.
39. Y. Morimoto, H. Natsume, K. Sugiboyashi and S. Fujimoto, Int. J. Pharm. **54**, 27, 1989.
40. H. Natsume, K. Sugibayashi, K. Juni, Y. Morimoto, T. Shibata and S. Fujimoto, Int. J. Pharm. **58**, 79, 1990.
41. J. Kreuter, Pharm. Acta Helv. **53**, 33, 1978; G. Birrenbach and P. P. Speiser, J. Pharm. Sci. **65**, 1763, 1976; P. P. Speiser, in *Microencapsulation: New Techniques and Applications*, T. Kondo, Ed., Techno Inc., Tokyo, Japan, 1979; J. Kreuter and E. Liehl, J. Pharm. Sci. **70**, 367, 1981.
42. P. C. Hiemenz, *Polymer Chemistry, The Basic Concepts*, Marcel Dekker, N.Y., 1984, Chapter 6; J. R. Robinson and V. H. L. Lee, Eds., *Controlled Drug Delivery*, Fundamentals and Applications, 2nd Edition, Marcel Dekker, N.Y., Chapter 3.
43. A. Rolland, B. Collet, R. Le Verge and L. Toujas, J. Pharm. Sci. **78**, 481, 1989.
44. N. Al Khouri Fallouh, L. Roblot-Treupel, H. Fessi, J. P. Devissaguet and F. Puisieux, Int. J. Pharm. **28**, 125, 1986; P. Couvreur, M. Roland and P. Speiser, U. S. Patent, 4329 332 1982.
45. E. M. Gipps, P. Groscurth, J. Kreuter and P. P. Speiser, J. Pharm. Sci. **77**, 208, 1988; E. M. Gipps, R. Arshady, J. Kreuter, P. Groscurth and P. P. Speiser, J. Pharm. Sci. **75**, 256, 1986.
46. B. Kante, P. Couvreur, G. Dubois-Krack, C. de Meester, P. Guiot, M. Roland, M. Mercier and P. Speiser, J. Pharm. Sci. **71**, 786, 1982.
47. P. Couvreur, B. Kante, L. Grislain, M. Roland and P. Speiser, J. Pharm. Sci. **71**, 790, 1982.
48. A. G. Thombre and K. J. Himmelstein, J. Pharm. Sci. **73**, 219, 1984.
49. A. Urtti, L. Salminen and O. Miinalainem, Int. J. Pharm. **23**, 147, 1985.
50. A. Hussain, S. Hirai and J. Sieg, J. Pharm. Sci. **69**, 738, 1980.
51. D. D.-S. Tang-Liu, S. Liu, J. Neff and R. Sandri, J. Pharm. Sci. **76**, 780, 1987.
52. R. E. Stratford, Jr., L. Wulf-Carson, S. Dodda-Kashi and V. H. L. Lee, J. Pharm. Sci. **77**, 838, 1988.
53. Y. Rojanasakul and J. R. Robinson, Int. J. Pharm. **55**, 237, 1989.
54. G. M. Grass and J. R. Robinson, J. Pharm. Sci. **77**, 3, 1988.
55. G. M. Grass and J. R. Robinson, J. Pharm. Sci. **77**, 15, 1988.
56. R. D. Schoenwald and S. H. Huang, J. Pharm. Sci. **72**, 1266, 1983.
57. T. F. Patton and J. R. Robinson, J. Pharm. Sci. **64**, 1312, 1975.
58. S. S. Chrai and J. R. Robinson, J. Pharm. Sci. **63**, 1218, 1974.
59. R. D. Schoenwald and P. Stewart, J. Pharm. Sci. **69**, 391, 1980.
60. H.-W. Hui and J. R. Robinson, J. Pharm. Sci. **75**, 280, 1986.
61. G. M. Grass, J. Cobby and M. C. Makoid, J. Pharm. Sci. **73**, 618, 1984.
62. J. Cobby, M. Mayersohn and G. C. Walker, J. Pharm. Sci. **63**, 725, 732, 1974.
63. B. A. Johnson and G. Zografi, J. Pharm. Sci. **75**, 529, 1986.
64. H. Gray and C. M. Moss, *Anatomy of the Human Body*, 29th Edition, Lea & Febiger, Philadelphia, 1972, pp. 1114–1119.
65. Y. W. Chien, K. S. E. Su and S-F. Chang, *Nasal Systemic Drug Delivery*, Marcel Dekker, N.Y., 1989, Chapter 1.

66. V. H. K. Li, J. R. Robinson and V. H. L. Lee, in *Controlled Drug Delivery*, 2nd Edition, J. R. Robinson and V. H. L. Lee, Eds., Marcel Dekker, N.Y., 1987, pp 44–45.

67. A. Hussain, S. Hirai and R. Bawarshi, J. Pharm. Sci. **69**, 1411, 1980.

68. A. A. Hussain, S. Hirai and R. Bawarshi, J. Pharm. Sci. **70**, 466, 1981; A. A. Hussain, R. Kimura and C. H. Huang, J. Pharm Sci. **73**, 1300, 1984.

69. S.-F. Chang, L. Moore and Y. W. Chien, Pharm. Res. **5**, 718, 1988.

70. C. H. Huang, R. Kimura, R. B. Nassar and A. Hussain, J. Pharm. Sci. **74**, 608, 1985.

71. Y. Maitani, Y. Machida and T. Nagai, Int. Pharm. J. **49**, 23, 1989.

72. Y. W. Chien, Ed., *Transdermal Systemic Medication*, Elsevier, N.Y., 1985, Chapters 7, 9.

73. Y. W. Chien, K. S. E. Su and S-F. Chang, *Nasal Systemic Drug Delivery*, Marcel Dekker, N.Y., 1989, Chapter 4.

74. M. A. Hussain, A. B. Shenvi, S. M. Rowe and E. Shefter, Pharm. Res. **6**, 186, 1989.

75. K. S. E. Su, K. M. Campanale, L. G. Mendelsohn, G. A. Kerchner and C. L. Gries, J. Pharm. Sci. **74**, 394, 1985.

76. S. C. Raehs, J. Sandow, K. Wirth and H. P. Merkle, Pharm. Res. **5**, 689, 1988; J. P. Longenecker, A. C. Moses, J. S. Flier, R. D. Silver, M. C. Carey and E. J. Dubovi, J. Pharm. Sci. **76**, 351, 1987.

77. W. A. J. J. Hermens and F. W. H. M. Merkus, Pharm. Res. **4**, 445, 1987.

78. A. S. Harris, I. M. Nilsson, Z. G.-Wagner and U. Alkner, J. Pharm. Sci. **75**, 1085, 1986.

79. A. S. Harris, M. Ohlin, S. Lethagen and I. M. Nilsson, J. Pharm. Sci. **77**, 337, 1988.

80. Y. Kurosaki, S. Hisaichi, L.-Z. Hong, T. Nakayama and T. Kimura, Int. J. Pharm. **49**, 47, 1989; K. W. Garren and A. J. Repta, J. Pharm. Sci. **78**, 160, 1989.

81. R. Anders and H. P. Merkle, Int. J. Pharm. **49**, 231, 1989.

82. A. E. Collins and P. B. Deasy, J. Pharm. Sci. **79**, 116, 1990.

83. M. A. Hussain, B. J. Aungst, C. A. Koval and E. Shefter, Pharm. Res. **5**, 615, 1988.

84. K. Park, Int. J. Pharm. **53**, 209, 1989.

85. K. V. R. Rao and P. Buri, Int. J. Pharm. **52**, 265, 1989.

86. P. R. Byron, Ed., *Respiratory Drug Delivery*, CRC, Boca Raton, Fla., 1990.

87. V. H. K. Li, J. R. Robinson and V. H. L. Lee, in *Controlled Drug Delivery*, 2nd Edition, J. R. Robinson and V. H. L. Lee, Eds., Marcel Dekker, N.Y., 1987, pp. 45–49.

88. R. L. Juliano, in *International Encyclopedia of Pharmacology and Therapeutics*, Section 120, Methods of Drug Delivery, G. M. Ihler, Ed., Pergamon Press, Oxford, 1986, p. 141.

89. P. R. Byron, J. Pharm. Sci. **75**, 433, 1986.

90. P. R. Byron, N. S. R. Roberts and A. R. Clark, J. Pharm. Sci. **75**, 168, 1986.

91. P. R. Byron, Ed., *Respiratory Drug Delivery*, CRC, Boca Raton, Fla., 1990, pp. 225–227.

92. L. Krowczynski, *Extended-Release Dosage Forms*, CRC, Boca Raton, Fla., 1987, Chapter 6.

93. P. J. Sinko and G. L. Amidon, Pharm. Res. **5**, 645, 1988.

94. M. Hu and G. L. Amidon, J. Pharm. Sci. **77**, 1007, 1988.

95. G. L. Amidon, P. J. Sinko and D. Fleisher, Pharm. Res. **5**, 651, 1988.

96. J. G. Prieto, L. Santos, J. P. Barrio and M. L. Alonso, J. Pharm. Sci. **76**, 596, 1987.

97. M. A. Hussain, B. J. Aungst and E. Shefter, Pharm. Res. **5**, 44, 1988.

98. G. E. Peters, l. E. F. Hutchinson, R. Hyde, C. McMartin and S. B. Metcalfe, J. Pharm. Sci. **76**, 857, 1987.

99. L. Krowczynski, *Extended-Release Dosage Forms*, CRC, Boca Raton, Fla., 1987, pp. 104–110; ibid. p. 105.

100. M. A. Hussain, R. C. Diluccio and E. Shefter, Pharm. Res. **6**, 49, 1989.

101. S. S. Ozturk, B. O. Palsson and J. B. Dressman, Pharm. Res. **5**, 272, 1988; ibid. p. 281.

102. H. C. Wilson and G. W. Cuff, J. Pharm. Sci. **78**, 582, 1989.

103. S. S. Jambhekar, and J. Cobby, J. Pharm. Sci. **74**, 991, 1985.

104. F. Theeuwes and S. I. Yum, Ann. Biomed. Eng. **4**, 343, 1976; Alzet Mini-Osmotic Pump Bibliography, Alza Corp. 1981; F. Theeuwes, in *Directed Drug Delivery*, R. T. Borchardt, A. J. Repta and V. J. Stella, Eds., Humana Press, Clifton, N.J., 1985, pp. 121–146.

105. F. Theeuwes, J. Pharm. Sci. **64**, 1987, 1975.

106. F. Theeuwes, D. Swanson, P. Wong, P. Bonsen, V. Place, K. Heimlich and K. C. Kwan, J. Pharm. Sci. **72**, 253, 1983.

107. G. L. Amidon, T. Higuchi and J. B. Dressman, U.S. Patent, 4 685 918 (1987).

108. J. L. Haslam, A. E. Merfeld and G. S. Rork, Int. J. Pharm. **56**, 227, 1989.

109. B. Lindstedt, G. Ragnarsson and J. Hjärtstam, Int. J. Pharm. **56**, 261, 1989.

110. R. Bodmeier and O. Paeratakul, J. Pharm. Sci. **79**, 925, 1990.

111. V. H. K. Li, J. R. Robinson and V. H. L. Lee, in *Controlled Drug Delivery*, 2nd Edition, J. R. Robinson and V. H. L. Lee, Eds., Marcel Dekker, N. Y., 1987, p. 43.

112. A. G. de Boer, D. D. Breimer, J. Pronk and J. M. Gubens-Stibbe, J. Pharm. Sci. **69**, 804, 1980.

113. G. G. Liversidge, T. Nishihata, K. K. Engle and T. Higuchi, Int. J. Pharm. **23**, 87, 1985.

114. T. Nishihata, S. Kim, S. Morishita, A. Kamada, N. Yata and T. Higuchi, J. Pharm. Sci. **72**, 280, 1983.

115. K. Morimoto, H. Akatsuchi, R. Aikawa, M. Morishita and K. Morisaka, J. Pharm. Sci. **73**, 1366, 1984.

116. W. M. Wu, T. Murakami, Y. Higashi and N. Yata, J. Pharm. Sci. **76**, 508, 1987; W. M. Wu, T. Murakami, A. Yamajo, Y. Higashi and N. Yata, J. Pharm. Sci. **78**, 499, 1989.

117. T. Nishihata, C.-S. Lee, M. Yamamoto, J. H. Rytting and T. Higuchi, J. Pharm. Sci. **73**, 1326, 1984.

118. T. Nishihata, J. H. Rytting and T. Higuchi, J. Pharm. Sci. **69**, 744, 1980.

119. T. Nishihata, J. H. Rytting and T. Higuchi, J. Pharm. Sci. **70**, 71, 1981.

120. J. A. Fix, P. S. Leppert, J. A. Porter and L. J. Caldwell, J. Pharm. Sci. **72**, 1134, 1983.

121. T. Nishihata, S. Kawabe, M. Miyake, S. Kim and A. Kamada, Int. J. Pharm. **22**, 147, 1984.

122. Y. Watanabe, E. J. van Hoogdalem, A. G. de Boer and D. D. Breimer, J. Pharm. Sci. **77**, 847, 1988; E. J. van Hoogdalem, M. A. Hardens, A. G. de Boer and D. D. Breimer, Pharm. Res. **5**, 453, 1988.

123. J. A. Fix, J. Alexander, M. Cortese, K. Engle, P. Leppert and A. J. Repta, Pharm. Res. **6**, 501, 1989.

124. A. Buur and H. Bundgaard, J. Pharm. Sci. **75**, 522, 1986.

125. M. Tomita, M. Shiga, M. Hayashi and S. Awazu, Pharm. Res. **5**, 341, 1988.

126. W. Curatolo, Pharm. Res. **4**, 271, 1987.

127. R. L. Bronaugh and R. F. Stewart, J. Pharm. Sci. **75**, 487, 1986.

128. R. H. Guy and J. Hadgraft, Pharm. Res. **5**, 753, 1988.

129. K. Tojo, J. Pharm. Sci. **76**, 889, 1987.

130. B. W. Barry, Int. J. Cosmet. Sci. **10**, 281, 1988.

131. M.-S. Wu, J. Pharm. Sci. **72**, 1421, 1983.

132. K. Tojo, C. C. Chiang and Y. W. Chien, J. Pharm. Sci. **76**, 123, 1987.

133. P. P. Sarpotdar and J. L. Zatz, J. Pharm. Sci. **75**, 176, 1986.

134. J. Swarbrick, G. Lee, J. Brom and N. P. Gensmantel, J. Pharm. Sci. **73**, 1352, 1984.

135. C. Fleeker, O. Wong and J. H. Rytting, Pharm. Res. **6**, 443, 1989.

136. P. S. Banerjee and W. A. Ritschel, Int. J. Pharm. **49**, 189, 1989.

137. D. B. Guzek, A. H. Kennedy, S. C. McNeill, E. Wakshull and R. O. Potts, Pharm. Res. **6**, 33, 1989.

138. R. O. Potts, S. C. McNeill, C. R. Desbonnet and E. Wakshull, Pharm. Res. **6**, 119, 1989.

139. S. Y. Chan and A. L. W. Po, Int. J. Pharm. **55**, 1, 1989.

140. E. M. Niazy, A. M. Molokhia and A. S. El Gorashi, Int. J. Pharm. **56**, 181, 1989.

141. T. Nishihata, J. H. Rytting, K. Takahashi and K. Sakai, Pharm. Res. **5**, 738, 1988.

142. J. W. Wiechers, B. F. H. Drenth, J. H. G. Joknman and R. A. de Zeeuw, Pharm. Res. **4**, 519, 1987.

143. P. K. Wotton, B. Møollgaard, J. Hadgraft and A. Hoelgaard, Int. J. Pharm. **24**, 19, 1985; R. A. Patel and R. C. Vasavada, Pharm. Res. **5**, 116, 1988; P. Agrawala and W. A. Ritschel, J. Pharm. Sci. **77**, 776, 1988; P. Catz and D. R. Friend, Int. J. Pharm. **55**, 17, 1989.

144. O. Wong, J. Huntington, T. Nishihata and J. H. Rytting,

Pharm. Res. **6**, 286, 1989; D. D.-S. Tang-Liu, J. Neff, H. Zolezio and R. Sandri, Pharm. Res. **5**, 477, 1988.

145. G. Gienger, A. Knoch and H. P. Merkle, J. Pharm. Sci. **75**, 9, 1986.
146. R. H. Guy and J. Hadgraft, J. Pharm. Sci. **73**, 883, 1984; R. H. Guy and J. Hadgraft, J. Pharm. Sci. **74**, 1016, 1985.
147. Y. W. Chien, in *Controlled Drug Delivery*, 2nd Edition, J. R. Robinson and V. H. L. Lee, Eds., Marcel Dekker, N.Y., 1987, p. 533, 534.
148. D. Arndts and K. Arndts, Eur. Clin. Pharmacol. **26**, 79, 1984;
149. P. K. Noonan, M. A. Gonzalez, R. Ruggirello, J. Tomlinson, E. Babcock-Atkinson, M. Ray, A. Golub and A. Cohen, J. Pharm. Sci. **75**, 688, 1986.
150. B. Berner, J. Pharm. Sci. **74**, 718, 1985.
151. R. R. Burnette and B. Ongpipattanakul, J. Pharm. Sci. **77**, 132, 1988.
152. P. Tyle, Pharm. Res. **3**, 318, 1986.
153. P. Glikfeld, C. Cullander, R. Hinz and R. H. Guy, Pharm. Res. **5**, 443, 1988.
154. O. Siddiqui, Y. Sun, J.-C. Liu and Y. W. Chien, J. Pharm. Sci. **76**, 341, 1987.
155. S. Del Terzo, C. R. Behl and R. A. Nash, Pharm. Res. **6**, 85, 1989.
156. R. R. Burnette and D. Marrero, J. Pharm. Sci. **75**, 738, 1986.
157. G. B. Kasting, E. W. Merrit and J. C. Keister, J. Membrane Sci. **35**, 137, 1988.
158. G. B. Kasting and J. C. Keister, J. Controlled Release **8**, 195, 1989.
159. R. R. Burnette and T. M. Bagniefski, J. Pharm. Sci. **77**, 492, 1988.
160. I. H. Pitman and S. J. Rostas, J. Pharm. Sci. **70**, 1181, 1981.
161. C. G. Pitt, Int. J. Pharm. **59**, 173, 1990.
162. V. H. K. Li, J. R. Robinson and V. H. L. Lee, in *Controlled Drug Delivery*, 2nd. Edition, J. R. Robinson and V. H. L. Lee, Eds., Marcel Dekker, N.Y., 1987, p. 37.
163. L. Krowczynski, *Extended-Release Dosage Forms*, CRC, Boca Raton, Fla., 1987, p. 59.
164. K. Hirano and H. Yamada, J. Pharm. Sci. **71**, 500, 1982.
165. L. Krowczynski, *Extended-Release Dosage Forms*, CRC, Boca Raton, Fla., 1987, p. 84.
166. S. Sato and S. W. Kim, Int. J. Pharm. **22**, 229, 1984.
167. L. A. Seminoff, G. B. Olsen and S. W. Kim, Int. J. Pharm. **54**, 241, 1989.
168. S. Y. Jeong, S. W. Kim, M. J. D. Eennink and J. Feijen, J. Controlled Release **1**, 57, 1984.
169. S. Benita, D. Babay, A. Hoffman and M. Donbrow, Pharm. Res. **5**, 178, 1988.
170. A. A. Hussain, R. Barawshi-Nassar and C. H. Huang, "Physicochemical Considerations of Intranasal Drug Administration," in *Transnasal Systemic Medication*, Y. C. Chien, Ed., Elsevier, New York, 1985, pp. 128–129.
171. B. Hoener and L. Z. Benet, *Modern Pharmaceutics*, Banker and Rhodes, Eds., Marcel Dekker, N.Y., 1990, p. 165.
172. D. S. Roy and G. L. Flynn, Pharm. Res., **6**, 147, 1989.

Additional References

A. C. Tanquary and R. E. Lacey, *Controlled Release of Biologically Active Agents*, Plenum Press, N.Y., 1974.

D. R. Paul and F. W. Harris, Eds., *Controlled Release Polymeric Formulations*, American Chemical Society, Washington, D.C., 1976.

S. K. Chandrasekaran and J. E. Shaw, "Design of Transdermal Systems, in *Contemporary Topics in Polymer Science*, Vol. 2, Plenum Press, N.Y., 1977.

G. Gregoriadis, Ed., *Drug Carriers in Biology and Medicine*, Academic Press, N.Y., 1979.

R. Baker, Ed., *Controlled Release of Bioactive Materials*, Academic Press, N.Y., 1980.

R. Juliano, Ed., *Drug Delivery Systems*, Oxford Press, N.Y., 1980.

A. F. Kydonieus, Ed., *Controlled Release Technologies: Methods, Theory and Applications*, CRC, Boca Raton, Fla., 1980.

S. Yolles and M. P. Sartori, *Drug Delivery Systems*, Oxford Press, N.Y., 1980.

H. Bundgaard, A. B. Hansen and H. Kofod, Eds., *Optimization of Drug Delivery*, Munksgaard, Copenhagen, 1981.

D. H. Lewis, Ed., *Controlled Release of Pesticides and Pharmaceuticals*, Plenum Press, N.Y., 1981.

L. F. Prescott and W. S. Nimmo, Eds., *Drug Absorption*, ADIS Press, Balgowlah, Australia and New York, 1981.

Y. W. Chien, *Novel Drug Delivery Systems*, Marcel Dekker, N.Y., 1982.

C. Gregoriadis, J. Senior and A Trouet, Eds., *Targeting of Drugs*, Plenum Press, N.Y., 1982.

M. Ostro, Ed., *Liposomes*, Marcel Dekker, New York, 1983.

T. J. Roseman and S. Z. Mansdorf, Eds., *Controlled Release Delivery Systems*, Marcel Dekker, N.Y., 1983.

S. S. Davis, L. Illum, J. G. McVie and E. Tomlinson, Eds., *Microspheres and Drug Therapy*, Elsevier, N.Y., 1984.

P. D. Deasy, *Microencapsulation and Related Drug Processes*, Marcel Dekker, N.Y., 1984.

R. S. Langer and D. L. Wise, Eds., *Medical Applications of Controlled Release*, Vol. I, *Classes of Systems*, Vol. II, *Applications and Evaluation*, CRC, Boca Raton, Fla., 1984.

R. T. Borchardt, A. J. Repta and V. J. Stella, Eds., *Directed Drug Delivery: A Multi-disciplinary Problem*, Humana Press, Clifton, N.J., 1985.

Y. W. Chien, Ed., *Transdermal Systemic Medications*, Elsevier, N.Y., 1985.

L. F. Prescott and W. S. Nimmo, Eds., *Rate Control in Drug Therapy*, Churchill Livingstone, N.Y., 1985.

V. Smolen, Ed., *Controlled Drug Bioavailability*, Wiley, N.Y., 1985.

P. Guiot and P. Couvreur, *Polymeric Nanoparticles and Microspheres*, CRC, Boca Raton, Fla., 1986.

G. M. Ihler, *Methods of Drug Delivery*, Pergamon Press, N.Y., 1986.

N. A. Peppas, Ed., *Hydrogels in Medicine and Pharmacy*, CRC, Boca Raton, Fla., 1986.

H. A. J. Struyker-Boudier, *Rate-Controlled Drug Administration and Action*, CRC, Boca Raton, Fla., 1986.

Y. W. Chien, Ed., *Transdermal Controlled Systemic Medications*, Marcel Dekker, N.Y., 1987.

A. F. Kydonieus and B. Berner, Eds., *Transdermal Delivery of Drugs*, Vols. I, II, and III, CRC, Boca Raton, Fla., 1987.

P. I. Lee and W. R. Good, Eds., *Controlled Release Technology*, ACS Symposium Series, No. 348, American Chemical Society, Washington, D.C., 1987.

J. R. Robinson and V. H. L. Lee, Eds., *Controlled Drug Delivery, Fundamentals and Applications*, 2nd Edition, Marcel Dekker, N.Y., 1987.

A. Rembaum and Z. A. Tokes, *Microspheres: Medical and Biological Applications*, CRC, Boca Raton, Fla., 1988.

P. Tyle, Ed., *Drug Delivery Devices, Fundamentals and Applications*, Marcel Dekker, N.Y., 1988.

P. R. Byron, *Respiratory Drug Delivery*, CRC, Boca Raton, Fla., 1989.

Y. W. Chien, K. S. E. Su and S.-F. Chang, *Nasal Systemic Drug Delivery*, Marcel Dekker, N.Y., 1989.

L. T. Fan and S. K. Singh, *Controlled Release—A Quantitative Treatment*, Springer-Verlag, New York, 1989.

U. Gundert-Remy and H. Möller, *Oral Controlled Release Products*, CRC, Boca Raton, Fla., 1989.

R. Gurney and H. E. Junginger, *Bioadhesion Possibilities and Future Trends*, CRC, Boca Raton, Fla., 1989.

J. Hadgraft and R. H. Guy, Eds., *Transdermal Drug Delivery*, Marcel Dekker, N.Y., 1989.

J. G. Hardy, S. S. Davis and C. G. Wilson, Eds., *Drug Delivery to the Gastrointestinal Tract*, Wiley, N.Y., 1989.

V. M. Lenaerts and R. Gurney, *Bioadhesive Drug Delivery Systems*, CRC, Boca Raton, Fla., 1989.

D. W. Osborne and A. H. Amann, Eds., *Topical Drug Delivery Formulations*, Marcel Dekker, N.Y., 1989.

J. Kost, Ed., *Pulsed and Self-Regulated Drug Delivery*, CRC, Boca Raton, Fla., 1990.

*Problems**

19–1. (a) Calculate the volume VW_3 of total water encapsulated in a three-lamella ($n = 3$) liposome having a radius $R = 0.0447$ μm and

---

*Note that the definition of the symbols of Lichtenberg and Markello in this problem are not the same as those of Pidgeon and Hunt *(Problem 19–1)*. For example, i of R_i does not have the same meaning for these authors.

a volume of phospholipid, VL_3 (which constitutes the three bilayers) of 15.2 μm^3. See *Example 19–1*, page 514.

(b) The liposomal preparation is found to contain a homogeneous population of $N = 52.7 \times 10^{14}$ liposome particles. The total volume of phospholipid, TVL_3 in the N liposomes of this three-lamellar preparation is calculated[10] knowing N and VL_3. The total volume of water TVW_3 entrapped in the N liposomes of this three-lamellar liposomal population is calculated using $N \times VW_3$.

(c) Calculate E, the *encapsulation ratio* of water to phospholipid (see p. 514, *Example 19–1*).

(d) Calculate the total surface area TSA_3 for the homogeneous population of three-lamella liposomes. The equation required is

$$TSA_3 = 4\pi N_3 R_3{}^2$$

The value for R_3 is 0.0447 and for N_3 is 52.7×10^{14}, as found in the accompanying table.

Data for *Problem 19–3*:

Parameters Used to Calculate Homogeneous Liposome Populations

n	1	2	3
R (μm)	0.0225	0.0336	0.0447
$VL_n \times 10^5$ μm^3	1.99	6.68	15.2
$LW_n \times 10^5$ μm^3	2.78	9.21	22.2
E	1.40	1.38	1.46
$N \times 10^{-14}$	404	120	52.7
$TSA \times 10^{-13}$ μm^2	25.7	17.0	13.2
$TVW \times 10^{-12}$ μm^3	1.12	1.11	1.17

**The table and equations in this problem are from reference 10.

Answers: **(a)** $VW_3 = 2.22 \times 10^{-4}$ μm^3; **(b)** $TVL_3 = 8.01 \times 10^{11}$ μm^3; **(c)** $E = 1.46$; **(d)** $TSA_3 = 1.32 \times 10^{14}$ μm^2

19–2. Lichtenberg and Markello[11] calculated the dimensions of a liposome in a way somewhat different from that used by Pidgeon and Hunt *(Problem 19–1)*. For a multilamellar vesicle—a liposome—of five bilayers (Fig. 19–29), the radius R_i of the outer surface of any of the bilayers, $i = 1$ to $i = 5$, is given by the equation of Lichtenberg and Markello[11]

$$R_i = R_1 - [(i-1)(45.7 + d)] \qquad (19-92)$$

in which R_1, the outermost radius of the liposome, is 5000 Å, the value 45.7 is the thickness in angstroms of each phospholipid bilayer, and $d = 60.0$ Å is the thickness of each aqueous shell separating the bilayers.

As observed in Figure 19–29, the serial number i of each bilayer is counted inward from the outermost bilayer, designated R_1.

(a) Using equation (19–92), obtain the values in angstroms for the radius of each of the phospholipid bilayers, R_2, R_3, R_4, and R_5.

PE, the *percent exposure*, is defined as the external surface area of the outermost bilayer, $4\pi R_1{}^2$, divided by the sum of the surface areas of the five bilayers, and multiplied by 100. The equation for *percent exposure* is

$$PE = \frac{R_1{}^2}{\sum\limits_{i=1}^{n} [R_1 - (i-1)(45.7 + d)]^2} \times 100 \qquad (19-93)$$

Counting from the outer phospholipid bilayer of radius R_1, the innermost bilayer radius is R_n, in which $n = 5$.

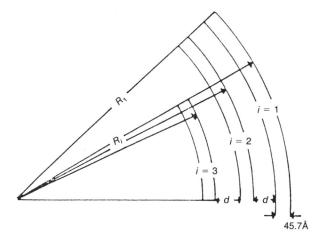

Fig. 19–29. Model of a liposome showing multilamellar (multilayer) structure of the lipid bilayers. R_1 stands for the outermost radius of the liposomal vesicle, i is the serial number of the bilayers running from $i = 1$ for the outermost bilayer, and d is the thickness of the aqueous layers interposed between the lipid bilayers. The authors have assumed that the thickness of each hydrated phospholipid bilayer is 45.7 Å, as shown at the bilayer labeled $i = 1$. (After D. Lichtenberg and T. Markello, J. Pharm. Sci. **73**, 122, 1984, reproduced with permission of the copyright owner.)

(b) Calculate the percent exposure PE for this liposome in which d is 60 Å. Note that a value 4π appears in both the numerator and denominator to obtain the surface area. These terms cancel and so do not appear in equation (19–93).

(c) The aqueous core of the liposome has a radius

$$R_n = R_5 = R_1 - [(45.7 \times n) + d(n-1)] \qquad (19-94)$$

in which $R_1 = 5000$ Å and $d = 60$ Å and the volume

$$V_n = V_5' = (4/3)\pi R_5^{3'}$$

Calculate the radius R_5' and the volume V_5' of the aqueous core of the liposome.

Answers: **(a)** $R_2 = 4894$ Å, $R_3 = 4789$ Å, $R_4 = 4683$ Å, $R_5 = 4577$ Å; **(b)** $PE = 4.36\%$; **(c)** $R_5' = 4532$ Å, $V_5' = 3.90 \times 10^{11}$ Å$^3 = 0.39$ μm^3

19–3. (a) The mean diameter of an ethylcellulose microsphere containing indomethacin was found by Benita et al.[169] using a projection microscope to be 340 μm (340×10^{-4} cm). What is the volume of the microsphere assuming it is roughly spherical?

(b) The density of the microsphere is 1.15 g/cm^3; calculate its mass in micrograms.

(c) The amount of indomethacin in the microsphere is 22.5% by weight. What is the total amount of the drug that can be released in 0.5 mL of buffer solution from the microsphere?

Answers: **(a)** 2.058×10^{-5} cm^3; **(b)** 23.67 μg; **(c)** 5.33 μg/0.5 mL or 10.66 μg/mL.

19–4. The polymer polylactide was used as a biodegradable controlled-release microcapsule for delivery of the narcotic antagonist cyclazocine. The molecular weight of polylactide in g/mole (daltons) may be determined using the Mark–Houwink equation

$$[\eta] = K M^a$$

in which $[\eta]$ is the intrinsic viscosity, 17.50 dL/g at 25° C, and the values of K and a for this class of polymers have been reported to be $K = 1.69 \times 10^{-3}$ dL/g and $a = 0.950$, respectively.

What is the molecular weight of the polylactide used to prepare the microcapsule? (*Note:* 1 dL = 0.1 liter = 100 mL.)

Answer: The molecular weight of this polylactide is 16,845 daltons = 16,845 g/mole ≅ 17,000 gram/mole.

19–5. The diffusion coefficient D of a new pilocarpine derivative in ocular fluid is 9.2×10^{-9} cm^2/sec. The surface area S of an Ocusert is

0.80 cm², the liquid-liquid partition coefficient K between the fluids of the Ocusert and the eye is 1.83, and the thickness of the Ocusert membrane, h, is 0.01 cm. The solubility of the drug in water, C_s, is 8.0 mg/cm³. Calculate the cumulative amount of pilocarpine released from an Ocusert in milligrams per 24-hour day. See *Example 19-8*.

Answer: 0.931 mg

19-6. The transcorneal permeation of pilocarpine at several pH values was studied at 34° C using an in vitro rabbit corneal preparation. The fraction of un-ionized pilocarpine, f_B, as a function of pH is found in the following table:

Data for *Problem 19-6**

pH	4.67	5.67	6.24	6.40
f_B	0.01	0.09	0.27	0.35

*Data from A. K. Mitra and T. J. Mikkelson, J. Pharm. Sci. **77**, 771, 1988.

The permeability coefficient of the nonionized form P_B is 9.733×10^{-6} cm/sec and the permeability coefficient of the ionized form is $P_{BH^+} = 4.836 \times 10^{-6}$ cm/sec. The concentration of pilocarpine in the donor compartment is constant, $C_d = 3.69 \times 10^{-5}$ mole cm⁻³.

(a) Compute the total permeability coefficient, $P = P_B f_B + P_{BH^+} f_{BH^+}$ and the total flux, $J = J_B + J_{BH^+} = PC_d$ for pilocarpine under steady-state conditions at the various pH values studied.

(b) Compute the amount of penetrant, M, through the corneal membrane at 30, 60, and 150 min at pH 6.4 for the ionized and the nonionized forms of pilocarpine. The diffusional area is $S = 0.95$ cm².

(c) Compute the lag time, t_L, in minutes at pH 4.67. The thickness of the membrane is $h = 0.022$ cm. *Hint:* Use the equations given in Chapter 13 to solve parts (b) and (c).

Partial Answer: **(a)** At pH 4.67, $P = 4.885 \times 10^{-6}$ cm/sec; $J = 1.80 \times 10^{-10}$ mole/(cm² sec); **(b)** At $t = 30$ min, $M_B = 2.15 \times 10^{-7}$ mole; $M_{BH^+} = 1.98 \times 10^{-7}$ mole; **(c)** $t_L = 13$ min

19-7. The nasal absorption of benzoic acid is influenced greatly by pH, the percent absorbed being large at low pH, i.e., pH 2 to 4, and the percent absorbed being small at high pH, i.e., pH 6 to 8. The observed absorption constant k_{obs} at low pH is given by equation (19-17), and at high pH values k_{obs} is given by equation (19-18). The ionization constant of benzoic acid $K_a = 6.30 \times 10^{-5}$, $pK_a = 4.2$. At a pH of 2.4, the observed first-order absorption rate constant,[170] k_{obs}, is 9.60×10^{-3} min⁻¹, and at pH 7.19, k_{obs} is 2.40×10^{-3} min⁻¹.

(a) Calculate k_{HA} and k_{A^-}, the specific first-order nasal absorption rate constants at pH 2.4 where benzoic acid is in the totally nonionized form, and at pH 7.19 where benzoic acid is in the totally ionized form.

(b) Using k_{HA} and k_{A^-} obtained in (a) above, calculate k_{obs} for the nasal absorption of benzoic acid at pH 8.2 and for absorption at pH = 3.0.

Answers: **(a)** $k_{HA} = 9.75 \times 10^{-3}$ min⁻¹; $k_{A^-} = 2.40 \times 10^{-3}$ min⁻¹; **(b)** k_{obs} at pH 3.0 = 9.17×10^{-3} min⁻¹; k_{obs} at pH 8.2 = 2.40×10^{-3} min⁻¹.

19-8. Nasal absorption has been considered to be facilitated by a carrier mechanism and therefore to follow the Michaelis-Menten scheme (pp. 293, 294). The Lineweaver-Burk equation (equation (12-68), p. 294),

$$\frac{1}{V} = \frac{1}{V_m} + \frac{K_m}{V_m}\frac{1}{S}$$

may be used for nasal absorption. V is the rate or velocity of absorption of a drug substance, V_m is the maximum velocity of absorption when the drug is at a high concentration and all the carrier is combined with it, S is the concentration of the drug, and K_m is the Michaelis constant that expresses the tendency of the carrier-drug to decompose.

The nasal absorption of the amino acid L-tyrosine was measured in a nasal in situ rat preparation at 37° C and a pH of 7.4; the data of Hussain et al.[170] as read from their graph is:

Data for *Problem 19-8*

$10^{-3} \times S^{-1}$ (concentration⁻¹)(M⁻¹)* of L-tyrosine	0.42	0.86	1.79	3.58
$10^{-3} \times V^{-1}$ (absorption rate⁻¹)(M⁻¹ hr)	3.19	4.62	5.72	8.00

*Note that the value 0.42, for example, expressed as $10^{-3} \times$ (concentration) is actually $0.42 \times 10^3 = 420$. And $3.580 \times 10^{-3} \times$ (concentration) means 3580. Likewise for the reciprocal concentration $S^{-1} = 3580$ in the table, V^{-1} is equal to 8.00×10^3 or 8000. That is to say, when the exponent on a unit in a table heading is negative, as in (mole/liter) $\times 10^{-3}$, the actual exponent is to be read 10^{+3}. When the exponent in the table heading is 10^{+3}, the actual exponent is read as 10^{-3}

(a) Using linear regression analysis, calculate V_m, the maximum rate of nasal absorption of L-tyrosine.

(b) Also from regression analysis, calculate the Michaelis constant K_m and give an interpretation of this constant in nasal absorption. (*Hint:* Return to the word-definition of K_m on page 294 and the formula $K_m = (k_2 + k_3)/k_1$.

(c) Plot the data on a rectangular coordinate graph and carry the straight line to a point where it intersects the *horizontal* axis, to the *left* of the vertical or *y*-axis. At this point, $-1/K_m$ may be read. Use the Lineweaver-Burk expression to show that this point on the horizontal axis provides the value, $-1/K_m$. (*Hint:* Set $1/V$, the value on the *y*-axis, equal to zero.) Finally, read the value $-1/K_m$ on the *x*-axis, invert it, and change the sign to obtain K_m. How does this value of K_m compare with K_m obtained from the slope of the line in (b) above?

(d) At a concentration $S = 4.26 \times 10^{-4}$ molar, such that $1/S = 2347$ M⁻¹, what is the absorption rate of L-tyrosine in molar concentration per hour?

Answers: **(a)** $V_m = 3.32 \times 10^{-4}$ M hr⁻¹; **(b)** $K_m = 4.75 \times 10^{-4}$ M; **(c)** $K_m = 4.74 \times 10^{-4}$ M; **(d)** $1/V = 6359.5$ M⁻¹ hr; $V = 1.57 \times 10^{-4}$ molar concentration per hour (mole/liter hr)

19-9.* An aerosol was administered to an isolated perfused rat lung preparation. Using equation (19-22), compute the particle transfer B at $t = 20$ min. The transferable amount, $A = 30$ μg, the respiratory frequency $RF = 14$ min⁻¹, the dose number $n = 20$ min $\times$ 14 cycles/min, and the rate constant $k = 0.058$ min⁻¹. (See *Example 19-11*.)

Answer: $B = 12.3$ μg

19-10. An aerosol was administered to an isolated perfused rat lung preparation. Compute the particle transfer B at $t = 40$ min. The transferable amount $A = 7.8$ μg, the respiratory frequency $RF = 14$ min⁻¹, the dose number $n = 280$, and the rate constant $k = 0.07$ min⁻¹. *Hint:* You will need equation (19-22) to compute B_{20} for $t = 20$ min, and use this value in equation (19-23) to obtain the value of B_{40} at $t = 40$ min.

Answer: $B_{40} = 3.61$ μg

19-11. A penicillin derivative has a K_a of 3.5×10^{-3} mole/liter at 25° C and a solubility C_s in the stationary layer of solvent in contact with the drug particle of 2.6×10^{-3} g/cm³. In the bulk phase of the solution, the concentration of drug, c_g is 1.7×10^{-4} g/cm³. The diffusion coefficient D of the drug in the medium is 6.8×10^{-7} cm²/sec, the total surface area S of the particles is 1.5×10^4 cm², and the thickness h of the stationary layer is 8.0×10^{-3} cm. Hoener and Benet[171] modified the Nernst-Brunner equation as follows:

$$\frac{dM}{dt} = \frac{DS}{h}\left\{ C_s\left(1 + \frac{K_a}{[H^+]}\right) - C_g \right\}$$

to calculate the dissolution rate of weak acids such as penicillin in solutions of increasing pH. Calculate the dissolution rate dM/dt of the penicillin derivative in solution of increasing pH that would occur in the stomach and the small intestine, viz., pH = 0, 1.0, 2.0, 3.0, 4.0,

*Problem 19-9 was prepared by Dr. P. R. Byron, Medical College of Virginia, Virginia Commonwealth University.

5.0, 6.0, and 7.0, and plot dM/dt versus pH on rectangular coordinate paper. You may also care to plot log (dM/dt) versus pH to obtain a much-improved curve.

Answer:

pH	0	1	2	3	4	5	6	7
(dM/dt) g/sec	0.003	.00321	.0042	.0147	0.119	1.163	11.6	116

19–12. A new drug, gastrogen, was developed to inhibit gastric acid secretion and was formulated into an osmotic gastrointestinal therapeutic system. The area S of the semipermeable membrane of the new dosage form is 2.0 cm^2, the membrane thickness h is 0.019 cm, the permeability coefficient K of the drug in gastric fluid is 5.0×10^{-6} cm^2/(atm hr), and the osmotic pressure π, provided by KCl in this osmotic pump-like dosage form, is 120 atm. The solubility of the drug in the gastric fluid C_s at 37° C is 750 mg/cm^3. What is the zero-order delivery rate of the drug in mg/hr from this system? Disregard any drug diffusion through the membrane. Use equation (19–50).

Answer: $(dM/dt)_z = 47.4$ mg/hr

19–13.* (a) A formulation scientist prepares a batch of 400-mg tablets (surface area $S = 2$ cm^2) and coats them to a 10% w/w loading with an enteric coating acidic polymer, HA. The pK_a of the polymer is 4.5 and its intrinsic solubility $[HA]_o = 6$ mg/mL. If these tablets are tested under simulated gastric conditions (pH = 1.5) and intestinal conditions (pH = 6.8) in well-buffered media, will they meet the specification criteria of staying intact in gastric conditions for at least 2 hours but disintegrating within 30 minutes in the intestine? Use equation (19–41) to compute the rate of dissolution, v of the polymer at sink conditions, where $C_{T,b} = 0$. The diffusion coefficient of the polymer is $D_p = 5 \times 10^{-8}$ cm^2/sec in aqueous media and the boundary layer thickness h is 50 μm. Assume that the coating remains intact until 90% has dissolved.

(b) If specification criteria are not accomplished with these tablets, what changes in the formulation can be used to meet specifications? *Hint:* The concentration of polymer at the surface–liquid interface, $C_{T,s}$, can be computed from equation (19–42) using the pH values given above.

Answers: (a) Polymer dissolution rate at gastric pH is 72×10^{-4} mg/min; at intestinal pH it is 1.44 mg/min. The time required for dissolution before the coating ruptures is 83 hr in the gastric medium and 25 minutes in the intestinal medium. The release meets specifications. (b) If release does not meet specifications, slightly less coating could be used. Or, a polymer that provides an enteric coating could be used with lower pK_a and/or higher solubility.

19–14. (a) Using equations (19–48) and (19–43), compute the surface pH value and the solubility, $C_{T,s}$, at the solid–liquid interface of papaverine, a weak base, in a matrix-type dosage form. The pH of the bulk is 3.0. The intrinsic solubility of the drug is $[B]_o = 3.08 \times 10^{-5}$ M, the dissociation constant of the conjugate acid is $K_a = 1.26 \times 10^{-6}$, and the diffusivities of the nonionized and ionized species are $D_B = D_{BH^-} = 6.8 \times 10^{-6}$ cm^2/sec, and $D_{H^+} = D_{OH^-} = 2.7 \times 10^{-5}$ cm^2/sec. Assume sink conditions, i.e., $[B] = [BH^+] = 0$. That is to say, in the sink the concentrations are reduced to zero. (Data from Ozturk et al.[101]). *Hint:* Use the values given in Table 19–1 for basic drugs to compute the terms a, b, and c in equation (19–48).

(b) Using equation (19–41), compute the in vitro rate of dissolution, v. The surface area of the matrix is 1.8 cm^2. The thickness of the aqueous layer is 100 μm. *Hint:* Use the diffusivity $D_B = 6.8 \times 10^{-6}$ cm^2/sec and the value $C_{T,s}$ obtained in part (a) in equation (19–41). Under sink conditions, $C_{T,b}$ in equation (19–41) is equal to zero. *Example 19–14* shows the calculations for an acidic drug.

Answers: (a) The pH at the surface is 3.85; $C_{T,s} = 3.47 \times 10^{-3}$ M; (b) $v = 4.25 \times 10^{-6}$ mole cm^{-2} sec^{-1}

19–15. The rate of delivery into a biologic system of a weak

electrolyte drug from an aqueous vehicle depends on the solubility and the ionization of the drug, which are functions of the pH. Roy and Flynn[173] studied the aqueous solubility of fentanyl, a synthetic analog of morphine, at 35° C and at various pH values. Fentanyl is a basic drug, and its equilibrium in water can be expressed as

$$BH^+ + H_2O \rightleftarrows B + H_3O^+$$

where B is the free base and BH$^+$ its conjugate acid. The pK_a of the conjugate acid is obtained from

$$pK_a = pH - \log \frac{[BH^+]}{[B]} \qquad (19\text{–}95)$$

Using the equation

$$pH = pK_a + \log \frac{S_o}{S - S_o} \qquad (19\text{–}96)$$

where S is the total solubility at a given pH value and S_o the solubility of the free base, B, independent of pH. Compute the solubility S of fentanyl at pH values 5.48 and 7.04. The pK_a value of the conjugate acid is 8.99 (obtained from solubility measurements), and the solubility S_o of the free base is 0.0099 mg/mL.

Answer: $S = 32$ mg/mL at pH 5.48, and $S = 0.89$ mg/mL at pH 7.04

19–16. From in situ perfusion experiments using the rat intestine, cephalexin, one of the cephalosporin antibiotics, is absorbed by a nonpassive mechanism involving a biochemical carrier that ferries the drug across the living membrane.[93] Michaelis–Menten kinetics, pages 293 to 294, was found useful in modeling the carrier-mediated absorption of the drug, as shown on pages 530 and 531.

(a) Compute the "intrinsic" (dimensionless) permeability $P_c^\star$ of the carrier, given that the maximum flux $J_{max}^\star$ is 9.1. The Michaelis constant, K_m is 7.2. Use equation (19–35).

(b) The following concentrations C_w of drug were found at the intestinal wall from a series of experiments: $C_w = 0.01, 0.05, 0.1, 5.0, 10.0, 50.0,$ and 100.0 mM. Compute the intrinsic intestinal wall permeability, $P_w^\star$, using equation (19–36) for a combination of carrier $P_c^\star$ and passive membrane $P_m^\star$ permeabilities, and the drug concentrations C_w given above. For cephalexin, $P_m^\star$ was found to be zero.

(c) Plot $P_w^\star$ (y-axis) against C_w. Is the relationship linear? Does a logarithmic relationship in C_w yield a straight line? How would you interpret the shape of this plot?

Partial Answer: (a) $P_c^\star = 1.264$; (b) $P_w^\star = 1.262$ for $C_w = 0.01$ mM; (c) Compare your graph with that given in Sinko and Amidon.[93]

19–17. (a) Calculate the intrinsic permeability $P_c^\star$ of the carrier-drug complex responsible for transporting the drug cephradine across the intestine. The values of $J_{max}^\star$ and K_m, obtained experimentally by Sinko and Amidon[93] for cephradine transport, are given as $J_{max}^\star = 1.60$; $K_m = 1.50$.

(b) Calculate the total permeability $P_w^\star$ of cephradine at the wall of the rat intestine when the gut wall concentration, C_w, has the values 0.10 mM, 7.2 mM, and 50 mM. The passive permeability $P_m^\star$ was found to be 0.30 for cephradine.

Answers: (a) $P_c^\star = 1.067$; (b) $P_w^\star = 1.300, 0.484, 0.331$

19–18. (a) Compute the Graetz number, Gz, for the human intestine using an intestinal length L of 500 cm, a volume flow rate V_m of 0.5 mL/min, and a diffusivity D of 5.0×10^{-6} cm^2/sec. What are the dimensions on Gz? The Graetz number is defined as $G_z = \pi DL/2V_m$, where π is the ratio of the circumference of a circle to its diameter.

(b) Compute the fractional dose F absorbed at the human intestine for the following wall permeability values. $\Gamma_w^\star = 0.5, 1, 1.5, 2, 2.5,$ and 3 (dimensionless quantities). The fractional dose absorbed is $F = 1 - ex(-4G_zP_w^\star)$.[95] Plot the results on a graph of F (y-axis) against $P_w^\star$. (Data from Amidon et al.[95])

Partial Answer: (a) $Gz = 0.47$; (b) For $P_w^\star = 0.50$, $F = 0.61$. See pages 530 to 531 to assist you in answering this problem.

19–19. Compute the pH at which the apparent absorption rate constant, K_{app}, of a cephalosporin is 0.173 min^{-1} as obtained by Prieto et al.[96] in the in situ rat intestinal technique. The weight of the rat is 248 g, the pK_a of the drug is 2.76, and the contributions of the nonionized and ionized forms of the drug to V_{app}, the apparent

---

**Problem 19–13* was prepared by Dr. J. B. Dressman, College of Pharmacy, University of Michigan.

absorption rate constant per metabolic weight unit, are $V_o = 57.312 \times 10^{-3}$ min^{-1} g^{-1} and $V_{-1} = 1.860 \times 10^{-3}$ min^{-1} g^{-1}, respectively. See *Example 19–13* and equations (19–38) and (19–39).

Answer: pH = 4.54

19–20. The approximate osmotic pressure π produced by a saturated phenobarbital sodium solution in an osmotic pump-like device is given by the equation

$$\pi = \nu \frac{C_s}{M} RT$$

in which ν is the number of particles into which a molecule of phenobarbital sodium ionizes, namely about 2. The saturation concentration (solubility) of phenobarbital at ordinary temperatures is $C_s = 100$ g/liter. The molecular weight of the drug M is 254.2 g/mole, R is 0.082 liter atm mole^{-1} deg^{-1}, and T is 310° K for body temperature on the Kelvin scale.

Calculate the osmotic pressure produced by the drug (exclusive of any added osmotic agent mixed with the drug) using the equation just given.

Answer: 20 atm

19–21. If the new drug, gastrogen, has a diffusion coefficient $D = 6.3 \times 10^{-6}$ cm^2/sec at 37° C, and the path length L of the orifice in the osmotic pump-type dosage form is 10×10^{-4} cm, what is the maximum size S_{max}, (diameter in μm) of the orifice for proper delivery of the drug from the device? $C_s = 750$ mg/cm^3 at 37° C in the gastric fluid. Assume the dimensionless sizing factor f has a value of 50, and the zero-order delivery rate $(dM/dt)_z$ is 35 mg/hr at body temperature. *Note:* D must be in cm^2/hr. See the calculations of S_{max} on p. 536 where $(dM/dt)_z$ is given.

Answer: 72.5 μm diameter

19–22. Compute the radius of the pores in the colonic mucosa after treatment with the enhancer, sodium laurate, at 37° C. The ratio of the osmotic water permeability coefficient to the permeability coefficient of tritiated water through the membrane, P_f/P_d, is 17.48. The viscosity and diffusion coefficient of water at 37° C are 6.915×10^{-3} poise and 3.24×10^{-5} cm^2/sec, respectively. The molar volume of water is 18.14 cm^3/mole at 37° C and the radius a_w of the water molecule is 1.5 Å. The gas constant R is 8.3143×10^7 erg deg^{-1} mole^{-1} (Data from Tomita et al.[125]). See *Example 19–16*, page 538 and equations (19–58) and (19–59).

Answer: Pore radius $r = 13.1$ Å

19–23. The total flux, J, of an acidic drug through the skin at several pH values is given by the equation

$$J = P_{HA}[HA] + P_{A^-}[A^-]$$

where P_{HA} and P_{A^-} are the permeability coefficients of the nonionized HA and ionized A$^-$ species, respectively. The concentration of the ionized species, [A$^-$], can be computed from the equation

$$[A^-] = \frac{10^{(pH - pK_a)}}{1 + 10^{(pH - pK_a)}} [T]$$

where [T] = [A$^-$] + [HA] is the total concentration of ionized A$^-$ and nonionized HA species.

Fleeker et al.[135] studied the diffusion of an acidic drug, indomethacin (see Fig. 11–6) through hydrated snake skin as a biologic membrane at pH 7.0 and 32° C. The pK_a of indomethacin is 4.5.

(a) Calculate the total flux J of indomethacin at pH 7. The total concentration [T] of indomethacin at pH 7 is 916.6 μg/mL and the permeability coefficients are $P_{HA} = 3.62 \times 10^{-3}$ cm/hr and $P_{A^-} = 2.19 \times 10^{-5}$ cm/hr.

(b) In a second experiment the snake skin was pretreated with dodecyl N, N-dimethylamino acetate, a new enhancer. The permeability coefficients of indomethacin were found to be $P_{HA} = 3.90 \times 10^{-3}$ cm/hr and $P_{A^-} = 7.97 \times 10^{-4}$ cm/hr in the presence of the enhancer. The total concentration of indomethacin and the pH were kept unchanged, [T] = 916.6 μg/mL and pH = 7. [A$^-$] is calculated using the equation above, together with the equation [HA] = [T] − [A$^-$]. Compute the total flux of indomethacin in the presence of the enhancer.

(c) Using the flux values obtained in (a) and (b) compute the amount of indomethacin penetrated per unit area, Q (μg/cm^2) = Jt, at $t = 5$ hr and $t = 20$ hr. Plot Q (y-axis) against time (x-axis).

Answers: **(a)** J (without enhancer) = 0.0305 μg/(cm^2 hr); **(b)** J (after treatment with enhancer) = 0.739 μg/(cm^{2}hr).

19–24. Compute the permeability coefficients P_{HA} and P_{A^-} for the nonionized and ionized forms of Chromocarb, a chromone-2-carboxylic acid, through excised human skin at 37° C. Chromocarb is under clinical trial as a capillary protectant is diabetes. The ratios of the flux to the concentration of ionized form, $J/[A^-]$ at three pH values, are:

Data for *Problem 19–24*

pH	5	6	7
$J/[A^-] \times 10^5$ (cm/hr)	158	48	7.3

The pK_a of the compound is 1.93. P_{HA} and P_{A^-} are computed using equation (19–75) together with linear regression of $J/[A^-]$ against [H$^+$]. Is the drug more liable to penetrate the skin in the ionized or nonionized form?

Answer: $P_{HA} = 1.639$ cm/hr; $P_{A^-} = 19.3 \times 10^{-5}$ cm/hr

19–25. Compute the solubility C of desoxycorticosterone in the stratum corneum using the following data obtained from in vitro experiments with intact and stripped mouse skin (data from Table II in reference 132). The lag times across the intact and stripped skin are $t_2 = 3.90$ hr and $t_1 = 1.20$ hr; the permeation rates are $(dQ/dt)_2 = 4.73$ μg/(cm^2 hr) and $(dQ/dt)_1 = 12.1$ μg/(cm^2 hr). The thickness, h$_2$, of the stratum corneum is 10 μm. See *Example 19–19*.

Answer: $C = 32.3$ mg/mL

19–26.* When a penetration enhancer was used, the lipid–protein partition coefficient of the new drug referred to in *Example 19–18* increased by 100-fold, the other properties remaining unchanged. Using the random brick model and the data given in *Example 19–18*, calculate the flux and the per cent increase in the flux due to the action of the enhancer.

Partial Answer: The flux J is 0.038 μg/(cm^2 sec)

19–27. The in vitro binding of vasopressin using rat skin at 30° C was analyzed according to the Langmuir approach (pp. 380–382). The following results were found (data calculated from the constants given in P. S. Banerjee and W. A. Ritschel[136]):

Data for *Problem 19–27*

$c/(x/m)$(mL^{-1} mg)	c (μg/mL)
21.32	10
21.46	20
21.60	30
21.87	50
22.15	70
22.57	100
23.27	150

(a) using equation (19–76) together with regression analysis, compute the *affinity constant b* (mL/μg) of vasopressin for adsorption on the skin, and the *maximum adsorption capacity* y_m (μg/mg).

(b) Do you believe that the authors were justified in using an

---

Problem 19–26 was prepared by Dr. K. Tojo, Kyushu Institute of Technology, Kyushu, Japan.

adsorption model and the Langmuir equation to study the binding of vasopressin to the proteins in the skin?

Answers: **(a)** $b = 6.56 \times 10^{-4}$ mL/µg; $Y_m = 71.94$ µg/mg; **(b)** Review the section on protein binding, Chapter 11, to answer this question.

19–28. K. Hirano and H. Yamada[164] studied the subcutaneous absorption of *p*-hydroxyazobenzene from aqueous suspensions. The ratios of the cube root of drug amount W at the subcutaneous injection site to the applied dose, W_o, at several times are given in the table:

Data for *Problem 19–28*

$(W/W_o)^{1/3}$	1	0.958	0.916	0.874	0.832
t (hr)	0	1.0	2.0	3.0	4.0

(a) Plot $(W/W_o)^{1/3}$ (y-axis) against t and compute the absorption rate constant, k, from the slope using equation (19–88). You can also use regression analysis to obtain k.

(b) Compute k from equation (19–89), (page 547) given the solubility of *p*-hydroxyazobenzene, $C_s = 0.034$ mg/mL, and substitute the k value into equation (19–88) to predict $(W/W_o)^{1/3}$. If the initial dose W_o is 2.5 mg, what is the remaining amount W after 5 hours?

(c) According to the authors, equation (19–89) allows one to compute the absorption rate constant for drugs in suspension having similar particle size and sedimentation volume. Using equation (19–89), calculate k for betamethasone ($C_s = 0.002$ mgmL), sulfamethoxazole ($C_s = 5.7$ mg/mL), and *p*-aminoazobenzene ($C_s = 0.049$ mg/mL). The experimental k values are 0.0096, 0.374, and 0.065 hr^{-1}, respectively. How well do your calculated k values agree with the experimental values?

Answers: **(a)** $k = 0.042$ hr^{-1}; **(b)** $k = 0.045$ hr^{-1}; after 5 hr, $W = 1.16$ mg; **(c)** betamethasone, $k = 0.010$; sulfamethoxazole, $k = 0.659$; *p*-aminoazobenzene, $k = 0.054$ hr^{-1}

20
Polymer Science*

HISTORICAL BACKGROUND

High polymers found technologic applications many years before their nature was understood. Early practical applications included the mercerization of cotton (treatment of yarn with cold strong caustic to produce shrinkage and increase its strength and affinity for dyes) (John Mercer, 1844); the nitration of cellulose to Pyroxylin USP (Braconnot, 1833) and to guncotton (Schoenbein, 1847); the molding of nitrated cellulose plasticized with camphor, called *celluloid*, into billiard balls and detachable collars (Hyatt, 1868); the extrusion of collodion through spinnerettes followed by denitrification of the resulting filaments (Chardonnet, 1886); the acetylation of cellulose (Schuetzenberger, 1870); and the formation of the water-soluble cellulose derivatives xanthate (Cross and Bevan, 1893) and cuprammonium cellulose (Schweizer, 1857), eventually leading to the production of regenerated cellulose fibers and films (viscose and Bemberg rayon, cellophane film).

Goodyear discovered the vulcanization of rubber by sulfur in 1839. Fully synthetic resins from phenol and formaldehyde, called *bakelite*, were manufactured by Baekeland beginning in 1910.

Recognition of the chemical nature of polymers began only in the early 1920s, when Staudinger concluded, from research on natural rubber, starch, and cellulose, that these compounds consisted of giant chains of carbon atoms (plus oxygen atoms in the case of the two polysaccharides) held together by covalent bonds. They were truly macromolecules. This notion was met with disbelief and even ridicule by many of his contemporaries. Not until the 1930s, when linear polymers were being synthesized, especially by W. H. Carothers in the Du Pont laboratories, did Staudinger's concept gain universal acceptance—a prime example of delayed recognition. The Nobel prize in chemistry was finally awarded to Staudinger in 1953.

Mark[1] and Flory,[2] pioneers in the physical chemistry of polymers in the solid state and in solution, were active until their recent deaths. The bulk of their work

*This chapter was prepared by Dr. Hans Schott, Professor of Pharmaceutical and Colloid Chemistry, Temple University, School of Pharmacy, Philadelphia, PA.

was done in the last 45 years, and Flory received the Nobel prize in chemistry in 1974. Likewise, nearly all of the information in this chapter was developed after 1940.

PHARMACEUTICAL APPLICATIONS OF POLYMERS

With the inclusion of tests and standards for high-density polyethylene and other plastics in the twentieth revision of the U.S. Pharmacopeia, polymers have officially entered the world of pharmacy. Actually, pharmacists have been employing polymers in every aspect of their work for many years. Typical examples are polyethylene and polyolefin bottles, polystyrene vials, rubber closures, rubber and plastic tubing for injection sets, and flexible bags of plasticized polyvinyl chloride to hold blood and intravenous solutions. Barrels and plungers of hypodermic syringes are made of polypropylene or, when optical clarity is required, of polycarbonate. Unit-dose packaging makes use of unplasticized polyvinyl chloride for cups and trays, laminates of polyethylene with aluminum or cellophane, and polyester film for strip-package or blister-package containers.

Among the water-soluble polymers used to coat tablets are hydroxypropyl methylcellulose and hydroxypropylcellulose, polyethylene glycol, povidone, and sodium carboxymethylcellulose. Some of these polymers are also used as binders for tabletting granulations, as are acacia, gelatin, and sodium alginate. Ethylcellulose, being insoluble in water, is combined with water-soluble polymers to influence the dissolution rate of the coating film. Cellulose acetate phthalate, hydroxypropyl methylcellulose phthalate, and copolymers of methacrylic acid and its esters, Eudragit, are used for enteric coating of tablets. Starch as a tablet disintegrant has been joined recently by carboxymethyl starch of low substitution and by cross-linked povidone. All three polymers are insoluble but swell rapidly and extensively in water.

A wide variety of synthetic and natural polymers are used to thicken suspensions and ophthalmic solutions, as protective colloids to stabilize emulsions and suspensions and to form water-soluble jellies and ointment bases. Gelatin has the widest range of applications in the pharmaceutical field. It is the major constituent of hard and soft capsules, in addition to being used as a suppository base, as an emulsifying and suspending agent, for absorbable films, powders and sponges, as a boot in combination with zinc oxide, and for microencapsulation in combination with acacia.

Sustained-release dosage forms employ polymers as shells for microencapsulated drugs, as erodible and nonerodible matrices, as barrier membranes to regulate the release of drugs by diffusion, as ion-exchange resins, as reagents to form slightly soluble salts with basic drugs (tannic and polygalacturonic acids), and as backbones for pendent drug molecules attached by labile bonds.

In addition to polymers being used as excipients, some drugs themselves are polymers, including insulin, heparin and its antagonist, protamine sulfate, the plasma expanders dextran and normal human serum albumin, and the bulk laxatives methylcellulose and sodium carboxymethylcellulose. In addition, there is polycarbophil, which binds fecal water to decrease the fluidity of diarrheal stools. The anion-exchange resins colestipol hydrochloride and cholestyramine bind and increase the fecal excretion of bile salts to lower the blood cholesterol level.

Thus, it is seen that polymers are essential to the dispensing pharmacist, to the manufacturing pharmacist, and to the research pharmacist.

DEFINITIONS[3-7]

As Staudinger recognized, carbon atoms can bond to one another, forming the backbone of linear polymers via long chains of covalently bonded carbon atoms. Silicon and sulfur possess the same ability. Such *homochain* polymers have the following backbone structures:

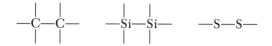

Heterochain polymers contain other atoms in the backbone. Examples include

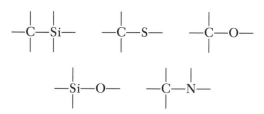

and even purely inorganic polymers such as polymetaphosphate (Calgon)

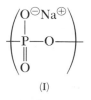

(I)

and polyphosphonitrilic chloride,

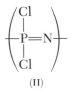

(II)

When vinylpyrrolidone, a *monomer*, is polymerized, it forms the *linear polymer* polyvinylpyrrolidone (Povidone USP), a protective colloid capable of complexing iodine and whose aqueous solutions form strong films on drying.

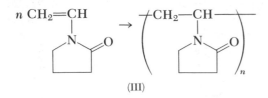

(III)

The structure between parentheses represents the *repeat unit* or *mer*. The number n of repeat units per macromolecule is called the *degree of polymerization* (*DP*).

The polymerization of such vinyl compounds is called an *addition* or *chain-reaction polymerization*. The process is most often started by a free radical formed by the thermal decomposition of an *initiator* such as benzoyl peroxide. Such a

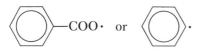

free radical adds to the double bond of a vinyl monomer, opening it and producing another compound with an unpaired electron:

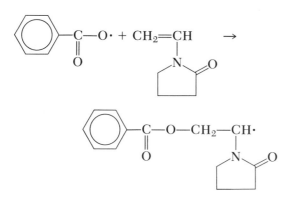

The free radical propagates rapidly as $n - 1$ other monomer molecules add successively to the growing chain, forming the polymer of Structure III.

Condensation or *stepwise polymerization* is illustrated by the formation of polyethylene terephthalate, a polyester used to form fibers and films:

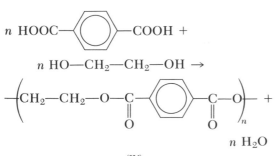

(IV)

This polyesterification reaction proceeds stepwise, and the molecular weight of the polymer increases gradually as the steam formed is vented from the reactor.

Homopolymers consist of a single monomer, such as Structures I to III; *copolymers* incorporate two or more monomers. Many naturally occurring polymers such as cellulose and natural rubber are homopolymers, but proteins are copolymers of different amino acids.

One of the many polyolefins is a resin for containers used to store parenteral solutions. It is a *random copolymer* of ethylene (*E*) and propylene (*P*): The two repeat units follow no particular sequence in the chain, for example, —*PPEPEEPEPP*—.

In *alternating copolymers* such as polypropylene sulfone, made by the copolymerization of propylene and sulfur dioxide, the two mers alternate:

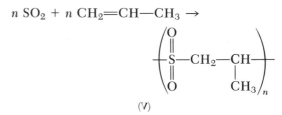

(V)

Block copolymers contain long sequences of the same mer. For instance, the fecal softener poloxalkol is a block copolymer of ethylene oxide and propylene oxide:

$$HO\text{---}(CH_2\text{---}CH_2O)_a\left(CH\text{---}CH_2O\right)_b(CH_2\text{---}CH_2O)_c H$$
$$\hspace{3cm} | \hspace{2cm} CH_3$$

(VI)

The *monomer functionality* determines whether a polymer is formed by a reaction and whether this polymer is linear, branched, or a network (or cross-linked) polymer. Acetic acid and ethanol are monofunctional, that is, each molecule possesses one reactive functional group. Their esterification produces only another monomer, ethyl acetate. Ethylene glycol and phthalic acid are bifunctional monomers, and their esterification produces the linear polymer IV. When ethylene glycol is partially or completely replaced by the trifunctional monomer glycerin, a cross-linked or network polymer is produced that is insoluble and infusible and is therefore called *thermosetting*. Small amounts of glycerin produce a branched structure.

Most linear and branched polymers are *thermoplastic*, that is, they can be softened or melted by heat and dissolved in appropriate solvents. Linear (a), branched (b), and network or cross-linked polymers (c) can be represented schematically as in Figure 20–1.

In network polymers, such as the polyesters produced by the condensation of *glyc*erin (trifunctional) and *phthal*ic anhydride (bifunctional), called *glyptals*, each macroscopic object consists of a single molecule because each atom in the object is bound to every other atom through covalent bonds.

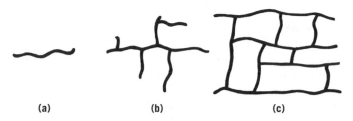

Fig. 20–1. Schematic illustration of branching and cross-linking.

Vinyl monomers are bifunctional since the carbon–carbon double bond can be considered to contain two unpaired electrons:

$$\cdot CH_2\!\!-\!\!CH\cdot$$
$$\underset{X}{|}$$

During free-radical chain polymerizations, a free radical can abstract a hydrogen atom from an existing chain, producing another free radical that can grow into a *branch* through the addition of monomer molecules. Ionizing radiation can also introduce such free radicals into a polymer, and a second monomer can be grafted onto a polymeric substrate after irradiation. For instance, irradiating polyethylene film or molded objects with gamma rays followed by exposure to acrylic acid results in the *grafting* of polyacrylic acid branches onto the polyethylene substrate, rendering the polyethylene surface hydrophilic:

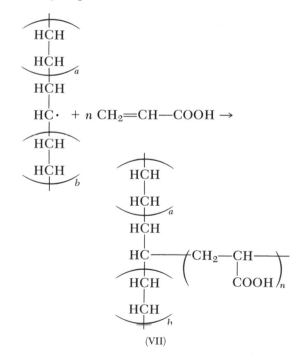

(VII)

This structure represents a *graft copolymer*.

Network copolymers that are monographs in the USP/NF include the cation–exchange resin sodium polystyrene sulfonate, used to remove excess potassium ions and the anion–exchange resin choles-

tyramine, used to remove bile salts, croscarmellose sodium, and crospovidone. The last two products are cross-linked carboxymethylcellulose sodium and povidone. Their linear analogs are water-soluble. The cross-linked polymers are insoluble but swell fast and extensively in aqueous media, including gastric juice. These powders, with average particle size of the order of 50 μm, are incorporated into tablets at about 2% as disintegrants.

Sodium polystyrene sulfonate, a polyelectrolyte, is soluble in water. To make it insoluble in water, styrene (a bifunctional monomer) is copolymerized with a small percentage of divinylbenzene (a tetrafunctional monomer). After sulfonation and neutralization, the structure of the resin is

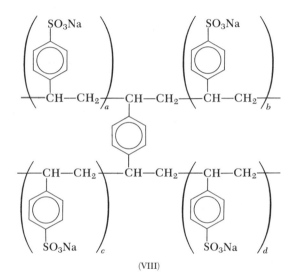

(VIII)

The two linear chains *ab* and *cd* are tied together by the phenylene cross-link. In a grain of ion-exchange resin, all polystyrene sulfonate chains are thus tied together into a single network. The influx of aqueous gastrointestinal fluid swells the grain until the phenylene cross-links are strained, so that the fluid freely permeates the swollen grain and exchanges its K^+ with the Na^+ of the resin. The grain does not dissolve because it consists of a network of covalent carbon–carbon bonds holding together all repeat units and chains.

Polycarbophil, a monograph (see calcium polycarbophil, in the U.S.P. XXII), is polyacrylic acid lightly cross-linked with divinyl glycol,

$$H_2C\!\!=\!\!CH\!\!-\!\!\underset{OH}{\overset{|}{CH}}\!\!-\!\!\underset{OH}{\overset{|}{CH}}\!\!-\!\!CH\!\!=\!\!CH_2$$

Each particle consists of a single molecule because of its network structure. Swelling in the acid gastric fluid is minimal because the carboxylic acid groups are not ionized. In the neutral to slightly alkaline intestinal fluids, particularly of the colon, the carboxylic acid groups become ionized, making the polymer a *polyelectrolyte*. The schematic structure of two chains of polyacrylic acid in the ionized form, tied together by one divinyl glycol cross-link, is as shown:

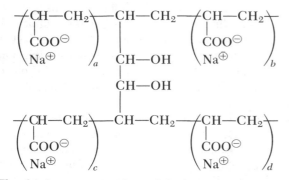

The high concentration of ionic groups inside the carbophil particles causes a large influx of water by osmosis, swelling the particles until the cross-links are strained. The cross-links prevent the dissolution of the sodium polyacrylate chains, however. Each grain, when fully swollen, absorbs 50 to 65 times its weight in water, decreasing the fluidity of liquid stool in diarrheal disorders.

Two definitions pertain to cellulose and starch derivatives. The anhydroglucose repeat unit has three hydroxyl groups, namely, the primary hydroxyl on the Number 6 carbon atom, which is the first to react during substitution reactions, and two secondary hydroxyls on the Number 2 and 3 carbon atoms. Cellulose is a linear polymer consisting of D(+)-glucose residues,

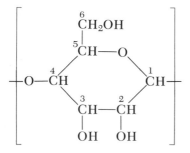

that are linked by β-1,4 glycosidic bonds.

The *degree of substitution (DS)* represents the number of hydroxyl groups per anhydroglucose repeat unit that have been substituted, for example, methylated, carboxymethylated, oxyethylated, acetylated, and so on. *DS* values range from 0 to 3.00 and are usually not integer numbers because they represent average values over an entire sample.

Molar substitution (MS) in hydroxyethyl cellulose is the average number of ethylene oxide molecules that have reacted with one anhydroglucose repeat unit. After an ethylene oxide molecule has added onto one of the three hydroxyl groups, the resulting hydroxyethyl group can add more ethylene oxide molecules in competition with the remaining two glucose hydroxyls. While the *MS* is known from the weight increase of the cellulose sample or from the consumption of ethylene oxide, the *DS* of hydroxyethyl cellulose is usually not known. For commercial hydroxyethyl cellulose, the *MS*

is usually in the range of 1.8 to 2.3. This value may correspond to a *DS* of 0.9 to 1.0, indicating that most of the ethoxylation took place on one hydroxyl group, probably the primary hydroxyl group of the Number 6 carbon atom, each of which added two ethylene oxide molecules on the average.

Molar substitution is used instead of degree of substitution whenever the substitution reaction in cellulose produces hydroxylated derivatives. *MS* values can exceed 3.00. Some grades of hydroxypropyl cellulose, produced by the ring-opening addition of propylene oxide to alkali cellulose, have an *MS* of 4.0 and above.

MOLECULAR WEIGHT AVERAGES[8,9]

Small molecules and many biopolymers are *monodisperse*, that is, all molecules of a given pure compound have the same molecular weight. All sucrose molecules weigh 342.30 g divided by Avogadro's number; all molecules of human serum albumin weigh 69,000 g divided by Avogadro's number.

In synthetic polymerization reactions such as III to V, no two chains grow equally fast or for the same length of time. The resultant macromolecules are *heterodisperse*, that is, they have different chain lengths and a range of molecular weights, which can be described by an average molecular weight and by a molecular weight distribution.

The problem of choosing a meaningful average value for the molecular weight is identical to that encountered in micromeritics (Chapter 16). Take the simple example of a batch of polystyrene made up of two monodisperse or homogeneous fractions, Fraction *A* with a molecular weight of 1000 and Fraction *B* with a molecular weight of 100,000. The low-molecular-weight fraction *A*, with a *DP* of 9 to 10, is called an *oligomer*. Assuming that the batch contains an equal number of molecules n or an equal mole fraction X of the two polystyrene fractions: $n_A = n_B$ and

$$X_A = \frac{n_A}{n_A + n_B} = X_B = \frac{n_B}{n_A + n_B} = 0.500$$

The average molecular weight $\overline{M}$, based on the number of molecules present, should be

$$\overline{M} = (0.500)(1000) + (0.500)(100,000)$$

$$= \frac{1000 + 100,000}{2} = 50,500 \qquad (20-1)$$

One can argue, however, that this averaging procedure gives an unrealistic value because each small molecule *A* affects $\overline{M}$ just as strongly as each large molecule *B* even though it weighs only 1% of *B*. Only 1% of the weight of the sample consists of molecules *A* with a molecular weight of 1000 while 99% of the weight consists of molecules *B* of molecular weight 100,000.

Therefore, based on the weight fraction w of A and B present, the average molecular weight should more realistically be expressed as

$$\overline{M} = (0.01)(1000) + (0.99)(100,000) = 99,010 \qquad (20-2)$$

The former molecular weight average is called the *number-average* molecular weight, $\overline{M}_n$. It is obtained by adding the molecular weight of each molecule or mole in the sample and dividing by the total number of molecules or moles. The latter molecular weight average is called the *weight-average* molecular weight, $\overline{M}_w$. It is an average weighted according to the weight fraction w (or the w/v concentration in solution) of each molecule or mole.

Mathematically, the general expression is

$$\overline{M}_b = \frac{\Sigma w_i M_i^b}{\Sigma w_i M_i^{b-1}} = \frac{\Sigma N_i M_i^{b+1}}{\Sigma N_i M_i^b} \qquad (20-3)$$

in which the weight fraction w_i of the ith monodisperse fraction, with the homogeneous molecular weight M_i, is equal to the number of molecules n_i or of moles N_i times M_i divided by the total weight of the sample, namely, by $\Sigma n_i M_i$ or $\Sigma N_i M_i$, respectively. b is an integer whose value specifies the particular average of M.

If $b = 0$, the number-average molecular weight results. Keeping in mind that $\Sigma w_i = 1$ and $\Sigma X_i = 1$, equation (3) becomes

$$\overline{M}_n = \frac{1}{\Sigma w_i/M_i} = \frac{\Sigma N_i M_i}{\Sigma N_i} = \Sigma X_i M_i \qquad (20-4)$$

This equation is comparable to the first equation in Table 16–3 and pertains to a number-average distribution.

To calculate $\overline{M}_n$ for the bimodal polystyrene sample, the most convenient term in equation (20–4) is the expression in X_i that was already used in equation (20–1). To use the expression in w_i, one must calculate w_A and w_B. Assume that the sample consists of two molecules of A and two of B. Then

$$w_A = \frac{(2)(1000)}{(2)(1000) + (2)(100,000)} = 0.009901$$

and

$$w_B = \frac{(2)(100,000)}{(2)(1000) + (2)(100,000)} = 0.990099$$

As a check, $w_A + w_B = 1.000000$. Then, from the term containing w_i in equation (20–4):

$$\overline{M}_n = \frac{1}{\dfrac{0.009901}{1000} + \dfrac{0.990099}{100,000}} = 50,500$$

The number-average molecular weight is influenced especially by the low-molecular-weight fraction in a polymer. Experimentally, it is determined by end-group analysis and from the colligative properties, especially osmotic pressure (Chapter 5).

If $b = 1$ in equation (20–3) the weight-average molecular weight results:

$$\overline{M}_w = \Sigma w_i M_i = \frac{\Sigma N_i M_i^2}{\Sigma N_i M_i} = \frac{\Sigma X_i M_i^2}{\Sigma X_i M_i} \qquad (20-5)$$

This equation is comparable to $\Sigma nd^2/\Sigma nd$ in Table 16–3 and pertains to the weight-average distribution. For the polystyrene sample, using the term in X_i from equation (20–5) gives

$$\overline{M}_w = \frac{(0.500)(1000)^2 + (0.500)(100,000)^2}{(0.500)(1000) + (0.500)(100,000)} = 99,020$$

Using the term in w_i gives

$$\overline{M}_w = (0.009901)(1000) + (0.990099)(100,000) = 99,020$$

Since the molecules contribute to the weight-average molecular weight of a polymer in direct proportion to their weight in the sample, this average is especially sensitive to high-molecular-weight fractions, for example, to a lightly cross-linked fraction in an otherwise linear polymer.

Another molecular weight average, the z-average, is obtained by setting $b = 2$ in equation (20–3):

$$\overline{M}_z = \frac{\Sigma w_i M_i^2}{\Sigma w_i M_i} = \frac{\Sigma N_i M_i^3}{\Sigma N_i M_i^2} = \frac{\Sigma X_i M_i^3}{\Sigma X_i M_i^2} \qquad (20-6)$$

$\overline{M}_z$ is obtained from sedimentation equilibrium measurements in the ultracentrifuge. For the bimodal polystyrene sample, $M_z = 99,990$.

There are number-average and weight-average degrees of polymerization to match the number-average and weight-average molecular weights. For instance, if a povidone sample has $\overline{M}_w = 70,000$, then $\overline{DP}_w = 70,000 \div 111.1 = 630$. The molecular weight of the repeat unit, which is also the molecular weight of the vinylpyrrolidone monomer, is 111.1.

From their definitions, it follows that $\overline{M}_z \geq \overline{M}_w \geq \overline{M}_n$ and $\overline{M}_w/\overline{M}_n = \gg 1$. This ratio is a measure of the polydispersity of a polymer sample. Many biopolymers are monodisperse; for them, the ratio $\overline{M}_w/\overline{M}_n$ is unity. For vinyl polymers made by solution polymerization to high conversion, the ratio is in the 2 to 5 range. For vinyl polymers made by bulk polymerization, the ratio is frequently about 10. Gel permeation chromatography is used for analytic and preparative polymer fractionation. Fractional precipitation, described in the following, is also used.

MOLECULAR WEIGHT DETERMINATION FROM SOLUTION VISCOSITY[10,11]

Staudinger predicted and found, with solutions of cellulose derivatives, that the reduced viscosity of a polymer is proportional to its molecular weight. Reduced viscosity is specific viscosity divided by concentration (equation (15–22)). His observations were modified by Mark and Houwink and by the theoretic analysis of W. Kuhn. The reduced viscosity was replaced by the intrinsic viscosity or limiting viscosity number [η], which is the reduced viscosity extrapolated to infinite dilution. The proportionality of [η] is to a power, a, of the molecular weight usually between 0.5 and 1.1. The most common a values are between 0.6 and 0.8.

$$[\eta] = \lim_{c \to 0} \frac{\eta_{12} - \eta_1}{c\eta_1} = \lim_{c \to 0} \frac{\eta_{sp}}{c} \qquad (20-7)$$

in which η_{12} is the viscosity of the solution of concentration c, η_1 is the viscosity of the solvent, and η_{sp} is the specific viscosity defined by equation (15–20). Since concentration in polymer viscometry is usually expressed in grams of polymer per deciliter of solution (1 dL = 0.1 liter = 100 mL or cm^3), corresponding to % w/v, [η] is given in units of dL/g. In colloid chemistry, [η] is usually expressed in mL/g.

If Einstein's law of viscosity is obeyed, [η] = 0.025 dL/g. This value is approximated by globular proteins at the isoelectric point and by polymer latexes. Most polymer molecules in solution, including denatured proteins, assume the shape of voluminous random coils. For them, [η] is one to four orders of magnitude larger.

The modified Staudinger equation, often called the Mark–Houwink equation (equation (15–24)) is

$$[\eta] = KM^a \qquad (20-8)$$

The parameters K and a are constant for a given polymer–solvent combination at a given temperature. The exponent a usually has values between 0.5 and 0.8. K values are in the 0.2×10^{-4} to 8×10^{-4} dL/g range. For instance, for polyvinyl alcohol in water at 30° C, $K = 4.28 \times 10^{-4}$ dL/g and $a = 0.64$. Extensive tabulations of K and a values for many polymers in different solvents at different temperatures have been published.[12]

The values of K and a are determined by calibration measurements, using polymer fractions of known molecular weight (see *Problem 20–6*). Thus, viscosity measurements do not afford absolute molecular weight determinations like osmometry, light scattering, or ultracentrifugation. Because of the simplicity of the equipment and speed and accuracy of the measurements, [η] determination is the method most widely and routinely used to determine polymer molecular weights.

The viscosity-average molecular weight, $\overline{M}_v$, lies between the weight-average and the number-average value. It is closer to the former, often being 10 to 20% below $\overline{M}_w$.

$$\overline{M}_v = (\Sigma w_i M_i^a)^{1/a} = \left(\frac{\Sigma N_i M_i^{a+1}}{\Sigma N_i M_i} \right)^{1/a} \qquad (20-9)$$

For a polydisperse sample, M in the Mark–Houwink equation, equation (20–8), is replaced by $\overline{M}_v$. For $a = 1$, $\overline{M}_v = \overline{M}_w$ as given by equation (20–5).

Viscosities of dilute solutions are measured in glass capillary viscometers. Experimental precautions include working in constant-temperature baths regulated to ±0.02° C and using efflux times of at least 200 seconds. Slow flow rates obviate the kinetic energy correction, minimize end effects, and give essentially zero-shear viscosities, that is, the flow occurs in the lower Newtonian region, and the solution viscosity is independent of the efflux time t. A special glass capillary viscometer with a series of bulbs permits measurement of the apparent viscosity at a series of shear rates and extrapolation to zero shear.

For accurate extrapolation to zero concentration, solution concentrations are usually chosen to give relative viscosities between 1.1 and 1.5. Because the polymer solutions used are so dilute, their density is practically identical with that of the solvent, simplifying equation (17–12) to

$$\eta_{rel} = \frac{\eta_{12}}{\eta_1} \cong \frac{t_{12}}{t_1} \qquad (20-10)$$

Extrapolation of reduced viscosities to zero concentration to obtain the intrinsic viscosity eliminates the effect of the buildup of the reduced viscosity due to intermolecular entanglements. The linear extrapolation is usually made by the Huggins equation:

$$\frac{\eta_{sp}}{c} = \eta_{red} = [\eta] + k_1[\eta]^2 c \qquad (20-11)$$

An alternate definition of intrinsic viscosity makes use of the inherent viscosity, namely, $\eta_{inh} = \ln \eta_{rel}/c$. According to this definition,

$$[\eta] = \lim_{c \to 0} \frac{\ln \eta_{rel}}{c} \qquad (20-12)$$

TABLE 20–1. *Viscosity Measurements of Dilute Solutions of Polymethyl Methacrylate in Ethylene Chloride at 25° C*[13]

c_2 (g/dL)	Efflux times (sec)	$\eta_{rel} = \dfrac{t_{12}}{t_1}$	$\eta_{inh} = \dfrac{\ln \eta_{rel}}{c_2}$	$\eta_{red} = \dfrac{\eta_{rel} - 1}{c_2}$
0	t_1 235.6	1.000	—	—
0.125	t_{12} 246.2	1.045	0.352	0.360
0.250	257.0	1.091	0.348	0.364
0.500	279.6	1.187	0.342	0.374
1.000	328.6	1.395	0.333	0.395

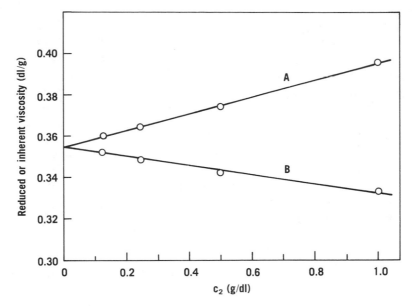

Fig. 20–2. Plots of reduced and inherent viscosity versus concentration for polymethyl methacrylate in ethyl chloride at 25° C for the determination of intrinsic viscosity. Line *A* represents reduced viscosity; line *B* represents inherent viscosity.

Another linear extrapolation to obtain [η], using the inherent viscosity, is based on the Kraemer equation:

$$\eta_{inh} = \frac{\ln \eta_{rel}}{c} = [\eta] - k_2[\eta]^2 c \qquad (20\text{--}13)$$

A set of experimental viscosity data illustrates the use of the Huggins and Kraemer equations to determine intrinsic viscosity from relative viscosities.

Example 20–1. From the data of Table 20–1, determine the intrinsic viscosity by means of the Huggins and Kraemer equations. Subscript 1 refers to the solvent, 2 to the polymer and 12 to the polymer solution. Efflux times are given with four significant figures because they are averages of four to five measurements. Linear regression analysis of the data plotted according to the Huggins equation (Fig. 20–2, line *A*), gives $\eta_{red} = 0.354 + 0.0404c$. Hence, [η] = 0.354 dL/g and

$$k_1 = slope/[\eta]^2 = 0.0404/(0.354)^2 = 0.322$$

Linear regression analysis according to the Kraemer equation (Fig. 20–2, line *B*) gives $\eta_{inh} = 0.354 - 0.0212c$. Hence, [η] = 0.354 dL/g and

$$k_2 = -slope/[\eta]^2 = -(-0.0212)/(0.354)^2 = 0.170$$

The two lines converge to their common intercept [η] at $c = 0$. Instead of using linear regression analysis, intercept and slopes of the two lines can be obtained from Figure 20–2. The sum of the Huggins and Kraemer slope constants, $k_1 + k_2 = 0.322 + 0.170 = 0.492 \cong 0.500$, as required by theory.

CONFORMATION OF DISSOLVED LINEAR MACROMOLECULES[2,5,6,8,14,15]

Because of a relatively large freedom of rotation around bonds between carbon and other atoms forming their backbone, polymer chains are quite flexible. This is illustrated in Figure 20–3 by depicting four successive carbon atoms in a chain, and fixing the bond (length = 1.54 Å) between carbon atoms Numbers 1 and 2 as reference in the plane of the paper.

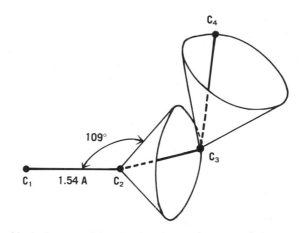

Fig. 20–3. Rotational freedom in a four-carbon atom chain sequence.

Atom Number 3 can be located anywhere on a circle around the base of a cone swept out by rotating the C_2—C_3 bond at the fixed tetrahedral bond angle of 109° relative to the C_1—C_2 bond. When locating C_4, every position of atom Number 3 on that circle gives rise to another cone with a circular base swept out by rotating the C_3—C_4 bond at a 109° angle. C_4 may be located on any point of any one of these many circles. This illustrates that the number of possible conformations[*] of a polymer chain of many carbon atoms is enormous, resulting in a high flexibility for that chain.

Because they are buffeted by surrounding solvent molecules engaged in thermal agitation, polymer chains in solution adopt ever-changing shapes of random coils

---

[*]Different geometric arrangements of polymer chains caused by rotation about single bonds in their backbone are designated as *conformations*. Different arrangements fixed by chemical bonding that involve isomerism are called *configurations*. Changes in configuration require breaking and reforming of primary valence bonds.[4,9]

in a writhing segmental Brownian motion. Most polymers have a bulk density of 1 g/cm³, but in solution, the randomly coiled chains are permeated by solvent and occupy a volume many times larger than their bulk volume. The average density of polymer segments within a randomly coiled chain is of the order of 10^{-5} to 10^{-3} g/cm³.

The dimensions of the coiled chain depend on the polymer–solvent interaction, being larger in a thermodynamically good solvent that solvates the chains extensively but more shrunken in a poor solvent. Bulky substituents (e.g., the phenyl group in polystyrene), ionized groups (e.g., sodium carboxylate groups in neutralized Carbomer USP), rings in the backbone (such as those in polyethylene terephthalate or cellulose), or unsaturation (as the partial double bond in polypeptide chains introduced by resonance) reduce the flexibility of the polymer chain and result in more open or larger coils and hence in larger intrinsic viscosities.

The shape of a randomly coiled polymer chain changes continuously owing to the random bombardment by solvent molecules, and no two chains have the same shape at a given time. Therefore, the dimensions of a random coil are averaged over all polymer molecules and over long periods of time by statistical techniques. The problem of predicting the distance between the two ends of a coiled chain is analogous to calculating the distance traveled by a diffusing particle in random Brownian motion, which is treated as a *random flight* (Fig. 20–4). In the case of a polymer chain, each step corresponds to adding another carbon atom to the chain. Three restrictions prevent treatment of the *end-to-end distance*, R, as a completely random flight: Each step can only proceed by the distance of the carbon–carbon bond length of 1.54 Å, the bond angle of 109 to 110° must be preserved, and there are steric hindrances.

The root-mean-square value of the end-to-end distance R is used for its average. For the four R values of 100, 200, 200, and 300 Å, the root-mean-square average is

$$\langle R^2 \rangle^{1/2} = \sqrt{\frac{100^2 + (2)(200)^2 + 300^2}{4}} = 212 \text{ Å}$$

In addition to the end-to-end distance, the *radius of gyration*, S, is also used to describe the dimensions of the randomly coiled chain. It is the root-mean-square distance of the chain segments from the center of gravity of the coiled chain and is more meaningful than R for branched polymers, in which there are more than two chain ends. For linear polymers, $\langle R^2 \rangle = 6\langle S^2 \rangle$.

As W. Kuhn calculated in 1934 by the *random flight* method, if a polymer molecule consists of a chain of n identical segments of length L that are freely jointed, that is, with no restriction as to the bond angle θ between segments,

$$\langle R^2 \rangle = nL^2 \qquad (20\text{--}14)$$

Thus, $\langle R^2 \rangle$ is directly proportional to the molecular weight. Introducing the tetrahedral bond angle $\theta = 110°$, with $\cos\theta = -\frac{1}{3}$, and assuming free rotation about that angle, the root-mean-square end-to-end distance is doubled:

$$\langle R^2 \rangle \cong \left(\frac{1 - \cos\theta}{1 + \cos\theta} \right) nL^2 = 2nL^2 \qquad (20\text{--}15)$$

The following factors further expand the dimensions of real polymer molecules in solution, increasing the end-to-end distance beyond the value given by equation (20–15): short-range interactions, namely, steric hindrance to free rotation about carbon–carbon bonds in the backbone of the chain caused by bulky substituents or by rings, or unsaturation in the backbone producing rigid planar conformations; ionic groups; and long-range intramolecular interactions, namely, the excluded volume (chain segments have finite thickness, and no two segments can occupy the same volume at the same time).

Example 20–2. For a polystyrene molecule with a molecular weight of 1,000,000, calculate the length of the fully extended chain (called the *contour length*), the root-mean-square end-to-end distance assuming a freely jointed chain, and the root-mean-square end-to-end distance and the radius of gyration for a bond angle of 110°.

The molecular weight of styrene and of the repeat unit is 104.16; hence, $DP = 1,000,000/104.16 = 9600$. The fully extended chain, in a planar, all-*trans*, zig-zag conformation, has the following dimensions:

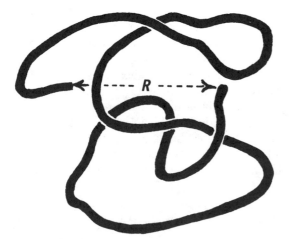

Fig. 20–4. Randomly coiled linear polymer chain showing end-to-end distance R.

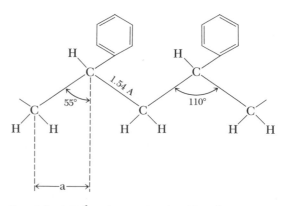

Projection of the 1.54 Å carbon–carbon bond length on the chain axis makes the contribution $a = (1.54 \text{ Å}) \sin(110°/2) = (1.54 \text{ Å}) \sin 55° =$

1.26 Å to the contour length of the chain. Each repeat unit adds 1.26 Å × 2 = 2.52 Å to that length; for 9600 repeat units, it is 2.52 Å × 9600 = 24,190 Å.

The polystyrene chain contains $n = 2\,DP = 2 \times 9600 = 19,200$ bonds in the backbone of the chain of $L = 1.54$ A. According to equation (20–14), if it is freely jointed, its root-mean-square end-to-end distance is $\langle R^2 \rangle^{1/2} = [(19.200)(1.54\ \text{Å})^2]^{1/2} = 213$ Å.

With the restriction of the tetrahedral bond angle but allowing free rotation, equation (20–15) gives $\langle R^2 \rangle^{1/2} = [(2)(19,200)(1.54\ \text{Å})^2]^{1/2} = 302$ Å, corresponding to $\langle S^2 \rangle^{1/2} = \langle R^2 \rangle^{1/2}/\sqrt{6} = 123$ Å.

The actual $\langle R^2 \rangle^{1/2}$ value for a polystyrene fraction with molecular weight of 10^6, deduced from intrinsic viscosity measurements in good solvents, is at least three times larger.[16] This discrepancy is chiefly due to the greater stiffness of the polystyrene chain brought about by hindered rotation around the carbon–carbon chain bonds, which in turn is ascribed to the bulky phenyl side groups and to solvation of the macromolecule.

For comparison, a latex sphere consisting of a polystyrene molecule with a molecular weight of 10^6 and a density of 1.06 g/cm^3 has a radius

$$R = \left[\left(\frac{10^6\ \text{g}}{\text{mole}} \right) \left(\frac{\text{mole}}{6.023 \times 10^{23}\ \text{molecules}} \right) \left(\frac{\text{cm}^3}{1.06\ \text{g}} \right) \left(\frac{10^{24}\ \text{Å}^3}{\text{cm}^3} \right) \left(\frac{3}{4\pi} \right) \right]^{\frac{1}{3}} = 72\ \text{Å}$$

The same molecule dissolved as a random coil, with a radius of about 1100 Å, occupies a volume $(1100/72)^3 = 3600$ times larger. The polymer segment density within the random coil is 1.06 g/cm^3/3600 = 2.9×10^{-4} g/cm^3. Thus, polymer molecules in solution spread throughout the solvent and occupy or fill the solution space effectively. Therefore, dissolved polymers are excellent thickening agents for solvents (see next section).

POLYMERS AS THICKENING AGENTS[1,2,17]

The extraordinary ability of dissolved macromolecules to build up the relative viscosity of their solutions is illustrated with high-viscosity, USP-grade methylcellulose. An aqueous 2.00% (*w/v*) solution has an apparent viscosity at low shear and room temperature of 80 poise. Since water has a viscosity of 0.01 poise, the relative viscosity of that solution is 8000, that is, the 2% of dissolved polymer increases the viscosity of water 8000-fold!

At a polymer molecular weight of 300,000 and a molecular weight of 187 for a methylcellulose repeat unit with a degree of substitution of 1.8, $DP = 300,000/187 = 1600$. If each of the macromolecules were cut up by hydrolysis into its building blocks, namely, 1600 molecules of methylglucose, a 2.19% solution of methylglucose would result. While the viscosity of methylglucose solutions has not been reported, the viscosity of a 2.19% (*w/v*) solution of glucose in water, which is probably about the same, is a mere 1.05 centipoise, that is, only 5% higher than the viscosity of water. Splitting the polymer into its building blocks reduces the relative viscosity from 8000 to 1.05. Even a 34% (*w/v*) solution of glucose in water has a relative viscosity of only 2.99. By contrast, the viscosity of polymer solutions increases almost exponentially with concentration. (The reader will note that the viscosity values in Figure 20–5 are plotted on an eighth-root scale that is almost as compressed as a logarithmic

scale.) Solutions of high polymers frequently set to gels at concentrations of 5% or higher.

The factors responsible for the thickening action of dissolved polymers are discussed in the following paragraphs, starting with considerations of single polymer molecules in solution and then considering the effect of intermolecular entanglements. The reasons for the pseudoplastic or shear-thinning behavior of polymer solutions (defined on p. 456) are also discussed.

Each repeat unit of methylcellulose has three to four ether groups and one to two hydroxyl groups that are extensively hydrated in aqueous solution. An ether oxygen has two unshared electron pairs and can therefore bind two water molecules by hydrogen bonding. Each of these water molecules can hydrogen-bond additional water molecules, thus surrounding the polymer chain with a sheath of water of hydration. Likewise, a polystyrene molecule dissolved in benzene is extensively solvated by van der Waals forces. When the chains move, their solvation layers are dragged along. The resultant increase in the size of the flow units increases the resistance to flow or the viscosity of the solution.

Solvation cannot account for the considerable increase in viscosity due to the dissolved polymer, however, because the 1600 molecules of methylglucose are as extensively hydrated as is the methylcellulose macromolecule. The chief difference is the cooperative nature of the flow of the latter, in which all 1600 repeat units plus their water of hydration must move together, resulting in a very large flow unit.

A very large amount of solvent is located within a randomly coiled polymer molecule. As mentioned previously, a random coil consists of approximately 0.01% polymer and 99.99% solvent. Only a small portion of that solvent is attached to the polymer by secondary valence forces. The bulk of the solvent is "free."

According to the *free-draining coil* model, the randomly coiled polymer chain in translational motion leaves the free solvent within it largely unperturbed. For this freely permeable coiled chain, theoretic calculations predict that the intrinsic viscosity is proportional to the molecular weight, making the exponent a in the Mark–Houwink equation (equation (20–8)) unity. At the other extreme, if the random coil were completely impenetrable to external solvent attempting to flow through it and all solvent molecules within the coil moved with the same velocity as the coil itself, a would equal 0.5.

The viscosity observed for dilute polymer solutions is far greater than that calculated for free-draining coils, indicating that a portion of the free solvent molecules inside a coiled macromolecule is mechanically trapped and is dragged along when the macromolecule moves. Some of the nonsolvating solvent forms part of the flow unit, further increasing its size and frictional resistance.

Newton postulated that a solvent is made up of a stack of parallel, very thin layers. Laminar flow in pure

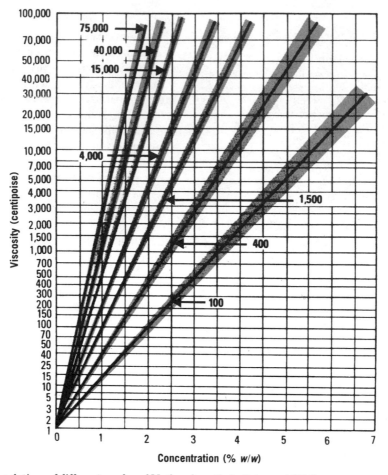

Fig. 20–5. Viscosity of aqueous solutions of different grades of Methocel, methylcellulose, at 20° C versus concentration. Numbers on the curves represent viscosities of 2% (*w/w*) solutions in centipoises. Representative number-average molecular weights corresponding to these numbers written in parentheses are: 26,000 (100 cps); 63,000 (1500 cps); 120,000 (15,000 cps). The vertical scale is eighth-root rather than logarithmic. (Reprinted with permission of The Dow Chemical Company.)

shear consists in the slippage of these layers past one another. Motion is transmitted by friction between adjacent layers. Layers near the source of the shear stress that promotes flow move faster than more distant layers or layers near a wall. There is a velocity gradient, shown by the difference in the length of the arrows representing the velocity of flow of individual layers in Figure 20–6. A randomly coiled macromolecule spans several adjacent solvent layers moving with different velocities. The upper portion of the random coil is subject to a greater shear stress than the lower portion because it is immersed in faster-moving layers. The resultant couple causes the random coil to rotate clockwise. This rotation further increases the frictional resistance of the solution.

The thermal agitation of the solvent molecules combined with the great chain flexibility causes dissolved linear macromolecules to become entangled even at moderate concentrations (Fig. 20–7A). Because each random coil extends through a relatively large volume of solution and because its segments are engaged in continuous Brownian motion, neighboring chains tend to interpenetrate and become entangled. During flow, chain entanglements act as temporary cross-links and pro-

mote the cooperative motion of adjacent, interpenetrating chains. The Huggins equation (equation (20–11)) is valid only for dilute solutions having relative viscosities of 2.0 or less, in which intermolecular entanglements are minimal. Chain entanglements cause the reduced

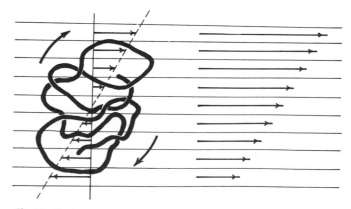

Fig. 20–6. A randomly coiled linear macromolecule in a laminar shear field exhibiting rotational motion. Arrows inside the coil indicate relative velocity of solvent layers. The solvent layer through the center of the coil is "stationary," i.e., moves with the same velocity as the coil. Arrows to the right of the coil indicate absolute velocity of solvent layers.

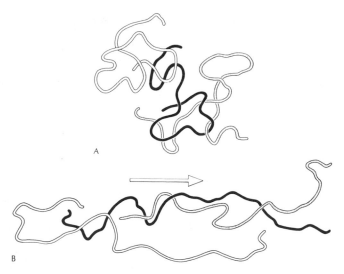

Fig. 20–7. Three randomly coiled linear polymer chains: (A) at rest; (B) in a shear field. (From H. Schott and A. Martin, *American Pharmacy*, 7th Edition, L. W. Dittert, Ed., Lippincott, Philadelphia, 1974.)

viscosity to increase faster with concentration than is predicted by equation (20–11). For the large thickening effects required in pharmaceutical formulations, semilogarithmic relationships between solution viscosity (or reduced viscosity) and concentration, such as those of Figure 20–5, are more representative.

The same factors that promote the unusually high viscosity of polymer solutions cause them to be pseudoplastic or shear-thinning, so that the apparent solution viscosity decreases continuously with increasing shear stress or rate of shear (see Chapter 17).

Under the influence of increasing shear, isolated randomly coiled polymer chains uncoil or unravel progressively, becoming more elongated and streamlined, and line up in the direction of flow. The reduced cross-sectional area of the coiled macromolecules in the flow direction causes smaller disturbances of fewer streamlines in the solvent, reducing the friction. The same coil deformation also reduces the amount of water trapped inside the chains that is dragged along as they move, reducing the size of the flow units and hence the frictional resistance or viscosity of the solution.

The tendency of the random coils to rotate in the shear field depicted in Figure 20–6 is reduced, because chains that are largely uncoiled and elongated in the direction of flow overlap fewer solvent layers, reducing the magnitude of the couple that produces rotation.

Interpenetrating polymer chains are gradually disentangled with increasing shear and tend to flow increasingly as separate units. Consequently, the size of the flow units drops as does the resistance to flow or viscosity. Figure 20–7B pictures the three previously interpenetrating chains largely disentangled, uncoiled, and lined up in the direction of flow.

Brownian motion of chain segments tends to produce roughly spherical random coils that interpenetrate one another and trap mechanically large amounts of sol-

vent. This effect is independent of the applied shear. The opposite effect of partial uncoiling, elongation, and alignment of the random coils, reduction in the amount of trapped solvent, and disentanglement in flow is proportional to the applied shear. Therefore, for each shear stress or rate of shear applied to a polymer solution, there is a corresponding average equilibrium degree of chain uncoiling, elongation, and disentanglement, resulting in a characteristic average size for the flow unit with a characteristic average amount of mechanically trapped solvent and, hence, a characteristic value for the apparent viscosity.

At low shear rates, the effects of Brownian motion prevail. The chains largely retain the conformation of random coils, trap large amounts of solvent, and remain extensively entangled, resulting in large flow units and high apparent viscosity. At high shear rates, the chains are largely uncoiled and elongated, trapping much less solvent, and are mostly disentangled, resulting in small flow units and low apparent viscosity.

Because the polymer chains are exceedingly thin and flexible, they adjust to changing shear rates almost instantaneously, that is, much faster than the response time of viscometers. These short relaxation times preclude hysteresis effects or thixotropy (see Chapter 17). The apparent viscosity of polymer solutions does not depend on the shear history (length of time and level of shear rate at which the polymer solution was stirred previously), but only on the current rate of shear (and on concentration and temperature, of course).

POLYMER SOLUTIONS—OVERVIEW

Some of the problems and questions encountered in the preparation, characterization, and use of polymer solutions are: what solvent to use; how to mix polymer and solvent; at what concentration to work; how temperature and molecular weight affect this use concentration; what thermodynamic factors govern dissolution, solution properties, and the solubility limit; how to prevent gelation or precipitation (or how to promote it if gels are desired). These and related topics are discussed in the following sections.

SOLVENT SELECTION[4,6a,18,19]

Just as for small molecules, polymers dissolve best or most extensively in solvents having similar solubility parameters (defined by equation (10–21)). For a liquid to dissolve a polymer, the difference between their solubility parameters should be less than about 2 $(cal/cm^3)^{1/2}$.* The heat of vaporization of polymers

---

*1 $(cal/cm^3)^{1/2}$ = 2.046 $(joule/cm^3)^{1/2}$.

cannot be determined because attempts to evaporate them cause thermal decomposition into low-molecular-weight fragments. Thus, indirect methods are required to determine δ_2 values for polymers.

An obvious method is to measure the solubility limit of a given polymer fraction at a given temperature in a variety of solvents. Maximum solubility is observed in the solvent whose δ_1 best matches δ_2. Alternatively, fixed amounts of a polymer sample are mixed with constant volumes of a series of solvents having gradually increasing δ_1 values to give final concentrations comparable to the intended use concentration. The polymer will be soluble at room temperature in a group of solvents covering a certain range of δ_1 values. Its δ_2 value is about midpoint in the range of δ_1 values of the solvents in which the polymer is completely soluble.[12] Polymers are most extensively solvated in solvents of the same δ value, resulting in stiffer chains with greater radii of gyration. Hence, plots of intrinsic viscosity of linear polymers dissolved in a variety of solvents versus δ_1 reach maxima at $\delta_1 = \delta_2$.[20]

Cross-linked polymers, for example, rubber vulcanizates, cannot dissolve but swell most extensively in solvents having the same δ value.[21] Plots of degree of swelling in different solvents (cm^3 solvent uptake/g dry polymer) versus δ_1 reach maxima at $\delta_1 = \delta_2$.

Estimates of the solubility parameter of polymers can be made by treating it as an additive and constitutive property based on the molar attraction constants F of the groups that make up their repeat units:

$$\delta_2 = \frac{\Sigma F}{V} = \frac{\rho_2 \Sigma F}{M} \qquad (20-16)$$

in which V and M are molar volume and molecular weight, respectively, of the repeat unit and ρ_2 is the polymer density.[22-24] Group contributions to the molar attraction constant of a repeat unit are listed in Table 20–2.

Example 20–3. Using the data of Table 20–2, calculate the solubility parameter of polymethyl methacrylate. The polymer (Lucite, Plexiglas) has a density of 1.18 g/cm^3.

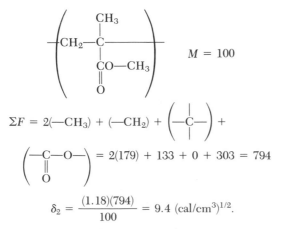

$$\Sigma F = 2(-CH_3) + (-CH_2-) + \left(\underset{|}{\overset{|}{-C-}}\right) +$$

$$\left(\underset{O}{\overset{\parallel}{-C-O-}}\right) = 2(179) + 133 + 0 + 303 = 794$$

$$\delta_2 = \frac{(1.18)(794)}{100} = 9.4 \ (cal/cm^3)^{1/2}.$$

This value agrees well with the experimentally determined value of 9.3 ± 0.2.

TABLE 20–2. *Molar Attraction Constants F of Groups in (cal/cm³)$^{1/2}$/mole repeat unit*[6a,22,23]

Group	F	Group	F
—CH$_3$	179	$-\overset{\parallel}{\underset{O}{C}}-O-$	303
—CH$_2$—	133		
$-\overset{\mid}{\underset{\mid}{CH}}$	67	—OH	240
		—OH aromatic	171
		—NH$_2$	230
$-\overset{\mid}{\underset{\mid}{C}}-$	0	—NH—	180
—CH=CH—	231		
—CH=CH— aromatic	237	$-\overset{\mid}{\underset{\mid}{N}}-$	61
		—C≡N	400
—O— ether, acetal	108	—Cl	206
		—Cl aromatic	161
$-\overset{\parallel}{\underset{O}{C}}-$	284		

Table 20–3 lists solubility parameters for a variety of polymers. The value for a given polymer may vary, depending on the polarity and/or hydrogen-bonding capacity of the solvents used to determine δ_2.

The methods outlined here for determining the solubility parameter of polymers fail when the predominant forces between solvent and polymer molecules are dipole forces or hydrogen bonds rather than London dispersion forces. In that case, a refinement consists in splitting the solubility parameter of the solvents into three partial parameters corresponding to the contribution of these three types of secondary valence forces, and plotting the component parameters in a three-dimensional system in which polymers are then located.[12,24,25]

TABLE 20–3. *Solubility Parameters of Polymers in (cal/cm³)$^{1/2}$* [12,21–24]

Polymer	δ_2
Polytetrafluoroethylene	6.2
Polydimethyl siloxane	7.6
Polyethylene	7.9
Polyisobutylene	8.0
Polyisoprene (natural rubber)	8.1
Polychloroprene	8.7
Polypropylene	8.7
Polystyrene	8.8–9.3
Polymethyl methacrylate	9.1–9.5
Polyvinyl chloride	9.4–9.8
Polyvinyl acetate	9.6
Polyethylene terephthalate	10.7
Cellulose diacetate	10.9
Polyvinylidene chloride	12.2
Polyvinyl alcohol	12.6–14.2
Polyhexamethylene adipamide (6,6 nylon)	13.6
Polyacrylonitrile	12.5–15.4
Cellulose	15.7

PREPARING POLYMER SOLUTIONS

The dissolution of solid polymers in solvents occurs in two overlapping stages. Upon contact, the solvent molecules start diffusing immediately into the solid particles, gradually swell them, and transform them into gel particles. The solvated polymer molecules in the swollen particle surface gradually become disentangled from one another and slowly diffuse out into the solvent. The latter stage can be speeded up considerably by stirring, which disentangles matted polymer chains and reduces the thickness of the stagnant liquid layer surrounding each particle.

Most polymers are available as powders or grains. When these are added to a solvent with stirring, the mixing conditions must result in complete wetting and separation of the particles before they can swell and become sticky or gelatinize. Otherwise, the particles tend to aggregate into lumps, in which a swollen, translucent outer layer sometimes even encloses dry powder particles. Because of their large size or small surface areas, these lumps dissolve very slowly.

To cause dispersal of the powders and avoid lumping, the initial solvent temperatures should be conducive to limited swelling and poor dissolution. For instance, methylcellulose is more soluble in cold than in hot water. Therefore, its powder should be dispersed with high shear in about one fourth the total amount of water heated to 80° to 90° C. Because of the poor solvent power of hot water for methylcellulose, the particles are dispersed before their surface layer becomes swollen and tacky. Once the particles are thoroughly wetted and dispersed, the rest of the water is added cold or even as ice to cool the suspension to about 5° C, at which temperature water is an excellent solvent and swells and dissolves the dispersed particles fast with moderate shear. The procedure is similar for hydroxypropylcellulose and hydroxypropyl methylcellulose.

Most water-soluble polymers, such as polyvinyl alcohol and sodium carboxymethylcellulose, are more soluble in hot than in cold water. Therefore, their powders are wetted out and dispersed in ice-cold water, followed by dissolution at 90° C or above for the former and 60° to 65° C for the latter. An alternative procedure to prevent agglomeration of polymer powders into lumps during dissolution consists in prewetting the powders with a water-miscible liquid that does not swell the polymer. For methylcellulose and sodium carboxymethylcellulose, anhydrous alcohol or propylene glycol is recommended.

Some polymers are used in mixed solvents. To dissolve ethylcellulose in an 80% toluene/20% ethyl alcohol mixture, the powder is first slurried in toluene until a uniform dispersion is obtained. The development of surface stickiness, swelling, and dissolution is slow because toluene by itself is only a poor solvent. The alcohol is then added to effect prompt dissolution.

Aqueous polymer solutions, especially of cellulose derivatives, are stored for approximately 48 hours after dissolution to promote full hydration, maximum viscosity and clarity. If salts are to be incorporated, they are added at this point rather than dissolved in the water before adding the polymer; otherwise, the solutions may not reach their full viscosity and clarity.

THERMODYNAMICS OF POLYMER SOLUTIONS[1,2,6,6a,9,18,26-28]

For the dissolution of a polymer (subscript 2) in a solvent (subscript 1) at constant temperature T, the free energy of mixing or solution (see Chapter 10) is

$$\Delta G_m = \Delta H_m - T \Delta S_m \qquad (20\text{–}17)$$

in which G, H, and S represent free energy, enthalpy or heat, and entropy, respectively (defined in Chapters 3 and 10); Δ indicates the changes in these parameters during mixing, that is, the differences between G, H, and S of the solution and of the polymer plus solvent prior to dissolution.

For dissolution to occur spontaneously, ΔG_m must be negative. This can be realized by a negative ΔH_m (exothermic mixing) or by a positive ΔS_m (increased randomness or disorder), preferably at a high temperature. Entropy effects are predominant in the dissolution of polymers at all temperatures.

To dissolve crystalline polymers, the secondary valence forces holding the chains together in the lattice, represented by the heat of fusion (see the following), must be overcome. Polyethylene, because of its high crystallinity, is soluble in solvents such as toluene only when heated within 25° C of its melting point. Cellulose is insoluble in water even though its monomer, dextrose, is very soluble. Attempts to dissolve cellulose in water by heating under pressure result instead in hydrolysis. The melting point of cellulose is so high that it undergoes thermal decomposition rather than melting when heated dry. The following discussion refers to the dissolution of polymers in the amorphous state.

Because the molecular weight and molar volume of polymers are so much greater than those of solvents, concentrations are expressed as volume fractions ϕ (defined in chapter 10) rather than as mole fractions X as is customary for small solute molecules. In comparatively dilute polymer solutions, X_1 is close to unity, whereas ϕ_1 is not.

Example 20–4. Calculate the mole fractions and volume fractions of the components in a 5% (*w/v*) solution of a polystyrene fraction ($M_2 = 80,000$) in toluene ($M_1 = 92$). The densities are: toluene, $\rho_1 = 0.87$; polystyrene, $\rho_2 = 1.08$; solution, $\rho_{12} = 0.88$ g/cm³. Using 100 cm³ solution as basis for the calculations,

$$(100 \text{ cm}^3 \text{ solution})\left(\frac{0.88 \text{ g}}{\text{cm}^3}\right) = 88 \text{ g solution}$$

The number of moles is

$$n_1 = (88 - 5 \text{ g})\left(\frac{\text{mole}}{92 \text{ g}}\right) = 0.902 \text{ mole}$$

and

$$n_2 = (5 \text{ g})\left(\frac{\text{mole}}{80,000 \text{ g}}\right) = 0.0000625 \text{ mole}$$

The mole fractions are

$$X_1 = \frac{0.902}{0.902 + 0.0000625} = 0.99993 \cong 1.000$$

and

$$X_2 = \frac{0.0000625}{0.902 + 0.0000625} \cong \frac{0.0000625}{0.902} = 0.00007 \cong 0.000$$

The volumes are

$$V_1 = (88 - 5 \text{ g})\left(\frac{\text{cm}^3}{0.87 \text{ g}}\right) = 95.4 \text{ cm}^3$$

and

$$V_2 = (5 \text{ g})\left(\frac{\text{cm}^3}{1.08 \text{ g}}\right) = 4.63 \text{ cm}^3$$

The volume fractions are

$$\phi_1 = \frac{95.4}{95.4 + 4.63} = 0.954$$

$$\phi_2 = \frac{4.63}{95.4 + 4.63} = 0.046$$

As a check, $0.954 + 0.046 = 1.000$.

Heat of Mixing. The dissolution of polymers is frequently endothermic, with the heat of mixing ΔH_m positive (which militates against dissolution because it tends to make ΔG_m positive) but small. In terms of the solubility parameter[18,19]:

$$\Delta H_m \cong V_{12}(\delta_1 - \delta_2)^2\phi_1\phi_2 \qquad (20\text{--}18)$$

in which V_{12} is the volume of the mixture.

In the *Flory–Huggins theory* of polymer solutions, published independently by these two polymer chemists between 1941 and 1944, ΔH_m is assumed to be positive and is given by the van Laar expression:

$$\Delta H_m = \chi R T n_1 \phi_2 \qquad (20\text{--}19)$$

in which χ is the Flory–Huggins interaction parameter.*

Deviations of polymer solutions from ideal behavior as represented by Raoult's law (see Chapters 5 and 10), for example, are ascribed mainly to the small entropies

---

*This dimensionless parameter, sometimes represented by μ, characterizes the interaction energy for a given polymer–solvent combination. It specifies, in multiples of RT, the excess free energy of transfer of a mole of solvent from the pure solvent to the pure polymer phase. Comparison of equations (20–18) and (20–19) gives

$$\chi = \left(\frac{V_1}{RT}\right)(\delta_1 - \delta_2)^2$$

in which V_1 is the molar volume of the solvent. The interaction parameter χ is related to the second virial coefficient A_2 of polymer solutions, which in turn is connected with the coefficient B of equation (15–12) by the relation[9,10] $B = RTA_2 = RT(v_2^2/V_1)(0.5 - \chi)$; v_2 is the partial specific volume of the dissolved polymer. A_2, B, and χ can be calculated from osmotic pressure, light scattering, or vapor pressure data. Ideal behavior occurs when $A_2 = B = 0$ or $\chi = 0.5$, making the plot of reduced osmotic pressure versus concentration a straight, horizontal line (Curve I of Figure 15–7).

of mixing, resulting from the enormous disparity in size of the molecules of the two components.

Entropy of Mixing. Flory and Huggins derived the entropy of mixing of polymer solutions from statistical calculations based on a pseudolattice model, depicted in two dimensions in Figure 20–8. Each lattice point or site can be occupied either by a solvent molecule or by a segment of the polymer chain. A linear polymer molecule is assumed to consist of a number of segments joined flexibly together, each having the same size as a solvent molecule. For polystyrene dissolved in toluene, a segment is identical with a repeat unit. The conformational entropy of mixing is calculated from Boltzmann's relationship $\Delta S_m = R \ln W$, in which W is the number of distinguishable arrangements of filling the lattice with polymer chains and solvent molecules. The result is

$$\Delta S_m = -R(n_1 \ln \phi_1 + n_2 \ln \phi_2) \qquad (20\text{--}20)$$

in which $\phi_2 = \dfrac{N n_2}{n_1 + N n_2}$ for n_2 moles of polymer molecules of N segments each, provided polymer and solvent have the same density, because each polymer segment occupies the same volume as one solvent molecule. N often represents DP. For polymer samples with a broad molecular weight distribution, $n_2 \ln \phi_2$ is summed over all fractions, becoming $\Sigma n_{2,i} \ln \phi_{2,i}$. As before, $\phi_1 + \Sigma \phi_{2,i} = 1.00$

Since both ϕ_1 and ϕ_2 are less than 1, their logarithms are negative and ΔS_m is positive, as one would expect,

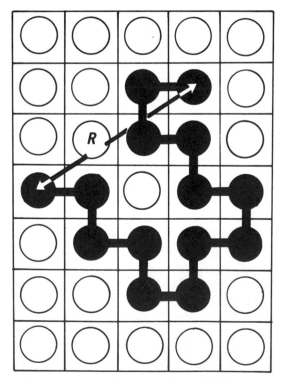

Fig. 20–8. Placement of a 14-segment, 13-link polymer chain occupying 14 lattice sites and of 21 solvent molecules on a 5 × 7 two-dimensional lattice. $\phi_1 = \frac{21}{35} = 0.60$; $\phi_2 = \frac{14}{35} = 0.40$.

because mixing causes an increase in disorder or randomness. A positive ΔS_m makes a negative contribution toward ΔG_m according to equation (20–17), promoting dissolution.

Example 20–5. Estimate the entropy change when dissolving 78 g of a polystyrene fraction with a molecular weight of 52,000 in 1090 cm^3 toluene (molecular weight, 92 g/mole). Densities are 1.07 g/cm^3 for the polystyrene and 0.87 for toluene. The numbers of moles are

$$n_1 = (1090 \text{ cm}^3)\left(\frac{0.87 \text{ g}}{\text{cm}^3}\right)\left(\frac{\text{mole}}{92 \text{ g}}\right) = 10.3 \text{ mole}$$

and

$$n_2 = (78 \text{ g})\left(\frac{\text{mole}}{52,000 \text{ g}}\right) = 0.0015 \text{ mole}$$

The polymer volume is

$$V_2 = (78 \text{ g})\left(\frac{\text{cm}^3}{1.07 \text{ g}}\right) = 72.9 \text{ cm}^3$$

and the volume fractions are

$$\phi_1 = \frac{1090}{1090 + 72.9} = 0.9373$$

and

$$\phi_2 = \frac{72.9}{1090 + 72.9} = 0.0627$$

As a check, $0.9373 + 0.0627 = 1.0000$. The entropy of mixing is

$$\Delta S_m = -\left(\frac{1.987 \text{ cal}}{\text{mole °K}}\right)(2.303)[(10.3 \text{ mole})$$
$$\times (\log 0.9373) + (0.0015 \text{ mole})(\log 0.0627)]$$
$$= 1.33 \text{ cal/°K}$$

If the styrene had not been polymerized, the entropy change of mixing 78 g or 0.75 mole liquid styrene monomer with 1090 cm^3 or 948 g or 10.3 mole toluene can be calculated by equation (1) of chapter 2 in reference 18 for ideal solutions as

$$\Delta S_m = -R(n_1 \ln X_1 + n_2 \ln X_2)$$
$$= -\left(\frac{1.987 \text{ cal}}{\text{mole °K}}\right)(2.303)\left[(10.3 \text{ mole})\right.$$
$$\times \log\left(\frac{10.3}{10.3 + 0.75}\right) + (0.75 \text{ mole})$$
$$\left.\times \log\left(\frac{0.75}{10.3 + 0.75}\right)\right]$$
$$= 5.45 \text{ cal/°K}$$

This equation for ΔS_m of two kinds of small molecules is quite similar to equation (20–20). The ΔS_m value for dissolving the monomer is four times larger than that for dissolving the same amount of polymer.

Free Energy of Mixing. Combining equations (20–17), (20–19), and (20–20) gives the overall free energy of dissolution per mole of lattice sites or of solvent:

$$\Delta G_m = RT(n_1 \ln \phi_1 + n_2 \ln \phi_2 + \chi n_1 \phi_2) \quad (20–21)$$

The first two terms in the parentheses, representing entropy contributions, are negative. The third term, representing the enthalpy contribution, is positive and militates against dissolution.

This equation shows why two or more molten polymers are, as a rule, incompatible. When the solvent in a polymer solution is replaced by an equal volume of a

second liquid polymer, n_1 decreases substantially at constant ϕ_1, making the first term in the parentheses very small. The sum of the first two terms, which are negative, would then be smaller than the third term, which is positive, making ΔG_m positive. The process occurring spontaneously, because its free energy change is negative, would be the opposite of mixing, namely, phase separation of the two liquid polymers. In fact, even dilute solutions of two different kinds of polymers in the same solvent frequently separate into two phases upon mixing, with each phase containing practically all of one of the polymers.

Differentiation of equation (20–21) with respect to n_1 gives the partial molar free energy of mixing (defined on p. 67):

$$\frac{\Delta \overline{G}_1}{RT} = \ln a_1 = \ln \phi_1 + \left(1 - \frac{1}{N}\right)\phi_2 + \chi \phi_2^2 \quad (20–22)$$

This is the basic equation of the Flory–Huggins theory. The activity of the solvent, a_1, is equal to $p_1/p_1°$ (see Raoult's law on pp. 107 and 218). Thus, equation (20–22) can be verified by measuring the vapor pressure of the solvent. The agreement between calculated and observed activities is generally fair to good. Alternative expressions are still being developed.

PHASE SEPARATION[1,4,5,6a,9,26,29,30]

Equation (20–22) predicts when phase separation will occur in a polymer solution: if χ and, hence, ΔH_m, is zero or negative, $\Delta \overline{G}_1$ is negative, and mixing occurs, over the entire range of compositions or ϕ values, helped by the mutual attraction between polymer and solvent. The interaction parameter χ is actually composed not only of the temperature-dependent enthalpy term (equation (20–19)) but also of a temperature-independent, entropy-related term. For most polymer-solvent combinations, χ is positive and increases with decreasing temperature as the solvent becomes progressively poorer, causing ΔG_m *and* $\Delta \overline{G}_1$ to become progressively less negative. When they change from negative to positive, at a critical value χ_c, phase separation begins.

In binary solvent–polymer systems, equilibrium between two phases requires that $\Delta \overline{G}_1$ be the same in both phases, which corresponds to the requirement that the first and second derivative of $\Delta \overline{G}_1$ with respect to ϕ_2 be zero. Applying this requirement to equation (20–22) results in the three equations, (20–23), (20–24), and (20–25), relating the χ_c and $\phi_{2,c}$ values at the critical solution temperature T_c, and T_c itself, to the polymer molecular weight:

$$\chi_c = \frac{(1 + \sqrt{N})^2}{2N} \cong \frac{1}{2} + \frac{1}{\sqrt{N}} \quad (20–23)$$

N, the number of polymer segments equivalent in size

to a solvent molecule, represents the ratio of the molar volumes of polymer to solvent and, frequently, the *DP*. The critical solution temperature (also called upper consolute temperature; cf. p. 40 and Figures 2–14 and 2–16) is the temperature above which complete solution occurs over the entire range of concentrations. Phase separation begins only below T_c. This equation indicates that, as the chain length N or DP increases, χ_c falls, and the temperature at which a polymer fraction first becomes completely soluble increases. This effect is small, however, because the minimum value of χ_c for very high molecular weights is 0.5.

The dependence of phase separation on molecular weight can be used for polymer *fractionation*. The temperature of a polymer solution at nearly critical conditions (χ only slightly below 0.5) is lowered progressively. Alternatively, the polymer sample is dissolved in a good solvent, and a liquid miscible with the solvent that does not dissolve the polymer ($\chi \geqslant 0.5$) is added in successive increments at constant temperature. Examples of polymer–solvent–precipitant systems are gelatin–water–ethanol and polystyrene–benzene–methanol.[12] Both processes render the solvent increasingly poorer and gradually increase the χ value of the system. The solution exceeds the χ_c value of the highest-molecular-weight fraction first, causing it to precipitate in a separate layer (see the following), which is removed from the main volume of the solution. With further cooling or nonsolvent addition, the χ_c values of progessively lower-molecular-weight fractions are exceeded, causing them to precipitate in turn. The oligomer or low-molecular-weight tail, possessing the highest χ_c, remains in solution the longest. Refractionation is usually used to obtain sharper fractions.

The critical volume fraction of the polymer is

$$\phi_{2,c} = \frac{1}{1 + \sqrt{N}} \cong \frac{1}{\sqrt{N}} \qquad (20-24)$$

As $N \cong DP \cong 10^3$ to 10^4 for typical polymers, $\phi_{2,c} \cong$ 0.03 to 0.01 or 3 to 1 volume percent. Polymer solubilities near the critical temperature generally amount to only a few percent (*v/v*).

Typical phase diagrams for four polystyrene fractions in cyclohexane[30] are shown in Figure 20–9. They resemble binary phase diagrams of low-molecular-weight solutes (e.g., Fig. 2–14), except that the present curves are highly asymmetric and nearly coincide with the temperature axis for low ϕ_2 values. The areas above the curves are single-phase regions representing complete miscibility; those beneath the curves represent two-phase regions or partial miscibility. The fraction with a molecular weight of 43,600 has a critical solution temperature of 19° C. Above that temperature, there is complete miscibility; below it, phase separation occurs. The 15° *tie line* (defined on p. 40) indicates that at 15° C, solutions of that polystyrene

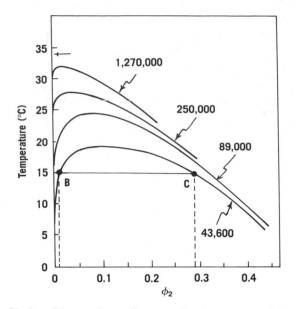

Fig. 20–9. Binary phase diagram of polystyrene–cyclohexane showing the precipitation temperature as a function of polymer concentration for four polystyrene fractions. Numbers represent viscosity-average molecular weights (From A. R. Shultz and P. J. Flory, J. Am. Chem. Soc. **74**, 4762, 1952, reprinted with permission from the Journal of the American Chemical Society. Copyright 1952, American Chemical Society.)

rene fraction separate into two phases: The one represented by Point *B*, with $\phi_2 = 0.007$, is almost pure solvent. Even the polymer-rich phase represented by Point *C* has $\phi_2 = 0.29$ only, that is, it contains 71% (*v/v*) solvent. These facts indicate that the solvent is much more soluble in the polymer than the polymer is in the solvent.

The coexistence of two liquid phases, one the nearly pure solvent and the other a moderately concentrated polymer solution, is called *coacervation*. The polymer-rich phase, called a *coacervate*, is a viscous liquid or sometimes a gelatinous semisolid, depending on the polymer concentration and molecular weight.

The critical solution temperature T_c is related to the molecular weight by

$$\frac{1}{T_c} \cong \frac{1}{\theta}\left(1 + \frac{D}{\sqrt{M}}\right) \qquad (20-25)$$

in which D is a constant for the polymer–solvent combination. The *Flory temperature* θ is the critical temperature, T_c, for a polymer of infinite molecular weight. The θ temperatures for some polymer–solvent systems are found in Table 20–4. According to equation (20–25), T_c increases as the molecular weight of the polymer fraction increases. Qualitatively, this is corroborated by Figure 20–9.

Example 20–6. Using the data obtainable from Figure 20–9, show that equation (20–25) is correct and evaluate D. For polystyrene in cyclohexane θ is 34.0° C (see Table 20–4). Rearranging equation (20–25) gives

TABLE 20–4. *Theta Temperatures for Various Polymer–Solvent Systems for Polymers of Infinite Molecular Weight*[12,27]

Polymer	Solvent	θ, °C
Polystyrene	Cyclohexane/toluene($\frac{87}{13}$)	15
	Cyclohexane	34.0
	Cyclohexanol	83.5
Polyethylene	n-Hexane	133
	n-Octanol	180
Polymethyl methacrylate	Toluene	−65
	Acetone	−55
	Methyl ethyl ketone/isopropanol($\frac{50}{50}$)	25.0
	n-Propanol	84.4
Polyvinyl alcohol	Water	~102
Povidone	Dioxane	−10
	Water/acetone($\frac{33}{67}$)	25
Polyoxyethylene	Isopropanol	30
Polydimethyl siloxane	n-Hexane	−173
	Toluene	−30
	Methyl ethyl ketone	20

$$D = \frac{(\theta - T_c)\sqrt{M}}{T_c}$$

The T_c values (highest temperatures reached by the curves) for the four polystyrene fractions listed in the following tabulation were read from Figure 20–9. D is then calculated for each of the fractions with this equation with T_c expressed in degrees Kelvin.

$M \times 10^{-3}$	T_c, °C	T_c, °K	D
∞	34.0	307.2	—
1,270	31.1	304.3	10.7
250	27.6	300.8	10.6
89	23.6	296.8	10.5
43.6	19.2	292.4	10.6
			mean $\overline{10.6} \pm 0.1$

Since all four fractions give D values that are identical within ±1%, D is constant, corroborating equation (20–25).

Alternatively, the plot of the reciprocal of T_c in degrees absolute versus $1/\sqrt{M}$ for the four polystyrene fractions is linear. Extrapolation to $1/\sqrt{M} = 0$ (corresponding to $M = \infty$) according to equation (20–25) gives $T_c = \theta = 307.2°$ K = 34.0° C, in perfect agreement with the experimental value of θ. The slope of that plot is 0.03429. According to equation (20–25), the slope equals D/θ. Since $\theta = 307.2$, $D = (0.03429)(307.2) = 10.5$, in agreement with the average D value calculated previously.

As the temperature of the polymer solutions is lowered, the solvent becomes progressively poorer until, at the Flory or θ-temperature, the solvent becomes what is known as a θ-solvent. At these conditions, the polymer–solvent interaction is so weak that it is balanced exactly by the polymer–polymer interaction, that is, by the attraction between polymer segments that are at some distance from one another along the chain but that approach each other during its writhing motion. The latter, long-range intramolecular interaction tends to contract the random coil while solvation tends to expand it, thereby increasing the end-to-end distance and radius of gyration. Because the two types of interactions are in exact balance at the

θ-temperature, polymer chains assume their *unperturbed dimensions:* The dimensions are governed only by bond lengths, bond angles, and the potential hindering bond rotation as caused, for instance, by bulky side groups, but not by segment–solvent nor by segment–segment attractions. The excluded volume vanishes at the θ-temperature, and the chains interpenetrate one another freely with no net interaction, as they do in the molten state. At temperatures a few degrees below the θ-temperature, the intermolecular attraction among polymer segments is sufficiently stronger than the attraction between polymer segments and solvent molecules to cause precipitation. Above the θ-temperature, solvation predominates.

At the θ-temperature, the partial molar free energy due to polymer–solvent interaction is zero, and the solution behaves ideally over a range of concentrations: The second virial coefficient becomes zero and $\chi = 0.5$. Hence, polymer solutions are often studied at the θ-temperature.

Since the polymer chain is tightly coiled and compact in a θ-solvent, the exponent a in the Mark–Houwink equation (equation (20–8)) becomes 0.5. The reason is as follows. At θ-conditions, the chain behaves ideally, that is, as if it were freely jointed and perfectly flexible so that its shape is described by the *random-flight model* (see p. 564). The chain dimensions are unperturbed by polymer–solvent and intramolecular polymer–polymer interactions (excluded volume effect), and the square of the root-mean-square end-to-end distance, $\langle R^2 \rangle$, is proportional to the molecular weight M (see equation (20–14)). The hydrodynamic volume of a randomly coiled chain, comprising the volume of the random coil plus that of the solvent inside it, is always proportional to the cube of the end-to-end distance. For the ideal random coil, it is also proportional to $M^{3/2}$ because $\langle R^2 \rangle$ is proportional to M. The anhydrous volume is always proportional to M. The hydrodynamic volume thus increases faster with increasing chain length than the anhydrous volume by the solvation factor $M^{3/2}/M = M^{1/2}$. Since the intrinsic viscosity depends on the size of the flow unit or the solvation factor, it is proportional to $M^{1/2}$ at θ-conditions where the random coil behaves ideally, making $a = 0.5$. Equation (20–8) then becomes

$$[\eta]_\theta = k_\theta M^{0.5} \qquad (20\text{–}8a)$$

If the random coil does not behave ideally because solvation and other factors that reduce chain flexibility expand it and increase $\langle R^2 \rangle$ beyond the unperturbed value corresponding to the θ-state, a will increase above 0.5.

θ-Temperatures for different polymer–solvent combinations extrapolated to infinite molecular weight are listed in Table 20–4. A more extensive list and a summary of the experimental methods used to determine θ-solvents are given in reference 12.

GEL FORMATION, COACERVATION, AND MICROENCAPSULATION[31]

Gels are semisolids characterized by relatively high yield values. Their plastic viscosity may be low, but they possess some elasticity. Gels consist of two interpenetrating continuous phases. One is solid, composed of highly asymmetric particles with a high surface area; the other is liquid. The solid phase extending throughout an aqueous gel may be a "house of cards" type built by bentonite clay platelets 10 to 50 Å thick whose positively charged edges attract their negatively charged faces, or it may consist of microscopic soap fibers produced by crystallization of soap molecules into ribbons. The liquid phase permeates the solid scaffolding, filling the voids.

Polymer solutions are prone to setting to gels because the solute consists of long and flexible chains of molecular thickness that tend to become entangled, attract each other by secondary valence forces, and even crystallize. When the three-dimensional polymerization of multifunctional monomers (functionality ≥ 3) reaches a given conversion, gelation occurs at a sharp "gel point." Cross-linking of dissolved polymer molecules also causes their solutions to gel. Both types of reaction produce permanent gels, held together by primary valence forces.

Reversible gel formation of polymer solutions, involving only secondary valence forces, occurs when the solvent becomes so poor that the polymer precipitates: Intermolecular contacts between polymer segments form in preference to contacts between polymer segments and solvent molecules, turning points of chain entanglements into physical cross-links. This kind of gel formation occurs when the temperature of the solution is lowered 10° C or more below the θ-temperature. For instance, aqueous gelatin solutions set to gels when cooled to temperatures in the vicinity of 30° C (the gel melting point). These temperatures decrease somewhat as the concentration increases. Aqueous methylcellulose solutions gel when heated above ~50° C (thermal gelation) because the polymer is less soluble in hot water and precipitates.

Because of its pronounced tendency to crystallize, polyethylene separates from solutions in organic solvents as a crystalline solid. Since single polyethylene chains extend through several crystalline regions and connect them, gels are formed when the polyethylene concentration is high enough to fill the entire solution with a continuous network of interconnected chains, held together by shared crystallites (see the following). Polyethylene resins dissolved in hot mineral oil at a 5% concentration crystallize on cooling to form the hydrocarbon ointment base called Plastibase or Jelene (see p. 500). Hot aqueous solutions of pectin and agar containing only 2 to 5% of these polysaccharides set to gels on cooling, immobilizing 95 to 98% of interstitial water.

Other polymers require higher concentrations to gel or solidify their entire solutions.

Gels often contract on standing, and some of the interstitial liquid is squeezed out. This phenomenon, called *syneresis*, is due to additional crystallization or to the formation of additional contact points between polymer segments on aging. In the case of irreversible gels formed by three-dimensional polymerization, continuing cross-linking or polycondensation reactions tighten the polymer network and shrink the solid phase.

If not enough polymer is present to form a fibrous network extending throughout the entire solution when phase separation occurs, gelatinous precipitates containing typically about 10 to 20% polymer separate from almost pure solvent (see previous discussion). The compositions of these two phases are given by Points C and B in Figure 20–9. Such phase separations can be brought about not only by cooling the solutions below T_c but also by adding a nonsolvent liquid and thereby raising χ above $χ_c$.

In the case of aqueous polymer solutions, the addition of salts can also cause phase separation, which is called *salting out*. Abstraction of water of hydration from polymers due to the addition of large amounts of salts (several molal), which require water for their own hydration, raises the effective ϕ_2 of polymer solutions above their critical value $\phi_{2,c}$. Polyelectrolytes are particularly prone to salting out. The electrostatic repulsion between approaching segments that, together with hydration, contributed to their solubility in water is swamped by the addition of large amounts of inorganic ions, further contributing to precipitation. Combinations of a water-miscible nonsolvent liquid and a salt produce synergistic salting-out effects.

The formation of such gels or gelatinous precipitates is reversible. Heating of gelatin gels or of Plastibase above their gel melting points, cooling of methylcellulose gels below the temperature of thermal gelation, and addition of more solvent after a nonsolvent liquid or a salt has produced phase separation, revert these two-phase systems to homogeneous solutions.

The same factors that bring about reversible gelation or separation of a gelatinous precipitate from polymer solutions may, under different conditions of composition and temperature, lead to *coacervation*, that is, the separation of small droplets of a polymer-rich, second liquid phase. On standing, these droplets eventually coalesce. This phenomenon has been studied extensively with gelatin by Bungenberg de Jong.[31] Maintaining a temperature of 50° C to avoid gel formation, the addition of alcohol or of sodium sulfate to isoelectric aqueous gelatin solutions produces coacervation. For instance, a system containing 13% gelatin, 38% water, and 49% alcohol separated a coacervate containing 27% gelatin, 37% water, and 36% alcohol. Another system with a composition of 9% gelatin, 80% water, and 11%

sodium sulfate separated a coacervate of 25% gelatin, 69% water, and 6% sodium sulfate.

Among the systems polymer–solvent–nonsolvent liquid capable of undergoing coacervation are natural rubber–benzene–methanol, polystyrene–xylene–petroleum ether, polyvinyl acetate–methyl ethyl ketone–*n*-hexane, polyvinyl acetate–chloroform–isopropanol, and ethylcellulose–dichloromethane–*n*-hexane. For instance, coacervation occurs when a 9% ethylcellulose solution in dichloromethane is combined with two to four times its volume of *n*-hexane.[32]

Coacervation is the basis for one method of *microencapsulation* of solid or liquid drugs that has wide commercial application, for instance, in the manufacture of sustained-release dosage forms.[33,34] The core material, that is, the drug to be encapsulated, must be available as a fine powder, preferably micronized, or as an immiscible liquid. It is dispersed (or, if it is a liquid, emulsified) in the polymer solution prior to coacervation and must therefore be insoluble in the liquid medium. The precipitant liquid or salting-out electrolyte is added with continuous stirring. The coacervate droplets form mainly around the core particles, which act as nuclei because, even prior to the addition of precipitants, the solid surfaces are coated with a layer of adsorbed polymer, albeit a very thin one. Stirring is maintained to prevent the coacervate droplets, which engulf the core particles, from coalescing. The coacervate phase must be fluid enough to wrap completely around the core particles but viscous enough to avoid being sheared off the surface of the particles during stirring. To transform the viscous liquid coacervate envelopes into solid, continuous polymer shells completely encasing the core particles, they must be dried and hardened. The first step usually consists in cooling the system, preferably to a temperature below the second-order transition temperature of the polymer (see the following). Cooling will concentrate, shrink, and harden the polymeric wall material. The polymer may also be cross-linked to shrink and harden the microcapsule shells further, causing them to tighten and collapse around the core particles. Gelatin walls are commonly cross-linked with formaldehyde, which forms intermolecular methylene bridges. The microencapsulated particles with their shells still swollen by solvents are washed by decantation and finally dried. Commercial microcapsules have diameters in the range between 5 and 500 μm, and wall thicknesses between 1 and 10 μm.

POLYMERS IN THE SOLID STATE—OVERVIEW

Some polymers are useful as elastic closures, others as strong packaging films or fibers, and still others as tough plastic containers. The end uses of solid polymers depend on their mechanical, permeability, electric, thermal, and optical properties, which in turn are governed by their chemical nature, processing variables, and morphologic characteristics.

Among the pertinent factors, besides molecular weight and molecular weight distribution, are the following. The chemical structure of the polymers depends on the nature of the atoms and bonds in the backbone, for example, the stereoregular configuration of chain atoms and the presence of rings or double bonds in the chain, and on the polarity, frequency, and size of the substituent or side groups. These factors determine the flexibility and symmetry of the chains, the closeness of chain packing in the solid state and, hence, the magnitude of the interchain attraction, cohesion, and strength of the polymers.

In addition to the factors just mentioned, the crystallinity of polymers depends on thermodynamic aspects. Crystallinity and orientation also depend on processing conditions such as the rate of extrusion or injection and especially on the rate of cooling when the polymer is processed in the molten state, and on drawing or other postextrusion treatment. Branching, especially short-chain branching, and random copolymerization interfere with crystallization. For amorphous polymers, cross-linking (vulcanization) or the use of fillers may be desirable. Polymer processing methods are described in the following section.

The chemical composition and processing variables together determine the molecular order and morphologic characteristics of polymeric objects, specifically, the degree of crystallinity, the degree of chain orientation or alignment, the number and size of crystallites and spherulites, and any preferred orientation of the crystallites, as well as the susceptibility to developing flaws (cracks, crazing). These and related topics are discussed in the following section.

MECHANICAL PROPERTIES[35–39]

Solids can be deformed by tension, bending, shear, torsion, and compression. The following discussion is limited to tension, which is the mode most widely tested. The cause of deformation is stress, that is, the applied force F per unit area of cross-section A. Stress in tension is called *tensile stress* σ. The most widely used units of stress are: lb/in.^{2} or psi, dyne/cm^2, and newton/m^2 or N/m^2. The conversion factors are 1 psi = 6.895×10^4 dyne/cm^2 = 6895 N/m^2. The effect of stress is deformation or strain. Strain in tension is called *elongation* ϵ. It is the increase in length $\Delta L = L - L_0$ relative to the original length L_0, that is, $\epsilon = (L - L_0)/L_0 = \Delta L/L_0$, in which L is the length under a given tensile stress. Elongation is dimensionless because it is expressed as a fraction of the original length. It can also be expressed as a percentage, $100\,\Delta L/L_0$.

Ideal or elastic solids are deformed when subjected to stress but regain their original shape and dimensions

TABLE 20-5. *Mechanical Properties of Some Solids[35,37,38]*

Material	Young's Modulus (psi × 10⁻⁵)	Tensile Strength (psi × 10⁻³)	(Tensile Strength / Specific Gravity) (psi × 10⁻³)
Glass	87	10	4
Steel	320	60	7.6
Copper	174	39	4.3
Aluminum	100	9	3.3
Polystyrene	5	7	6.6
Polymethyl methacrylate	4.6	9	7.6
Polyvinyl chloride	4.7	7	5
6,6 Nylon	2.9	10	8.8
Cellulose acetate (secondary)	2.9	6.6	5.1
High-density polyethylene	1.7	5.3	5.5
Low-density polyethylene	0.36	2.2	2.4
Natural rubber (vulcanized, unfilled)	0.0019	2.9	3.1
Tendon	0.19	—	—
Gelatin gel, 30% solids	0.00022	—	—

when the stress is released. According to *Hooke's law*, the stress is directly proportional to the strain. In tension:

$$\frac{F}{A} = E\left(\frac{L - L_0}{L_0}\right) \qquad (20-26)$$

The proportionality constant E, called *Young's modulus* or *modulus of elasticity*, is a measure of the hardness, stiffness, or rigidity (or softness, flexibility, or pliability) of the solid, that is, of its resistance to deformation: $E = \Delta\sigma/\Delta\epsilon$. Characteristic values are listed in Table 20–5, in which glass, metals, and tendon are included for comparison. Steel has an elastic modulus $320/2.9 = 110$ times greater than 66 nylon, indicating that it is 110 times stiffer or harder and that the force required to stretch a steel wire by, say, 1% is 110 times greater than that required to stretch an equally thick nylon filament by the same amount. Nylon is 1500 times stiffer than pure gum rubber because the ratio of their moduli is $2.9/0.0019 \cong 1500$.

Representative *stress-strain curves* in tension or load-elongation curves are plotted in Figure 20–10 for steel, a typical tough plastic such as high-density polyethylene, a thermoplastic cellulose derivative or a nylon, and a typical elastomer. The curve for the plastic is discussed in detail. Along the linear portion LO, the elongation is directly proportional to the applied stress, following Hooke's law, equation (20–26). Young's modulus is the slope of LO or the tangent of the angle LOC. The linear portion of the curve for steel is about 100 times steeper than for the plastic while the one for the rubber is about 1000 times flatter, reflecting the magnitude of their moduli of elasticity. Beyond L, the plot curves and Hooke's law no longer applies.

Point R is the *yield point*, and the corresponding stress M is the *yield stress*. The plastic behaves elastically when subjected to stresses below M. When stresses up to the yield stress are applied and then removed, a plastic specimen that had stretched along OLR retracts along the same curve RLO and assumes

its original length. The curve shows no hysteresis, and the sample undergoes no permanent elongation. Beyond R, where the applied stresses exceed M, the specimen exhibits plasticity, becoming ductile and flowing or creeping under nearly constant stress, resembling a highly viscous liquid. The corresponding portion RAH of the stress-strain curve is nearly horizontal. This phenomenon is called *cold flow* or *creep*. If the stress is released at A, the sample retracts along AC. The nonrecoverable deformation OC is called *permanent set*. Cold flow causes a change in the structure of the plastic. Crystalline domains may melt and reform with an orientation parallel to the direction of flow. Disordered, randomly coiled chains lined up parallel to one another during cold flow may crystallize, and flaws may heal. Thus, the curve may turn up after H because the structural rearrangement stiffened the specimen, increasing its modulus and resistance to

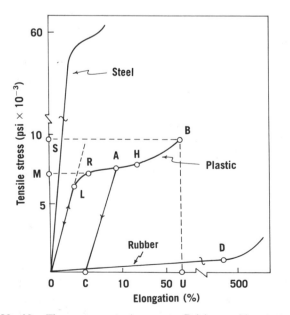

Fig. 20–10. Three stress-strain curves. Psi is an abbreviation of lbs/in². See the text for discussion of the curves.

deformation. This phenomenon is called *strain harden-ing*. At *B*, the sample ruptures: *U* is the ultimate elongation or the *elongation to* (or at) *break; S* is the *tensile strength* or ultimate strength. See Table 20–5 for representative values.

Since tensile strength measures the ability of solids to withstand rupture, plastics are generally weaker than metals. Because plastics are also lighter, they have approximately the same tensile strength as metals when compared on an equal weight basis (as is done in the last column of Table 20–5, headed Tensile Strength/Specific Gravity) rather than on an equal volume basis (as is done in the third column, headed Tensile Strength). Even though elastomers are much softer than plastics, their tensile strength is not much lower.

The time during which solids are subjected to stress may affect their behavior. Stresses smaller than the yield stress, if applied for long periods of time, may produce creep (see p. 468 for creep of pharmaceutical solids). Faster testing speeds, that is, higher rates of elongation, result in higher tensile strength and lower elongation to break. Another related fact is that the tensile strength determined at low speeds, which is closest to an equilibrium value, is usually smaller by at least an order of magnitude than the tensile strength calculated from the cohesion of the polymer, using data such as those of Table 20–7. The explanation for these two facts is the existence of cracks, notches, or voids in the piece of plastic or strip of film being tested. These flaws represent weak spots where failure or rupture will occur. The cracks or voids grow and propagate under stress; if the specimen is stretched slowly, their rate of propagation keeps up with the rate of elongation of the entire specimen. Extensive propagation of cracks or voids lowers the tensile strength of the specimen because the intact material next to these flaws bears the entire load distributed over a reduced area and ruptures.

Temperature has a profound effect on the mechanical properties of polymers. All data in this chapter refer to room temperature unless stated otherwise. Young's modulus and the tensile strength of plastics are reduced by raising the temperature, while their elongation to break is increased. Elastomers, on the other hand, become stiffer when the temperature is raised, that is, their modulus of elasticity increases. Joule observed in 1859 that a rubber band, stretched to a given length by a weight suspended from it, contracted upon heating and stretched upon cooling. The increase in tension of a stretched rubber band on heating resembles the increase in pressure of a gas with increasing temperature.

The areas under the stress-strain curves of Figure 20–10 represent the product, stress × elongation, which is the energy or work necessary to break the polymeric material. It is equal to

$$\int_0^{\epsilon=B} \sigma \, d\epsilon$$

and constitutes a measure of its toughness or brittleness. In Table 20–6, polymers are divided into five categories according to a qualitative description of their mechanical behavior and the corresponding stress-strain characteristics. Hard or stiff polymers, as opposed to soft ones, are characterized by high moduli. Strong (as opposed to weak) polymers have high tensile strengths. Tough (as opposed to brittle) polymers have large areas under their stress-strain curves and require large amounts of energy to break under stress, combining high or at least moderate tensile strength with high elongation.

Stiff and brittle plastics such as polystyrene and

TABLE 20–6. *Qualitative Description and Stress-Strain Characteristics of Various Polymers at Room Temperature*[37,40]

| Polymer Description | Characteristics of Stress-Strain Curve | | | | Examples |
	Young's Modulus	Yield Stress	Tensile Strength	Elongation to Break	
Soft, weak	Low	Low	Low	Low to moderate	Soft gels
Soft, tough	Low	Low	Moderate	Very high (20–1000%)	Elastomers, plasticized polyvinyl chloride
Hard, brittle	High	None (break around yield point)	Moderate to high	Very low (<2%)	Polystyrene, polymethyl methacrylate, phenol-formaldehyde resins
Hard, strong	High	High	High	Moderate (~5%)	Rigid polyvinyl chloride, impact-resistant polystyrene polyblends
Hard, tough	High	High	High	High (cold drawing or "necking")	Nylons, ethyl cellulose, cellulose nitrate, cellulose acetate

polymethyl methacrylate have high moduli and high tensile strength, that is, their stress-strain curves rise steeply. They break at elongations of only about 2%, however, undergoing little or no cold flow: their breaking point *B* occurs at about the same point at which other polymers of comparable modulus have a yield point *R*. Their stress-strain curves extend over narrow areas, indicating that the work required to break them is small and that they have low impact resistance. Some commercial grades of polystyrene are toughed considerably by incorporating 5 to 10% of an elastomer. Elastomers are soft, and their stress-strain curves are shallow at low elongations. The curves frequently turn up rather sharply at elongations of about 200 or 300%, however, and extend to ultimate elongations as high as 700% or more, so that the areas under the curves are large and the elastomers tough.

Most hard and tough polymers such as thermoplastic cellulose derivatives, nylons, and the engineering plastics acetal, polycarbonate, and polysulfone owe their high elongation to *cold drawing* or "necking": The specimens do not elongate uniformly but, after the yield point, develop a constricted region or neck that undergoes large, permanent elongation. As the stretching continues, the constricted region propagates in both directions toward the specimen clamps. The cross-sectional area of the drawn portion or neck remains constant during the stretching. Not all polymers fit into the five categories. For instance, low-density polyethylene (LDPE) has a moderate modulus, yield stress, and tensile strength and a high elongation. It is moderately hard and tough.

The end use of polymers is governed largely by their mechanical properties at room temperature. Elastomers fall into the "soft, tough" category, whereas plastics fall into one of the three "hard" categories (hard, brittle; hard, strong; hard, tough). Table 20–7 lists the distinctive mechanical properties of commercial elastomers, plastics, packaging films, and textile fibers. The latter two have similar properties and are grouped together. They are stronger and stiffer than plastics because, after extrusion, they are cold drawn, which brings their chains into alignment, promotes more extensive crystallization, and preferentially orients the crystallites (see the following sections).

The properties of plastics listed in Table 20–7 are those of thermoplastic resins that are processed in the molten state rather than those of highly cross-linked, thermosetting resins such as melamine–formaldehyde. Plastics are generally intermediate in mechanical properties between the weaker and softer elastomers and the stronger and stiffer films or fibers, overlapping both groups. Some polymers such as 66 nylon and polypropylene can function both as plastics and as films or fibers. Cold drawing produces orientation and higher crystallinity, which increases their tensile strength about ten times and doubles or triples their modulus, bringing them from the plastics to the film/fiber range.

INTERCHAIN COHESIVE FORCES

The forces responsible for the mechanical strength of packaging films and plastic containers are the secondary valence forces between adjacent polymer chains rather than the primary valence forces joining together the backbone atoms of single chains. This fact is corroborated by three observations. First, mechanical stresses causing failure are usually much smaller than the strength of covalent bonds. When a solid polymeric object is ruptured by an external stress, the weak secondary valence forces between chains are the ones to yield and break because they are the weakest links in the object; these weak forces cause chains to slip and move past one another and produce deformation, flow, and failure. Second, primary valence bonds are not generally broken when a packaging film tears or a plastic container ruptures, and the molecular weight of the polymer is not reduced. Thirdly, the energy or strength of the covalent bonds between carbon–carbon, carbon–oxygen, and carbon–nitrogen atoms forming the backbones of the chains of most commercial films, fibers, plastics, and elastomers are all in the 70 to 85 kcal/mole range. This range is much too narrow to account for the vast differences in mechanical strength of the four categories of polymeric objects shown in Table 20–7.

Two models showing the need for lateral attraction between chains are a parallel bundle of pencils and a bowl of cooked spaghetti, with the pencils and noodles representing polymer chains. The individual pencils are strong, and even the individual noodles are much stronger than the mass in the bowl. Without some glue or lateral adhesion, the bundle of pencils would fall apart and the mass of spaghetti could be pulled apart without breaking any noodles, that is, the assemblies

TABLE 20–7. *Typical Mechanical Properties of Commercial Elastomers, Plastics, and Films/Fibers*

End Use	Tensile Strength (psi $\times 10^{-3}$)	Young's Modulus (psi)	Ultimate Elongation (%)
Elastomers	1–4	10–400	300–900
Plastics	2–12	10^4–5×10^5	2–200
Films/fibers	20–100	10^5–10^6	10–50

would have negligible mechanical strength and would be much weaker than the component elements or chains.

Table 20–8 lists individual polymers, the structure of their repeat units, and the magnitude of their interchain attraction energy or cohesion. The latter values were calculated by summing the attractive energies for all groups in 5-Å lengths of polymer chains, assuming that each chain is surrounded by four other chains. The polymers are listed in order of increasing polarity corresponding to increasing attraction between chains. They fall into three categories.

Cohesive energies between 1.0 and 2.0 kcal/mole are the lowest. These polymers are primarily hydrocarbons and only dispersion forces, the weakest of the secondary valence forces, are involved in interchain attraction. The solid polymers in this category are elastomers, with the lowest mechanical strength. Plastics are stronger. Their cohesive energies range from 2 to 5 kcal/mole and involve dipole–dipole attraction in addition to dispersion forces. The highest interchain attraction, above 5 kcal/mole, produces materials with the highest strength, suitable for use as films and fibers. The high cohesion is due to interchain attraction by

TABLE 20–8. *Energy of Interchain Attraction or Cohesion for Different Polymers[1]*

Polymer	Repeat Unit	Cohesion (kcal/mole)	
Polyethylene	CH_2-CH_2-	1.0	
Polyisobutylene	$-CH_2-\underset{CH_3}{\overset{CH_3}{C}}-$	1.2	ELASTOMERS
cis-Polyisoprene (natural rubber)	$-CH_2-\underset{}{\overset{CH_3}{C}}=CH-CH_2-$	1.3	
Polychloroprene	$-CH_2-\underset{}{\overset{Cl}{C}}=CH-CH_2-$	1.6	
Polyvinyl chloride	$-CH_2-\underset{Cl}{CH}-$	2.6	
Polyvinyl acetate	$-CH_2-\underset{O-CO-CH_3}{CH}-$	3.2	
Polystyrene	$-CH_2-CH-$ (phenyl)	4.0	
Polyvinyl alcohol	$-CH_2-\underset{OH}{CH}-$	4.2	PLASTICS
Cellulose acetate (secondary)	(ring structure with $CH_2O-CO-CH_3$, OH, $O-CO-CH_3$)	4.8	
Cellulose	(ring structure with CH_2OH, OH, OH)	6.2	
6 Nylon	$-\underset{O}{\overset{}{C}}-NH-(CH_2)_5-$	5.6	FILMS and FIBERS
Silk fibroin	$-\underset{O}{\overset{}{C}}-NH-\underset{R}{CH}-$	9.8	

hydrogen bonds, the strongest secondary valence forces, in addition to dispersion and dipole–dipole attractive forces.

Since the solubility parameter and the energy of interchain attraction are both a measure of the polarity of the polymers, they should be related. Comparison of the δ_2 values of Table 20–3 and the cohesion values of Table 20–8 gives the following linear regression,[41] with a correlation coefficient of 0.93:

$$\text{cohesion} = -3.90 + 0.676\,\delta_2 \qquad (20\text{--}27)$$

There are two exceptions in Table 20–8. Polyethylene, according to its calculated cohesion, belongs after the elastomers, but according to its actual mechanical strength belongs among the stronger plastics. Polyvinyl alcohol has the strength of fiber- or film-forming polymers even though its calculated cohesion places it among the plastics, which are weaker. The chains of these two polymers are smooth and symmetric, permitting them to pack or fit together closely.[1] Van der Waals intermolecular attraction forces fall off with the seventh power of the interchain distance. Interchain distances in angstroms for amorphous polymers at room temperature, obtained from the halos in their x-ray diffraction patterns, are as follows: polyethylene, 5.5; *cis*-polyisoprene, 5.9; polyisobutylene, 7.8. The kinky configuration of the natural rubber chain and the two bulky methyl side groups in polyisobutylene produce larger interchain distances and, hence, smaller interchain attraction and lower mechanical strength than those of polyethylene, which has a straight and smooth chain.

In summary, for polymers to be mechanically strong, they should have smooth and symmetric chains capable of fitting together closely, without bulky side groups, and a high concentration of polar functional groups.

CRYSTALLINITY

Maximum interchain attraction, resulting in greatest mechanical strength, requires that the polymer chains be packed as densely as possible and that the polar groups of adjacent chains be in registry, so that there is an efficient geometric matching-up of interacting dipoles or hydrogen-bonding groups between chains. Thus, to be mechanically strong, a polymer should be highly crystalline. Conversely, a weaker and softer polymer for use as an elastomer can be obtained by preventing crystallization, for example, by random copolymerization.

Polyvinyl alcohol crystallizes in a fully extended zigzag conformation. The repeat distance along the chain axis, 2.52 Å, corresponds to layers of hydroxyl groups largely hydrogen bonded. This arrangement, plus the relatively small size of the hydroxyl groups resulting in smooth chains, produces a highly crystalline polymer.[4] Polyvinyl alcohol is manufactured by the hydrolysis of polyvinyl acetate. Commercial products are available with varying degrees of hydrolysis and, hence, a wide range of solubilities and strengths. Hydrolysis is a random process, leaving residual acetyl groups randomly distributed along the polymer chains. A partially hydrolyzed product:

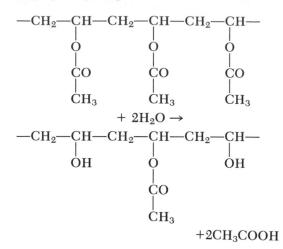

is in effect a random copolymer of polyvinyl alcohol and polyvinyl acetate. Residual acetyl groups, because of their bulk, keep adjacent chains apart and lower the density and crystallinity of the product. They reduce the interchain dispersion forces and interrupt the matching of hydrogen-bonding hydroxyl groups between adjacent chains, resulting in lower mechanical strength and higher gas permeability.

Polyethylene crystallizes with the chains in the fully extended planar zigzag conformation packed side by side with their axes parallel to one another. Isotactic polypropylene (see the following section) crystallizes with the chains in a helical conformation, three repeat units per turn. In random copolymers of ethylene and propylene in the 40/60 to 60/40 range, the chains can fit into neither the zigzag lattice of polyethylene nor the helical lattice of polypropylene. On cooling from the melt, the chains remain disordered and the copolymers, called *polyolefins*, are amorphous. In addition to being virtually free of extractables, they contain no spherulites (see under *Morphology*) because they lack crystallinity, which increases their translucency. Furthermore, their modulus or stiffness (see under *Mechanical Properties*) is low. The resultant higher impact resistance compared with that of the two crystalline homopolymer resins, combined with the low water vapor transmission rate common to all hydrocarbon plastics, makes the polyolefins useful as containers for purified water and parenteral solutions.

Short-chain branching disrupts the crystallinity of solid polymers and weakens them mechanically. Depending on the polymerization process, polyethylene can be mostly linear (high-density polyethylene, HDPE), producing a tough plastic that crystallizes well and is mechanically strong, or it can be branched, with *n*-butyl or pentyl side chains, which result in lower

TABLE 20-9. *Effect of Short-Chain Branching on Crystallinity and Other Properties of Polyethylene*[12]

Property	Polyethylene Resin of:		
	Low Density (LDPE)	Medium Density	High Density (HDPE)
Methyl groups per 1000 C atoms	83–46	46–8	0
Density (g/cm³)	0.910–0.925	0.926–0.940	0.941–0.965
Crystallinity (%)	37–50	50–62	62–75
Tensile modulus (psi × 10⁻³)	8–25	25–55	60–150
Permeability* to:			
Oxygen	3.4–1.5	1.4–0.9	0.8–0.5
Carbon dioxide	12.5–5.4	5.1–3.0	2.8–1.0
Water vapor	65–42	39–29	26–15

*Transmission rate, $\dfrac{(cm^3 \text{ gas, STP})(cm \text{ thickness})}{(cm^2 \text{ area}) \sec (cm \text{ Hg}) 10^{10}}$

crystallinity, lower density, and a weaker, softer, and more permeable plastic (low-density polyethylene, LDPE). HDPE is used in containers, LDPE in packaging films. There are also polyethylene resins of intermediate density. Table 20–9 shows the effect of branching in polyethylene resins on some of their properties. The extent of branching is measured by IR as the number of methyl groups per 1000 carbon atoms: each methyl group represents one branch. Since branching interferes with the close packing or crystallization of the chains, it results in polymers with fewer and smaller crystalline domains and a large fraction of amorphous or disordered domains having therefore lower density. The greater softness of LDPE compared with HDPE is reflected in a lower modulus. Diffusion through polymers occurs primarily in the amorphous regions, whereas the crystalline domains are comparatively impervious to penetrants. Thus, the permeability toward gases and vapors increases with decreasing crystallinity or density, being lowest for HDPE.

By measuring the density ρ_{obs} of a polymer sample or its reciprocal, the specific volume v_{obs}, one can calculate how crystalline it is, that is, the weight fraction α of crystalline domains or $1 - \alpha$ of amorphous domains; 100α represents percent crystallinity. Specific volumes are additive. If v_{am} is the specific volume of the completely amorphous polymer, extrapolated from the specific volume of the molten polymer at different temperatures above the melting point to room temperature, and v_{cr} is the specific volume of the perfectly crystalline polymer, calculated from its unit cell dimensions obtained from x-ray diffraction, then

$$v_{obs} = \alpha v_{cr} + (1 - \alpha)v_{am}$$

Hence,

$$\alpha = \frac{v_{am} - v_{obs}}{v_{am} - v_{cr}} \qquad (20\text{–}28)$$

Example 20–7. For polyethylene, $\rho_{cr} = 1.000$ and $\rho_{am} = 0.861$ g/cm³ at 25° C; hence $v_{cr} = 1.000$ and $v_{am} = 1.161$ cm³/g. Calculate the percent crystallinity for a low-density sample with $\rho_{obs} = 0.912$ and a medium-density sample with $\rho_{obs} = 0.933$ gcm³. For LDPE,

$$\alpha = \frac{1.161 - 1/0.912}{1.161 - 1.000} = 0.401$$

For the medium-density sample,

$$\alpha = \frac{1.161 - 1/0.933}{1.161 - 1.000} = 0.554$$

The LDPE is 40% crystalline and 60% amorphous; the medium-density sample is 55% crystalline and 45% amorphous.

TACTICITY[6a]

Commercial polystyrene used for manufacturing plastic vials and other vinyl homopolymers such as polymethyl methacrylate or polyvinyl acetate cannot crystallize, even though their chains have little or no branching. In vinyl polymers, every other chain carbon atom is essentially asymmetric without, however, producing optical activity.

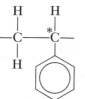

Three different types of homopolymers with different configurations and different physical properties can be produced, depending on the method and conditions of polymerization. With the main chain of a polystyrene molecule in the planar zigzag conformation, the phenyl groups can all be on the same side of the main chain, that is, they are all either above or below the plane of the main chain:

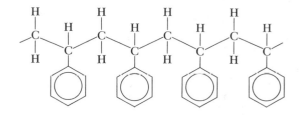

In this arrangement, all tertiary carbon atoms have the same configuration, that is, all are *d*- (or *l*-): -*dddddd*-. This is the *isotactic* form. In the *syndiotactic* configuration, the phenyl groups lie alternatively above and below the plane of the backbone:

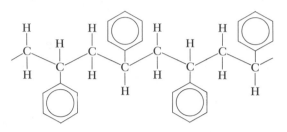

Syndiotactic polymers are alternating -*dldldl*- copolymers. Both classes of polymers are produced through stereospecific, stereoregular, or coordination polymerization generally employing Ziegler–Natta catalysts, such as mixtures of an aluminum alkyl and a titanium chloride. Isotactic and syndiotactic polymers crystallize owing to their regular structures. Because of the theoretic importance of these structures and the commercial importance of the polymers, Ziegler and Natta were jointly awarded the 1963 Nobel prize in chemistry.

In *atactic* polymers, there is no regularity in the configuration of the asymmetric carbon atoms. The substituent groups lie randomly above and below the plane of the backbone. Atactic polymers are random -*dlddldll*- copolymers and, because of their lack of stereoregularity, cannot crystallize. Free-radical addition polymerization generally produces atactic polymers. The effect of stereoregularity on selected physical properties is shown in Table 20–10.

MORPHOLOGY[6a]

Crystalline domains are called *crystallites*. They alternate with more disordered, "amorphous" regions. Single polymer chains often run through several contiguous crystallites and amorphous regions. When polymers are processed from the melt or from solution into films or molded objects, crystallization starts when nuclei develop here and there in the evaporating solution or in the cooling melt. The nuclei form as a few chain segments in the randomly coiled and entangled mass line up, and arrange themselves into an orderly lattice. Crystallization proceeds as these nuclei grow into crystallites until all the solvent has evaporated or all the melt has solidified.

When neighboring crystallites grow, quite a few segments of the chains forming these crystallites cannot be incorporated into them but remain outside in a disordered state. Being trapped between crystallites immobilizes such segments and prevents them from aligning and fitting into a lattice. When the mass cools, these segments are frozen into their disordered conformations as amorphous regions. If the molten polymer is cooled slowly or annealed, more chain segments have the opportunity to arrange or incorporate themselves into crystallites. Quenching freezes more segments into amorphous regions because the solidification is too sudden to permit extensive ordering and results in lower crystallinity. These considerations explain why even objects of HDPE, a polymer possessing smooth, symmetric chains without branches or side groups, are seldom more than 80% crystalline.

Single crystals of HDPE, visible in the electron microscope as thin, flat, rhombohedral platelets, form when very dilute solutions (~0.1%) of the polymer are slowly cooled. Electron diffraction measurements indicate that the polymer chains in single crystals of HDPE and other polymers are oriented perpendicularly to the faces of these lamellae. Since polymer molecules in extended conformation are at least 1000 Å long, whereas the platelets are only about 100 Å thick, the chains in these single crystals are folded and double back over themselves repeatedly. Chain folding occurs in the crystallites of many synthetic polymers.

Spherulites. Crystallization in synthetic polymers often produces polycrystalline aggregates called *spherulites*. These are spherical, radially symmetric arrays of fibrillar crystallites ranging in diameter from less than one micron to several millimeters. Microtome sections examined under the microscope show fibers or feathers radiating from the center of a spherulite like spokes of a wheel (see Fig. 20–11). Spherulites are quite common in plastics. It is not known exactly why they form, but they grow from their centers outward until they meet other growing spherulites. Individual polymer chains are folded and oriented perpendicularly to the fiber axes or spherulitic radii.

Slow cooling or annealing of molten plastics produces fewer but large spherulites; quenching or the addition of nucleating agents produces more and small spherulites. Because the boundaries between spherulites are weak regions prone to failure under stress, spherulites, especially large ones, reduce the strength and toughness of plastics and tend to make them brittle. Fortu-

TABLE 20–10. *Effect of Stereoregularity on Some Polymer Properties*

	Density (g/cm³)	Melting Point or Softening Temperature (°C)
Polypropylene		
Atactic, amorphous	0.85	75
Isotactic, crystalline	0.93	160
Syndiotactic, crystalline	0.90	138
Polystyrene		
Atactic, amorphous	1.06	100
Isotactic, crystalline	1.11	235

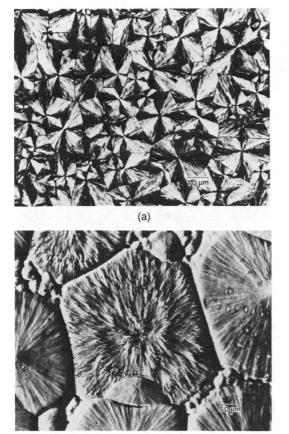

(a)

(b)

Fig. 20–11. (a) Spherulites of polyethylene crystallized from a thin film of melt. Transmission photomicrograph between crossed polarizers showing characteristic extinction crosses. (b) Spherulites of isotactic polypropylene crystallized from a thin film of melt. Photomicrograph with oblique reflected light showing radiating fibrous texture. (Courtesy of Dr. H. D. Keith, Bell Laboratories.)

nately, there is some overlapping and interpenetration between fibers of adjacent spherulites across their boundaries, providing mechanical interlocking and reinforcing the boundaries. One visible effect of spherulites is the opacity of polyethylene bottles.

Microcrystalline Cellulose. This form of cellulose consists entirely of crystalline material. Its manufacture involves the following steps. Native cellulose is treated with dilute mineral acid, which penetrates the amorphous, disordered regions relatively fast because of their lower density and hydrolyzes the accessible cellulose chain segments located there into water-soluble fragments. The acid is washed out before it penetrates the ordered and dense crystalline regions appreciably, leaving the crystallites intact. Washing also removes the soluble degradation products of the cellulose that constituted the amorphous regions. The remaining mass consists of the "unhinged" crystallites, which are no longer connected by the chain segments from the amorphous regions. Wet milling of the mass of crystallites, followed by spray-drying of their aqueous suspension, results in spongy, porous aggregates of fibrillar bundles that are used as tablet additives.

Additional shear breaks up the aggregated bundles into the individual needle- or rod-shaped crystallites averaging 0.3 μm in length and 0.02 μm in width. These colloidal particles thicken water and other liquids to thixotropic vehicles and, at higher concentrations, to semisolids.

ORIENTATION

Drawing fibers with or without the application of heat causes permanent elongation or cold flow and promotes the alignment or orientation of polymer chains and crystallites in the direction of stretch, that is, parallel to the fiber axis. This orientation process, called cold drawing, is carried out at a temperature below the melting point but above the glass transition temperature of the polymer (see the following). Cold drawing often causes crystallites to melt and to reform with parallel orientation. Even noncrystallizing polymers can be oriented by drawing. Polymers capable of crystallization crystallize more extensively when their chains are lined up parallel to each other. Drawing increases the strength and stiffness of fibers.

When films are extruded through a flat die and drawn in the direction of extrusion, alignment causes increased strength in that direction but reduced strength and the tendency to split in the transverse direction. Films are therefore oriented biaxially, that is, they are drawn simultaneously in the direction of extrusion and in the transverse direction. This is easily accomplished by extruding the film through a die with a circular slit and stretching the tubular film with air pressure applied from the inside to the zone where it is solidifying (cf. p. 591 and Fig. 20–15).

THERMODYNAMICS OF FUSION AND CRYSTALIZATION[6a]

Equation (20–17), previously applied to the binary system solvent–polymer, is now applied to the one-component system consisting of the polymer alone, to describe the reversible process:

$$\text{liquid amorphous polymer} \underset{\text{melting or fusion}}{\overset{\text{solidification and crystallization}}{\rightleftharpoons}} \text{solid crystalline polymer}$$

$$\Delta G_f = \Delta H_f - T \Delta S_f \qquad (20\text{–}17a)$$

The subscripts are changed from m (for mixing) to f (fusion) or cr (crystallization).

Heats of Crystallization and Fusion. The latent heat of crystallization or solidification, ΔH_{cr}, is negative because the process is exothermic. It represents the bond energies released during crystallization by the increased interchain attraction through secondary valence forces. When the polymer solidifies, the chains arrange themselves into an orderly lattice. The polar groups of adjacent chains are matched and the inter-chain distances reduced (i.e., the density increases). Both factors maximize the formation of secondary valence bonds between adjacent chains by dispersion and dipole forces. Dipole forces depend on the presence of polar groups as measured, for instance, by the solubility parameter. Heat of fusion, ΔH_f, represents the energy that must be supplied to break a large fraction of the secondary valence forces between neighboring chains as the polymer melts. High-density polyethylene has a heat of crystallization of -1850 cal/mole mer and a heat of fusion of $+1850$. The corresponding values for low-density polyethylene are about one half of these because of its lower crystallinity.

For crystalline and semicrystalline polymers, the heats of fusion and crystallization have the same absolute values only if the solid sample whose ΔH_f is being measured during melting and the solidifying sample whose ΔH_{cr} is being measured during solidification and crystallization have the same degree of crystallinity. If either process involves a higher degree of crystallinity, the corresponding enthalpy change will have a higher absolute value. Most thermodynamic data reported for polymers refer to the fusion process rather than to crystallization.

Transition temperatures (temperature of solidification and melting, glass transition temperature, temperature of thermal degradation), specific heat and heat of fusion and, for crystalline polymers, heat of crystallization are measured by differential thermal analysis (DTA) or differential scanning calorimetry (DSC). In DTA, the sample and a thermally inert reference material are heated or cooled at a programmed rate. The temperature difference between the two materials is recorded as a function of temperature. In DSC, the amount of heat required to maintain the temperature of the sample at the value given by the temperature program is measured either as the power input or as the heat flow[11] (see pp. 46–49).

Additional ΔH_f values are listed in Table 20–11. The data are given in cal/g rather than in cal/mole repeat unit to be more closely comparable: The repeat units of polyethylene and polyethylene terephthalate have molecular weights of 28 and 192, respectively. Their heats of fusion in cal/g, relating approximately to equal volumes or chain lengths, are 66 and 30, that is, the ΔH_f value for polyethylene is over twice that for polyethylene terephthalate. On a cal/mole repeat unit basis, the values are 1850 and 5760, with the latter having a ΔH_f value over three times larger than the former.

Polyethylene has a high heat of fusion even though it lacks polar groups because its chains are smooth and symmetric and can pack together closely. Since van der Waals forces fall off with the seventh power of the distance, small interchain distances result in large interchain attraction and high ΔH_{cr}.

Entropies of Crystallization and Fusion. The entropies of mixing and of fusion are quite similar if the former is considered only for the polymer. The Boltzmann relationship, $S = R \ln W$, applied to the fusion process, is

$$\Delta S_f = S_l - S_s = R \ln W_l - R \ln W_s$$

$$= R \ln \frac{W_l}{W_s} \cong R \ln W_l$$

$$(20\text{–}29)$$

Subscript l refers to the liquid, molten, or amorphous polymer, and subscript s refers to the solid, crystalline polymer. W, the number of possible chain conformations, is unity for the crystalline polymer, which has only one stable lattice conformation. By contrast, W_l is enormously large because of the freedom of rotation about the bonds in the backbone of the chains of molten or liquid polymers, making $W_l \gg W_s$, $W_l/W_s \gg 1$, and ΔS_f positive. According to equation (20–17a), a positive entropy change contributes to making the free energy change for the process negative and thereby tends to make that process occur spontaneously. This is an example of the universal tendency toward randomization or disorder. The reverse process of ordering or

TABLE 20–11. *Melting Points, Heats and Entropies of Fusion, and Glass Transition Temperatures for Various Polymers[5,12,24]*

Polymer	T_{MP} (°C)	ΔH_f (cal/g)	ΔS_f (cal/g °K)	T_g (°C)	$\left(\dfrac{T_g, °K}{T_{MP}, °K}\right)$
Polydimethyl siloxane (silicone rubber)	-40	4.3	0.02	-121	0.65
Polybutadiene (1,4-*cis*)	2	40.6	0.15	-95	0.65
Polyisoprene (*cis*, natural rubber)	26	15	0.05	-68	0.68
Polyethylene (HDPE)	139	66	0.16	-70	0.49
Polypropylene (isotactic)	186	62	0.13	-18	0.55
Polystyrene (isotactic)	240	20.5	0.04	85	0.69
Polyethylene terephthalate	265	30	0.06	69	0.64
Polyhexamethylene adipamide (66 nylon)	265	48	0.09	53	0.61
Polytetrafluoroethylene (Teflon)	325	13.7	0.023	126	0.67

crystallization is opposed by freedom of rotation through fusion and its increase in entropy. For polyethylene,

$$\Delta S_f = +4.5 \text{ cal/mole mer-}°K \text{ and}$$

$$\Delta S_{cr} = -4.5.$$

The magnitude of S_l and ΔS_f depends on W_l, which in turn depends on the flexibility of the chains or the freedom of rotation around chain bonds within the constraint of the tetrahedral carbon–carbon bond angle. As is seen in Table 20–11, ΔS_f is high for polyethylene. The methyl and especially the much larger phenyl side groups on every other carbon atom in the polypropylene and polystyrene chains hinder free rotation about the chain bonds and reduce the number of conformations that these chains can assume in the molten or liquid state. Therefore, the entropies of fusion of polypropylene and polystyrene are lower than that of polyethylene, by 19 and 75%, respectively. An olefinic double bond and a phenylene ring in the polymer backbone render the chains of polyisoprene and of polyethylene terephthalate relatively stiff, reducing W_l and ΔS_f considerably. Resonance between

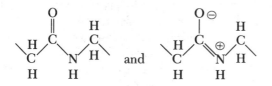

confers partial double bond character to the C—N bond and coplanarity to the amide group and the two carbon atoms, accounting for the stiffness and low ΔS_f of polyamides, including polypeptides. The potential energy barrier hindering rotation about a F_2C—CF_2 bond is more than an order of magnitude higher than that about a H_2C—CH_2 bond, resulting in considerable chain stiffness and a low entropy of fusion for polytetrafluoroethylene.

Melting Point. The transition between solid, crystalline, and liquid, amorphous polymers occurs at their crystalline melting point. Two opposing factors affect the free energy change and the melting point, one favoring fusion and the other crystallization.

Fusion occurs spontaneously if ΔG_f is negative. According to equation (20–17a) ΔG_f depends on ΔH_f, ΔS_f, and temperature. Since fusion is endothermic, ΔH_f is positive, and a high heat of fusion tends to make ΔG_f positive, opposing fusion and favoring crystallization. ΔS_f is also positive but, since the product $T \Delta S_f$ in equation (20–17a) is preceded by a minus sign, it makes a negative contribution to ΔG_f. Thus, a high entropy of fusion and a high temperature tend to promote fusion and oppose crystallization.

Below the melting point, the absolute value of ΔH_f (which is positive) is greater than the absolute value of $T \Delta S_f$ (which is also positive but makes a negative

contribution to ΔG_f because of the minus sign preceding it). On balance, ΔG_f is positive, and fusion does not occur spontaneously. Solidification and crystallization of molten polymers occur spontaneously below their crystalline melting points, however, and the equilibrium state is the solid, crystalline state because ΔG_{cr} is negative.

Neither the ΔH_f nor the ΔS_f values depend markedly on temperature. Thus, as T and $T \Delta S_f$ increase, ΔG_f becomes increasingly smaller. At the melting point, $\Delta G_f = 0$, and above the melting point, it becomes negative. Therefore, fusion occurs spontaneously above the melting point and the equilibrium state of the polymer is the molten, liquid, or amorphous state.

At the crystalline melting point, solid and liquid polymers are in equilibrium, and $\Delta G_{cr} = \Delta G_f = 0$. Hence, from equation (20–17a),

$$T_{MP} = \frac{\Delta H_f}{\Delta S_f} \qquad (20-30)$$

High melting points in polymers can be achieved by high values of ΔH_f and/or by low values of ΔS_f. Polarity, indicated by a high solubility parameter, tends to increase ΔH_f and the melting point by increasing the secondary valence forces between chains. Chain stiffness lowers ΔS_f and raises the melting point.

Example 20–8. High-density polyethylene has a latent heat of fusion of 1850 cal/mole mer and a crystalline melting point of 139° C. Calculate its entropy of fusion.

$$T_{MP} = 139° \text{ C} + 273 = 412° \text{ K}$$

From equation (20–30),

$$\Delta S_f = \Delta H_f/T_{MP}$$

$$= \left(\frac{1850 \text{ cal}}{\text{mole mer}}\right)\left(\frac{1}{412° \text{ K}}\right) = 4.49 \text{ cal/mole mer-}°K$$

To compare this value with that of Table 20–11, note that the molecular weight of a mer or repeat unit, —CH_2—CH_2—, is 28. Therefore,

$$\Delta S_f = \left(\frac{4.49 \text{ cal}}{\text{mole mer }°K}\right)\left(\frac{\text{mole mer}}{28 \text{ g}}\right) = 0.16 \text{ cal/g-}°K$$

Decreases in either the molecular weight or the size of the crystallites lower the melting point of a polymer somewhat. Since most commercial polymers have a range of molecular weights and crystallites of different sizes, their melting point is not as sharp as that of low-molecular-weight crystalline compounds.

Practical considerations often dictate the choice of polymers according to their melting point. Many resins are extruded in the molten state. Since thermal degradation is much more extensive at higher temperatures, low melting points and low processing temperatures are desirable from the fabricator's viewpoint. End-use preferences are for high melting points. For instance, steam sterilization carried out at 121° C and sterilization by dry heat at even higher temperatures would soften or melt polyethylene containers. Polypropylene containers, on the other hand, can be steam sterilized since their melting point is 173° to 186° C and their heat distortion temperature is 145° C.

GLASS–RUBBER TRANSITION[6,6a]

Neither atactic polystyrene nor SBR (styrene–butadiene rubber, a random copolymer of 76% butadiene/24% styrene) can crystallize. Yet, at room temperature, amorphous polystyrene is hard and brittle, whereas SBR is soft and extensible. The former is in the "glassy" state, the latter in the "rubbery" state. Upon lowering the temperature, SBR reversibly turns glassy (hard and brittle) over a narrow temperature range centered at −62° C. Upon heating, polystyrene reversibly turns rubbery (soft and extensible) over a narrow temperature range centered at 90° C. The temperature at which a glassy polymer becomes rubbery on heating and a rubbery polymer reverts to a glassy one on cooling is called the *glass transition temperature, T_g*.

The mechanical properties of SBR and polystyrene in their rubbery state (SBR above −62° C and polystyrene above 90° C) are rather similar. Their consistency is that of chewing gum. The major constituent of chewing gum, a gummy substance called chicle, is an impure form of *trans*-polyisoprene, another rubber. Both rubbery polymers have low tensile strength, low modulus of elasticity (ca. 10^2 psi, where psi represents lbs/in.^{2}), and very high elongation. The mechanical properties of the two polymers in their glassy state (at temperatures below their respective glass transition temperatures) are also rather similar: Both have comparatively high tensile strength, high modulus of elasticity (ca. 10^5 psi), and very low elongation. The effect of temperature on the modulus of elasticity of the two polymers is illustrated in Figure 20–12. The values change little with temperature except near the glass transition temperature, where they change abruptly. A shift along the temperature axis by 152° C nearly superim-

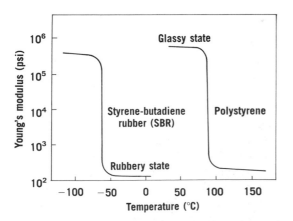

Fig. 20–12. Schematic plot of Young's modulus versus temperature for two amorphous polymers. Polystyrene is in the glassy state (brittle solid), while SBR is in the rubbery state (soft, very viscous semisolid) at room temperature.

poses the two curves.[7] The major difference between the two polymers is that, at room temperature, polystyrene, like most plastics, is below its T_g and is therefore in the glassy state, while SBR, like all elastomers, is above its T_g and is therefore in the rubbery state.

Polymers in the rubbery state are very viscous liquids, with relatively high freedom of rotation around the carbon–carbon bonds in the backbone within the constraint of the tetrahedral bond angle. The temperature is high enough so that most bonds can overcome the potential energy barrier against rotation. Rotational freedom results in very flexible chains, segmental or micro-Brownian motion, and changing chain conformations, as discussed for polymer solutions. Segmental mobility is considerably smaller in rubbery, liquid bulk polymers than in their solutions because of the much higher viscosity of the former.

As the temperature is lowered progressively, the number of bonds capable of overcoming the potential energy barrier to rotation diminishes, as does the segmental mobility. At the glass transition temperature, rotational or micro-Brownian motion ceases altogether, that is, the chain conformations are frozen in. Below T_g, the only motion left is the vibration of atoms about their equilibrium positions. When a polymer is stressed at temperatures below its T_g, the frozen, randomly coiled chains have largely lost their ability to slip past one another. Because rupture is not preceded by cold flow, elongations to break are small, and the polymer is brittle.

The amorphous domains in partly crystalline polymers undergo glass–rubber transitions just as purely amorphous polymers do. Many commercial grades of crystallizable polymers are about half crystalline and half amorphous. Two characteristic transition temperatures are associated with such semicrystalline polymers, the glass transition temperature with the amorphous portion, and the crystalline melting point with the crystalline portion. T_g is always lower than T_{MP}. Factors that restrict the rotation around carbon–carbon backbone bonds, such as the bulky phenyl side groups in polystyrene, render the chain stiffer. They raise the glass transition temperature by restricting the segmental mobility in the amorphous regions and increase the crystalline melting point by reducing the segmental mobility in the melt and, hence, the entropy of fusion (see previous discussion). Polar, especially hydrogen-bonding, groups that increase the interchain attraction or cohesion also raise T_g and T_{MP}, the latter by increasing the heat of fusion.

Since the two transition temperatures are affected by the same factors, their values are related. As is seen in Table 20–11, the ratio T_g/T_{MP} is equal to 1/2 for polymers with symmetric chains like polyethylene (also for polyvinylidene chloride and dimethylsilicones) and to 2/3 for polymers whose main-chain carbon atoms do not have two identical substituents, provided both

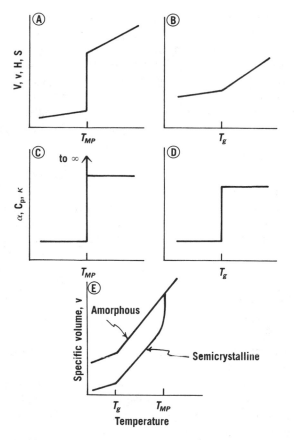

Fig. 20–13. Effect of melting point T_{MP} and glass transition temperature T_g on thermodynamic functions of crystalline, amorphous, and semicrystalline polymers. See text for definition of symbols.

temperatures are expressed on the absolute temperature scale.

From the thermodynamic viewpoint, melting as a phase change is a *first-order transition:* $\Delta G_f = 0$ at the melting point. Primary thermodynamic functions, that is, properties such as volume V or density and its reciprocal, specific volume v, entropy, and enthalpy undergo a sharp discontinuity at the melting point of a crystalline polymer, which, in the case of enthalpy, is the latent heat of fusion (Fig. 20–13A). The glass transition is identified as a *second-order transition.* At the glass transition temperature of an amorphous polymer, the primary functions merely undergo a change in slope when plotted against temperature (Fig. 20–13B). The derived thermodynamic functions: heat capacity

$$C_p = \left(\frac{\partial H}{\partial T}\right)_P$$

cubic thermal expansion coefficient

$$\alpha_v = \frac{1}{V}\left(\frac{\partial V}{\partial T}\right)_P$$

or

$$\alpha = \left(\frac{\partial v}{\partial T}\right)_P$$

and isothermal compressibility

$$\kappa = -\frac{1}{V}\left(\frac{\partial V}{\partial P}\right)_T$$

go to infinity at a first-order transition such as occurs at the melting point of a crystalline polymer (Fig. 20–13C) and show a sharp discontinuity at a second-order transition such as occurs at the glass transition temperature of an amorphous polymer (Fig. 20–13D). Figure 20–13E shows the dependence on temperature of the specific volume of an amorphous and of a partly crystalline polymer. Both plots undergo a change in slope at T_g corresponding to the glass transition in the amorphous polymer and in the amorphous portion of the semicrystalline polymer. When the temperature is increased to the melting point, the crystalline portion of the semicrystalline polymer melts, resulting in an abrupt increase in the specific volume and a discontinuity in the specific volume–temperature plot as the compact crystallites suddenly change into the less dense melt.

The initial slope of the plot below T_g, which represents the thermal expansion coefficient of the solid polymer, is smaller than the slope above the melting point, which represents the thermal expansion coefficient of the molten polymeric liquid. For atactic polymethyl methacrylate and polystyrene, which are completely amorphous plastics, and for the elastomer SBR, $\alpha = dv/dT$ at atmospheric pressure is 2.15, 2.5, and 1.8×10^{-4} cm^3/g-°K in the glassy state and 4.6, 5.5, and 6.6×10^{-4} cm^3/g-°K in the liquid–rubbery state, respectively.

From a kinetic viewpoint, the glass transition temperature is the temperature at which the relaxation time for segmental motion in the polymer backbone is comparable to, or at least of the same order of magnitude as, the time scale of the temperature change during the measurement. Therefore, the glass transition of a polymer is not as sharp and well defined as the melting point and depends much more on the method of measurement and on the rate of heating or cooling during the measurement. Thermal expansion coefficient, elastic modulus or hardness, heat capacity, thermal conductivity, isothermal compressibility, broad-line NMR, dielectric constant, and refractive index, which are used to measure the glass transition temperature, may give values that vary by as much as 20° C for a single sample. The experimentally measured T_g depends on the rate of heating or cooling. Fast cooling of a rubbery polymer during the measurement gives a higher value for the T_g than slow cooling, whereas fast heating of a glassy polymer gives a lower value than slow heating. These observations indicate that the glass transition is not a genuine thermodynamic transition but a kinetic phenomenon.

The glass transition temperature decreases somewhat with the molecular weight of a polymer. Many polymers have two or three glass transitions corresponding to the freezing-in of the rotational motions that occur in the main chain and in side chains as well as those of entire side groups.

The glass–rubber transition occurs in amorphous polymers and in the amorphous domains of partly crystalline polymers. Therefore, the properties of highly crystalline polymers, with about 20% or less of amorphous regions, undergo little if any change at the T_g. The profound effect of the glass transition on the mechanical properties of amorphous polymers or polymers with low crystallinity (below 10%) is illustrated by Figure 20–12 for the elastic modulus. Within a temperature range of about 10° C, the modulus changes more than 1000-fold. Polymers of intermediate crystallinity (10 to 80%) are hornlike and tough in texture below their T_g and leathery and tough between their T_g and T_{MP}. They may retain their good impact resistance in part even below the T_g.

The diffusivity (see Chapter 13) of small molecules through amorphous or semicrystalline polymers is considerably lower below than above their glass transition temperatures. The segmental mobility in the amorphous regions above the T_g greatly facilitates the transport of penetrants.

PLASTICIZATION

The glass transition temperature of a random copolymer on the Kelvin scale is frequently the weighted average of the glass transition temperatures of the two homopolymers on a weight (or, sometimes, volume) fraction basis.

Example 20–9. Polyvinyl chloride and polyvinyl acetate have T_g values of 81° and 29° C, respectively. Calculate the glass transition temperature of a random copolymer of 80% *w/w* vinyl chloride and 20% *w/w* vinyl acetate.

$$T_g = (0.8)(81 + 273) + (0.2)(29 + 273) = 344° \text{ K} = 71° \text{ C}$$

This process, by which T_g of rigid polyvinyl chloride is lowered through copolymerization, is called *internal plasticization*. It extends the lower end of the temperature range over which polyvinyl chloride is flexible. *External plasticizers* are high-boiling liquids that, at room temperature, have low vapor pressures and are not volatile. Their role is to lower the T_g of a polymer below room temperature, rendering it softer and more flexible. They must be soluble in the polymer. External

plasticizers act as lubricants between the polymer chains, facilitating the slippage of chain past chain under stress and extending the temperature range for segmental rotation to lower temperatures. If these liquids solvate the polymer extensively, they stiffen its chains and render them less flexible. Therefore, they should be poor solvents that are just compatible with the polymer. Plasticizers are liquids with low glass transition temperatures, in the range of −50° to −150° C, at which they freeze to glasses rather than crystallize on cooling. Their diffusion coefficients in the polymer should be comparatively low to minimize migration. Plasticizer migration from the walls of containers may contaminate the contents. Internal plasticizers do not migrate at all. External plasticizers are only effective with amorphous polymers or in the amorphous regions of semicrystalline polymers.

The effect of di-(2-ethylhexyl)phthalate, also called dioctyl phthalate, on the properties of polyvinyl chloride is shown in Table 20–12. The pure polymer is rigid at room temperature because it is in the glassy state. The plasticizer has a glass transition temperature of about −100° C and, at the 30% level, lowers that of the polymer to 5° C. At room temperature, plasticized polyvinyl chloride is therefore in the rubbery state. In the form of bags, it is used in containers for parenteral solutions and plasma because of its flexibility and transparency. A problem associated with the high level of di-(2-ethylhexyl)phthalate in flexible polyvinyl chloride bags containing intravenous solutions or plasma is the release of the liquid plasticizer, which exists in the infusion liquids as colloidal droplets,[42] especially upon agitation.[43] The released plasticizer may also become molecularly associated with lipid or protein components of stored plasma or whole blood.[44]

ELASTOMERS[45]

Elastomers or rubbers are polymers characterized by low glass transition temperatures. Those that are homopolymers capable of crystallizing also have low melting temperatures, mostly below room temperature (see the first three entries in Table 20–11). Elastomers are characterized by low solubility parameters (see Table 20–3) and low interchain attractive forces (Table 20–8). Like most crystalline polymers at temperatures

TABLE 20–12. *Effect of Plasticizer on Mechanical Properties of Polyvinyl Chloride*

Property	Rigid Polyvinyl Chloride	Polyvinyl Chloride (70% *w/w*) + Dioctyl Phthalate (30%)
Tensile strength (psi)	8000	3600
Young's modulus (10^5 psi)	4.6	0.2
Elongation to break (%)	30	200
Glass transition temperature (°C)	81	5

above their melting points and amorphous polymers above their glass transition temperatures, raw rubbers are viscous liquids of taffy-like consistency. They flow under stress, are tacky, and have little snap-back or elasticity. The appropriate model is a bowl of spaghetti.

Moderate cross-linking, called *vulcanization*, ties the chains together by primary valence bonds at a few points, preventing slippage of chain past chain under stress. Mechanical stresses are generally too weak to break primary valence bonds. The randomly coiled, lightly cross-linked chains of vulcanized elastomers are uncoiled and extended by stress, but this elongation stops when cross-links and backbone bonds become strained. The extended chains resume their original random conformations rapidly when the stress is released, causing the object to snap back to its original shape. Thus, the cross-links impart elasticity, minimize creep and permanent set, and eliminate tackiness. The high segmental mobility or micro-Brownian motion at room temperature is preserved because vulcanization raises the glass transition temperature by only a few degrees.

The cross-links are spaced widely apart, on the average about 1 per 100 repeat units, and do not prevent the reversible crystallization of homopolymer elastomers when stretched to high elongations. Stresses producing high elongations forcibly line up the randomly coiled elastomer chains in spite of the resultant decrease in entropy. This chain alignment or orientation leads to crystallization in stretched homopolymer elastomers, which thereby lowers their free energy by an amount equal to the heat of crystallization.

The stress-strain curves turn up at these elongations (Point *D* in Figure 20–10) because crystallization increases the modulus of elasticity. Once the stress is released, the elastomers "melt" because the absolute value of the positive $T \Delta S_f$ term is larger than the absolute value of the positive ΔH_f. According to equation (20–17a), ΔG_f is negative, and the elastomers that had crystallized under stress revert spontaneously to the more stable, contracted state in which the chains are randomly coiled. The latent heat of fusion or crystallization of elastomers is comparatively small because most elastomers are hydrocarbons, lacking polar groups. Furthermore, many have kinky chains owing to olefinic unsaturation in the *cis* configuration in their backbone and/or bulky side groups that prevent close packing and increase the distance between adjacent chains. These factors reduce the interchain cohesion and, hence, ΔH_f. While solvents of low polarity dissolve raw gums, they merely swell vulcanized rubbers.

Vulcanization or curing of natural rubber and other polybutadiene-type elastomers is carried out by mixing 2 to 5% sulfur plus a vulcanization accelerator (a mercaptobenzothiazole, a thiuram sulfide or disulfide, or a dithiocarbamate) and an activator (a zinc, lead, or calcium soap) into the raw gum and heating to 130° to 150° C. The olefinic unsaturation activates the hydrogen

on the α-carbon, and sulfide or disulfide cross-links are introduced:

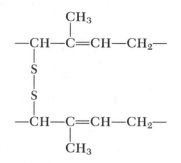

Extensive cross-linking, using 30% or more of sulfur based on the weight of raw natural rubber, produces a hard plastic with an ultimate elongation of only about 4% called *ebonite*.

Elastomers without olefinic unsaturation may be vulcanized by added peroxides that, on heating, decompose and abstract protons from the chains, producing free radicals. The combination or coupling of free radicals from adjacent chains produces cross-links between them.

Even vulcanization does not improve the mechanical properties of most elastomers sufficiently for certain end uses. *Reinforcing fillers* are powders of small particle size, 200 to 500 Å, such as carbon blacks and colloidal silicon dioxide. They are incorporated into the raw rubber together with the vulcanizing ingredients by milling, at levels of 20 to 75% of the weight of raw gum. The small particle size produces a large rubber–filler interfacial area; the degree of reinforcement increases with decreasing particle size.[38]

Incorporation of reinforcing fillers into homopolymer elastomers capable of crystallizing on stretching, such as natural rubber, polychloroprene, and polyisobutylene, usually increases their tensile strength and reduces their elongation to break only moderately but may improve their tear and abrasion resistance greatly. On the other hand, elastomers that cannot crystallize on stretching, such as the random copolymers of styrene with butadiene, butadiene with acrylonitrile, and ethylene with propylene, must be compounded with reinforcing fillers to attain satisfactory tensile strength and Young's modulus as well as abrasion and tear resistance. Their pure-gum vulcanizates are weak and soft, but reinforcing fillers can raise the mechanical properties to the levels developed in homopolymers by crystallization on stretching.

The reinforcing particles must be well wetted by the rubber to promote intimate dispersion during milling and good adhesion after vulcanization. The elastomer chains are strongly adsorbed on the colloidal filler particles and adhere to them even at large deformations. The composite thus acquires some of the strength, stiffness, and abrasion resistance of the disperse phase because the solid particles are mechanically integrated with the rubber.

Inert fillers and pigments such as clay, calcium carbonate, and talc do not improve the mechanical properties but facilitate molding and extruding and lower the price.

FABRICATION TECHNOLOGY[38,46-49]

Thermoplastic resins are fabricated in the molten state by extrusion into films or fibers and by molding into three-dimensional objects.

Extrusion.[38,46,47] A single-screw extruder is a conveyor similar to a meat grinder. It consists of a screw, driven by a motor connected to its shaft through a gear reducer, rotating inside a cylindric barrel. The rotating screw moves the resin pellets forward and generates by shear most of the heat required to melt the pellets, as well as the hydrostatic pressure to force the molten plastic through the die (Fig. 20–14).

The size of the extruder is described by the inside diameter of the barrel, which ranges from 1 inch for extruders with a capacity of about 5 lb/hr to 8 inches for a capacity of about 1000 lb/hr. The length of the barrel is about 18 to 24 times its diameter for the extrusion of thermoplastics. Shorter barrels are used to extrude rubber.

The screw consists of three zones, namely, a feed section, a transition section, and a metering section. The screw usually has the same pitch or helical angle in the three sections but decreasing channel depth. The process variables—temperature and speed of revolution of the screw—do not afford a range of conditions wide enough for the effective extrusion of different polymers. For instance, polyamides have lower melt viscosities than polyethylene resins, while polyvinyl chloride resins degrade readily at high temperatures. Therefore, different screws are available for a single extruder, having different lengths for the three zones,

different channel depths, and different compression ratios (channel depth in the feed section to channel depth in the metering section, that is, volumetric displacement in the feed section to that in the metering section.)

Resin pellets, granules, or flakes are fed from the hopper into the feed section of the extruder, from where they are conveyed to the transition section. Here the pellets are compressed and melted. A large portion of the heat required to melt the resin is generated by viscous friction as the pellets are sheared between the rotating screw and the stationary wall of the barrel. Another portion of the heat is supplied externally through the barrel, usually by electric band heaters mounted on the barrel. As the resin advances through the transition zone, it is plasticated, melted, and mixed. By the time it reaches the metering section, it is a homogeneous, very viscous liquid. The metering section of the screw has the shallowest channel depth. It pumps the melt through a screen-pack filter into the die cavity. The filter removes solid impurities and lumps of unmelted resin. If the extruded film is to have uniform thickness, it is essential that the melt exits through the die slit at a constant flow rate, free of sudden surges. The metering section ensures a constant delivery rate.

Flat film is extruded downward through a die with a long slit for an opening onto highly polished chill rolls that are water-cooled. From there, the sheet is rolled up on a windup roll. *Tubular film* is produced by extruding the melt upward through an annular die around a mandrel (Fig. 20–15). As the tube is pulled upward, it is blown up to a bubble by air injected through the mandrel, stretched, and biaxially oriented. The hot tubular film is cooled by air issuing through the holes of a hollow ring surrounding the tube near the point where it leaves the die, below the zone where it is inflated to a bubble. As the inflated, solidifying film moves upward, it is gradually deformed into the layflat

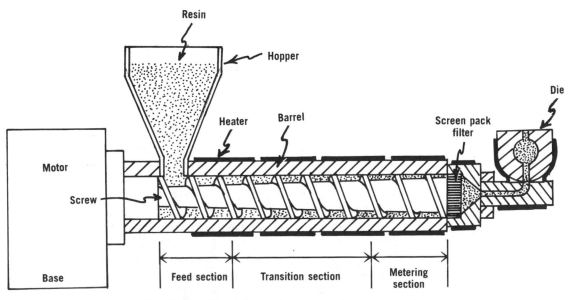

Fig. 20–14. Schematic drawing of a single-screw extruder.

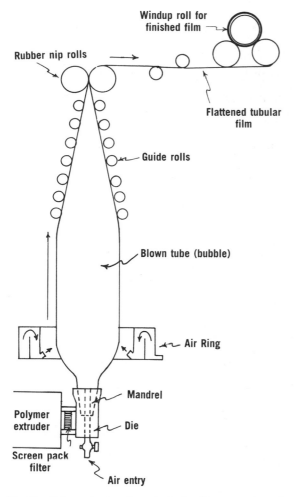

Windup roll for
finished film

Rubber nip rolls

Flattened tubular
film

Guide rolls

Blown tube (bubble)

Air Ring

Mandrel

Polymer
extruder

Die

Screen pack
filter

Air entry

Fig. 20–15. Schematic drawing of tubular film extrusion, showing film being pulled upwards and expanded into a bubble.

form by the action of guide rolls. A pair of rubber-covered nip rolls collapses the film completely and thereby seals in the inflating air that expanded the molten film issuing from the die into a bubble. A windup roll then rolls the flattened film up, pulling it upward continuously away from the die.

Injection molding.[38,46–49] Of the various molding processes, injection molding is the most widely used. The following three operations are carried out successively. The thermoplastic resin, in the form of pellets, is heated, melted, and pushed into the die cavity, which is filled with the melt. The molten plastic cools and solidifies in the mold while under pressure. Finally, the mold is opened and the part is ejected. Molds may have several cavities for the simultaneous molding of several parts, or a single cavity.

Two types of machines are used to melt and inject the resin into the mold, a *plunger injection molding machine* and a *reciprocating screw injection molding machine*. The plunger molding machine is fitted with a hydraulic ram that compresses the resin pellets at the same time that they are heated and melted. The molten resin is pushed through a nozzle into the mold cavities and is cooled under pressure to below its melting or glass transition temperature. The molten resin shrinks

on cooling, the mold is opened, and the solidified plastic parts are ejected.

The second molding machine, consisting of a reciprocating screw, mixes and homogenizes the melting resin. The screw resembles that of the single screw extruder depicted in Figure 20–14, except that it is moved forward and backward in the barrel by a hydraulic mechanism. The resin is fed from a hopper into the barrel, plasticized and melted by the rotating screw. The screw, then acting as a plunger, forces the melt into the mold cavities, where the plastic cools and solidifies. The molded plastic is then ejected from the mold cavities.

The molten resin shrinks on cooling and solidifying because its density decreases with rising temperature. Amorphous plastics shrink far less on solidifying than semicrystalline plastics owing to crystallization of the latter (see equation (20–28) and (Fig. 20–13). Molds are filled under high pressure. By compressing the melt, more material is made to flow into the mold cavity, reducing the *shrinkage on cooling*. The average linear shrinkage of polystyrene on cooling from 500° F to room temperature ranges from 3.5% at atmospheric pressure to 1.4% at 10,000 psi and 0.3% at 20,000 psi. Percent refers to the linear dimension at room temperature and atmospheric pressure. The corresponding linear shrinkage of polyethylene is 7.0%, 5.1%, and 3.6%, respectively. These values are higher because polyethylene is semicrystalline whereas polystyrene is amorphous. Mold pressures in commercial injection machines range from 6000 to 60,000 psi.

FUTURE TRENDS IN PHARMACEUTICAL AND OTHER BIOMEDICAL USES OF POLYMERS

This chapter illustrates some of the pharmaceutical applications of polymers. In the past, wider use of polymers in the health sciences field was limited by economic consideration: The pharmaceutical industry uses polymers in much smaller amounts than do other industries such as the textile, packaging, and tire industries. Therefore, the manufacturers of plastics and elastomers found no economic incentive to tailor-make polymers for the special needs of the pharmaceutical industry, or to seek clearance from the Food and Drug Administration for pharmaceutical applications of existing commercial polymers.

Presently, health scientists, commercial laboratories, and some pharmaceutical companies design, prepare, manufacture, and process or fabricate their own polymers in accordance with their specialized requirements. The following areas of polymer research and development are being actively pursued by academic and industrial investigators and health science practitioners. In addition to sutures, implants of plastics and elastomers in human and animal bodies are widely used for repair or replacement of tissues, organs, or parts of organs. Some of the problems encountered with implants are degeneration of adjoining tissues and formation of blood clots and thrombi on the surfaces of implanted synthetic polymers; enlargement of implants through sorption of lipids or moisture, which constitutes a problem with precision parts; and corrosion and weakening of implants due to interaction with enzymes and other physiologic compounds and/or mechanical stresses. Considerable research is in progress to achieve biocompatibility of synthetic polymers through surface modification to prevent blood clotting, to make porous implants that permit ingrowth of adjoining tissue, and to search for stronger and more durable polymers.

A skin substitute to cover burns has been introduced. It is a composite made of an outer layer of silicone elastomer to protect the wound from infection and dehyration, bonded to a porous bottom layer that is adhesive and biodegradable consisting of cross-linked collagen combined with glycosaminoglycan. After the skin has grown back underneath this composite film, the bottom layer is biodegraded and the elastomeric top layer sloughed off.[50]

Sustained-release dosage forms are a fertile area for the application of plastics, elastomers, and film-forming polymers (see Chapters 13 and 19). The synthesis and evaluation of macromolecular prodrugs is in full swing. Medical and pharmaceutical journals publish increasing numbers of articles dealing with polymers, while polymer journals publish increasing numbers of articles dealing with pharmaceutical and biomedical uses of polymers. Three specialized publications, "Journal of Biomedical Materials Research," "Biomaterials, Medical Devices and Artificial Organs," and "Biomaterials," started in 1967, 1973, and 1980, respectively, cover polymeric as well as other biomaterials, for example, ceramics and metals.

References and Notes

1. H. Mark and A. V. Tobolsky, *Physical Chemistry of High Polymeric Systems*, Interscience, New York, 1950.
2. P. J. Flory, *Principles of Polymer Chemistry*, Cornell University, Ithaca, 1953.
3. A. X. Schmidt and C. A. Marlies, *Principles of High-Polymer Theory and Practice*, McGraw-Hill, New York, 1948.
4. F. W. Billmeyer, *Textbook of Polymer Science*, 3rd Edition, Wiley, New York, 1984.
5. H.-G. Elias, *Macromolecules I, Structure and Properties*, translated by J. W. Stafford, 2nd Edition Plenum, New York, 1984.
6. P. C. Hiemenz, *Polymer Chemistry*, Dekker, New York, 1984.
6a. L. H. Sperling, *Introduction to Physical Polymer Science*, Wiley, New York, 1992.
7. L. Mandelkern, *An Introduction to Macromolecules*, Springer-Verlag, New York, 1972.
8. B. Vollmert, *Polymer Chemistry*, translated by E. H. Immergut, Springer-Verlag, New York, 1973.
9. M. L. Miller, *The Structure of Polymers*, Reinhold, New York, 1966.
10. P. W. Allen (Ed.), *Techniques of Polymer Characterization*, Butterworths, London, 1959.
11. E. A. Collins, J. Bares and F. W. Billmeyer, *Experiments in Polymer Science*, Wiley, New York, 1973.
12. J. Brandrup and E. H. Immergut (Eds.), *Polymer Handbook*, 3rd Edition, Wiley, New York, 1989.
13. F. W. Billmeyer and C. B. de Than, J. Am. Chem. Soc. **77**, 4763, 1955.
14. C. Tanford, *Physical Chemistry of Macromolecules*, Wiley, New York, 1961.
15. P. J. Flory, *Statistical Mechanics of Chain Molecules*, Wiley-Interscience, New York, 1969.
16. T. G. Fox and P. J. Flory, J. Am. Chem. Soc. **73**, 1915, 1951.
17. F. Bueche, *Physical Properties of Polymers*, Interscience, New York, 1962.
18. J. H. Hildebrand and R. L. Scott, *The Solubility of Nonelectrolytes*, 3rd Edition, Dover, New York, 1964.
19. J. H. Hildebrand, J. M. Prausnitz and R. L. Scott, *Regular and Related Solutions*, Van Nostrand Reinhold, New York, 1970.
20. D. Mangaraj et al., Makromol. Chem. **65**, 39, 1963; **67**, 75, 84, 1963; **84**, 225, 1965.
21. G. M. Bristow and W. F. Watson, Trans. Faraday Soc. **54**, 1731, 1742, 1958.
22. P. A. Small, J. Appl. Chem. **3**, 71, 1953.
23. K. L. Hoy, J. Paint Technol. **42**, 76, 1970.
24. D. W. van Krevelen, *Properties of Polymers, Their Estimation and Correlation with Chemical Structure*, 2nd Edition, Elsevier, New York, 1976.
25. C. M. Hansen, J. Paint Technol. **39**, 104, 505, 511, 1967; I & EC Prod. Res. Dev. 8(1), 2, 1969.
26. E. M. Frith and R. F. Tuckett, *Linear Polymers*, Longmans, Green, London, 1951.
27. H. Morawetz, *Macromolecules in Solution*, 2nd Edition, Wiley, New York, 1975.
28. H. Tompa, *Polymer Solutions*, Butterworths, London, 1956.
29. K. Shinoda, *Principles of Solution and Solubility*, Marcel Dekker, New York, 1978.
30. A. R. Shultz and P. J. Flory, J. Am. Chem. Soc. **74**, 4760, 1952; **75**, 3888, 1953.
31. H. R. Kruyt (Ed.), *Colloid Science II, Reversible Systems*, Elsevier, New York, 1949.
32. S. Kasai and M. Koishi, Chem. Pharm. Bull. **25**, 314, 1977.
33. C. Thies, Polymer-Plast. Technol. Eng. 5(1), 1, 1975.
34. P. L. Madan, Drug Dev. Ind. Pharm. 4, 95, 1978; Asian J. Pharm. Sci. **1**, 1, 1979.
35. R. Houwink, *Elasticity, Plasticity and Structure of Matter*, 2nd Edition, Harren Press, Washington, D.C., 1953.
36. T. Alfrey, *Mechanical Behavior of High Polymers*, Interscience, New York, 1948.
37. L. E. Nielsen, *Mechanical Properties of Polymers and Composites*, Reinhold, New York, 1974.
38. F. Rodriguez, *Principles of Polymer Systems*, 2nd Edition, Hemisphere Publishing, Washington, D.C., 1982.
39. H. Schott, in *Remington's Pharmaceutical Sciences*, 18th Edition, A. R. Gennaro (Ed.), Mack Publishing Co., Easton, Pa., 1990, Chapter 20.
40. T. S. Carswell and H. K. Nason, Modern Plastics, **21**, 121, June, 1944.
41. H. Schott, Biomaterials 3, 195, 1982.
42. J. H. Corley, T. E. Needham, E. D. Sumner and R. Mikeal, Am. J. Hosp. Pharm. **34**, 259, 1977.
43. M. Horioka, T. Aoyama and H. Karasawa, Chem. Pharm. Bull. **25**, 1791, 1977.
44. I. J. Stern, J. E. Miripol, R. S. Izzo and J. D. Lueck, Toxicol. Appl. Pharmacol. **41**, 507, 1977.
45. M. Morton (Ed.), *Rubber Technology*, 2nd Edition, Van Nostrand Reinhold, New York, 1973.
46. E. C. Bernhardt (Ed.), *Processing of Thermoplastic Materials*, Reinhold, New York, 1959.
47. J. M. McKelvey, *Polymer Processing*, Wiley, New York, 1962.
48. I. I. Rubin, *Injection Molding—Theory and Practice*, Wiley, New York, 1972.
49. H. S. Kaufman and J. J. Falcetta (Eds.), *Introduction to Polymer Science and Technology*, Wiley, New York, 1977.
50. T. Jaksic and J. F. Burke, Ann. Rev. Med. 38, 107, 1987.

Problems

20–1. Consider the following three combinations of reagents:

(a) $C_2H_5OH + HOOC—(CH_2)_4—COOH$;

(b) $H_2N—(CH_2)_6—NH_2 + Cl—CO—(CH_2)_8—CO—Cl$ + enough Na_2CO_3 to neutralize the hydrochloric acid formed;

(c) In a mixture of 50 mole-% propylene glycol + 50 mole-% phthalic anhydride, replace 20 mole-% of the propylene glycol with 10 mole-% pentaerythritol, $C(CH_2OH)_4$.

What type of polymer will be formed by the three condensation reactions?

Partial Answer: (**a**) Diethyl adipate will be formed. Since one of the two monomers is monofunctional, no polymer results.

20-2. When $a = 1$ in the Mark–Houwink equation, equation (20-8) becomes

$$\frac{\eta_{sp}}{c} = K\,M$$

the original Staudinger equation, for very dilute polymer solutions. The statement is made in the text that the molecular weight average obtained in that case is the weight–average molecular weight. Prove it.

20-3. When determining the molecular weight of a sample of 6-nylon or poly(ϵ-caprolactam), $H[NH—(CH_2)_5—CO]_nOH$, 2.500 g dry polymer consumed 2.21 cm³ of 0.1 N NaOH. What is the number–average degree of polymerization, i.e., the value of n? Note that each polymer chain or molecule has one amine and one carboxylic acid end-group.

Answer: $n = 100$

20-4. A polymer sample was fractionated into three homogeneous or monodisperse fractions as follows:

Data for *Problem 20-4*

Fraction	Weight, grams	Molecular weight
A	10	100,000
B	20	
C	100	10,000

Given that the weight–average molecular weight of the entire sample is 23,000, calculate the molecular weight of fraction B.

Answer: 50,000 (49,500 has three significant figures, which is more than the M values of the input).

20-5. A sample of polyvinyl chloride was fractionated from its solution in tetrahydrofuran. The weight-percent (based on the weight of the entire sample) and the molecular weight (g/mole) of successive fractions were as follows:

Data for *Problem 20-5*

Fraction no.	Weight-%	Molecular weight
1	6	7×10^3
2	9	1.7×10^4
3	15	3.8×10^4
4	20	7.5×10^4
5	23	1.4×10^5
6	16	2.5×10^5
7	8	4.5×10^5
8	3	1.05×10^6

Assuming that the fractions are essentially monodisperse, calculate $\overline{M}_z$, $\overline{M}_w$, $\overline{M}_n$, and $\overline{M}_w/\overline{M}_n$ of the polyvinyl chloride sample.

Answer: $\overline{M}_z = 401,000$; $\overline{M}_w = 162,000$; $\overline{M}_n = 43,500$; and $\overline{M}_w/\overline{M}_n = 3.73$

20-6. The polymethyl methacrylate sample of Table 20-1 was one of four fractions of very narrow molecular weight distribution, essentially monodisperse, that had been studied by light scattering and by viscosity in ethylene chloride solution at 25° C.[13] The molecular weights and intrinsic viscosities of these fractions are as follows:

Data for *Problem 20-6*

Fraction no.	Molecular weight	Intrinsic viscosity (dL/g)
1	393,000	1.084
2	168,000	0.571
3	117,000	0.430
4	91,000	0.354

Determine the values of K and a in the Mark–Houwink equation, (20-8), for polymethyl methacrylate in ethylene chloride at 25° C.

Answer: Linear regression analysis of equation (20-8) gives $a = 0.765$, $K = 5.74 \times 10^{-5}$ dL/g

20-7. Calculate the solubility parameter of polyvinyl chloride. The unplasticized polymer has a density of 1.42 g/cm³.

Answer: $\delta = 9.2$ (cal/cm³)$^{1/2}$

20-8. Pyroxylin USP (cellulose dinitrate) has a solubility parameter of 10.8 (cal/cm³)$^{1/2}$. It is insoluble in ethyl alcohol [$\delta = 12.7$ (cal/cm³)$^{1/2}$] and in ethyl ether [$\delta = 7.4$ (cal/cm³)$^{1/2}$], but it is soluble in a mixture of these two solvents. Explain briefly.

20-9. Will the intrinsic viscosity of polyethylene oxide increase, decrease, or remain unaffected as the temperature of its aqueous solution is increased?

Hint: Express your answer in terms of hydration.

20-10. Which solution of polyethylene oxide has the higher reduced viscosity in water at 25° C, one of 0.001% (w/v) or one of 1.00%? Explain your answer in terms of the Huggins equation.

20.11. Consider the crystalline melting points of the following polymers:

Polymer	Melting point, °C
$A{+}0—(CH_2)_2—0—CO—(CH_2)_6—CO{+}$	45
$B{+}0—(CH_2)_2—0—CO—$$—CO{+}$	265
$C{+}CH_2—CH_2{+}$	135
$D{+}CH_2—$$—CH_2{+}$	380

(**a**) Explain the increased melting point in going from A to B.

(**b**) Explain the increased melting point in going from C to D.

20-12. The melting points of some isotactic polyolefins ${+}\;CH_2—CH{+}$ are as follows:

$$|$$
$$R$$

	R	Melting point, °C
E	$—CH_3$	165
F	$—C_2H_5$	125
G	$—CH_2—CH_2—CH_3$	75

Explain the trend in melting point when going from E to F to G.

20-13. The glass transition temperatures of polyacrylonitrile, polybutadiene, and of a nitrile rubber (a copolymer of butadiene and acrylonitrile) are 104°, −95°, and −25° C, respectively. Estimate the composition of the nitrile rubber.

Answer: 37% (w/w) acrylonitrile and 63% (w/w) butadiene. *Note:* The solvent resistance increases in proportion with the acrylonitrile content; 40% acrylonitrile is about the upper limit in nitrile rubbers.

20–14. Load-elongation data for a fiber of secondary cellulose acetate, obtained with a tensile tester at 25° C, are given below.

Data for *Problem 20–14*

Stress (pound/square inch, psi)	Strain or elongation (%)
2000	0.94
4000	1.88
5000	2.35
5630	2.80
6000	3.13
6360	4.22
6200	5.00
6000	6.88
5880	10.0
5880	15.0
5880	20.0
5880	22.0 (rupture)

(a) Plot the strain-stress curve. **(b)** Calculate Young's modulus from the slope of the initial linear portion of the plot (which includes the origin). *Note:* To obtain the modulus in psi, the strain or elongation should have no units. Therefore, the percent elongation must be changed into fractional values. For instance, use 0.0188 instead of 1.88%. **(c)** What is the yield stress and the tensile strength? **(d)** What is the permanent deformation at 20% elongation, and what is the elongation to break?

Answers: **(b)** 213,000 psi; **(c)** 6360 psi and 5880 psi; **(d)** 20% − 4.22% = 15.78%, and the elongation to break is 22%.

20–15. The load-elongation data below were obtained by stretching a specimen of vulcanized natural rubber without filler (pure gum) in a tensile tester until it ruptured.

Data for *Problem 20–15*

Stress (psi)	Elongation (in./in.)
26.3	0.15
49.0	0.28
80	0.60
90	0.75
116	1.00
142	2.00
178	3.0
263	4.0
410	5.0
660	6.0
1120	7.0
2010	8.0

(a) Plot the stress-strain curve. **(b)** Calculate the (initial) Young's modulus. Note that only the initial two points are on a straight line with the origin and give the same initial modulus. *Note:* At elongations > 0.28 or 28%, the plot tends to level off and the modulus decreases. At elongations ≥ 2.00 or 200%, the curve turns up, which corresponds to an increase in modulus.

Answer: **(b)** 175 psi

20–16. (a) Using the data of *Problem 20–15*, calculate the tensile strength and the elongation to break. **(b)** The stress-strain curve is sigma-shaped. What causes the upturn at strains ≥ 2.0, which corresponds to an increase in modulus?

Answer: **(a)** 2010 psi and 8.0 (i.e., 800%). In the previous problem, the elongation was expressed in percent because it was quite low, less than 1.0 in./in. or 100%. The tensile strength is given in pounds per square inch of original cross-section of the tensile specimen. Since the specimen is stretched to 9 times its original length, the cross-sectional area decreases considerably in the course of the extension. The true tensile strength would be the load to break the specimen divided by the cross-sectional area at the elongation to break. It is approximately 10 times greater than the apparent value calculated above. Tensile strength and Young's modulus, calculated in *Problems 20–15* and *20–16*, are somewhat lower than the corresponding values in Table 20–5, indicating that the specimen of *Problems 20–15* and *20–16* was somewhat less vulcanized or cross-linked than the specimen of Table 20–5. The latter sample was presumably compounded with more sulfur.

(b) The rubber crystallizes at extensions ≥ 2.0, as the extended chains are progressively lined up parallel to one another. Crystallization causes the specimen to stiffen.

20–17. A filament of HDPE has a diameter of 2 mm. By how many percent will a 30-kg weight stretch it reversibly? Use Table 20–5 for Young's modulus.

Answer: 8.0%

20–18. The specific volume of molten polypropylene, in cm^3/g, is a linear function of the temperature T (in degrees centigrade) according to the following equation:

$$v_{am} = 1.156 + 0.000841\ T$$

The density of completely crystalline polypropylene at 25° C, as calculated from x-ray diffraction data, is 0.936 g/cm^2. Estimate the density at 25° C of a sample of solid polypropylene that is two-thirds crystalline.

Answer: 0.907 g/cm^3

20–19. Hydroxypropyl methylcellulose, type 2190, USP contains (on a dry basis) 7 to 12% (w/w) hydroxypropyl groups, OH—CH—CH_2—O—, and 28 to 30% (w/w) methoxy groups,
|
CH_3
CH_3—O—. Using the average values of 9.5% and 29% for the weight percentages of the two substituent groups, calculate the degree of substitution (DS) for hydroxypropoxy and methoxy, by means of algebra.

Answer: DS for hydroxypropoxy = 0.33; DS for methoxy = 2.42

20–20. A polypeptide containing lysine and benzyl glutamate as the sole monomers has been synthesized. The following data were obtained by analysis: 4.632 g polymer consumes 1.65 mL of 0.10 N NaOH when titrated against thymol blue, and 2.087 g polymer generates 183.3 mL nitrogen STP when analyzed according to the Van Slyke method (treatment with $NaNO_2$ + acetic acid produces 1 molecule N_2 for each NH_2 group by diazotization). STP means standard temperature (273.15°K or 0°C) and pressure (1 atmosphere or 76 cm Hg). Calculate the average molecular weight. What type of average is it? Calculate the mole-% lysine and benzyl glutamate.

Answer: $\overline{M}_n$ = 28,070; mole-% lysine = 62.9, mole-% benzyl glutamate = 37.1

Appendix: Calculus Review

The rules for some useful derivatives are found in Table A–1. The reader will notice in rule (a) that the rate of change of a constant k with respect to a change in x is zero since it is evident that a constant, by definition, does not change. As noted in rule (d), the base of the natural logarithm raised to the power x has the strange property of remaining unchanged on differentiation.

TABLE A–1. *Rules of Differentiation*

Function	Derivative	Rule
$y = k$	$dy/dx = 0$	(a)
$y = kx$	$dy/dx = k$	(b)
$y = kx^n$	$dy/dx = knx^{n-1}$	(c)
$y = ke^x$	$dy/dx = ke^x$	(d)
$y = k \ln x$	$dy/dx = k/x$	(e)
$y = u + v + w$	$dy/dx = du/dx + dv/dx + dw/dx$	(f)
$y = uv$	$dy/dx = u(dv/dx) + v(du/dx)$	(g)
$y = u/v$	$dy/dx = \dfrac{v(du/dx) - u(dv/dx)}{v^2}$	(h)

Several examples are given here to illustrate the use of the rules of Table A–1.

Example A–1. Differentiate $y = 2x^5 - \dfrac{4}{\sqrt[3]{x^2}} + 4x + 6$. According to rule (f), the derivative of y with respect to x is the sum of the derivatives of the separate terms. The separate functions are differentiated by the application of rule (c). Hint: The second right-hand term may be written $-4x^{-2/3}$.

$$\frac{dy}{dx} = (2 \times 5)x^{5-1}$$

$$- \left(-\frac{4 \times 2}{3} \right) x^{-(2/3 + 3/3)} + 4x^{1-1} + 0$$

$$\frac{dy}{dx} = 10x^4 + \frac{8}{3\sqrt[3]{x^5}} + 4$$

Example A–2. Differentiate the product

$$y = 3x^4(x^2 + 2)$$

Applying rule (g), in which, in this case, $u = 3x^4$ and $v = (x^2 + 2)$, one obtains

$$\frac{dy}{dx} = 12x^3 \text{ and } \frac{dv}{dx} = 2x$$

then

$$\frac{dy}{dx} = u\frac{dv}{dx} + v\frac{du}{dx} = 3x^4(2x) + (x^2 + 2)12x^3$$

$$\frac{dy}{dx} = 6x^5 + 12x^5 + 24x^3 = 18x^5 + 24x^3$$

This particular problem is actually solved more simply by first multiplying out the terms on the right-hand side of the equation to give

$$y = 3x^6 + 6x^4$$

and then differentiating by rule (f) in Table A–1 to obtain directly

$$\frac{dy}{dx} = 18x^5 + 24x^3$$

Example A–3. Differentiate the quotient $y = \dfrac{2 \ln x}{\ln x + 1}$. Using rules (e) and (h), one proceeds as follows. Let $u = 2 \ln x$ and $v = \ln x + 1$. Then

$$\frac{du}{dx} = \frac{2}{x} \text{ and } \frac{dv}{dx} = \frac{1}{x}$$

$$\frac{dy}{dx} = \frac{v(du/dx) - u(dv/dx)}{v^2}$$

$$= \frac{(\ln x + 1)\dfrac{2}{x} - (2 \ln x)\dfrac{1}{x}}{(\ln x + 1)^2}$$

and, upon simplifying,

$$\frac{dy}{dx} = \frac{2}{x(\ln x + 1)^2}$$

At times an expression may appear too complicated to differentiate directly. When y is some function not of x but of u, or $y = f(u)$, which in turn is a function of x, or $u = f(x)$, three steps are used in the differentiation. For example, if

$$y = (x^2 + 1)^2$$

this is the form $y = f(u)$, in which $u = (x^2 + 1)$ is in turn some function of x.

(1) Let $u = x^2 + 1$, and first differentiate y with respect to u: $y = u^2$;

$$dy/du = 2u = 2(x^2 + 1)$$

(2) Then differentiate u with respect to x:

$$u = x^2 + 1; \quad du/dx = 2x$$

(3) Now, it is observed that when the differential equations of steps *(1)* and *(2)* are multiplied together, du is eliminated and dy/dx is obtained:

$$dy/dx = dy/du \times du/dx = 2u \times 2x$$

$$dy/dx = 2(x^2 + 1)2x = 4x(x^2 + 1)$$

Example A–4. If $y = \ln (x^2 + 5)$, find dy/dx. First, let $u = x^2 + 5$.

$$y = \ln u; \quad dy/du = \frac{1}{u}; \quad du/dx = 2x$$

Therefore, $dy/dx = dy/du \times du/dx = 2x/(x^2 + 5)$

Example A–5. If $y = e^{ax}$, find dy/dx.
Let $u = ax$, then $y = e^u$ and $dy/du = e^u = e^{ax}$, $du/dx = a$ and $dy/dx = ae^{ax}$.

SUCCESSIVE DIFFERENTIATION

In addition to serving as a necessary tool in integral calculus, differentiation allows one to compute the rate of change of the dependent variable, for example, distance in a falling body problem, with respect to the independent variable, for example, time. It is also useful for computing maxima and minima of various functions. These two applications are illustrated in the examples of the following sections.

We know from physics that the derivative of distance with respect to time ds/dt gives the velocity v of a body. It will also be recalled from physics that acceleration a is defined as the rate of change of velocity with time, v/t, or distance divided by the square of time, s/t^2. In incremental notation, the *average acceleration* over the distance Δs can be written as

$$a_{\text{aver}} = \frac{\Delta v}{\Delta t} \equiv \frac{\Delta s}{(\Delta t)^2} \qquad (A-1)$$

The *instantaneous acceleration* at any time during the fall of a body is expressed by writing the limit of the ratio of the increments in equation (A–1). The change in velocity with respect to time dv/dt may be expressed as ds/dt taken a second time with respect to time, or $d(ds/dt)/dt$. This is known as the *second derivative with respect to time* and is written in the short-hand symbol d^2s/dt^2. Hence,

$$\lim_{\Delta t \to 0} \frac{\Delta v}{\Delta t} \equiv \frac{dv}{dt} \equiv \frac{d^2s}{dt^2}$$

In general, beginning with the function $y = f(x)$ and differentiating y with respect to x gives the *first derivative* dy/dx. Differentiating again with respect to x gives the *second derivative*, d^2y/dx^2, and successive differentiations give the *third derivative* d^3y/dx^3, the *fourth derivative* d^4y/dx^4, and so on.

Example A–6. The equation from general physics relating the distance and time of fall of a body beginning at rest is $s = \frac{1}{2}gt^2$. The velocity after 4 seconds is given by

$$v = \frac{ds}{dt} = gt = 981 \times 4 = 3924 \text{ cm/sec.}$$

in which g is the acceleration of gravity, 981 cm/sec^2. What is the acceleration a at this time?
Taking the second derivative of distance with respect to time simply involves differentiating the result just given a second time:

$$a = \frac{d^2s}{dt^2} = \frac{dv}{dt} = g$$

$$a = 981 \text{ cm/sec}^2$$

This result expresses the fact that the acceleration is constant at 981 cm/sec^2 throughout the fall. Taking the third derivative of distance with respect to time yields

$$\frac{d^3s}{dt^3} = 0$$

which shows that the rate of change of acceleration with time is zero. This is another way of saying that the acceleration is constant. See Problem 14 in Chapter 1.

From a geometric point of view, on a graph of y plotted against x, the first derivative dy/dx gives the slope of the line at any point, and the second derivative d^2y/dx^2 gives the rate of change of the slope with respect to x. The slope of the curve is equal to two times the value of x at any point, since $dy/dx = 2x$. The rate of change of the slope of the curve is constant at a value of 2 since $d^2y/dx^2 = 2$.

Maxima and Minima. Within the region where a curve slopes up to the right, dy/dx is positive. Where it slopes up to the left, dy/dx is negative. Where the curve is flat, exhibiting a maximum, a minimum, or a horizontal point of inflection, dy/dx is zero, and the tangent to the curve is a horizontal line.

The second derivative expresses the difference between these three possibilities. If the second derivative is positive for the value of x at the *critical value*, that is, at the point in qustion, the point represents a minimum; if the second derivative is negative, the point represents a maximum; and if the second derivative is zero, there may be a point of inflection (or there may be an unusually flat maximum or minimum or none of these).

Example A–7. Does the curve of the equation $y = x^2$ show a minimum or a maximum, and if so, what is its value?
The problem is solved by taking the first derivative and setting the result equal to zero.

$$\frac{dy}{dx} = 2x$$

$$2x = 0$$

Hence the curve shows a critical value at $x = 0$. The second derivative $d^2y/dx^2 = 2$ is positive, so that y has a *minimum* value at $x = 0$. By such a calculation, it can be shown that the buffer capacity of an acid buffer exhibits a maximum at pH = pK_a where the concentrations of the salt and the acid are equivalent, as seen on page 174.

The Differential. Before considering the topic of partial differentiation, it is necessary to introduce the *differential*. The differential of y is dy and the differential of x is dx. If $y = \ln x$, $dy/dx = 1/x$ or, written as the differential of y,

$$dy = \frac{1}{x} dx$$

Beginning with the function, $y = 3x^2 + 4x - 3$, the differential of y is written,

$$dy = 6x \, dx + 4 \, dx$$

Partial Differentiation. In these examples and all previous discussions, y has depended on only one variable, x. When y is a function of several variables, for example, $y = f(u,v,w)$, the total change in y, that is, the total differential dy, is the sum of the individual changes in y with respect to each of the variables. In partial differentiation, v and w are held constant while u is allowed to change, u and w are held constant while v changes, and u and v are held constant while w changes.

The symbol ∂ is used for partial differentiation, and the fundamental equation for the *total differential* of y is written,

$$dy = \left(\frac{\partial y}{\partial u}\right) du + \left(\frac{\partial y}{\partial v}\right) dv + \left(\frac{\partial y}{\partial w}\right) dw \quad (A\text{-}2)$$

in which $\partial y/\partial u$, $\partial y/\partial v$, and $\partial y/\partial w$ are the partial derivatives of y with respect to the three variables.

Example A–8. Find the total differential of y for the function, $y = 2u^3 + 3uv^2 + 4w$, in which y is a function of the variables u, v, and w.

$$\frac{\partial y}{\partial u} = 6u^2 + 3v^2$$

$$\frac{\partial y}{\partial v} = 6uv$$

$$\frac{\partial y}{\partial w} = 4$$

$$\therefore dy = (6u^2 + 3v^2)\, du + 6uv\, dv + 4\, dw$$

Equation (A–2) is used in thermodynamics and may be applied here to the relationship between the volume V, temperature T, and pressure P of a gas. According to the ideal gas equation, the volume of a gas depends on the temperature and pressure, that is, $V = f(T,P)$, and the change of volume is given by the equation

$$dV = \left(\frac{\partial V}{\partial T}\right)_P dT + \left(\frac{\partial V}{\partial P}\right)_T dP \quad (A\text{-}3)$$

which expresses the fact that an infinitesimal change dV in V is obtained from the temperature coefficient of volume $\partial V/\partial T$ multiplied by the change in temperature dT plus the pressure coefficient of volume $\partial V/\partial P$ multiplied by the change in pressure dP. The partial

derivatives are written as $(\partial V/\partial T)_P$ and $(\partial V/\partial P)_T$ to show that P is held constant while differentiating V with respect to T, and T is held constant while differentiating V with respect to P.

Figure A–1a is meant to be an infinitesimally small section of a surface representing the function, $V = f(T,P)$. The projection of this three-dimensional diagram to a V vs. T and a V vs. P plot are shown in Figures A–1b and A–1c. The general shapes of the curves in Figure A–1 agree with the ideal gas laws, that is, the volume increases linearly with temperature, and volume decreases as the pressure increases. The slope of the line ab or cd in Figure A–1b is the temperature coefficient of volume $(\partial V/\partial T)_P$, and the change in volume in going from a to b, $(V_b - V_a)$, is equal to the slope multiplied by the change in temperature dT, or $(\partial V/\partial T)_P\, dT$. The slope of the line bd or ac in Figure A–1c is $(\partial V/\partial P)_T$, and the change in volume in going from b to d, $(V_d - V_b)$, is $(\partial V/\partial P)_T\, dP$.

It is equally proper to carry out the pressure change first, proceeding in Figure A–1a from a to c, and then bring about the temperature change, passing from c to d. The total change in volume in going from a to d, viz., $V_d - V_a \equiv dV$, may be represented by a diagonal curve on the surface of the figure, A–1a. According to the method of partial differentiation, the total change is obtained by the two-step process:

$$V_d - V_a = (V_b - V_a) + (V_d - V_b)$$

or

$$dV = \left(\frac{\partial V}{\partial T}\right)_P dT + \left(\frac{\partial V}{\partial P}\right)_T dP$$

The path by which we arrive at V_d from V_a has no influence on the value of dV. The differential depends only on the initial and final values V_a and V_d; thus, dV is said to be an *exact differential* and V is referred to as a *thermodynamic property*. These terms are used in the chapter on thermodynamics. Since V, T, and P are all independent variables, the change in any one can be

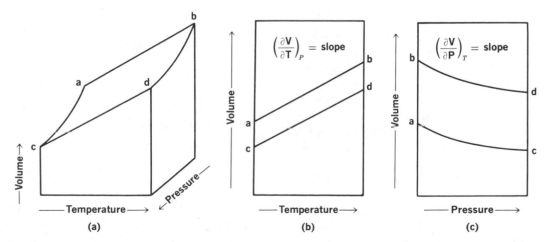

Fig. A–1. Graphical demonstration of the fundamental equation of partial differentiation. (After F. Daniels, *Mathematical Preparation for Physical Chemistry*, McGraw-Hill, New York, 1928, p. 179.)

obtained in terms of the others. For example, $P = f(T,V)$ and thus the infinitesimal change in P with changes in temperature and volume is

$$dP = \left(\frac{\partial P}{\partial T}\right)_V dT + \left(\frac{\partial P}{\partial V}\right)_T dV \qquad \text{(A–4)}$$

INTEGRAL CALCULUS

Integration. Integration can be considered as the summation of infinitesimal elements, such as dy. The symbol for integration is an elongated s, written $\int$, and $\int dy = y$ means that the summation of the infinitesimal elements of y gives the whole value y. Integration is also considered as the reverse of differentiation in the same sense that division is the reverse of multiplication. When we divide 15 by 3, we obtain the answer by thinking of the number by which 3 is multiplied to yield 15. Similarly in calculus when we are asked to integrate $2x$, we attempt to recall the value that, when differentiated, yielded $2x$. The function $y = x^2$ and the more general expression $y = x^2 + C$ come to mind as possible answers, since, in either case,

$$\frac{dy}{dx} = 2x \qquad \text{(A–5)}$$

The symbol C stands for a constant. Equation (A–5) may also be written in the differential form for the purpose of integration where dy can be summed to give y:

$$dy = 2x \, dx$$

and we signify our intention to integrate by adding the integral sign to both sides of the equation.

$$\int dy = \int 2x \, dx$$

Both *integral signs must always be followed by differentials*, this being the reason for separating dy and dx in the previous step. The final result after integration is written:

$$y = x^2 + C \qquad \text{(A–6)}$$

This process of finding the function when the differential is given is known as *integration*. Thus, if the rate of change of y with x is known, it is possible by integration to obtain the functional relationship between the variables y and x. The constant of integration C has been added to "play safe," since it is quite possible that the value we are seeking in the integration process contained a constant that dropped out on differentiation.

The constant can be evaluated from the *boundary conditions* of the problem, that is, from the values of y for known values of x. If the function does not contain a constant term, the value of C will turn out to be zero, and no harm has been done by its inclusion. If, in the example just given, the boundary condition is given as $y = 5$ when $x = 3$, one obtains the following result by substituting the boundary condition into equation (A–6):

$$5 = 9 + C$$

or

$$C = 5 - 9 = -4$$

and substituting this value of C in equation (A–6) the final result becomes

$$y = x^2 - 4$$

Rules of Integration. The rules of integration are not obtained by mathematical derivations as were those of differentiation. Instead, the integration rules follow from a consideration of examples, such as the following

(a) If $y = x^5 + C$, $\dfrac{dy}{dx} = 5x^4$, or

$$dy = 5x^4 \, dx$$

then

$$\int 5x^4 \, dx = x^5 + C$$

(b) If $y = \dfrac{x^3}{3} + C$, $\dfrac{dy}{dx} = \dfrac{3x^2}{3} = x^2$, or

$$dy = x^2 \, dx;$$

then

$$\int x^2 \, dx = \frac{x^3}{3} + C$$

(c) If $y = x^{(n+1)} + C$, $\dfrac{dy}{dx} = (n + 1)x^n$

then

$$\int (n + 1)x^n \, dx = x^{(n+1)} + C$$

or in general $\displaystyle\int x^n \, dx = \dfrac{x^{(n+1)}}{n + 1} + C$

The integral $x^{-1} \, dx$ is a special case to which the general formula in (c) does not apply. This case is treated in (d)

(d) If $y = \ln x + C$, $\dfrac{dy}{dx} = \dfrac{1}{x}$ from Table A–1,

$$dy = dx/x;$$

then

$$y = \int \frac{dx}{x} = \ln x + C$$

The student should take particular note of the integral under (d), since it is frequently used in science. The

TABLE A–2. *Summary of Several Important Derivatives and Integrals*

Function	Derivative	Integral
$y = x^n$	$\dfrac{dy}{dx} = nx^{n-1}$	$\displaystyle\int x^n \, dx = \dfrac{x^{n+1}}{n+1} + C; \; n \neq -1$
$y = e^x$	$\dfrac{dy}{dx} = e^x$	$\displaystyle\int e^x \, dx = e^x + C$
$y = \ln x$	$\dfrac{dy}{dx} = \dfrac{1}{x}$	$\displaystyle\int \ln x \, dx = x(\ln x - 1) + C*$
$y = \dfrac{1}{x}$	$\dfrac{dy}{dx} = -\dfrac{1}{x^2}$	$\displaystyle\int \dfrac{1}{x} \, dx = \ln x + C$

*This integration is done by the method illustrated in *Example A–11*.

most important derivatives and integrals are summarized in Table A–2. The integration of sums and differences and the treatment of constants, not shown in these examples, are best learned by studying the following problems.

Example A–9. Find y when the *differential equation,* as it is called, $dy/dx = 4x^3 + 6x^2 - 3$, is given.

$$\int dy = \int (4x^3 + 6x^2 - 3)\, dx$$
$$= 4\int x^3 \, dx + 6\int x^2 \, dx - 3\int dx$$

The constants are taken outside the integral signs since they are not changed by integration. Applying (c) to each term, the integration results in

$$y = 4\frac{x^4}{4} + 6\frac{x^3}{3} - 3x + C = x^4 + 2x^3 - 3x + C$$

Example A–10. Integrate $dy/dx = -2/x^{1/2}$ with $y = 2$ when $x = 4$

$$y = -2\int \frac{dx}{x^{1/2}} = -2\int x^{-1/2} \, dx$$

and by use of the general formula (c), above,

$$y = -2\int x^{-1/2} \, dx = \frac{-2x^{(-1/2 + 2/2)}}{(-\frac{1}{2} + \frac{2}{2})} + C = -4x^{1/2} + C$$

Then, employing the boundary conditions: $2 = -4 \times (4)^{1/2} + C$

$$C = 2 + 8 = 10$$

and finally

$$y = -4x^{1/2} + 10$$

If one is not sure of the answer, he or she should check it by differentiating the result:

$$y = -4x^{1/2} + 10$$
$$\frac{dy}{dx} = -\frac{4}{2}x^{(1/2 - 2/2)} = -2x^{-1/2} = -\frac{2}{x^{1/2}}$$

Example A–11. Integrate

$$dy = (3 + x^4)^{-1/2}x^3 \, dx$$

Problems of this type are solved by introducing the function u. Let

$$u = 3 + x^4$$

then

$$du = 4x^3 \, dx$$

It should therefore be possible to substitute

$$dy = u^{-1/2} \, du$$

for this function, except for the fact that

$$u^{-1/2} \, du = (3 + x^4)^{-1/2}4x^3 \, dx$$

which differs from the original differential by a factor of 4. Therefore, we write

$$dy = \tfrac{1}{4}u^{-1/2} \, du = (3 + x^4)^{-1/2}x^3 \, dx$$

The left-hand side is easily integrated to give

$$y = \tfrac{1}{4}\frac{u^{1/2}}{1/2} + C = \frac{(3 + x^4)^{1/2}}{2} + C$$

and this is obviously the solution of the original problem.

Exercises. Integrate the following expressions.

1. $dy = (5 - x^2)x \, dx$; with $y = 9$ when $x = 2$
Answer: $y = \tfrac{5}{2}x^2 - \tfrac{1}{4}x^4 + 3$

2. $dy = \dfrac{5 - x}{x^2} \, dx$

Answer: $y = C - \dfrac{5}{x} - \ln x$

[Hint: Write as

$$y = \int (5 - x)x^{-2} \, dx = \int (5x^{-2} - x^{-1}) \, dx]$$

3. $dy = (3 + x^2)^3 x \, dx$

Answer: $y = \dfrac{(3 + x^2)^4}{8} + C$

[Hint: Let $u = (3 + x^2)$; $du = 2x \, dx$. Then $(3 + x^2)^3 2x \, dx = u^3 \, du$ and $\tfrac{1}{2}u^3 \, du = (3 + x^2)^3 x \, dx.$]

The Definite Integral. All previous formulas of integration have involved an arbitrary constant C, and these are known as *indefinite integrals.* When the integration is carried out between two definite values of x, the integration constant drops out of the result and the integral is called a *definite integral.* The process by which the definite integral is obtained is known as *integration between limits.* The definite integral of $f(x)$ dx is written

$$\int_a^b f(x)dx \tag{A–7}$$

in which a and b represent the limits between which the integration is carried out. The process is described as follows. After $f(x) \, dx$ is integrated in the usual way, the limits b and a are substituted successively for x in the result, and the second quantity is subtracted from the first. The constant of integration disappears when the subtraction is carried out. The details of the method are illustrated in *Example A–12*. Notice that y is integrated between limits in the same manner as x.

Example A–12. Find the solution of the *differential equation*, as it is called, $dy/dx = 2x$, given that $y = 0$ when $x = 2$ and $y = a$ when $x = 3$.

$$\int_0^a dy = 2\int_2^3 x\, dx$$

$$[y]_0^a = [x^2 + C]_2^3$$

$$a - 0 = (9 + C) - (4 + C)$$

$$a = 5$$

Example A–13. The velocity of a body falling freely from rest is expressed by the equation $v = gt$. What is the distance (in cm) that the body has fallen between the third and the fourth second? The problem is solved by integration.

$$v = \frac{ds}{dt} = gt$$

The distance at $t = 3$ sec is given the symbol s_3 and the corresponding distance traveled at $t = 4$ sec is written s_4. The distance traveled between the third and fourth second is therefore $s_4 - s_3 = \Delta s$. It is solved by integration as follows.

$$\int_{s_3}^{s_4} ds = g\int_3^4 t\, dt$$

$$[s]_{s_3}^{s_4} = \tfrac{1}{2}g[(t^2)]_3^4 = \tfrac{1}{2}g(16 - 9) = \tfrac{7}{2}g$$

$$s_4 - s_3 = \Delta s = \tfrac{7}{2} \times 981 = 3434 \text{ cm}$$

Applications. The rate of disintegration of a radioactive element may be expressed as

$$\text{Rate} = \lambda N$$

$$-\frac{dN}{dt} = \lambda N$$

in which λ is the specific reaction rate and N the number of atoms remaining undecomposed at time t. The rate of decrease of radioactive atoms with time is written as $-dN/dt$, the negative sign being included because the number of atoms is decreasing with increasing time. Radioactive disintegration is one case of what is called *first-order* decomposition. The general expression for a first-order rate, which will be discussed in Chapter 12, is ordinarily written in the form of a differential equation

$$-\frac{dc}{dl} = kc \qquad (A–8)$$

in which c is the concentration of the substance decomposing at any time. It is desirable to integrate this equation so that k can be computed conveniently. The limits of the definite integrals are obtained by writing the initial concentration, i.e., the concentration at $t = 0$, as c_0 and the concentration at some other time t as c. Equation (A–8) is put into a convenient form for integration by separating the variables, that is, by collecting c and dc on one side of the equation and dt on the other side. The boundary limits are added, and the equation is ready for integration:

$$-\int_{c_0}^c \frac{dc}{c} = k\int_0^t dt$$

$$-[(ln\ c)]_{c_0}^c = k[(t)]_0^t$$

$$(-\ln c) - (-\ln c_0) = k(t - 0)$$

$$kt = \ln \frac{c_0}{c} = 2.303 \log \frac{c_0}{c}$$

$$k = \frac{2.303}{t} \log \frac{c_0}{c}$$

Based on the rules of logarithms, the solution may also be written

$$c = c_0 e^{-kt}$$

or

$$c = c_0 10^{-kt/2.303}$$

The rate of growth of bacteria frequently may be expressed by a similar equation, $dN/dt = \alpha N$, in which N is the number of cells present at any moment t, and α is the *rate* constant. On integration between the limits N_0 at $t = L$ and N at time t, the equation is written,

$$\alpha = \frac{2.303}{(t - L)} \log \frac{N}{N_0}$$

in which L is the lag or induction period before the bacteria begin to follow the logarithmic growth law.

As an illustration of both differentiation and integration, we may consider a derivation of the ideal gas law. It follows from Boyle's law and Charles' law that the volume of one mole of an ideal gas is a function of the pressure and the temperature

$$V = f(P,T) \qquad (A–9)$$

and the total differential can be written.

$$dV = \left(\frac{\partial V}{\partial P}\right)_T dP + \left(\frac{\partial V}{\partial T}\right)_P dT \qquad (A–10)$$

Now, at a fixed temperature, according to Boyle's law,

$$V = \frac{k_1}{P}; \ k_1 = PV \qquad (A–11)$$

and at a fixed pressure, according to Charles' law,

$$V = k_2 T; \ k_2 = \frac{V}{T} \qquad (A–12)$$

The partial derivative of equation (A–11) is given by the expression

$$\left(\frac{\partial V}{\partial P}\right)_T = -\frac{k_1}{P^2} = -\frac{PV}{P^2} = -\frac{V}{P} \qquad (A–13)$$

and the partial derivative of (A–12) is

$$\left(\frac{\partial V}{\partial T}\right)_P = k_2 = \frac{V}{T} \qquad (A-14)$$

Substituting these values into equation (A–10) gives

$$dV = -\left(\frac{V}{P}\right)dP + \left(\frac{V}{T}\right)dT$$

or by factoring V from the right-hand terms and dividing both sides by V, we have

$$\frac{dV}{V} + \frac{dP}{P} = \frac{dT}{T} \qquad (A-15)$$

Integration of equation (A–15) then yields

$$\ln V + \ln P = \ln T + \ln R \qquad (A-16)$$

The ln R term has been written in place of C, the integration constant. R is the molar gas constant.

The *equation of state*, that is, the equation relating P, V, and T for an ideal gas, is finally obtained by taking the antilogarithms of the terms in equation (A–16),

$$PV = RT$$

which, for n moles of gas, becomes

$$PV = nRT \qquad (A-17)$$

Index

Page numbers in *italics* indicate illustrations; numbers followed by "t" indicate tables; numbers followed by "n" indicate notes.

LOGARITHMS

Natural Numbers	0	1	2	3	4	5	6	7	8	9	PROPORTIONAL PARTS								
											1	2	3	4	5	6	7	8	9
10	0000	0043	0086	0128	0170	0212	0253	0294	0334	0374	4	8	12	17	21	25	29	33	37
11	0414	0453	0492	0531	0569	0607	0645	0682	0719	0755	4	8	11	15	19	23	26	30	34
12	0792	0828	0864	0899	0934	0969	1004	1038	1072	1106	3	7	10	14	17	21	24	28	31
13	1139	1173	1206	1239	1271	1303	1335	1367	1399	1430	3	6	10	13	16	19	23	26	29
14	1461	1492	1523	1553	1584	1614	1644	1673	1703	1732	3	6	9	12	15	18	21	24	27
15	1761	1790	1818	1847	1875	1903	1931	1959	1987	2014	3	6	8	11	14	17	20	22	25
16	2041	2068	2095	2122	2148	2175	2201	2227	2253	2279	3	5	8	11	13	16	18	21	24
17	2304	2330	2355	2380	2405	2430	2455	2480	2504	2529	2	5	7	10	12	15	17	20	22
18	2553	2577	2601	2625	2648	2672	2695	2718	2742	2765	2	5	7	9	12	14	16	19	21
19	2788	2810	2833	2856	2878	2900	2923	2945	2967	2989	2	4	7	9	11	13	16	18	20
20	3010	3032	3054	3075	3096	3118	3139	3160	3181	3201	2	4	6	8	11	13	15	17	19
21	3222	3243	3263	3284	3304	3324	3345	3365	3385	3404	2	4	6	8	10	12	14	16	18
22	3424	3444	3464	3483	3502	3522	3541	3560	3579	3598	2	4	6	8	10	12	14	15	17
23	3617	3636	3655	3674	3692	3711	3729	3747	3766	3784	2	4	6	7	9	11	13	15	17
24	3802	3820	3838	3856	3874	3892	3909	3927	3945	3962	2	4	5	7	9	11	12	14	16
25	3979	3997	4014	4031	4048	4065	4082	4099	4116	4133	2	3	5	7	9	10	12	14	15
26	4150	4166	4183	4200	4216	4232	4249	4265	4281	4298	2	3	5	7	8	10	11	13	15
27	4314	4330	4346	4362	4378	4393	4409	4425	4440	4456	2	3	5	6	8	9	11	13	14
28	4472	4487	4502	4518	4533	4548	4564	4579	4594	4609	2	3	5	6	8	9	11	12	14
29	4624	4639	4654	4669	4683	4698	4713	4728	4742	4757	1	3	4	6	7	9	10	12	13
30	4771	4786	4800	4814	4829	4843	4857	4871	4886	4900	1	3	4	6	7	9	10	11	13
31	4914	4928	4942	4955	4969	4983	4997	5011	5024	5038	1	3	4	6	7	8	10	11	12
32	5051	5065	5079	5092	5105	5119	5132	5145	5159	5172	1	3	4	5	7	8	9	11	12
33	5185	5198	5211	5224	5237	5250	5263	5276	5289	5302	1	3	4	5	6	8	9	10	12
34	5315	5328	5340	5353	5366	5378	5391	5403	5416	5428	1	3	4	5	6	8	9	10	11
35	5441	5453	5465	5478	5490	5502	5514	5527	5539	5551	1	2	4	5	6	7	9	10	11
36	5563	5575	5587	5599	5611	5623	5635	5647	5658	5670	1	2	4	5	6	7	8	10	11
37	5682	5694	5705	5717	5729	5740	5752	5763	5775	5786	1	2	3	5	6	7	8	9	10
38	5798	5809	5821	5832	5843	5855	5866	5877	5888	5899	1	2	3	5	6	7	8	9	10
39	5911	5922	5933	5944	5955	5966	5977	5988	5999	6010	1	2	3	4	5	7	8	9	10
40	6021	6031	6042	6053	6064	6075	6085	6096	6107	6117	1	2	3	4	5	6	8	9	10
41	6128	6138	6149	6160	6170	6180	6191	6201	6212	6222	1	2	3	4	5	6	7	8	9
42	6232	6243	6253	6263	6274	6284	6294	6304	6314	6325	1	2	3	4	5	6	7	8	9
43	6335	6345	6355	6365	6375	6385	6395	6405	6415	6425	1	2	3	4	5	6	7	8	9
44	6435	6444	6454	6464	6474	6484	6493	6503	6513	6522	1	2	3	4	5	6	7	8	9
45	6532	6542	6551	6561	6571	6580	6590	6599	6609	6618	1	2	3	4	5	6	7	8	9
46	6628	6637	6646	6656	6665	6675	6684	6693	6702	6712	1	2	3	4	5	6	7	7	8
47	6721	6730	6739	6749	6758	6767	6776	6785	6794	6803	1	2	3	4	5	5	6	7	8
48	6812	6821	6830	6839	6848	6857	6866	6875	6884	6893	1	2	3	4	4	5	6	7	8
49	6902	6911	6920	6928	6937	6946	6955	6964	6972	6981	1	2	3	4	4	5	6	7	8
50	6990	6998	7007	7016	7024	7033	7042	7050	7059	7067	1	2	3	3	4	5	6	7	8
51	7076	7084	7093	7101	7110	7118	7126	7135	7143	7152	1	2	3	3	4	5	6	7	8
52	7160	7168	7177	7185	7193	7202	7210	7218	7226	7235	1	2	2	3	4	5	6	7	7
53	7243	7251	7259	7267	7275	7284	7292	7300	7308	7316	1	2	2	3	4	5	6	6	7
54	7324	7332	7340	7348	7356	7364	7372	7380	7388	7396	1	2	2	3	4	5	6	6	7